CHAPTER 1

Introduction

1.1 Introduction 2

1.2 Apoptosis and Neurodegeneration 4

1.3 The Role of Oxidative Mechanisms in Neurodegenerative Diseases 8

1.4 Abnormal Protein-Protein Interactions: Underlying Mechanisms of Diverse Neurodegenerative Diseases 11

1.5 The Ubiquitin Pathway, Neurodegeneration and Brain Function 14

1.6 The Genetics of Neurodegeneration 17

Introduction

Dennis W. Dickson

Despite their clinical and pathologic diversity, neurodegenerative diseases share certain basic processes, as is true of basic pathologic processes in any organ system. Unique to nervous system degenerative disorders is the selective loss of specific populations of neurones. The particular population of neurones that are vulnerable in each disorder determines the clinical presentation. The distribution of the pathology is in fact more predicative of the clinical presentation than the molecular nature of the pathology. One of the best examples of this is the variety of pathologic entities that can present clinically with a frontal lobe dementia (chapters 2, 7). It remains one of the major unattained goals of modern research on the degenerative diseases to determine the molecular basis for neuronal selective vulnerability.

A complete review of all the basic processes that are shared by neurodegenerative disorders is beyond the scope of this book, but some of the more important are discussed in this Chapter. The basic processes discussed include oxidative stress, programmed cell death, protein aggregation and protein degradation. Virtually all of the neurodegenerative disorders are complex disorders that involve interaction between environmental and genetic factors. In some cases, genetic factors are the driving force, but in others they are merely risk factors for the disorder. Given the importance of genetics to understanding the neurodegenerative disorders, an introduction to basic genetic principles is also included in this section. In addition, each chapter of this book provides information about clinical genetics in addition to presentations on clinical, pathologic and molecular aspects of the disorders.

While much of the focus in studies of neurodegeneration is rightly placed on understanding neuronal changes, the role of glia in neurodegenerative disorders is increasingly recognised (7). While glia, especially astrocytes, display reactive changes as a part of virtually every neurodegenerative disorder, the changes are usually considered secondary rather than primary events. More recently astrocytes and oligodendroglia have been implicated in fundamental abnormalities of certain neurodegenerative disorders. Among the neurodegenerative disorders where neuroglia have been directly implicated are multiple system atrophy (chapter 3) and in several of the tauopathies (chapter 2), where a diversity of tau-immunoreactive glial inclusions have been described.

The other glial cells that play a role in virtually all neurodegenerative disorders are microglia. Microglia are cells of the mononuclear phagocytic system that respond to virtually all forms of cellular injury. They are also the cells most clearly linked to inflammatory processes in the brain. A comprehensive discussion of neuroinflammation, especially as it relates to Alzheimer's disease, can be found in several recent reviews (1, 4, 5). Briefly, neuroinflammation is a term for a locally induced, nonimmune-mediated, chronic inflammatory response without any apparent influx of leukocytes from the blood. It is characterised by activated microglia, which is a term used for both morphologic and antigenic changes in microglia that differentiate them from the resting and ramified microglia that populate the neural parenchyma. Neuroinflammation has been studied most extensively in Alzheimer's disease (chapter 2) and Parkinson's disease (chapter 3), but some degree of microglial activation is common to virtually all neurodegenerative disorders. In almost all cases, it is considered a secondary or reactive disease process, since it follows the distribution of the neurodegeneration. There is little evidence to suggest that microglial changes precede neuronal changes. Nevertheless, neuroinflammation may amplify or accelerate the neurodegenerative process.

Basic Mechanisms of Neurodegeneration

Programmed cell death is an attractive mechanism to explain selective vulnerability of neuronal populations since most neurodegeneration is not associated with frank inflammation, and this form of cell death does not provoke inflammatory reactions. Chapter 1.2 by Kevin Roth presents a balanced discussion of the role that apoptosis and other mechanisms of cell death may play in neurodegeneration. The chapter provides background information about molecular pathways involved in intrinsic and extrinsic pathways of activation of apoptosis. Intrinsic pathways act through changes in mitochondrial permeability, and the role of mitochondria in neurodegeneration is increasingly recognised. The linkage between programmed cell death and cellular energy metabolism linked to mitochondrial function is being explored. Mitochondria are also one of the major sources of reactive oxygen species generated as byproducts of oxidative phosphorylation. A topic that is not discussed in this overview is the role of mitochondrial metabolism in neurodegeneration (8). This topic is covered thoroughly in the ISN book on muscle disease, since many of the mitochondrial cytopathies are associated with muscle pathology (2).

Accumulation of reactive oxygen species and the cellular defenses against oxidative stress are reviewed in chapter 1.3 by George Perry and co-

Neurodegeneration

The Molecular Pathology of Dementia and Movement Disorders

Volume Editor

Dennis Dickson

Chapter Editors

Catherine Bergeron

Jean-Jacques Hauw

Kurt A. Jellinger

Peter L. Lantos

Hidehiro Mizusawa

Advisory Editors

John A. Hardy

Yoshikuni Mizuno

To be cited as: Dickson DW, *Neurodegeneration: The Molecular Pathology of Dementia and Movement Disorders*, ISN Neuropath Press, Basel 2003, 414 pages.

Neurodegeneration: The Molecular Pathology of Dementia and Movement Disorders

Volume Editor	Dennis W. Dickson, Jacksonville, Fla, United States
Chapter Editors	Catherine Bergeron, Toronto, Canada Jean-Jacques Hauw, Paris, France Kurt A. Jellinger, Vienna, Austria Peter L. Lantos, London, United Kingdom Hidehiro Mizuzawa, Tokyo, Japan
Advisory Editors	John A. Hardy, Bethesda, Md, United States Yoshikuni Mizuno, Tokyo, Japan
Production Editors	Yngve Olsson, Uppsala, Sweden
Layout	Duncan MacRae, Los Angeles, Calif, United States
Editorial Assistants	Margaritka Dikova-Sorge, Munich, Germany Angelica Tibbling, Uppsala, Sweden
Printed by	Allen Press, Inc. Lawrence, Kan, United States
Publisher	ISN Neuropath Press International Society of Neuropathology Institute of Pathology Schönbeinstrasse 40 CH - 4003 Basel Switzerland
ISBN	3-9522313-1-2

Pathology & Genetics

Pathology & Genetics is a book series published by the International Society of Neuropathology (ISN) in collaboration with other international organisations. The first volume on tumours of the nervous system, initiated by Dr Paul Kleihues, Lyon, France was published 1997 together with WHO. A second edition of this volume published by WHO in 2000 can be purchased from IARC Press, Lyon, France (Fax: +33 4 7273 8302).

The ISN General Council elected in 2000 Dr Yngve Olsson, Uppsala, Sweden to serve as a Series Editor for additional volumes. This book on muscle diseases is volume 2 in the ISN Book Series.

Preface

Neurodegenerative diseases share the common property of neuronal loss of specific populations of neurones. The neuronal loss in many of these conditions involves nuclei that are anatomically related to functional systems, such as the extrapyramidal and pyramidal motor systems or the higher order association and limbic cortices. The particular system affected determines the clinical presentation, with many of the most common neurodegenerative disorders presenting with cognitive or motoric deficits or both. The focus of this volume is on disorders that produce dementia or movement disorders.

The basic mechanisms of neuronal loss and the basis for selective vulnerability, while previously largely a matter of speculation, are increasingly understood based upon fundamental molecular abnormalities that have been discovered in these disorders. While the conceptual classification of neurodegenerative disorders in the past has been based upon either the clinical syndromes or anatomical distribution of pathology, it is only in recent years that a molecular classification of neurodegeneration has been seriously considered. This book takes a bold approach to classify neurodegenerative disorders along molecular, rather than clinical terms. The major advances in molecular genetics and application of biochemical and immunochemical studies to neurodegenerative disorders are credited with this new approach. Many neurodegenerative disorders are associated with mutations or genetic variants in specific genes that cause or confer increased risk for the disorder, and in some cases the same molecules or abnormal variants of these molecules can be detected within degenerating neurones and glia.

The major molecules that provide the conceptual framework for the organisation of this book are as follows:

Amyloid. The most common of the neurodegenerative disorders is Alzheimer's disease (AD) in which mutations in β-amyloid precursor protein (APP) gene or genes related to APP metabolism strongly implicate amyloid in the pathogenesis of AD. In addition to β-amyloid deposits, AD is also associated with neurofibrillary degeneration characterized by accumulation of aggregates of the microtubule associated protein tau within vulnerable neurons. While the amyloid deposits are composed of different molecules in familial British dementia and some forms of familial Creutzfeldt-Jakob disease, these are also disorders associated with both amyloid deposits and neurofibrillary tangles. Given the differences in the genetic basis of these disorders, in the present classification, these disorders are separated, but could arguably be grouped in this chapter.

Tau. In addition to AD, neurofibrillary pathology has been noted in a wide range of disorders, which previously suggested that tau pathology might be a relatively nonspecific response of neurones to diverse insults. This view has changed in recent years with the discovery of mutations in the Tau gene in frontotemporal dementia and Parkinsonism linked to chromosome 17 (FTDP-17). Disorders in which abnormalities in tau are considered to play a critical role in disease pathogenesis have been referred to as tauopathies. This group of disorders includes both genetically determined and sporadic conditions, including FTDP-17, Pick's disease, progressive supranuclear palsy and others.

Synuclein. The second most common neurodegenerative disorder is Parkinson's disease, which has long been associated with Lewy bodies in vulnerable neurones. The discovery of mutations in the gene for α-synuclein lead to the recognition that synuclein was a major component of Lewy bodies. Moreover, biochemical and structural alterations in synuclein have been detected in several disorders, including Parkinson's disease, dementia with Lewy bodies and multiple system atrophy. These disorders are grouped together under the term synucleinopathy.

Trinucleotide repeat diseases. Huntington's disease (HD) is one of the most extensively studied hereditary neurodegenerative diseases. The discovery that the mutation in HD was an expansion of a trinucleotide repeat, specifically CAG, in the coding region of the HD gene revealed a common molecular mechanism in a group of disorders that are grouped in this book as the trinucleotide repeat diseases. Not all trinucleotide repeat diseases are associated with CAG repeats in the coding region of affected genes, but the discovery that CAG repeats lead to formation of polyglutamine stretches within the protein suggested common pathogenetic mechanisms involving protein aggregation and inclusion body formation, a phenomenon seen repeatedly in various neurodegenerative disorders.

Prion diseases. A common theme for many of the degenerative disorders is the formation of abnormal conformers of normal cellular proteins that are directly related to pathogenesis of neurodegeneration. Prion disorders are the archetypal example of conformational disorders, in that the only difference known between the pathogenic and normal cellular form of PrP is conformation. Yet this is sufficient to lead to a fulminant and invariably fatal neurodegeneration. Prion diseases, like many of the other neurodegenerative disorders, include sporadic and familial forms. Even the sporadic forms may have a genetic predisposition, specifically polymorphisms in the prion protein gene (PRNP).

Separate chapters in this book are devoted to frontotemporal dementia (FTD) and motor neurone disease, but as science progresses these chapters may be merged in future editions given the increased frequency of motor neurone disease in FTD and the fact that there are shared histopathologic features, such as ubiquitinated neuronal inclusions in both. Except in some of the rare genetic forms of ALS, the proteins that make up the inclusion bodies in these disorders have evaded detection. Once they are discovered, disorders in this category will have a rational classification.

Motor neurone diseases. A section in this book is devoted to motor neurone degenerations that are specifically associated with central nervous system pathology. Rather than separate the motor neurone diseases by the various molecules that are felt to play critical roles in degeneration, this is the chapter of the book that most closely follows a traditional approach. In part this is because so many different molecules have been implicated in the various disorders. A complete discussion of other disorders of the motor unit not associated with neurodegeneration can be found in a companion ISN text, *Structural and Molecular Basis of Skeletal Muscle Diseases*.

The last chapter is a collection of relatively newly described entities or neurodegenerative disorders that do not fit well into the current classification. The choice of disorders to include in this section was necessarily selective and based in part upon the frequency of the condition, but also on disorders in which molecular methods have unraveled the mystery of the disorder. These entities are included as a paradigm to follow in the study of other rare neurodegenerative disorders.

The organisation of this book puts clear emphasis on biochemical and genetics aspects of neurodegenerative diseases and sometimes includes disorders with quite different clinical presentations in the same chapter. It is the assumption of the editors that discovery of treatments that act at these fundamental levels will lead to improvement regardless of the clinical phenotype. Obviously, time will tell if this approach was reasonable. Each chapter includes a discussion of the genetics and molecular pathogenesis of the disorder, but not omitted are also discussions of clinical presentation, diagnostic evaluation and epidemiology for each entity as far as it is possible.

Finally, there are several other features that we hope will make this book valuable, including generous use of high quality illustrations, frequent use of graphs and tables to summarise clinical and pathologic concepts, relatively rapid publication and a modest cost. The authors are excited about the project and hope that this book provides a useful reference to students of neurodegenerative disorders.

Dennis Dickson

Contents

Preface iii

Chapter 1: Introduction **1**
Introduction 2
Apoptosis and Neurodegeneration 4
The Role of Oxidative Mechanisms in Neurodegenerative Diseases 8
Abnormal Protein-Protein Interactions: Underlying Mechanisms of Diverse Neurodegenerative Diseases 11
The Ubiquitin Pathway, Neurodegeneration and Brain Function 14
The Genetics of Neurodegeneration 17
Alzheimer's Disease and Ageing 23

Chapter 2: Alzheimer's Disease and Ageing **23**
Alzheimer Type Dementia 24
Genetics of Alzheimer's Disease 40
Neuropathology of Alzheimer's Disease 47
Plaque-predominant and Tangle-predominant Variants of Alzheimer's Disease 66
Molecular Pathogenesis of Alzheimer's Disease 69
Alzheimer Animal Models: Models of Ab Deposition in Transgenic Mice 74
Tauopathies 81

Chapter 3: Tauopathies **81**
Introduction to the Tauopathies 82
Frontotemporal Dementia and Parkinsonism Linked to Chromosome 17 Associated with Tau Gene Mutations (FTDP-17T) 86
Progressive Supranuclear Palsy (PSP) or Steele-Richardson-Olszewski Disease 103
Corticobasal Degeneration 115
Pick's Disease 124
Argyrophilic Grain Disease 132
Parkinsonism-dementia Complex of Guam 137
Postencephalitic Parkinsonism 143
Transgenic Animal Models of Tauopathies 150
Synucleinopathies 155

Chapter 4: Synucleinopathies **155**
Introduction to Synucleinopathies 156
Lewy Body Disorders
Parkinson's Disease 159
Dementia with Lewy Bodies 188
Lewy Bodies in Conditions Other Than Disorders of α-Synuclein 200
Multiple System Atrophy 203
Experimental Models of Synucleinopathies 215
Trinucleotide Repeat Disorders 225

Chapter 5: Trinucleotide Repeat Disorders **225**
Introduction to Trinucleotide Repeat Disorders 226
Huntington's Disease 229
Spinocerebellar Ataxias 242
Friedreich's Ataxia 257
Dentatorubral-pallidoluysian Atrophy 269
Spinal and Bulbar Muscular Atrophy 275
Prion Disorders 281

Chapter 6: Prion Disorders **281**
Introduction to Prion Diseases 282
Creutzfeldt-Jakob Disease
Sporadic Creutzfeldt-Jakob Disease 287
Familial Creutzfeldt-Jakob Disease 298
Iatrogenic Prion Disorders 307
Variant Creutzfeldt-Jakob Disease 310
Gerstmann-Sträussler-Scheinker Disease 318
Fatal Insomnia: Familial and Sporadic 326
Kuru 333
In Vivo and In Vitro Models of Prion Disease 335
Frontotemporal Degeneration 339

Chapter 7: Frontotemporal Degeneration **339**
Frontotemporal Degeneration: Introduction 340
Frontotemporal Lobar Degeneration 342

Chapter 8: Motor Neurone Disorders **349**
Amyotrophic Lateral Sclerosis 350
Primary Lateral Sclerosis 369
Spinal Muscular Atrophy 372
Other Neurodegenerative Disorders 377

Chapter 9: Other Neurodegenerative Disorders **377**
Other Neurodegenerative Disorders: Introduction 378
Inherited Amyloidoses and Neurodegeneration: Familial British Dementia and Familial Danish Dementia 380
Neuroaxonal Dystrophies
Neuroaxonal Dystrophies 386
Infantile Neuroaxonal Dystrophy (Seitelberger Disease) 390
Neurodegeneration with Brain Iron Acculation, Type 1 (Hallervorden-Spatz Disease) 394
Familial Encephalopathy with Neuroserpin Inclusion Bodies 400
Neuronal intranuclear inclusion disease 404

Contributors **407**

Acknowledgments **412**

Index **413**

workers. One consequence of cellular oxidative stress is post-translational modification (eg, nitration) of proteins. These proteins take on abnormal properties that may lead to changes in their solubility and promote aggregation. Aggregation of abnormal conformers of neuronal and glial proteins is increasingly recognised as a common mechanism of a number of neurodegenerative disorders. The role of protein-protein interaction, *protein aggregation* and changes in structural properties of proteins that favour interaction and aggregation is the topic reviewed by John Trojanowski (chapter 1.4).

Accompanying protein aggregation and accumulation is usually evidence of aberration of the normal cellular mechanisms for *protein degradation*. While two major pathways exist for protein degradation, including lysosomal and non-lysosomal, much current research in neurodegenerative disease is focussed on the role of non-lysosomal pathways mediated by ubiquitin and the proteasome, which is reviewed in chapter 1.5 by John Mayer (see also reference 3). Lysosomal pathways may also be involved in neurodegenerative processes and the reader is referred to reviews by Nixon and co-workers for a discussion of the role of lysosomes in neurodegeneration (6).

Genetics of Neurodegeneration

Chapter 1.6 by John Hardy provides background on modern genetic mechanisms and some examples of how genetics has contributed to providing a conceptual framework for investigating the pathogenesis of certain neurodegenerative diseases. The review also provides practical guidelines for the pathologist confronted with a degenerative condition that may have genetic underpinnings. Finally, the rapid pace of studies on the human genome and the impact that this will increasingly have on our understanding and ability to decipher the role of genetics in neurodegeneration is discussed.

References

1. Eikelenboom P, Rozemuller AJ, Hoozemans JJ, Veerhuis R, van Gool WA (2000) Neuroinflammation and Alzheimer disease: clinical and therapeutic implications. *Alzheimer Dis Assoc Dis* 14 (suppl 1): S54-S61.

2. Karpati G (2002) *Structural and molecular basis of skeletal muscle diseases.* ISN Neuropath Press, Basel.

3. Mayer RJ, Tipler C, Arnold J, Laszlo L, Al-Khedhairy A, Lowe J, Landon M. (1996) Endosome-lysosomes, ubiquitin and neurodegeneration. *Adv Exp Med Biol* 389: 261-269.

4. McGeer PL, McGeer EG (2001) Inflammation, autotoxicity and Alzheimer disease. *Neurobiol Aging* 22: 799-809.

5. Mrak RE, Griffin W (2001) Interleukin-1, neuroinflammation, and Alzheimer's disease. *Neurobiol Aging* 22: 903-908.

6. Nixon RA, Cataldo AM, Mathews PM (2000) The endosomal-lysosomal system of neurons in Alzheimer's disease pathogenesis: a review. *Neurochem Res* 25: 1161-1172.

7. Schipper HM (1996)Astrocytes, brain aging, and neurodegeneration. *Neurobiol Aging* 17: 467-480.

8. Wallace DC (2001) A mitochondrial paradigm for degenerative diseases and ageing. *Novartis Fnd Symp* 235: 247-263.

Apoptosis and Neurodegeneration

Kevin A. Roth

Bcl-2	B-cell CLL/lymphoma 2
IAP	inhibitor of apoptosis protein
NAIP	neuronal apoptosis inhibitor protein

Introduction

Loss of neurones is a hallmark feature of most, if not all, neurodegenerative diseases. Given the limited neurogenic capacity of the adult nervous system, neuronal cell death marks an irreversible and catastrophic phase of the neurodegenerative process. Consequently, tremendous scientific effort has been focused on the cellular and molecular pathways regulating neurone death. Cell death can be roughly divided into necrotic and non-necrotic types (3). Necrotic cell death is typically characterised by cell swelling and requires no active participation of the degenerating cell. In contrast, non-necrotic cell death is regulated by cell autonomous processes and typically produces distinctive ultrastructural changes. Several types of regulated cell death have been described including apoptotic and autophagic death (2). Apoptosis is characterised by specific cytological features including chromatin condensation and margination, nuclear fragmentation, and cytoplasmic blebbing (15). Autophagic death is characterised by the presence of large numbers of autophagic vacuoles in the cytoplasm of cells displaying additional cytological features of apoptotic and/or necrotic degeneration (38). In the developing nervous system, apoptosis is by far the most common and well-investigated form of programmed cell death (defined as developmentally and genetically regulated cell death) and apoptotic cell death has been implicated in a variety of neurodegenerative disorders.

Bcl-2 and Caspases

Investigations over the last 10 years have revealed particularly significant roles for members of the Bcl-2 and caspase families in neuronal apoptosis. The Bcl-2 family can be divided into pro- and anti-apoptotic groups (16). Bcl-2 is the prototypical anti-apoptotic family member and along with other highly homologous anti-apoptotic members such as Bcl-X_L, acts to decrease cellular sensitivity to death promoting stimuli. The pro-apoptotic Bcl-2 family members can be subdivided into 2 groups based on their extent of Bcl-2 homology. Multi-domain members, such as Bax and Bak, contain multiple Bcl-2 homologous domains and act in large part by regulating mitochondrial cytochrome c release and function (35). BH3 domain-only pro-apoptotic molecules such as Bid and Bad have limited homology with Bcl-2 and appear to act upstream of Bax and Bak, perhaps by interfering with the action of anti-apoptotic Bcl-2 family members (11). Targeted gene disruptions of several pro- and anti-apoptotic Bcl-2 family members have revealed significant roles for these genes in regulating naturally-occurring neuronal death during nervous system development (23).

Caspases are cysteine-containing, aspartate-specific proteases and represent a second major family of cell death regulators (22). There are approximately 15 mammalian caspases that can be divided into three major groups. One group, including caspases 1, 4, and 5, is largely involved in cytokine processing and probably plays only an indirect role in neuronal apoptosis. The second group consists of initiator caspases (eg, caspase-2, -8, and -9), that transduce apoptotic signals to the third group of caspases, including caspases 3, 6 and 7, which act as true apoptosis "effector" molecules. Caspases exist at baseline as inactive proenzymes and are cleaved into two active subunits in response to apoptotic stimuli, typically by self-initiation or trans-caspase activation. The apoptotic phenotype is dependent upon effector caspase activity and caspase-3 is the predominant effector caspase in the nervous system (5). Although the apoptotic neuronal phenotype requires caspase-3-like activity, upstream cellular events may commit neurones to cell death prior to or coincident with caspase-3 activation. Thus, engagement of an apoptotic death pathway may result in neuronal cell death prior to emergence of the cytological features that originally defined the term "apoptosis." This fact has led to confusion as investigators have used various definitions of apoptotic death (28). As we learn more about the molecules regulating neuronal cell death, morphological descriptions of regulated cell death will likely be replaced by molecular ones.

In most, but not all, neuronal cell death paradigms, caspases act downstream of the Bcl-2 family. For example, the increased neuronal cell death observed in the Bcl-X_L-deficient embryonic mouse nervous system is completely blocked by concomitant deficiency in caspase-9 or caspase-3 (24, 37). A variety of other molecules including Apaf-1, Smac/Diablo, and inhibitor of apoptosis protein (IAP) family members play significant roles in neuronal cell death regulation, largely through their effects on Bcl-2 family function and caspase activity. Neuronal apoptosis inhibitor protein (NAIP) is a member of the IAP family and a direct inhibitor of the effector caspases 3 and 7 (20). Deletions in the NAIP gene have been associated with childhood spinal muscular atrophy and NAIP has been proposed to modify the severity of this disease (25). In total, a

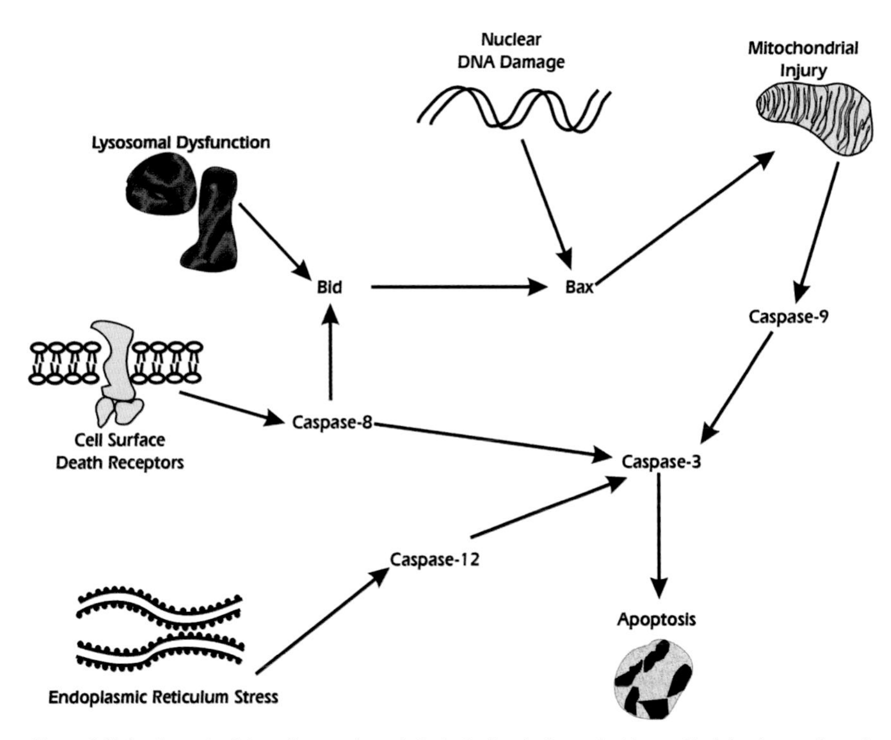

Figure 1. Molecular and cellular pathways of apoptotic death. Apoptosis may be triggered by injury to any of a variety of organelles. If the apoptotic stimulus is sufficiently large, Bcl-2 family mediated caspase activation occurs and the degenerating neurone displays apoptotic cytological features. However, the persistent presence of acutely sublethal injurious stimuli may induce anti-apoptotic compensatory changes that inhibit caspase function. Under such circumstances, neurone injury may result in organelle dysfunction and neurodegeneration in the absence of caspase-mediated apoptotic death.

complex set of molecular checks and balances tightly controls the extent and significance of neuronal caspase activation.

Apoptosis-associated Molecules and Processes in Neurodegenerative Diseases

Since selective neuronal cell death is a consistent feature of human neurodegenerative disease, the possibility that apoptosis-associated molecules and processes underlie neurodegenerative disease pathogenesis has received increasing attention (10, 36). This hypothesis requires a critical analysis of several questions. First, is the neuronal cell death observed in the most common neurodegenerative diseases such as Alzheimer's disease, Parkinson's disease, and Huntington's disease apoptotic? Second, what are the etiological stimuli that lead to engagement of the apoptotic death pathway? Third, if neurone death in these diseases can be classified as "apoptotic," is neurological dysfunction a direct consequence of neurone loss or does it occur prior to caspase-dependent neurone death? Unfortunately, definitive answers to these questions are not yet available. Caspase activation and/or apoptotic degeneration has been reported in Alzheimer's, Parkinson's, and Huntington's disease brain (1, 6, 30); however, other investigators have failed to detect convincing morphological or biochemical evidence for apoptotic death in these diseases (8, 32, 38). Experimental models have also generated mixed results on the presence and significance of caspase activation and apoptotic cell death in neurodegenerative diseases. To date, there is not compelling evidence for or against the hypothesis that neurones die by caspase-mediated apoptosis in human neurodegenerative disease.

The stimuli that produce neurone death in Alzheimer's and Parkinson's disease are unknown in the vast majority of cases. Familial Alzheimer's and Parkinson's disease clearly point to an etiological role for amyloid precursor protein, presenilins, and α-synuclein in these cases and altered huntingtin protein function causes Huntington's disease. In none of these diseases however, have genetic abnormalities in Bcl-2 or caspase family members been implicated in disease pathogenesis. The absence of defined mutations in these genes does not rule out an important role for apoptosis-associated molecules in neurodegenerative diseases, yet it strongly suggests that genetically dysregulated apoptosis is not the primary defect. Even in the case of childhood spinal muscular atrophy in which deletions of NAIP may modify disease severity, the disease itself is caused by mutations in the survival motor neurone (SMN) gene (18). Defining the stimuli that produce neurodegeneration and how they engage regulated cell death pathways in both hereditary and sporadic neurodegenerative diseases represents a significant challenge. Unlike programmed cell death in the developing nervous system or in vitro models of neuronal apoptosis, neurone loss in most human neurodegenerative diseases is a slowly progressive chronic process that invokes compensatory changes in a wide variety of pro-survival molecules and pathways. For example, although in vitro application of Aβ produces Bcl-2 and/or caspase family-dependent neuronal apoptosis (27), transgenic models of in vivo Aβ overproduction have failed to demonstrate significant caspase activation or neuronal loss (12). Similarly, pro-apoptotic effects of mutated Huntington have been demonstrated in vitro, but neurone loss in transgenic models of Huntington's disease is non-apoptotic (33). Evidence has now accumulated that damage to any of a variety cell organelles can trigger Bcl-2 and caspase-mediated apoptosis (Figure 1). It is also clear that organelle dysfunction can lead to cell death independently of caspase activation and cytological evidence of apoptosis. In chronic neurodegenerative diseases, a fine balance may exist between organelle dysfunction, engagement of apoptotic death pathways, and pro-survival compensatory changes in gene expression and cell function. More significant than whether neurones in neurodegenerative diseases die by apoptotic or non-apoptotic pathways is determining whether neuronal dysfunction precedes neurone death and if so, do apoptosis-associated molecules play a critical role in causing dysfunction?

Caspases in Synaptic Degeneration

Increasing attention is being placed on the earliest histopathological findings in human neurodegenerative disease brain tissue and experimental animal models of these diseases. Interestingly, several studies suggest that alterations in synaptic structure or function precede neurone loss in Alzheimer's, Parkinson's, and Huntington's disease and that these changes correlate with neurological dysfunction in animal models of neurodegenerative disease. Significant changes in synapse density and structure have been observed in transgenic mouse models of Alzheimer's disease and synapse loss has been cited as the major correlate of cognitive decline in human Alzheimer's disease patients (9, 31). In Parkinson's disease models, mutant α-synuclein production produced loss of dopamine-containing dense core granules and non-apoptotic cell death and caspase inhibitors retarded cell death but not neuritic loss or functional impairment in 6-hydroxydopamine treated mesencephalic dopaminergic neurones (29, 34). Neuritic alterations and reduced synaptic responsiveness have been reported in in vivo models of Huntington's disease and these changes preceded neurone loss which appeared to occur through a non-apoptotic process (14, 17, 19). Considering a number of studies that have implicated caspases in neurodegenerative disease, the possibility that caspases play a role in synaptic degeneration, independent of their pro-apoptotic action, must be considered.

Localised synaptic caspase activation has been demonstrated in response to death-promoting stimuli, and this signal can be propagated retrogradely to the neuronal cell body triggering apoptotic death (4, 13, 21). Caspases, however, are not necessary for non-apoptotic neuritic and synaptic degeneration, and Bcl-2 overexpression inhibits neurone loss, but not axonal degeneration, in a mouse model of neurodegenerative disease (7, 26). It remains possible that localised caspase activation plays an important role in the synaptic alterations observed early in neurodegenerative disease, but data in support of this hypothesis are not yet compelling. If caspases can be demonstrated to play a significant role in the early synaptic pathology observed in neurodegenerative diseases, administration of caspase inhibitors at the onset of neurological symptoms could prove to have substantial clinical benefit. In contrast, if caspases are involved only in the final execution of dysfunctional neurones, caspase inhibitors will be of little clinical value.

The tremendous scientific interest in both apoptosis and neurodegenerative disease has produced significant advances in our understanding of the cellular and molecular processes controlling neurone life and death. Despite the fact that numerous questions remain about the precise role of apoptosis-associated molecules in human neurodegenerative disease, there is no disputing that a dead neurone is a dysfunctional neurone. Future investigations are necessary to devise strategies for restoring function to injured neurones before they become committed to death, apoptotic or otherwise.

References

1. Anderson JK (2001) Does neuronal loss in Parkinson's disease involve programmed cell death. *BioEssays* 23: 640-646.

2. Clarke PGH (1990) Developmental cell death: morphological diversity and multiple mechanisms. *Anat Embryol* 181: 195-213.

3. Clarke PGH (1999) Apoptosis versus necrosis. How valid a dichotomy for neurons? In *Cell Death and Diseases of the Nervous System*, VE Koliatsos, RR Ratan (eds). Humana Press: Totowa, New Jersey. pp. 3-28.

4. Cowan CM, Thai J, Krajewski S, Reed J, Nicholson DW, Kaufmann SH, Roskams AJ (2001) Caspases 3 and 9 send a pro-apoptotic signal from synapse to cell body in olfactory receptor neurons. *J Neurosci* 21: 7099-7109.

5. D'Mello SR, Kuan C-Y, Flavell RA, Rakic P (2000) Caspase-3 is required for apoptosis-associated DNA fragmentation but not for cell death in neurons deprived of potassium. *J Neurosci Res* 59: 24-31.

6. Evert BO, Wüllner U (2000) Cell death in polyglutamine diseases. *Cell Tiss Res* 301: 189-204.

7. Finn JT, Weil M, Archer F, Siman R, Srinivasan A, Raff MC (2000) Evidence that Wallerian degeneration and localized axon degeneration induced by local neurotrophin deprivation do not involve caspases. *J Neurosci* 20: 1333-1341.

8. Graeber MB, Grasbon-Frodl E, Abell-Aleff P, Kösel S (1999) Nigral neurons are likely to die of a mechanism other than classical apoptosis in Parkinson's disease. *Parkinsonism and Related Disorders* 5: 187-192.

9. Holtzman DM, Bales KR, Tenkova T, Fagan AM, Parsadanian M, Sartorius LJ, Mackey B, Olney J, McKeel D, Wozniak D, et al (2000) Apoliproprotein E isoform-dependent amyloid deposition and neuritic degeneration in a mouse model of Alzheimer's disease. *Proc Natl Acad Sci USA* 97: 2892-2897.

10. Honig LS, Rosengerg RN (2000) Apoptosis and neurologic disease. *Am J Med* 108: 317-330

11. Huang DCS, A. S (2000) BH3-only proteins - essential initiators of apoptotic cell death. *Cell* 103: 839-842.

12. Irizarry MC, McNamara M, Fedorchak K, Hsiao K, Hyman BT (1997) APPSw transgenic mice develop age-related Ab deposits and neuropil abnormalities, but no neuronal loss in CA-1. *J Neuropathol Exp Neurol* 56: 965-973.

13. Ivins KJ, Bui ETN, Cotman CW (1998) b-amyloid induces local neurite degeneration in cultured hippocampal neurons: evidence for neuritic apoptosis. *Neurobiol Dis* 5: 365-378.

14. Kegel KB, Kim M, Sapp E, McIntyre C, Castaño JG, Aronin N, DiFiglia M (2000) Huntingtin expression stimulates endosomal-lysosomal activity, endosome tubulation, and autophagy. *J Neurosci Res* 20: 7268-7278.

15. Kerr JFR, Wyllie AH, Currie AR (1972) Apoptosis: a basic biological phenomenon with wide-ranging implications in tissue kinetics. *Br J Cancer* 26: 239-257.

16. Korsmeyer SJ (1999) BCL-2 gene family and the regulation of programmed cell death. *Cancer Res* 59 suppl: 1693s-1700s.

17. Laforet GA, Sapp E, Chase K, McIntyre C, Boyce FM, Campbell M, Cadigan BA, Warzecki L, Tagle DA, Reddy PH, et al (2001) Changes in cortical and striatal neurons predict behavioral and electrophysical abnormalities in a transgenic murine model of Huntington's disease. *J Neurosci* 21: 9112-9123.

18. Lefebvre S, Burglen L, Reboullet S, Clermont O, Burlet P, Viollet L, Benichou B, Cruaud C, Millasseau P, Zeviani M (1995) Identification and characterization of a spinal muscular atrophy-determining gene. *Cell* 80.

19. Li H, Li S-H, Yu Z-X, Shelbourne P, Li X-J (2001) Huntingtin aggregate-associated axonal degeneration is an early pathological event in Huntington's Disease mice. *J Neurosci* 21: 8473-8481.

20. Maier JKX, Lahoua Z, H GN, Fetni R, Johnston A, Davoodi J, Rasper D, Roy S, Slack RS, Nicholson DW, et al (2002) The neuronal apoptosis inhibitory protein is a direct inhibitor of Caspases 3 and 7. *J Neurosci Res* 22: 2035-2043.

21. Mattson MP, Keller JN, Begley JG (1998) Evidence for synaptic apoptosis. *Exp Neurol* 153: 35-48.

22. Nicholson DW (1999) Caspase structure, proteolytic substrates, and function during apoptotic cell death. *Cell Death and Differentiation* 6: 1028-1042.

23. Roth KA, D'Sa C (2001) Apoptosis and brain development. *Mental Retardation and Developmental Disabilities* 7: 261-266.

24. Roth KA, Kuan C-Y, Haydar TF, D'Sa-Eipper C, Shindler KS, Zheng TS (2000) Epistatic and independent apoptotic functions of Caspase-3 and Bcl-XL in the developing nervous system. *Proc Natl Acad Sci U S A* 97: 466-471.

25. Roy N, Mahadevan MS, McLean M, Shutler G, Yaraghi Z, Farahani R, Baird S, Besner-Johnston A, Lefebvre C, Kang X, et al (1995) The gene for neuronal apoptosis inhibitory protein is partially deleted in individuals with spinal muscular atrophy. *Cell* 80: 167-178.

26. Sagot Y, Dubois-Dauphin M, Tan H, DeBilbao F, Aebischer P, Martinou JC, Kato AC (1995) Bcl-2 overexpression prevents motoneuron cell body loss but not axonal degeneration in a mouse model of a neurodegenerative disease. *J Neurosci* 15: 7727-7733.

27. Selznick LA, Zheng TS, Flavell RA, Rakic P, Roth KA (2000) Amyloid beta-induced death is Bax-dependent but caspase-independent. *J Neuropathol Exp Neurol* 59: 271-279.

28. Sloviter RS (2002) Apoptosis: a guide for the perplexed. *Trends Pharmacol Sci* 23: 19-24.

29. Stefanis L, Larsen KE, Rideout HJ, Sulzer D, Greene LA (2001) Expression of A53T mutant but not wild-type a-synuclein in PC12 cells induces alterations of the ubiquitin-dependent degradation system, loss of dopamine release, and autophagic cell death. *J Neurosci* 21: 9549-9560.

30. Su JH, Anderson AJ, Cummings BJ, Cotman CW (1994) Immunohistochemical evidence for apoptosis in Alzheimer's disease. *NeuroReport* 5: 2529-2533.

31. Terry RD, Masliah E, Salmon DP, Butters N, DeTeresa R, Hill R, Hansen LA, Katzman R (1991) Physical basis of cognitive alterations in Alzheimer's disease: synapse loss is the major correlate of cognitive impairment. *Ann Neurol* 30: 572-580.

32. Tobin AJ SE (2000) Huntington's disease: the challenge for cell biologists. *Trends Cell Biol* 10: 531-536.

33. Turmaine M, Raza A, Mahal A, Mangiarini L, Bates GP, Davies SW (2000) Nonapoptotic neurodegeneration in a transgenic mouse model of Huntington's disease. *Proc Natl Acad Sci U S A* 97: 8093-8097.

34. von Coelln R, Kügler S, Bähr M, Weller M, Dichgans J, Schulz JB (2001) Rescue from death but not from functional impairment: caspase inhibition protects dopaminergic cells against 6-hydroxydopamine-induced apoptosis but not against the loss of their terminals. *J Neurochem* 77: 263-273.

35. Wei MC, Zong W-X, Cheng EHY, Lindsten T, Panoutsakopoulou V, Ross AJ, Roth KA, MacGregor GR, Thompson CB, Korsmeyer SJ (2001) Proapoptotic BAX and BAK: A requisite gateway to mitochondrial dysfunction and death. *Science* 292: 727-730.

36. Wellington CL, Hayden MR (2000) Caspases and neurodegeneration: on the cutting edge of new therapeutic approaches. *Clin Genet* 57: 1-10.

37. Zaidi AU, D'Sa-Eipper C, Brenner J, Kuida K, Zheng TS, Flavell RA, Rakic P, Roth KA (2001) Bcl-XL-Caspase-9 interactions in the developing nervous system: evidence for multiple death pathways. *J Neurosci Res* 21: 169-175.

38. Zaidi AU, McDonough JS, Klocke BJ, Latham CB, Korsmeyer SJ, Flavell RA, Schmidt RE, Roth KA (2001) Chloroquine-induced neuronal cell death is p53 and Bcl-2 family-dependent but caspase-independent. *J Neuropathol Exp Neurol* 60: 937-945.

The Role of Oxidative Mechanisms in Neurodegenerative Diseases

George Perry
Ravi Srinivas
Akihiko Nunomura
Mark A. Smith

AD	Alzheimer's disease
NFH	neurofilament heavy subunit
SOD	superoxide dismutase

Oxidative damage is a major feature of the cytopathology of a number of chronic neurodegenerative diseases, such as Alzheimer's disease and Parkinson's disease. Historically, the concept of oxidative stress has been used to indicate an excess of oxygen free radicals that breach oxidant defences with consequent detriment. By this definition, detection of damage resulting from reactive oxygen species is indicative of oxidative stress (3). Reactive oxygen species are a by-product of cellular oxidative metabolism and are generated in the mitochondria during oxidative phosphorylation with production of molecules with unpaired electrons, such as superoxide (O_2^-). Superoxide is a short-lived molecule that is reduced by the family of superoxide dismutases (SODs) to generate hydrogen peroxide (H_2O_2). Reduction of H_2O_2, for example through the action of redox-active divalent cations such as iron, generates hydroxyl radicals ($^{\cdot}OH$), which are potent free radicals that lead to oxidative damage of proteins, lipids and nucleic acids. Nitric oxide is another short-lived free radical with limited toxicity that is produced by a family of nitric oxide synthases. After interaction with superoxide, nitric oxide forms peroxynitrite (ONOO-), which is another powerful reactive species that can lead to damage of cellular macromolecules through nitration or generation of additional free radicals. Cells have evolved an elaborate array of anti-oxidant defences, including SOD, glutathione reductase and catalase (3).

Detection of Cellular Oxidative Damage

Cellular oxidative damage can be detected in a variety of ways. Widely used markers of oxidative damage to lipids include 4-hydroxynonenal and isoprostanes; to nucleic acids include 8-hydroxy-2′-deoxyguanosine; and to proteins include nitration and glycation. Indirect evidence of cellular oxidative stress is increased expression of molecules involved in oxidant defence, such as heme-oxygenases, SODs, glutathione transferases and catalase (3). It is important to note that neurones displaying signs of oxidative stress are not necessarily succumbing to oxidative stress, but may be adapting by way of oxidant defences. These findings suggest that neurodegenerative disorders where oxidative stress is postulated to play a role, such as Parkinson's disease and Alzheimer's disease, are associated with mechanisms that maintain a balance between oxidative stress and adaptation to this stress, reflecting the ability of living systems to dynamically regulate their defence mechanisms in response to oxidants. Therefore, mere evidence of oxidative damage does not necessarily indicate cell death by way of oxidative stress given that the cell may have successfully increased its defences sufficiently to compensate for the increased flux of reactive oxygen responsible for the damage. It does, however, indicate that the normal balance between production and defences of oxidative stress has been challenged.

Consequences and Mechanisms of Cellular Oxidative Damage

Evidence suggests that cells that fail to compensate for oxidative stress enter apoptosis, which in turn leads to death within hours. Therefore, cells can only experience oxidative stress for short periods of time without rapidly dying (7, 8). This is particularly germane to the discussion of degenerative diseases that have a course of years.

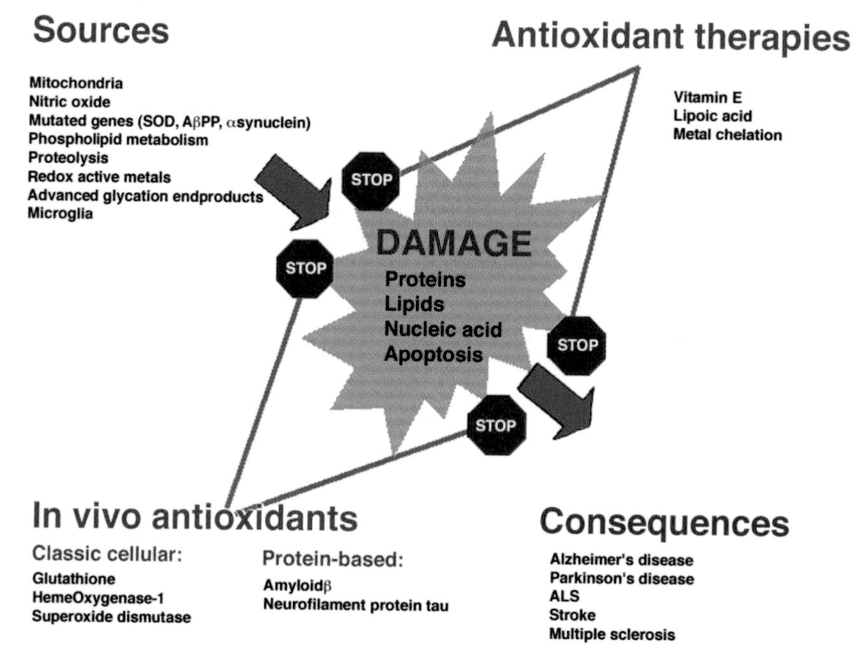

Figure 1. Schematic presentation of sources of products causing oxidative cellular damage influencing various CNS diseases. In vivo antioxidants and various therapeutic agents may reduce the consequences.

Those cells experiencing increased oxidative damage, by their continued existence, testify to their increased compensatory response to reactive oxygen.

This is certainly the case for Alzheimer disease (AD), where oxidative damage is evident in every category of macromolecule examined, including presence of increased sulfhydryls, induction of heme-oxygenase-1, and increased expression of Cu/Zn superoxide dismutase (5, 6, 9). Even those aspects of AD thought most deleterious, the pathological lesions, senile plaques and neurofibrillary tangles, may play an important aspect in oxidant defence (2). Quantitative analysis of the extent of oxidative damage in AD shows the oxidative damage is actually reduced in those neurones with the most cytopathology (5). This suggests that oxidative defences extend beyond the classical antioxidant enzymes and low molecular weight reductants. A prominent role may also be played by the distinct structural and biochemical changes that are associated with, and considered part of, the spectrum of the disease.

The importance of this aspect is seen when taking into consideration that protection of critical cellular components from oxidants can be through the incorporation of damage to less critical cellular components. At the present time, the exhaustion of cellular reductants (which are incidentally the same category of agents most often used as therapeutics) is used as a measure of antioxidant potential; however, cellular macromolecules may share a similar function. Consistent with this view is the physiological modification of neurofilament heavy subunit (NFH) by carbonyls (2). Intriguingly, although NFH has a long half-life, the same extent of carbonyl modification is found throughout the normal ageing process, as well as along the length of the axon. Therefore, NFH may be uniquely adapted as a carbonyl scavenger due to a high lysine content. For example, the sequence, lysine-serine-proline, is repeated approximately 50 times in the sidearm portion of the molecule, a domain that is exposed on the surface of a neurofilament structure.

While more studies are required to understand the role of NFH modifications in neuronal homeostasis, it is tempting to consider them as additional neuronal defences important in protecting the axon, the major location of neurofilaments, from some of the most toxic products of oxidation, reactive aldehydes. The slow turnover rate of proteins in the axon, which can take years, may necessitate this protection. Maintenance of steady state levels of carbonyl adduction suggests the existence of a mechanism for metabolic regeneration of the neurofilament lysines analogous to the scavenging of reactive oxygen shown by methionine on the surface of many proteins and subsequent regeneration of methionine catalysed by methionine sulfoxide reductase (2).

RNA is extensively modified in AD and, while clearly damaged, the rapid turnover of RNA may also serve a protective function. With the formation of hydroxyl-radicals, every macromolecule would be potentially susceptible to attack, but the most critical aspect for the cell is to reduce damage to systems, such as enzyme active sites, the compromise of which leads to cell death. While RNA alteration may lead to protein sequence anomalies (8), RNA destruction can more easily be accommodated in cellular metabolism than damage to DNA (1, 4) or enzyme active site destruction. The large pool of neuronal RNA may even mean that errors in protein synthesis, resulting from oxidatively modified RNA, can be corrected by the metabolic turnover of abnormal proteins. Certainly, renewal of components is a common theme in biology, and although energetically wasteful, rids the cells of the consequences of damage.

In sum, the simple concept that oxidative damage is deleterious to cells and amenable by therapeutic increases in antioxidants may be far too simplistic. The proposed concept of homeostatic balance between oxidant stress and defences is a possible explanation for why efforts to increase oxidative defences by therapeutic use of antioxidants has produced, at most, moderate benefits. It is imperative that the overall homeostatic system be considered before decisions are made about the short-term and long-term consequences of therapeutic antioxidants. If cells survive and function with evidence of oxidative damage, it is unlikely that the oxidant stress has damaged critical systems. Augmentation of antioxidants may only have marginal benefit or even detrimental effects by upsetting the homeostatic balance. Instead, oxidative damage should be considered a window to view both the homeostatic compensations necessary for survival and as a means to design therapeutics to modify the more fundamental abnormalities responsible for altering oxidative balance in neurodegenerative disorders.

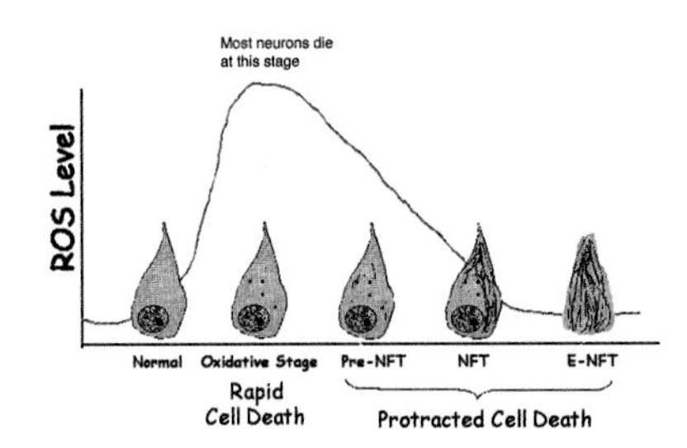

Figure 2. Chronology of neuronal pathology in Alzheimer's disease. Metabolic and oxidative alterations precede tau phosphorylation. The pathological lesions, neurofibrillary tangles and senile plaques, are late events.

References

1. Gabbita SP, Lovell MA, Markesbery WR (1988) Increased nuclear DNA oxidation in the brain in Alzheimer's disease. *J Neurochem* 7: 2034-2040.

2. Levine RL, Mosoni L, Berlett BS, Stadtman ER (1996) Methionine residues as endogenous antioxidants in proteins. *Proc Natl Acad Sci U S A* 93: 15036-15040.

3. Markesbery WR, Carney JM (1999) Oxidative alterations in Alzheimer's disease. *Brain Pathol* 9:133-146.

4. Mecocci P, MacGarvey J, Beal MF (1994) Oxidative damage to mitochondrial DNA is increased in Alzheimer's disease. *Ann Neurol* 36:747-751.

5. Nunomura A, Perry G, Hirai K, Aliev G, Takeda A, Chiba S, Smith MA (1999) Neuronal RNA oxidation in Alzheimer disease and Down's syndrome. *Ann NY Acad Sci* 893: 362-364.

6. Pappolla MA, Omar RA, Kim KS, Robalds N K (1992) Immunohistochemical evidence of oxidative stress in Alzheimer's disease. *Am J Pathol* 140: 621-628.

7. Perry G, Nunomura A, Smith MA (1998) A suicide note from Alzheimer disease neurons? *Nat Med* 4: 897-898.

8. Perry G, Nunomura A, Lucassen P, Lassmann H, Smith MA (1998) Apoptosis and Alzheimer's disease. *Science* 282:1268-1269.

9. Smith MA, Rudnicka Nawrot M, Richey PL, Praprotnik D, Mulvihill P, Miller CA, Sayre LM, Perry G (1995) Carbonyl-related posttranslational modification of neurofilament protein in the neurofibrillary pathology of Alzheimer's disease. *J Neurochem* 64: 2660-2666.

10. van Leeuwen FW, de Kleiju DP, van den Hurk HH, Neubauer A, Sonnemans MA, Sluijs JA, Koycu S, Ramdjielal RDJ, Salehi A, Martens GJM, Grosveld FG, Peter J, Burbach H, Hol EM (1998) Frameshift mutants of beta amyloid precursor protein and ubiquitin-B in Alzheimer's and Down patients. *Science* 279: 242-247.

Abnormal Protein-Protein Interactions: Underlying Mechanisms of Diverse Neurodegenerative Diseases

J. Q. Trojanowski

Aβ	beta-amyloid peptides
AD	Alzheimer's disease
ALS	amyotrophic lateral sclerosis,
CNS	central nervous system
DLB	dementia with Lewy bodies
DS	Down's syndrome
FAD	familial Alzheimer's disease
FTDP	frontotemporal dementia and Parkinsonism
GCI	glial cytoplasmic inclusion
LB	Lewy body
LBVAD	Lewy body variant of Alzheimer's disease
MSA	multiple system atrophy
NBIA 1	meurodegeneration with brain iron accumulation type 1 (Hallervorden-Spatz disease)
NF	neurofilament
NFT	neurofibrillary tangle
NIID	neuronal intranuclear inclusion disease
PD	Parkinson's disease
PHFtau	paired helical filament tau,
PAF	progressive autonomic failure
RBD	REM sleep behavior disorder
SOD1	superoxide dismutase 1
SP	senile plaque

Abnormal interactions between proteins result in the aggregation of proteinaceous fibrils that are common neuropathological features of many neurodegenerative disorders including Alzheimer's disease (AD) (chapter 2), Parkinson's disease (PD) (chapter 4) and prion encephalopathies (chapter 6). Increasing evidence provides compelling support for the hypothesis that abnormal protein-protein interactions and the lesions that result from them play mechanistic roles in the dysfunction and death of brain cells in neurodegenerative diseases. This hypothesis predicts that the abnormal interaction between normal brain proteins alters their conformation and promotes the assembly of these pathological conformers into filaments that progressively accumulate as intracellular or extracellular fibrous deposits in the central nervous system (CNS). Further, the transformation of the normal proteins into pathological conformers is predicted to result in losses of functions, and the disease proteins or aggregates thereof are predicted to acquire neurotoxic properties culminating in the dysfunction and death of affected brain cells. Thus, the "abnormal protein-protein interactions" hypothesis describes plausible unifying mechanisms to account for the onset/progression of a large number of seemingly unrelated neurodegenerative disorders characterised neuropathologically by filamentous brain lesions formed by different proteins including AD, PD and other brain diseases discussed in this volume.

Recognition of a common mechanistic theme shared by a number of seemingly unrelated neurodegenerative disorders began to emerge in the last decade. As a result, the pessimistic notion that each degenerative disorder of the ageing brain would require a disease-specific therapeutic intervention may be incorrect, since a large number of these disorders are characterised neuropathologically by aggregates of proteinaceous fibrils that may share similar targets for drug discovery (Table 1). Thus, despite differences in the molecular composition of the structural elements of these filamentous lesions as well as the brain regions and cell types they affect, growing evidence supports the hypothesis that similar pathological mechanisms may underlie these disorders. More specifically, the onset and/or progression of many neurodegenerative disorders may be linked mechanistically to abnormal interactions between brain proteins that lead to their assembly into filaments and the aggregation of these filaments within brain cells or in the extracellular space as inclusions or deposits, respectively.
These filamentous lesions are exemplified by intranuclear neuronal inclusions formed by diverse proteins harboring mutant or abnormally expanded polyglutamine tracts in hereditary trinucleotide repeat disorders, intracytoplasmic neurofibrillary tangles (NFTs), extracellular amyloid or senile plaques (SPs) in sporadic and familial AD (FAD), and by prion protein deposits in sporadic or genetic forms of transmissible spongiform encephalopathies.

Sporadic and familial AD illustrate some of the enigmatic overlap among these neurodegenerative diseases. For example, the heterogeneous dementing disorders classified as AD overlap with a large group of distinct neurodegenerative disorders known as tauopathies (8). These are characterised by prominent filamentous tau neuropathology throughout the brain as well as with another diverse group of disorders known as synucleinopathies (11) that are characterised by prominent filamentous α-synuclein brain pathology. Thus, the diagnostic hallmarks of AD are numerous SPs composed of Aβ fibrils and intraneuronal NFTs formed by tau filaments, but these NFTs are similar to the tau inclusions characteristic of neurodegenerative tauopathies, many of which do not show evidence of other disease specific brain lesions. Although *tau* gene mutations were shown to cause hereditary tauopathies known as familial frontotemporal dementia and Parkinsonism linked to chromosome 17 (FTDP-17) in many kindreds, some of these kindreds were thought to have FAD prior to the discovery of *tau* gene mutations pathogenic for FTDP-17 (8). Moreover, while Lewy bodies (LBs) are hallmark neuronal inclusions of PD, LBs together with SPs and NFTs define a common subtype of AD known as the LB variant of AD (LBVAD), while numerous cortical LBs are the defining brain lesions of dementia with LBs (DLB), which may be difficult to clinically differentiate from AD. Further, *α-synu-*

Disease	Lesion/components	Location
AD*†#	SPs/Aβ NFTs/PHFtau	Extracellular Intracytoplasmic
ALS*	Spheroids/NF subunits, SOD1	Intracytoplasmic
DLB‡	LBs/α-synuclein	Intracytoplasmic
DS*†‡	SPs/Aβ NFTs/PHFtau LBs/α-synuclein	Extracellular Intracytoplasmic Intracytoplasmic
NBIA 1‡	LBs/α-synuclein GCIs/α-synuclein	Intracytoplasmic Intracytoplasmic
LBVAD (AD+DLB)‡	SPs/Aβ NFTs/PHFtau LBs/α-synuclein	Extracellular Intracytoplasmic Intracytoplasmic
MSA‡	GCIs/α-synuclein	Intracytoplasmic
NIID	Inclusions/Expanded poly-glutamine tracts	Intranuclear
PD*‡	LBs/α-synuclein	Intracytoplasmic
PAF‡	LBs/α-synuclein	Intracytoplasmic
Prion diseases*	Amyloid plaques/Prions	Extracellular
RBD‡	LBs/α-synuclein	Intracytoplasmic
Tauopathies*†	Tangles/Abnormal tau	Intracytoplasmic
Tri-nucleotide repeat diseases	Inclusions/Expanded poly-glutamine tracts	Intranuclear and Intradendritic

Table 1. Abnormal protein-protein interactions: mechanisms of disease in diverse neurodegenerative disorders. The table lists hereditary and sporadic neurodegenerative disorders of the CNS characterized neuropathologically by prominent filamentous lesions. Most of these lesions arise within one or more compartments (ie, nuclei, cell bodies, processes) of one or more cell types of the CNS (neurons, astrocytes, oligodendroglia), but some are extracellular deposits of aggregated filaments.

* Both hereditary and sporadic forms of these disorders occur.

† Neurodegenerative diseases with prominent tau pathology are grouped together and referred to as tauopathies. Examples of tauopathies are: progressive supranuclear palsy, Pick's disease, corticobasal degeneration, hereditary frontotemporal dementia with parkinsonism linked to chromosome 17 (FTDP-17) and Guam amyotrophic lateral sclerosis/parkinsonism dementia complex. AD can be included among the tauopathies because of the prominent tau pathology in almost all sporadic and familial forms of this disorder, but LBVAD is one of the most common subtypes of sporadic AD and the distinctive lesions in this form of AD are abundant cortical a-synuclein positive LBs, while similar lesions are common in the brains of many patients with familial AD and DS.

‡ Neurodegenerative diseases with prominent synuclein pathology are synucleinopathies.

clein gene mutations cause familial PD, albeit in rare kindreds, but it also is known that FAD mutations and trisomy 21 lead to abundant accumulations of LBs composed of α-synuclein filaments in the brains of most FAD and elderly Down's syndrome (DS) patients, respectively. While it is unclear how abnormalities in other genes promote the formation of LBs from wild type α-synuclein proteins, the accumulation of α-synuclein into filamentous inclusions now appears to play a mechanistic role in the pathogenesis of a number of progressive neurological disorders including PD, DLB, DS, FAD, LBVAD, sporadic AD, multiple system atrophy (MSA), neurodegeneration with brain iron accumulation type 1 (NBIA 1) and other synucleinopathies (11).

Thus, the aggregation of brain proteins into potentially toxic lesions is a common mechanistic theme in a diverse group of neurodegenerative diseases that share an enigmatic symmetry. Specifically, mutations in the gene encoding the disease protein cause a familial variant of the disorder as well as its hallmark brain lesions, but the same brain lesions also can be formed by the corresponding wild-type protein in sporadic forms of the disease. Clarification of this enigmatic symmetry in any one of these disorders is likely to have a profound impact on understanding the mechanisms that underlie all of these disorders as well as on efforts to develop novel therapies to treat them. For example, it appears that there may be interactions between tau, α-synuclein and Aβ or its precursor protein that might "cross-seed" or promote protein fibrillization and deposition, while other proteins may have the effect of ameliorating neurodegeneration in experimental animal models (3, 6, 9, 10, 14). Thus, further insight into the role homeostatic and pathological chaperones play in abnormal protein-protein interactions and neurodegeneration could lead to new targets for drug discovery. Indeed, compounds have been identified that prevent the conversion of normal proteins into abnormal conformers or variants with conformations that predispose the pathological proteins to form potentially toxic filamentous aggregates (12), and it is plausible to speculate that some of these agents may have therapeutic efficacy in more than one disorder listed in Table 1. Moreover, novel therapeutic approaches that utilize peptide building blocks of the abnormal fibrils that form amyloid to prevent or reverse AD, prion diseases or other amyloidoses by immunological or alternative mechanism could be extended to treat other of the disorders reviewed elsewhere in this monograph (1, 2, 4, 5, 13). While there also may be therapies that emerge from understanding the consequences of specific losses of function by a disease protein (7) as the full implications of abnormal protein-protein interactions in mechanisms of brain degeneration coalesce into coherent insights into their role in this group of disorders, this is likely to lead to the discovery of new and better therapies for neurodegenerative diseases of the elderly caused by abnormal filamentous aggregates of different brain proteins.

References

1. DeMattos RB, Bales KR, Cummins DJ, Dodart JC, Paul SM, Holtzman DM (2001) Peripheral anti-A beta antibody alters CNS and plasma A beta clearance and decreases brain A beta burden in a mouse model of Alzheimer's disease. *Proc Natl Acad Sci U S A* 98: 8850-8855.

2. Enari M, Flechsig E, Weissmann C (2001) Scrapie prion protein accumulation by scrapie-infected neuroblastoma cells abrogated by exposure to a prion protein antibody. *Proc Natl Acad Sci U S A* 98: 9295-9299.

3. Gotz J, Chen F, van Dorpe J, Nitsch RM (2001) Formation of neurofibrillary tangles in P301l tau transgenic mice induced by Abeta 42 fibrils. *Science* 293: 1491-1495.

4. Hammarstrom P, Schneider F, Kelly JW (2001) Trans-suppression of misfolding in an amyloid disease. *Science* 293: 2459-2462.

5. Heppner FL, Musahl C, Arrighi I, Klein MA, Rulicke T, Oesch B, Zinkernagel RM, Kalinke U, Aguzzi A (2001) Prevention of scrapie pathogenesis by transgenic expression of anti- prion protein antibodies. *Science* 294: 178-182.

6. Ishihara T, Higuchi M, Zhang B, Yoshiyama Y, Hong M, Trojanowski JQ, Lee VM (2001) Attenuated neurodegenerative disease phenotype in tau transgenic mouse lacking neurofilaments. *J Neurosci* 21: 6026-6035.

7. Lee VM, Daughenbaugh R, Trojanowski JQ (1994) Microtubule stabilizing drugs for the treatment of Alzheimer's disease. *Neurobiol Aging* 15: S87-89.

8. Lee VM, Goedert M, Trojanowski JQ (2001) Neurodegenerative tauopathies. *Annu Rev Neurosci* 24: 1121-1159

9. Lewis J, Dickson DW, Lin WL, Chisholm L, Corral A, Jones G, Yen SH, Sahara N, Skipper L, Yager D, Eckman C, Hardy J, Hutton M, McGowan E (2001) Enhanced neurofibrillary degeneration in transgenic mice expressing mutant tau and APP. *Science* 293: 1487-1491.

10. Masliah E, Rockenstein E, Veinbergs I, Sagara Y, Mallory M, Hashimoto M, Mucke L (2001) beta -Amyloid peptides enhance alpha -synuclein accumulation and neuronal deficits in a transgenic mouse model linking Alzheimer's disease and Parkinson's disease. *Proc Natl Acad Sci U S A* 98: 12245-12250.

11. Murray IVJ, Lee VM-Y, Trojanowski JQ (2001) Synucleinopathies: a pathological and molecular review. *Clin Neurosci Res* 1/6: 445-455.

12. Priola SA, Raines A, Caughey WS (2000) Porphyrin and phthalocyanine antiscrapie compounds. *Science* 287: 1503-1506.

13. Schenk D, Barbour R, Dunn W, Gordon G, Grajeda H, Guido T, Hu K, Huang J, Johnson-Wood K, Khan K, Kholodenko D, Lee M, Liao Z, Lieberburg I, Motter R, Mutter L, Soriano F, Shopp G, Vasquez N, Vandevert C, Walker S, Wogulis M, Yednock T, Games D, Seubert P (1999) Immunization with amyloid-beta attenuates Alzheimer-disease-like pathology in the PDAPP mouse. *Nature* 400: 173-177.

14. Shin RW, Bramblett GT, Lee VM, Trojanowski JQ (1993) Alzheimer disease A68 proteins injected into rat brain induce codeposits of beta-amyloid, ubiquitin, and alpha 1-antichymotrypsin. *Proc Natl Acad Sci U S A* 90: 6825-6828.

The Ubiquitin Pathway, Neurodegeneration and Brain Function

R. John Mayer
Khosrow Rezvani
Robert Layfield
Simon Dawson

ALS	amyotrophic lateral sclerosis
ARJP	autosomal recessive juvenile parkinsonism
DUB	deubiquitylating
UbL	ubiquitin-like domain
UCHL	ubiquitin carboxyl hydrolase

Introduction

This chapter is driven by the notion that the significance of our understanding of the ubiquitin pathway of regulated intracellular proteolysis is of the same magnitude as the discovery of protein phosphorylation and dephosphorylation. There is scarcely a biochemical pathway in the cell that does not involve a contribution from the ubiquitin-dependent pathway or one controlled by ubiquitin paralogues. The processes include cell division, DNA repair, transcription, translation, signal transduction, autophagy, endocytosis and antigen processing (14). Furthermore, ubiquitin and related ubiquitons (15) are not only attachable and removable from proteins, but can also be genetically built into proteins as a ligand for numerous downstream recognition proteins in key cellular processes.

The Ubiquitin Pathway

Ubiquitin is a small basic protein that can be activated in an ATP-dependent set of reactions to become conjugated to target proteins destined to be recognised and degraded by a large supramacromolecular complex, the 26S proteasome. This exquisitly-regulated protease degrades multiubiquitylated target proteins to small peptides and releases ubiquitin for further rounds of ubiquitylation reactions. The proteasome is the cellular counterpart of the ribosome, which synthesises proteins. Ubiquitin is activated by a ubiquitin activating enzyme (E1), conjugated to target proteins by ubiquitin conjugating enzymes (E2s) under the direction of the arbiters of protein life and death, the ubiquitin protein ligases (E3s). Ubiquitin can also be removed from target proteins by deubiquitylating enzymes (DUBs). The interplay between these enzymes determines the fate of key regulatory proteins in all of the major cellular physiologic pathways that control eukaryotic life (4). Genome sequencing reveals the complexity of the system by showing that there are many E2s, E3s and DUBs indicating that functional specificity must be at the hub of the ubiquitin pathway. Specific E2s, E3s, DUBs and possibly proteasomes control the degradative fate of individual proteins in the cell.

The Nervous System

The first inkling that the ubiquitin pathway was involved in the central nervous system came from the neuropathologic observation that inclusions in the major human neurodegenerative diseases contain multiubiquitylated proteins (for review, see 4). The application of ubiquitin immunocytochemistry is now routine in molecular neuropathology; however, the question of why *tau* should be ubiquitylated in Alzheimer's disease or why synuclein should be ubiquitylated in Parkinson's diseases or indeed which proteins are ubiquitylated in inclusions in motor neurone disease remains to be elucidated. An appreciation of the fundamental roles of the ubiquitin pathway in development and homeostasis in the nervous system is emerging, as contributions from clinical and experimental findings indicate that the ubiquitin system is used in controlling widespread nerve cell functions.

Mutations in Proteins of the Ubiquitin Pathway in Neurologic Disorders

Angelman's syndrome is a developmental neurological syndrome characterised by microcephaly and mental retardation that is caused by mutations in an E3 ligase, E6-AP (7). An E3 recognizes its substrates based on specific ubiquitination signals. Recent findings reveal that all known E3s utilize one of 2 catalytic domains—a HECT domain or a RING finger domain (18).

E6-AP is the archetype of the HECT-domain (HECT is homologous to the E6-AP carboxyl-terminus) ubiquitin protein ligases (7). There are many more HECT-domain ubiquitin protein ligases, some of which are predominately expressed in the brain. Further neurological and neuropsychiatric disorders involving defects in HECT-domain E3 ligases will almost certainly be described.

Ubiquitin Pathway in Chronic Neurodegenerative Disease

Ubiquitin protein ligases of the RING finger family are an even larger group of E3 ligases. These zinc-dependent enzymes are increasingly seen to be involved in controlling many aspects of celular biology, including apoptosis and signal transduction (26). Genomic walking to find the gene responsible for juvenile onset autosomal recessive juvenile parkinsonism (ARJP) identified *parkin*, a RING finger E3 ubiquitin protein ligase (8). Several mutations in *parkin* are associated with ARJP. The subtrates of parkin are not fully characterised, but include a synaptic vesicle-associated protein and possibly α-synuclein (23, 28). In idiopathic Parkinson's disease it is reported that a post-translationally modified form of α-synuclein is ubiquitylated by *parkin* and that loss of *parkin* function contributes to the accumulation of this form of α-synuclein (23). Very rarely, idiopathic Parkinson's disease is associated with mutation in the DUB ubiquitin carboxyl hydrolase (UCHL-1, also known as PGP 9.5) (11). Interestingly, PGP 9.5 is also mutated in the gracile axonal mouse (21), a model associated with neuraxonal dystrophy. Very recently another RING finger ubiquitin ligase, dorfin, has been described in inclusion bodies in ALS (16).

Molecular misreading, whereby normal genetic information is misread during transcription is an age-related process in the brain that results in mutant proteins, including a carboxyl-terminal extended form of ubiquitin (25). This mutant ubiquitin cannot be conjugated to target proteins, but can be incorporated into multiubiquitin chains that are refractory to disassembly by DUBs and are potent inhibitors of the degradation of multiubiquitylated proteins by the 26S proteasome (10). Compounding this age-related inhibition of the proteasome is the observation that aggregates of ubiquitylated proteins can also inhibit the 26S proteasome (2). A combination of age-related genetic and proteomic changes within individual neurones could serve to block the ubiquitin pathway and cause cell death by apoptotic or other mechanisms.

Age is the major risk factor for the most common chronic neurodegenerative diseases, such as Alzheimer's disease and Parkinson's disease. Therefore, age-related inhibition of the ubiquitin pathway, which prevents normal degradation of the precursors of the intraneuroneal ubiquitylated inclusions that characterise neurodegenerative diseases, will lead to neurodegeneration. By way of proof, outside of the nervous system, is the experimental finding in transgenic mice that targeted deletion of the gene for one of 2 cytokeratins, which normally form heterodimers, gives rise to a partnerless liver cytokeratin that is produced and degraded during approximately two-thirds of the mouse life span. Then, and within a very short period of time, the partnerless cytokeratin accumulates in hepatic ubiquitylated inclusions indistinguishable from human Mallory bodies with concomitant hepatic cell death (12). The single partnerless cytokeratin is degraded until some change in a down-stream element of the ubiquitin pathway causes the pathway to malfunction or become overwhelmed resulting in the formation of ubiquitylated aggregates of the previously soluble cytokeratin molecules, inclusion body accumulation and liver cell death.

The age-related progression towards overt pathologic change and morbidity in this mouse model is not dissimilar to prion strains, which propagate and produce ubiquitin-related neuropathology (6) prion protein aggregates, vacuolar changes and mortality at precise times in the life of the infected mice (19). A similar mechanism would account for the occurence of hyperphosphorylated tau in neurofibrillary tangles, α-synuclein in Lewy bodies and polyglutamine expansion proteins in nuclear inclusions in the triplet expansion diseases (eg, Huntington's disease).

Ubiquitin Pathway and Neurotransmission

There have been several discoveries that show that the ubiquitin pathway plays fundamental roles in the development and function of the nervous system. One of the first was the demonstration that a DUB controls eye development (5) and that similarly an E2 controls neuroneal growth and neuromuscular junction formation in *Drosophila* (17). Recently, the yeast 2-hybrid genetic screen with a GABA receptor subunit has identified a ubiquiton called PLIC-1 (1), a protein that has an N-terminal ubiquitin-like domain (UbL) and a C-terminal UBA domain. The UbL domain of ubiquitons can bind to the 26S proteasome (22) and to E3s (9). The UbA domain binds to ubiquitin (3) and polyubiquitin chains (27). PLIC-1 binds to and stabilises GABA receptors, possibly acting in a dominant-negative fashion to stabilise GABA receptors (1). Likewise another PLIC-related ubiquiton called "ubiquilin" binds to and stabilises presenillins, which are critical for the generation of the amyloidogenic versions of Aβ from the Alzheimer precursor protein (13). Finally, metabotropic glutamate receptors bind via proline-containing motifs in their C-termini to members of the Homer family of proteins (24). This sub-family of Homer proteins interacts via their carboxyl-terminal tails with the proteasome, presumably to control metabotropic glutamate receptor degradation (20).

The significance of these findings becomes more apparent when set in the context of pre- and post-synaptic elements of the synapse. The establishment of functioning synapses in development and remodelling during synaptic plasticity include protein changes in the multi-protein post-synaptic densities that depend on the synaptic ubiquitin pathway. For example, a subset of 26S proteasomes associated with post-synaptic densities could control synaptic remodelling as part of synaptic plasticity by degrading receptors or associated proteins, which are replaced by the synthesis of new proteins controlling and consolidating synaptic function.

References

1. Bedford FK, Kittler JT, Muller E, Thomas P, Uren JM, Merlo D, Wisden W, Triller A, Smart TG, Moss SJ (2001) GABAA receptor cell surface number and subunit stability are regulated by the ubiquitin-like protein Plic-1. *Nature Neurosci* 4: 908-916.

2. Bence NF, Sampat RM, Kopito RR (2001) Impairment of the ubiquitin-proteasome system by protein aggregation. *Science* 292: 1552-1555.

3. Bertolaet BL, Clarke DJ, Wolff M, Watson MH, Henze M, Divita G, Reed SI (2001) UBA domain of DNA damage-inducible proteins interact with ubiquitin. *Nature Struct Biol* 8: 417-422.

4. Hershko A, Ciechanover A (1998) The ubiquitin system. *Ann Rev Biochem* 671998: 425-480.

5. Huang Y, Baker RT, Fischer-Vase JA (1995) Control of cell fate by a deubiquitinating enzyme encoded by the fat facets gene. *Science* 270: 1828-1831.

6. Kenward N, Landon M, Laszlo L, Mayer RJ (1996) Heat shock proteins, molecular chaperones and the prion encephalopathies. *Cell Stress Chaperones* 1: 18-26.

7. Kishino T, Lalande M, Wagstaf J (1997) UBE3A/E6-AP mutations cause Angelman's syndrome. *Nature Genetics* 15: 70-73.

8. Kitada T, Asakawa S, Hattori N, Matsumine H, Yamamura Y, Minoshima S, Yokochi M, Mizuno Y, Shimizu N (1998) Mutations in the parkin gene cause autosomal recessive juvenile parkinsonism. *Nature* 392: 605-608.

9. Kleijnen MF, Shih AH, Zhou P, Kumar S, Scoccio RE, Kedersha NL, Gill G, Howley PM (2000) The hPLIC proteins may provide a link between the ubiq-

uitination machinery and the proteasome. *Mol Cell* 6: 409-419.

10. Lam YA, Pickart CM, Alban A, Landon M, Jamieson C, Ramage R, Mayer RJ, Layfield R (2000) Inhibition of the ubiquitin-proteasome system in Alzheimer's disease. *Proc Natl Acad Sci U S A* 97: 9902-9906.

11. Leroy E, Boyer R, Auberger G, Leube B, Ulm G, Mezey E, Harta G, Brownstein MJ, Jonnalagada S, Chernova T, Dehejia A, Lavedan C, Gasser T, Steinbach PJ, Wilkinson KD, Polymeropoulos MH (1998) The ubiquitin pathway in Parkinson's disease. *Nature* 395: 451-452.

12. Magin TM, R. S, Leitgeb S, Wanninger F, Zatloukal K, Grund C, Melton DW (1998) Lesions form in keratin 18 knockout mice: formation of novel keratin filaments, secondary loss of keratin 7 and accumulation of liver-specific keratin 8-positive aggregates. *J Cell Biol* 140: 1441-1451.

13. Mah AL, Perry G, Smith M, Monteiro MJ (2000) Identification of ubiquilin, a novel presenilin interactor that increases presenilin protein accumulation. *J Cell Biol* 151: 847-862.

14. Mayer RJ (2000) The meteoric rise of regulated intracellular proteolysis. *Nature Rev Mol Cell Biol* 1: 145-148.

15. Mayer RJ, Landon M, Layfield R (1998) Ubiquitin superfolds: intrinsic and attachable regulators of cellular activities? *Folding & Design* 3: R97-R99.

16. Niwa JI, Ishigaki S, Hishikawa N, Yamamoto M, Doyu M, Murata S, Tanaka K, Taniguchi N, Sobue G (2002) Dorfin ubiquitylates mutant SOD1 and prevents mutant SOD1-mediated neurotoxicity. *J Biol Chem* (published on line):

17. Oh CE, McMahon R, Benzer S, Tanouye MA (1994) Bendless, a Drosophila gene affecting neuronal connectivity, encodes a ubiquitin-conjugating enzyme homolog. *J Neurosci* 14: 3166-3179.

18. Pickart CM (2001) Mechanisms underlying ubiquitination. *Ann Rev Biochem* 70: 503-533.

19. Prusiner SB (1992) Chemistry and biology of prions. *Biochemistry* 31: 12277-12288.

20. Rezvani K, Dawson S, Mee M, Mayer RJ (2001) *The S8 ATPase of the 26S proteasome interacts with Homer-3 proteins: implications for metabotropic glutamate receptor signaling (abstract).* Presented at FASEB Ubiquitin Meeting, Saxtons River, Vermont, USA.

21. Saigoh K, Wang YI, Suh J, Yamanishi T, Sakai Y, Kiyosawa H, Harada T, Ichihara N, Wakana S, Kikuchi T, Wada K (1999) Intragenic deletion in the gene encoding ubiquitin carboxy-terminal hydrolase in gad mice. *Nature Genetics* 23: 47-51.

22. Schauber C, Chen L, Tongaonkar P, Vega I, Lambertson D, Potts W, Madura K (1998) Rad23 links DNA repair to the ubiquitin/proteasome pathway. *Nature* 391: 715-718.

23. Shimura H, Sclossmacher MG, Hattori N, Frosch MP, Trockenbacher A, Schneider R, Mizuno Y, Kosik KS, Selkoe DJ (2001) Ubiquitination of a new form of a-synuclein by parkin from human brain: implications for Parkinson's disease. *Science* 293: 263-269.

24. Tu JC, Xiao B, Yuan JP, Lanahan AA, Leoffer K, Li M, Linden DJ, Worley PF (1998) Homer binds a novel proline-rich motif and links Group I metabotrpic glutamate receptors with IP3 receptors. *Neuron* 21: 717-726.

25. van Leeuwen FW, de Kleijn DPV, van den Hurk HH, Neubauer A, Sonnemans MAF, Sluijs JA, Koycu S, Ramdjielal RDJ, Salehi A, Martens GJM, Grosveld FG, Peter J, Burbach H, Hol EM (1998) Frameshift mutations of beta amyloid precursor protein and ubiquitin-B in Alzheimer's and Down patients. *Science* 279: 242-247.

26. Weissman AM (2001) Themes and variations on ubiquitylation. *Nature Rev Mol Cell Biol* 2: 169-178.

27. Wilkinson CRM, Seeger M, Hartmann-Petersen R, Stone M, Wallace M, Semple C, Gordon C (2001) Proteins containing the UBA domain are able to bind to multi-ubiquitin chains. *Nature Cell Biol* 3: 1-5.

28. Zhang Y, Gao J, Chung KKK, Huang H, Dawson VL, Dawson T (2000) Parkin functions as an E2-dependent ubiquitin-dependent ligase and promotes the degradation of the synaptic vesicle-associated protein, CDCrel-1. *Proc Natl Acad Sci U S A* 97: 13354-13359.

The Genetics of Neurodegeneration

John Hardy

AD	Alzheimer's disease
ALS	amyotrophic lateral sclerosis
APP	amyloid precurso protein
FTDP	frontotemporal degeneration and parkinsonism
PD	Parkinson's disease

Evolution has protected the brain from the environment: it is largely behind the blood brain barrier and is immunologically privileged. Therefore, it is not surprising that genetics has a major role in neurodegenerative disease. Of course, at some level, all diseases have a genetic component, as recent work on the influence of genetics on survival after head injury shows. Until the last 20 years, however, knowledge of inheritance was considered an almost useless piece of information and so practicing clinicians and pathologists rarely considered it since it did not impact on their clinical care. Even now, it is surprising how frequently detailed family histories are not taken. More recently, however, especially over the last 10 years with the advent of the human genome project, it has become clear that molecular genetic analysis is the most effective route to develop an understanding of disease. It is also clear that, especially with completion of the draft human genome (27, 48), that this process will accelerate and increasingly underpin therapeutic approaches.

In this chapter, I have several aims: *i)* to summarise the history of molecular genetic approaches to neurological disease, *ii)* to discuss how a clinician and pathologist can approach a familial disorder, *iii)* to discuss how molecular genetics complements and subverts the notions of clinicopathologic entities, *iv)* to review the genetics of the major adult neurodegenerative diseases, and *v)* to outline how genetics can guide treatments aimed at disease pathogenesis.

Molecular Genetics, Positional Cloning and Genetic Analysis

Positional cloning relies on a very simple principle: DNA sequences that are close together tend to be inherited together. The closer they are together, the more frequently this will occur. If therefore, an experimenter can follow the inheritance of variable DNA sequences though families with disease, and they find a sequence that co-inherits more often with disease than by chance, then they can surmise that the DNA sequence is in the same chromosomal region as the mutation causing the disease. This is called "genetic linkage" and the DNA sequence is said to be "linked" to the disease. Note that the term "linked" does not mean that the DNA sequence has anything to do with the disease anymore than living next to a bank robber would imply you were a petty thief. While the statistics of this analysis are outside the scope of this chapter, suffice to say that any family with 5 or more living affected individuals is very useful for genetic analysis of this sort, and a working rule for many genetic laboratories is that any family with 3 or more living affected individuals is worth collecting.

Identification of linkage is the first real step towards finding a gene. When linkage has been found, the next step is to define precisely the position of the gene by examining the inheritance of many DNA sequences from the region in many similar families. Stage two then begins with sequencing gene after gene from that region until mutations are found in affected family members. This outline describes the path taken, for example, in the cloning of the presenilin 1 gene (*PSEN1*) in Alzheimer's disease (41, 44). It is sometimes the case that once linkage has been identified, a gene from that region immediately stands out as a candidate for the pathogenic gene. This is called the "positional candidate" approach, and describes the identification of the α-synuclein gene for Parkinson's disease (37) and tau for frontotemporal degeneration and parkinsonism linked to chromosome 17 (FTDP-17) (38). In these cases and many others, the breakthroughs came because of the identification and characterisation of large families with multiply affected individuals with a simple (eg, autosomal dominant) inheritance pattern. While those of us interested in neurodegenerative disease awoke to the possibility of this approach to disease with the identification of linkage to Huntington's disease (15), the hunts for the genes for Duchenne dystrophy (32, 34) and cystic fibrosis (25) were of particular importance in defining the strategies for this approach to disease. Also, of course, the notion of "positional candidates" depends on the cloning of disease-related genes such as the prion gene and the APP gene by molecular pathologists (2, 24).

Now, however, most (though not all) neurodegenerative diseases with simple patterns of heredity have been worked out, and increasingly molecular geneticists are starting to try and analyse diseases which are familial, but which don't have simple patterns of inheritance. In these conditions, slightly different approaches are taken to elucidate the disease. In diseases with clear inheritance patterns, the approach taken is to find which chromosomal segment unambiguously inherits with disease and thus, using many families, the gene can be precisely localised. When the inheritance mode is less clear, the approach taken is to collect a large number of families and determine which areas of the genome are inherited with the disease more often that one would expect by chance. While this may seem a subtle change, it is a much weaker approach—the former invites a "yes/no" answer, while the latter offers a probability statement. As such, the localisation is much poorer and identifying genes has been correspondingly slower. In neurodegenerative disease, the apolipoprotein E gene in Alzheimer's disease is currently the only universally accepted risk-factor locus identified by this method (46).

Another way to identify genes for complex conditions is to guess them and then test variants of the gene for association with the disease. One asks whether a particular gene variant occurs more often in cases of disease than in controls, such as their spouse. An enormous number of such studies have been performed with disappointing results. Many positive results have been reported, but very few have been replicated. In large part this is probably because of the problem of multiple testing, compounded by publication bias. Thus, if a lab tests 20 gene variants for association with disease and finds one "p" value of 0.05, this is not surprising, but if journals only accept for publication the positive reports, clearly problems will arise. This area, however, has had some successes with identification of the prion gene as a risk factor locus for sporadic prion diseases (6, 8, 36) and with the identification of the tau gene as a risk factor locus for progressive supranuclear palsy and corticobasal degeneration (1, 22).

As we begin to understand the pathophysiology of neurodegenerative diseases more completely and as more genetic variability is identified throughout relevant genes, it is to be hoped that more risk factor loci will be identified by pure "guessing" or through guessing informed by genetic linkage information (11, 35).

How Should a Clinician or Pathologist Approach a Familial Disorder?

It is remarkable how infrequently a detailed family history is taken. Any individual with a neurologic condition should have a detailed family history taken that should include the current ages and age of death of all descendants of their grandparents, and this family history should include, not only the suspected disease of the proband, but should include all other neurologic conditions. It should also include any information concerning consanguinity between parents and information about ethnic origin. For diseases in which genes are known, testing can, of course be done on a single fresh or frozen sample (it is exceedingly difficult to do this on fixed and paraffin embedded specimens). For diseases in which genes are not known, samples should be stored so that when genes for diseases are found, the descendants of the proband can have the benefit of knowing the precise disease their antecedents suffered from.

From a research perspective deciding which families may be useful for genetic linkage studies is a complex issue, but a simple rule of thumb is that families with 3 or more affected individuals from whom samples can be collected are worth following up, and a family with 6 or more such individuals could be used, on its own, to localize a genetic defect.

Molecular Genetics Complements and Subverts the Notions of Clinicopathologic Entities

The notion of neurologic diseases being clinicopathologic entities has been so central to Western thought about these diseases for the last 100 years that we sometimes forget it is only one way of looking at disease. It has been such an extraordinarily successful concept that its weaknesses have been largely overlooked. However, it has several weaknesses: *i)* while the clinician sees the disease progressing, the pathologist usually sees the final outcome, *ii)* humans are exquisitely sensitive to peculiarities in each others' behavior and in clinicians, this natural attribute is trained to higher levels. Thus, if the same disease process hits different brain regions in different individuals, leading to different symptoms, different diagnostic labels may be attached to them. For example, a stroke, no matter what area of the brain it afflicts is always called a stroke, but Lewy body disease in the substantia nigra is given a different name than Lewy body disease in the cortex. *iii)* Pathologists often implicitly assume that lesions (for example, the plaques and tangles of Alzheimer's disease) are permanent; that they wait to be counted. This assumption (which underpins studies correlating clinical features with the quantity of pathological lesions) is unwarranted and probably wrong, and *iv)* pathologists can only see what is there. This hampers enormously the understanding of diseases that leave no visible lesion.

Molecular genetic understanding of diseases both complements and subverts the clinicopathologic approach to disease. It complements it because molecular genetics is a uniquely powerful tool to understand where pathogenesis begins (with APP processing and Aβ metabolism for example, in Alzheimer's disease [19]). It subverts it because it shows disease entities are not always what they seem. To give some examples, prion mutations can give rise to widely different pathologies even in the same families (7); Parkinson's disease and Lewy body dementia can appear as alternate phenotypes of the same lesion (20); tau mutations give rise to diseases previously thought to be unrelated (40, 47); the same presenilin mutation can give rise to widely differing forms of Alzheimer's disease (9); Lewy bodies occur in kindreds with APP, presenilin and prion mutations (28, 31), and so on. As a general rule, when the genetic lesions underlying a disease are discovered, the phenotype range is found to be larger than was previously suspected.

A Brief Review of Genetic Findings in Mendelian Neurodegenerative Diseases

The genetic bases of most major Mendelian neurodegenerative diseases have been elucidated. The major exception is Parkinson's disease, where progress was hampered by the belief that genetics did not play a role in this disorder, but even in this area, progress is now rapid.

Alzheimer's disease. Three genes have been shown to carry mutations that cause autosomal dominant Alzheimer's disease: the APP gene (14), and the presenilin 1 (44) and presenilin 2 (30) genes. APP gene mutations typically cause disease onset in the mid-50s (33), whereas presenilin 1 gene mutations lead to onset in the 30s and 40s (18). Presenilin 2 mutations lead to a variable onset age (3). All mutations affect APP processing such that a more amyloidogenic form of Aβ is produced (43).

Parkinson's disease. The genetics of Parkinson's disease is very complex with 9 reported genetic linkages (16). Two genes have been discovered so far: the α-synuclein gene (38) and the parkin gene (26). The former acts as an autosomal dominant locus, and the latter is an autosomal recessive locus. The biochemical relationship between the cognate proteins of this loci is not yet clear, but one plausible, but unproven suggestion is that parkin, a ubiquitin ligase (45) is responsible for degrading misfolded synuclein (29).

Frontal temporal dementia. Mutations in the tau gene are a major cause of FTD (23); however, there are at least 2 other genetic linkages to be found (4, 21).

Familial amyotrophic lateral sclerosis. Mutations in superoxide dismutase and *alsin* are 2 known causes of ALS (17, 39, 49), although there are several extant and unresolved genetic linkages.

Prion disease. Mutations in the prion gene are the only known cause of familial prion diseases, with wide phenotypic diversity encompassing diseases as disparate as Creutzfeldt-Jakob disease, fatal familial insomnia and Gerstmann-Straussler syndrome (5).

Huntington's disease, dentatorubropallidoluysial atrophy and spinocerebellar ataxias. There are now 18 genes in which CAG expansions encoding polyglutamine tracts, have been discovered and this number is growing steadily (12).

How Genetics Guides Treatments Aimed at Pathogenesis

Genetics identifies the molecular lesion that initiates a disease process; in this was it identifies where pathogenesis begins. It helps guide treatment strategies in several interconnected ways—it allows the creation of transgenic models of the disease in which therapies can be easily tested and it allows the creation of cellular and animal models of pathogenesis which can be used to dissect more precisely that pathogenic processes. Furthermore, it often sheds unexpected light on commonalities between diseases that may eventually aid in therapeutic design. In diseases where multiple genes have been found, it often proves the case that the products from these genes outline a common pathogenic biochemical pathway.

Perhaps the best example of this approach has been in Alzheimer's disease, where all the known mutations were shown to alter APP processing such that more amyloidogenic Aβ was produced. Animal models replicating these features were made (13) and were then used to develop treatment strategies based upon this understanding of pathogenesis (42). Similar approaches have been used successfully with the polyglutamine diseases (10). These gene-knowledge-based treatment strategies are now about to reach the clinic. We do not yet know whether all the genes involved in Parkinson's disease, ALS or FTD will similarly map out pathogenic biochemical pathways or whether the situation will be more complicated.

The Present Situation and Our Tasks

This chapter is written at a time of great optimism. Genetic knowledge is helping us understand diseases that have been mysterious since their descriptions, typically at the turn of the last century. Therapies based on this understanding is just about to reach the clinic for several of these diseases, and we hope that this will be a new dawn and a revolution in the treatment of these diseases to the same or greater extent that the introduction of L-dopa by Hornykiewicz was in the early 1960s. We will know whether this approach is going to be successful in the next few years.

However, there is still much to do. For the most part, we don't understand "sporadic" diseases. The cause of typical sporadic Alzheimer's disease and Parkinson's disease, as well as many other diseases, remains mysterious. Over the next few years, the task of geneticists will be to try to understand the causes of these disorders and to understand the interaction between genetic and environmental factors.

This genetic progress will have societal impact, too. If we are able to genuinely massively reduce the burden of neurological disease, and if other areas of health research make similar progress, how will society deal with the increasing elderly population?

References

1. Baker M, Litvan I, Houlden H, Adamson J, Dickson D, Perez-Tur J, Hardy J, Lynch T, Bigio E, Hutton M (1999) Association of an extended haplotype in the tau gene with progressive supranuclear palsy. *Hum Mol Genet* 4: 711-715.

2. Basler K, Oesch B, Scott M, Westaway D, Walchli M, Groth DF, McKinley MP, Prusiner SB, Weissmann C (1986) Scrapie and cellular PrP isoforms are encoded by the same chromosomal gene. *Cell* 46: 417-428.

3. Bird TD, Levy-Lahad E, Poorkaj P, Sharma V, Nemens E, Lahad A, Lampe TH, Schellenberg GD (1996) Wide range in age of onset for chromosome 1-related familial Alzheimer's disease. *Ann Neurol* 40: 932-936.

4. Brown J, Ashworth A, Gydesen S, Sorensen A, Rossor M, Hardy J, Collinge J (1995) Familial non-specific dementia maps to chromosome 3. *Hum Mol Genet* 4: 1625-1628.

5. Collinge J (2001) Prion diseases of humans and animals: their causes and molecular basis. *Ann Rev Neurosci* 24: 519-550.

6. Collinge J, Beck J, Campbell T, Estibeiro K, Will RG (1996) Prion protein gene analysis in new variant cases of Creutzfeldt-Jakob disease. *Lancet* 348: 56-57.

7. Collinge J, Owen F, Poulter M, Leach M, Crow TJ, Rossor MN, Hardy J, Mullan MJ, Janota I, Lantos PL (1990) Prion dementia without characteristic pathology. *Lancet* 336: 7-9.

8. Collinge J, Palmer MS, Dryden AJ (1991) Genetic predisposition to iatrogenic Creutzfeldt-Jakob disease. *Lancet* 337: 1441-1442.

9. Crook R, Verkkoniemi A, Perez-Tur J, Mehta N, Baker M, Houlden H, Farrer M, Hutton M, Lincoln S, Hardy J, Gwinn K, Somer M, Paetau A, Kalimo H, Ylikoski R, Poyhonen M, Kucera S, Haltia M (1998) A variant of Alzheimer's disease with spastic paraparesis and unusual plaques due to deletion of exon 9 of presenilin 1. *Nat Med* 4: 452-455.

10. Davies SW, Turmaine M, Cozens BA, DiFiglia M, Sharp AH, Ross CA, Scherzinger E, Wanker EE, Mangiarini L, Bates GP (1997) Formation of neuronal intranuclear inclusions underlies the neurological dysfunction in mice transgenic for the HD mutation. *Cell* 90: 537-548.

11. Ertekin-Taner N, Graff-Radford N, Younkin LH, Eckman C, Baker M, Adamson J, Ronald J, Blangero J, Hutton M, Younkin SG (2000) Linkage of plasma Abeta42 to a quantitative locus on chromosome 10 in late-onset Alzheimer's disease pedigrees. *Science* 290: 2303-2304.

12. Evidente VG, Gwinn-Hardy KA, Caviness JN, Gilman S (2000) Hereditary ataxias. Mayo Clin Proc 75: 475-490.

13. Games D, Adams D, Alessandrini R, Barbour R, Berthelette P, Blackwell C, Carr T, Clemens J, Donaldson T, Gillespie F (1995) Alzheimer-type neuropathology in transgenic mice overexpressing V717F beta-amyloid precursor protein. *Nature* 373: 523-527.

14. Goate A, Chartier-Harlin MC, Mullan M, Brown J, Crawford F, Fidani L, Giuffra L, Haynes A, Irving N, James L, et al. (1991) Segregation of a missense mutation in the amyloid precursor protein gene with familial Alzheimer's disease. *Nature* 349: 704-706.

15. Gusella JF, Wexler NS, Conneally PM, Naylor SL, Anderson MA, Tanzi RE, Watkins PC, Ottina K, Wallace MR, Sakaguchi AY (1983) A polymorphic DNA marker genetically linked to Huntington's disease. *Nature* 306: 234-238.

16. Gwinn-Hardy K, Farrer M (2002) Parkinson's genetics: an embarrassment of riches. *Ann Neurol* 51: 7-8.

17. Hadano S, Hand CK, Osuga H, Yanagisawa Y, Otomo A, Devon RS, Miyamoto N, Showguchi-Miyata J, Okada Y, Singaraja R, Figlewicz DA, Kwiatkowski T, Hosler BA, Sagie T, Skaug J, Nasir J, Brown RHJ, Scherer SW, Rouleau GA, Hayden MR, Ikeda JE (2001) A gene encoding a putative GTPase regulator is mutated in familial amyotrophic lateral sclerosis 2. *Nat Genet* 29: 166-173.

18. Haltia M, Viitanen M, Sulkava R, Ala-Hurula V, Poyhonen M, Goldfarb L, Brown P, Levy E, Houlden H, Crook R, et al. (1994) Chromosome 14-encoded Alzheimer's disease: genetic and clinicopathological description. *Ann Neurol* 36: 362-367.

19. Hardy J (1997) Amyloid, the presenilins and Alzheimer's disease. *Trends Neurosci* 20: 154-159.

20. Hardy J, Perez-Tur J, Baker M, Farrer M, Crook R, Hutton M, Johnson WG, Gwinn K, Muenter M, Rocca WA, Maraganore D (1998) Exclusion of genetic linkage to 4q21-23 and 17q21 in a family with Lewy body parkinsonism. *Am J Med Genet* 81: 166-171.

21. Hosler BA, Siddique T, Sapp PC, Sailor W, Huang MC, Hossain A, Daube JR, Nance M, Fan C, Kaplan J, Hung WY, McKenna-Yasek D, Haines JL, Pericak-Vance MA, Horvitz HR, Brown RHJ (2000) Linkage of familial amyotrophic lateral sclerosis with frontotemporal dementia to chromosome 9q21-q22. *JAMA* 284: 1664-1669.

22. Houlden H, Baker M, Morris HR, MacDonald N, Pickering-Brown S, Adamson J, Lees AJ, Rossor MN, Quinn NP, Kertesz A, Khan MN, Hardy J, Lantos PL, St George-Hyslop P, Munoz DG, Mann D, Lang AE, Bergeron C, Bigio EH, Litvan I, Bhatia KP, Dickson D, Wood NW, Hutton M (2001) Corticobasal degeneration and progressive supranuclear palsy share a common tau haplotype. *Neurology* 56: 1702-1706.

23. Hutton M, Lendon CL, Rizzu P, Baker M, Froelich S, Houlden H, Pickering-Brown S, Chakraverty S, Isaacs A, Grover A, Hackett J, Adamson J, Lincoln S, Dickson D, Davies P, Petersen RC, Stevens M, de Graaff E, Wauters E, van Baren J, Hillebrand M, Joosse M, Kwon JM, Nowotny P, Heutink P, et al. (1998) Coding and splice donor site mutations in tau cause autosomal dominant dementia (FTDP-17). *Nature* 393: 702-705.

24. Kang J, Lemaire HG, Unterbeck A, Salbaum JM, Masters CL, Grzeschik KH, Multhaup G, Beyreuther K, Muller-Hill B (1987) The precursor of Alzheimer's disease amyloid A4 protein resembles a cell-surface receptor. *Nature* 325: 733-736.

25. Kerem B, Rommens JM, Buchanan JA, Markiewicz D, Cox T, Chakravarti A, Buchwald M, Tsui LC (1989) Identification of the cystic fibrosis gene: genetic analysis. *Science* 245: 1073-1080.

26. Kitada T, Asakawa S, Hattori N, Matsumine H, Yamamura Y, Minoshima S, Yokochi M, Mizuno Y, Shimizu N (1998) Mutations in the parkin gene cause autosomal recessive juvenile parkinsonism. *Nature* 392: 605-608.

27. Lander ES, Linton LM, Birren B, Nusbaum C, Zody MC, Baldwin J, et.al (2001) Initial sequencing and analysis of the human genome. *Nature* 409: 860-921.

28. Lantos PL, Ovenstone IM, Johnson J, Clelland CA, Roques P, Rossor MN (1994) Lewy bodies in the brain of two members of a family with the 717 (Val to Ile) mutation of the amyloid precursor protein gene. *Neurosci Lett* 172: 77-79.

29. Leroy E, Boyer R, Auburger G, Leube B, Ulm G, Mezey E, Harta G, Brownstein MJ, Jonnalagada S, Chernova T, Dehejia A, Lavedan C, Gasser T, Steinbach PJ, Wilkinson KD, Polymeropoulos MH (1998) The ubiquitin pathway in Parkinson's disease. *Nature* 395: 451-452.

30. Levy-Lahad E, Wasco W, Poorkaj P, Romano DM, Oshima J, H. PW, Yu CE, Jondro PD, Schmidt SD, Wang K (1995) Candidate gene for the chromosome 1 familial Alzheimer's disease locus. *Science* 269: 973-977.

31. Lippa CF, Fujiwara H, Mann DM, Giasson B, Baba M, Schmidt ML, Nee LE, O'Connell B, Pollen DA, St George-Hyslop P, Ghetti B, Nochlin D, Bird TD, Cairns NJ, Lee VM, Iwatsubo T, Trojanowski JQ (1998) Lewy bodies contain altered alpha-synuclein in brains of many familial Alzheimer's disease patients with mutations in presenilin and amyloid precursor protein genes. *Am J Pathol* 153: 1365-1370.

32. Monaco AP, Neve RL, Colletti-Feener C, Bertelson CJ, Kurnit DM, Kunkel LM (1986) Isolation of candidate cDNAs for portions of the Duchenne muscular dystrophy gene. *Nature* 323: 646-650.

33. Mullan M, Tsuji S, Miki T, Katsuya T, Naruse S, Kaneko K, Shimizu T, Kojima T, Nakano I, Ogihara T (1993) Clinical comparison of Alzheimer's disease in pedigrees with the codon 717 Val→Ile mutation in the amyloid precursor protein gene. *Neurobiol Aging* 14: 407-419.

34. Murray JM, Davies KE, Harper PS, Meredith L, Mueller CR, Williamson R (1982) Linkage relationship of a cloned DNA sequence on the short arm of the X chromosome to Duchenne muscular dystrophy. *Nature* 300: 69-71.

35. Myers A, Holmans P, Marshall H, Kwon J, Meyer D, Ramic D, Shears S, Booth J, DeVrieze FW, Crook R, Hamshere M, Abraham R, Tunstall N, Rice F, Carty S, Lillystone S, Kehoe P, Rudrasingham V, Jones L, Lovestone S, Perez-Tur J, Williams J, Owen MJ, Hardy J, Goate AM (2000) Susceptibility locus for Alzheimer's disease on chromosome 10. *Science* 290: 2304-2305.

36. Palmer MS, Dryden AJ, Hughes JT, Collinge J (1991) Homozygous prion protein genotype predisposes to sporadic Creutzfeldt-Jakob disease. *Nature* 352: 340-342.

37. Polymeropoulos MH, Lavedan C, Leroy E, Ide S, Dehejia A, Dutra A, Pike B, Root H, Rubenstein J, Boyer R, Stenroos ES, Chandrasekharappa S, Athanassiadou A, Papapetropoulos T, Johnson WG, Lazzarini AM, Duvoisin RC, Di Iorio G, Golbe LI, Nussbaum RL (1997) Mutation in the alpha-synuclein gene identified in families with Parkinson's disease. *Science* 276: 2045-2047.

38. Poorkaj P, Bird TD, Wijsman E, Nemens E, Garruto RM, Anderson L, Andreadis A, Wiederholt WC, Raskind M, Schellenberg GD (1998) Tau is a candidate gene for chromosome 17 frontotemporal dementia. *Ann Neurol* 43.

39. Rosen DR, Siddique T, Patterson D, Figlewicz DA, Sapp P, Hentati A, Donaldson D, Goto J, O'Regan JP, Deng HX (1993) Mutations in Cu/Zn superoxide dismutase gene are associated with familial amyotrophic lateral sclerosis. *Nature* 362: 59-62.

40. Rosso SM, van Herpen E, Deelen W, Kamphorst W, Severijnen LA, Willemsen R, Ravid R, Niermeijer MF, Dooijes D, Smith M, Goedert M, Heutink P, van Swieten JC (2002) A novel tau mutation, S320F, causes a tauopathy with inclusions similar to those in Pick's disease. *Ann Neurol* 51: 373-376.

41. Schellenberg GD, Bird T, Wijsman EM, Orr H, Anderson L, Nemens E, White JA, Bonnycastle L, Weber JL, Alonso ME (1992) Genetic linkage evidence for a familial Alzheimer's disease locus on chromosome 14. *Science* 258: 668-671.

42. Schenk D, Barbour R, Dunn W, Gordon G, Grajeda H, Guido T, Hu K, Huang J, Johnson-Wood K, Khan K, Kholodenko D, Lee M, Liao Z, Lieberburg I, Motter R, Mutter L, Soriano F, Shopp G, Vasquez N, Vandevert C, Walker S, Wogulis M, Yednock T, Games D, Seubert P (1999) Immunization with amyloid-beta attenuates Alzheimer-disease-like pathology in the PDAPP mouse. *Nature* 400: 173-177.

43. Scheuner D, Eckman C, Jensen M, Song X, Citron M, Suzuki N, Bird TD, Hardy J, Hutton M, Kukull W,

Larson E, Levy-Lahad E, Viitanen M, Peskind E, Poorkaj P, Schellenberg G, Tanzi R, Wasco W, Lannfelt L, Selkoe D, Younkin S (1996) Secreted amyloid beta-protein similar to that in the senile plaques of Alzheimer's disease is increased in vivo by the presenilin 1 and 2 and APP mutations linked to familial Alzheimer's disease. *Nat Med* 2: 864-870.

44. Sherrington R, Rogaev EI, Liang Y, Rogaeva EA, Levesque G, Ikeda M, Chi H, Lin C, Li G, Holman K (1995) Cloning of a gene bearing missense mutations in early-onset familial Alzheimer's disease. *Nature* 375: 754-760.

45. Shimura H, Hattori N, Kubo S, Mizuno Y, Asakawa S, Minoshima S, Shimizu N, Iwai K, Chiba T, Tanaka K, Suzuki T (2000) Familial Parkinson disease gene product, parkin, is a ubiquitin-protein ligase. *Nat Genet* 25: 302-305.

46. Strittmatter WJ, Saunders AM, Schmechel D, Pericak-Vance M, Enghild J, Salvesen GS, Roses AD (1993) Apolipoprotein E: high-avidity binding to beta-amyloid and increased frequency of type 4 allele in late-onset familial Alzheimer disease. *Proc Natl Acad Sci U S A* 90: 1977-1981.

47. Tsuboi Y, Uitti RJ, Delisle MB, Ferreira JJ, Brefel-Courbon C, Rascol O, Ghetti B, Murrell JR, Hutton M, Baker M, Wszolek ZK (2002) Clinical features and disease haplotypes of individuals with the N279K tau gene mutation: a comparison of the pallidopontonigral degeneration kindred and a French family. *Arch Neurol* 59: 943-950.

48. Venter JC, Adams MD, Myers EW, Li PW, Mural RJ, Sutton GG et al (2001) The sequence of the human genome. *Science* 291: 1304-1351.

49. Yang Y, Hentati A, Deng HX, Dabbagh O, Sasaki T, Hirano M, Hung WY, Ouahchi K, Yan J, Azim AC, Cole N, Gascon G, Yagmour A, Ben-Hamida M, Pericak-Vance M, Hentati F, Siddique T (2001) The gene encoding alsin, a protein with three guanine-nucleotide exchange factor domains, is mutated in a form of recessive amyotrophic lateral sclerosis. *Nat Genet* 29: 160-165.

CHAPTER 2

Alzheimer's Disease and Ageing

Chapter Editor: Dennis Dickson

2.1 Alzheimer Type Dementia 24

2.2 Genetics of Alzheimer's Disease 40

2.3 Neuropathology of Alzheimer's Disease 47

2.4 Plaque-predominant and Tangle-predominant Variants of Alzheimer's Disease 66

2.5 Molecular Pathogenesis of Alzheimer's Disease 69

2.6 Alzheimer Animal Models: Models of Aβ Deposition in Transgenic Mice 74

Alzheimer Type Dementia

David Knopman

AAN	American Academy of Neurology
AD	Alzheimer's disease
ADCS	Alzheimer's disease co-operative study
APOE	apolipoprotein E
CBC	complete blood count
CDR	clinical dementia rating scale
ChEI	cholinesterase inhibitor
CT	computer tomography
GDS	global deterioration scale
ERT	estrogen replacement therapy
MR	magnetic resonance tomography
NSAID	nonsteroidal anti-inflammatory agent
MCI	mild cognitive impairment
MMSE	mini-mental state examination
NSAID	nonsteroidal anti-inflammatory drug
PET	positron emission tomography

Introduction

Alzheimer's disease (AD) is the most common cause of dementia with prominent anterograde amnesia. Dementia is a syndrome defined by subacute or insidious decline in cognition from a previously higher level (6). Dementia, in contrast to disorders defined by deficits in only one cognitive or behavioural domain, is diagnosed when there are deficits in multiple domains. Some diagnostic criteria require 3 dysfunctional areas (48), whereas the DSM -IV (6) and NINCDS-ADRDA (171) criteria require only memory impairment plus one other cognitive or behavioural deficit to diagnose dementia. Besides memory dysfunction, the other manifestations of dementia include abnormalities in speech/language, visuospatial function, abstract reasoning/executive function and mood/personality. The specificity of the diagnosis of dementia is enhanced by also requiring that the patient's cognitive and behavioural deficits interfere "significantly" with daily function and independence.

Major criteria for clinical diagnosis of AD from DSM-IV (6) (Table 1) and NINCDS-ADRDA (Table 2) (171) are highly concordant with one another. Both emphasise the primacy of deficits in learning new material among core cognitive deficits while requiring evidence for deficits in other domains and impairment of daily functioning. Both definitions of AD require the clinical syndrome to be insidious in onset and gradually progressive with an inexorable decline.

Synonyms and Historical Annotations

The concept of dementia in the elderly arose in antiquity, but it wasn't until the 20th century that any insight into its nature was forthcoming. Even after Alzheimer's original description of the pathological nature of the illness in 1907 (5), it was decades until the relationships between pathology and clinical features were understood. Pioneering work of Blessed, Tomlinson and Roth (24) indicated that there was a relationship between dementia and the number of lesions in the brains; however, the clinical manifestations of AD has been the focus of study in only the last third of the century.

The gradual onset and continuing decline of cognitive function from a previously higher level, resulting in impairment in social or occupational function.

Impairment of recent memory (the inability to learn new information), and at least one of the following:

- disturbances of language (word-finding difficulties)
- disturbances of praxis (inability to execute skilled motor activities in the absence of weakness)
- disturbances of visual processing (visual agnosia and constructional disturbances)
- disturbances of executive function (including abstract reasoning and concentration)

The cognitive deficits are not due to other psychiatric disease, neurological diseases or systemic diseases.

The deficits do not exclusively occur in the setting of delirium.

Table 1. DSM-IV criteria for dementia, from (6).

Definition of dementia
"A decline in memory and other cognitive functions in comparison with the patient's previous level of function as determined by a history of decline in performance and by abnormalities noted from clinical examination and neuropsychological tests."

Criteria for the clinical diagnosis of probable AD
Dementia established by clinical examination and documented by (mental status tests) and confirmed by neuropsychological tests;
deficits in 2 or more areas of cognition;
progressive worsening of memory and other cognitive functions;
no disturbances in consciousness;
onset between ages 40 and 90;
absence of systemic disorders or other brain disease that in and of themselves could account for the progressive deficits in memory and cognition.

Features that make AD uncertain or unlikely
Sudden, apoplectic onset;
focal neurological findings such as hemiparesis, sensory loss, visual field deficits, and incoordination early in the course of the illness;
seizures or gait disturbances at the onset or very early in the course of the illness.

Criteria for clinical diagnosis of possible AD
May be made on the basis of the dementia syndrome, in the absence of other neurological, psychiatric or systemic disorders sufficient to cause dementia, and in the present of variations in the onset, presentation or clinical course;
may be made in the presence of a second systemic or brain disorder sufficient to produce dementia, which is not considered to be the cause of the dementia; and
when a single, gradually progressive severe cognitive deficit is identified in the absence of other identifiable cause.

Table 2. The essentials of the NINCDS-ADRDA criteria for the clinical diagnosis of AD, from (171).

Epidemiology

Prevalence of AD. The prevalence, which is the number of cases in a population at any one time, of dementia and AD increases with advancing age (1, 11, 54, 58, 81, 98, 104, 138, 190, 201, 271). There is considerable consistency across recent prevalence surveys in North America and Europe, especially when similar case-finding methods for mild dementia are used (109). In 65 to 69 year olds the prevalence of dementia is approximately 1 per 100 individuals. With each subsequent 5-year increment, the prevalence of dementia and AD doubles (109) (Figure 1). Over age 85 years, estimates of the prevalence of dementia vary between 20% to nearly 50% (1, 11, 54, 58, 81, 98, 104, 138, 190, 201, 271). Beyond age 85, it appears that dementia prevalence continues to rise. Some earlier studies found a decrease above this age, but recent studies have confirmed that the proportion of individuals with dementia continues to rise over this age.

Incidence of AD. The incidence, which is the number of newly diagnosed cases in a certain time interval, also rises dramatically with advancing age (12, 58, 74, 91, 120, 191, 218, 246). The number of new cases of dementia, mainly AD, exceeds 1 per 100 individuals per year from 70 to 80 years of age. It is not until 80 years of age and above that the rate reaches 2 per 100 individuals per year. Differences in definitions of dementia account for variability in estimates of incidence rates between studies; studies using definitions that admit milder cases show higher incidence rates. Because patients with dementia tend to live for a number of years, incidence rates are considerably lower than prevalence rates.

Proportion of AD in representative samples of dementia. At least 50% to as many as 80% of dementia patients in epidemiological surveys have AD (1, 11, 54, 58, 81, 98, 104, 138, 271). Table 3 shows the breakdown of diagnoses of demented individuals in one epidemiologically valid population from Framingham, Massachusetts. AD is also the most common diagnosis in clinic (146, 257) and autopsy samples (25, 72, 115, 117, 216, 265). From the 3 different methods of case identification (clinical, epidemiological and autopsy), there is consistency in the proportion of dementia cases due to AD. Both the epidemiological and neuropathological studies show that diagnoses other than AD often coexist with AD.

Diagnosis	Percent of cases
Probable AD	55.6
Probable vascular dementia	8.9
Dementia with stroke, relationship unknown	5.6
Dementia with Parkinson's disease	3.3
Dementia and parkinsonism, relationship unknown	4.4
Nonprogressive dementia due to single episode of brain injury	4.4
Dementia due to other known aetiology	2.2
Dementia due to multiple aetiologies	12.2
Unclassifiable dementia	3.3

Table 3. Dementia diagnoses in an epidemiological sample (n = 90) (11).

Lifetime risk of AD. The effects of competing mortality temper the lifetime risk for developing AD. In the Framingham study (237), a non-demented 65-year-old man had a 6.3%, and a 65-year-old woman, a 12% chance of subsequently developing AD in their remaining lifetimes. The gender differences reflect the greater longevity of women. These lower values for lifetime risk should be contrasted to the much higher prevalence estimates for those over age 85 years old.

Gender. Prevalence and incidence studies have shown a consistently higher rate of dementia in women compared to men (74). Whether this represents a true biological effect or merely reflects excess premature mortality of males beginning at approximately age 45 years is not clear. Large genetic studies also suggest that women are at greater risk for AD than men (148). In any case, the male to female differences are modest, after correcting for the number of individuals at risk of either gender.

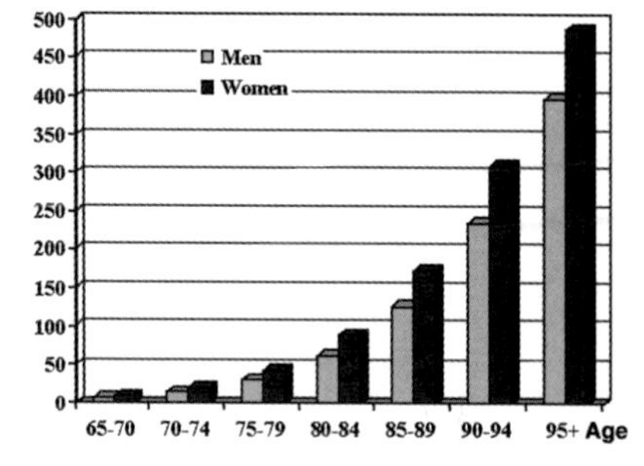

Figure 1. Prevalence (per 1000) of AD of mild severity or greater, in men and women, plotted by 5-year age brackets, data from reference (109).

Ethnicity. No geographic isolates of AD exist. No striking racial differences appear in the prevalence or incidence of AD; however, the number of ethnic groups that have been well studied outside of European, European-American, Japanese and, most recently, African-American groups (58, 98, 255) is quite limited. Studies in Shanghai, China (276) have revealed a strong relationship between educational attainment and risk of AD.

The differences, if any, between European-Americans and African-Americans, is currently a matter of controversy, as conflicting estimates of dementia prevalence and incidence have emerged in the few studies that examined African-American populations (58, 59, 98, 231, 255). Diagnostic methods could explain the different results; alternatively, biological and sociocultural diversity within one ethnic group can be very large.

Studies in Native American populations are few (97, 220). A study of

Risk factors
Age
Family history
Low educational attainment
Head injury
Atherosclerosis
Elevated serum homocysteine
Protective factors
NSAIDS
Estrogen replacement therapy
statin drugs

Table 4. Proposed risk and protective factors for AD.

Cherokees from Oklahoma found an interesting relationship between the extent of an individual's non-Cherokee heritage and risk for AD. The greater the degree of pure Cherokee heritage, the lower the odds of AD (220).

Risk factors and protective factors for AD. *Risk factors.* Putative risk factors are presented in Table 4. Despite a large number of studies devoted to detection of risk factors for AD, only a few characteristics clearly increase an individual's risk for developing dementia. The two most prominent are advancing age and a family history of dementia.

Family history of dementia increases the risk for AD (100, 148). A large multicenter study that involved nearly 1700 patients found that the lifetime risk to first-degree relatives of clinically diagnosed AD patients was approximately 15% by age 80 years and 39% by age 96 years (148). A considerable portion of that risk is mediated by the apolipoprotein E (APOE) gene. Bearing a child with Down's syndrome is associated with an increased risk for AD in the mothers if they were under age 35 at the birth of the Down's syndrome child (232).

Very low educational achievement (<eighth grade education) has been a consistently observed, but modestly potent, risk factor that increases a person's odds of developing AD by 2- to 3-fold (35, 42, 65, 126, 190, 246, 249, 276). There may be a threshold effect for education so that studies that do not include large numbers of subjects with less than an eighth grade education may not detect the association (14). Even when diagnostic methods are specifically modified to reduce educational or cultural biases, the education effect remains (249).

In a study of a teaching order of Catholic sisters, Snowdon and colleagues (242) have shown that cognitive performance at age 20 years was predictive of the subsequent development of dementia roughly 50 years later. Their hypothesis is that early life experiences contribute to the development of "brain reserve." Increased numbers of neurones or synapses presumably acts as a buffer in ameliorating the deleterious effects of AD pathology. In general, enriched childhood environments are associated with higher educational attainment, but in Snowdon's view it is the sum of all enriching experiences, not the least of which is good childhood nutrition, that protects from the subsequent development of dementia.

Cardiovascular disease confers a small to moderate increased risk for AD (36, 53, 104, 121, 147, 206). The cardiovascular risk factors associated with AD include atherosclerosis broadly defined, history of stroke, history of mid-life hypertension and carotid artery disease.

Several studies have shown that elevated homocysteine is associated with AD (40, 122, 167, 236). The most compelling study to date measured homocysteine levels in initially non-demented individuals (236). Those individuals who subsequently became demented had higher levels of homocysteine at baseline. It is not clear how homocysteine elevations are linked to AD. There are several possibilities. It is possible that elevated homocysteine levels increase the burden of cerebrovascular lesions. Another possibility is that homocysteine is a marker for sub-clinical vitamin B12 or folate deficiency, which in turn has other impacts on AD. Third, higher levels of homocysteine could indicate lower levels of methionine, which in turn could affect pathways downstream from methionine such as polyamine synthesis.

The relationship between head injury and AD (37, 64, 83, 183) has been the subject of serious concerns about recall bias among caregivers of diagnosed dementia patients. Because the putative head injury could have occurred 30 years prior to the development of dementia, prospective studies that allow minimisation of recall bias have not yet been done. However, because of the link between boxing and AD (119, 217), the importance of non-sports-related head trauma to AD seems plausible. Mayeux and colleagues have proposed that the risk of head trauma for AD is mediated by APOE ϵ4 genotype (165).

Occupational exposure to industrial solvents and agricultural chemicals have not shown consistent increases in risk for AD (144). The evidence against aluminium (22, 82, 89, 223) as a risk factor for AD outweighs suggestions (46, 78) of a possible role for aluminium. Recent neuropathological studies find no difference between AD and control brains in aluminium content, especially when exquisite attention is paid to analytic techniques (22, 157). In case-control studies comparing regions with high versus low aluminium levels in drinking water, the risk for AD in the high aluminium region was only trivially increased (61, 161, 223) except for one study (172).

Protective factors. Several protective factors have been observed in incidence cohorts; however, epidemiological associations do not prove causality. Each of the following associations between medication use and AD risk reduction could have been driven by indication bias. The factor that indicated need for medication may actually mediate the risk of AD.

Estrogen replacement therapy (ERT) has received considerable attention and has been consistently associated with reductions in risk for AD (28, 114, 130, 193, 254). There is a strong socio-economic bias in the use of ERT, with women in higher classes using ERT at much higher levels. Even when this bias is taken into account statistically, the ERT effect on AD risk remains. Basic biochemical and pathological studies have shown that estrogen plays a role in survival of hippocampal and cholinergic neurones

(158, 169) thus providing a credible explanation for the ERT observations.

The use of nonsteroidal anti-inflammatory agents (NSAIDs) (7, 27, 170, 208, 250) has also consistently been observed to offer protection. In addition to simply showing an association with any use, a prospective, population-based epidemiological study has shown that longer usage of NSAID use decreased risk for AD (110). In general, there seems to be some specificity for the observation in that neither aspirin nor acetaminophen shows the same associations with AD risk reduction as do the NSAIDs. On the other hand, a survey of the effect of various NSAIDs on Aβ peptide production has revealed that some NSAIDs have rather dramatic effects whereas others have none (267). Thus, it is possible that the NSAID association is not mediated through inflammation, but rather through interference in β-amyloid (Aβ) production (267).

The use of statin-type cholesterol lowering drugs has been added to this list (116, 275). Whether the effect is mediated through serum cholesterol or another mechanisms is unknown. There is some evidence that dietary fat and serum lipids are related to dementia. In an incidence study from the Netherlands (123), dietary total fat intake (RR = 2.4) was associated with incident dementia. On the other hand, serum LDL cholesterol levels were not associated with risk for AD, but rather only for dementia with stroke (180). Experimental evidence supports the use of cholesterol-lowering drugs as a means of lowering brain Aβ peptide levels (57). Both epidemiological studies supporting the association between statins and AD risk reduction were prevalence studies. The possibility of indication bias is considerable under such circumstances.

Cigarette smoking may be a protective factor for AD (29, 60, 81, 92), although in some studies it has been a risk factor (67, 192, 207). Intuitively, it would appear more likely to be a risk factor because of its association with vascular disease. However, a putative mechanism by which smoking could be protective is via stimulation of nicotinic receptors in the brain. Nicotinic receptors on cholinergic neurones might mediate the production of trophic factors that promote survival of key neuronal populations in AD (272).

Clinical Features

Presentation of AD. Disturbances in recent memory function are the typical symptoms that lead to the suspicion and eventual diagnosis of AD. Patients repeat themselves in conversation, repeat the same question, or forget recent conversations (140, 188, 198, 222) (Table 5). The symptoms may be so insidious in onset that they may be ignored or misinterpreted by family caregivers or physicians as insignificant, "normal ageing," or depression. Patients with AD usually ignore their own shortcomings and deny or minimise their deficits (88, 155, 235, 244). Symptoms are typically present for 1 to 3 years before family members bring the patient to medical attention. Loss of the ability to carry out key daily tasks such as shopping, handling money or doing chores around the house may be more powerful triggers than forgetfulness for seeking medical attention. Neuropsychiatric symptoms also are more likely to prompt an evaluation than forgetfulness itself.

Cognitive deficits in AD. A deficit in recent memory is the hallmark of the cognitive disorder in AD. More precisely it is a deficit in new learning and encoding of information (86, 137, 198, 251, 270). While the ability to retrieve information from long-term memory is eventually impaired in AD, the important diagnostic feature is the deficit in new learning. It is sometimes referred to as "short-term" memory. Operationally, recall of information after a delay of 5 to 30 minutes is the measure of new learning in AD patients. In the majority of patients with AD, memory complaints will be the dominant set of symptoms. Memory complaints account for many of the symptoms that caregivers report (263).

Deficits in learning and retaining new information
- Re-asking the same question several times over a 5-10 minute period
- forgetting recent events that happened a few hours or days before
- forgetting recent conversations
- misplacing items repeatedly
- forgetting names of familiar friends or of family members
- temporal or geographic disorientation

Language deficits
- Problems with finding words
- Loss of conversational skills

Deficits in spatial ability and orientation
- Getting lost in familiar places
- Difficulties in dressing
- Difficulties in object or person recognition

Deficits in reasoning or handling complex tasks
- Loss of interest or inability to perform hobbies or chores
- Use of telephone
- Dealing with finances, checkbook, taxes, bills
- Shopping
- Meal preparation
- Housekeeping
- Driving, as in accidents, getting lost
- Impairment of occupational activities

Alterations in mood or behavior
- Subtle changes in interpersonal relationships
- New onset anxiety
- New onset depression
- Agitation in the form of paranoia, irritability, delusional or illogical thinking

Alterations in basic activities of daily living
- Bathing
- Dressing
- Toileting
- Feeding

Table 5. Symptoms of dementia due to AD. Major domains from AHCPR guidelines.

Orientation is clearly impaired in patients with in AD. Given the ubiquitous nature of impairment of orientation in dementia, as well as its ease of assessment, reference to orientation among the core deficits of dementia would seem warranted. To the extent that orientation is mediated by memory, attention, language, visuospatial function and even executive functions, its impairment is a proxy for dysfunction in one or more of those domains. Disturbances of language function, "aphasia," are frequently seen in AD. Observational studies show that dementia patients exhibit deficits in naming (56, 239) and word fluency at mild stages of disease (56, 84).

Disturbances of visuospatial synthesis are well recognised and may be the predominant symptom in AD in some patients (47, 76, 79, 103, 150, 176, 261). On occasion, the visual symptoms are the presenting ones. Impairment of "executive" functions and attention may be demonstrable neuropsychologically in early AD (125, 139), and the consequences of deficits in problem-solving, judgement, foresight and mental agility lead to loss of competence in daily living (159). Both the DSM-IV and NINCDS-ADRDA definitions of AD fail to include changes in personality, impairment of affect and disturbances of behaviour among the core symptoms of dementia, even though, empirically, these entities are common in early dementia of diverse aetiologies. The spectrum of changes is protean, ranging from increased apathy and social withdrawal to disinhibition or irritability (51, 77, 173, 194, 212, 214, 256). Recognition of the affective and behavioural symptoms of dementia should increase diagnostic sensitivity. So long as some other cognitive deficits are present, the inclusion of this domain should not reduce specificity of the diagnosis of dementia.

On occasion, AD presents in ways other than as a disorder of recent memory. Sometimes, impaired judgement, social misbehaviour and other manifestations of a fronto-temporal dementia may be as prominent as the memory disorder (31, 177, 186). Another rare alternative presentation of AD is that of a visual disturbance, visual agnosia that is more bothersome to the patient's functions than the memory problems. The visual agnosia manifests as impaired figure-ground perceptions, impaired reading, impaired face recognition and impaired object recognition occurs (47, 76, 79, 103, 150, 176, 261). Rarely will AD patients present with anomia or expressive language deficits (84).

Diagnostic accuracy for AD. Many clinical-pathological studies have addressed the diagnostic accuracy of the clinical diagnosis of AD (20, 23, 72, 75, 105, 118, 132, 152, 166, 260, 265). The mean sensitivity of the diagnosis of probable AD in these studies was 81% with a range of 49 to 100%. The mean specificity of the diagnosis of probable AD was 70% with a range of 47 to 100% (135). The combination of the "possible" and "probable" categories has had higher sensitivity but lower specificity compared to the "probable" category alone. The restrictiveness of "probable AD" and its lower sensitivity in the studies that enrolled dementia cases suggests that neuropathologically definite AD has a more pleomorphic clinical picture than is depicted in the description of "probable AD." On the other hand, the lower specificity of "probable" plus "possible" AD definitions reflects the reality that non-AD dementias share many features with AD. Because AD with coexistent pathology is common, specificity improves when the pathological diagnosis of AD is broadened to allow the diagnosis to be made in the presence of other pathology.

In most instances in routine clinical practice, the diagnostic criteria of the NINCDS-ADRDA workgroup yield an accurate view of the diagnosis of AD. In comparison to the autopsy gold standard, the most important deficiencies in the clinical diagnosis are: *i)* failure to recognise that AD is the principal diagnosis in the setting of alternative medical or neurological diagnoses, and *ii)* failing to recognise relevant coexistent pathologies when most of the clinical picture looks like typical AD.

Age of onset. Historically, a great deal was made out of distinguishing between a "presenile" and a "senile" form of AD. In the past 20 years, that distinction has been largely abandoned, but the fact remains that there are some clinical features of the disease that co-vary with age. For example, the autosomal dominant form of AD occurs almost exclusively among those with very young age of onset. The effects of some susceptibility genes such as APOE, have a strong age dependence. Clinically, several studies have shown that patients under age 65 to 70 years tend to have slightly different clinical presentations, either in terms of faster rates of progression or more language deficits at the time of diagnosis (16, 99, 107, 149, 210). However, even if such differences are present in group analyses, age-related differences are hardly ever detectable on an individual basis (107).

Natural history. The natural history of AD is considerably variable from one individual to the next, but there are some approximate values that can be applied to the different phases of the illness. The average length of time from onset of symptoms until diagnosis is about 2 to 3 years (73, 136, 182, 257, 266). The average duration of time from diagnosis to nursing home placement (a marker of severe dementia) is roughly 3 to 6 years (30, 43, 102, 134, 136, 234, 238, 248). Alzheimer patients spend 3 years in nursing homes prior to death (269). Thus, the total duration of AD is roughly 9 to 12 years.

A large number of studies have examined rate of progression of AD within the symptomatic phase using mental status examinations such as the MMSE. Across patients whose initial MMSE scores ranged from 10 to 26, the average rate of change per year is about 3 points (70, 128, 141, 189, 224, 230, 259). The variability is considerable as indicated by the standard deviation of ~4 of this value (133, 259). The rate of decline obeys a curvilinear relationship to the cognitive test scores (181, 246). Faster rates of decline occur in the mid-portions of the scales, and slower rates occur among milder and more severe patients. Moreover, a decline over one 6-month or 1-year period does not predict the rate of decline over a subsequent time interval (224).

There are few predictors of rate of progression, but parkinsonian signs, hallucinations and delusions have been shown to be associated with more rapid decline (38, 156, 247). This set of observations is consistent with recent findings that patients with dementia with Lewy bodies have a faster rate of decline than comparably demented AD patients (187).

Another way of conceptualising the progression of AD is to look at the time to reach key milestones of the disease such as deteriorating to a CDR of 3 or losing basic activities of daily living skills. Estimates of the time to reach a CDR stage of 3, enter a nursing home, or lose basic activity of daily living functions is given in Table 6 (71). The table shows how variable the rate of decline is among a rather homogeneous cohort of patients with clinical AD, a high proportion of whom were shown to have AD neuropathologically (75).

Mortality in AD averages under 10% per year (13, 26, 30, 55, 101, 129, 136, 143, 160, 266). Median survival for patients with AD is roughly 5 to 6 years (2, 3, 94, 101, 178, 274). Causes of death in AD include pneumonia, sepsis and other common causes of mortality in the elderly such as cardiovascular disease and stroke (15, 143).

Milestone	N of subjects at entry	Cumulative probability year 1	year 2	year 3
Reached CDR* 2	203 CDR <2	44	71	81
Reached CDR 3	336 CDR <3	13	34	54
lost ≥ 5 IADL†	304 IADL <5	23	53	68
Lost feeding ability	343 with ability	1	9	15
Lost dressing ability	343 with ability	5	17	37
Lost toileting ability	342 with ability	3	11	21

* CDR - Clinical Dementia Rating Scale

† Items (n=7) from IADL scale (24): performing household tasks, coping with small sums of money, remembering short lists of items, finding one's way indoors, finding one's way around familiar streets, understanding situations or explanations, and recalling recent events.

Table 6. Cumulative probability of reaching milestones of AD over 3 years in CERAD cohort (71).

Clinical stages of AD. *Presymptomatic phase.* Presymptomatic individuals who are at risk to develop AD cannot be identified prospectively except for those very rare individuals from families with known autosomal dominant AD. Several studies have shown that, in retrospect, individuals destined to develop AD are cognitively inferior, as a group, to those not destined to develop AD (52, 106, 113, 127, 164, 199, 258). The group differences are not distinctive enough to be of use in prediction in individual instances, however.

Two studies that have combined PET imaging and assessment of genetic susceptibility for AD conferred by APOE genotype (213, 241) have shown that non-demented individuals who are homozygous for the ϵ4 allele have the pattern of reduced parietal lobe metabolism that is seen in patients with established AD. These intriguing findings support the belief that biochemical dysfunction is occurring in presymptomatic AD. However, from a clinical diagnostic perspective, an abnormal PET scan in a non-demented individual has no proved predictive value for subsequent AD at this time.

Mild cognitive impairment. Mild cognitive impairment (MCI) is now recognised as an important diagnostic group encompassing the spectrum between normal and demented (199). Others have referred to this state as possible dementia prodrome, or very mild AD (222). The term age-associated memory impairment appears to describe a similar group of patients, but the memory impairment is not "age-associated," but rather is "disease-associated." MCI is often a precursor of AD, but not always (90, 199). Approximately 15% of MCI patients deteriorate and qualify for a diagnosis of AD per year (199). Patients with mild cognitive impairment are sometimes identified because they are discovered coincidentally to have poor performance on mental status testing. Sometimes patients with MCI refer themselves to physicians because of concerns about their own memory.

Diagnostic criteria (199) for MCI include a memory complaint, objective evidence of impaired recent memory, intact daily function and intact non-memory cognitive functions. The lack of significant impairment in functioning in daily affairs is perhaps the major distinction between early dementia and MCI. Individuals with MCI defined as above show memory impairment comparable to AD patients, but have scores on most non-memory neuropsychological tests that are comparable to normal elderly individuals (200).

As implied by the statistic of rate of conversion, not all MCI patients go on to develop AD. Thus, some individuals with the features of MCI have a static condition, rather than a deteriorating one. Some of these individuals presumably have had impaired memory on a life-long basis. Others may have sustained brain injuries at an earlier age that have produced static dysfunction. Thus, the category of MCI, as currently conceptualised, is heterogeneous with respect to prognosis for future decline. MCI is also heterogeneous with respect to the cognitive deficit most impaired. Some individuals may have predominantly language, visuospatial or executive deficits, though memory deficits characterise the majority of MCI individuals (197). Attempts are ongoing to identify the subset of MCI patients who will invariably go on to AD. One predictor that has emerged is an increasing level of dysfunction in daily affairs as reported by an informant but not by the patient (252). Hippocampal atrophy on MR imaging together with neuropsychological features hold considerable promise for identifying MCI patients who are at risk to progress to AD within a few years (112, 262). A study of patients with a syndrome nearly identically defined as MCI showed that PET imaging abnormalities of the Alzheimer type (ie parietal hypometabolism) was usually seen in MCI patients who converted to AD during the follow-up period (19).

Mild AD. The syndrome of mild AD (which is CDR stage 1 [108] or GDS stages 3 or 4 [215]) is characterised by clear-cut deficits in recent memory, deficits in at least one of the other cognitive domains and loss of functional independence. Functional loss might take the form of difficulties with financial affairs, difficulties with geographic orientation in their own homes and other familiar places (95), or an inability to do tasks such as those in one's job or around the home. Their ability to recall information from the past is often only minimally impaired at this stage of the illness. Changes in personality frequently are part of the presentation of mild AD. The spectrum of personality changes is protean, ranging from increased apathy and social withdrawal to disinhibition or irritability (51, 77, 173, 194, 212, 214, 256). Depression also is common, and can exacerbate cognitive deficits (85, 142, 151). Paranoia and obsessions may become evident, although these are more likely to occur in later stages of the disease. Frank hallucinations and delusions occasionally occur in mild AD.

On mental status examination, patients with mild AD score between 20 and 26 on the MMSE. Memory performance may be the most abnormal portion of the cognitive examination. Patients recall nil after a short delay (34, 86, 137, 198, 270). A mild AD patient may have largely intact conversational comprehension and spontaneous speech. However, mild patients and their families report word finding difficulties, that can be observed with naming tests that use less common objects (56, 239). Abstract reasoning deficits may be detectable with more difficult tasks that require mental agility to manipulate sequential mental tasks. However, prior intellectual and occupational achievement strongly affects how well a mild AD patient will do with naming or abstract reasoning. Most patients with mild AD have some constructional difficulties. On more detailed neuropsychological testing, widespread deficits in visuospatial processing are often observed (21, 176).

The motor neurological examination is typically normal in patients with mild AD. Some subtle extrapyramidal signs may be seen (66, 73, 247).

Moderate AD. Patients with moderate AD (CDR stage 2) not only are dependent on others for higher level daily living activities such as finances, shopping or transportation, but may on occasion need to be reminded to bathe and to dress appropriately. Moderate AD patients may fail to recognise acquaintances that are not part of the patient's daily retinue. Patients at this stage of AD should no longer operate motor vehicles or devices such as lawn movers, power saws or probably even stoves and ranges. Neuropsychiatric disturbances may become prominent. Delusions and hallucinations are common. Patients often begin to misrecognise their own homes as "home." Irritability and paranoia are common symptoms of moderate AD. Disrupted sleep may also occur.

On mental status examinations with the MMSE, moderately severe AD patients will score between 10 and 19. Patients at this stage have word- and name-finding deficits that are obvious in conversation. Information or recent events are often almost instantly forgotten. Motor apraxia may be evident at this stage of AD (209). If patients with moderate AD have reasonably competent spouse or child caregivers, they can often remain in the family residence. If not, moderate AD patients may need supervised living situations. Some assistance almost always becomes needed for solo caregivers in the later stages of moderate AD. Even at this stage of the illness, the motor neurological examination may be normal except for signs of mild rigidity or bradykinesia (73, 247).

Severe AD. Patients with severe AD (CDR stage 3) need 24-hour supervision. They have negligible memory for events, conversations and unfortunately, even close family members. They have substantial word finding difficulties. Their spontaneous speech is impoverished. They may be virtually mute, or they may use jargon-filled speech that conveys no meaningful information (195). They need extensive assistance with bathing, dressing, eating and toileting. They are more likely than milder patients to become aggressive when offered assistance with undressing or toileting, although some severe patients are very docile. Despite their fragmentary cognition, severely demented patients may experience depression, anxiousness and fear. They typically score below 10 on the MMSE (195, 264).

A minority of AD patients experience generalised seizures (175, 219), often in the severe stage of the disease. Patients may also exhibit marked rigidity, bradykinesia, gait and balance difficulties and masked facies (39, 73).

Imaging. Structural neuroimaging with magnetic resonance imaging is of potential use in the diagnosis of AD (62, 111, 131, 145, 213, 228). Hippocampal atrophy (63, 111) is increased substantially in AD, but there is overlap with non-impaired elderly. Serial measurements of brain volume on neuroimaging may differentiate normal elderly from those with AD (62). The high degree of technical precision needed to carry out such measurements may not be practical in the routine clinical diagnosis of AD. Magnetic resonance imaging can detect small infarctions that may have been clinically silent (32, 154). It is not clear whether identification of small infarctions has diagnostic value for estimating the burden of vascular pathology relevant to dementia.

Laboratory diagnostic assessment. *Routine assessments.* In keeping with the general focus of the assessment of dementia in the elderly, where AD is the most prevalent disorder, the laboratory diagnostic tests are used to rule out disorders other than AD, for there are no established laboratory markers for AD. Consensus guidelines provide a framework for choosing the proper laboratory tests (10, 135) (Table 7). The new guidelines for the diagnosis of dementia by the American Academy of Neurology (AAN) (135) have expanded upon the prior recommendations.

The new guidelines of the AAN (135) are very clear on the necessary role of imaging at the time of initial diagnosis of a dementing illness. A metaanalysis suggested that imaging was appropriate (160). The view among neurologists who work with dementia patients is that a CT or MR scan should be part of the routine initial assessment of dementia patients unless there is some compelling argument to the contrary. There are some circumstances in dementia patients that should unequivocally prompt an imaging study such as the presence of neurological signs or symptoms—headaches, seizures, abnormal motor exam findings. In instances where the onset could be shorter than approximately 6 months but is unclear given deficiencies in the information available to the physician, an imaging study is justified to rule out neoplasms and chronic subdural haematomas. The importance of imaging studies rises as the duration of the dementia decreases, or when the clinician is uncertain about the duration of the dementia. Later in this chapter and elsewhere in this volume, the initial presentations as cognitive disorders of brain structural lesions are discussed. There are few circumstances that argue against the need for an imaging study. One would be the situation of a patient with a documented multi-year history of now advanced dementia. In such a patient, an imaging study would have a very low yield of useful information.

A number of blood studies are usually indicated in the routine assessment of AD patients (10, 204). These include CBC, electrolytes, serum calcium, thyroid function tests and serum cobalamin level. The yield of these tests for medically important information, in the setting of the assessment of a dementia patient, is usually low (240). The rationale for CBC and electrolytes is to use abnormalities in these values as evidence for serious underlying medical disease. Thyroid function testing and cobalamin levels have a more specific purpose, namely to rule out deficiency states that may be associated with dementia.

The AAN guidelines call for the selective use of the serum VDRL. In many places in the United States where neurosyphilis is rare, there is probably little justification. However, in the southeastern United States, a number of urban areas and a few other locales with known concentrations of neurosyphilis (243), a VDRL should be obtained in a dementia assessment.

Measure	Recommendation
*Neurologic history and examination	Required
*Laboratory studies: complete blood count, electrolytes, calcium, glucose, blood urea nitrogen, creatinine, liver function tests, thyroid function tests, serum B12 level	Required
*Neuroimaging studies, CT or MRI	Required
*Other tests, such as syphilis serology, human immunodeficiency virus testing, chest radiography, urinalysis, toxicology screen	When indicated
*Lumbar puncture	When indicated
*Neuropsychological testing	When indicated
*PET or SPECT	When indicated

Table 7. Recommended diagnostic assessment for suspected dementia, adapted from (135, 204).

The electroencephalogram (EEG) should not be routinely ordered in a dementia assessment (10, 45, 204). Its use is justified when the patient has evidence of fluctuations in cognitive status that could represent seizures. It is not useful in the diagnosis of AD as EEG findings in early AD range from normal to diffuse slowing (93). It is only when Creutzfeldt-Jakob disease is in the differential diagnosis that an EEG might play a role in a patient who otherwise was suspected of having AD.

Cerebrovascular assessments, in particular cerebral angiography or carotid ultrasonography should be limited to those patients with specific evidence for cerebrovascular disease. These might include patients with transient ischaemic attacks or the very rare patients where cerebral vasculitis is a serious consideration.

Lumbar punctures for cerebrospinal fluid examinations are also not routinely indicated (45) as their yield is quite low (17). Patients with subacute dementia syndromes might be considered suspects for chronic meningitides or meningeal carcinomatosis; in such patients, CSF examinations for cell counts, cytology, glucose and protein are justified.

AD-specific diagnostic markers. The diagnosis of AD cannot be verified with a laboratory test at present. A variety of methods have been proposed, including CSF tests (8, 68, 69, 124, 179), various tests involving the eyes (80, 87, 153, 233), magnetic resonance neuroimaging approaches (63, 111, 131, 213, 228) and functional neuroimaging (41, 163, 203, 228, 253). To a greater or lesser degree with each proposed diagnostic test, there is either clear evidence of overlap between normal elderly and AD, or there is insufficient data available to prove that the procedure is useful clinically. In part, some of the failures may be due to the inaccuracies of the clinical diagnosis, as discussed above, as well as the difficulties in obtaining autopsy confirmation of the diagnosis in a large representative sample of patients. There is also a problem with determining the proper comparison group. It is not clear whether cognitively normal subjects, patients with non-AD dementias or both should be the primary "not-AD" comparison. A reliable non-invasive or minimally invasive marker of the brain neuropathology of AD is sorely needed. Criteria for evaluating future diagnostic markers have recently been formulated (44).

Cerebrospinal fluid markers lack diagnostic precision at present, but there may be instances where abnormalities that appear specific for AD such as depressed levels of Aβ-42 and increased levels of tau or the AD7C protein will increase diagnostic certainty (8, 68, 69, 124, 179).

Genotyping for diagnostic purposes mainly revolves around the APOE gene. In a study of 1170 patients with neuropathologically confirmed diagnoses (166), APOE genotyping marginally improved diagnostic accuracy. Ninety percent of those patients with a clinical diagnosis of AD who had an APOE ε4 allele proved to have AD neuropathologically, in contrast to patients diagnosed with AD clinically but who were APOE ε4 negative, 69% of those also had AD neuropathologically. Assuming that a competent clinical diagnostic assessment has already been completed, this study suggests that the addition of APOE testing increases diagnostic accuracy for a diagnosis of AD by about 4% if an APOE ε4 allele is present (from 90% to 94%), and for a diagnosis of not-AD if an APOE ε4 is absent by 8% (from 64% to 72%). The absence of APOE ε4 allele increased specificity from 55% to 70.6% compared to the clinical diagnosis. For some patients, families and physicians, this increase in diagnostic certainty may be desirable whereas in most instances, it will be unnecessary. APOE testing also raises a number of other management issues such as genetic counselling that may complicate, rather than complement, the initial diagnostic approach (9, 168, 202, 245).

Therapy for AD

Cholinesterase inhibitors. Initial autopsy-based neurochemical studies in the late 1970s demonstrated deficits in the enzymes responsible for synthesis of AD (49, 196). Subsequent studies demonstrated the principal locations of the cholinergic projection neurones—the septum, diagonal band and nucleus basalis—lateral and anterior to the hypothalamus exhibited marked cell loss in AD (196, 211, 226). The cholinergic deficit, at the time of death in patients with clinically mild AD when evaluated shortly before death, has been quite modest (50). In contrast, other investigators have marked reductions in cholinergic neurones of the nucleus basalis in individuals with mild cognitive impairment (184). While the neurochemical findings appear to detract from the rationale for early treatment of the cholinergic deficit in AD, the results are consistent with the clinical observations of the modest effects of the cholinesterase inhibitor (ChEI) drugs. Moreover, it is reassuring that the deficits are mild enough in early AD in order for the ChEI drugs to have a substrate upon which to act. Pivotal trials for three AchEI drugs, donepezil (33), rivastigmine (221) and galantamine (273), have all shown similar effects on cognition and daily function with modest, but clinically relevant, effects.

Estrogen replacement therapy. Despite a sound basis in epidemiological studies and basic neuroscience, expectations for estrogen as a treatment for symptomatic AD suffered serious blows with the publication of 2 negative studies. The larger of the 2 involved over 120 women with mild AD (185). In a study was of a year's duration carried out by the NIH funded AD Co-operative study, estrogen (in the form of orally administered equine estrogens) had no effect on cognitive function or any other measure of the disease. A smaller study from a few centres similarly found no benefits for estrogen in AD (96).

Anti-inflammatory drugs. A one-year trial of low dose prednisone (1 month of 20 mg/d followed by 11 months of 10 mg/d) versus placebo in 138 symptomatic mild to moderate AD patients (4) conducted by the ADCS failed to show any beneficial effects for this agent on cognitive test scores, global ratings, or behavioural ratings. Similarly, a small study with a nonsteroidal anti-inflammatory drug (diclofenac) failed to demonstrate any differences between placebo- and drug-treated patients (227). A multinational one-year trial of celecoxib also proved to be negative (273).

Anti-oxidants. Although the evidence from epidemiological studies is equivocal, some positive (162), and others negative (174) on the impact of antioxidant substances on reduction of risk for AD, the biochemical evidence favouring a role for oxidative injury in the AD brain is strong. Oxidative damage to lipids, nucleic acids and proteins has been demonstrated repeatedly. Isoprostanes, markers of peroxidation of arachidonic acid, are elevated in AD brain (205) Vitamin E (α-tocopherol) is a fat-soluble substance that blocks lipid peroxidation and is the most widely used anti-oxidant. There is an extensive literature on α-tocopherol supporting its role as an antioxidant, with in vitro evidence of improved cell survival in the presence of Aβ (18). A clinical trial using the antioxidants selegiline and vitamin E was the first to report convincing benefits of this modality (225). In this study, the median delay in appearance of the study endpoints of severe dementia was about 8 months, compared to the placebo group. There was no indication of superior improvement with the combination of vitamin E and selegiline. These findings suggest that it can be recommended to most patients with AD.

Statins. As previously mentioned, several studies have suggested that lipid-lowering strategies might be of value in the treatment of AD, but results of beneficial effects of treatment in prospective trials have yet to be published.

Secretase inhibitors. Initial human studies of α-secretase or γ-secretase inhibitors have yet to be reported.

Beta-amyloid immunisation. Schenk and colleagues (229) showed that monthly intraperitoneal injections of Aβ into transgenic mice that carried the mutant APP prevented amyloid deposition. Schenk et al also showed that immunisations at 11 months of age produced nearly as dramatic results. In another study Aβ was delivered via intranasal administration.Weiner et al administered synthetic human Aβ peptide via the nasal mucosa and treated mice had a lower plaque burden (268). These preclinical trials prompted initiation of clinical studies in humans, but a number of instances of an apparent allergic encephalitis appeared, terminating the study.

Future Directions

Finding effective therapies that arrest or reverse existing dementia due to AD is an obvious and challenging goal for the field. Equally ambitious is the goal of discovering, testing and validating preventive therapies. Prevention studies aimed at preventing the development of dementia involve thousands of healthy subjects followed for several years. Such studies are expensive and intensely resource-demanding. In addition to identifying as many of the best potential agents for such a study, the judgement about selecting the best few candidates to pursue.

Research in prevention of AD would be greatly facilitated by advances in our knowledge of biomarkers of risk for future AD. Such studies are similarly expensive and probably require longitudinal follow-up of a large series of patients all the way to autopsy.

References

1. A Canadian study of health and aging: study methods and prevalence of dementia (1994) *CMAJ* 150: 899-913.

2. Aevarsson O, Svanborg A, Skoog I (1998) Seven-year survival rate after age 85 years: relation to Alzheimer disease and vascular dementia. *Arch Neurol* 55: 1226-1232.

3. Aguero-Torres H, Fratiglioni L, Guo Z, Viitanen M, Winblad B (1999) Mortality from dementia in advanced age: a 5-year follow-up study of incident dementia cases. *J Clin Epidemiol* 52: 737-743.

4. Aisen PS, Davis KL, Berg JD, Schafer K, Campbell K, Thomas RG, Weiner MF, Farlow MR, Sano M, Grundman M, Thal LJ (2000) A randomized controlled trial of prednisone in Alzheimer's disease. Alzheimer's Disease Cooperative Study. *Neurology* 54: 588-593.

5. Alzheimer A (1987) Über eine eignartige Erkrankung der Hirnrinde (About a peculiar disease of the cerebral cortex; English translation in Alz Dis Ass Dis 1:7-8, 1987. *Allgemeine Zeitschrift fur Psychiatrie und Psychisch-Gerichtliche Medizin* 1: 7-8.

6. American Psychiatric Association (1994) *Diagnostic and Statistical Manual of Mental Disorders*, American Psychiatric Association, Washington DC.

7. Andersen K, Launer LJ, Ott A, Hoes AW, Breteler MM, Hofman A (1995) Do nonsteroidal anti-inflammatory drugs decrease the risk for Alzheimer's disease? The Rotterdam Study. *Neurology* 45: 1441-1445.

8. Andreasen N, Vanmechelen E, Van de Voorde A, Davidsson P, Hesse C, Tarvonen S, Raiha I, Sourander L, Winblad B, Blennow K (1998) Cerebrospinal fluid tau protein as a biochemical marker for Alzheimer's disease: a community based follow up study. *J Neurol Neurosurg Psychiatry* 64: 298-305.

9. Apolipoprotein (1996) Apolipoprotein E genotyping in Alzheimer's disease. National Institute on Aging/Alzheimer's Association Working Group. *Lancet* 347: 1091-1095.

10. Assessing dementia (1991) The Canadian consensus. Organizing Committee, Canadian Consensus Conference on the Assessment of Dementia. *CMAJ* 144: 851-853.

11. Bachman DL, Wolf PA, Linn R, Knoefel JE, Cobb J, Belanger A, D'Agostino RB, White LR (1992) Prevalence of dementia and probable senile dementia of the Alzheimer type in the Framingham Study. *Neurology* 42: 115-119.

12. Bachman DL, Wolf PA, Linn RT, Knoefel JE, Cobb JL, Belanger AJ, White LR, D'Agostino RB (1993) Incidence of dementia and probable Alzheimer's disease in a general population: the Framingham Study. *Neurology* 43: 515-519

13. Barclay LL, Zemcov A, Blass JP, Sansone J (1985) Survival in Alzheimer's disease and vascular dementias. *Neurology* 35: 834-840.

14. Beard CM, Kokmen E, Offord KP, Kurland LT (1992) Lack of association between Alzheimer's disease and education, occupation, marital status, or living arrangement. *Neurology* 42: 2063-2068.

15. Beard CM, Kokmen E, Sigler C, Smith GE, Petterson T, O'Brien PC (1996) Cause of death in Alzheimer's disease. *Ann Epidemiol* 6: 195-200.

16. Becker JT, Huff FJ, Nebes RD, Holland A, Boller F (1988) Neuropsychological function in Alzheimer's disease. Pattern of impairment and rates of progression. *Arch Neurol* 45: 263-268.

17. Becker PM, Feussner JR, Mulrow CD, Williams BC, Vokaty KA (1985) The role of lumbar puncture in the evaluation of dementia: the Durham Veterans Administration/Duke University Study. *J Am Geriatr Soc* 33: 392-396.

18. Behl C, Davis J, Cole GM, Schubert D (1992) Vitamin E protects nerve cells from amyloid beta protein toxicity. *Biochem Biophys Res Commun* 186: 944-950.

19. Berent S, Giordani B, Foster N, Minoshima S, Lajiness-O'Neill R, Koeppe R, Kuhl DE (1999) Neuropsychological function and cerebral glucose utilization in isolated memory impairment and Alzheimer's disease. *J Psychiatr Res* 33: 7-16.

20. Berg L, McKeel DW, Jr., Miller JP, Storandt M, Rubin EH, Morris JC, Baty J, Coats M, Norton J, Goate AM, Price JL, Gearing M, Mirra SS, Saunders AM (1998) Clinicopathologic studies in cognitively healthy aging and Alzheimer's disease: relation of histologic markers to dementia severity, age, sex, and apolipoprotein E genotype. *Arch Neurol* 55: 326-335.

21. Binetti G, Cappa SF, Magni E, Padovani A, Bianchetti A, Trabucchi M (1998) Visual and spatial perception in the early phase of Alzheimer's disease. *Neuropsychology* 12: 29-33.

22. Bjertness E, Candy JM, Torvik A, Ince P, McArthur F, Taylor GA, Johansen SW, Alexander J, Gronnesby JK, Bakketeig LS, Edwardson JA (1996) Content of brain aluminum is not elevated in Alzheimer disease. *Alzheimer Dis Assoc Disord* 10: 171-174.

23. Blacker D, Albert MS, Bassett SS, Go RC, Harrell LE, Folstein MF (1994) Reliability and validity of NINCDS-ADRDA criteria for Alzheimer's disease. The National Institute of Mental Health Genetics Initiative. *Arch Neurol* 51: 1198-1204.

24. Blessed G, Tomlinson BE, Roth M (1968) The association between quantitative measures of dementia and of senile change in the cerebral grey matter of elderly subjects. *Br J Psychiatry* 114: 797-811.

25. Boller F, Lopez OL, Moossy J (1989) Diagnosis of dementia: clinicopathologic correlations. *Neurology* 39: 76-79.

26. Bowen JD, Malter AD, Sheppard L, Kukull WA, McCormick WC, Teri L, Larson EB (1996) Predictors of mortality in patients diagnosed with probable Alzheimer's disease. *Neurology* 47: 433-439.

27. Breitner JC, Gau BA, Welsh KA, Plassman BL, McDonald WM, Helms MJ, Anthony JC (1994) Inverse association of anti-inflammatory treatments and Alzheimer's disease: initial results of a co-twin control study. *Neurology* 44: 227-232.

28. Brenner DE, Kukull WA, Stergachis A, van Belle G, Bowen JD, McCormick WC, Teri L, Larson EB (1994) Postmenopausal estrogen replacement therapy and the risk of Alzheimer's disease: a population-based case-control study. *Am J Epidemiol* 140: 262-267.

29. Brenner DE, Kukull WA, van Belle G, Bowen JD, McCormick WC, Teri L, Larson EB (1993) Relationship between cigarette smoking and Alzheimer's disease in a population-based case-control study. *Neurology* 43: 293-300.

30. Brodaty H, McGilchrist C, Harris L, Peters KE (1993) Time until institutionalization and death in patients with dementia. Role of caregiver training and risk factors. *Arch Neurol* 50: 643-650.

31. Brun A (1993) Frontal lobe degeneration of non-Alzheimer type revisited. *Dementia* 4: 126-131.

32. Bryan RN, Wells SW, Miller TJ, Elster AD, Jungreis CA, Poirier VC, Lind BK, Manolio TA (1997) Infarctlike lesions in the brain: prevalence and anatomic characteristics at MR imaging of the elderly—data from the Cardiovascular Health Study. *Radiology* 202: 47-54.

33. Burns A, Rossor M, Hecker J, Gauthier S, Petit H, Moller HJ, Rogers SL, Friedhoff LT (1999) The effects of donepezil in Alzheimer's disease—results from a multinational trial. *Dement Geriatr Cogn Disord* 10: 237-244.

34. Buschke H, Sliwinski MJ, Kuslansky G, Lipton RB (1997) Diagnosis of early dementia by the Double

Memory Test: encoding specificity improves diagnostic sensitivity and specificity. *Neurology* 48: 989-997.

35. Callahan CM, Hall KS, Hui SL, Musick BS, Unverzagt FW, Hendrie HC (1996) Relationship of age, education, and occupation with dementia among a community-based sample of African Americans. *Arch Neurol* 53: 134-140.

36. Carmelli D, Swan GE, Reed T, Miller B, Wolf PA, Jarvik GP, Schellenberg GD (1998) Midlife cardiovascular risk factors, ApoE, and cognitive decline in elderly male twins. *Neurology* 50: 1580-1585.

37. Chandra V, Kokmen E, Schoenberg BS, Beard CM (1989) Head trauma with loss of consciousness as a risk factor for Alzheimer's disease. *Neurology* 39: 1576-1578.

38. Chui HC, Lyness SA, Sobel E, Schneider LS (1994) Extrapyramidal signs and psychiatric symptoms predict faster cognitive decline in Alzheimer's disease. *Arch Neurol* 51: 676-681.

39. Clark CM, Ewbank D, Lerner A, Doody R, Henderson VW, Panisset M, Morris JC, Fillenbaum GG, Heyman A (1997) The relationship between extrapyramidal signs and cognitive performance in patients with Alzheimer's disease enrolled in the CERAD Study. Consortium to Establish a Registry for Alzheimer's Disease. *Neurology* 49: 70-75.

40. Clarke R, Smith AD, Jobst KA, Refsum H, Sutton L, Ueland PM (1998) Folate, vitamin B12, and serum total homocysteine levels in confirmed Alzheimer disease. *Arch Neurol* 55: 1449-1455.

41. Claus JJ, van Harskamp F, Breteler MM, Krenning EP, de Koning I, van der Cammen TJ, Hofman A, Hasan D (1994) The diagnostic value of SPECT with Tc 99m HMPAO in Alzheimer's disease: a population-based study. *Neurology* 44: 454-461.

42. Cobb JL, Wolf PA, Au R, White R, D'Agostino RB (1995) The effect of education on the incidence of dementia and Alzheimer's disease in the Framingham Study. *Neurology* 45: 1707-1712.

43. Colerick EJ, George LK (1986) Predictors of institutionalization among caregivers of patients with Alzheimer's disease. *J Am Geriatr Soc* 34: 493-498.

44. Consensus Consensus report of the Working Group on: "Molecular and Biochemical Markers of Alzheimer's Disease" (1998) The Ronald and Nancy Reagan Research Institute of the Alzheimer's Association and the National Institute on Aging Working Group. *Neurobiol Aging* 19: 109-116.

45. Corey-Bloom J, Thal LJ, Galasko D, Folstein M, Drachman D, Raskind M, Lanska DJ (1995) Diagnosis and evaluation of dementia. *Neurology* 45: 211-218.

46. Crapper DR, Krishnan SS, De Boni U, Tomko GJ (1975) Aluminum: a possible neurotoxic agent in Alzheimer's disease. *Trans Am Neurol Assoc* 100: 154-156.

47. Crystal HA, Horoupian DS, Katzman R, Jotkowitz S (1982) Biopsy-proved Alzheimer disease presenting as a right parietal lobe syndrome. *Ann Neurol* 12: 186-188.

48. Cummings JL, Benson DF (1992) *Dementia: A Clinical Approach.* Butterworths: Boston.

49. Davies P, Maloney AJ (1976) Selective loss of central cholinergic neurons in Alzheimer's disease. *Lancet* 2: 1403.

50. Davis KL, Mohs RC, Marin D, Purohit DP, Perl DP, Lantz M, Austin G, Haroutunian V (1999) Cholinergic markers in elderly patients with early signs of Alzheimer disease. *JAMA* 281: 1401-1406.

51. Devanand DP, Jacobs DM, Tang MX, Del Castillo-Castaneda C, Sano M, Marder K, Bell K, Bylsma FW, Brandt J, Albert M, Stern Y (1997) The course of psychopathologic features in mild to moderate Alzheimer disease. *Arch Gen Psychiatry* 54: 257-263.

52. Elias MF, Beiser A, Wolf PA, Au R, White RF, D'Agostino RB (2000) The preclinical phase of alzheimer disease: A 22-year prospective study of the Framingham Cohort. *Arch Neurol* 57: 808-813.

53. Elias MF, Wolf PA, D'Agostino RB, Cobb J, White LR (1993) Untreated blood pressure level is inversely related to cognitive functioning: the Framingham Study. *Am J Epidemiol* 138: 353-364.

54. Evans DA, Funkenstein HH, Albert MS, Scherr PA, Cook NR, Chown MJ, Hebert LE, Hennekens CH, Taylor JO (1989) Prevalence of Alzheimer's disease in a community population of older persons. Higher than previously reported. *JAMA* 262: 2551-2556.

55. Evans DA, Smith LA, Scherr PA, Albert MS, Funkenstein HH, Hebert LE (1991) Risk of death from Alzheimer's disease in a community population of older persons. *Am J Epidemiol* 134: 403-412

56. Faber-Langendoen K, Morris JC, Knesevich JW, LaBarge E, Miller JP, Berg L (1988) Aphasia in senile dementia of the Alzheimer type. *Ann Neurol* 23: 365-370.

57. Fassbender K, Simons M, Bergmann C, Stroick M, Lutjohann D, Keller P, Runz H, Kuhl S, Bertsch T, von Bergmann K, Hennerici M, Beyreuther K, Hartmann T (2001) Simvastatin strongly reduces levels of Alzheimer's disease beta - amyloid peptides Aβ 42 and Aβ 40 in vitro and in vivo. *Proc Natl Acad Sci U S A* 98: 5856-5861.

58. Fillenbaum GG, Heyman A, Huber MS, Woodbury MA, Leiss J, Schmader KE, Bohannon A, Trapp-Moen B (1998) The prevalence and 3-year incidence of dementia in older Black and White community residents. *J Clin Epidemiol* 51: 587-595.

59. Folstein MF, Bassett SS, Anthony JC, Romanoski AJ, Nestadt GR (1991) Dementia: case ascertainment in a community survey.*J Gerontol* 46: 132-138.

60. Ford AB, Mefrouche Z, Friedland RP, Debanne SM (1996) Smoking and cognitive impairment: a population-based study. *J Am Geriatr Soc* 44: 905-909.

61. Forster DP, Newens AJ, Kay DW, Edwardson JA (1995) Risk factors in clinically diagnosed presenile dementia of the Alzheimer type: a case-control study in northern England. *J Epidemiol Community Health* 49: 253-258.

62. Fox NC, Freeborough PA, Rossor MN (1996) Visualisation and quantification of rates of atrophy in Alzheimer's disease. *Lancet* 348: 94-97

63. Fox NC, Warrington EK, Freeborough PA, Hartikainen P, Kennedy AM, Stevens JM, Rossor MN (1996) Presymptomatic hippocampal atrophy in Alzheimer's disease. A longitudinal MRI study. *Brain* 119: 2001-2007.

64. French LR, Schuman LM, Mortimer JA, Hutton JT, Boatman RA, Christians B (1985) A case-control study of dementia of the Alzheimer type. *Am J Epidemiol* 121: 414-421.

65. Friedland RP (1993) Epidemiology, education, and the ecology of Alzheimer's disease. *Neurology* 43: 246-249.

66. Funkenstein HH, Albert MS, Cook NR, West CG, Scherr PA, Chown MJ, Pilgrim D, Evans DA (1993) Extrapyramidal signs and other neurologic findings in clinically diagnosed Alzheimer's disease. A community-based study. *Arch Neurol* 50: 51-56.

67. Galanis DJ, Petrovitch H, Launer LJ, Harris TB, Foley DJ, White LR (1997) Smoking history in middle age and subsequent cognitive performance in elderly Japanese-American men. The Honolulu-Asia Aging Study. *Am J Epidemiol* 145: 507-515.

68. Galasko D, Chang L, Motter R, Clark CM, Kaye J, Knopman D, Thomas R, Kholodenko D, Schenk D, Lieberburg I, Miller B, Green R, Basherad R, Kertiles L, Boss MA, Seubert P (1998) High cerebrospinal fluid tau and low amyloid beta42 levels in the clinical diagnosis of Alzheimer disease and relation to apolipoprotein E genotype. *Arch Neurol* 55: 937-945.

69. Galasko D, Clark C, Chang L, Miller B, Green RC, Motter R, Seubert P (1997) Assessment of CSF levels of tau protein in mildly demented patients with Alzheimer's disease. *Neurology* 48: 632-635.

70. Galasko D, Corey-Bloom J, Thal LJ (1991) Monitoring progression in Alzheimer's disease. *J Am Geriatr Soc* 39: 932-941.

71. Galasko D, Edland SD, Morris JC, Clark C, Mohs R, Koss E (1995) The Consortium to Establish a Registry for Alzheimer's Disease (CERAD). Part XI. Clinical milestones in patients with Alzheimer's disease followed over 3 years. *Neurology* 45: 1451-1455.

72. Galasko D, Hansen LA, Katzman R, Wiederholt W, Masliah E, Terry R, Hill LR, Lessin P, Thal LJ (1994) Clinical-neuropathological correlations in Alzheimer's disease and related dementias. *Arch Neurol* 51: 888-895.

73. Galasko D, Kwo-on-Yuen PF, Klauber MR, Thal LJ (1990) Neurological findings in Alzheimer's disease and normal aging. *Arch Neurol* 47: 625-627.

74. Gao S, Hendrie HC, Hall KS, Hui S (1998) The relationships between age, sex, and the incidence of dementia and Alzheimer disease: a meta-analysis. *Arch Gen Psychiatry* 55: 809-815.

75. Gearing M, Mirra SS, Hedreen JC, Sumi SM, Hansen LA, Heyman A (1995) The Consortium to Establish a Registry for Alzheimer's Disease (CERAD). Part X. Neuropathology confirmation of the clinical diagnosis of Alzheimer's disease. *Neurology* 45: 461-466.

76. Giannakopoulos P, Gold G, Duc M, Michel JP, Hof PR, Bouras C (1999) Neuroanatomic correlates of visual agnosia in Alzheimer's disease: a clinicopathologic study. *Neurology* 52: 71-77.

77. Gilley DW, Wilson RS, Beckett LA, Evans DA (1997) Psychotic symptoms and physically aggressive

behavior in Alzheimer's disease. *J Am Geriatr Soc* 45: 1074-1079.

78. Good PF, Perl DP, Bierer LM, Schmeidler J (1992) Selective accumulation of aluminum and iron in the neurofibrillary tangles of Alzheimer's disease: a laser microprobe (LAMMA) study. *Ann Neurol* 31: 286-292.

79. Graff-Radford NR, Bolling JP, Earnest Ft, Shuster EA, Caselli RJ, Brazis PW (1993) Simultanagnosia as the initial sign of degenerative dementia. *Mayo Clin Proc* 68: 955-964.

80. Graff-Radford NR, Lin SC, Brazis PW, Bolling JP, Liesegang TJ, Lucas JA, Uitti RJ, O'Brien PC (1997) Tropicamide eyedrops cannot be used for reliable diagnosis of Alzheimer's disease. *Mayo Clin Proc* 72: 495-504.

81. Graves AB, Larson EB, Edland SD, Bowen JD, McCormick WC, McCurry SM, Rice MM, Wenzlow A, Uomoto JM (1996) Prevalence of dementia and its subtypes in the Japanese American population of King County, Washington state. The Kame Project. *Am J Epidemiol* 144: 760-771.

82. Graves AB, White E, Koepsell TD, Reifler BV, van Belle G, Larson EB (1990) The association between aluminum-containing products and Alzheimer's disease. *J Clin Epidemiol* 43: 35-44.

83. Graves AB, White E, Koepsell TD, Reifler BV, van Belle G, Larson EB, Raskind M (1990) The association between head trauma and Alzheimer's disease. *Am J Epidemiol* 131: 491-501.

84. Green J, Morris JC, Sandson J, McKeel DW, Jr., Miller JW (1990) Progressive aphasia: a precursor of global dementia? *Neurology* 40: 423-429.

85. Greenwald BS, Kramer-Ginsberg E, Marin DB, Laitman LB, Hermann CK, Mohs RC, Davis KL (1989) Dementia with coexistent major depression. *Am J Psychiatry*146: 1472-1478.

86. Grober E, Kawas C (1997) Learning and retention in preclinical and early Alzheimer's disease. *Psychol Aging* 12: 183-188.

87. Growdon JH, Graefe K, Tennis M, Hayden D, Schoenfeld D, Wray SH (1997) Pupil dilation to tropicamide is not specific for Alzheimer disease. *Arch Neurol* 54: 841-844.

88. Grut M, Jorm AF, Fratiglioni L, Forsell Y, Viitanen M, Winblad B (1993) Memory complaints of elderly people in a population survey: variation according to dementia stage and depression. *J Am Geriatr Soc* 41: 1295-1300.

89. Hachinski V (1998) Aluminum exposure and risk of Alzheimer disease. *Arch Neurol* 55: 742.

90. Hanninen T, Hallikainen M, Koivisto K, Helkala EL, Reinikainen KJ, Soininen H, Mykkanen L, Laakso M, Pyorala K, Riekkinen PJ, Sr. (1995) A follow-up study of age-associated memory impairment: neuropsychological predictors of dementia. *J Am Geriatr Soc* 43: 1007-1015.

91. Hebert LE, Scherr PA, Beckett LA, Albert MS, Pilgrim DM, Chown MJ, Funkenstein HH, Evans DA (1995) Age-specific incidence of Alzheimer's disease in a community population. *JAMA* 273: 1354-1359.

92. Hebert LE, Scherr PA, Beckett LA, Funkenstein HH, Albert MS, Chown MJ, Evans DA (1992) Relation of smoking and alcohol consumption to incident Alzheimer's disease. *Am J Epidemiol* 135: 347-355.

93. Helkala EL, Laulumaa V, Soininen H, Partanen J, Riekkinen PJ (1991) Different patterns of cognitive decline related to normal or deteriorating EEG in a 3-year follow-up study of patients with Alzheimer's disease. *Neurology* 41: 528-532.

94. Helmer C, Joly P, Letenneur L, Commenges D, Dartigues JF (2001) Mortality with dementia: results from a French prospective community- based cohort. *Am J Epidemiol* 154: 642-644.

95. Henderson VW, Mack W, Williams BW (1989) Spatial disorientation in Alzheimer's disease. *Arch Neurol* 46: 391-394.

96. Henderson VW, Paganini-Hill A, Miller BL, Elble RJ, Reyes PF, Shoupe D, McCleary CA, Klein RA, Hake AM, Farlow MR (2000) Estrogen for Alzheimer's disease in women: randomized, double-blind, placebo-controlled trial. *Neurology* 54: 295-301.

97. Hendrie HC, Hall KS, Pillay N, Rodgers D, Prince C, Norton J, Brittain H, Nath A, Blue A, Kaufert J, et al. (1993) Alzheimer's disease is rare in Cree. *Int Psychogeriatr* 5: 5-14.

98. Hendrie HC, Osuntokun BO, Hall KS, Ogunniyi AO, Hui SL, Unverzagt FW, Gureje O, Rodenberg CA, Baiyewu O, Musick BS (1995) Prevalence of Alzheimer's disease and dementia in two communities: Nigerian Africans and African Americans. *Am J Psychiatry*152: 1485-1492.

99. Heston LL, Mastri AR (1982) Age at onset of Pick's and Alzheimer's dementia: implications for diagnosis and research. *J Gerontol* 37: 422-424.

100. Heston LL, Mastri AR, Anderson VE, White J (1981) Dementia of the Alzheimer type. Clinical genetics, natural history, and associated conditions. *Arch Gen Psychiatry* 38: 1085-1090.

101. Heyman A, Peterson B, Fillenbaum G, Pieper C (1996) The consortium to establish a registry for Alzheimer's disease (CERAD). Part XIV: Demographic and clinical predictors of survival in patients with Alzheimer's disease. *Neurology* 46: 656-660.

102. Heyman A, Peterson B, Fillenbaum G, Pieper C (1997) Predictors of time to institutionalization of patients with Alzheimer's disease: the CERAD experience, part XVII. *Neurology* 48: 1304-1309.

103. Hof PR, Bouras C, Constantinidis J, Morrison JH (1990) Selective disconnection of specific visual association pathways in cases of Alzheimer's disease presenting with Balint's syndrome.*J Neuropathol Exp Neurol* 49: 168-184.

104. Hofman A, Ott A, Breteler MM, Bots ML, Slooter AJ, van Harskamp F, van Duijn CN, Van Broeckhoven C, Grobbee DE (1997) Atherosclerosis, apolipoprotein E, and prevalence of dementia and Alzheimer's disease in the Rotterdam Study. *Lancet* 349: 151-154.

105. Holmes C, Cairns N, Lantos P, Mann A (1999) Validity of current clinical criteria for Alzheimer's disease, vascular dementia and dementia with Lewy bodies. *Br J Psychiatry* 174: 45-50.

106. Howieson DB, Dame A, Camicioli R, Sexton G, Payami H, Kaye JA (1997) Cognitive markers preceding Alzheimer's dementia in the healthy oldest old. *J Am Geriatr Soc* 45: 584-589.

107. Huff FJ, Growdon JH, Corkin S, Rosen TJ (1987) Age at onset and rate of progression of Alzheimer's disease. *J Am Geriatr Soc* 35: 27-30.

108. Hughes CP, Berg L, Danziger WL, Coben LA, Martin RL (1982) A new clinical scale for the staging of dementia. *Br J Psychiatry* 140: 566-572.

109. Hy LX, Keller DM (2000) Prevalence of AD among whites: a summary by levels of severity. *Neurology* 55: 198-204.

110. int' Veld BA, Ruitenberg A, Hofman A, Launer LJ, van Duijn CM, Stijnen T, Breteler MM, Stricker BH (2001) Nonsteroidal antiinflammatory drugs and the risk of Alzheimer's disease. *N Engl J Med* 345: 1515-1521.

111. Jack CR, Jr., Petersen RC, O'Brien PC, Tangalos EG (1992) MR-based hippocampal volumetry in the diagnosis of Alzheimer's disease. *Neurology* 42: 183-188.

112. Jack CR, Jr., Petersen RC, Xu YC, O'Brien PC, Smith GE, Ivnik RJ, Boeve BF, Waring SC, Tangalos EG, Kokmen E (1999) Prediction of AD with MRI-based hippocampal volume in mild cognitive impairment. *Neurology* 52: 1397-1403.

113. Jacobs DM, Sano M, Dooneief G, Marder K, Bell KL, Stern Y (1995) Neuropsychological detection and characterization of preclinical Alzheimer's disease. *Neurology* 45: 957-962.

114. Jacobs DM, Tang MX, Stern Y, Sano M, Marder K, Bell KL, Schofield P, Dooneief G, Gurland B, Mayeux R (1998) Cognitive function in nondemented older women who took estrogen after menopause. *Neurology* 50: 368-373.

115. Jellinger K, Danielczyk W, Fischer P, Gabriel E (1990) Clinicopathological analysis of dementia disorders in the elderly. *J Neurol Sci* 95: 239-258.

116. Jick H, Zornberg GL, Jick SS, Seshadri S, Drachman DA (2000) Statins and the risk of dementia. *Lancet* 356: 1627-1631.

117. Joachim CL, Morris JH, Selkoe DJ (1988) Clinically diagnosed Alzheimer's disease: autopsy results in 150 cases. *Ann Neurol* 24: 50-56.

118. Jobst KA, Barnetson LP, Shepstone BJ (1998) Accurate prediction of histologically confirmed Alzheimer's disease and the differential diagnosis of dementia: the use of NINCDS-ADRDA and DSM- III-R criteria, SPECT, X-ray CT, and Apo E4 in medial temporal lobe dementias. Oxford Project to Investigate Memory and Aging. *Int Psychogeriatr* 10: 271-302.

119. Jordan BD, Relkin NR, Ravdin LD, Jacobs AR, Bennett A, Gandy S (1997) Apolipoprotein E epsilon4 associated with chronic traumatic brain injury in boxing. *JAMA* 278: 136-140.

120. Jorm AF, Jolley D (1998) The incidence of dementia: a meta-analysis. *Neurology* 51: 728-733.

121. Kalmijn S, Feskens EJ, Launer LJ, Kromhout D (1996) Cerebrovascular disease, the apolipoprotein e4 allele, and cognitive decline in a community-based study of elderly men. *Stroke* 27: 2230-2235.

122. Kalmijn S, Launer LJ, Lindemans J, Bots ML, Hofman A, Breteler MM (1999) Total homocysteine and cognitive decline in a community-based sample of elderly subjects: the Rotterdam Study. *Am J Epidemiol* 150: 283-289.

123. Kalmijn S, Launer LJ, Ott A, Witteman JC, Hofman A, Breteler MM (1997) Dietary fat intake and the risk of incident dementia in the Rotterdam Study. *Ann Neurol* 42: 776-782.

124. Kanai M, Matsubara E, Isoe K, Urakami K, Nakashima K, Arai H, Sasaki H, Abe K, Iwatsubo T, Kosaka T, Watanabe M et al (1998) Longitudinal study of cerebrospinal fluid levels of tau, Ab1-40, and Ab1-42(43) in Alzheimer's disease: a study in Japan. *Ann Neurol* 44: 17-26.

125. Kanne SM, Balota DA, Storandt M, McKeel DW, Jr., Morris JC (1998) Relating anatomy to function in Alzheimer's disease: neuropsychological profiles predict regional neuropathology 5 years later. *Neurology* 50: 979-985.

126. Katzman R (1993) Education and the prevalence of dementia and Alzheimer's disease. *Neurology* 43: 13-20.

127. Katzman R, Aronson M, Fuld P, Kawas C, Brown T, Morgenstern H, Frishman W, Gidez L, Eder H, Ooi WL (1989) Development of dementing illnesses in an 80-year-old volunteer cohort. *Ann Neurol* 25: 317-324.

128. Katzman R, Brown T, Thal LJ, Fuld PA, Aronson M, Butters N, Klauber MR, Wiederholt W, Pay M, Xiong RB et al (1988) Comparison of rate of annual change of mental status score in four independent studies of patients with Alzheimer's disease. *Ann Neurol* 24: 384-389.

129. Katzman R, Hill LR, Yu ES, Wang ZY, Booth A, Salmon DP, Liu WT, Qu GY, Zhang M (1994) The malignancy of dementia. Predictors of mortality in clinically diagnosed dementia in a population survey of Shanghai, China. *Arch Neurol* 51: 1220-1225.

130. Kawas C, Resnick S, Morrison A, Brookmeyer R, Corrada M, Zonderman A, Bacal C, Lingle DD, Metter E (1997) A prospective study of estrogen replacement therapy and the risk of developing Alzheimer's disease: the Baltimore Longitudinal Study of Aging. *Neurology* 48: 1517-1521.

131. Killiany RJ, Moss MB, Albert MS, Sandor T, Tieman J, Jolesz F (1993) Temporal lobe regions on magnetic resonance imaging identify patients with early Alzheimer's disease. *Arch Neurol* 50: 949-954.

132. Klatka LA, Schiffer RB, Powers JM, Kazee AM (1996) Incorrect diagnosis of Alzheimer's disease. A clinicopathologic study. *Arch Neurol* 53: 35-42.

133. Knopman D, Gracon S (1994) Observations on the short-term 'natural history' of probable Alzheimer's disease in a controlled clinical trial. *Neurology* 44: 260-265.

134. Knopman D, Schneider L, Davis K, Talwalker S, Smith F, Hoover T, Gracon S (1996) Long-term tacrine (Cognex) treatment: effects on nursing home placement and mortality, Tacrine Study Group. *Neurology* 47: 166-177.

135. Knopman DS, DeKosky ST, Cummings JL, Chui H, Corey-Bloom J, Relkin N, Small GW, Miller B, Stevens JC (2001) Practice parameter: diagnosis of dementia (an evidence-based review). Report of the Quality Standards Subcommittee of the American Academy of Neurology. *Neurology* 56: 1143-1153.

136. Knopman DS, Kitto J, Deinard S, Heiring J (1988) Longitudinal study of death and institutionalization in patients with primary degenerative dementia. *J Am Geriatr Soc* 36: 108-112.

137. Knopman DS, Ryberg S (1989) A verbal memory test with high predictive accuracy for dementia of the Alzheimer type. *Arch Neurol* 46: 141-145.

138. Kokmen E, Beard CM, Offord KP, Kurland LT (1989) Prevalence of medically diagnosed dementia in a defined United States population: Rochester, Minnesota, January 1, 1975. *Neurology* 39: 773-776.

139. Kopelman MD (1991) Frontal dysfunction and memory deficits in the alcoholic Korsakoff syndrome and Alzheimer-type dementia. *Brain* 114: 117-137.

140. Koss E, Patterson MB, Ownby R, Stuckey JC, Whitehouse PJ (1993) Memory evaluation in Alzheimer's disease. Caregivers' appraisals and objective testing. *Arch Neurol* 50: 92-97.

141. Kraemer HC, Tinklenberg J, Yesavage JA (1994) 'How far' vs 'how fast' in Alzheimer's disease. The question revisited. *Arch Neurol* 51: 275-279.

142. Kramer SI, Reifler BV (1992) Depression, dementia, and reversible dementia. Clin Geriatr Med 8: 289-297.

143. Kukull WA, Brenner DE, Speck CE, Nochlin D, Bowen J, McCormick W, Teri L, Pfanschmidt ML, Larson EB (1994) Causes of death associated with Alzheimer disease: variation by level of cognitive impairment before death. *J Am Geriatr Soc* 42: 723-726.

144. Kukull WA, Larson EB, Bowen JD, McCormick WC, Teri L, Pfanschmidt ML, Thompson JD, O'Meara ES, Brenner DE, van Belle G (1995) Solvent exposure as a risk factor for Alzheimer's disease: a case- control study. *Am J Epidemiol* 141: 1059-1071; discussion 1072-1079.

145. Laakso MP, Soininen H, Partanen K, Lehtovirta M, Hallikainen M, Hanninen T, Helkala EL, Vainio P, Riekkinen PJ, Sr. (1998) MRI of the hippocampus in Alzheimer's disease: sensitivity, specificity, and analysis of the incorrectly classified subjects. *Neurobiol Aging* 19: 23-31.

146. Larson EB, Reifler BV, Sumi SM, Canfield CG, Chinn NM (1985) Diagnostic evaluation of 200 elderly outpatients with suspected dementia. *J Gerontol* 40: 536-543.

147. Launer LJ, Masaki K, Petrovitch H, Foley D, Havlik RJ (1995) The association between midlife blood pressure levels and late-life cognitive function. The Honolulu-Asia Aging Study. *JAMA* 274: 1846-1851.

148. Lautenschlager NT, Cupples LA, Rao VS, Auerbach SA, Becker R, Burke J, Chui H, Duara R, Foley EJ, Glatt SL, Green RC, Jones R, Karlinsky H, Kukull WA, Kurz A, Larson EB, Martelli K, Sadovnick AD, Volicer L, Waring SC, Growdon JH, Farrer LA (1996) Risk of dementia among relatives of Alzheimer's disease patients in the MIRAGE study: What is in store for the oldest old? *Neurology* 46: 641-650.

149. Lawlor BA, Ryan TM, Schmeidler J, Mohs RC, Davis KL (1994) Clinical symptoms associated with age at onset in Alzheimer's disease. *Am J Psychiatry*151: 1646-1649.

150. Levine DN, Lee JM, Fisher CM (1993) The visual variant of Alzheimer's disease: a clinicopathologic case study. *Neurology* 43: 305-313.

151. Levy ML, Cummings JL, Fairbanks LA, Bravi D, Calvani M, Carta A (1996) Longitudinal assessment of symptoms of depression, agitation, and psychosis in 181 patients with Alzheimer's disease. *Am J Psychiatry*153: 1438-1443.

152. Lim A, Tsuang D, Kukull W, Nochlin D, Leverenz J, McCormick W, Bowen J, Teri L, Thompson J, Peskind ER, Raskind M, Larson EB (1999) Clinico-neuropathological correlation of Alzheimer's disease in a community-based case series. *J Am Geriatr Soc* 47: 564-569.

153. Litvan I, FitzGibbon EJ (1996) Can tropicamide eye drop response differentiate patients with progressive supranuclear palsy and Alzheimer's disease from healthy control subjects? *Neurology* 47: 1324-1326.

154. Longstreth WT, Jr., Bernick C, Manolio TA, Bryan N, Jungreis CA, Price TR (1998) Lacunar infarcts defined by magnetic resonance imaging of 3660 elderly people: the Cardiovascular Health Study. *Arch Neurol* 55: 1217-1225.

155. Lopez OL, Becker JT, Somsak D, Dew MA, DeKosky ST (1994) Awareness of cognitive deficits and anosognosia in probable Alzheimer's disease. *Eur Neurol* 34: 277-282.

156. Lopez OL, Wisnieski SR, Becker JT, Boller F, DeKosky ST (1997) Extrapyramidal signs in patients with probable Alzheimer disease. *Arch Neurol* 54: 969-975.

157. Lovell MA, Ehmann WD, Markesbery WR (1993) Laser microprobe analysis of brain aluminum in Alzheimer's disease. *Ann Neurol* 33: 36-42.

158. Luine VN (1985) Estradiol increases choline acetyltransferase activity in specific basal forebrain nuclei and projection areas of female rats. *Exp Neurol* 89: 484-490.

159. Marson DC, Cody HA, Ingram KK, Harrell LE (1995) Neuropsychologic predictors of competency in Alzheimer's disease using a rational reasons legal standard. *Arch Neurol* 52: 955-959.

160. Martin DC, Miller J, Kapoor W, Karpf M, Boller F (1987) Clinical prediction rules for computed tomographic scanning in senile dementia. *Arch Intern Med* 147: 77-80.

161. Martyn CN, Barker DJ, Osmond C, Harris EC, Edwardson JA, Lacey RF (1989) Geographical relation between Alzheimer's disease and aluminum in drinking water. *Lancet* 1: 59-62.

162. Masaki KH, Losonczy KG, Izmirlian G, Foley DJ, Ross GW, Petrovitch H, Havlik R, White LR (2000) Association of vitamin E and C supplement use with cognitive function and dementia in elderly men. *Neurology* 54: 1265-1272.

163. Masterman DL, Mendez MF, Fairbanks LA, Cummings JL (1997) Sensitivity, specificity, and positive predictive value of technetium 99-HMPAO SPECT in

discriminating Alzheimer's disease from other dementias. *J Geriatr Psychiatry Neurol* 10: 15-21.

164. Masur DM, Sliwinski M, Lipton RB, Blau AD, Crystal HA (1994) Neuropsychological prediction of dementia and the absence of dementia in healthy elderly persons. *Neurology* 44: 1427-1432.

165. Mayeux R, Ottman R, Maestre G, Ngai C, Tang MX, Ginsberg H, Chun M, Tycko B, Shelanski M (1995) Synergistic effects of traumatic head injury and apolipoprotein-epsilon 4 in patients with Alzheimer's disease. *Neurology* 45: 555-557.

166. Mayeux R, Saunders AM, Shea S, Mirra S, Evans D, Roses AD, Hyman BT, Crain B, Tang MX, Phelps CH (1998) Utility of the apolipoprotein E genotype in the diagnosis of Alzheimer's disease. Alzheimer's Disease Centers Consortium on Apolipoprotein E and Alzheimer's Disease. *N Engl J Med* 338: 506-511.

167. McCaddon A, Davies G, Hudson P, Tandy S, Cattell H (1998) Total serum homocysteine in senile dementia of Alzheimer type. *Int J Geriatr Psychiatry* 13: 235-239.

168. McConnell LM, Koenig BA, Greely HT, Raffin TA (1998) Genetic testing and Alzheimer disease: has the time come? Alzheimer Disease Working Group of the Stanford Program in Genomics, Ethics & Society. *Nat Med* 4: 757-759.

169. McEwen BS, Alves SE, Bulloch K, Weiland NG (1997) Ovarian steroids and the brain: implications for cognition and aging. *Neurology* 48: S8-15.

170. McGeer PL, Schulzer M, McGeer EG (1996) Arthritis and anti-inflammatory agents as possible protective factors for Alzheimer's disease: a review of 17 epidemiologic studies. *Neurology* 47: 425-432.

171. McKhann G, Drachman D, Folstein M, Katzman R, Price D, Stadlan EM (1984) Clinical diagnosis of Alzheimer's disease: report of the NINCDS-ADRDA Work Group under the auspices of Department of Health and Human Services Task Force on Alzheimer's Disease. *Neurology* 34: 939-944.

172. McLachlan DR, Bergeron C, Smith JE, Boomer D, Rifat SL (1996) Risk for neuropathologically confirmed Alzheimer's disease and residual aluminum in municipal drinking water employing weighted residential histories. *Neurology* 46: 401-405.

173. Mega MS, Cummings JL, Fiorello T, Gornbein J (1996) The spectrum of behavioral changes in Alzheimer's disease. *Neurology* 46: 130-135.

174. Mendelsohn AB, Belle SH, Stoehr GP, Ganguli M (1998) Use of antioxidant supplements and its association with cognitive function in a rural elderly cohort: the MoVIES Project. Monongahela Valley Independent Elders Survey. *Am J Epidemiol* 148: 38-44.

175. Mendez MF, Catanzaro P, Doss RC, R AR, Frey WH, 2nd (1994) Seizures in Alzheimer's disease: clinicopathologic study. *J Geriatr Psychiatry Neurol* 7: 230-233.

176. Mendez MF, Mendez MA, Martin R, Smyth KA, Whitehouse PJ (1990) Complex visual disturbances in Alzheimer's disease. *Neurology* 40: 439-443.

177. Miller BL, Ikonte C, Ponton M, Levy M, Boone K, Darby A, Berman N, Mena I, Cummings JL (1997) A study of the Lund-Manchester research criteria for frontotemporal dementia: clinical and single-photon emission CT correlations. *Neurology* 48: 937-942.

178. Molsa PK, Marttila RJ, Rinne UK (1995) Long-term survival and predictors of mortality in Alzheimer's disease and multi-infarct dementia. *Acta Neurol Scand* 91: 159-164.

179. Monte SM, Ghanbari K, Frey WH, Beheshti I, Averback P, Hauser SL, Ghanbari HA, Wands JR (1997) Characterization of the AD7C-NTP cDNA expression in Alzheimer's disease and measurement of a 41-kD protein in cerebrospinal fluid.*J Clin Invest* 100: 3093-3104.

180. Moroney JT, Tang MX, Berglund L, Small S, Merchant C, Bell K, Stern Y, Mayeux R (1999) Low-density lipoprotein cholesterol and the risk of dementia with stroke. *JAMA* 282: 254-260.

181. Morris JC, Edland S, Clark C, Galasko D, Koss E, Mohs R, van Belle G, Fillenbaum G, Heyman A (1993) The consortium to establish a registry for Alzheimer's disease (CERAD). Part IV. Rates of cognitive change in the longitudinal assessment of probable Alzheimer's disease. *Neurology* 43: 2457-2465.

182. Morris JC, Heyman A, Mohs RC, Hughes JP, van Belle G, Fillenbaum G, Mellits ED, Clark C (1989) The Consortium to Establish a Registry for Alzheimer's Disease (CERAD). Part I. Clinical and neuropsychological assessment of Alzheimer's disease. *Neurology* 39: 1159-1165.

183. Mortimer JA, van Duijn CM, Chandra V, Fratiglioni L, Graves AB, Heyman A, Jorm AF, Kokmen E, Kondo K, Rocca WA et al (1991) Head trauma as a risk factor for Alzheimer's disease: a collaborative re-analysis of case-control studies. EURODEM Risk Factors Research Group. *Int J Epidemiol* 20: S28-35.

184. Mufson EJ, Ma SY, Cochran EJ, Bennett DA, Beckett LA, Jaffar S, Saragovi HU, Kordower JH (2000) Loss of nucleus basalis neurons containing trkA immunoreactivity in individuals with mild cognitive impairment and early Alzheimer's disease. *J Comp Neurol* 427: 19-30.

185. Mulnard RA, Cotman CW, Kawas C, van Dyck CH, Sano M, Doody R, Koss E, Pfeiffer E, Jin S, Gamst A, Grundman M, Thomas R, Thal LJ (2000) Estrogen replacement therapy for treatment of mild to moderate Alzheimer disease: a randomized controlled trial. Alzheimer's Disease Cooperative Study. *JAMA* 283: 1007-1015.

186. Neary D, Snowden JS, Northen B, Goulding P (1988) Dementia of frontal lobe type. *J Neurol Neurosurg Psychiatry* 51: 353-361.

187. Olichney JM, Galasko D, Salmon DP, Hofstetter CR, Hansen LA, Katzman R, Thal LJ (1998) Cognitive decline is faster in Lewy body variant than in Alzheimer's disease. *Neurology* 51: 351-357.

188. Oppenheim G (1994) The earliest signs of Alzheimer's disease. *J Geriatr Psychiatry Neurol* 7: 116-1620.

189. Ortof E, Crystal HA (1989) Rate of progression of Alzheimer's disease. *J Am Geriatr Soc* 37: 511-514.

190. Ott A, Breteler MM, van Harskamp F, Claus JJ, van der Cammen TJ, Grobbee DE, Hofman A (1995) Prevalence of Alzheimer's disease and vascular dementia: association with education. The Rotterdam study. *BMJ* 310: 970-973.

191. Ott A, Breteler MM, van Harskamp F, Stijnen T, Hofman A (1998) Incidence and risk of dementia. The Rotterdam Study. *Am J Epidemiol* 147: 574-580.

192. Ott A, Slooter AJ, Hofman A, van Harskamp F, Witteman JC, Van Broeckhoven C, van Duijn CM, Breteler MM (1998) Smoking and risk of dementia and Alzheimer's disease in a population- based cohort study: the Rotterdam Study. *Lancet* 351: 1840-1843.

193. Paganini-Hill A, Henderson VW (1996) Estrogen replacement therapy and risk of Alzheimer disease. *Arch Intern Med* 156: 2213-2217.

194. Patterson MB, Mack JL, Mackell JA, Thomas R, Tariot P, Weiner M, Whitehouse PJ (1997) A longitudinal study of behavioral pathology across five levels of dementia severity in Alzheimer's disease: the CERAD Behavior Rating Scale for Dementia. The Alzheimer's Disease Cooperative Study. *Alzheimer Dis Assoc Disord* 11: S40-44.

195. Peavy GM, Salmon DP, Rice VA, Galasko D, Samuel W, Taylor KI, Ernesto C, Butters N, Thal L (1996) Neuropsychological assessment of severely demeted elderly: the severe cognitive impairment profile. *Arch Neurol* 53: 367-372.

196. Perry EK, Tomlinson BE, Blessed G, Bergmann K, Gibson PH, Perry RH (1978) Correlation of cholinergic abnormalities with senile plaques and mental test scores in senile dementia. *Br Med J* 2: 1457-1459.

197. Petersen RC, Doody R, Kurz A, Mohs RC, Morris JC, Rabins PV, Ritchie K, Rossor M, Thal L, Winblad B (2001) Current concepts in mild cognitive impairment. *Arch Neurol* 58: 1985-1992.

198. Petersen RC, Smith GE, Ivnik RJ, Kokmen E, Tangalos EG (1994) Memory function in very early Alzheimer's disease. *Neurology* 44: 867-872.

199. Petersen RC, Smith GE, Ivnik RJ, Tangalos EG, Schaid DJ, Thibodeau SN, Kokmen E, Waring SC, Kurland LT (1995) Apolipoprotein E status as a predictor of the development of Alzheimer's disease in memory-impaired individuals. *JAMA* 273: 1274-1278.

200. Petersen RC, Smith GE, Waring SC, Ivnik RJ, Tangalos EG, Kokmen E (1999) Mild cognitive impairment: clinical characterization and outcome. *Arch Neurol* 56: 303-308.

201. Pfeffer RI, Afifi AA, Chance JM (1987) Prevalence of Alzheimer's disease in a retirement community. *Am J Epidemiol* 125: 420-436.

202. Post SG, Whitehouse PJ, Binstock RH, Bird TD, Eckert SK, Farrer LA, Fleck LM, Gaines AD, Juengst ET, Karlinsky H, Miles S, Murray TH, Quaid KA, Relkin NR, Roses AD, St George-Hyslop PH, Sachs GA, Steinbock B, Truschke EF, Zinn AB (1997) The clinical introduction of genetic testing for Alzheimer disease. An ethical perspective. *JAMA* 277: 832-836.

203. Powers WJ, Perlmutter JS, Videen TO, Herscovitch P, Griffeth LK, Royal HD, Siegel BA, Morris JC, Berg L (1992) Blinded clinical evaluation of positron emission tomography for diagnosis of probable Alzheimer's disease. *Neurology* 42: 765-770.

204. Practice p (1994) Practice parameter for diagnosis and evaluation of dementia. (summary statement) Report of the Quality Standards Subcommittee of the American Academy of Neurology. *Neurology* 44: 2203-2206.

205. Pratico D, Clark CM, Lee VM, Trojanowski JQ, Rokach J, FitzGerald GA (2000) Increased 8,12-iso-iPF2alpha-VI in Alzheimer's disease: correlation of a noninvasive index of lipid peroxidation with disease severity. *Ann Neurol* 48: 809-812.

206. Prince M, Cullen M, Mann A (1994) Risk factors for Alzheimer's disease and dementia: a case-control study based on the MRC elderly hypertension trial. *Neurology* 44: 97-104.

207. Prince M, Lewis G, Bird A, Blizard R, Mann A (1996) A longitudinal study of factors predicting change in cognitive test scores over time, in an older hypertensive population. *Psychol Med* 26: 555-568.

208. Prince M, Rabe-Hesketh S, Brennan P (1998) Do antiarthritic drugs decrease the risk for cognitive decline? An analysis based on data from the MRC treatment trial of hypertension in older adults. *Neurology* 50: 374-379.

209. Rapcsak SZ, Croswell SC, Rubens AB (1989) Apraxia in Alzheimer's disease. *Neurology* 39: 664-668.

210. Raskind MA, Carta A, Bravi D (1995) Is early-onset Alzheimer disease a distinct subgroup within the Alzheimer disease population? *Alzheimer Dis Assoc Disord* 9: S2-6.

211. Rasool CG, Svendsen CN, Selkoe DJ (1986) Neurofibrillary degeneration of cholinergic and non-cholinergic neurons of the basal forebrain in Alzheimer's disease. *Ann Neurol* 20: 482-488.

212. Reichman WE, Coyne AC, Amirneni S, Molino B, Jr., Egan S (1996) Negative symptoms in Alzheimer's disease. *Am J Psychiatry*153: 424-426.

213. Reiman EM, Uecker A, Caselli RJ, Lewis S, Bandy D, de Leon MJ, De Santi S, Convit A, Osborne D, Weaver A, Thibodeau SN (1998) Hippocampal volumes in cognitively normal persons at genetic risk for Alzheimer's disease. *Ann Neurol* 44: 288-291.

214. Reisberg B, Borenstein J, Salob SP, Ferris SH, Franssen E, Georgotas A (1987) Behavioral symptoms in Alzheimer's disease: phenomenology and treatment. *J Clin Psychiatry* 48 Suppl: 9-15.

215. Reisberg B, Ferris SH, de Leon MJ, Crook T (1982) The Global Deterioration Scale for assessment of primary degenerative dementia. *Am J Psychiatry*139: 1136-1139.

216. Risse SC, Raskind MA, Nochlin D, Sumi SM, Lampe TH, Bird TD, Cubberley L, Peskind ER (1990) Neuropathological findings in patients with clinical diagnoses of probable Alzheimer's disease. *Am J Psychiatry*147: 168-172.

217. Roberts GW, Allsop D, Bruton C (1990) The occult aftermath of boxing. *J Neurol Neurosurg Psychiatry* 53: 373-378.

218. Rocca WA, Cha RH, Waring SC, Kokmen E (1998) Incidence of dementia and Alzheimer's disease: a reanalysis of data from Rochester, Minnesota, 1975-1984. *Am J Epidemiol* 148: 51-62.

219. Romanelli MF, Morris JC, Ashkin K, Coben LA (1990) Advanced Alzheimer's disease is a risk factor for late-onset seizures. *Arch Neurol* 47: 847-850.

220. Rosenberg RN, Richter RW, Risser RC, Taubman K, Prado-Farmer I, Ebalo E, Posey J, Kingfisher D, Dean D, Weiner MF, Svetlik D, Adams P, Honig LS, Cullum CM, Schaefer FV, Schellenberg GD (1996) Genetic factors for the development of Alzheimer disease in the Cherokee Indian. *Arch Neurol* 53: 997-1000.

221. Rosler M, Anand R, Cicin-Sain A, Gauthier S, Agid Y, Dal-Bianco P, Stahelin HB, Hartman R, Gharabawi M (1999) Efficacy and safety of rivastigmine in patients with Alzheimer's disease: international randomised controlled trial. *BMJ* 318: 633-638.

222. Rubin EH, Morris JC, Grant EA, Vendegna T (1989) Very mild senile dementia of the Alzheimer type. I. Clinical assessment. *Arch Neurol* 46: 379-382.

223. Salib E, Hillier V (1996) A case-control study of Alzheimer's disease and aluminium occupation. *Br J Psychiatry* 168: 244-249.

224. Salmon DP, Thal LJ, Butters N, Heindel WC (1990) Longitudinal evaluation of dementia of the Alzheimer type: a comparison of 3 standardized mental status examinations. *Neurology* 40: 1225-1230.

225. Sano M, Ernesto C, Thomas RG, Klauber MR, Schafer K, Grundman M, Woodbury P, Growdon J, Cotman CW, Pfeiffer E, Schneider LS, Thal LJ (1997) A controlled trial of selegiline, alpha-tocopherol, or both as treatment for Alzheimer's disease. The Alzheimer's Disease Cooperative Study. *N Engl J Med* 336: 1216-1222.

226. Saper CB, German DC, White CL, 3rd (1985) Neuronal pathology in the nucleus basalis and associated cell groups in senile dementia of the Alzheimer's type: possible role in cell loss. *Neurology* 35: 1089-1095.

227. Scharf S, Mander A, Ugoni A, Vajda F, Christophidis N (1999) A double-blind, placebo-controlled trial of diclofenac/misoprostol in Alzheimer's disease. *Neurology* 53: 197-201.

228. Scheltens P, Launer LJ, Barkhof F, Weinstein HC, Jonker C (1997) The diagnostic value of magnetic resonance imaging and technetium 99m- HMPAO single-photon-emission computed tomography for the diagnosis of Alzheimer disease in a community-dwelling elderly population. *Alzheimer Dis Assoc Disord* 11: 63-70.

229. Schenk D, Barbour R, Dunn W, Gordon G, Grajeda H, Guido T, Hu K, Huang J, Johnson-Wood K, Khan K, Kholodenko D, Lee M, Liao Z, Lieberburg I, Motter R, Mutter L, Soriano F, Shopp G, Vasquez N, Vandevert C, Walker S, Wogulis M, Yednock T, Games D, Seubert P (1999) Immunization with amyloid-beta attenuates Alzheimer-disease-like pathology in the PDAPP mouse. *Nature* 400: 173-177.

230. Schneider LS (1992) Tracking dementia by the IMC and the MMSE. *J Am Geriatr Soc* 40: 537-538.

231. Schoenberg BS, Anderson DW, Haerer AF (1985) Severe dementia. Prevalence and clinical features in a biracial US population. *Arch Neurol* 42: 740-743.

232. Schupf N, Kapell D, Lee JH, Ottman R, Mayeux R (1994) Increased risk of Alzheimer's disease in mothers of adults with Down's syndrome. *Lancet* 344: 353-356.

233. Scinto LF, Daffner KR, Dressler D, Ransil BI, Rentz D, Weintraub S, Mesulam M, Potter H (1994) A potential noninvasive neurobiological test for Alzheimer's disease. *Science* 266: 1051-1054.

234. Scott WK, Edwards KB, Davis DR, Cornman CB, Macera CA (1997) Risk of institutionalization among community long-term care clients with dementia. *Gerontologist* 37: 46-51.

235. Seltzer B, Vasterling JJ, Yoder JA, Thompson KA (1997) Awareness of deficit in Alzheimer's disease: relation to caregiver burden. *Gerontologist* 37: 20-24.

236. Seshadri S, Beiser A, Selhub J, Jacques PF, Rosenberg IH, D'Agostino RB, Wilson PW, Wolf PA (2002) Plasma homocysteine as a risk factor for dementia and Alzheimer's disease. *N Engl J Med* 346: 476-483.

237. Seshadri S, Wolf PA, Beiser A, Au R, McNulty K, White R, D'Agostino RB (1997) Lifetime risk of dementia and Alzheimer's disease. The impact of mortality on risk estimates in the Framingham Study. *Neurology* 49: 1498-1504.

238. Severson MA, Smith GE, Tangalos EG, Petersen RC, Kokmen E, Ivnik RJ, Atkinson EJ, Kurland LT (1994) Patterns and predictors of institutionalization in community-based dementia patients. *J Am Geriatr Soc* 42: 181-185.

239. Shuttleworth EC, Huber SJ (1988) The naming disorder of dementia of Alzheimer type. *Brain Lang* 34: 222-234.

240. Siu AL (1991) Screening for dementia and investigating its causes. *Ann Intern Med* 115: 122-132.

241. Small GW, Mazziotta JC, Collins MT, Baxter LR, Phelps ME, Mandelkern MA, Kaplan A, La Rue A, Adamson CF, Chang L et al (1995) Apolipoprotein E type 4 allele and cerebral glucose metabolism in relatives at risk for familial Alzheimer disease. *JAMA* 273: 942-947.

242. Snowdon DA, Kemper SJ, Mortimer JA, Greiner LH, Wekstein DR, Markesbery WR (1996) Linguistic ability in early life and cognitive function and Alzheimer's disease in late life. Findings from the Nun Study. *JAMA* 275: 528-532.

243. St Louis ME, Wasserheit JN (1998) Elimination of syphilis in the United States. *Science* 281: 353-354.

244. Starkstein SE, Sabe L, Chemerinski E, Jason L, Leiguarda R (1996) Two domains of anosognosia in Alzheimer's disease. *J Neurol Neurosurg Psychiatry* 61: 485-490.

245. Statement (1995) Statement on use of apolipoprotein E testing for Alzheimer disease. American College of Medical Genetics/American Society of Human Genetics Working Group on ApoE and Alzheimer disease. *JAMA* 274: 1627-1629.

246. Stern RG, Mohs RC, Davidson M, Schmeidler J, Silverman J, Kramer-Ginsberg E, Searcey T, Bierer L, Davis KL (1994) A longitudinal study of Alzheimer's disease: measurement, rate, and predictors of cognitive deterioration. *Am J Psychiatry*151: 390-396.

247. Stern Y, Albert M, Brandt J, Jacobs DM, Tang MX, Marder K, Bell K, Sano M, Devanand DP, Bylsma F et al (1994) Utility of extrapyramidal signs and psychosis as predictors of cognitive and functional decline, nursing home admission, and death in Alzheimer's disease: prospective analyses from the Predictors Study. *Neurology* 44: 2300-2307.

248. Stern Y, Tang MX, Albert MS, Brandt J, Jacobs DM, Bell K, Marder K, Sano M, Devanand D, Albert SM, Bylsma F, Tsai WY (1997) Predicting time to nursing home care and death in individuals with Alzheimer disease. *JAMA* 277: 806-812.

249. Stern Y, Tang MX, Denaro J, Mayeux R (1995) Increased risk of mortality in Alzheimer's disease patients with more advanced educational and occupational attainment. *Ann Neurol* 37: 590-595.

250. Stewart WF, Kawas C, Corrada M, Metter EJ (1997) Risk of Alzheimer's disease and duration of NSAID use. *Neurology* 48: 626-632.

251. Storandt M, Botwinick J, Danziger WL, Berg L, Hughes CP (1984) Psychometric differentiation of mild senile dementia of the Alzheimer type. *Arch Neurol* 41: 497-499.

252. Tabert MH, Albert SM, Borukhova-Milov L, Camacho Y, Pelton G, Liu X, Stern Y, Devanand DP (2002) Functional deficits in patients with mild cognitive impairment: prediction of AD. *Neurology* 58: 758-764.

253. Talbot PR, Lloyd JJ, Snowden JS, Neary D, Testa HJ (1998) A clinical role for 99mTc-HMPAO SPECT in the investigation of dementia? *J Neurol Neurosurg Psychiatry* 64: 306-313.

254. Tang MX, Jacobs D, Stern Y, Marder K, Schofield P, Gurland B, Andrews H, Mayeux R (1996) Effect of oestrogen during menopause on risk and age at onset of Alzheimer's disease. *Lancet* 348: 429-432.

255. Tang MX, Stern Y, Marder K, Bell K, Gurland B, Lantigua R, Andrews H, Feng L, Tycko B, Mayeux R (1998) The APOE-epsilon4 allele and the risk of Alzheimer disease among African Americans, whites, and Hispanics. *JAMA* 279: 751-755.

256. Teri L, Larson EB, Reifler BV (1988) Behavioral disturbance in dementia of the Alzheimer's type. *J Am Geriatr Soc* 36: 1-6.

257. Thal LJ, Grundman M, Klauber MR (1988) Dementia: characteristics of a referral population and factors associated with progression. *Neurology* 38: 1083-1090.

258. Tierney MC, Szalai JP, Snow WG, Fisher RH (1996) The prediction of Alzheimer disease. The role of patient and informant perceptions of cognitive deficits. *Arch Neurol* 53: 423-427.

259. van Belle G, Uhlmann RF, Hughes JP, Larson EB (1990) Reliability of estimates of changes in mental status test performance in senile dementia of the Alzheimer type. *J Clin Epidemiol* 43: 589-595.

260. Victoroff J, Mack WJ, Lyness SA, Chui HC (1995) Multicenter clinicopathological correlation in dementia. *Am J Psychiatry*152: 1476-1484.

261. Victoroff J, Ross GW, Benson DF, Verity MA, Vinters HV (1994) Posterior cortical atrophy. Neuropathologic correlations. *Arch Neurol* 51: 269-274.

262. Visser PJ, Verhey FR, Hofman PA, Scheltens P, Jolles J (2002) Medial temporal lobe atrophy predicts Alzheimer's disease in patients with minor cognitive impairment. *J Neurol Neurosurg Psychiatry* 72: 491-497.

263. Vitaliano PP, Russo J, Breen AR, Vitiello MV, Prinz PN (1986) Functional decline in the early stages of Alzheimer's disease. *Psychol Aging* 1: 41-46.

264. Volicer L, Hurley AC, Lathi DC, Kowall NW (1994) Measurement of severity in advanced Alzheimer's disease. *J Gerontol* 49: M223-226.

265. Wade JP, Mirsen TR, Hachinski VC, Fisman M, Lau C, Merskey H (1987) The clinical diagnosis of Alzheimer's disease. *Arch Neurol* 44: 24-29.

266. Walsh JS, Welch HG, Larson EB (1990) Survival of outpatients with Alzheimer-type dementia. *Ann Intern Med* 113: 429-434.

267. Weggen S, Eriksen JL, Das P, Sagi SA, Wang R, Pietrzik CU, Findlay KA, Smith TE, Murphy MP, Bulter T, Kang DE, Marquez-Sterling N, Golde TE, Koo EH (2001) A subset of NSAIDs lower amyloidogenic Abeta42 independently of cyclooxygenase activity. *Nature* 414: 212-216.

268. Weiner HL, Lemere CA, Maron R, Spooner ET, Grenfell TJ, Mori C, Issazadeh S, Hancock WW, Selkoe DJ (2000) Nasal administration of amyloid-beta peptide decreases cerebral amyloid burden in a mouse model of Alzheimer's disease. *Ann Neurol* 48: 567-579.

269. Welch HG, Walsh JS, Larson EB (1992) The cost of institutional care in Alzheimer's disease: nursing home and hospital use in a prospective cohort. *J Am Geriatr Soc* 40: 221-224.

270. Welsh K, Butters N, Hughes J, Mohs R, Heyman A (1991) Detection of abnormal memory decline in mild cases of Alzheimer's disease using CERAD neuropsychological measures. *Arch Neurol* 48: 278-281.

271. White L, Petrovitch H, Ross GW, Masaki KH, Abbott RD, Teng EL, Rodriguez BL, Blanchette PL, Havlik RJ, Wergowske G, Chiu D, Foley DJ, Murdaugh C, Curb JD (1996) Prevalence of dementia in older Japanese-American men in Hawaii: The Honolulu-Asia Aging Study. *JAMA* 276: 955-960.

272. Whitehouse PJ, Kalaria RN (1995) Nicotinic receptors and neurodegenerative dementing diseases: basic research and clinical implications. *Alzheimer Dis Assoc Disord* 9: 3-5.

273. Wilcock GK, Lilienfeld S, Gaens E (2000) Efficacy and safety of galantamine in patients with mild to moderate Alzheimer's disease: multicentre randomised controlled trial. Galantamine International-1 Study Group. *BMJ* 321: 1445-1449.

274. Wolfson C, Wolfson DB, Asgharian M, M'Lan CE, Ostbye T, Rockwood K, Hogan DB (2001) A reevaluation of the duration of survival after the onset of dementia. *N Engl J Med* 344: 1111-1116.

275. Wolozin B, Kellman W, Ruosseau P, Celesia GG, Siegel G (2000) Decreased prevalence of Alzheimer disease associated with 3-hydroxy-3- methyglutaryl coenzyme A reductase inhibitors. *Arch Neurol* 57: 1439-1443.

276. Zhang MY, Katzman R, Salmon D, Jin H, Cai GJ, Wang ZY, Qu GY, Grant I, Yu E, Levy P et al (1990) The prevalence of dementia and Alzheimer's disease in Shanghai, China: impact of age, gender, and education. *Ann Neurol* 27: 428-437.

Genetics of Alzheimer's Disease

Lars Bertram
Rudy Tanzi

A2M	alpha2-macroglobulin gene
ACT	α-1-antichymotrypsin gene
AD	Alzheimer's disease
APOE	apolipoprotein E gene
APP	amyloid precursor protein
BACE	β-secretase cleave enzyme gene
EOFAD	early onset familial Alzheimer's disease
IDE	insulin-degrading enzyme gene
IL1A	interleukin-1 alpha gene
LOAD	late onset Alzheimer's disease
LRP1	low density lipoprotein receptor-related protein-1 gene
NCSTN	nicastrin gene
PSEN1	presenilin gene
TFCP2	transcriptional factor LBP-1c/CP2/LSF gene
VLDL-R	very low density lipoprotein receptor gene
QTL	quantitative trait locus

Introduction

While the complete etiological picture of AD remains unresolved, there is now consensus that disease onset and progression are strongly influenced by genetic factors. Similar to many other common diseases like diabetes, coronary artery disease or breast-cancer, AD is a genetically *complex* and heterogeneous disorder. It is complex because there is no single (or simple) mode of inheritance that accounts for its heritability and *heterogeneous* because mutations and polymorphisms in multiple genes are involved together with non-genetic factors. Adding to this complexity is an age-related dichotomy, because early onset familial AD (EOFAD) is caused by rare and highly penetrant mutations that are transmitted in an autosomal dominant fashion, while risk and/or onset age variation for late onset AD (LOAD) is probably conferred by common polymorphisms with relatively low penetrance but high prevalence (51).

Several additional features aggravate the identification of genetic risk factors (or modifiers) for LOAD: *i)* locus and/or allelic heterogeneity, ie, one or more loci and/or alleles are contributing to disease risk in any given population; *ii)* only minor to modest effect of associated genetic variants, making replication of marginally significant findings difficult; *iii)* unknown—and difficult to model—interaction patterns between genes and/or environmental factors; *iv)* population differences and stratification (or "admixture"), which is a potential problem in case-control, but not in family-based association studies; and *v)* inadequate sample sizes and/or sampling strategies. Although the first 3 of these factors are fundamental to the disease itself, the latter 2 can be addressed to a substantial extent through the analysis of larger samples and the employment of family-based association methods.

Despite these complexities, tremendous progress has been made over the past 2 decades in deciphering AD genetics, which has laid the foundation for our current understanding of the etiological and pathogenic mechanisms leading to AD as well as for the development of novel approaches for treatment and prevention.

Genetics of Early-onset AD

Initial attempts to understand the role of genes in AD in the early 1980s focused on rare multi-generational families with EOFAD (onset less than 60 years of age), autosomal dominant, fully penetrant forms of the disease using conventional linkage analysis and subsequent positional cloning. In 1987, initial results showed linkage of EOFAD to the long arm of chromosome 21 encompassing a region which harbored a compelling candidate gene for AD mutations: the amyloid precursor protein (*APP*) gene (53). In 1990, the first *APP* mutation was discovered in a pedigree with Dutch type hereditary cerebral haemorrhage with amyloidosis shortly followed by a missense mutation occurring in the same *APP* exon (exon 17) in patients with EOFAD (for review, see 17, 51). Since then, a total of 12 different pathogenic mutations have been identified in *APP,* all of which are missense mutations lying within or close to the domain encoding the Aβ peptide, the major component of β-amyloid in AD (for an overview of all EOFAD mutations see the "AD Mutation Database" at http://molgen-www. uia.ac.be/ADMutations/). Although the *APP* mutations account for less than 0.1% of all AD cases (51) they carry virtually complete penetrance leading to AD between the fourth and seventh decades of life.

One year after the first EOFAD mutation was found in *APP*, a second EOFAD locus was reported to reside on chromosome 14q (49); however, it took 3 more years until the underlying gene was identified and named presenilin 1 (*PSEN1*) (for review, see 17, 51). *PSEN1* encodes a highly conserved polytopic membrane protein that is required for γ-secretase activity necessary to liberate Aβ from APP (16). EOFAD mutations in this gene as well as those in *APP* and the *PSEN1* homologue on chromosome 1 (*PSEN2*) led to an increase of secreted $A\beta_{42}$, the primary component of β-amyloid plaques in the brain (16, 40). Over the last 5 years, it has become clear that the majority of EOFAD mutations identified to date reside in *PSEN1* (currently more than 100; see also the "AD Mutation Database"), while only 7 mutations have been found in *PSEN2*. On average, EOFAD mutations in *PSEN1* confer an earlier onset age than those in *APP* or *PSEN2*, suggesting a more aggressive disease course in individuals affected by changes in the latter protein (6, 7).

Recent reports suggest that γ-secretase activity depends on the presence of other proteins besides the prese-

Chromosome	Pericak-Vance, 1997 (36)	Pericak-Vance, 2000 (38)	Myers, 2002* (32)	Li, 2002 (26)	Zubenko, 1998 (60)	Hiltunen, 2001 (19)
1p36	-	-	TLS=1.7	-	-	P=0.006
5p13-15	-	TLS=2.2	TLS=2.8	-	-	P=0.001
6p21	TLS>1.0	-	MLS=2.0*	-	-	P=0.003
q15	TLS>1.5	-	TLS=1.9	-	-	-
9p21	-	**MLS=4.3**	**TLS=1.8**	-	-	-
q22	-	TLS=2.0	MLS=2.4*	-	-	-
10q26	-	-	**TLS=4.1**	**MLS=2.4**	-	-
12p11	MLS=3.7	-	MLS=1.4	-	-	-
19q13	-	**TLS=3.6**	**MLS=1.8***	**MLS=3.3**	**P<0.0001**	-
Xq21-26	-	-	MLS=1.9*	-	P=0.0002	-

Table 1. *Overview of concordant linkage/association regions observed in full genome screens published to date.* Only results reflecting a *P*-value ≤0.01 (ie, TLS or MLS≥1.4) in at least 2 studies were considered. TLS=2-point lod score, MLS=multi-point lod score. Shading indicates chromosomes with significant findings using published criteria (Lander & Kruglyak, 1995 (25)). Note that samples in references (26, 32, 38) partly overlap. *Stage I linkage results from this group (21) were used whenever they exceeded the results of the Stage II findings.

nilins. In particular, a novel type 1 transmembrane glycoprotein (nicastrin; gene: *NCSTN*) was identified as a component of the γ-secretase complex that cleaves APP and Notch (58). In addition, there is also some genetic evidence that points to the chromosomal location of *NCSTN* on chromosome 1q22-23 as a region to contain a novel AD locus (19); however, subsequent analyses aimed at identifying functionally important sequence variants in early-onset as well as late-onset AD patients were largely unsuccessful. The only sequence variant predicted to change the amino acid sequence of the gene (N417Y) was present in AD cases as well in controls and, more importantly, did not lead to any changes in $A\beta_{40}$ and $A\beta_{42}$ levels (12). The same study did, however, identify a 4-locus haplotype that appears to be associated with EOFAD, especially when no ϵ4 allele of *APOE* is present. No effect was observed in LOAD patients, despite the positive association results with LOAD on 1q23 in previous studies. Further research is needed to clarify whether or not variants in *NCSTN* play a significant role in contributing to the population-wide risk for AD.

Genetics of Late-onset AD

As outlined above, the genetics of LOAD is considerably more difficult to disentangle, because this form of the disease is more often characterized by incomplete family data (eg, relatives who died before the family-specific age of risk and/or the lack of genotypic information for parents). Another complication is the unknown number of "phenocopies," ie, subjects with a non-genetic form of the disease or subjects suffering from other forms of age-related cognitive decline. In this case, even linkage studies with reasonable sample sizes (ie, 500-1000 families) either lead to broad, ill-defined peak regions or may not at all be sufficiently powerful to identify genetic factors of moderate or especially small effect. It has been suggested that such loci may be more readily pinpointed through studies of association or linkage disequilibrium, ie, testing for co-segregation of particular alleles/haplotypes and disease phenotype *across* families or individual cases (41), ideally in proteins that have a proven or at least plausible functional role in AD neuropathogenesis and that map to regions of established or suggestive linkage. It was this type of *positional candidate gene* strategy that in 1993 led to the discovery of a common variant—ϵ4—of the gene encoding apolipoprotein E (protein: apoE; gene: *APOE*) as a risk factor for AD (45, 50).

Over the last decade, more than 3 dozen association findings have been reported between AD and candidate genes on nearly every chromosome in the genome (6, 7).With the exception of *APOE*, none of these findings has been consistently replicated. A recent study modeling AD as a quantitative trait locus (QTL), ie, using a continuous rather than a binary (affected/unaffected) phenotype definition, reported evidence for the existence of at least four additional AD susceptibility loci (or genetic risk-factors) besides *APOE*, with one of these predicted to exert an even greater effect (11). In addition to association studies of AD with candidate genes chosen on the basis of pathobiological arguments, complete and unbiased genome screens have been performed in attempts to find genetic linkage to novel AD loci (Table 1). These studies have revealed candidate AD regions on several different chromosomes, most notably on chromosomes 12, 10, and 9. Because these latter genomic regions meet the critical criteria: *i)* of having been replicated in subsequent, independent studies and *ii)* of being characterised by both positive linkage and/or association findings, they are more likely than others to represent authentic signals from novel AD genes (52).

APOE. Preceding the first reports of significant association of *APOE* ϵ4 with AD was not only the evidence of

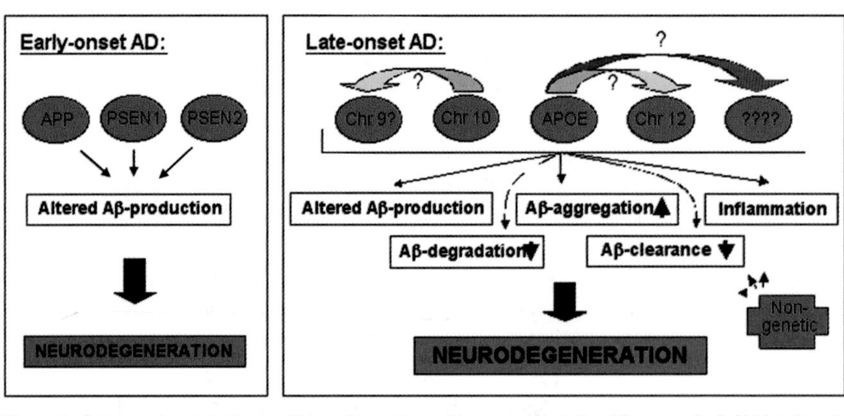

Figure 1. *Scheme of contribution and interaction pattern of known and putative AD genes.* **A.** (left) Mutations in the *early-onset* AD genes *APP, PSEN1, PSEN2* all lead to an increase in Aβ-production without any known interaction with other factors. **B.** (right) Simplified scheme of the interaction pattern of known and proposed *late-onset* AD genes. Likely, these risk-factor genes each affect one or more of the known pathogenic mechanisms leading to neurodegeneration in AD. Their effects are further influenced by gene-gene interactions and the contribution of non-genetic risk-factors. Note that none of the interaction patterns outlined here for didactic purposes has actually been established.

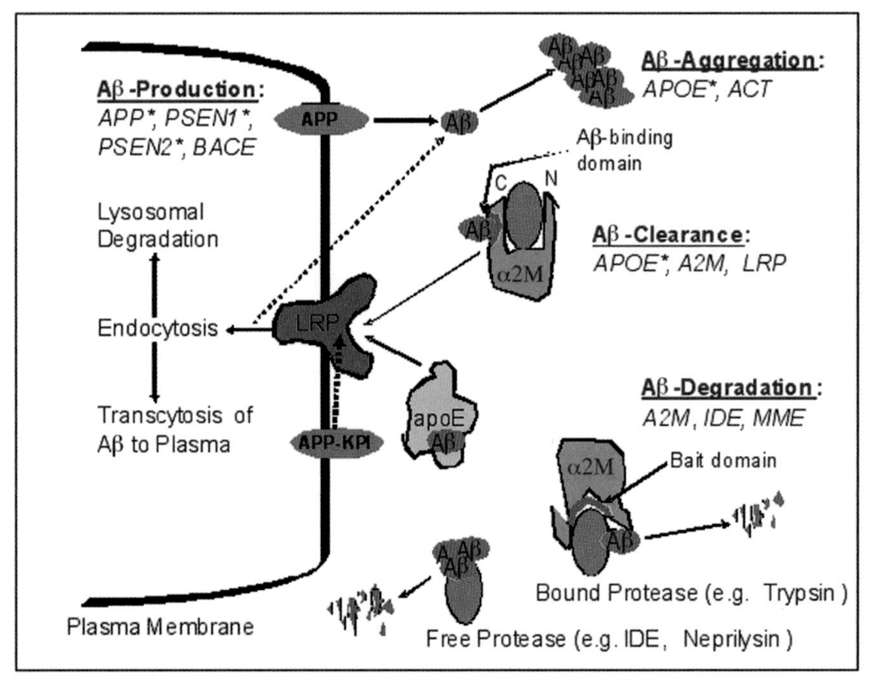

Figure 2. *Possible pathogenetic routes of Ab production, clearance, and degradation.* Early-onset AD genes *APP, PSEN1*, and *PSEN2* along with *BACE* (β-secretase) are involved in the production of Aβ. The late-onset AD gene *APOE* and the putative AD gene, α-1-antichymotrypsin (*ACT*) have been proposed to play roles in the aggregation and fibrillogenesis of Aβ. *APOE* and putative AD genes, *LRP* and *A2M* may play roles in the clearance of Aβ as follows: Once α2M-Aβ or apoE-Aβ complexes are internalized by LRP they may be targeted for endosomal recycling, lysosomal degradation, or undergo trancytosis across the blood-brain barrier to the plasma. Membrane APP containing an alternatively-spliced Kunitz protease inhibitor (KPI) domain may also undergo internalization by LRP and generate Aβ (dotted-arrows) via the endocytic pathway (Note: APP has also been shown to undergo LRP-independent endocytosis). Extracellular degradation of Aβ can occur via binding of the peptide to α2M followed by degradation by an active protease (eg, trypsin) bound to the bait region of α2M. Alternatively, Aβ may be degraded by 'free' proteases such as the insulin degrading enzyme (*IDE*) or neprilysin (*MME*). Asterisk (*) denotes established AD genes.

suggestive linkage to chromosome 19 (37), but also the observation that apoE binds Aβ (50). Testing this bona fide positional candidate gene for genetic association with the disease yielded—in contrast to all other association-based findings in AD—the only observation that to date has been consistently replicated in a large number of studies across several ethnic groups (for a recent meta analysis, see 15). In addition to the increased risk exerted by the ϵ4-allele, several studies have also reported a weak, albeit significant, protective effect for the least frequent allele, ϵ2.

Regardless of its established association, the APOE ϵ4-allele is neither necessary nor sufficient to cause AD, but instead most likely operates as a genetic risk-modifier by decreasing the age of onset in a dose-dependent manner (8, 30). Contradicting earlier estimates that APOE-ϵ4 accounts for 50% of the "predicted total genetic effect" in AD, a recent and more systematic study suggested the actual contribution of this polymorphism to onset of AD to be only 7 to 9% (11).

Despite the overwhelming support from genetic data suggesting an important contribution of this gene to AD risk or onset age variation, the potential biological consequences of the *APOE* polymorphisms are only poorly understood. The most straightforward hypothesis proposes that the different variants directly influence Aβ-accumulation (see also Figures 1, 2) (50). Several lines of evidence support this notion, showing an increased number of Aβ-plaques in the brain of ϵ4-allele carriers and marked differences in the deposition of Aβ-plaques depending on the presence or absence of human *APOE* in transgenic mice overexpressing APP (for a recent review on *APOE* function, see 39), Furthermore, there is evidence for an *APOE* dependent onset age variation in EOFAD caused by *PSEN1* mutations (33). On the other hand, no consensus has yet been reached regarding the predominant *mechanism(s)* underlying these effects, although systemic dysfunction in lipid transport, and more specifically cholesterol homeostasis are likely pathways, especially since high plasma cholesterol levels are associated with increased β-amyloid in the brain (18). Interestingly, cholesterol has also been shown to both increase Aβ-production and to stabilize the peptide in the brains of transgenic AD mice. Thus, it is possible that *APOE*-ϵ4 confers risk for AD via mechanisms that are shared with its effects on cardiovascular disease, eg, by increasing a carrier's risk for hypercholesterolemia, as this would also elevate accumulation of Aβ.

Finally, evidence from several association studies on polymorphisms in the regulatory regions of *APOE* suggest that protein expression, either alone or in conjunction with the different ε2/3/4 isoforms, could also be responsible for the observed biological effects (10, 23). These findings, however, have been refuted in a number of follow-up reports, indicating that the observed genetic association may reflect population-specific linkage disequilibrium with *APOE*-ε4, rather than indicating that the promoter polymorphisms are independent AD risk factors.

Chromosome 12. In the late 90s, three independent laboratories almost simultaneously identified AD linkage regions on the short arm and in the vicinity of the centromeric region of chromosome 12 (36, 42, 57). Subsequent analyses found strong evidence for association with 2 biologically highly plausible and related candidate genes: *A2M*, encoding alpha2-macroglobulin (A2M) (9, 27) and LRP1, encoding the low density lipoprotein receptor-related protein-1 (LRP) (20). Both A2M and LRP have been found to play roles in mediating endogenous Aβ-binding and clearance. LRP also serves as a receptor for the apoE, APP, and A2M proteins (Figure 2).

In the case of *A2M*, the combination of promising linkage *and* association findings has initiated a huge set of follow-up investigations—only exceeded in number by the studies on *APOE*. Most subsequent attempts to corroborate the original finding in independent laboratories, mainly employing the classical case-control design, were negative. A recent meta-analysis even concluded that "*A2M* is not genetically associated with LOAD in white patients or mixed populations as found in the United States" (22). This conclusion stands against at least 11 independent reports demonstrating significant association between polymorphisms in A2M and AD in U.S. whites and other ethnic groups, using both case-control and family-based designs (for recent reviews, see 6, 7). Although over time only more detailed and sufficiently sized analyses will indicate the extent to which variation in *A2M* confers risk for AD, the growing number of confirmatory reports, even amidst multiple refutations, make it unlikely that the initial findings are due to type I (false-positive) error alone. In fact, further analyses in a greatly enlarged sample of NIMH families, including those for which the initial association was described, revealed novel exonic and intronic polymorphisms in *A2M* that appear to be equally or stronger associated with disease than the 5 bp deletion upstream of exon 18 (Saunders et al; unpublished data). More interestingly, haplotype analyses including all or only subsets of these polymorphisms, showed at least as strong an association than any of the polymorphisms alone. Along these lines, recent case-control as well as family-based studies using haplotypes of SNPs in or around *APOE* revealed strongly positive findings for polymorphisms that, individually, were either not or only weakly associated with AD (14, 29). It is noteworthy that the only haplotype-based study on *A2M* in the AD literature to date supports an association of this locus and AD (56).

LRP1, the second candidate to be associated with AD on chromosome 12, resides approximately 50 million base-pairs (Mb) from *A2M* towards the q-telomere. After the initial reports showing significant association of polymorphisms in this gene and AD (20), follow-up results have been inconsistent (6, 7). Interestingly, it was again the study of multi-locus haplotypes that recently led to significant positive findings in a set of samples (46) that yielded only negative results analyzing polymorphisms individually (47). Mapping only ~7 Mb proximal of *LRP1* is the gene encoding the transcriptional factor LBP-1c/CP2/LSF (*TFCP2*), which has recently been associated in 2 case-control studies (24, 54). Suggested roles for this protein in AD pathogenesis are the regulation of transcription/expression of other AD-related proteins, APP binding and internalization (via Fe65) or the regulation of inflammatory processes.

Although the findings on chromosome 12 require further investigation, it is unlikely that the positive associations reported for these genes (*A2M*, *LRP*, and *TFCP2*) reflect linkage disequilibrium between the 2 loci, ie, *A2M* on the one and *LRP1* and/or *TFCP2* on the other end, given the huge chromosomal distance in between the implicated regions (ie, ~50 Mb). More likely, these results suggest the existence of 2 separate AD genes on chromosome 12, one near *A2M*, or *A2M* itself, and one near *LRP1*. Along these lines, neither *LRP1* (4, 5) nor *TFCP2* (Bertram et al, unpublished data) appear to be associated in a family-based sample which, on the other hand, continues to show strong association with *A2M*.

Chromosome 10. Recently, 3 research groups, reported significant linkage of predominantly late-onset AD to the long arm of chromosome 10 (4, 5, 13, 31). The study by Myers and colleagues (31) followed up on their own prior suggestive linkage results in this chromosomal region by genotyping additional markers and increasing their sample size. The linkage peak in the enlarged sample occurred near 65 Mb and—in the same sample—was found to be stronger than the linkage signal around *APOE*. A second study (13) showed that a quantitative phenotype (ie, elevated plasma $A\beta_{42}$ levels) yielded strong evidence for linkage in a very similar region on chromosome 10 when analyzing 5 large and multi-generational pedigrees. Interestingly, this study found no evidence of linkage to the APOE region at all. Finally, an hypothesis-driven linkage analyses was performed on 6 genetic markers (4, 5), using markers chosen because they mapped close to the gene encoding insulin-degrading enzyme (*IDE*), for which several studies have suggested a principal role in the degradation and clearance of Aβ (for a recent review, see 48). Two of the 6 markers showed significant linkage to AD by parametric and non-parametric analyses. In addition, there was evidence for significant association of the best-linked marker in the full and unstratified sample (ie, *D10S583*), a finding that was very recently replicated in an independent case-control study (1). These association results could be an indication of linkage disequilibrium with the actual disease modifying variant which is located nearby.

Support for an AD locus on the more distal portion of chromosome 10 comes from yet another linkage study published almost 2 years after the initial reports, and the peak region of this study coincides almost precisely with the distal bounds of the region implied by one of the previous analyses, ie, ~110 Mb (26). Instead of using a conventional binary phenotype definition, the authors of this study chose a QTL approach based on age at onset. Interestingly, the linkage signal around 110 Mb was not only the strongest observed in their full genome screen (excluding linkage at the *APOE* locus), but also emerged as an onset age modifying locus for Parkinson's disease, which was evaluated simultaneously (26). At this point, it cannot be excluded that methodological or sampling/stratification differences across studies are responsible for the discrepant localization of linkage peaks which, in fact, could all be caused by the same gene. Another possible explanation is the presence of 2 loci, of which one primarily influences *disease risk*, while the other acts more like a modifier of *onset age* (26). In any regard, even though the actual disease gene(s) and its function still remains elusive, the fact that several independent laboratories have observed similar findings using different methodologies considerably increase the likelihood of at least one major late-onset AD locus on chromosome 10.

Finally, 3 case-control studies (28, 59, 60) reported evidence for association of AD with an anonymous microsatellite marker (*D10S1423*, at ~19 Mb) on the *short* arm of chromosome 10, while a fourth report failed to confirm these findings (34). The authors of the original study hypothesized this to reflect linkage disequilibrium with an AD gene nearby, a notion that is also supported by a recent full genome screen observing some evidence of association in this region (19); however, the results of these reports are mostly nominal (ie uncorrected for multiple comparisons) and stem from fairly small samples (case populations <100 individuals), requiring further follow-up in independent samples of sufficient size and more stable estimates of effect size. Of note, the analysis of this and two adjacent microsatellite markers on chromosome 10p in the NIMH dataset, did not reveal any evidence of association (5a), indicating that the population-wide effect of a putative gene in this area is—if at all present—only minor. Moreover, this marker maps too far proximal to be explained by the linkage evidence of the four studies detailed above.

Chromosome 9. Four years before any evidence of linkage to AD was reported on chromosome 9, a case-control study from Japan (35) reported significant association with a common polymorphism in the gene encoding the very low density lipoprotein receptor (*VLDL-R*). This gene maps to the p-telomere of chromosome 9 at ~3 Mb. As for most other genetic associations in AD, this report was followed by a series of replications as well as refutations (for review, see 6, 7), including one family-based report from our group (4, 5). Later, the full genome scan by Kehoe and colleagues reported evidence for "suggestive" linkage on this chromosome at ~26 Mb and, more pronounced, at ~100 Mb (21), findings that were generally confirmed in a second stage analysis using an extended dataset (32). While the proximal linkage region (near marker *D9S171*) was later reported to be "significantly" linked to autopsy-confirmed AD in a meeting report using an overlapping set of NIMH families (38), this region did not show evidence for suggestive linkage in the genome screen including the full NIMH dataset (7a); however, in this latter analysis the evidence for linkage to the more distal peak was strengthened, with most pronounced findings in late-onset families. Thus, even though there is growing evidence for linkage of AD to chromosome 9 (Table 1), the discrepant results with respect to peak *localization* across studies resemble the situation on chromosomes 10 and 12. Similarly, it remains unclear whether the observed signals on chromosome 9 are due to one or 2 (or more) underlying loci. Although it is possible that *VLDL-R* is responsible for the linkage evidence on chromosome 9p, further studies focusing on both refining the linkage region(s) as well as assessing truly *positional* candidate genes are needed to resolve this issue. For instance, one interesting candidate, the gene encoding member 1 of the family of APP-binding proteins (X11, gene: *APBA1*) is located roughly halfway between the 2 peaks, but its potential association with AD remains unresolved.

Findings on other chromosomes. As mentioned earlier, there are well over 30 reports in the literature suggesting an association with novel genetic risk-factors and AD (6, 7, 52). Many of these investigated *positional* candidate genes and were discussed in the sections above; however, a good portion of investigations selected their targets solely on biological grounds, ie, testing functionally plausible candidates that *do not* map near any of the proposed linkage peaks. Examples of these cases are the genes encoding cathepsin D (located on chromosome 11p15, proposed to display γ-secretase like activities), α-synuclein (chromosome 4q22, involved in the binding and aggregation of Aβ), members of the interleukin-1 cluster genes (chromosome 2, involved in inflammatory processes) and the angiotensin-converting enzyme (chromosome 17, possibly also involved in inflammation and the regulation of the brain's renin-angiotensin system). None of these risk-factors has yet been shown to play a more than minor role in contributing to population-wide AD risk, and it is likely that many of the initial results will in fact prove to be false-positive findings (ie, type I errors).

One of the more promising candidates both on the grounds of independent confirmatory reports as well as biological function is a member of the interleukin-1 genes on chromosome 2q13, the gene encoding interleukin-1 alpha (*IL1A*). There is growing evidence that neuroinflammatory processes significantly contribute to AD neuropathology (2, 43). Genetically, variants in *IL1A* have been associated with AD in 4 case-control studies (for review, see 3), In 2 of these studies the effect was limited to early-onset AD patients. On the other hand, a total of 4 independent case-control studies failed to observe this evidence (3). Notably, 3 of these studies were quite small (ie, less than 200 individuals in the case and/or control group), and only one study included more than 600 individuals.

Finally, 2 more biologically very important AD candidate genes should not go unmentioned in this overview: the genes encoding the β-secretase cleavage enzymes (*BACE1* and *BACE2*). In particular, *BACE1*, located on chromosome 11q23, is the major β-secretase activity in humans with abundant expression in the CNS (for a recent review, see 55), while its homologue *BACE2*, which resides in the obligatory Down-syndrome region on chromosome 21q22 (44) predominantly displays α-secretase activity and shows only minor expression in brain. Both genes are located in chromosomal regions that show evidence for linkage in some studies, but not in others. Moreover, none of the published sequencing and association analyses were able to find any meaningful DNA variant for either enzyme. Future studies will reveal whether or not these proteins are actually involved in AD pathogenesis on a genetic level.

References

1. Ait-Ghezala G, Abdullah L, Crescentini R, Crawford F, Town T, Singh S, Richards D, Duara R, Mullan M (2002) Confirmation of association between D10S583 and Alzheimer's disease in a case—control sample. *Neurosci Lett* 325: 87-90.

2. Akiyama H, Barger S, Barnum S, Bradt B, Bauer J, Cole GM, Cooper NR, Eikelenboom P, Emmerling M, Fiebich BL, Finch CE et al (2000) Inflammation and Alzheimer's disease. *Neurobiol Aging* 21: 383-421.

3. Bertram L, et al (submitted) Genetic analyses of the interleukin-1 cluster on chromosome 2 in Alzheimer's disease families.:

4. Bertram L, Blacker D, Crystal A, Mullin K, Keeney D, Jones J, Basu S, Yhu S, Guenette S, McInnis M, Go R, Tanzi R (2000) Candidate genes showing no evidence for association or linkage with Alzheimer's disease using family-based methodologies. *Exp Gerontol* 35: 1353-1361.

5. Bertram L, Blacker D, Mullin K, Keeney D, Jones J, Basu S, Yhu S, McInnis MG, Go RC, Vekrellis K, Selkoe DJ, Saunders AJ, Tanzi RE (2000) Evidence for genetic linkage of Alzheimer's disease to chromosome 10q. *Science* 290: 2302-2303.

5a. Bertram L, Saunders AJ, Mullin K, Sampson A, Moscarillo TJ, Basset SS, Go RCP, Blacker D, Tanzi RE (2003) No association between marker D10S14234 and Alzheimer's disease. *Mol Psychiatry* in press.

6. Bertram L, Tanzi RE (2001) Dancing in the dark? The status of late-onset Alzheimer's disease genetics. *J Mol Neurosci* 17: 127-136.

7. Bertram L, Tanzi RE (2001) Of replications and refutations: the status of Alzheimer's disease genetic research. *Curr Neurol Neurosci Rep* 1: 442-450.

7a. Blacker D, Bertram L, Saunders J, Moscarillo TJ, Albert M, Wiener H, Perry RT, Collins JS, Harrell LE, Go RCP, Mahoney A et al (2003) Results of a high-resolution genome screen of 437 Alzheimer's disease families. *Hum Mol Genet* 12: 23-32.

8. Blacker D, Haines JL, Rodes L, Terwedow H, Go RC, Harrell LE, Perry RT, Bassett SS, Chase G, Meyers D, Albert MS, Tanzi R (1997) ApoE-4 and age at onset of Alzheimer's disease: the NIMH genetics initiative. *Neurology* 48: 139-147.

9. Blacker D, Wilcox MA, Laird NM, Rodes L, Horvath SM, Go RC, Perry R, Watson B, Jr., Bassett SS, McInnis MG, Albert MS, Hyman BT, Tanzi RE (1998) Alpha-2 macroglobulin is genetically associated with Alzheimer disease. *Nat Genet* 19: 357-360.

10. Bullido MJ, Artiga MJ, Recuero M, Sastre I, Garcia MA, Aldudo J, Lendon C, Han SW, Morris JC, Frank A, Vazquez J, Goate A, Valdivieso F (1998) A polymorphism in the regulatory region of APOE associated with risk for Alzheimer's dementia. *Nat Genet* 18: 69-71.

11. Daw EW, Payami H (2000) The number of trait loci in late-onset Alzheimer disease. *Am J Hum Genet* 66: 196-204

12. Dermaut B, Theuns J, Sleegers K, Hasegawa H, Van den Broeck M, Vennekens K, Corsmit E, St George-Hyslop P, Cruts M, van Duijn CM, Van Broeckhoven C (2002) The gene encoding nicastrin, a major gamma-secretase component, modifies risk for familial early-onset Alzheimer disease in a Dutch population-based sample. *Am J Hum Genet* 70: 1568-1574.

13. Ertekin-Taner N, Graff-Radford N, Younkin LH, Eckman C, Baker M, Adamson J, Ronald J, Blangero J, Hutton M, Younkin SG (2000) Linkage of plasma Abeta42 to a quantitative locus on chromosome 10 in late-onset Alzheimer's disease pedigrees. *Science* 290: 2303-2304.

14. Fallin D, Cohen A, Essioux L, Chumakov I, Blumenfeld M, Cohen D, Schork NJ (2001) Genetic analysis of case/control data using estimated haplotype frequencies: application to APOE locus variation and Alzheimer's disease. *Genome Res* 11: 143-151.

15. Farrer LA, Cupples LA, Haines JL, Hyman B, Kukull WA, Mayeux R, Myers RH, Pericak-Vance MA, Risch N, van Duijn CM (1997) Effects of age, sex, and ethnicity on the association between apolipoprotein E genotype and Alzheimer disease. A meta-analysis. APOE and Alzheimer Disease Meta Analysis Consortium. *JAMA* 278: 1349-1356.

16. Haass C, De Strooper B (1999) The presenilins in Alzheimer's disease—proteolysis holds the key. *Science* 286: 916-919.

17. Hardy J (1997) Amyloid, the presenilins and Alzheimer's disease. *Trends Neurosci* 20: 154-159.

18. Hartmann T (2001) Cholesterol, A beta and Alzheimer's disease. *Trends Neurosci* 24: S45-48.

19. Hiltunen M, Mannermaa A, Thompson D, Easton D, Pirskanen M, Helisalmi S, Koivisto AM, Lehtovirta M, Ryynanen M, Soininen H (2001) Genome-wide linkage disequilibrium mapping of late-onset Alzheimer's disease in Finland. *Neurology* 57: 1663-1668.

20. Kang DE, Saitoh T, Chen X, Xia Y, Masliah E, Hansen LA, Thomas RG, Thal LJ, Katzman R (1997) Genetic association of the low-density lipoprotein receptor-related protein gene (LRP), an apolipoprotein E receptor, with late-onset Alzheimer's disease. *Neurology* 49: 56-61.

21. Kehoe P, Wavrant-De Vrieze F, Crook R, Wu WS, Holmans P, Fenton I, Spurlock G, Norton N, Williams H, Williams N, Lovestone S et al (1999) A full genome scan for late onset Alzheimer's disease. *Hum Mol Genet* 8: 237-245.

22. Koster MN, Dermaut B, Cruts M, Houwing-Duistermaat JJ, Roks G, Tol J, Ott A, Hofman A, Munteanu G, Breteler MM et al (2000) The alpha2-macroglobulin gene in AD: a population-based study and meta-analysis. *Neurology* 55: 678-684.

23. Lambert JC, Berr C, Pasquier F, Delacourte A, Frigard B, Cottel D, Perez-Tur J, Mouroux V, Mohr M, Cecyre D, Galasko D et al (1998) Pronounced impact of Th1/E47cs mutation compared with -491 AT mutation on neural APOE gene expression and risk of developing Alzheimer's disease. *Hum Mol Genet* 7: 1511-1516.

24. Lambert JC, Goumidi L, Vrieze FW, Frigard B, Harris JM, Cummings A, Coates J, Pasquier F, Cottel D, Gaillac M, St Clair D, Mann DM, Hardy J, Lendon

CL, Amouyel P, Chartier-Harlin MC (2000) The transcriptional factor LBP-1c/CP2/LSF gene on chromosome 12 is a genetic determinant of Alzheimer's disease. *Hum Mol Genet* 9: 2275-2280.

25. Lander E, Kruglyak L (1995) Genetic dissection of complex traits. guidelines for interpreting and reporting linkage results. *Nat Genetics* 11: 241-247

26. Li YJ, Scott WK, Hedges DJ, Zhang F, Gaskell PC, Nance MA, Watts RL, Hubble JP, Koller WC, Pahwa R, Stern MB et al (2002) Age at onset in two common neurodegenerative diseases is genetically controlled. *Am J Hum Genet* 70: 985-993.

27. Liao A, Nitsch RM, Greenberg SM, Finckh U, Blacker D, Albert M, Rebeck GW, Gomez-Isla T, Clatworthy A, Binetti G, Hock C, Mueller-Thomsen T, Mann U, Zuchowski K, Beisiegel U, Staehelin H, Growdon JH, Tanzi RE, Hyman BT (1998) Genetic association of an alpha2-macroglobulin (Val1000Ile) polymorphism and Alzheimer's disease. *Hum Mol Genet* 7: 1953-1956.

28. Majores M, Bagli M, Papassotiropoulos A, Schwab SG, Jessen F, Rao ML, Maier W, Heun R (2000) Allelic association between the D10S1423 marker and Alzheimer's disease in a German population. *Neurosci Lett* 289: 224-226.

29. Martin ER, Lai EH, Gilbert JR, Rogala AR, Afshari AJ, Riley J, Finch KL, Stevens JF, Livak KJ, Slotterbeck BD, Slifer SH, Warren LL, Conneally PM, Schmechel DE, Purvis I, Pericak-Vance MA, Roses AD, Vance JM (2000) SNPing away at complex diseases: analysis of single-nucleotide polymorphisms around APOE in Alzheimer disease. *Am J Hum Genet* 67: 383-394.

30. Meyer MR, Tschanz JT, Norton MC, Welsh-Bohmer KA, Steffens DC, Wyse BW, Breitner JC (1998) APOE genotype predicts when--not whether--one is predisposed to develop Alzheimer disease. *Nat Genet* 19: 321-322.

31. Myers A, Holmans P, Marshall H, Kwon J, Meyer D, Ramic D, Shears S, Booth J, DeVrieze FW, Crook R, Hamshere M et al (2000) Susceptibility locus for Alzheimer's disease on chromosome 10. *Science* 290: 2304-2305.

32. Myers A, Wavrant De-Vrieze F, Holmans P, Hamshere M, Crook R, Compton D, Marshall H, Meyer D, Shears S, Booth J et al (2002) Full genome screen for Alzheimer disease: stage II analysis. *Am J Med Genet* 114: 235-244.

33. Nacmias B, Latorraca S, Piersanti P, Forleo P, Piacentini S, Bracco L, Amaducci L, Sorbi S (1995) ApoE genotype and familial Alzheimer's disease: a possible influence on age of onset in APP717 Val-->Ile mutated families. *Neurosci Lett* 183: 1-3.

34. Nishimura AL, Oliveira JR, Otto PA, Matioli SR, Brito-Marques PR, Bahia VS, Nitrini R, Zatz M (2001) No evidence of association between the D10S1423 locus and Alzheimer disease in Brazilian patients. *J Neural Transm* 108: 305-310

35. Okuizumi K, Onodera O, Namba Y, Ikeda K, Yamamoto T, Seki K, Ueki A, Nanko S, Tanaka H, Takahashi H, et al. (1995) Genetic association of the very low density lipoprotein (VLDL) receptor gene with sporadic Alzheimer's disease. *Nat Genet* 11: 207-209.

36. Pericak-Vance MA, Bass MP, Yamaoka LH, Gaskell PC, Scott WK, Terwedow HA, Menold MM, Conneally PM, Small GW, Vance JM, Saunders AM, Roses AD, Haines JL (1997) Complete genomic screen in late-onset familial Alzheimer disease. Evidence for a new locus on chromosome 12. *JAMA* 278: 1237-1241.

37. Pericak-Vance MA, Bebout JL, Gaskell PC, Jr., Yamaoka LH, Hung WY, Alberts MJ, Walker AP, Bartlett RJ, Haynes CA, Welsh KA et al (1991) Linkage studies in familial Alzheimer disease: evidence for chromosome 19 linkage. *Am J Hum Genet* 48: 1034-1050.

38. Pericak-Vance MA, Grubber J, Bailey LR, Hedges D, West S, Santoro L, Kemmerer B, Hall JL, Saunders AM, Roses AD, Small GW, Scott WK, Conneally PM, Vance JM, Haines JL (2000) Identification of novel genes in late-onset Alzheimer's disease. *Exp Gerontol* 35: 1343-1352.

39. Poirier J (2000) Apolipoprotein E and Alzheimer's disease. A role in amyloid catabolism. *Ann N Y Acad Sci* 924: 81-90

40. Price DL, Tanzi RE, Borchelt DR, Sisodia SS (1998) Alzheimer's disease: genetic studies and transgenic models. *Annu Rev Genet* 32: 461-493

41. Risch N, Merikangas K (1996) The future of genetic studies of complex human diseases. *Science* 273: 1516-1517.

42. Rogaeva E, Premkumar S, Song Y, Sorbi S, Brindle N, Paterson A, Duara R, Levesque G, Yu G, Nishimura M, Ikeda M et al (1998) Evidence for an Alzheimer disease susceptibility locus on chromosome 12 and for further locus heterogeneity. *JAMA* 280: 614-618.

43. Rothwell NJ, Luheshi GN (2000) Interleukin 1 in the brain: biology, pathology and therapeutic target. *Trends Neurosci* 23: 618-625.

44. Saunders AJ, Kim T-W, al. e (1999) BACE maps to chromosome 11 and a BACE homolog, BACE2, reside in the obligate Down syndrome region of chromosome 21. *Science* 286: 1255a

45. Schmechel DE, Saunders AM, Strittmatter WJ, Crain BJ, Hulette CM, Joo SH, Pericak-Vance MA, Goldgaber D, Roses AD (1993) Increased amyloid beta-peptide deposition in cerebral cortex as a consequence of apolipoprotein E genotype in late-onset Alzheimer disease. *Proc Natl Acad Sci U S A* 90: 9649-9653.

46. Scott WK, Grubber J (2000) Fine-mapping of the chromosome 12 Alzheimer disease locus using family-based association tests of microsatellite markers. *Neurobiol Aging* 21 ((abstract)): S129

47. Scott WK, Yamaoka LH, Bass MP, Gaskell PC, Conneally PM, Small GW, Farrer LA, Auerbach SA, Saunders AM, Roses AD, Haines JL, Pericak-Vance MA (1998) No genetic association between the LRP receptor and sporadic or late- onset familial Alzheimer disease. *Neurogenetics* 1: 179-183.

48. Selkoe DJ (2001) Clearing the brain's amyloid cobwebs. *Neuron* 32: 177-180.

49. St George-Hyslop P, Haines J, Rogaev E, Mortilla M, Vaula G, Pericak-Vance M, Foncin JF, Montesi M, Bruni A, Sorbi S, et al. (1992) Genetic evidence for a novel familial Alzheimer's disease locus on chromosome 14. *Nat Genet* 2: 330-334.

50. Strittmatter WJ, Saunders AM, Schmechel D, Pericak-Vance M, Enghild J, Salvesen GS, Roses AD (1993) Apolipoprotein E: high-avidity binding to beta-amyloid and increased frequency of type 4 allele in late-onset familial Alzheimer disease. *Proc Natl Acad Sci U S A* 90: 1977-1981.

51. Tanzi RE (1999) A genetic dichotomy model for the inheritance of Alzheimer's disease and common age-related disorders. *J Clin Invest* 104: 1175-1179.

52. Tanzi RE, Bertram L (2001) New frontiers in Alzheimer's disease genetics. *Neuron* 32: 181-184.

53. Tanzi RE, Gusella JF, Watkins PC, Bruns GA, St George-Hyslop P, Van Keuren ML, Patterson D, Pagan S, Kurnit DM, Neve RL (1987) Amyloid beta protein gene: cDNA, mRNA distribution, and genetic linkage near the Alzheimer locus. *Science* 235: 880-884.

54. Taylor AE, Yip A, Brayne C, Easton D, Evans JG, Xuereb J, Cairns N, Esiri MM, Rubinsztein DC (2001) Genetic association of an LBP-1c/CP2/LSF gene polymorphism with late onset Alzheimer's disease. *J Med Genet* 38: 232-233.

55. Vassar R (2001) The beta-secretase, BACE: a prime drug target for Alzheimer's disease. *J Mol Neurosci* 17: 157-170.

56. Verpillat P, Bouley S, Hannequin D, Belliard S, Puel M, Thomas-Anterion C, Dubois B, Agid Y, Campion D, Clerget-Darpoux F, Brice A (2000) Alpha2-macroglobulin gene and Alzheimer's disease: confirmation of association by haplotypes analyses. *Ann Neurol* 48: 400-402.

57. Wu WS, Holmans P, Wavrant-DeVrieze F, Shears S, Kehoe P, Crook R, Booth J, Williams N, Perez-Tur J, Roehl K, Fenton I, Chartier-Harlin MC, Lovestone S, Williams J, Hutton M, Hardy J, Owen MJ, Goate A (1998) Genetic studies on chromosome 12 in late-onset Alzheimer disease. *JAMA* 280: 619-622.

58. Yu G, Nishimura M, Arawaka S, Levitan D, Zhang L, Tandon A, Song YQ, Rogaeva E, Chen F, Kawarai T, Supala A et al (2000) Nicastrin modulates presenilin-mediated notch/glp-1 signal transduction and betaAPP processing. *Nature* 407: 48-54.

59. Zubenko GS, Hughes HB, 3rd, Stiffler JS (2001) D10S1423 identifies a susceptibility locus for Alzheimer's disease in a prospective, longitudinal, double-blind study of asymptomatic individuals. *Mol Psychiatry* 6: 413-419.

60. Zubenko GS, Hughes HB, Stiffler JS, Hurtt MR, Kaplan BB (1998) A genome survey for novel Alzheimer disease risk loci: results at 10-cM resolution. *Genomics* 50: 121-128.

Neuropathology of Alzheimer's Disease

Charles Duyckaerts
Dennis W. Dickson

AD	Alzheimer's disease
AMPA	alpha-amino-3-hydroxy-5-methylisoxazole-4-proprionc acid
APOE	apolipoprotein E
APP	amyloid precursor protein
CAA	congophilic angiopathy
CERAD	consortium to establish a registry of Alzheimer's disease
CT	computer tomography
EOAD	early onset Alzheimer's disease
GFAP	glial fibrillary acidic protein
ICAM	intercellular adhesion molecule
LOAD	late onset Alzheimer's disease
NFT	neurofibrillar tangle
PSEN	presenilin
PHF	paired helical filament

Macroscopy

On external examination the brain in Alzheimer's disease (AD) may look relatively unremarkable, but often shows some degree of atrophy, especially of the medial temporal lobe. (Figure 1). The olfactory bulb is consistently smaller than expected in AD (Figure 2). On coronal sections of the brain there is usually enlargement of the lateral and third ventricles. The cortical ribbon may be thinner than usual, but this may be subtle and best appreciated in the medial temporal lobe (Figure 2). The brainstem sections usually show the expected degree of pigmentation in the substantia nigra unless other pathologic processes, most often Lewy body pathology, are present. In advanced cases, the locus coeruleus may be pale (Figure 2) (227). The cerebellum is usually grossly unremarkable. Gross examination will exclude some of the other causes of dementia that may sometimes clinically mimic AD, such as vascular disease, frontal tumours or hydrocephalus. The presence of these changes, especially vascular disease, does not preclude a diagnosis of AD, since mixed dementia is frequent, especially in the very old. On the other hand, the clinical significance of small lesions (such as a lacunar infarct or a small meningioma) is doubtful, since such lesions rarely cause dementia by themselves (48, 78).

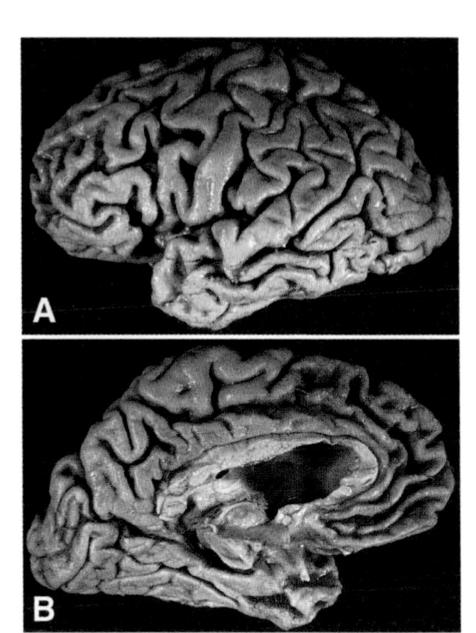

Figure 1. Lateral and medial views of Alzheimer brain. **A.** The lateral view shows diffuse atrophy that is most marked in the frontal and temporal pole, with notable sparing of pre- and postcentral gyri. **B.** On medial view the atrophy is most marked in medial temporal lobe (uncus) and frontal pole. Note marked widening of the rhinal sulcus.

Cerebral atrophy. *Loss of brain weight and volume.* Brain atrophy, producing brain weights lower than normal, is almost always present in AD. Although it is not commonly practised or even possible in some cases, the degree of brain atrophy is best assessed by comparing the volume of the brain to that of its own cranial capacity (47). The brain fills about 92% of the intracranial cavity in the sixth decade of life, 83% in the ninth, and 81% in the tenth. The loss of brain weight is particularly severe in early onset AD (EOAD), while departure from the norm may be subtle in late onset AD (LOAD). Brain weight in LOAD frequently overlaps with age-matched controls. On the other hand, large series have shown clear differences between the mean weight of brains with AD and those without, whatever the age, but these group differences cannot be used for the diagnosis of individual cases (for review, see 78, 130, 235). The weight of individual lobes of the brain has been evaluated in AD compared to controls. The decrease in weight is 41% for the temporal lobe, 30% for the parietal lobe and 14% for the frontal lobe (182).

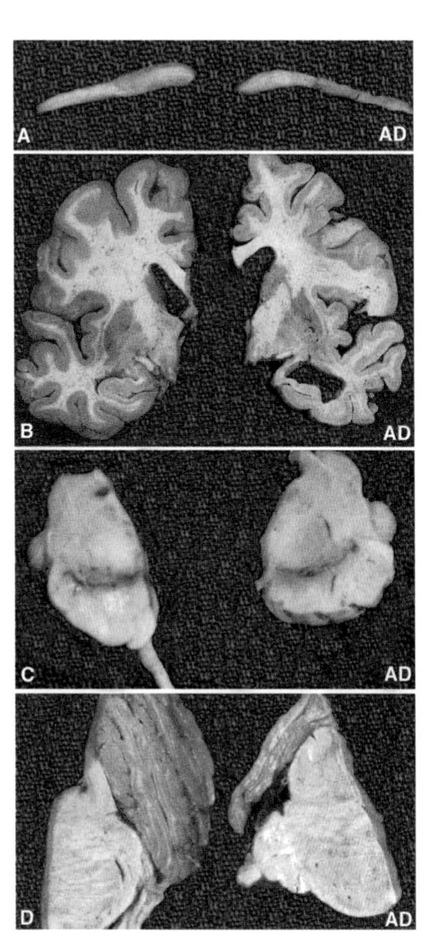

Figure 2. Side-by-side comparison of normal (left side) and AD. **A.** The olfactory bulb is consistently smaller than normal in AD. **B.** The coronal sections show thinning of the cortical ribbon that is most marked in the medial temporal lobe, with particular atrophy of the anterior sections of the hippocampus. **C.** The midbrain sections show normal pigment in the substantia nigra, but **B.** pontine sections show loss of pigment in the locus coeruleus.

Gyral atrophy. Gyral atrophy is usually less marked in LOAD than in EOAD (120) and is absent in up to

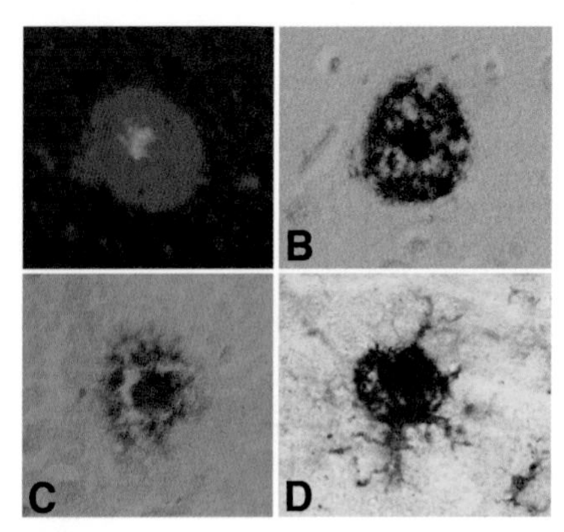

Figure 3. Classical senile plaques. Thioflavin-S fluorescent microscopy (**A**), as well as immunostains for Aβ (**B**) and amyloid-associated molecules such as β1-antichymotrypsin (**C**) show a dense central core, a clear zone and a peripheral halo of non-compact amyloid. Double staining for Aβ and HLA-DR (**D**) to detect microglia, shows that the clear zone in classical plaques is occupied by cellular elements, including microglia.

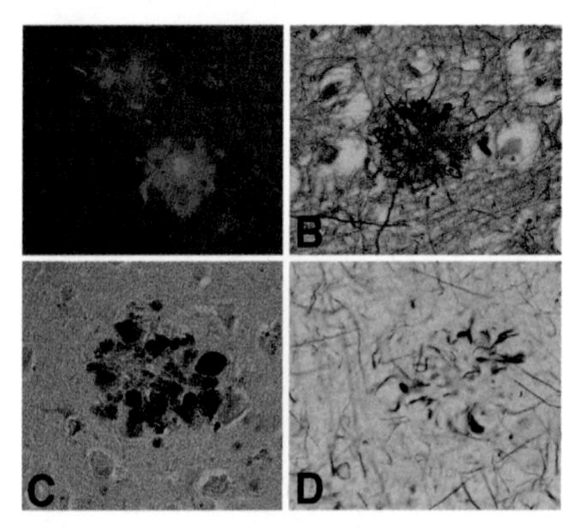

Figure 4. Neuritic plaques. Thioflavin (**A**) and Bielschowsky (**B**) stains show both amyloid deposits and neuritic elements in neuritic plaques, while immunostains for dystrophic neurites, such as ubiquitin (**C**) and Bodian's silver stain (**D**) detect only the neuritic elements of neuritic plaques.

40% of AD brains (236). When present, gyral atrophy is prominent in the temporal lobes, especially the temporal pole and the medial temporal lobe (153) (Figure 1). The frontal lobe may have more obvious atrophy than the parietal lobe, while the occipital lobe is generally preserved (192). On sectioning the brain, the gyral atrophy is due to contributions from both grey and white matter. The most severely affected areas are usually the temporal pole, the anterior part of the hippocampal gyrus and the amygdala (Figure 2). Occasionally, atrophy may be asymmetric or focal, mimicking primary lobar atrophies, such as Pick's disease (59, 227, 235). AD cases with focal

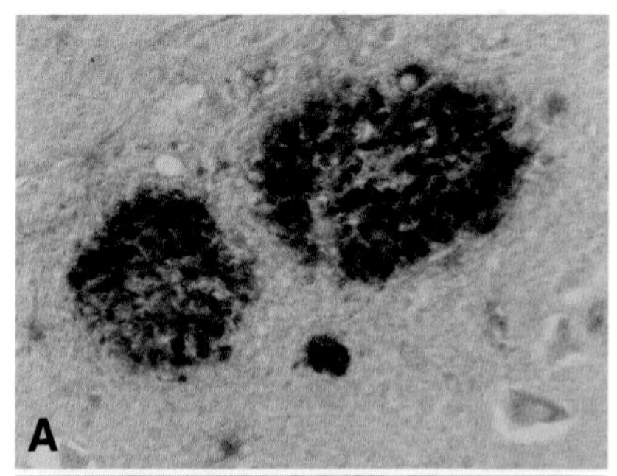

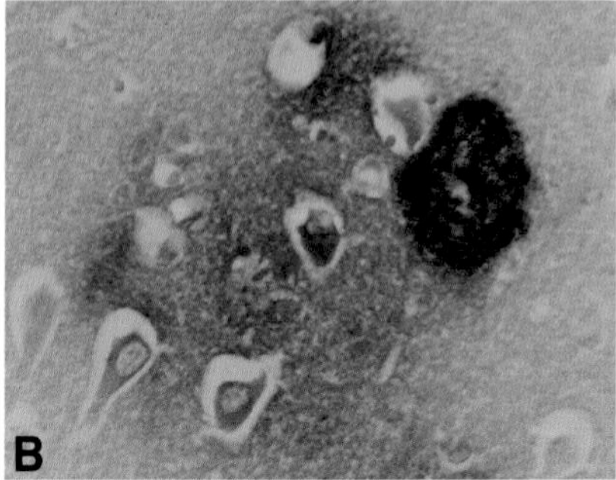

Figure 5. Aβ immunostaining in AD. Sections of AD (**A**) and elderly control (**B**) brains are immunostained with two antibodies to Aβ, one that detects an amino-terminal epitope (6E10, brown chromogen) and one that detects a carboxyl-terminal epitope (4G8, blue). Dense deposits in AD and controls are double labelled, but diffuse deposits in controls show only blue carboxyl-terminal immunoreactivity consistent with deposition of peptides with truncated or modified amino terminal domains.

atrophy may be associated with focal cognitive deficits such as progressive aphasia (166, 190), agnosia (17), Balint's syndrome (116) or frontal lobe dementia (128).

Thickness and length of the cortical ribbon. Decrease in the thickness of the isocortex is moderate in AD (130, 226, 237), whereas the length of the cortical ribbon is decreased, and the amount of decrease correlates with cognitive status (76). These results suggest that AD is associated with loss of columns of neurones, arranged perpendicularly to the surface of the cortex (34).

Ventricular dilation. Ventricles are larger in AD, but the degree of ventricular enlargement correlates poorly with cognitive impairment. Slightly more than half (57%) of AD patients have ventricular volumes greater than normal (121). Ventricular enlargement evaluated by CT scan or MRI has low sensitivity as a marker for AD (sensitivity: 46%±20%), but greater specificity (90%±7%) (49). The yearly rate of lateral ventricular enlargement, on the contrary, has been found to be both sensitive (100%) and specific (100%) (147).

Microscopy

The cardinal histopathologic lesions of AD are senile plaques composed of extracellular Aβ deposits and neurofibrillary tangles composed of intraneuronal tau protein aggregates. There are also pervasive microscopic changes that are less apparent with routine histopathologic methods, including neuronal and synaptic loss. The cardinal histopathologic lesions are necessary for the pathologic diagnosis of AD, while the latter, although important in terms of pathogenesis and clinical manifestations of the disease, lack specificity and are not generally useful for pathologic diagnosis.

Amyloid deposits—senile plaques and amyloid angiopathy. The extracellular deposits that make the core of the senile plaque may be inconspicuous with usual histopathologic staining methods such as haematoxylin and eosin. They are revealed with amyloid stains such as Congo red or thioflavin S, but also readily detected with silver stains such as the Bielschowsky stain (Figures 3, 4). Amyloid refers to extracellular deposits of relatively insoluble fibrillar proteins or peptides with a high content of β-pleated sheet secondary structure, the feature that is responsible for characteristic staining properties (91).

The major amyloid peptide isolated from CAA (92, 93) is similar to the major peptide isolated from parenchymal amyloid deposits (162). The peptide is known under various names, including "β peptide," "A4 peptide," "amyloid β protein," "amyloid peptide" or "Aβ." The latter will be used in this chapter. The qualifier "amyloid" may be inappropriate for some of the Aβ deposits in the brain, because some of the deposits are not visualised by Congo red or thioflavin S stains. These deposits have been referred to as "pre-amyloid" deposits (223), and they may not be fibrillar at the electron microscopic level although this has been discussed (33). More refined biochemical analyses have revealed that Aβ in brain tissue and CAA is actually a heterogenous mixture of peptides with various amino- and carboxyl-terminal modifications and the types of deposits labeled with antibodies to various Aβ epitopes varies (Figure 5). In addition to amino-terminal modifications and truncations, 2 major carboxyl-terminal conformers—Aβ40 and Aβ42—have been recognised and have been linked to the pathogenesis of AD (chapter 2.5).

Focal deposits. Immunostaining of Aβ reveals a large number of spherical, dense deposits in the cerebral cortex (Figure 3), usually exhibiting amyloid properties and appearing as fibrils on electron microscopy, hence the term "fibrillised Aβ" (263) (Figure 6). Most of these lesions contain both Aβ40 and Aβ42 based upon immunohistochemistry with antibodies specific to the carboxyl-terminus of Aβ (15), with Aβ40 within the centre and Aβ42 at the periphery of these focal deposits (Figure 7). Focal deposits often have a dense central core surrounded by a ring devoid of immuno-reactivity and composed of cellular processes, surrounded in turn by a faintly positive more diffuse rim of amyloid (Figures 3, 7). These lesions are referred to as "classic plaques," "cored plaques," or "type 1 plaques" (125). Some focal deposits have only a dense central core and no peripheral rim of cell processes or diffuse amyloid. These lesions have been referred to as "compact" or "burned-out" plaques (56, 259, 262); plaques in cerebellum and globus pallidus often have these characteristics (Figure 8). Some plaques have less compact or reticular amyloid deposits without a definite core and have been referred to as "primitive," "immature," or "type 2 plaques" (125) (Figures 5A, 9).

Diffuse deposits. Non-compact amyloid deposits vary in size from a few microns to more than a hundred microns in diameter (259) (Figure 5B). They have irregular contours and are not surrounded by degenerating neurites. They are often either weakly

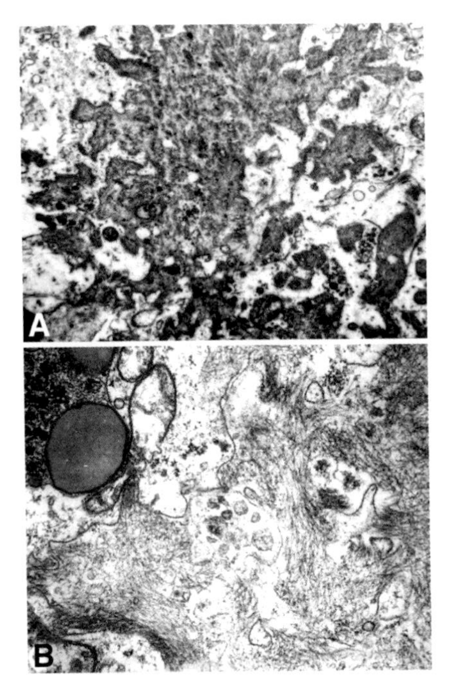

Figure 6. Electron microscopy of dense amyloid cores. There are radiating bundles of fibrils, about 5 to 10-nm in diameter and closely apposed to cell membranes of microglial cells. From the Neuropathology files of Albert Einstein College of Medicine, courtesy of Robert D. Terry, MD.

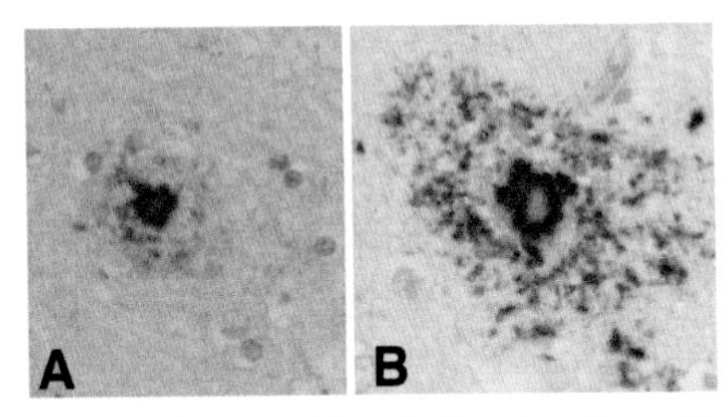

Figure 7. Immunostaining of adjacent sections with antibodies specific to Aβ40 and Aβ42. Plaque cores are enriched in Aβ40 (**A**), while Aβ42 (**B**) tends to be more abundant in the periphery of the core and the surrounding non-compact amyloid.

stained or completely negative with amyloid stains; however, they are visible with modified Bielschowsky stain and Aβ immunostains. They have been referred to as "preamyloid deposits" (223), "non-fibrillised Aβ deposits" (263), "diffuse deposits" (57) or "type 3 plaques" (125). Whether they contain fibrillar forms of Aβ has been debated (33). Diffuse plaques may be traversed by abnormal neurites in advanced AD (209), but generally they lack dystrophic neurites (56). Diffuse plaques should be clearly distinguished from neuritic plaques, since they do not have the same clinical significance (Figure 10). Diffuse plaques

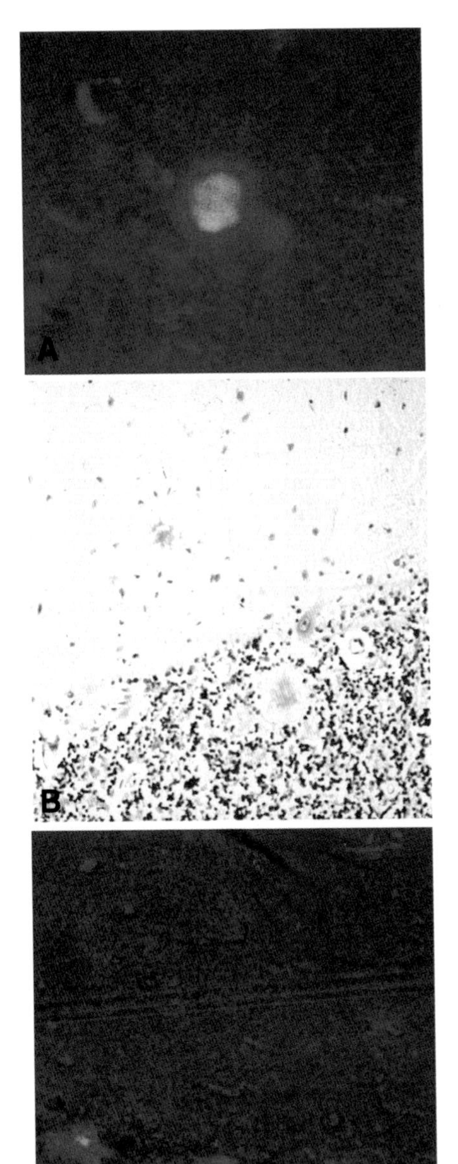

Figure 8. Burned-out plaques. **A.** Thioflavin-S reveals a dense amyloid core in the cortex of AD without significant peripheral non-compact amyloid or obvious neuritic degeneration. Similar lesions are common in the cerebellar Purkinje cell layer (**B**—H&E, **C**—thioflavin-S).

are present, sometimes in very large numbers, in elderly non-demented individuals (57, 58). Given this observation, they have been called "benign" plaques (263) and have been thought to characterise "pathological ageing," a form of senile cerebral parenchymal amyloidosis (63). In the cerebral cortex, diffuse deposits may be considered an early stage of plaque formation (61), but this is not always the

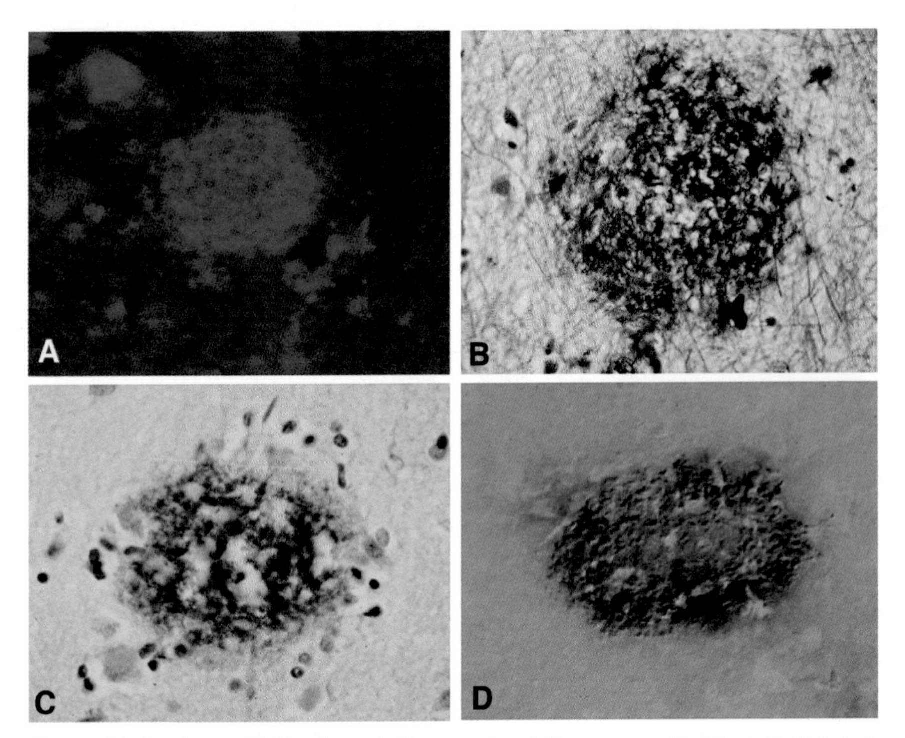

Figure 9. Primitive plaques. Primitive plaques lacking compact amyloid cores are weakly stained with thioflavin-S (**A**). On Bielschowsky stain (**B**) and Aβ immunostains (**C**) amyloid has a reticular appearance. Non-amyloid components, such as complement factor C1q (**D**) are also present (double stain with Aβ – brown chromogen and C1q – blue chromogen).

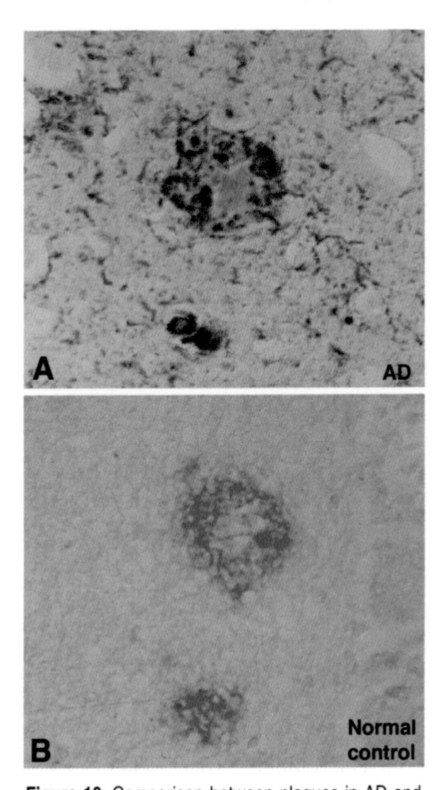

Figure 10. Comparison between plaques in AD and in normal controls. Neuritic plaques in AD (**A**), which contain tau-immunoreactive neurites, are distinctly different from non-neuritic plaques in normal controls (**B**). Both sections from prospectively studied individuals, double immunostained for tau (brown chromogen) and Aβ (blue chromogen).

case. As previously mentioned, amino-terminal-truncated or modified Aβ has been shown in diffuse plaques (61) (Figure 5). There are regions, such as the striatum and the molecular layer of the cerebellar cortex, where diffuse deposits are abundant, but neuritic plaques are rare or absent. The proportion of total surface area of a cortical section occupied by Aβ deposits (so-called "amyloid load" or "amyloid burden") (43.) may reach 25 percent in AD (171), with focal deposits (dense cored plaques) accounting for no more than half this value.

Fleecy and lake-like deposits. These amyloid deposits are unusually large, ill-defined clouds of Aβ in the internal entorhinal layers and are made of amino-terminal truncated fragments of Aβ. Lake-like deposits are similar lesions found in the superficial layers of the presubiculum (261). A continuous subpial band of Aβ immunoreactivity is frequently seen in severely involved cortical areas outside of the medial temporal lobe and sometimes in juxtaposition with meningocerebral vessels with CAA. They are Congo red negative similar to diffuse plaques and are mainly immunoreactive for Aβ42. In some cases Aβ has been detected in the cytoplasm of astrocytes in fleecy (233) and diffuse (2) deposits where they have been speculated to participate in clearance of Aβ.

Other deposits. Some deposits are made of a single (or of a few) intensely stained granules (less than 5 μm in diameter). They have been called punctate or stellate deposits (56) and are usually associated with focal and diffuse deposits. Cotton-wool plaques are particularly large plaques that are readily visible on routine haematoxylin and eosin stains. They are ball-like lesions that are poorly stained with amyloid stains, but visualised with antibodies to Ab42. Cotton wool plaques are often associated with moderate to severe CAA, and they contain only sparse glial and neuritic elements. In these respects they have similarities to diffuse plaques; however, diffuse plaques are invisible with routine histologic stains. Cotton wool plaques were first described in cases of familial AD due to deletion of exon 9 of the PSEN1 gene (119, 151). Recently, cotton wool plaques have also been detected in sporadic cases of AD, but in this circumstance they are virtually always associated with more typical senile plaques (142).

Vascular deposits. Deposition of Aβ in the walls of the cerebral blood vessels in CAA is common in AD (for review, see 108, 250). Vascular deposits are segmental rather than continuous and often situated close to branch points of vessels (133). CAA occurs mainly in small arteries of the leptomeninges and penetrating arteries of the cerebral and cerebellar (84) cortices (Figure 11). Vessels in the white matter only rarely have CAA, with sometimes abrupt termination of CAA in penetrating vessels as they cross the cortical grey-white junction. CAA may also affect veins and capillaries, especially in lamina IV of the primary visual cortex, where dyshoric angiopathy is also common (Figure 11). In the parenchyma, some plaques, especially in the primary visual cortex in cases with CAA, may be angiocentric appearing as if amyloid was coming out of the vessel into the parenchyma (Figure 12). This form of amyloid plaque was first described by Scholz (211), who attributed it to a disturbance of the blood-brain barrier, and termed it dyshoric angiopathy. The degenerating neurites may converge to the vascular deposit (194), and in some familial forms of AD the majority of the dense amyloid deposits are angiocentric (137). CAA is very frequent in AD (on the order of 80% of cases), but not inevitable. The factors that influence the balance between parenchymal and vascular deposition of amyloid are not known, but APOE genotype is one contributing factor with APOE ϵ4 homozygous patients more prone to CAA (247). Biochemical studies of brains with abundant CAA have shown more Aβ40 than Aβ42 (although this has been discussed, 198) and immunohistochemistry with carboxyl-terminal specific antibodies confirms that CAA is preferentially composed of Aβ40 (38, 221).

At the electron microscopic level, fibrils of Aβ in CAA appear to accumulate initially on the external side of the basal membrane of vascular smooth muscle cells located at the border of the media and the adventitia (264). In cerebral capillaries, small Aβ deposits are seen in the endothelial basal lamina itself (269).

CAA is frequently associated with aneurysmal dilatation and arteriolosclerosis, which may be responsible for lobar haemorrhages or small infarcts (126, 252). The balance between CAA and parenchymal Aβ deposits is quite variable. Among APP mutations, one (a substitution of glutamine by glutamic acid at codon 693 of APP770) causes a predominantly vascular disease (hereditary cerebral haemorrhage with amyloidosis of Dutch origin) (144).

Non-amyloid Components of Senile Plaques

Activated microglia (165) (Figure 3D), early components of the complement cascade (77, 164) (Figure 9D), alpha 1 antichymotrypsin (1) (Figure 3C), and proinflammatory cytokines (65) have been identified in senile plaques, indicating an ongoing inflammation. Activated microglia are most evident in dense cored plaques, especially those with Aβ40 (4, 253) (Figure 3D). The role of microglia in clearance or production of amyloid has been debated. Experimental evidence suggests that microglia are capable of phagocytosis of Aβ through a number of well-defined surface receptors for Aβ (272). In addition to their association with senile plaques, microglia are activated throughout the brain in AD. Microglial activation correlates with the degree of neurofibrillary degeneration in the hippocampus (69), where microglia may be responding to neuronal and synaptic degeneration and loss.

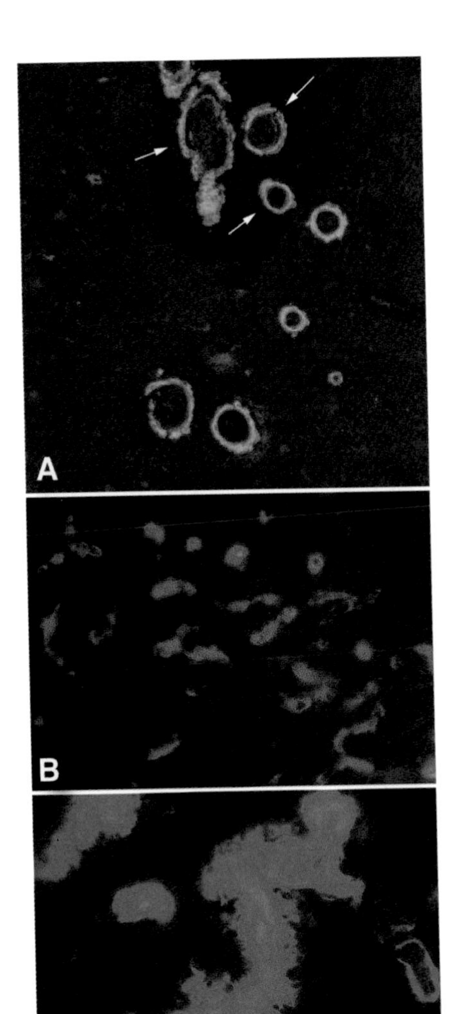

Figure 11. Cerebral amyloid angiopathy. Leptomeningeal (arrows) and parenchymal vessels are affected (**A**), including capillaries especially in layer IV of the visual cortex (**B** and **C**). Note extension of amyloid into the adjacent tissue, so-called dyshoric angiopathy (**C**).

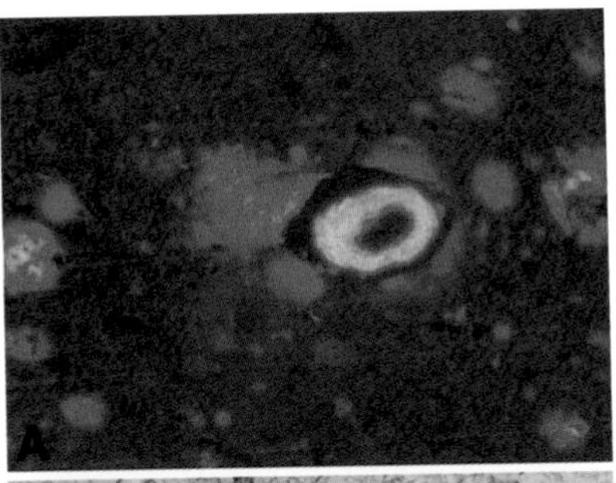

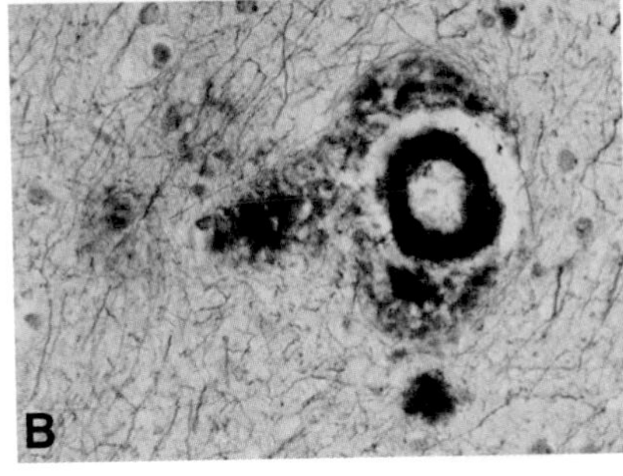

Figure 12. Cerebral amyloid angiopathy (CAA) and perivascular plaques. Thioflavin-S shows CAA of parenchymal vessel with amyloid deposits in the adjacent parenchyma seemingly emanating from the vessel wall.

Various non-amyloid components have been localised to senile plaques, including components of the extracellular matrix, such as proteoglycans (216). Amyloid P component, a serum-derived protein, is present in virtually all types of amyloid deposits and has also been shown to accumulate in cerebral amyloid deposits, possibly due to alterations in the blood brain barrier (188). Other components that have been demonstrated in senile plaques with immunohistochemistry include ICAM1 (244), thrombospondin (32), and others (for review, see 61). ApoE, which in the brain is astrocyte-derived, is also present in senile plaques, especially those with dense amyloid cores (68, 239) (Figure 13). Its deposition appears to be a secondary event (239). It may play the role of chaperone protein and facilitate amyloid clearance (265). Given that ApoE is a cholesterol transport lipoprotein, it is of interest that cholesterol has also recently been demonstrated in the core of senile plaques (173).

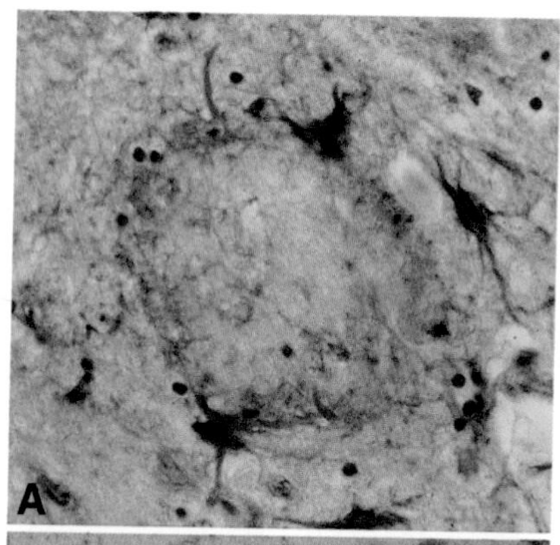

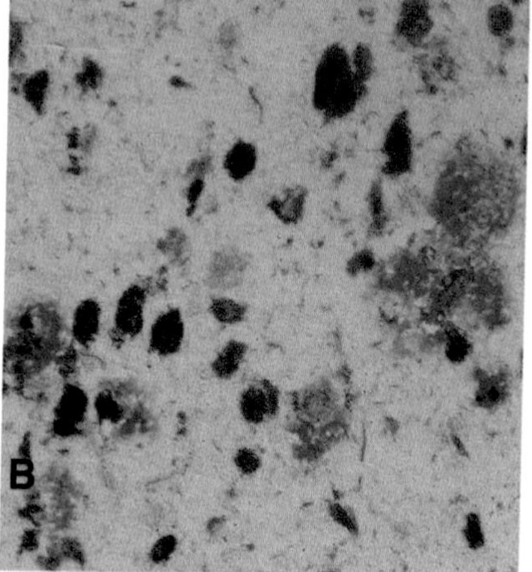

Figure 13. Astrocytes in AD. Astrocytes demonstrated with glial fibrillary acidic protein immunostaining are typically located at the periphery of senile plaques (A). They are the source of apolipoprotein-E (APOE), which is present in plaques and less often in neurofibrillary tangles. B. Double immunostain for APOE (blue chromogen) and tau (brown chromogen).

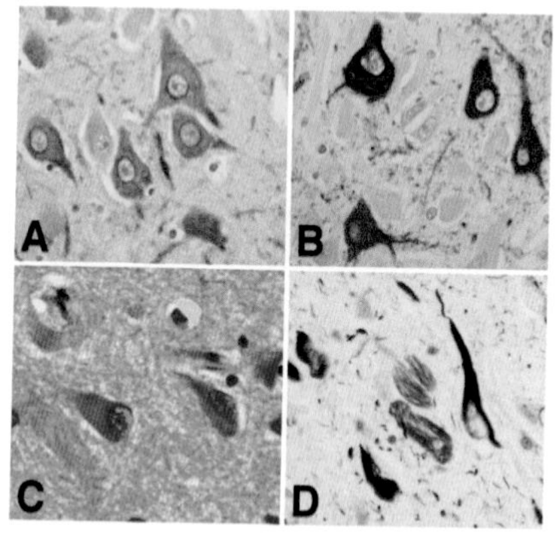

Figure 14. Neurofibrillary degeneration. Tau immunostains show a range of lesions, including pretangles (A and B) as well as intracellular and extracellular NFT. Extracellular NFT are eosinophilic on H&E (C) and weakly stained with dispersed fibrils on Gallyas stain (D). Intracellular tangles are dense and fibrillar on tau immunostains (B), basophilic on H&E (C) and intensely argyrophilic on Gallyas.

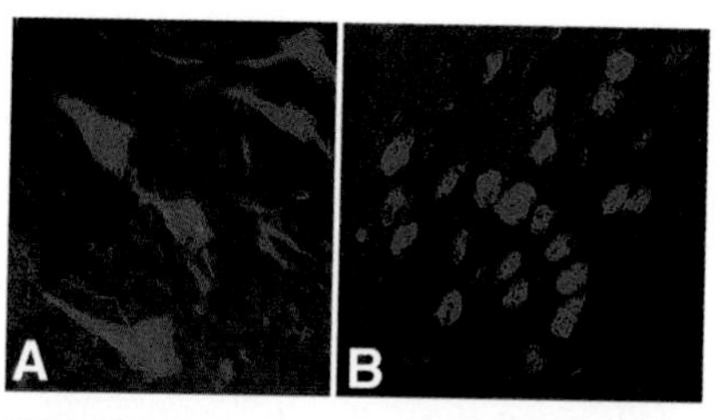

Figure 15. Thioflavin S staining of NFT. Note that flame-shaped lesions (A) are typical of NFT in pyramidal neurons, such as in the hippocampus, while globose NFT are more common in subcortical neurones, such as the basal nucleus of Meynert (B).

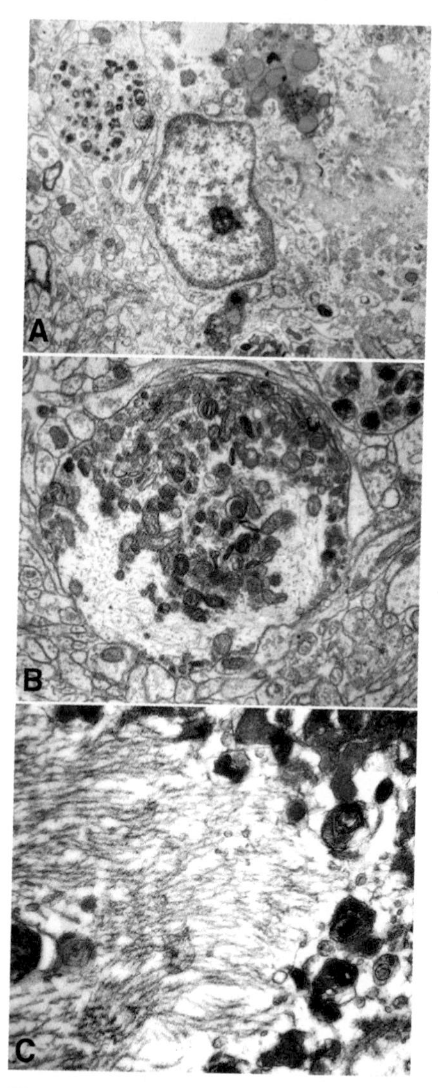

Figure 16. Electron microscopic appearance of neuritic elements in senile plaques in AD. There are swollen cell processes with heterogenous dense bodies and vesicular structures (A and B), characteristically mixed with paired helical filaments (C) that are also the major structural component of NFT. From the Neuropathology files of Albert Einstein College of Medicine, courtesy of Robert D. Terry, MD.

Neurofibrillary Degeneration

Neurofibrillary degeneration in advanced cases of AD is widespread in the neocortex, especially in multimodal association cortices. In the earliest stages of the disease, it is most prominent in the limbic cortices. Common histopathologic methods, such as haematoxylin and eosin can reveal neurofibrillary tangles (NFT), particularly in the hippocampus (Figure 14), but routine histology is insufficient to estimate the actual extent of neurofibrillary degeneration, which includes not only inclusions within perikarya (ie, NFT), but also tau inclusions in neuronal processes, so-called "neuropil threads" (28) (Figure 14). Silver impregnation methods such as modified Bielschowsky (271), Gallyas (25) and Bodian stains (138) are useful to varying degrees in revealing neurofibrillary degeneration (Figure 14), but there is considerable variability from one laboratory to the next in application of silver staining techniques (75). Amyloid stains such as Congo red and thioflavin-S can also be used to detect neurofibrillary pathology (Figure 15), but immunohistochemistry for tau protein, a microtubule-associated protein that promotes microtubule polymerisation and stabilisation, is the most sensitive and specific method for detecting neurofibrillary pathology (Figure 14), and it also offers the possibility for greater standardisation between laboratories.

Neurofibrillary pathology takes several forms in the AD brain, including NFT, neuropil threads and dystrophic neurites in the corona of senile plaques, a feature that defines the neuritic plaque (Figures 4, 10, 16). The proportion of volume occupied by neurofibrillary pathology (up to 37% in severe cases) may be high, and sometimes exceeds the burden of Aβ (43).

NFT are argyrophilic fibrillar lesions in the perikarya and proximal dendrites of neurones. There are several morphologic variants ("flame-shaped" and "globose") of NFT that are in part due to the nature of the neurones in which they form (Figure 15). Flame-shaped NFT are characteristic of pyramidal neurones and globose NFT are found in large non-pyramidal neurones, especially in basal forebrain and brainstem nuclei. On routine haematoxylin and eosin stains NFT are amphophilic to basophilic, but when the neurones harbouring NFT die and NFT become extracellular, they are eosinophilic (113) (Figure 15).

The composition of NFT was controversial when immunohistochemical methods were used for their study, but biochemical and molecular cloning methods have clearly demonstrated that the major structural component of NFT is tau protein. The tau in NFT is abnormal in a number of ways, including truncation, glycation and phosphorylation. The latter is the most thoroughly studied (54, 101, 134). Tau is a phosphoprotein, and its phosphorylation state affects its biologic activity, with better binding to microtubules in the non-phosphorylated state. Normal tau has been shown to undergo rapid dephosphorylation, but tau in NFT is resistant to dephosphorylation (163). It has been suggested that abnormal phosphorylation of tau in AD is due to a disturbance in the balance between activities of specific tau protein kinases and protein phosphatases (101).

Given the evidence that tau is the major structural component of NFT, it is not surprising that antibodies to tau strongly label neurofibrillary pathology in AD (30), not only NFT, but also neuropil threads and dystrophic neurites in senile plaques (55, 135). The sensitivity of tau immunostaining also reveals non-fibrillary precursors to NFT in neurones that are vulnerable to NFT (243). Lesions characterised by diffuse or granular cytoplasmic tau immunoreactivity, often concentrated in a peri-nuclear rim, have been referred to as "pretangles" (10) (Figure 15). A proportion of NFT are ubiquitinated (12, 243).

Given the highly insoluble and structurally stable nature of NFT, when neurones with NFT die, the NFT persists in the extracellular space, often invested by astrocytic processes. These lesions are referred to as extracellular NFT (Figure 15). Extracellular or ghost tangles have slightly different antigenic properties from intracellular NFT, in part due to proteolytic degradation of tau and to the association of tau fibrils with extracellular constituents. In particular, extracellular NFT contain epitopes of amyloid P component and some complement factors (C1q) (212). The frequency of extracellular NFT varies according to the region. They are common in Ammon's horn, rare in the isocortex and absent in the hypothalamus. Clusters of dystrophic neurites that contain fibrillar tau may form a dense plexus around extracellular NFT, a lesion referred to as a tangle-associated neuritic clusters (TANCs) (179) (Figure 17). TANCs are particularly common in the hippocampus, but have not been described in other regions vulnerable to NFT.

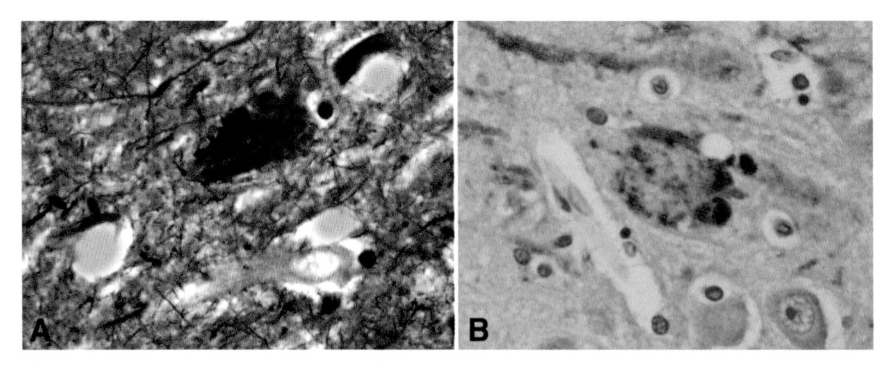

Figure 17. Tangle associated neuritic clusters (TANCs). These are clusters of argyrophilic neurites (**A**) as seen on a Bielschowsky stain associated with an extracellular NFT. The neurites in TANCs are composed of phospho-tau (**B**).

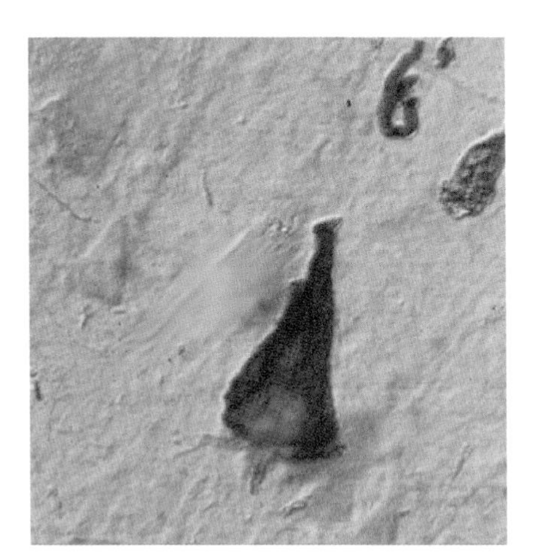

Figure 18. NFT are composed of phospho-tau and several kinases, which are capable of phosphorylating tau, such as cdc2, seen in NFT with immunohistochemistry.

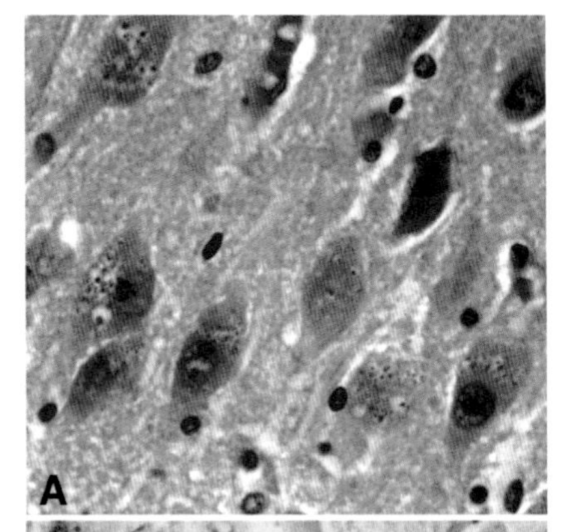

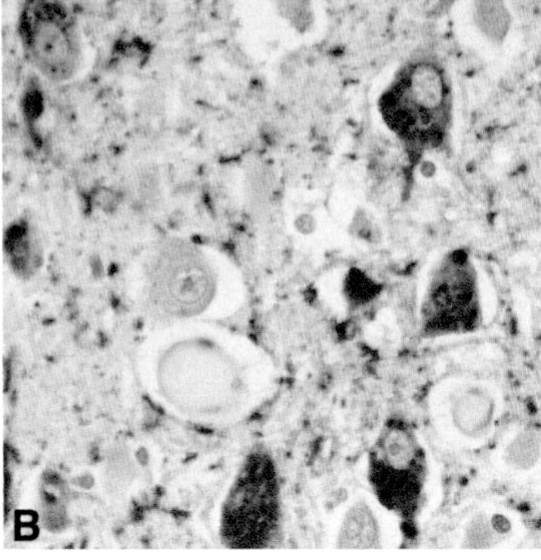

Figure 19. Granulovacuolar degeneration. This is characterized by basophilic granules with clear vacuoles (**A**). The granules have phospho-tau immunoreactivity (**B**).

In addition to tau, other molecules have been detected in NFT. Among the most common are antigens related to protein involved in phosphorylation. Antibodies to several different protein kinases, most of which have also been shown to phosphorylate tau in vitro, are associated with NFT. Among these are kinases involved in cell cycle regulation, such as cyclin dependent kinases (145, 224, 248). The cyclin dependent kinases have been shown to be present in pre-tangles and intracellular NFT, but not extracellular NFT (Figure 18). Another candidate kinase is glycogen-synthase 3 beta (GSK3β). The active form of the enzyme is immunohistochemically present in NFT (187). Antibodies to molecules involved in

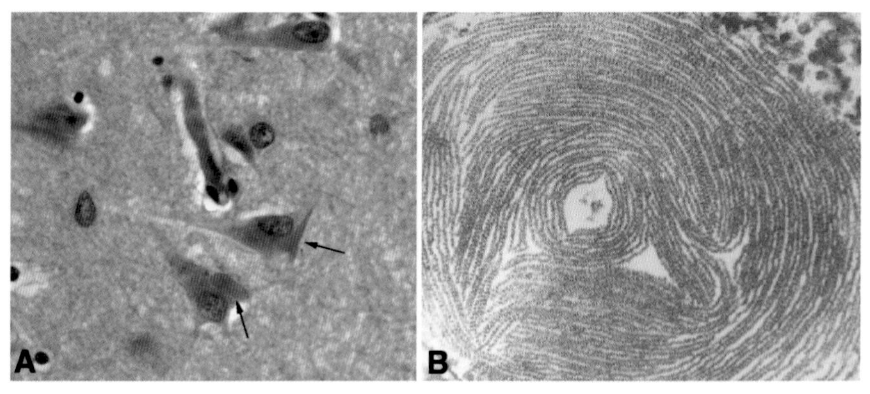

Figure 20. Hirano bodies. These are eosinophilic inclusions that are often rod shaped, but may take other configurations and are most often adjacent to pyramidal neurones (**A**). At the EM level (**B**) they are paracrystalline arrays of f-actin that appear as "beads-on-a-string." From the Neuropathology files of Albert Einstein College of Medicine, courtesy of Robert D. Terry, MD.

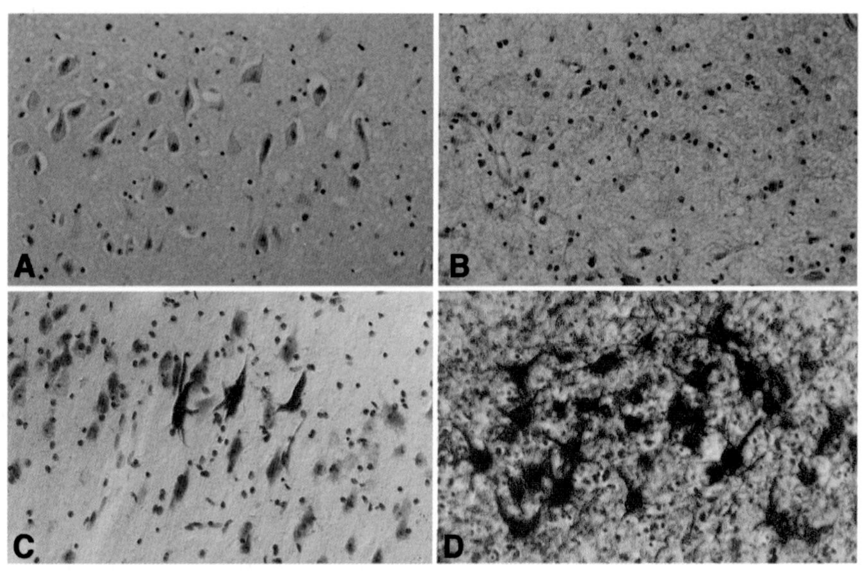

Figure 21. Comparison between normal elderly controls and AD. The neurones in the superficial layers of the entorhinal cortex are relatively well preserved in a normal elderly control (**A**), but show almost complete neuronal loss in advanced AD (**B**). A few mostly intracellular NFT are common in elderly controls (**C**), but NFT, including many extracellular NFT, are common in advanced AD (**D**). Note also numerous neuropil threads in AD, but their virtual absence in normal elderly controls.

oxidative processes, such as heme-oxygenase, nitric oxide and glycation have also been reported in NFT (98, 204, 214). The density of neurotubules is decreased in the tangle-bearing neurones (82, 99) as is the immunoreactivity to acetylated alpha-tubulin (111). The sequestration of tau in NFT seems thus to be accompanied by changes in neurotubules to which they are functionally linked.

At the ultrastructural level, NFT are composed of bundles of 22-nm diameter filaments helically arranged and referred to as paired helical filaments or "PHF" (Figure 16) (132, 229, 260). More recent atomic force microscopy suggests that a twisted ribbon may be a more accurate model for PHF (191, 203). In addition to PHF, 15-nm diameter straight filaments are present in some NFT, mixed with PHF or composing the entire NFT (170).

Neuropil threads. Neuropil threads (28) are short and tortuous argyrophilic neurites that are immunoreactive for tau and contain PHF. They have been speculated to be related to somatodendritic sprouting (123). Most neuropil threads are probably derived from dendritic processes (21), but up to 10% have been identified as myelinated axons with electron microscopy (184, 189). The density of neuropil threads is significantly greater in AD than in other neurodegenerative disorders with tau pathology (46).

The corona of neuritic senile plaques contains degenerating neuronal processes, some of which contain PHF. The neuritic elements associated with senile plaques are heterogeneous (67). Some have immunoreactivity with APP, ubiquitin (Figure 4C) or lysosomal markers. A subset has only tau immunoreactivity similar to neuropil threads (Figure 10). A third type has immunoreactivity for both APP and tau. Perhaps the type of plaque neurite that is clinically most significant is tau immunopositive, while plaque neurites that are positive for APP or ubiquitin can be seen in cortical regions whose function appears clinically normal. In contrast, even a few neuritic plaques in higher order association cortices, when having tau-immunoreactive processes, are associated with cognitive impairment. Other markers that have been used to detect dystrophic neurites in senile plaques include lectin histochemistry for concanavalin A, chromogranin, synaptic markers and neurofilament (61).

Ultrastructurally, plaques contain pre- and post-synaptic elements. Some plaque neurites show features that are characteristic of presynaptic axonal terminal with synaptic vesicles (229). These neurites may contain abnormal lamella dense bodies, some of which are derived from degenerating lysosomes (97). Some neurites contain PHF similar to NFT and others contain aggregates of normal neurofilaments. In addition to dystrophic neurites and amyloid, electron microscopy also demonstrated other cellular elements in senile plaques, including microglia in close apposition to amyloid and astrocytic processes at the periphery.

Relative Importance of Amyloid Deposits and Neurofibrillary Pathology

By convention, the pathologic diagnosis of AD requires both NFT and senile plaques (see later, diagnostic criteria) (234, 267). The balance between these 2 types of alterations is, however, variable. In some cases, the plaques are abundant in the isocortex in the absence of isocortical neurofibrillary pathology. Those so-called "plaque only" cases usually have neurofibrillary degeneration in the entorhinal cortex and hippocampus (226). Some plaque-only AD cases also have Lewy body disease (105). In general when plaque-only pathology is detected in a demented individual, it is important to determine if other types of pathology (eg, Lewy body, tangle, or vascular) may account for dementia.

On the other hand, in some cases, Aβ peptide deposition is minimal and the neurofibrillary pathology predominates. Such a pattern of involvement defines the "tangle predominant form of Alzheimer disease" (14, 23) or "senile dementia of the tangle type" (124), which is most common in very old subjects. In some series APOE ϵ4 allele is underrepresented in this patients (11). See chapter 2.4 on AD variants.

Other Lesions

Granulo-vacuolar degeneration. Granulo-vacuolar degeneration (GVD) is a neuronal intracytoplasmic vesicle containing a central basophilic granule that is argyrophilic with silver stains (Figure 19). It is most common in hippocampal pyramidal cells, especially in the CA2, CA1 and the subiculum, and usually found in association with NFT. It can also be found more widespread and has also been noted in ballooned or swollen neurones. Electron microscopy shows that a vacuole bound by a unit membrane, and enzyme histochemical studies suggest the vacuole may be derived from lysosomes. A dense finely granular mass makes up the granule. The granule of GVD is immunolabelled by antibodies to tubulin (193), ubiquitin (66) and neurofilament (64, 129), but the most consistent immune marker for GVD is tau protein (64, 66, 101, 127, 176) (Figure 21). Evidence suggests that tau in GVD is highly phosphorylated and possibly truncated (66). Antibodies to mitotic phospho-epitopes interestingly label GVD (249), as well as antibodies to activated caspase-3, an enzyme implicated in apoptosis (218).

GVD is not specific to AD and is also seen in "normal" ageing. It is constant in centenarians (109). It has also been noticed in Guam ALS-Parkinsonism dementia complex, Pick's disease, Down's syndrome. GVD is rare in the isocortex, amygdala, hypothalamus and in paramedian nuclei of the midbrain. Other areas of the brain are usually spared (for review, see 78, 227).

Hirano bodies. Hirano Bodies, eosinophilic rod-like structures (Figure 20), are located almost exclusively in the Sommer's sector of the hippocampal pyramidal layer, adjacent to neuronal cell bodies and occasionally within them. At the electron microscopic level they are paracrystalline arrays resembling "beads on a string" (Figure 20). When compared to age matched controls, AD brains have more Hirano bodies than controls (89). They are found in other conditions as well, especially Pick's disease and Guam-Parkinson-dementia complex. They have a paracrystalline appearance in electron microscopy and are composed of actin and actin-associated proteins (85, 94), tau (86), middle molecular weight neurofilaments subunit (210) and a C-terminal fragment of β-amyloid precursor protein (180) (for review, see 114). The presence of antigens of advanced glycation end products suggests that proteins in Hirano bodies are subjected to oxidative stress and subsequent posttranslational modification (178).

Perisomatic granules of hippocampal CA1 neurones. Ubiquitin immunopositive small (1-5 μm in diameter) granules are commonly found around neuronal perikarya in CA1. They contain epitopes of AMPA glutamine receptors GluR1 and 2 (8). They are visible in cases at Braak stage III or higher (195). They may represent a type of localised synaptic degeneration, but their clinical significance is unknown.

Spongiform changes. Spongiform or microvacuolar change is frequently found in the upper layers of the isocortex and rarely in deeper lamina, especially in the severe cases of AD (31, 82, 215). Some vacuolar change may be related to disconnection (74). It is nonspecific and can be found in many degenerative conditions, most notably frontotemporal degenerations (chapter 7.2). Superficial cortical spongiosis must be distinguished from the more intense and diffuse lesions of transmissible spongiform encephalopathies such as Creutzfeldt-Jakob disease. When spongiform changes are detected in the limbic gray matter, especially the amygdala and entorhinal cortex, of a brain that also has histopathologic features of AD, it is important to exclude Lewy body disease where this type of change is common (106).

Astrocytosis. The density of fibrous astrocytes is notably increased in the cortex of AD, in layers II through VI (206). The concentration of glial fibrillary acidic protein (GFAP) is increased (more than 10 times on average) not only in the cortex, but also in the thalamus, cerebellum, and brainstem (52). The increase in the density of GFAP-positive cells is correlated both with the density of Aβ deposits and the density of NFT (37). Mature senile plaques are wrapped by astrocytic processes (Figure 13), which may also penetrate the core (150).

Neuronal and synaptic loss in AD. *Neuronal loss.* Neuronal loss is well documented in AD (for review, see 107). In the hippocampus, the decrease in density of neurones may reach 57% (9). The most vulnerable neuronal populations in the hippocampus may be different in ageing and AD. While the hilus of the dentate gyrus and the subiculum show neuronal loss in ageing, CA1 is mainly affected in AD (254, 255). Neuronal loss in the hippocampus is highly correlated with the number of NFT (9, 42). Marked neuronal loss has also been documented in the entorhinal cortex (96) (Figure 21). It reaches 90% in advanced AD and correlates well with even the earliest stages of cognitive decline. In the isocortex, the loss mainly involves large neurones (228, 231) and is more severe in EOAD than LOAD (104, 158, 175). The detection of cortical neuronal loss has mostly been demonstrated with biased morphometric methods (228, 231). With unbiased stereologic methods using the disector technique (197), global neuronal loss was not apparent in the cortex in AD. Using the same methodology, but focusing on only one gyrus, the superior temporal sulcus, Gomez-Isla and Hyman found a 50% neuronal loss in the cortex of AD (95). In another study, an average difference of 98 millions neurones per parietal lobe was found between the cases with less than 5 neurofibrillary tangles/mm^2 and those with more (100). The neuronal loss predominated in lamina II and III, a population of neurones involved in cortico-cortical connections (51, 100, 122).

Neuronal loss has also been documented in the anterior olfactory nucleus (79, 225). It can reach 75% of the total number of neurones in the younger patients, while the olfactory bulb is relatively spared. The neuronal loss in the hypothalamic nuclei are heterogeneous (83, 136, 157, 222, 251).

All subdivisions of the amygdaloid complex appear to be affected to a varying degree (23-52% decrease). The cell loss is most marked in medial, medial central and cortical nuclei (112). The neuronal loss has been confirmed in another study using the disector method (246) and reached 56%. Several studies have emphasised the importance of the involvement of the nucleus basalis of Meynert in Alzheimer disease (6, 117, 256, 257). The neuronal loss, however, is variable and may be mild (117) or absent (90). The involvement of the various subnuclei is heterogeneous in the least affected cases (71, 143). A severe cell loss (50% decrease) has been found in the locus coeruleus with the disector technique (35). It affects mainly the rostral, cortical-projecting part, of the nucleus and spares the caudal, noncortical-projecting, part (87, 159). The serotoninergic raphe nuclei are also affected (3, 39, 44, 270). A 40% total loss has been found with the disector method (3). The loss of aminergic neurones has been correlated with the depression, which sometimes occurs in the course of AD (274) a finding that has not been confirmed (118). The medial subnuclei of the substantia nigra, projecting to the limbic cortex, may have NFT and show neuronal loss (88, 241, 242). Severe neuronal loss in the substantia nigra is not a feature of AD and suggests another disease process, most often Lewy body disease (88) (for review, see 152).

Although neuronal loss has been documented in AD, the mechanism that leads to the death of the cell has not been determined; however, apoptosis is an attractive candidate for several reasons (chapter 1.2). Several degenerative processes are indeed thought to trigger the apoptotic cascade, and the Aβ peptide has been found to exhibit some apoptotic effects in culture (41). A 2-fold increase in the number of DNA-breaks has been detected in AD compared to controls (177). Moreover, histochemical methods based on the use of terminal deoxynucleotidyl transferase (TdT) incorporating nucleotides at the free ends of the DNA strand (in situ end labelling) has revealed an abundance of DNA breaks in neuronal and glial nuclei in AD (72, 140, 146). On the other hand, contradictory results have also been reported (167) and moreover, the nuclear lesions associated with apoptosis (fragmentation and condensation of the nucleus) are either rare or absent in AD. The expression of proteins associated with the activation of the apoptotic cascade, such as the inducible transcription factor C-Jun and activated caspase 3, have been sought with disputable results (148, 218). The conclusion has been drawn that the increase in DNA fragmentation was not associated with apoptosis (217) and was the consequence of an abnormal sensitivity of the DNA to the metabolic disturbances in the post-mortem period. The density of neurones expressing activated caspase 3 (1 in 1100-5000 neurones) is more compatible with the putative frequency of neuronal death in a chronic disease than the prevalence of DNA breaks (218). Activated caspase 3 immunoreactivity was found in NFT in another study (220). The expression of various cyclins, cyclin-dependent kinases, and cyclin inhibitors in neurones during AD has lead to the suggestion that neuronal death in AD is a consequence of uncontrolled re-entry of postmitotic neurones in the cell cycle (181, 196, 248). The expression of the oncogenes c-myc and N-myc has also been documented in dystrophic neurites and in Aβ deposits (81).

Synaptic loss. Golgi methods have been used to study changes in dendritic morphology in AD. Post-mortem delay was shown to alter unavoidably dendritic shape (20, 258). Some abnormal processes ("filopodia") were sometimes observed on reticular neurones (5). A meshwork of abnormal dendrites was described (in EOAD, 80) and showed to be associated with the plaque (194).

The concentration of synaptophysin, located within small presynaptic vesicles, is decreased in the cerebral cortex in correlation with the intellectual status (13, 103, 160, 230, 273). The concentration of chromogranin A located in large dense core vesicles appears, on the contrary, to increase (141). Electron microscopy observation has shown that the synapses decrease in number but are enlarged, the total apposition length remaining unchanged (19, 50, 207, 208). It has been shown more recently that presynaptic membrane components (synaptoagmin, SNAP-25, and syntaxin 1/HPC-1) are little affected (less than 10% the value of the controls) compared to the vesicular components (synaptobrevin and synaptophysin—30% of the controls) (213). Results obtained with SNAP 25 immunohistochemistry tends to reveal a much smaller synaptic loss than synaptophysin (40, 60). All the mentioned synaptic markers are presynaptic and depend on the metabolism of cell bodies that are sometimes located far away. It is thus difficult to determine if the pre-synaptic alterations appear early (110) or late (139) in the cascade of pathological events, and if it is a major (230) or a minor correlate (62) of dementia. It has been shown that the decrease in synaptophysin immunoreactivity was not linked to the presence of Aβ deposits, especially diffuse plaques (161) and in the entorhinal-dentate gyrus system that it could on the contrary be related to the density of neurofibrillary tangles in the entorhinal cortex (103).

Topography of the Lesions

Neurofibrillary pathology. The distribution of neurofibrillary pathology (neurofibrillary tangles, neuropil threads, and neuritic plaques) differs from the distribution of parenchymal and vascular Aβ peptide. The most vulnerable regions for neurofibrillary pathology are limbic and association cortices, with primary cortices affected only in advanced AD (7, 115) (Figure 22). The cortical involvement may be ranked in a hierarchical order, with involvement of a given area only observed if areas of a lower rank are also involved (53, 73). For example, hippocampal NFT are not seen in the absence of entorhinal NFT and isocortical NFT are generally not seen in the absence of hippocampal NFT. This observation strongly suggests a progression of the lesions from the entorhinal cortex to the hippocampus and from the hippocampus to the isocortex. The hierarchical order of involvement is helpful in staging the severity of AD (eg, Braak and Braak staging) (26, 29).

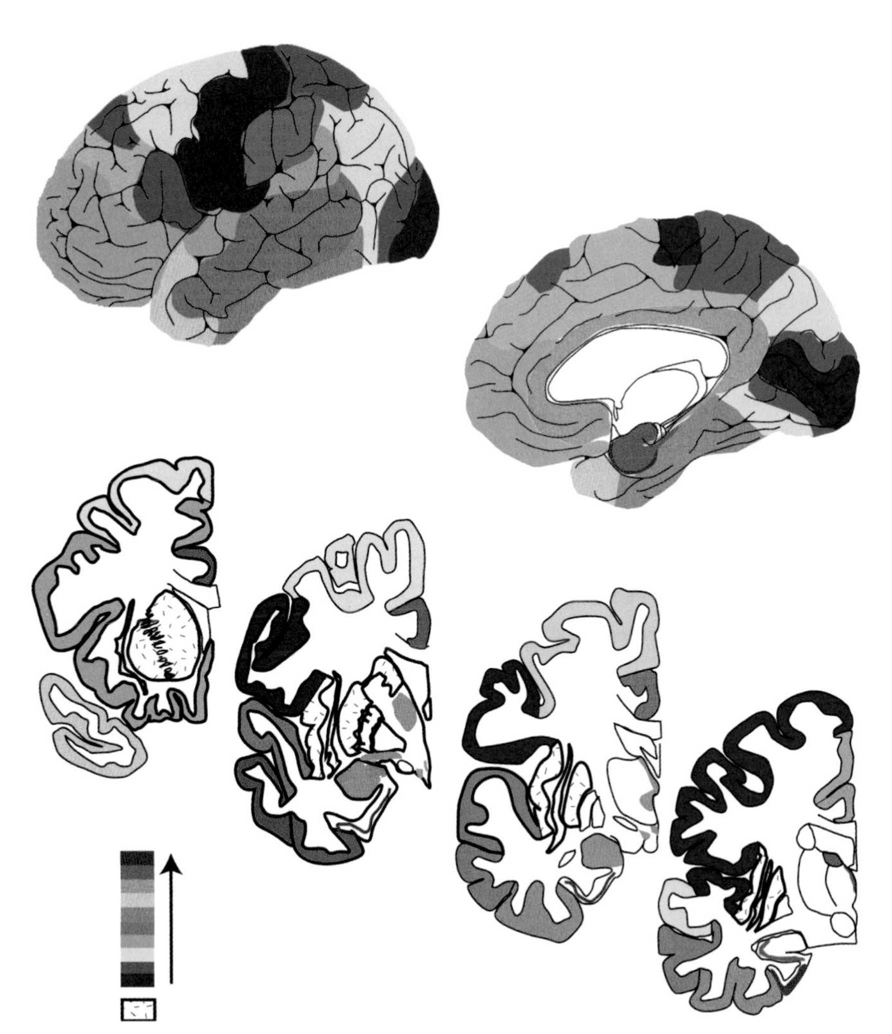

Figure 22. Colour scale indicates the severity of the neurofibrillary pathology. Dotted areas indicate a region for which the chronology of the neurofibrillary lesions is not fully documented. The most affected regions are also those that are involved at the earliest time in the course of the disease. The diagram is an average view of the progression of the lesions. The interindividual variability has not been specifically estimated. The figure is a compendium of data from several references.

In the subcortical areas, NFT are abundant in nuclei that project directly to the cortex, but not all of nuclei are equally affected (87). Most of the thalamic nuclei, for instance, are spared. The NFT are abundant, however, in the limbic nuclei of the thalamus (24). They are found in the magnocellular basal complex (medial septal nuclei, nucleus of the diagonal band of Broca, nucleus basalis of Meynert). In the nucleus basalis, NFT are present even in the early stages of the disease while ghost tangles are numerous in the late stages (205). In the amygdala, the corticomedial nuclei are more severely involved than the laterobasal nuclei. The lesions predominate in the ventromedial region of the amygdala (122, 238, 244) which receives projections from the hippocampus (122, 244). In the brainstem, the locus coeruleus (35), raphe nuclei (39, 200, 270) and the medial part of the substantia nigra (242) are selectively involved. In the lower brainstem, NFT are present at an early stage in "autonomic higher order processing nuclei" (medial and lateral parabrachial nuclei, subpeduncular nucleus in the pons; intermediate zone of the reticular formation in the medulla oblongata) (201). NFT are also found in the tegmental pontine reticular nucleus, that controls horizontal saccades (202) and in the rostral interstitial nucleus of the medial longitudinal fascicle (riMLF) involved in the vertical saccades (199).

Aβ deposits. Aβ peptide deposits are more diffusely and less predictably distributed than NFT (26, 36), but again higher order association cortices are more vulnerable than primary cortices. Temporal and occipital association cortices have the highest density, limbic and frontal association cortices the lowest, and parietal intermediate (7). The deposits are usually more abundant at the depths of sulci than over the crests of gyri. Aβ peptide deposits may relatively spare the hippocampal formation (36). Numerous deposits may be present in the striatum (22, 266) and in the cerebellum (266) where most are diffuse amyloid deposits that lack neuritic elements (155).

Cerebral amyloid angiopathy. CAA is most frequent in the occipital cortex, where it sometimes selectively affects the primary visual cortex, especially the small vessels in lamina IVb and IVc (172). It is less frequent in the frontal cortex. It is also found in the molecular layer of the cerebellum (185). It is rarely found in the white matter (149) where it can be associated with myelin pallor, and exceptionally in the spinal cord (250).

Progression of the Lesions

The progression of the lesions cannot be directly studied except for exceptional cases, in which a cortical biopsy and a post-mortem study, performed months or years later, are available on the same patient (16, 70, 156). These studies have shown either no change or at most a small increase in the density of senile plaques and NFT when followed for up to 11 years. In one study, the neuronal density of pyramidal neurones decreased between biopsy and autopsy (156). These data suggest that the disease progression in AD is slow. The same conclusions have been reached from cross-sectional studies of lesion distribution in autopsies of a wide range of ages (27). In such studies NFT are detected in the transentorhinal and entorhinal cortex in individuals as young as the third decade of life, while consistent isocortical NFT are not found until decades later.

The progression of Aβ deposits is less clear, but cross-sectional studies would suggest that amyloid deposits may precede NFT in the isocortex by a number of years. Diffuse deposits, in particular, may be detected in nondemented individuals (63, 268) or those with mild cognitive impairment (174) years before isocortical NFT are common. In Down syndrome patients, diffuse plaques are present at a very early age (in the second decade of life) (219) and may be preceded by the accumulation of Aβ peptide within neurones (102); diffuse deposits of Aβ peptide, sometimes in a columnar distribution in the isocortex, may be the only detectable lesions (154, 219). Formation of dense amyloid deposits with dystrophic neurites, microglial activation and deposition of complement factors are later events (4, 219).

Diagnostic Criteria

Senile plaques and NFT are found in aged persons who were not considered demented during their life (18, 45, 58). This observation has led to the idea that a certain threshold of lesions must be reached before AD is clinically apparent. These studies suggest that lesions accumulate in the brain for a long time before producing symptoms. In other words, AD is probably asymptomatic for years before dementia is detected. Should then any NFT or any Aβ deposits be considered evidence of a progressive disease that will lead inevitably to dementia? The question remains open. In a clinicopathological, community-based study, it was found that no clear threshold of pathological features could accurately predict dementia (45, 183). The minimal number of lesions necessary for the diagnosis can probably vary from one individual to the next (267).

Khachaturian criteria. Khachaturian, representing a panel of neuropathologists (131) proposed criteria based on the density of senile plaques stained by modified Bielschowsky method, thioflavin S or Congo red technique. The counts of senile plaques were to be performed in a field encompassing 1 mm^2. In any patient less than 50 years of age, the diagnosis was warranted if the count exceeded 2 to 5 plaques per field. Between 50 and 65 years of age the number of plaques had to be ≥8 per field. Between 66 and 75 years of age, plaques had to exceed 10 per field and over 75 years of age, 15 per field. These quantitative thresholds could be lowered when the patients were clinically demented. Problems with the Khachaturian criteria stem from the lack of distinction between various plaque types (eg, neuritic versus diffuse) and significant variability in plaque counts between laboratories due in part to differences in staining and counting methods (75, 168). Moreover, NFT are not included in these criteria.

CERAD criteria. The neuropathological protocol proposed by the Consortium to Establish a Registry of Alzheimer Disease (CERAD) relies on a semiquantitative assessment of the neuritic plaque density rather than on its direct evaluation (169). Samples from the middle frontal gyrus, superior and middle temporal gyri, inferior parietal lobule are assessed. Samples from the hippocampus and entorhinal cortex, as well as midbrain including substantia nigra should also be examined. Cartoons are provided illustrating representative microscopic fields with "sparse," "moderate" and "frequent" plaques. Only neuritic plaques are to be taken into account. While it is stated that neuritic plaques are those "with thickened silver-positive neurites" in practice and as illustrated in the cartoons plaques with dense amyloid cores without obvious neurites were also included in this category. Problems with these criteria stem from the lack of a requirement that the neurites in plaques display tau immunoreactivity.

The highest value of this semiquantitative evaluation is then compared with the age of the patient to yield an "age-related plaque score" with the following possibilities: 0—no histologic evidence of AD; A—histologic findings that are uncertain evidence of AD; B—histologic findings suggesting AD; and C—histologic findings indicating the diagnosis of AD. The age-related plaque score is finally integrated with the clinical history to reach a final diagnosis of definite AD, neuropathologically probable, neuropathologically possible and normal (169).

NIA-Reagan Institute criteria. The most recent criteria consider all lesions (amyloid deposits, neuritic plaques, neuropil threads and NFT) as abnormal. They are not thought to be the consequence of normal ageing. The density of the lesions helps to determine the probability linking the cognitive symptoms with the pathological observations (267). The criteria include both an "age-related plaque score" according to a procedure such as CERAD and a topographic staging of NFT such as the Braak and Braak staging system (25). A probabilistic approach is proposed for diagnosis of dementia recognising the clinical uncertainty of the pathologic lesions. Dementia has "a high likelihood" to be due to AD when the plaque score of the CERAD is "frequent" and Braak stage reaches V/VI. The likelihood is intermediate with CERAD "moderate" plaque score and Braak Stage III/IV. The likelihood is low with CERAD "infrequent" and Braak stage I/II. Criteria for the recognition of "incipient" dementia due to Alzheimer's disease are not proposed. Problems with the proposed criteria stem from the fact that other possible combinations of the scores (such as CERAD moderate and Braak stage VI) are not considered and there is uncertainty how the criteria can be applied to cases that lack clinical information about presence or absence of dementia.

References

1. Abraham CR, Selkoe DJ, Potter H (1988) Immunochemical identification of the serine protease inhibitor α-1 antichymotrypsin in the brain amyloid deposits of Alzheimer's disease. *Cell* 52: 487-501.

2. Akiyama H, Mori H, Saido T, Kondo H, Ikeda K, McGeer PL (1999) Occurrence of the diffuse amyloid β-protein (Aβ) deposits with numerous Aβ-containing glial cells in the cerebral cortex of patients with Alzheimer's disease. *Glia* 25: 324-331.

3. Aletrino MA, Vogels OJ, Van Domburg PH, Ten Donkelaar HJ (1992) Cell loss in the nucleus raphes dorsalis in Alzheimer's disease. *Neurobiol Aging* 13: 461-468.

4. Arends YM, Duyckaerts C, Rozemuller JM, Eikelenboom P, Hauw J-J (2000) Microglia, amyloid and dementia in Alzheimer disease. A correlative study. *Neurobiol Aging* 21: 39-47.

5. Arendt T, Zvegintseva HG, Leontovich TA (1986) Dendritic changes in the basal nucleus of Meynert and in the diagonal band nucleus in Alzheimer's disease—a quantitative Golgi investigation. *Neuroscience* 19: 1265-1278.

6. Arendt T, Bigl V, Arendt A, Tennstedt A (1983) Loss of neurones in the nucleus basalis of Meynert in Alzheimer's disease, paralysis agitans and Korsakoff's disease. *Acta Neuropathol (Berl)* 61: 101-108.

7. Arnold SE, Hyman BT, Flory J, Damasio AR, van Hoesen GW (1991) The topographical and neuroanatomical distribution of neurofibrillary tangles and neuritic plaques in the cerebral cortex of patients with Alzheimer's disease. *Cerebral Cortex* 1: 103-116.

8. Aronica E, Dickson DW, Kress Y, Morrison JH, Zukin RS (1998) Non-plaque dystrophic dendrites in Alzheimer hippocampus: A new pathological structure revealed by glutamate receptor immunocytochemistry. *Neuroscience* 82: 979-991.

9. Ball MJ (1977) Neuronal loss, neurofibrillary tangles and granulovacuolar degeneration in the hippocampus with ageing and dementia. *Acta Neuropathol (Berl)* 37: 111-118.

10. Bancher C, Brunner C, Lassmann H, Budka H, Jellinger K, Wiche G, Seitelberger F, Grundke-Iqbal I, Iqbal K, Wisniewski HM (1989) Accumulation of abnormally phosphorylated tau precedes the formation of neurofibrillary tangles in Alzheimer's disease. *Brain Res* 477: 90-99.

11. Bancher C, Egensperger R, Kosel S, Jellinger K and Graeber M B (1997) Low prevalence of apolipoprotein E epsilon 4 allele in the neurofibrillary tangle predominant form of senile dementia. *Acta Neuropathol (Berl)* 94: 403-409.

12. Bancher C, Grundke-Iqbal I, Iqbal K, Fried VA, Smith HT, Wisniewski HM (1991) Abnormal phosphorylation of tau precedes ubiquitination in neurofibrillary pathology of Alzheimer disease. *Brain Res* 539: 11-18.

13. Bancher C, Jellinger K, Lassmann H, Fischer P, Leblhuber F (1996) Correlations between mental state and quantitative neuropathology in the Vienna Longitudinal Study on Dementia. *Eur Arch Psychiat Clin Neurosci* 246: 137-146.

14. Bancher C, Jellinger KA (1994) Neurofibrillary tangle predominant form of senile dementia of Alzheimer type: a rare subtype in very old subjects. *Acta Neuropathol (Berl)* 88: 565-570.

15. Barelli H, Lebeau A, Vizzavona J, Delaere P, Chevallier N, Drouot C, Marambaud P, Ancolio K, Buxbaum JD, Khorkova O, Heroux J, Sahasrabudhe S, Martinez J, Warter JM, Mohr M, Checler F (1997) Characterization of new polyclonal antibodies specific for 40 and 42 amino acid-long amyloid β peptides: their use to examine the cell biology of presenilins and the immunohistochemistry of sporadic Alzheimer's disease and cerebral amyloid angiopathy cases. *Mol Med* 3: 695-707.

16. Bennett DA, Cochran EJ, Saper CB, Leverenz JB, Gilley DW, Wilson RS (1993) Pathological changes in frontal cortex from biopsy to autopsy in Alzheimer's disease. *Neurobiol Aging* 14: 589-596.

17. Benson DF (1989) Posterior cortical atrophy: a new entity or Alzheimer's disease? *Arch Neurol* 46: 843-844.

18. Berg L, McKeel DW Jr, Miller JP, Storandt M, Rubin EH, Morris JC, Baty J, Coats M, Norton J, Goate AM, Price JL, Gearing M, Mirra SS, Saunders AM (1998) Clinicopathologic studies in cognitively healthy aging and Alzheimer's disease: relation of histologic markers to dementia severity, age, sex, and apolipoprotein E genotype. *Arch Neurol* 55: 326-335.

19. Bertoni-Freddari C, Fattoretti P, Casoli T, Caselli U, Meier-Ruge W (1996) Deterioration threshold of synaptic morphology in aging and senile dementia of Alzheimer's type. *Anal Quant Cytol Histol* 18: 209-213.

20. Braak H, Braak E (1985) Golgi preparation as a tool in neuropathology with particular reference to investigations of the human telencephalic cortex. *Prog Neurobiol* 25: 93.

21. Braak H, Braak E (1988) Neuropil threads occur in dendrites of tangle-bearing nerve cells. *Neuropathol Appl Neurobiol* 14: 39-44.

22. Braak H, Braak E (1990) Alzheimer's disease: striatal amyloid deposits and neurofibrillary changes. *J Neuropathol Exp Neurol* 49: 215-224.

23. Braak H, Braak E (1990) Neurofibrillary changes confined to the entorhinal region and abundance of cortical amyloid in cases of presenile and senile dementia. *Acta Neuropathol (Berl)* 80: 479-486.

24. Braak H, Braak E (1991) Alzheimer's disease affects limbic nuclei of the thalamus. *Acta Neuropathol (Berl)* 81: 261-268.

25. Braak H, Braak E (1991) Demonstration of amyloid deposits and neurofibrillary changes in whole brain sections. *Brain Pathol* 1: 213-216.

26. Braak H, Braak E (1991) Neuropathological stageing of Alzheimer-related changes. *Acta Neuropathol (Berl)* 82: 239-259.

27. Braak H, Braak E (1997) Frequency of stages of Alzheimer-related lesions in different age categories. *Neurobiol Aging* 18: 351-357.

28. Braak H, Braak E, Grundke-Iqbal I, Iqbal K (1986) Occurrence of neuropil threads in the senile human brain and in Alzheimer's disease. A third location of paired helical filaments outside of neurofilament tangles and neuritic plaques. *Neurosci Lett* 65: 351-355.

29. Braak H, Duyckaerts C, Braak E, Piette F (1993) Neuropathological staging of Alzheimer-related changes correlates with psychometrically assessed intellectual status. In *Alzheimer's disease: advances in clinical and basic research*, B Corain, K Iqbal K, M Nicolini, B Winblad, H Wisniewski, P Zatta (eds). John Wiley & Sons: Chichester, pp. 131-137.

30. Brion JP, Passareiro H, Nunez J, Flament-Durand J (1985) Mise en évidence immunologique de la protéine tau au niveau des lésions de dégénérescence neurofibrillaire de la maladie d'Alzheimer. *Arch Biol (Brux)* 95: 229-235.

31. Brion S, Masse G, Plas J (1983) Histopathologie de la spongiose dans la maladie de Creutzfeldt-Jakob et dans les démences séniles et préséniles. In *Virus non conventionnels et affections du système nerveux central*, LA Court, F Cathala (eds). Masson; Paris pp. 227-234.

32. Buée L, Hof PR, Roberts DD, Delacourte A, Morrison JH, Fillit HM (1992) Immunohistochemical Identification of thrombospondin in normal human brain and in Alzheimer's disease. *Am J Pathol* 141: 783-788.

33. Bugiani O, Tagliavini F, Giaccone G, Verga L, El Hachimi K, Foncin JF, Frangione B (1995) Diffuse senile plaques: amorphous or fibrous? *Am J Pathol* 146: 777-778.

34. Buldyrev SV, Cruz L, Gomez-Isla T, Gomez-Tortosa E, Havlin S, Le R Stanley HE, Urbanc B, Hyman BT (2000) Description of microcolumnar ensembles in association cortex and their disruption in Alzheimer and Lewy body dementias. *Proc Natl Acad Sci U S A* 97: 5039-5043.

35. Busch C, Bohl J, Ohm TG (1997) Spatial, temporal and numeric analysis of Alzheimer changes in the nucleus coeruleus. *Neurobiol Aging* 18: 401-416.

36. Cairns NJ, Chadwick A, Luthert PJ, Lantos PL (1991) β-Amyloid protein load is relatively uniform throughout neocortex and hippocampus in elderly Alzheimer's disease patients. *Neurosci Lett* 129: 115-118.

37. Cairns NJ, Chadwick A, Luthert PJ, Lantos PL (1992) Astrocytosis, β A4-protein deposition and paired helical filament formation in Alzheimer's disease. *J Neurol Sci* 112: 68-75.

38. Castano EM, Prelli F, Soto C, Beavis R, Matsubara E, Shoji M, Frangione B (1996) The length of amyloid-β in hereditary cerebral hemorrhage with amyloidosis, Dutch type. Implication for the role of amyloid β 1-42 in Alzheimer's disease. *J Biol Chem* 271: 32185-32191.

39. Chen CP, Eastwood SL, Hope T, McDonald B, Francis PT, Esiri MM (2000) Immunocytochemical study of the dorsal and median raphe nuclei in patients with Alzheimer's disease prospectively assessed for behavioural changes. *Neuropathol Appl Neurobiol* 26: 347-355.

40. Clinton J, Blackman SE, Royston MC, Roberts GW (1994) Differential synaptic loss in the cortex in Alzheimer's disease: a study using archival material. *Neuroreport* 5: 497-500.

41. Cotman CW, Anderson AJ (1995) A potential role for apoptosis in neurodegeneration and Alzheimer's disease. *Mol Neurobiol* 10: 19-45.

42. Cras P, Smith MA, Richey PL, Siedlak SL, Mulvihill P, Perry G (1995) Extracellular neurofibrillary tangles reflect neuronal loss and provide further evidence of extensive protein cross-linking in Alzheimer disease. *Acta Neuropathol (Berl)* 89: 291-295.

43. Cummings BJ, Pike CJ, Shankle R, Cotman CW (1996) ß-amyloid deposition and other measures of neuropathology predict cognitive status in Alzheimer's disease. *Neurobiol Aging* 17: 921-933.

44. Curcio CA, Kemper T (1984) Nucleus raphe dorsalis in dementia of the Alzheimer type: neuronal changes and neuronal packing density. *J Neuropathol Exp Neurol* 43: 359-368.

45. Davis DG, Schmidt FA, Wekstein DR, Markesbery WR (1999) Alzheimer neuropathologic alterations in aged cognitively normal subjects. *J Neuropathol Exp Neurol* 58: 376-388.

46. Davis DG, Wang HZ, Markesbery WR (1992) Image analysis of neuropil threads in Alzheimer's, Pick's, Lewy body disease and in Progressive supranuclear palsy. *J Neuropathol Exp Neurol* 51: 594-600.

47. Davis PJM, Wright EA (1977) A new method for measuring cranial capacity volume and its application to the assessment of cerebral atrophy at autopsy. *Neuropathol Appl Neurobiol* 3: 341-358.

48. DeArmond SJ, Dickson DW, DeArmond B (1997) Degenerative diseases of the central nervous system. In *Textbook of Neuropathology*, RL Davis, DM Robertson (eds), 3rd ed, Baltimore: Williams & Wilkins, Baltimore, pp. 1063-1178.

49. DeCarli C, Kaye JA, Horwitz B, Rapoport SI (1990) Critical analysis of the use of computer-assisted transverse axial tomography to study human brain in aging and dementia of the Alzheimer type. *Neurology* 40: 872-883.

50. DeKosky ST, Scheff W (1990) Synapse loss in frontal cortex biopsies in Alzheimer's disease: correlation with cognitive severity. *Ann Neurol* 27: 457-464.

51. Delacoste MC, White CL (1993) The role of connectivity in Alzheimer's disease pathogenesis. A review and model system. *Neurobiol Aging* 14: 1-16.

52. Delacourte A (1990) General and dramatic glial reaction in Alzheimer brains. *Neurology* 40: 33-37.

53. Delacourte A, David JP, Sergeant N, Buee L, Wattez A, Vermersch P, Ghozali F, Fallet-Bianco C, Pasquier F, Lebert F, Petit H, Di Menza C (1999) The biochemical pathway of neurofibrillary degeneration in aging and Alzheimer's disease. *Neurology* 52 : 1158-1165.

54. Delacourte A, Defossez A (1986) Alzheimer's disease: Tau proteins, the promoting factors of microtubule assembly are major components of paired helical filaments. *J Neurol Sci* 76: 173-186.

55. Delaère P, Duyckaerts C, Brion JP, Poulain V, Hauw J-J (1989) Tau, paired helical filaments and amyloid in the neocortex: a morphometric study of 15 cases with graded intellectual status in aging and senile dementia of Alzheimer type. *Acta Neuropathol (Berl)* 77: 645-653.

56. Delaère P, Duyckaerts C, He Y, Piette F, Hauw J-J (1991) Subtypes and differential laminar distributions of ßA4 deposits in Alzheimer's disease: relationship with the intellectual status of 26 cases. *Acta Neuropathol (Berl)* 81: 328-335.

57. Delaère P, Duyckaerts C, Masters C, Piette F, Hauw J-J (1990) Large amounts of neocortical ßA4 deposits without Alzheimer changes in a nondemented case. *Neurosci Lett* 116: 87-93.

58. Delaère P, He Y, Fayet G, Duyckaerts C, Hauw J-J (1993) ßA4 deposits are constant in the brain of the oldest old: an immunocytochemical study of 20 French centenarians. *Neurobiol Aging* 14: 191-194.

59. Delay J, Brion S (1962) *Les démences tardives*, Masson: Paris, pp. 1-234.

60. Dessi F, Colle MA, Hauw J-J, Duyckaerts C (1997) Accumulation of SNAP-25 immunoreactive material in axons of Alzheimer's disease. *Neuroreport* 8: 3685-3689.

61. Dickson DW (1997) The pathogenesis of senile plaques. *J Neuropathol Exp Neurol* 56: 321-339.

62. Dickson DW, Crystal HA, Bevona C, Honer W, Vincent I, Davies P (1995) Correlations of synaptic and pathological markers with cognition of the elderly. *Neurobiol Aging* 16: 285-304.

63. Dickson DW, Crystal HA, Mattiace LA, Masur DM, Blau AD, Davies P, Yen SH, Aronson MK (1991) Identification of normal and pathological aging in prospectively studied nondemented elderly humans. *Neurobiol Aging* 13: 179-189.

64. Dickson DW, Ksiezak-Reding H, Davies P, Yen SH (1987) A monoclonal antibody that recognizes a phosphorylated epitope in Alzheimer's neurofibrillary tangles, neurofilaments and tau proteins immunostains granulovacuolar degeneration. *Acta Neuropathol (Berl)* 73: 254-258.

65. Dickson DW, Lee SC, Mattiace LA, Yen S-HC, Brosnan CF (1993) Microglia and cytokines in neurological disease, with special reference to AIDS and Alzheimer's disease. *Glia* 7: 75-83.

66. Dickson DW, Liu WK, Kress Y, Ku J, DeJesus O, Yen SH (1993) Phosphorylated tau immunoreactivity of granulovacuolar bodies (GVB) of Alzheimer's disease: localization of two amino terminal tau epitopes in GVB. *Acta Neuropathol (Berl)* 85: 463-470.

67. Dickson TC, King CE, McCormack GH, Vickers JC (1999) Neurochemical diversity of dystrophic neurites in the early and late stages of Alzheimer's disease. *Exp Neurol* 156: 100-110.

68. Dickson TC, Saunders HL, Vickers JC (1997) Relationship between apolipoprotein E and the amyloid deposits and dystrophic neurites of Alzheimer's disease. *Neuropathol Appl Neurobiol* 23: 483-491.

69. Di Patre PL, Gelman BB (1997) Microglial cell activation in aging and Alzheimer disease: partial linkage with neurofibrillary tangle burden in the hippocampus. *J Neuropathol Exp Neurol* 56: 143-149.

70. Di Patre PL, Read SL, Cummings JL, Tomiyasu U, Vartavarian LM, Secor DL, Vinters HV (1999) Progression of clinical deterioration and pathological changes in patients with Alzheimer disease evaluated at biopsy and autopsy. *Arch Neurol* 56: 1254-1261.

71. Doucette R, Fishman M, Hachinski VC, Mershkey H (1986) Cell loss from the nucleus basalis of Meynert in Alzheimer's disease. *Can J Neurol Sci* 13: 435-440.

72. Dragunow M, Faull RL, Lawlor P, Beilharz EJ, Singleton K, Walker EB, Mee E (1995) In situ evidence for DNA fragmentation in Huntington's disease striatum and Alzheimer's disease temporal lobes. *Neuroreport* 6: 1053-1057.

73. Duyckaerts C, Bennecib M, Grignon Y, Uchihara T, He Y, Piette F, Hauw J-J (1997) Modeling the relation between neurofibrillary tangles and intellectual status. *Neurobiol Aging* 18: 267-273.

74. Duyckaerts C, Colle MA, Seilhean D, Hauw J-J (1998) Laminar spongiosis of the dentate gyrus: a sign of disconnection, present in cases of Alzheimer disease. *Acta Neuropathol (Berl)* 95: 413-420

75. Duyckaerts C, Delaère P, Hauw J-J, Abbamondi-Pinto AL, Sorbi S, Allen I, Brion J-P, Flament-Durand J, Duchen L, Kauss J, Sclote W, Lowe J, Probst A, Ravid R, Swaab DF, Renkawek K, Tomlinson B (1990) Rating of the lesions in senile dementia of the Alzheimer type: concordance between laboratories. A

European multicenter study under the auspices of Eurage. *J Neurol Sci* 97: 295-323.

76. Duyckaerts C, Hauw J-J, Piette F, Rainsard C, Poulain V, Berthaux P, Escourolle R (1985) Cortical atrophy in senile dementia of the Alzheimer type is mainly due to a decrease in cortical length. *Acta Neuropathol (Berl)* 66: 72-74.

77. Eikelenboom P, Stam FC (1984) An immunohistochemical study on cerebral vascular and senile plaque amyloid in Alzheimer's dementia. *Virchows Arch (Cell Pathol)* 47: 17-25.

78. Esiri MM, Hyman BT, Beyreuther K, Masters Cl (1997) Ageing and dementia. In *Greenfield's neuropathology*, DI Graham, P Lantos (eds) , 6th ed. Arnold: London, pp. 153-234.

79. Esiri MM, Wilcock GK (1984) The olfactory bulbs in Alzheimer's disease. *J Neurol Neurosurg Psychiatry* 47: 56-60.

80. Ferrer I, Aymami A, Rovira A, Grau-Veciana JM (1983) Growth of abnormal neurites in atypical Alzheimer's disease. A study with the Golgi method. *Acta Neuropathol (Berl)* 59: 167-170.

81. Ferrer I, Blanco R (2000) N-myc and c-myc expression in Alzheimer disease, Huntington disease and Parkinson disease. *Mol Brain Res* 77: 270-276.

82. Flament-Durand J, Couck AM (1979) Spongiform alterations in brain biopsies of presenile dementia. *Acta Neuropathol (Berl)* 46: 159-162.

83. Fliers E, Swaab DF, Pool CW, Verwer RW (1985) The vasopressin and oxytocin neurons in the human supraoptic and paraventricular nucleus, changes with aging and in senile dementia. *Brain Res* 342: 45-53.

84. Fukutani Y, Cairns NJ, Rossor MN, Lantos PL (1997) Cerebellar pathology in sporadic and familial Alzheimer's disease including APP 717 (Val→Ile) mutation cases: a morphometric investigation. *J Neurol Sci* 149: 177-184.

85. Galloway PG, Perry G, Gambetti P (1987) Hirano body filaments contain actin and actin-associated proteins. *J Neuropathol Exp Neurol* 46: 185-199.

86. Galloway PG, Perry G, Kosik KS, Gambetti P (1987) Hirano bodies contain tau protein. *Brain Res* 403: 337.

87. German DC, Manaye KF, White CL 3d, Woodward DJ, McIntire DD, Smith WK, Kalaria RN, Mann DM (1992) Disease-specific patterns of locus coeruleus cell loss. *Ann Neurol* 32: 667-676.

88. Gibb WR, Mountjoy CQ, Mann DM, Lees AJ (1989) The substantia nigra and ventral tegmental area in Alzheimer's disease and Down's syndrome. *J Neurol Neurosurg Psychiatry* 52: 193-200.

89. Gibson PH, Tomlinson BE (1977) Numbers of Hirano bodies in the hippocampus of normal and demented people with Alzheimer's disease. *J Neurol Sci* 33: 199-206.

90. Gilmor, ML, Erickson, JD, Varoqui, H, Hersh, LB, Bennett, DA, Cochran, EJ, Mufson, EJ, Levey, AI (1999) Preservation of nucleus basalis neurons containing choline acetyltransferase and the vesicular acetylcholine transporter in the elderly with mild cognitive impairment and early Alzheimer's disease. *J Comp Neurol* 411: 693-704.

91. Glenner GG (1980) Amyloid deposits and amyloidosis. The β-fibrilloses. *New Engl J Med* 302: 1283-1292.

92. Glenner GG, Wong CW (1984) Alzheimer's disease and Down's syndrome: sharing of a unique cerebrovascular amyloid fibril protein. *Biochem Biophys Res Comm* 122: 1131-1135.

93. Glenner GG, Wong CW (1984) Alzheimer's disease: Initial report of the purification and characterization of a novel cerebrovascular amyloid protein. *Biochem Biophys Res Comm*un 120: 885-890.

94. Goldman JE (1983) The association of actin with Hirano bodies. *J Neuropathol Exp Neurol* 42: 146-152.

95. Gomez-Isla T, Hollister R, West H, Mui S, Growdon JH, Petersen RC, Parisi JE, Hyman, BT (1997) Neuronal loss correlates with but exceeds neurofibrillary tangles in Alzheimer's disease *Ann Neurol* 41: 17-24.

96. Gomez-Isla T, Price JL, McKeel DW, Morris JC, Growdon JH, Hyman BT (1996) Profound loss of layer II entorhinal cortex neurons occurs in very mild Alzheimer's disease. *J Neurosci* 16: 4491-4500.

97. Gonatas NK, Anderson W, Evangelista I (1967) The contribution of altered synapses in the senile plaque: an electron microscopic study in Alzheimer's dementia. *J Neuropathol Exp Neurol* 26: 25-39.

98. Good PF, Werner P, Hsu A, Olanow CW, Perl DP (1996) Evidence of neuronal oxidative damage in Alzheimer's disease. *Am J Pathol* 149: 21-28.

99. Gray EG (1986) Spongiform encephalopathy: a neurocytologist's viewpoint with a note on Alzheimer's disease. *Neuropathol Appl Neurobiol* 12: 149-172.

100. Grignon Y, Duyckaerts C, Bennecib M, Hauw J-J (1998) Cytoarchitectonic alterations in the supramarginal gyrus of late onset Alzheimer's disease. *Acta Neuropathol (Berl)* 95: 395-406.

101. Grundke-Iqbal I, Iqbal K, Tung YC, Quinlan H, Wiesniewski HM (1986) Abnormal phosphorylation of the microtubule associated protein (tau) in Alzheimer cytoskeletal pathology. *Proc Natl Acad Sci U S A* 83: 4913-4917.

102. Gyure KA, Durham R, Stewart WF, Smialek JE, Troncoso JC (2001) Intraneuronal aβ-amyloid precedes development of amyloid plaques in Down syndrome. *Arch Pathol Lab Med* 125: 489-492.

103. Hamos JE, DeGennaro LJ, Drachman DA (1989) Synaptic loss in Alzheimer's disease and other dementias. *Neurology* 39: 355-361.

104. Hansen LA, DeTeresa R, Davies P, Terry RD (1988) Neocortical morphometry, lesion counts, and choline acetyltransferase levels in the age spectrum of Alzheimer's disease. *Neurology* 38: 48-54.

105. Hansen LA, Masliah E, Galasko D, Terry RD (1993) Plaque-only Alzheimer disease is usually the Lewy body variant and vice versa. *J Neuropathol Exp Neurol* 52: 648-654.

106. Hansen LA, Masliah E, Terry RD, Mirra SS (1989) A neuropathological subset of Alzheimer's disease with concomitant Lewy body disease and spongiform change. *Acta Neuropathol (Berl)* 78: 194-201.

107. Hauw J-J, Duyckaerts C (2001) Alzheimer disease. In *Pathology of the aging nervous system* (2nd ed.) Duckett S, De La Torre JC (Eds.), Oxford University Press (New York) pp. 207-263.

108. Hauw J-J, Seilhean D, Duyckaerts C (1998) Cerebral amyloid angiopathy. In *Cerebrovascular disease. Pathophysiology, diagnosis and management*, MD Ginsberg, J Bogousslavsky (eds) Blackwell Scientific: Cambridge, pp. 1772-1795.

109. Hauw J-J, Vignolo P, Duyckaerts C, Beck M, Forette F, Henry JF, Laurent M, Piette F, Sachet A, Berthaux P (1986) Etude neuropathologique de 12 centenaires: la fréquence de la démence sénile de type Alzheimer n'est pas particulièrement élevée dans ce groupe de personnes très agées. *Rev Neurol (Paris)* 142: 107-115.

110. Heinonen O, Soininen H, Sorvari H, Kosunen O, Paljarvi L, Koivisto E, Riekkinen PJ Sr (1995) Loss of synaptophysin-like immunoreactivity in the hippocampal formation is an early phenomenon in Alzheimer's disease. *Neuroscience* 64: 375-384.

111. Hempen B, Brion JP (1996) Reduction of acetylated alpha-tubulin immunoreactivity in neurofibrillary tangle-bearing neurons in Alzheimer's disease. *J Neuropathol Exp Neurol* 55: 964-972.

112. Herzog AG, Kemper TL (1980) Amygdaloid changes in aging and dementia. *Arch Neurol* 37: 625-629.

113. Hirano A (1984) *Atlas of Neuropathology*. Lippincott: Philadelphia pp. 97-107 .

114. Hirano A (1994) Hirano bodies and related neuronal inclusions. *Neuropathol Appl Neurobiol* 20: 3-11.

115. Hirano A, Zimmerman HM (1962) Alzheimer's neurofibrillary changes. A topographical study. *Arch Neurol* 7: 227-242.

116. Hof PR, Archin N, Osmand AP, Dougherty JH, Wells C, Bouras C, Morrison JH (1993) Posterior cortical atrophy in Alzheimer's disease: analysis of a new case and re-evaluation of a historical report. *Acta Neuropathol (Berl)* 86: 215-223.

117. Höhman C, Antuono P, Coyle JT (1988) Basal forebrain cholinergic neurons and Alzheimer's disease. In *Psychopharmacology of the aging nervous system*, Iversen LL, Iversen SD, SH Snyder (eds). Plenum Press: New-York, pp. 69-106.

118. Hoogendijk WJ, Sommer IE, Pool CW, Kamphorst W, Hofman MA, Eikelenboom P, Swaab DF (1999) Lack of association between depression and loss of neurons in the locus coeruleus in Alzheimer disease. *Arch Gen Psychiatry* 56: 45-51.

119. Houlden H, Baker M, McGowan E, Lewis P, Hutton M, Crook R, Wood NW, Kumar-Singh S, Geddes J, Swash M, Scaravilli F, Holton JL, Lashley T, Tomita T, Hashimoto T, Verkkoniemi A, Kalimo H, Somer M, Paetau A. Martin JJ, Van Broeckhoven C, Golde T, Hardy J, Haltia M, Revesz T (2000) Variant Alzheimer's disease with spastic paraparesis and cotton wool plaques is caused by PS-1 mutations that lead to exceptionally high amyloid-b concentrations. *Ann Neurol* 48: 806-808.

120. Hubbard BM, Anderson JM (1981) A quantitative study of cerebral atrophy in old age and senile dementia. *J Neurol Sci* 50: 135-145.

121. Hubbard BM, Anderson JM (1981) Age, senile dementia and ventricular enlargement. *J Neurol Neurosurg Psychiat* 44: 631-635.

122. Hyman BT, van Hoesen GW, Damasio AR (1990) Memory-related neural systems in Alzheimer's disease: an anatomical study. *Neurology* 40: 1721-1730.

123. Ihara Y (1988) Massive somato-dendritic sprouting of cortical neurons in Alzheimer's disease. *Brain Res* 459: 138-144.

124. Ikeda K, Akiyama H, Arai T, Oda T, Kato M, Iseki E, Kosaka K, Wakabayashi K, Takahashi H (1999) Clinical aspects of 'senile dementia of the tangle type'— a subset of dementia in the senium separable from late-onset Alzheimer's disease. *Dement Geriatr Cogn Disord* 10: 6-11.

125. Ikeda S, Allsop D, Glenner GG (1989) Morphology and distribution of plaque and related deposits in the brains of Alzheimer's disease and control cases. An immunohistochemical study using amyloid β-protein antibody. *Lab Invest* 60: 113-122.

126. Jellinger K (1977) Cerebral hemorrhage in amyloid angiopathy. *Ann Neurol* 1: 604.

127. Joachim CL, Morris JH, Selkoe DJ, Kosik KS (1987) Tau epitopes are incorporated into a range of lesions in Alzheimer's disease. *J Neuropathol Exp Neurol* 46: 611-622.

128. Johnson J K, Head E, Kim R, Starr A and Cotman C W (1999). Clinical and pathological evidence for a frontal variant of Alzheimer disease. *Arch Neurol* 56: 1233-1239.

129. Kahn J, Anderton BH, Probst A, Ulrich J, Esiri M (1985) Immunologic studies of granulovacuolar degeneration using monoclonal antibodies to neurofilaments. *J Neurol Neurosurg Psychiatry* 48: 926-927.

130. Kemper T (1984) Neuroanatomical and neuropathological changes in normal aging and dementia. In *Clinical Neurology of Aging*, LM Albert (ed). Oxford University Press: New York, pp. 9-52.

131. Khachaturian ZS (1985) Diagnosis of Alzheimer's disease. *Arch Neurol* 42: 1097-1105.

132. Kidd M (1964) Alzheimer's disease. An electron microscopical study. *Brain* 87: 307-320.

133. Kimchi EY, Kajdasz S, Bacskai BJ, Hyman BT (2001) Analysis of cerebral amyloid angiopathy in a transgenic mouse model of Alzheimer disease using in vivo multiphoton microscopy. *J Neuropathol Exp Neurol* 60: 274-279.

134. Kosik KS, Joachim CL, Selkoe, DJ (1986) Microtubule-associated protein tau is a major component of paired helical filaments in Alzheimer disease. *Proc Natl Acad Sci U S A* 83: 4044-4048.

135. Kowall NW, Kosik KS (1987) Axonal disruption and aberrant localization of tau protein characterize the neuropil pathology of Alzheimer's disease. *Ann Neurol* 22: 639-643.

136. Kremer B, Swaab D, Bots G, Fisser B, Ravid R, Roos R (1991) The hypothalamic lateral tuberal nucleus in Alzheimer's disease. *Ann Neurol* 29: 279-284.

137. Kumar-Singh S, Cras P, Wang R, Kros JM, van Swieten J, Lubke U, Ceuterick C, Serneels S, Vennekens K, Timmermans JP, Van Marck E, Martin JJ, van Duijn CM, Van Broeckhoven C (2002) Dense-core senile plaques in the Flemish variant of Alzheimer's disease are vasocentric. *Am J Pathol* 161: 507-520.

138. Lamy C, Duyckaerts C, Delaère P, Payan C, Fermanian J, Poulain V, Hauw J-J (1989) Comparison of seven staining methods for senile plaques and neurofibrillary tangles in a prospective study of 15 elderly patients. *Neuropath Appl Neurobiol* 15: 563-578.

139. Lassmann H (1996) Patterns of synaptic and nerve cell pathology in Alzheimer's disease. *Behav Brain Res* 78: 9-14.

140. Lassmann H, Bancher C, Breitschopf H, Wegiel J, Bobinski M, Jellinger K, Wisniewski, HM (1995) Cell death in Alzheimer's disease evaluated by DNA fragmentation in situ. *Acta Neuropathol (Berl)* 89: 35-41.

141. Lassmann H, Weiler R, Fischer P, Bancher C, Jellinger K, Floor E, Danielczyk W, Seitelberger F, Winkler H (1992) Synaptic pathology in Alzheimer's disease: immunological data for markers of synaptic and large dense-core vesicles. *Neuroscience* 46: 1-8.

142. Le TV, Crook R, Hardy J, Dickson DW (2001). Cotton wool plaques in non-familial late-onset Alzheimer disease. *J Neuropathol Exp Neurol* 60: 1051-1061.

143. Lehéricy S, Hirsch EC, Cervera-Piérot P, Hersh LB, Bakchine S, Piette F, Duyckaerts C, Hauw JJ, Javoy-Agid F, Agid Y (1993) Heterogeneity and selectivity of the degeneration of cholinergic neurons in the basal forebrain of patients with Alzheimer's disease. *J Comp Neurol* 330: 15-31.

144. Levy E, Carman MD, Fernandez-Madrid IJ, Power MD, Lieberburg I, van Duinen SG, Bots GT, Luyendijk W, Frangione B (1990) Mutation of the Alzheimer's disease amyloid gene in hereditary cerebral hemorrhage, Dutch type. *Science* 248: 1124-1126.

145. Liu W-K, Williams RT, Hall FL, Dickson DW, Yen S-H (1995) Detection of a cdc2-related kinase associated with Alzheimer paired helical filaments. *Am J Pathol* 146: 228-238.

146. Lucassen PJ, Chung WC, Kamphorst W, Swaab DF (1997) DNA damage distribution in the human brain as shown by in situ end labeling, area-specific differences in aging and Alzheimer disease in the absence of apoptotic morphology. *J Neuropathol Exp Neurol* 56: 887-900.

147. Luxenberg JS, Haxby JV, Creasey H, Sundaram M, Rapoport SI (1987) Rate of ventricular enlargement in dementia of the Alzheimer type correlates with rate of neuropsychological deterioration. *Neurology* 37: 1135-1140.

148. MacGibbon GA, Lawlor PA, Walton M, Sirimanne E, Faull RL, Synek B, Mee E, Connor B, Dragunow M (1997) Expression of Fos, Jun, and Krox family proteins in Alzheimer's disease. *Exp Neurol* 147: 316-332.

149. Mandybur TI, Bates SRD (1978) Fatal massive intracerebral hemorrhage complicating cerebral amyloid angiopathy. *Arch Neurol* 35: 246-248.

150. Mandybur TI, Chuirazzi CC (1990) Astrocytes and the plaques of Alzheimer's disease. *Neurology* 40: 635-639.

151. Mann DM, Takeuchi A, Sato S, Cairns NJ, Lantos PL, Rossor MN, Haltia M, Kalimo H, Iwatsubo T (2001) Cases of Alzheimer's disease due to deletion of exon 9 of the presenilin-1 gene show an unusual but characteristic β-amyloid pathology known as 'cotton wool' plaques. *Neuropathol Appl Neurobiol* 27: 189-196.

152. Mann DMA (1988) Neuropathology and neurochemical aspects of Alzheimer's disease. In *Psychopharmacology of the Aging Nervous System, Handbook of Psychopharmacology.* LL Iversen, SD Iversen, SH Snyder (eds) Plenum Press: New York, pp. 1-67.

153. Mann DMA (1991) The topographic distribution of brain atrophy in Alzheimer's disease. *Acta Neuropathol (Berl)* 83: 81-86.

154. Mann DMA, Esiri MM (1989) The pattern of acquisition of plaques and tangles in the brains of patients under 50 years of age with Down's syndrome. *J Neurol Sci* 89: 169-179.

155. Mann DMA, Iwatsubo T, Snowden J S (1996) Atypical amyloid (Aβ) deposition in the cerebellum in Alzheimer's disease: an immunohistochemical study using end-specific A beta monoclonal antibodies. *Acta Neuropathol (Berl)* 91: 647-653.

156. Mann DMA, Marcyniuk B, Yates PO, Neary D, Snowden JS (1988) The progression of the pathological changes of Alzheimer's disease in frontal and temporal neocortex both at biopsy and autopsy. *Neuropathol Appl Neurobiol* 14: 177-195.

157. Mann DMA, Yates PO, Marcyniuk B (1985) Changes in Alzheimer's disease in the magnocellular neurones of the supraoptic and paraventricular nuclei of the hypothalamus and their relationship to the noradrenergic deficit. *Clin Neuropathol* 4: 127-134.

158. Mann DMA, Yates PO, Marcyniuk B (1985) Some morphometric observations on the *Cerebral Cortex* and hippocampus in presenile Alzheimer's disease, senile dementia of Alzheimer type and Down's syndrome in middle age. *J Neurol Sci* 69: 139-159.

159. Marcyniuk B, Mann DMA, Yates PO (1986) The topography of cell loss from locus coeruleus in Alzheimer's disease. *J Neurol Sci* 76: 335-345.

160. Masliah E, Terry RD, DeTeresa RM, Hansen LA (1989) Immunohistochemical quantification of the synapse-related protein synaptophysin in Alzheimer disease. *Neurosci Lett* 103: 234-239.

161. Masliah E, Terry RD, Mallory M, Alford M, Hansen LA (1990) Diffuse plaques do not accentuate synapse loss in Alzheimer's disease. *Am J Pathol* 137: 1293-1297.

162. Masters CL, Simms G, Weinman NA, Multhaup G, McDonald BL, Beyreuter K (1985) Amyloid plaque core protein in Alzheimer disease and Down syndrome. *Proc Natl Acad Sci U S A* 82: 4245-4249.

163. Matsuo ES, Shin RW, Billingsley ML, van deVoorde A, O'Connor M, Trojanowski JQ, Lee VMY (1994) Biopsy-derived adult human tau is phosphorylated at many of the same sites as Alzheimer's disease paired helical filament tau. *Neuron* 13: 989-1002.

164. McGeer PL, Akiyama H, Itagaki S, McGeer EG (1989) Complement activation in amyloid plaques in Alzheimer's dementia. *Neurosci Lett* 107: 341-346.

165. McGeer PL, Kawamata T, Walker DG, Akiyama H, Tooyama I, McGeer E (1993) Microglia in degenerative neurological diseases. *Glia* 7: 84-92.

166. Mesulam MM (1987) Primary progressive aphasia: differentiation from Alzheimer's disease. *Ann Neurol* 22: 533-534.

167. Migheli A, Cavalla P, Marino S, Schiffer D (1994) A study of apoptosis in normal and pathologic nervous tissue after in situ end-labeling of DNA strand breaks. *J Neuropathol Exp Neurol* 53: 606-616.

168. Mirra SS, Gearing M, McKeel DW, Crain BJ, Hughes JP, Van Belle G, Heyman A (1994) Inter-laboratory comparison of neuropathology assessments in Alzheimer's disease: a study of the consortium to establish a registry for Alzheimer's disease (CERAD). *J Neuropathol Exp Neurol* 53: 303-315.

169. Mirra SS, Heyman A, McKeel D, Sumi SM, Crain BJ, Brownlee LM, Vogel FS, Hughes JP, van Belle G, Berg L (1991) The consortium to establish a registry for Alzheimer's disease (CERAD). Part II. Standardization of the neuropathological assessment of Alzheimer's disease. *Neurology* 41: 479-486.

170. Miyakawa T, Katsuragi S, Yamashita K, Ohuchi K (1994) Morphological investigation of neurofibrillary tangles in Alzheimer's disease. *Jap J Psychiatry Neurol* 48: 43-47.

171. Mochizuki A, Peterson JW, Mufson EJ, Trapp BD (1996) Amyloid load and neural elements in Alzheimer's disease and nondemented individuals with high amyloid plaque density. *Exp Neurol* 142: 89-102.

172. Morel F, Wildi E (1952) General and cellular pathochemistry of senile and presenile alterations of the brain. In *Proceedings of the First International Congress of Neuropathology* Torino, Rosenberg, Sellier (eds) , vol 2, pp. 347-374.

173. Mori T, Paris D, Town T, Rojiani AM, Sparks DL, Delledonne A, Crawford F, Abdullah LI, Humphrey JA, Dickson DW, Mullan MJ (2001) Cholesterol accumulates in senile plaques of Alzheimer disease patients and in transgenic APP(SW) mice. *J Neuropathol Exp Neurol* 60: 778-785.

174. Morris JC, Storandt M, McKeel DW Jr, Rubin EH, Price JL, Grant EA, Berg L (1996) Cerebral amyloid deposition and diffuse plaques in "normal" aging: evidence for presymptomatic and very mild Alzheimer's disease. *Neurology* 46: 707-719.

175. Mountjoy CQ (1986) Correlations between neuropathological and neurochemical changes. *Brit Med Bull* 42: 81-85.

176. Mukaetova-Ladinska EB, Harrington CR, Roth M, Wischik CM (1993) Biochemical and anatomical redistribution of tau protein in Alzheimer's disease. *Am J Pathol* 143: 565-578.

177. Mullaart E, Boerrigter ME, Ravid R, Swaab DF, Vijg J (1990) Increased levels of DNA breaks in *Cerebral Cortex* of Alzheimer's disease patients. *Neurobiol Aging* 11: 169-173.

178. Munch G, Cunningham AM, Riederer P, Braak E (1998) Advanced glycation endproducts are associated with Hirano bodies in Alzheimer's disease. *Brain Res* 796: 307-310.

179. Munoz DG, Wang D (1992) Tangle-associated neuritic clusters. A new lesion in Alzheimer's disease and aging suggests that aggregates of dystrophic neurites are not necessarily associated with β/A4. *Am J Pathol* 140: 1167-1178.

180. Munoz DG, Wang D, Greenberg BD (1993) Hirano bodies accumulate C-Terminal sequence of β-amyloid precursor protein (β-APP) epitopes. *J Neuropathol Exp Neurol* 52: 14-21.

181. Nagy Z, Esiri MM, Smith AD (1998) The cell division cycle and the pathophysiology of Alzheimer's disease. *Neuroscience* 87: 731-739.

182. Najlerahim A, Bowen DM (1989) Regional weight loss in the *Cerebral Cortex* and some subcortical nuclei in senile dementia of the Alzheimer type. *Acta Neuropathol (Berl)* 75: 509-512.

183. Neuropathology Group of the Medical research Council Cognitive Function and Ageing Study (MRC CFAS) (2001) Pathology correlates of late-onset dementia in a multicentre, community-based population in England and Wales. *Lancet* 357: 169-175.

184. Ohtsubo K, Izumiyama N, Kuzuhara S, Mori H, Shimada H (1990) Curly fibers are tau-positive strands in the pre- and post-synaptic neurites, consisting of paired helical filaments: observations by the freeze-etch and replica method. *Acta Neuropathol (Berl)* 81: 111-115.

185. Pantelakis S (1954) Un type particulier d'angiopathie sénile du système nerveux central: L'angiopathie congophile. Topographie et fréquence. *Monatsschr Psychiatr Neurol* 128: 219-256.

186. Peers MC, Lenders MB, Defossez A, Delacourte A, Mazzuca M (1988) Cortical angiopathy in Alzheimer's disease: the formation of dystrophic perivascular neurites is related to the exudation of amyloid fibrils from the pathological vessels. *Virchow Arch A Pathol Anat* 414: 15-20.

187. Pei JJ, Braak E, Braak H, Grundke-Iqbal I, Iqbal K, Winblad B, Cowburn RF (1999) Distribution of active glycogen synthase kinase 3b (GSK-3b) in brains staged for Alzheimer disease neurofibrillary changes. *J Neuropathol Exp Neurol* 58: 1010-1019.

188. Perlmutter LS, Barron E, Myers M, Saperia D, Chui HC (1995) Localization of amyloid P component in human brain: vascular staining patterns and association with Alzheimer's disease lesions. *J Comp Neurol* 352: 92-105.

189. Perry G, Kawai M, Tabaton M, Onrato M, Mulvihill P, Richey P, Morandi A, Connolly JA, Gambetti P (1991) Neuropil threads of Alzheimer's disease show a marked alteration of the normal cytoskeleton. *J Neurosci* 11: 1748-1755.

190. Pogacar S, Williams RS (1984) Alzheimer's disease presenting as slowly progressive aphasia. *R I Med J* 67: 181-185.

191. Pollanen MS, Markiewicz P, Goh MC (1997) Paired helical filaments are twisted ribbons composed of two parallel and aligned components : image reconstruction and modeling of filament structure using atomic force microscopy. *J Neuropathol Exp Neurol* 56: 79-85.

192. Poppe W, Tennstedt A (1969) Studie über hirnatrophische Prozesse unter besondere Berücksichtigung des Morbus Pick und des Morbus Alzheimer. Fischer Verlag: Jena.

193. Price DL, Altschuler RJ, Struble RG, Casanova MF, Cork LC, Murphy DB (1986) Sequestration of tubulin in neurons in Alzheimer's disease. *Brain Res* 385: 305-310.

194. Probst A, Basler V, Bron B, Ulrich J (1983) Neuritic plaques in senile dementia of the Alzheimer type: a Golgi analysis in the hippocampal region. *Brain Res* 268: 249-254.

195. Probst A, Herzig MC, Mistl C, Ipsen S, Tolnay M (2001) Perisomatic granules (non-plaque dystrophic neurites) of hippocampal CA1 in Alzheimer's disease and Pick's disease: a lesion distinct from granulovacuolar degeneration. *Acta Neuropathol (Berl)* 102: 636-644.

196. Raina AK, Zhu X, Monteiro M, Takeda A, Smith MA (2000) Abortive oncogeny and cell cycle-mediated events in Alzheimer disease. *Prog Cell Cycle Res* 4: 235-242.

197. Regeur L, Badsberg Jensen G, Pakkenberg H, Evans SM, Pakkenberg B (1994) No global neocortical nerve cell loss in brains from patients with senile dementia of Alzheimer's type. *Neurobiol Aging* 15: 347-352.

198. Roher AE, Lowenson JD, Clarke S, Wood AS, Cotter RJ, Gowing E, Ball M. (1993) β-Amyloid-(1-42) is a major component of cerebrovascular amyloid deposits: Implications for the pathology of Alzheimer disease. *Proc Natl Acad Sci U S A* 90: 10836-10840.

199. Rüb U, Del Tredici K, Schultz C, Buttner-Ennever JA, Braak H (2001) The premotor region essential for rapid vertical eye movements shows early involvement in Alzheimer's disease-related cytoskeletal pathology. *Vision Res* 41: 2149-2156.

200. Rüb U, Del Tredici K, Schultz C, Thal DR, Braak E, Braak H (2000) The evolution of Alzheimer's disease-related cytoskeletal pathology in the human raphe nuclei. *Neuropathol Appl Neurobiol* 26: 553-567.

201. Rüb U, Del Tredici K, Schultz C, Thal DR, Braak E, Braak H (2001) The autonomic higher order processing nuclei of the lower brain stem are among the early targets of the Alzheimer's disease-related cytoskeletal pathology. *Acta Neuropathol (Berl)* 101: 555-564.

202. Rüb U, Schultz C, Del Tredici K, Braak H (2001) Early involvement of the tegmentopontine reticular nucleus during the evolution of Alzheimer's disease-related cytoskeletal pathology. *Brain Res* 908: 107-112.

203. Ruben GC, Iqbal K, Grundke-Iqbal I (1995) Helical ribbon morphology in neurofibrillary tangles of paired helical filaments. In *Research Advances in Alzheimer's Disease and Related Disorders*, K Iqbal, JA Mortimer, B Winblad, HM Wisniewski (eds). John Wiley & Son Ltd: Chichester, pp. 477-485.

204. Sasaki N, Fukatsu R, Tsuzuki K, Hayashi Y, Yoshida T, Fujii N, Koike T, Wakayama I, Yanagihara R, Garruto R, Amano N, Makita Z (1998) Advanced glycation end products in Alzheimer's disease and other neurodegenerative diseases. *Am J Pathol* 153: 1149-1155.

205. Sassin I, Schultz C, Thal DR, Rub U, Arai K, Braak E, Braak H (2000) Evolution of Alzheimer's disease-related cytoskeletal changes in the basal nucleus of Meynert. *Acta Neuropathol (Berl)* 100: 259-269.

206. Schechter R, Yen SH, Terry RD (1981) Fibrous astrocytes in senile dementia of the Alzheimer type. *J Neuropathol Exp Neurol* 40: 95-101.

207. Scheff SW, DeKosky ST, Price DA (1990) Quantitative assessment of cortical synaptic density in Alzheimer's disease. *Neurobiol Aging* 11: 29-37.

208. Scheff SW, Price DA (1993) Synapse loss in the temporal lobe in Alzheimer's disease *Ann Neurol* 33: 190-199.

209. Schmidt ML, DiDario AG, Lee VM, Trojanowski JQ (1994) An extensive network of PHF tau-rich dystrophic neurites permeates neocortex and nearly all neuritic and diffuse amyloid plaques in Alzheimer disease. *FEBS Letters* 344: 69-73.

210. Schmidt ML, Lee VM-Y, Trojanowski JQ (1989) Analysis of epitopes shared by Hirano bodies and neurofilament protein in normal and Alzheimer's disease hippocampus.*Lab Invest* 60: 513-522.

211. Scholz W (1938) Studien zur Pathologie der Hirngefässe II. Die drusige Entartung der Hirnarterien und Capillaren *Z gesamte Neurol Psychiatr* 162: 694-715.

212. Schwab C, Steele JC, McGeer EG, McGeer PL (1997) Amyloid P immunoreactivity precedes C4d deposition on extracellular neurofibrillary tangles. *Acta Neuropathol (Berl)* 93: 87-92.

213. Shimohama S, Kamiya S, Taniguchi T, Akagawa K, Kimura J (1997) Differential involvement of synaptic vesicle and presynaptic plasma membrane proteins in Alzheimer's disease. *Biochem Biophys Res Commun* 236: 239-242.

214. Smith MA, Kutty RK, Richey PL, Yan SD. Stern D, Chader GJ, Wiggert B, Petersen RB, Perry G (1994) Heme oxygenase-1 is associated with the neurofibrillary pathology of Alzheimer's disease. *Am J Pathol* 145: 42-47 .

215. Smith TW, Anwer U, DeGirolami U, Drachman DA (1987) Vacuolar change in Alzheimer's disease. *Arch Neurol* 44: 1225-1228.

216. Snow AD, Sekiguchi R, Nochlin D, Fraser P, Kimata K, Mizutani A, Arai M, Schreier WA, Morgan DG (1994) An important role of heparan sulfate proteoglycan (Perlecan) in a model system for the deposition and persistence of fibrillar A β-amyloid in rat brain. *Neuron* 12: 219-234.

217. Stadelmann C, Bruck W, Bancher C, Jellinger K, Lassmann H (1998) Alzheimer disease: DNA fragmentation indicates increased neuronal vulnerability, but not apoptosis. *J Neuropathol Exp Neurol* 57: 456-464.

218. Stadelmann C, Deckwerth TL, Srinivasan A, Bancher C, Bruck W, Jellinger K, Lassmann H (1999) Activation of caspase-3 in single neurons and autophagic granules of granulovacuolar degeneration in Alzheimer's disease. Evidence for apoptotic cell death. *Am J Pathol* 155: 1459-1466.

219. Stoltzner SE, Grenfell TJ, Mori C, Wisniewski KE, Wisniewski TM, Selkoe DJ, Lemere CA (2000) Temporal accrual of complement proteins in amyloid plaques in Down's syndrome with Alzheimer's disease. *Am J Pathol* 156: 489-499.

220. Su JH, Zhao M, Anderson AJ, Srinivasan A, Cotman CW (2001) Activated caspase-3 expression in Alzheimer's and aged control brain: correlation with Alzheimer pathology. *Brain Res* 898: 350-357.

221. Suzuki N, Iwatsubo T, Odaka A, Ishibashi Y, Kitada C, Ihara Y (1994) High tissue content of soluble A,1-40 is linked to cerebral amyloid angiopathy. *Am J Pathol* 145: 452-460.

222. Swaab DF, Fliers E, Partiman TS (1985) The suprachiasmatic nucleus of the human brain in relation to sex, age and senile dementia. *Brain Res* 342: 37-44.

223. Tagliavini F, Giaccone G, Frangione B, Bugiani P (1988) Preamyloid deposits in the *Cerebral Cortex* of patients with Alzheimer's disease and nondemented individuals. *Neurosci Lett* 93: 191-196.

224. Takahashi M, Iseki E, Kosaka K (2000) Cdk5 and munc-18/p67 co-localization in early stage neurofibrillary tangles-bearing neurons in Alzheimer type dementia brains. *J Neurol Sci* 172: 63-69.

225. ter Laak HJ, Renkawek K, van Workum FP (1994) The olfactory bulb in Alzheimer disease: a morphologic study of neuron loss, tangles, and senile plaques in relation to olfaction. *Alzheimer Dis Assoc Disord* 8: 38-48.

226. Terry RD, Hansen L A, DeTeresa R, Davies P, Tobias H and Katzman R (1987). Senile dementia of the Alzheimer type without neocortical neurofibrillary tangles. *J Neuropathol Exp Neurol* 46: 262-268.

227. Terry RD (1985) Alzheimer's disease. In *Neuropathology*, L Davis, DM Robertson (eds). Williams & Wilkins: Baltimore, pp. 824-841.

228. Terry RD, DeTeresa R, Hansen LA (1987) Neocortical cell counts in normal human adult aging. *Ann Neurol* 21: 530-539.

229. Terry RD, Gonatas JK, Weiss M (1964) Ultrastructural studies in Alzheimer presenile dementia. *Am J Pathol* 44: 269-297.

230. Terry RD, Masliah E, Salmon DP, Butters N, DeTeresa R, Hill R, Hansen LA, Katzman R (1991) Physical basis of cognitive alterations in Alzheimer's disease: synapse loss is the major correlate of cognitive impairment. *Ann Neurol* 30: 572-580.

231. Terry RD, Peck A, DeTeresa R, Schechter R (1981) Some morphometric aspects of the brain in senile dementia of the Alzheimer type. *Ann Neurol* 10: 184-192.

232. Thal DR, Sassin I, Schultz C, Haass C, Braak E, Braak H (1999) Fleecy amyloid deposits in the internal layers of the human entorhinal cortex are comprised of N-terminal truncated fragments of Aβ. *J Neuropathol Exp Neurol* 58: 210-216.

233. Thal DR, Schultz C, Dehghani F, Yamaguchi H, Braak H, Braak E (2000) Amyloid β-protein (Aβ)-containing astrocytes are located preferentially near N-terminal-truncated Aβ deposits in the human entorhinal cortex. *Acta Neuropathol (Berl)* 100: 608-617.

234. Tomlinson BE (1989) The neuropathology of Alzheimer's disease. Issues in need of resolution (Second Dorothy S. Russel Memorial Lecture). *Neuropathol Appl Neurobiol* 15: 491-512.

235. Tomlinson BE (1992) Ageing and the dementias. In *Greenfield's neuropathology*, JH Adams, LW Duchen (eds), 5th ed. Edward Arnold: London, pp. 1284-1410.

236. Tomlinson BE, Blessed G, Roth M (1970) Observation on the brains of demented old people. *J Neurol Sci* 11: 205-242.

237. Tomlinson BE, Corsellis JAN (1984) Ageing and the dementias. In *Greenfield's neuropathology*, JH Adams, JAN Corsellis, LW Duchen (eds), 4th ed. Edward Arnold: London, pp. 951-1025.

238. Tsuchiya K, Kosaka K (1990) Neuropathological study of the amygdala in presenile Alzheimer's disease. *J Neurol Sci* 100: 165-173.

239. Uchihara T, Duyckaerts C, Lazarini F, Mokhtari K, Seilhean D, Amouyel P, Hauw J-J (1996) Inconstant apolipoprotein E (ApoE)-like immunoreactivity in amyloid β protein deposits: Relationship with APOE genotype in aging brain and Alzheimer's disease. *Acta Neuropathol (Berl)* 92: 180-185.

240. Uchihara T, Elhachimi HK, Duyckaerts C, Foncin JF, Fraser PE, Levesque L, St George-Hyslop PH, Hauw J-J (1996) Widespread immunoreactivity of presenilin in neurons of normal and Alzheimer's disease brains: Double-labeling immunohistochemical study. *Acta Neuropathol (Berl)* 92: 325-330.

241. Uchihara T, Kondo H, Ikeda K, Kosaka K (1995) Alzheimer-type pathology in melanin-bleached sections of substantia nigra. *J Neurol* 242: 485-489.

242. Uchihara T, Kondo H, Kosaka K, Tsukagoshi H (1992) Selective loss of nigral neurons in Alzheimer's disease: a morphometric study. *Acta Neuropathol (Berl)* 83: 271-276.

243. Uchihara T, Nakamura A, Yamazaki M, Mori O (2001) Evolution from pretangle neurons to neurofibrillary tangles monitored by thiazin red combined with Gallyas method and double immunofluorescence. *Acta Neuropathol (Berl)* 101: 535-539.

244. Unger JW, Lapham LW, McNeill TH, Eskin TA, Hamill RW (1991) The amygdala in Alzheimer's disease: neuropathology and Alz 50 immunoreactivity. *Neurobiol Aging* 12: 389-399.

245. Verbeek MM, Otte-Höller I, Westphal JR, Wesseling P, Ruiter DJ, de Waal RMW (1994) Accumulation of intercellular adhesion molecule-1 in senile plaques in brain tissue of patients with Alzheimer's disease. *Am J Pathol* 144: 104-116.

246. Vereecken TH, Vogels OJ, Nieuwenhuys R (1994) Neuron loss and shrinkage in the amygdala in Alzheimer's disease. *Neurobiol Aging* 15: 45-54.

247. Vidal R, Calero M, Piccardo P, Farlow MR, Unverzagt FW, Mendez E, Jimenez-Huete A, Beavis R, Gallo G, Gomez-Tortosa E, Ghiso J, Hyman BT, Frangione B, Ghetti B (2000) Senile dementia associated with amyloid β protein angiopathy and tau perivascular pathology, but not neuritic plaques in patients homozygous for the APOE-epsilon4 allele. *Acta Neuropathol (Berl)* 100: 1-12.

248. Vincent I, Jicha G, Rosado M, Dickson DW (1997) Aberrant expression of mitotic cdc2/cyclin B1

kinase in degenerating neurons of Alzheimer's disease brain. *J Neurosci* 17: 3588-3598.

249. Vincent I, Zheng JH, Dickson DW, Kress Y, Davies P (1998) Mitotic phosphoepitopes precede paired helical filaments in Alzheimer's disease. *Neurobiol Aging* 19: 287-296.

250. Vinters HV (1987) Cerebral amyloid angiopathy: a critical review. *Stroke* 18: 311-324.

251. Vogels OJ, Broere CA, Nieuwenhuys R (1990) Neuronal hypertrophy in the human supraoptic and paraventricular nucleus in aging and Alzheimer's disease. *Neurosci Lett* 109: 62-67.

252. Vonsattel JP, Myers RH, Hedley-White ET, Ropper AH, Bird ED, Richardson EP Jr (1991) Cerebral amyloid angiopathy without and with cerebral hemorrhage: a comparative histologic study. *Ann Neurol* 30: 637-649.

253. Wegiel J, Wang KC, Tarnawski M, Lach B (2000) Microglia cells are the driving force in fibrillar plaque formation, whereas astrocytes are a leading factor in plaque degradation. *Acta Neuropathol (Berl)* 100: 356-364.

254. West MJ (1993) Regionally specific loss of neurons in the aging human hippocampus. *Neurobiol Aging* 14: 287-293.

255. West MJ, Coleman PD, Flood DG, Troncoso JC (1994) Differences in the pattern of hippocampal neuronal loss in normal aging and Alzheimer disease. *Lancet* 344: 769-772.

256. Whitehouse PJ, Hedreen JC, White CL, Clark AW, Price DL (1983) Neuronal loss in the basal forebrain cholinergic system is more marked in Alzheimer's disease than in senile dementia of Alzheimer type. *Ann Neurol* 13: 243-248.

257. Whitehouse PJ, Price DL, Clark AW, Coyle JT, DeLong MR (1981) Alzheimer disease: evidence for selective loss of cholinergic neurons in the nucleus basalis. *Ann Neurol* 13: 243-248.

258. Williams RS, Ferrante RJ, Caviness VS (1978) The Golgi rapid method in clinical neuropathology: the morphologic consequences of suboptimal fixation. *J Neuropathol Exp Neurol* 37: 13-33.

259. Wisniewski HM, Bancher C, Barcilowska M, Wen GY, Currie J (1989) Spectrum of morphological appearance of amyloid deposits in Alzheimer's disease. *Acta Neuropathol (Berl)* 78: 337-347.

260. Wisniewski HM, Merz PA, Iqbal K (1984) Ultrastructure of paired helical filaments of Alzheimer's neurofibrillary tangle. *J Neuropathol Exp Neurol* 43: 643-656.

261. Wisniewski HM, Sadowski M, Jakubowska-Sadowska K, Tarnawski M, Wegiel J (1998) Diffuse, lake-like amyloid-β deposits in the parvopyramidal layer of the presubiculum in Alzheimer disease. *J Neuropathol Exp Neurol* 57: 674-683.

262. Wisniewski HM, Terry RD (1973) Reexamination of the pathogenesis of the senile plaques. In *Progress in Neuropathology*, HM Zimmerman (ed) vol. 2. Grune & Stratton: New York, pp. 1-15.

263. Wisniewski HM, Wegiel J, Kotula L (1996) Some neuropathological aspects of Alzheimer's disease and its relevance to other disciplines. *Neuropathol Appl Neurobiol* 22: 3-11.

264. Wisniewski HM, Wegiel J, Wang KC, Lach B (1992) Ultrastructural studies of the cells forming amyloid in the cortical vessel wall in Alzheimer's disease. *Acta Neuropathol (Berl)* 84: 117-127.

265. Wisniewski T, Frangione B (1992) Apolipoprotein E. A pathological chaperone protein in patients with cerebral and systemic amyloid. *Neurosci Lett* 135: 235-238.

266. Wolf DS, Gearing M, Snowdon DA, Mori H, Markesbery WR, Mirra SS (1999) Progression of regional neuropathology in Alzheimer disease and normal elderly: findings from the Nun study. *Alzheimer Dis Assoc Disord* 13: 226-231.

267. Working Group (1997) Consensus recommendations for the postmortem diagnosis of Alzheimer's disease. The National Institute on Aging, and Reagan Institute Working Group on Diagnostic Criteria for the Neuropathological Assessment of Alzheimer's Disease. *Neurobiol Aging* 18(4 suppl): S1-S2.

268. Yamaguchi H, Sugihara S, Ogawa A, Oshima N, Ihara Y (2001) Alzheimer β amyloid deposition enhanced by apoE epsilon4 gene precedes neurofibrillary pathology in the frontal association cortex of nondemented senior subjects. *J Neuropathol Exp Neurol* 60: 731-739.

269. Yamaguchi H, Yamazaki T, Lemere CA, Frosch MP, Selkoe DJ (1992) β amyloid is focally deposited within the outer basement membrane in the amyloid angiopathy of Alzheimer's disease. *Am J Pathol* 141: 249-259.

270. Yamamoto T, Hirano A (1985) Nucleus raphe dorsalis in Alzheimer's disease: neurofibrillary tangles and loss of large neurons. *Ann Neurol* 17: 573-577.

271. Yamamoto T, Hirano A (1986) A comparative study of modified Bielschowsky, Bodian and thioflavin S stain on Alzheimer's neurofibrillary tangles. *Neuropathol Appl Neurobiol* 12: 3-9.

272. Yan SD, Zhu H, Fu J, Yan SF, Roher A, Tourtellotte WW, Rajavashisth T, Chen X, Godman GC, Stern D, Schmidt AM (1997) Amyloid-β peptide-receptor for advanced glycation endproduct interaction elicits neuronal expression of macrophage-colony stimulating factor: a proinflammatory pathway in Alzheimer disease. *Proc Natl Acad Sci U S A* 94: 5296-5301.

273. Zhan SS, Beyreuther K, Schmitt HP (1993) Quantitative assessment of the synaptophysin immuno-reactivity of the cortical neuropil in various neurodegenerative disorders with dementia. *Dementia* 4: 66-74.

274. Zweig RM, Ross CA, Hedreen JC, Steele C, Cardillo JE, Whitehouse PJ, Folstein MF, Price DL (1988) The neuropathology of aminergic nuclei in Alzheimer's disease. *Ann Neurol* 24: 233-242.

Plaque-predominant and Tangle-predominant Variants of Alzheimer's Disease

Kurt A. Jellinger

AD	Alzheimer's disease
APOE	apolipoprotein E
CBD	corticobasal degeneration
ChaT	cholinacethyl transferase
DNTC	diffuse neurofibrillary tangles with calcification
DRS	dementia rating scale
MMSE	mini-mental state examination
NFT	neurofibrillar tangle
NT	neuropil thread
PSP	progressive supranuclear palsy

Definition

The brains of some demented elderly individuals lack some of the classical histologic markers of "plaque and tangle" Alzheimer's disease (AD) and have been referred to as "plaque-only" or "plaque-predominant" AD (18). A "tangle predominant" form of senile dementia with no or only few amyloid deposits and no neuritic plaques has also been recognized (10, 21). Whereas 75% of the plaque-predominant AD often have Lewy body disease (5), a high frequency of concurrent Lewy body disease is not characteristic of tangle-only dementia (10).

Epidemiology

Around 25% of a consecutive autopsy series of AD cases were plaque-predominant AD (5). The incidence of tangle-only dementia in several autopsy series ranged from 0.7 to 7.7 % and was 5.5% in a personal consecutive autopsy series of 500 cases of clinically probable AD. While no such cases have been reported in other autopsy series of very old people (14), among non-demented or mildly demented centenarians, numerous hippocampal and scarce neocortical NFTs in the absence of senile plaques are observed in 8 to 10 % (8).

Genetics

The frequency of apolipoprotein (APOE) ε4 in plaque-predominant AD (21%) and tangle-only dementia (3-11%) is considerably less than in typical AD (38-43%). In some series of tangle-only dementia, the frequency of APOE ε2 was increased, but in others it was comparable to very old controls (1, 7), AD in nonagenarians, PSP (10) or dementia with argyrophilic grains (19, 20).

Clinical Features

While no gender differences have been reported for plaque-predominant AD, some series show a female preponderance (3:1) for tangle-only dementia. The mean age of onset for both groups is 83±6 years and the average duration of illness is 4 years (range 1-15 years), with an age range at death of 87 to 93 years. Clinically, both types show progressive dementia, ranging from mild to severe. Cognitive scales such as the Mini-Mental State Exam (MMSE) and the Dementia Rating Scale (DRS) are usually higher in plaque-predominant AD (MMSE: 15.5 ±8.7 and DRS: 92±25) and tangle-only dementia (MMSE: 12-13±7 and DRS: 90±7) than in typical AD (MMSE: 6.2±7.3 and DRS: 55±35), while there are no significant differences in the prevalence of depression, psychosis or extrapyramidal signs (6).

Neuroimaging in plaque-predominant AD does not significantly differ from typical AD, while in tangle-only dementia medial temporal lobe may show severe atrophy (9).

Neuropathology

Gross examination of the brain in both plaque-predominant AD and tangle-only dementia shows moderate to severe cerebral atrophy, with brain weights ranging from 1080 to 1090 grams, and not different from typical AD. Histologically, plaque-predominant AD brains show numerous amyloid plaques with variable numbers (sometimes sparse or absent) of neuritic plaques in multimodal association cortices of frontal, temporal and parietal lobes and lack of neocortical NFTs. With regards to many histological features (for example, cortical synaptophysin levels), there are no significant differences between plaque-predominant AD and typical AD, except that typical AD has increased numbers of neocortical NFTs, more severe neuronal loss and a higher average Braak stage (6, 18).

Tangle-only dementia shows abundant NFTs and often some neuropil threads (NTs) predominantly in the allocortex (hippocampus, pre- and prosubiculum, parahippocampal region and amygdala). A high proportion of the NFTs are extracellular. Hippocampal atrophy, neuronal and synaptic loss, as well as astrocytic and microglial proliferation are usually milder in tangle-only dementia than in typical AD, but significantly more severe than in clinically normal elderly controls (22). The pattern of NFTs in the hippocampus, glial changes and synaptic loss in centenarians without obvious dementia are similar to those in tangle-only dementia, but different from typical AD (8). In 20 to 30% of tangle-only dementia cases, a few NFTs are seen in frontal, temporal and parietal isocortices, but usually not in the primary cortices or the occipital lobe. Argyrophilic grains in CA1 subfield of hippocampus occur in 20 to 66% of tangle-only dementia cases, but never in neocortex. Argyrophilic, tau-positive oligodendroglial inclusions ("coiled bodies") in temporal and less in frontal white matter are seen in about half of the cases, while "tufted astrocytes" and "astrocytic plaques" are absent (11). Given these findings, the relation between tangle-only dementia and argyrophilic grain disease warrants further investigation. NFTs in subcortical nuclei (eg, locus ceruleus and substantia nigra) are seen in 20 to 30%, but are absent or rare in basal ganglia and other brainstem nuclei, and thus comparable to aged controls. Amorphous amyloid plaques are observed in around 25% of the cases, while cortical neuritic plaques are not found. Amyloid angiopathy of meningeal and cortical vessels is seen in 10 to 20%, and additional minor cerebrovascular lesions are occasionally present. Hippocampal sclerosis was seen in 10% of tangle-only dementia (10).

Immunohistochemistry and Biochemistry

There are no significant differences between tangle-only dementia and typical AD in the immunoreactivity of NFTs with different anti-tau antibodies, but detailed biochemical analysis of the tau isoform composition and immunohistochemistry with exon-10-specific tau antibodies in a large series of tangle-only dementia cases remains to be reported. To date no mutations have be found in the tau gene in tangle-only dementia (22); however, some reported cases of FTDP-17 have had pathologic features of tangle-only dementia (16).

Mean choline acetyl transferase (ChAT) activity in midfrontal and temporal cortices is significantly higher in both plaque-predominant AD and tangle-only dementia than in typical AD ($p=0.0015$), while somatostatin levels show mild, but not significant, reduction in tangle-only dementia (6, 18).

Differential Diagnosis

The occurrence of either tangles or plaques in isolation can result in dementing syndromes that despite strikingly different pathology are relatively indistinguishable clinically. Both plaque-predominant AD and tangle-only dementia are generally characterized by a less severe dementia than typical AD with a slower rate of cognitive progression and, pathologically, by lower Braak stages and less cholinergic deficit, despite similar density of neocortical synapses (6). Since AD without neocortical NFTs does not appear to differ significantly from AD with neocortical NFTs, both types might be considered as variants of the same disease (19). On the other hand, the greater severity of the latter might be associated with to-be-determined environmental or genetic factors, such as higher frequency of APOE ε4 (6).

Plaque-predominant AD is to be distinguished from a subgroup of very aged subjects with preserved mental status and numerous neocortical plaques and NFTs restricted to hippocampus (11). These clinically normal elderly have cholinergic marker levels (ChAT) and somatostatin levels significantly higher than demented AD patients (11).

Tangle-only dementia is to be distinguished from other tauopathies with variable involvement of the cortex and subcortical structures in the absence of significant amyloid:

Progressive supranuclear palsy has by widespread NFTs and NTs in basal ganglia and brainstem nuclei, while tangle-only dementia has little subcortical pathology. In addition, neocortical involvement is different, with the highest density of NFTs in prefrontal and motor cortices and relative sparing of medial temporal lobe structures in PSP (2). Tau-positive tufted astrocytes are found in PSP, but are not a feature of tangle-only dementia. There are also differences in the biochemistry of tau-protein and the ultrastructure of NFTs in PSP compared to tangle-only dementia. In PSP the tau is predominantly 4-repeat tau and the filaments are straight, while in tangle-only dementia there is a mixture of 3-repeat and 4-repeat tau and the filaments are paired helical filaments.

Corticobasal degeneration is associated with lobar frontal or parietal atrophy, swollen achromatic, cortical neurons, widespread NFT-like neuronal inclusions and tau-positive astrocytic plaques in gray and white matter (4). The latter are not a feature of tangle-only dementia. Difficulties may arise in cases of CBD with coexistent AD pathology (10).

Diffuse neurofibrillary tangles with calcification (DNTC) is a sporadic atypical dementia with localized temporal atrophy, Fahr-type pallidal calcification, and abundant NFTs and NTs. NFTs are more widespread in cerebral cortex than in tangle-only dementia and NFTs are also found in subcortical nuclei (12). Similar to tangle-only dementia there are few or no cortical amyloid plaques. On immunoblots, the tau in DNTC is similar to AD (17). Calcification is the major distinguishing feature from tangle-only dementia.

Autosomal dominant dementia with neurofibrillary tangles linked to chromosome 17 (FTDP-17). This form of FTDP-17 shows clinical and pathologic heterogeneity, but includes cases with widespread NFTs overlapping with PSP (15) and other cases with NFT relatively restricted to medial temporal lobe more closely resembling tangle-only dementia. Cases with medial temporal NFTs have been reported to have an atypical clinical phenotype, suggestive of familial schizophrenia (3).

Future Directions and Therapy

Tangle-only dementia is a sporadic form of late-onset dementia and needs to be differentiated from the "limbic form" of AD. It has no or very little subcortical tau pathology, thus being distinct from PSP and other tauopathies. The paucity of amyloid deposition and the absence of APOE ε4 in most cases raises the possibility that APOE ε2 might be protective, but this requires further investigation. Although morphologically and genetically different from typical AD, it may represent a variant of AD or alternatively a form of pathological aging. Its nosological position within the spectrum of AD pathologies and its possible relationship to other tauopathies remains to be elucidated, particularly by further analysis of the tau isoform composition. A specific therapy is unknown, and animal and cellular models wait to be developed.

References

1. Bancher C, Egensperger R, Kösel S, Jellinger K, Graeber MB (1997) Low prevalence of apolipoprotein E ε4 allele in the neurofibrillary tangle predominant

form of senile dementia. *Acta Neuropathol* 94: 403-409.

2. Bigio EH, Vono MB, Satumtira S, Adamson J, Sontag E, Hynan LS, White CL 3rd, Baker M, Hutton M (2001) Cortical synapse loss in progressive supranuclear palsy. *J Neuropathol Exp Neurol* 60: 403-410.

3. Bird TD, Wijsman EM, Nochlin D, Leehey M, Sumi SM, Payami H, Poorkaj P, Nemens E, Rafkind M, Schellenberg GD (1997) Chromosome 17 and hereditary dementia: linkage studies in three non-Alzheimer families and kindreds with late-onset FAD. *Neurology* 48: 949-954.

4. Dickson DE (2001) Progressive supranuclear palsy and corticobasal degeneration. In *Functional Neurobiology of Aging*, RR Hof, LCK Mobbs (eds). Academic Press, pp. 155-171.

5. Hansen LA, Masliah E, Galasko D, Terry RD (1993) Plaque-only Alzheimer disease is usually the Lewy body variant and vice versa. *J Neuropathol Exp Neurol* 52: 648-654.

6. Ho GJ, Hansen LA, Alford MF, Schoos B, Tiraboschi P, Foster K, Thal LJ, Corey-Bloom J (1999) Dementia associated with tangles or plaques in isolation. *Neurology* 52: A477-478.

7. Ikeda K, Akiyama H, Arai T, Sahara N, Mori H, Usami M, Sakata M, Mizutani T, Wakabayashi K, Takahashi H (1997) A subset of senile dementia high incidence of the ApoE ϵ2 allele. *Ann Neurol* 41: 693-695.

8. Itoh Y, Yamada M, Suematsu N, Matsushita M, Otomo E (1998) An immunohistochemical study of centenarian brains: a comparison. *J Neurol Sci* 157: 73-81.

9. Jack CR Jr, Dickson DW, Parisi JE, Xu YC, Cha RH, O'Brien PC, Edland SD, Smith GE, Boeve BF, Tangalos EG, Kokmen E, Petersen RC (2002) Antemortem MRI findings correlate with hippocampal neuropathology in typical aging and dementia. *Neurology* 58: 750-757.

10. Jellinger K, Bancher C (1998) Senile dementia with tangles (Tangle predominant form of senile dementia). *Brain Pathol* 8: 367-376.

11. Katzman R, Terry R, DeTeresa R, Brown T, Davies P, Fuld P, Renbing X, Peck A (1988) Clinical, pathological, and neurochemical changes in dementia: a subgroup with preserved mental status and numerous neocortical plaques. *Ann Neurol* 23: 138-144.

12. Kosaka K (1994) Diffuse neurofibrillary tangles with calcification: a new presenile dementia. *J Neurol Neurosurg Psychiatry* 57: 594-596.

13. Morris HR, Janssen JC, Bandmann O, Daniel SE, Rossor MN, Lees AJ, Wood NW (1999) The tau gene A0 polymorphism in progressive supranuclear palsy and related neurodegenerative diseases. *J Neurol Neurosurg Psychiatry* 66: 665-667.

14. Polvikoski T, Sulkava R, Myllykangas L, Notkola IL, Niinisto L, Verkkoniemi A, Kainulainen K, Kontula K, Perez-Tur J, Hardy J, Haltia M (2001) Prevalence of Alzheimer's disease in very elderly people: A prospective neuropathological study. *Neurology* 56: 1690-1696.

15. Reed LA, Grabowski TJ, Schmidt ML, Morris JC, Goate A, Solodkin A, Van Hoesen GW, Schelper RL, Talbot CJ, Wragg MA, Trojanowski JQ (1997) Autosomal dominant dementia with widespread neurofibrillary tangles. *Ann Neurol* 42: 564-572.

16. Spillantini MG, Bird TD, Ghetti B (1998) Frontotemporal dementia and Parkinsonism linked to chromosome 17: a new group of tauopathies. *Brain Pathol* 8: 387-402.

17. Tanabe Y, Ishizu H, Ishiguro K, Itoh N, Terada S, Haraguchi T, Kawai K, Kuroda S (2000) Tau pathology in diffuse neurofibrillary tangles with calcification (DNTC): biochemical and immunohistochemical investigation. *Neuroreport* 11: 2473-2477.

18. Terry RD, Hansen LA, DeTeresa R, Davies P, Tobias H, Katzman R (1987) Senile dementia of the Alzheimer type without neocortical neurofibrillary tangles. *J Neuropathol Exp Neurol* 46: 262-268.

19. Tolnay M, Probst A, Monsch AU, Staehelin HB, Egensperger R (1998) Apolipoprotein E allele frequencies in argyrophilic grain disease. *Acta Neuropathol* 96: 225-227.

20. Tolnay M, Villoz N, Probst A, Miserez AR (2003) Apoliprotein E genotype in senile dementia with tangles differs from Alzheimer's disease. *Neuropathol Appl Neurobiol* 29: 80-84.

21. Ulrich J, Spillantini MG, Goedert M, Dukas L, Staehelin HB (1992) Abundant neurofibrillary tangles without senile plaques in a subset of patients with senile dementia. *Neurodegeneration* 1: 257-284.

22. Yamada M, Itoh Y, Sodeyama N, Suematsu N, Otomo E, Matsushita M, Mizusawa H (2001) Senile dementia of the neurofibrillary tangle type: a comparison with Alzheimer's disease. *Dement Geriatr Cogn Disord* 12: 117-126.

Molecular Pathogenesis of Alzheimer's Disease

Colin L Masters
Konrad Beyruether

AD	Alzheimer's disease
APP	amyloid precursor protein
ER	endoplasmatic reticulum
IDE	insulin degrading enzyme
NEP	neprolysin
PSEN1	presenilin 1 gene

Introduction

The Aβ-amyloid theory of Alzheimer's disease (AD) has driven much of the current research effort in identifying rational therapeutic targets (for recent reviews, see 5, 44). The theory is now sufficiently developed in molecular terms to allow a number of drug targets to be defined and validated. Final proof or confirmation of this theory will only emerge with successful therapeutic approaches, preferably in the earliest stages of AD, or even before the cognitive changes are symptomatic (11).

The Aβ-amyloidogenic pathway begins with the biogenesis of Aβ, a mixture of proteolytic cleavage products from the amyloid precursor protein (APP). The balance between 2 principal forces leads to AD: biogenesis versus catabolism of Aβ (Figure 1). The overproduction of Aβ through some enhancement of β- or γ-secretase activity has been only a theoretical possibility, for which some preliminary evidence is now emerging (28). An increase in substrate supply, or an altered conformation of substrate is found in Down's syndrome and in some of the inherited pathogenic mutations of APP. In contrast, the failure to adequately degrade or clear Aβ from any of its intracellular or extracellular compartments in the brain may lead to the toxic oligomerisation of Aβ, resulting in neurodegeneration.

The Normal Structure and Function of the Amyloid Precursor Protein

The amyloid precursor protein (APP) has the structural characteristics of a cell surface receptor. As a type 1 transmembrane protein, the large extra-cytoplasmic domain probably interacts with a ligand that has as yet not been defined. Transduction of this signal occurs through the smaller cytoplasmic domain, which is known to interact with a variety of cytoplasmic factors such as Fe 65, X11, (2). Recent evidence suggests that the proteolytic release of the cytoplasmic domain may allow this signal to translocate to the nucleus, where an important end-point event occurs (12, 21). Analogous to the Notch signalling pathway, the evolutionary forces, which have shaped this system, will therefore have been reliant on the mechanisms of ligand-mediated ectodomain shedding and the subsequent proteolytic processing of the transmembrane regions of APP. Our current ideas on the normal function of APP suggest that it plays a role in cell adhesion, based upon studies in an artificial Drosophila expression system (20), normal platelets (27) and in genetically-manipulated mouse brain models (18). Thus, as originally suspected, APP may turn out to be involved in the molecular processes underlying synaptic plasticity, but more in the sense of a "forgetting" molecule in which the strength of synaptic contacts are weakened (19).

The Secretase Enzymes that Process the Juxtamembranous Domains of APP

A disparate and distinct series of at least 5 proteolytic steps are now known to surround the processing of APP (Figure 2). α-Secretases (metalloenzymes of the ADAM class) release the ectodomain, possibly into an internal cellular compartment, which allows for the packaging of the ectodomain for subsequent regulated vesicular release (as exemplified in the platelet APP system). In neurones however, β-secretase appears to be a

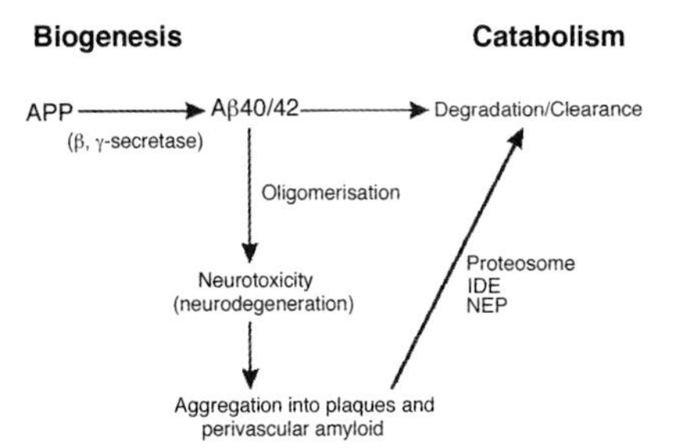

Figure 1. Biogenesis and catabolism of Aβ: the 2 principal forces which drive the AD pathway. APP undergoes proteolytic cleavages from β- and γ-secretases to generate the Aβ fragment of 40 or 42 residues. These fragments may undergo degradation within the proteosomal or lysozomal pathways of neurons, or through the action of degradative enzymes such as insulin degrading enzyme (IDE), neprolysin (NEP). Clearance of Aβ from the extracellular spaces of the brain may occur with the bulk flow of interstitial fluid towards the peri-arteriolar, peri-vascular, subependymal or subpial spaces. Depending on micro-environmental conditions (eg, pH or free zinc ions), the Aβ may aggregate or penetrate the lipid membranes of bystander cells, and acquire a toxic gain-of-function. Amyloid plaques and pervascular deposits are the hallmark of Alzheimer's disease, but may represent only the insoluble pool which is in equilibirum with the toxic oligomeric species of Aβ.

major pathway, which in conjunction with a γ-secretase activity may serve to determine axonal targeting (30).

The functional consequences of α-, β- and δ-cleavages remain uncertain, but the biogenesis of the full-length Aβ fragment clearly depends on β-secretase activity. The β-secretase has now been cloned and turns out to be a GPI-anchored aspartyl protease, and is currently the subject of intense scrutiny as a drug target (23).

The γ-secretases have proven to be most elusive, yet their identification has been a vindication of a combined clinical, pathological, and molecular biological approach. Gene linkage in pedigrees with early onset AD disclosed mutations in the presenilin 1 and presenilin 2 genes (*PSEN1*, *PSEN2*). The *PSEN1* and *PSEN2* genes encode multi-pass membrane proteins that may have the properties of a novel class of aspartyl protease

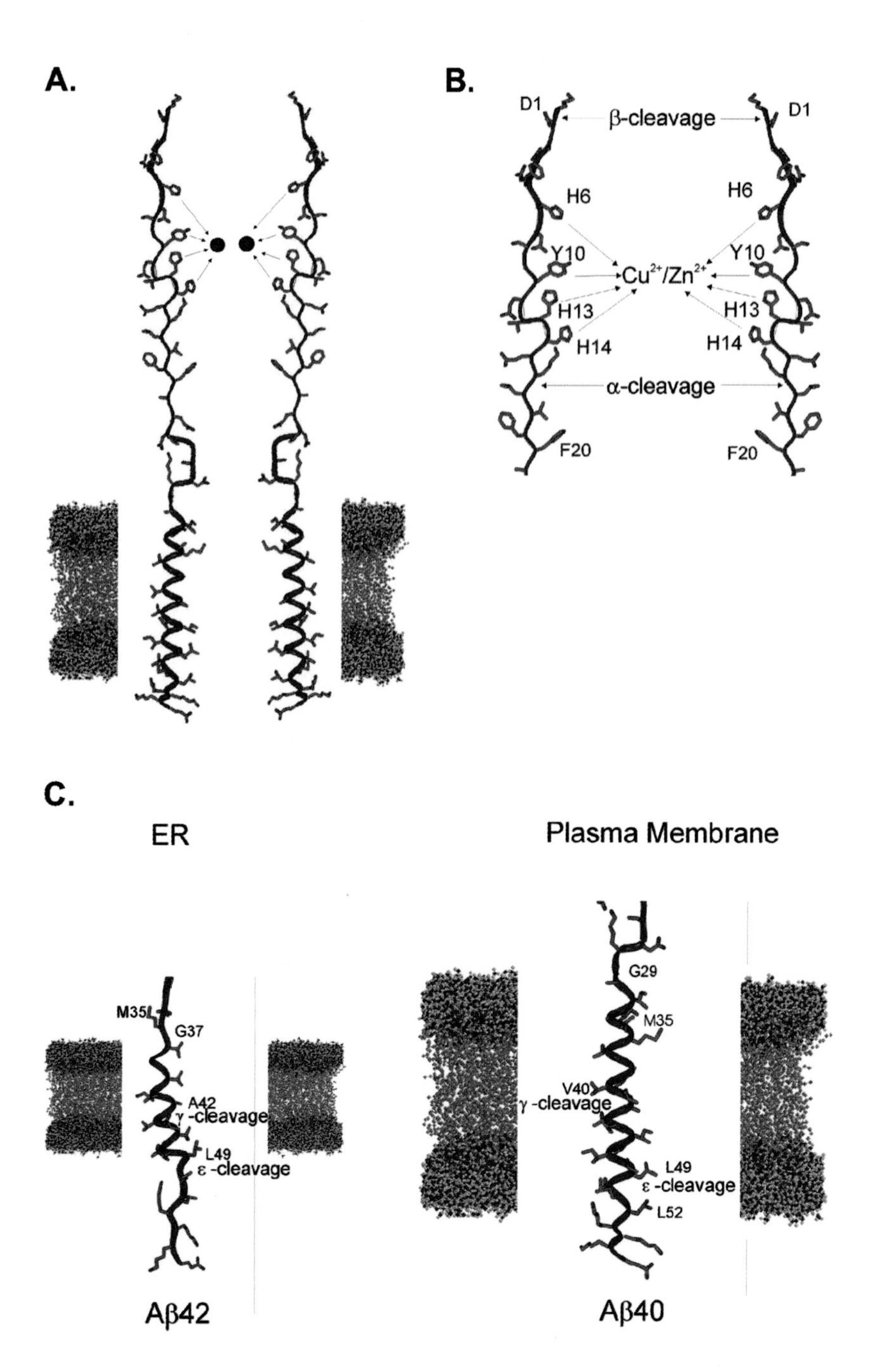

Figure 2. A. A schematic model of two Aβ molecules in the cell membrane. The metal binding domains and the transmembrane domains are shown in more detail in B and C. Two metal ions may help coordinate 2 or more Aβ molecules. Dimerisation may also occur through other sites of the APP molecule, particularly the copper-binding domain in the N-terminal region. **B.** The N-terminal domains of $A\beta_{1\text{-}20}$. While it is reasonably certain that the histidines (6, 13, 14) participate in metal coordination, the role of tyrosine (Y10) is far from clear. The principal sites of α- and β-cleavage are shown. **C.** The C-terminal cleavage of Aβ may be determined by the thickness and rigidity of the lipid membrane. In the thinner membranes of the ER (and pre-Golgi compartments), which are poor in cholesterol, the γ-cleavage event occurs at Alanine 42, situated halfway between Glycine 37 and Threonine 48. In this membranous environment, Methionine 35 would lie outside the lipid bilayer, and thereby be subject to oxidative modifications. Also, Leucine 49, the site of ϵ-cleavage, would lie outside the lipid bilayer. In contrast, in the thicker, rigid membranes near the cell surface (plasma membranes, early endosomes), the γ-cleavage event may be more likely to occur at Valine 40, halfway between Glycine 29 and Leucine 52. Note that in these thicker membranes, redox-active Methionine 35 is buried, the Leucine 49 ϵ-cleavage site is also within the bilayer, and the triple Lysine membrane anchor (residues 53, 54, 55) would be available for stabilisation. (Models kindly provided by K. Barnham).

(16). Further components of the γ-secretase activity are being identified, including nicastrin (9). Remarkably, the Notch processing pathway utilises a similar set of proteolytic machinery, serving to complicate the search for selective inhibitors of γ-secretase activity. More remarkable still has been the discovery of an analogous ϵ-cleavage of APP that parallels the Notch pathway of cytoplasmic domain release (26, 42, 47).

In Figure 2, current thoughts on the mechanisms of β- and γ-cleavage are summarised. It appears that the γ-cleavage occurs in the middle of the transmembrane domain of thinner, cholesterol-poor, membranes (such as the endoplasmic reticulum and pre-Golgi apparatus) to release the C-terminus of Aβ at position 42 (25, 36). In contrast, in thicker membranes (such as cell surface plasma membrane or endosomes), cleavage in the middle of the membrane releases the Aβ ending at position 40. Whether the thickness of the membrane also determines the ϵ-cleavage at position 49 remains to be determined, but at last the molecular basis of APP signalling through release of the intracellular domain is beginning to emerge. These events surround the biogenesis of $A\beta_{40}$ and $A\beta_{42}$ and are central to the amyloidogenic theory of AD. A clear picture of how the mutations in *PSEN1* and *PSEN2* affect Aβ production is yet to emerge (8). Selective inhibitors of β- and γ-activity are now available, and are at varying stages of preclinical and clinical development (4, 23).

Factors Modulating β- and γ-Secretase Function

In addition to cellular compartmentation (including axonal targeting and synapse release), the composition of the membranes in which APP is processed will clearly prove to be an important variable. Cholesterol content, for example, appears to affect most of the various secretase activities (17, 31, 40, 41), Small molecules such as indomethacin or insulin may affect $A\beta_{40}$ and $A\beta_{42}$ processing through pathways that remain to be elucidated

(22, 46). Dimerisation of APP or Aβ itself may have a profound effect on the various secretase activities, and therefore it is increasingly important to understand the structural basis of APP and Aβ self-association (43)

Aβ Aggregation and Accumulation in the Extracellular Space

It is likely that the tendency for Aβ to aggregate and accumulate in the extracellular space of the brain is to a large degree determined by its innate propensity for inter-molecular aggregation within the lipid bilayer (6). As an intra-membranous α-helix, Aβ might only self-associate after γ-cleavage, which would allow transformation into a β-sheet conformation. There are several experiments that show that the conversion from α-helix to β-sheet are subject to factors as diverse as metal ions (Cu, Zn ions in particular), lipid composition, and pH (38). Our studies in recent years have focused on the role of metal ions and lipids, not only because they are factors relevant to aggregation, but because they might lie at the heart of the central enigma: How does Aβ cause damage to neurons?

Aβ neurotoxicity. For reasons that are still unclear, nerve cells degenerate in topographically selected areas in the AD brain, and the *sine qua non* of this particular aspect of neuronal damage appears to be related to the presence of increased amounts of Aβ. The physical forms of Aβ are important, since the levels of "soluble" Aβ correlate best with the degree of neuronal damage (37). We have speculated that the topographic selectivity of Aβ aggregation is related to local micro-environmental factors, such as the concentration of free extracellular Zn^{++} ions (7). The inherent toxicity of Aβ is still not fully understood, but the major theories revolve around Aβ-Cu^{++} interactions causing oxidative damage or Aβ-lipid interactions which affect the stability and integrity of cellular membranes (13, 32, 39). Therapies targeting these interactions (such as compounds that prevent Aβ-Cu^{++} interactions, [10]) are now also in clinical trials.

Aβ degradation and clearance from the brain. In late onset sporadic AD (the most common form) there are compelling reasons to believe that a failure of degradation or clearance of Aβ from the ageing brain underlies its accumulation. Degradative pathways are now being elucidated, but remain untested in the context of brain ageing (Figure 1). Clearance of aggregated Aβ from the brain is undoubtedly a complex process (45), but its accumulation around the peri-arteriolar spaces as an amyloid congophilic angiopathy must provide a powerful clue. Similarly, the results of immunisation of a host with the Aβ peptide itself, which results in an increased clearance of Aβ suggests that cellular factors such as microglia, macrophages, and bulk flow across the brain-blood barrier are important variables (14, 29). Unfortunately, preliminary trials of immunisation with normal Aβ epitopes have proven problematical, as anticipated autoimmune responses caused serious adverse effects. Neo-epitopes or novel pathways of increased clearance (eg, enhanced proteosome function) may provide future avenues of therapeutic intervention.

Diagnostic assays based on the Aβ pathways in AD. If the Aβ theory of AD is correct, it should be possible to diagnose AD through some quantitative evaluation of some constituents of the APP/Aβ pathway. At the crudest level, simple imaging of Aβ in the brain through the use of Aβ-ligands should be possible. Early attempts at this process are now being reported, with a reasonable prospect that some form of in vivo whole brain imaging of Aβ will eventually yield useful results (1, 33, 34).

The CSF pool of Aβ species should also reflect the amounts of Aβ present in the extracellular spaces of the brain (3), but the contribution of Aβ from the choroid plexus, a site of high APP metabolism, needs to be taken into consideration. Studies to date suggest that CSF Aβ levels may be increased in the early stages of AD, yet decline below normal values as the disease progresses. This decline may be the result of either decreased Aβ production by degenerating neurons or a "sink" effect of Aβ entering into a large insoluble pool of aggregated Aβ in the AD-affected brain.

Plasma Aβ levels could also represent a useful window on cerebral Aβ turnover. Studies to date have provided conflicting results, but refinement of assay technologies and their application to clinically defined populations may yet reveal the utility of blood Aβ assays (15).

Downstream Events in the Evolution of AD

Neurofibrillary tangles have always been at the forefront of neuropathologic criteria for the diagnosis of AD, yet their causative role in the neurodegenerative process remains unclear. The tangles are composed of polymerised tau, but the mechanisms by which the tau protein accumulates remain enigmatic. Drawing on the discoveries of mutations in the tau gene that lead to abnormal tau assemblies in certain forms of frontotemporal dementia, it seems that the tau accumulations in AD-affected neurons are not necessarily the result of tau over-production, but rather may be a consequence of APP/Aβ-related neuronal damage (24, 35).

A similar relationship may also exist between Aβ toxicity and α-synuclein aggregation in Lewy body disease. The molecular pathways linking these phenomena are still poorly defined, but are worthy of continued pursuit since they may underlie the degenerative changes associated with these diseases.

References

1. Agdeppa ED, Kepe V, Liu J, Flores-Torres S, Satyamurthy N, Petric A, Cole GM, Small GW, Huang SC, Barrio JR (2001) Binding characteristics of radiofluorinated 6-dialkylamino-2- naphthylethylidene derivatives as positron emission tomography imaging probes for β-amyloid plaques in Alzheimer's disease. *J Neurosci* 21: RC189.

2. Ando K, Iijima KI, Elliott JI, Kirino Y, Suzuki T (2001) Phosphorylation-dependent regulation of the interaction of amyloid precursor protein with Fe65 affects the production of β-amyloid. *J Biol Chem* 276: 40353-40361.

3. Andreasen N, Minthon L, Davidsson P, Vanmechelen E, Vanderstichele H, Winblad B, Blennow K (2001) Evaluation of CSF-tau and CSF-Aβ42 as diagnostic markers for Alzheimer disease in clinical practice. *Arch Neurol* 58: 373-379.

4. Beher D, Wrigley JD, Nadin A, Evin G, Masters CL, Harrison T, Castro JL, Shearman MS (2001) Pharmacological knock-down of the presenilin 1 heterodimer by a novel γ-secretase inhibitor: implications for presenilin biology. *J Biol Chem* 276: 45394-45402.

5. Beyreuther K, Christen Y, Masters CL (2001) *Neurodegenerative Disorders: Loss of Function Through Gain of Function.* Springer: Berlin.

6. Bitan G, Lomakin A, Teplow DB (2001) Amyloid β-protein oligomerization: prenucleation interactions revealed by photo-induced cross-linking of unmodified proteins. *J Biol Chem* 276: 35176-35184.

7. Bush AI, Pettingell WH, Jr., Paradis MD, Tanzi RE (1994) Modulation of A β adhesiveness and secretase site cleavage by zinc. *J Biol Chem* 269: 12152-12158.

8. Cervantes S, Gonzalez-Duarte R, Marfany G (2001) Homodimerization of presenilin N-terminal fragments is affected by mutations linked to Alzheimer's disease. *FEBS Lett* 505: 81-86.

9. Chen F, Yu G, Arawaka S, Nishimura M, Kawarai T, Yu H, Tandon A, Supala A, Song YQ, Rogaeva E, Milman P, Sato C, Yu C, Janus C, Lee J, Song L, Zhang L, Fraser PE, St George-Hyslop PH (2001) Nicastrin binds to membrane-tethered Notch. *Nat Cell Biol* 3: 751-754.

10. Cherny RA, Atwood CS, Xilinas ME, Gray DN, Jones WD, McLean CA, Barnham KJ, Volitakis I, Fraser FW, Kim Y, Huang X, Goldstein LE, Moir RD, Lim JT, Beyreuther K, Zheng H, Tanzi RE, Masters CL, Bush AI (2001) Treatment with a copper-zinc chelator markedly and rapidly inhibits β-amyloid accumulation in Alzheimer's disease transgenic mice. *Neuron* 30: 665-676.

11. Collie A, Maruff P, Shafiq-Antonacci R, Smith M, Hallup M, Schofield PR, Masters CL, Currie J (2001) Memory decline in healthy older people: implications for identifying mild cognitive impairment. *Neurology* 56: 1533-1538.

12. Cupers P, Orlans I, Craessaerts K, Annaert W, De Strooper B (2001) The amyloid precursor protein (APP)-cytoplasmic fragment generated by γ-secretase is rapidly degraded but distributes partially in a nuclear fraction of neurones in culture. *J Neurochem* 78: 1168-1178.

13. Curtain CC, Ali F, Volitakis I, Cherny RA, Norton RS, Beyreuther K, Barrow CJ, Masters CL, Bush AI, Barnham KJ (2001) Alzheimer's disease amyloid-β binds copper and zinc to generate an allosterically ordered membrane-penetrating structure containing superoxide dismutase-like subunits. *J Biol Chem* 276: 20466-20473.

14. DeMattos RB, Bales KR, Cummins DJ, Dodart JC, Paul SM, Holtzman DM (2001) Peripheral anti-A β antibody alters CNS and plasma A β clearance and decreases brain A β burden in a mouse model of Alzheimer's disease. *Proc Natl Acad Sci U S A* 98: 8850-8855.

15. Ertekin-Taner N, Graff-Radford N, Younkin LH, Eckman C, Adamson J, Schaid DJ, Blangero J, Hutton M, Younkin SG (2001) Heritability of plasma amyloid β in typical late-onset Alzheimer's disease pedigrees. *Genet Epidemiol* 21: 19-30.

16. Evin G, Sharples RA, Weidemann A, Reinhard FB, Carbone V, Culvenor JG, Holsinger RM, Sernee MF, Beyreuther K, Masters CL (2001) Aspartyl protease inhibitor pepstatin binds to the presenilins of Alzheimer's disease. *Biochemistry* 40: 8359-8368.

17. Fassbender K, Simons M, Bergmann C, Stroick M, Lutjohann D, Keller P, Runz H, Kuhl S, Bertsch T, von Bergmann K, Hennerici M, Beyreuther K, Hartmann T (2001) Simvastatin strongly reduces levels of Alzheimer's disease β-amyloid peptides Aβ 42 and Aβ 40 in vitro and in vivo. *Proc Natl Acad Sci U S A* 98: 5856-5861.

18. Feng R, Rampon C, Tang YP, Shrom D, Jin J, Kyin M, Sopher B, Miller MW, Ware CB, Martin GM, Kim SH, Langdon RB, Sisodia SS, Tsien JZ (2001) Deficient neurogenesis in forebrain-specific presenilin-1 knockout mice is associated with reduced clearance of hippocampal memory traces. *Neuron* 32: 911-926.

19. Fitzjohn SM, Morton RA, Kuenzi F, Rosahl TW, Shearman M, Lewis H, Smith D, Reynolds DS, Davies CH, Collingridge GL, Seabrook GR (2001) Age-related impairment of synaptic transmission but normal long-term potentiation in transgenic mice that overexpress the human APP695SWE mutant form of amyloid precursor protein. *J Neurosci* 21: 4691-4698.

20. Fossgreen A, Brückner B, Czech C, Masters CL, Beyreuther K, Paro R (1998) Transgenic Drosophila expressing human amyloid precursor protein show γ-secretase activity and a blistered-wing phenotype. *Proc Natl Acad Sci U S A* 95: 13703-13708.

21. Gao Y, Pimplikar SW (2001) The γ-secretase-cleaved C-terminal fragment of amyloid precursor protein mediates signaling to the nucleus. *Proc Natl Acad Sci U S A* 98: 14979-14984.

22. Gasparini L, Gouras GK, Wang R, Gross RS, Beal MF, Greengard P, Xu H (2001) Stimulation of β-amyloid precursor protein trafficking by insulin reduces intraneuronal β-amyloid and requires mitogen-activated protein kinase signaling. *J Neurosci* 21: 2561-2570.

23. Ghosh AK, Bilcer G, Harwood C, Kawahama R, Shin D, Hussain KA, Hong L, Loy JA, Nguyen C, Koelsch G, Ermolieff J, Tang J (2001) Structure-based design: potent inhibitors of human brain memapsin 2 (β-secretase). *J Med Chem* 44: 2865-2868.

24. Götz J, Chen F, van Dorpe J, Nitsch RM (2001) Formation of neurofibrillary tangles in P301l tau transgenic mice induced by Aβ 42 fibrils. *Science* 293: 1491-1495.

25. Grziwa B, Grimm MOW, Masters CL, Beyreuther K, Hartmann T, Lichtenthaler SF. The transmembrane domain of the amyloid precursor protein in microsomal membranes is on both sides shorter than predicted. *J Biol Chem* in press.

26. Gu Y, Misonou H, Sato T, Dohmae N, Takio K, Ihara Y (2001) Distinct intramembrane cleavage of the β-amyloid precursor protein family resembling γ-secretase-like cleavage of Notch. *J Biol Chem* 276: 35235-35238.

27. Henry A, Li QX, Galatis D, Hesse L, Multhaup G, Beyreuther K, Masters CL, Cappai R (1998) Inhibition of platelet activation by the Alzheimer's disease amyloid precursor protein. *Br J Haematol* 103: 402-415.

28. Holsinger RM, McLean CA, Beyreuther K, Masters CL, Evin G (2002) Increased expression of the amyloid precursor β-secretase in Alzheimer's disease. *Ann Neurol* 51: 783-786.

29. Iwata N, Tsubuki S, Takaki Y, Shirotani K, Lu B, Gerard NP, Gerard C, Hama E, Lee HJ, Saido TC (2001) Metabolic regulation of brain Aβ by neprilysin. *Science* 292: 1550-1552.

30. Kamal A, Almenar-Queralt A, LeBlanc JF, Roberts EA, Goldstein LS (2001) Kinesin-mediated axonal transport of a membrane compartment containing β-secretase and presenilin-1 requires APP. *Nature* 414: 643-648.

31. Kojro E, Gimpl G, Lammich S, Marz W, Fahrenholz F (2001) Low cholesterol stimulates the nonamyloidogenic pathway by its effect on the α-secretase ADAM 10. *Proc Natl Acad Sci U S A* 98: 5815-5820.

32. Kremer JJ, Sklansky DJ, Murphy RM (2001) Profile of changes in lipid bilayer structure caused by β-amyloid peptide. *Biochemistry* 40: 8563-8571.

33. Kung HF, Lee CW, Zhuang ZP, Kung MP, Hou C, Plossl K (2001) Novel stilbenes as probes for amyloid plaques. *J Am Chem Soc* 123: 12740-12741.

34. Lee CW, Zhuang ZP, Kung MP, Plossl K, Skovronsky D, Gur T, Hou C, Trojanowski JQ, Lee VM, Kung HF (2001) Isomerization of (Z,Z) to (E,E)1-bromo-2,5-bis-(3-hydroxycarbonyl-4- hydroxy)styrylbenzene in strong base: probes for amyloid plaques in the brain. *J Med Chem* 44: 2270-2275.

35. Lewis J, Dickson DW, Lin WL, Chisholm L, Corral A, Jones G, Yen SH, Sahara N, Skipper L, Yager D, Eckman C, Hardy J, Hutton M, McGowan E (2001) Enhanced neurofibrillary degeneration in transgenic mice expressing mutant tau and APP. *Science* 293: 1487-1491.

36. Lichtenthaler SF, Beher D, Grimm HS, Wang R, Shearman MS, Masters CL, Beyreuther K (2002) The intramembrane cleavage site of the amyloid precursor protein depends on the length of its transmembrane domain. *Proc Natl Acad Sci U S A* 99: 1365-1370.

37. McLean CA, Cherny RA, Fraser FW, Fuller SJ, Smith MJ, Beyreuther K, Bush AI, Masters CL (1999) Soluble pool of Aβ amyloid as a determinant of severity of neurodegeneration in Alzheimer's disease. *Ann Neurol* 46: 860-866.

38. Michikawa M, Gong JS, Fan QW, Sawamura N, Yanagisawa K (2001) A novel action of alzheimer's amyloid β-protein (Aβ): oligomeric Aβ promotes lipid release. *J Neurosci* 21: 7226-7235.

39. Pratico D, Uryu K, Leight S, Trojanoswki JQ, Lee VM (2001) Increased lipid peroxidation precedes

amyloid plaque formation in an animal model of Alzheimer amyloidosis. *J Neurosci* 21: 4183-4187.

40. Refolo LM, Pappolla MA, LaFrancois J, Malester B, Schmidt SD, Thomas-Bryant T, Tint GS, Wang R, Mercken M, Petanceska SS, Duff KE (2001) A cholesterol-lowering drug reduces β-amyloid pathology in a transgenic mouse model of Alzheimer's disease. *Neurobiol Dis* 8: 890-899.

41. Runz H, Rietdorf J, Tomic I, de Bernard M, Beyreuther K, Pepperkok R, Hartmann T (2002) Inhibition of intracellular cholesterol transport alters presenilin localization and amyloid precursor protein processing in neuronal cells. *J Neurosci* 22: 1679-1689.

42. Sastre M, Steiner H, Fuchs K, Capell A, Multhaup G, Condron MM, Teplow DB, Haass C (2001) Presenilin-dependent γ-secretase processing of β-amyloid precursor protein at a site corresponding to the S3 cleavage of Notch. *EMBO Rep* 2: 835-841.

43. Scheuermann S, Hambsch B, Hesse L, Stumm J, Schmidt C, Beher D, Bayer TA, Beyreuther K, Multhaup G (2001) Homodimerization of amyloid precursor protein and its implication in the amyloidogenic pathway of Alzheimer's disease. *J Biol Chem* 276: 33923-33929.

44. Selkoe DJ (2001) Alzheimer's disease: genes, proteins, and therapy. *Physiol Rev* 81: 741-766.

45. Shirotani K, Tsubuki S, Iwata N, Takaki Y, Harigaya W, Maruyama K, Kiryu-Seo S, Kiyama H, Iwata H, Tomita T, Iwatsubo T, Saido TC (2001) Neprilysin degrades both amyloid β peptides 1-40 and 1-42 most rapidly and efficiently among thiorphan- and phosphoramidon-sensitive endopeptidases. *J Biol Chem* 276: 21895-21901.

46. Weggen S, Eriksen JL, Das P, Sagi SA, Wang R, Pietrzik CU, Findlay KA, Smith TE, Murphy MP, Bulter T, Kang DE, Marquez-Sterling N, Golde TE, Koo EH (2001) A subset of NSAIDs lower amyloidogenic Aβ42 independently of cyclooxygenase activity. *Nature* 414: 212-216.

47. Weidemann A, Eggert S, Reinhard FB, Vogel M, Paliga K, Baier G, Masters CL, Beyreuther K, Evin G (2002) A novel ϵ-cleavage within the transmembrane domain of the Alzheimer amyloid precursor protein demonstrates homology with Notch processing. *Biochemistry* 41: 2825-2835.

Alzheimer Animal Models: Models of Aβ Deposition in Transgenic Mice

Eileen McGowan
Fiona Pickford
Dennis W. Dickson

AD	Alzheimer's disease
APOE	apolipoprotein E
APP	amyloid precursor protein
COX	cyclooxygenase
GSK	glycogen synthase kinase
HPrP	hamster prion protein promotor
LTP	long term potentiation
PDGF	platelet derived growth factor
PS1	presenilin 1
YAC	yeast artificial chromosome

Transgenic mouse models have been used extensively to investigate the molecular mechanisms of Alzheimer's disease (AD) (17). Since the identification of the first familial AD-linked mutation in amyloid precursor protein (APP) was discovered (15), many groups have used transgenic approaches to attempt to generate models of AD that develop amyloid deposits in the brain.

A complete model of AD would exhibit all of the behavioural, biochemical and pathological hallmarks of the disease, including not only amyloid plaques, but also neurofibrillary tangles (NFTs) and neuronal loss. While a definitive model remains elusive, transgenic mice that replicate various aspects of AD pathology have been developed and they have proven invaluable in understanding the pathogenesis of AD. These models are currently being used to develop potential diagnostic and therapeutic approaches to AD. Current transgenic models of AD are summarised in Table 1.

Early Models of APP Transgenic Mice

Early attempts at generating mice expressing human APP were only partially successful. Overexpression of the murine homologue of the Aβ peptide, driven by the NF-L promoter in FVB/N mice was neurotoxic, with apoptotic cell death in the cerebral cortex, hippocampus and amygdala (30). The Aβ peptide was expressed intraneuronally, and neurotoxicity of control peptides expressed at similar levels was not investigated. A transgenic mouse expressing the C100 fragment of APP resulted in extracellular amyloid deposits, gliosis, cell loss in the hippocampus, as well as spatial learning deficits and abnormal long-term potentiation (LTP) (45). In a similar model, the C100 fragment of APP was expressed under the human dystrophin promoter (26). Severe hippocampal degeneration was noted, but Aβ aggregates were detected only intraneuronally, not extracellularly (46, 47).

To test the hypothesis that APP overexpression was sufficient for amyloid deposition, C57Bl/6J embryonic stem cells were transfected with yeast artificial chromosomes (YACs) containing 400 kb of human APP gene and 250 kb of flanking sequences (33). Human APP mRNA and protein expression was detected in both the brain and peripheral tissue at levels similar to the endogenous mouse APP gene. Although the transgene contained all the regulatory sites required for faithful spatio-temporal expression, no upregulation of APP was noted, no amyloid deposits formed and no cognitive or behavioural deficits were detected. Nevertheless, brains of mutant YAC $APPK_{670N,\ M671L}$ Swedish mutation mice had higher levels of total Aβ than wild-type YAC APP mice (32), and homozygous YAC $APPK_{670N,\ M671L}$ mice did develop diffuse and fibrillar Aβ deposition at 14 months in the olfactory cortex and olfactory bulb (28).

Given that cellular models of APP_{V717I} show selective increase of Aβ42 over Aβ40 (51), which is also characteristic of AD, Malherbe et al (37) used a rat neurone specific enolase promoter (NSE) to drive expression of human $APP695_{V717I}$ (London mutation). Transgene expression was 1.3-fold over endogenous APP in the hippocampus and neocortex, brain regions severely affected in AD. Aβ was not detected in any of the transgenic mouse lines, and in some cases αAPP was also upregulated, indicating a general upregulation of APP expression rather than a shift in processing towards the generation of the amyloidogenic fragment. No pathology or behavioural deficits were observed.

PDAPP Mice

Games et al (14) described the first APP transgenic model with robust amyloid pathology. The platelet derived growth factor-β (PDGF-β) promoter was used to drive expression of human APP_{V717F} (Indiana mutation). The cDNA minigene contained introns 7 and 8, allowing alternate splicing of exons 7 and 8 and hence generation of the 3 major isoforms of APP (APP695, APP751, and APP770). PDAPP mice had approximately 40 copies of the transgene and mutant APP expression at least a 10-fold over endogenous APP levels. Brain Aβ concentration was shown to increase with age with a disproportionate increase in Aβ42, from 27% at 4 months to 99% of total Aβ at 10 months of age (25). At 6 to 9 months, hemizygous transgenic PDAPP mice developed Aβ plaques in the hippocampus and cerebral cortex, and both the number and density of plaques increased with age. Many plaques in PDAPP mice were fibrillar (thioflavin S- positive and Congo red birefringent), recapitulating properties of dense core amyloid plaques found in AD, where it has been speculated that diffuse plaques evolve into compact plaques over time (49). The high level of expression of mutant APP and the consequent high levels of Aβ presumably exceeded a threshold required for deposition not reached in previous models. On the other hand, Aβ degra-

Transgenic line	Transgene	Level	Features	Deficits	References
PDAPP	hPDGF-β APP (695,751,770) V717F	10x	Aβ deposits at 6-9 months, gliosis, phospho-tau positive dystrophic neurites. Decrease in synapse and dendrite density surrounding plaques. Learning deficits. Plaque distribution altered by disruption of APOE	No NFTs or neuronal loss.	9, 14, 21, 23, 24
Tg2576	hPrP APP (695) K670N, M671L	5-6x	Aβ deposits at 9-12 months. Gliosis, dystrophic neurites containing phospho-tau. Localized neuron and synapse loss. Cognitive abnormalities. Impaired synaptic plasticity and age-dependent memory deficits. Aβ42 production elevated by 40% and deposition accelerated to 10-12 weeks by crossing with mutant PS1 mice.	No NFTs. Aβ peptides may be modified/processed differently to those in AD brains.	7, 8, 19, 20, 22, 55
Tg APP23	moThy-1 APP (751) K670N, M671L	7x	Aβ deposits at 6 months associated with dystrophic neurites and phospho-tau. Up to 25% neuronal loss, proportional to plaque burden.	No NFTs or behavioural studies reported to date.	6, 50
TgC3-3	moPrP Humanized mouse APP (695) K670N, M671L	2x	Aβ deposits at 18 months, and 9 months when crossed with mutant PS1 transgenic mice.	No NFTs or neuronal loss.	3, 4, 5
TgCRND-8	hPrP APP (695) K670N, M671L + V717I	5x	Aβ deposits at 3 months. Dense-cored plaques, activated microglia and dystrophic neurites from 5 months. Behavioural deficits from 11 weeks. Pathology accelerated when crossed with mutant PS1 mice, with deposits as early as 1 month.	No NFTs. Rapid progression does not mirror typical AD time course.	10
TgAPP/Ld/2	moThy-1 APP (695) V717I	25x (RNA)	Aβ deposits at 12 months, correlates with Aβ levels. Behavioural deficits from 3 months. Mice crossed with PS1 null mice lack Aβ deposits. LTP was unimpaired, but cognitive deficits remained.	No NFTs or neuronal loss.	11, 41
TgAPP/Sw/1	MoThy-1 APP (770) K670N, M671L	7x (RNA)	Rare Aβ deposits at 18 months. Behavioural deficits, premature death, extensive neurodegeneration and apoptosis.	No NFTs.	41, 42, 43, 44
APP/Fl/1	MoThy-1 APP (770) A692G	14x (RNA)	Behavioural disturbances, premature death, astrogliosis and microvacuolation.	No amyloid deposits or NFTs.	29
APP/Du/4	MoThy-1 APP (770) E693Q	5x (RNA)	Behavioural disturbances, premature death, astrogliosis and microvacuolation.	No amyloid deposits or NFTs.	29
APP-C100	Neural dystrophin APP (695) bp 1769 - 2959	20x (RNA)	Occasional spontaneous seizures and variable premature death; increased b-secretase processing. Low Aβ levels. Intracellular accumulation. Severe hippocampal degeneration after 18 months.	No amyloid deposits or NFTs.	26, 46, 47
TgAPPSwe-KI	Mouse genomic APP K670N, M671L	0.5x	Increased Aβ levels.	No neuropathology or behavioural studies reported to date.	48
TgR1.40-YAC	Human genomic APP K670N, M671L	2-3 hemi, 4-6 homo	Aβ deposits at 24 months (hemi), 14 months (homo).	No NFTs. Amyloid plaques developed at such late age as to correspond to aging, rather than AD.	31, 32, 33

Table 1. Summary of APP transgenic mice.

dation has not been thoroughly studied in this model.

Phosphorylated neurofilament-immunoreactive dystrophic neurites were detected in the rim of plaques at 10 to 12 months of age, while phosphorylated tau-immunoreactive dystrophic neurites were observed after 14 months of age (38). The dystrophic plaque neurites did not contain filamentous tau, and no NFT were detected. Although there was significant amyloid deposition, with gliosis and decreased synaptic and dendritic densities in PDAPP mice, no neuronal loss has been described (24).

PDAPP mice have both age-independent and age-dependent memory deficits. Significant impairments in radial-maze spatial discrimination tests have been described at all ages compared to non-transgenic mice (12). These deficits began prior to amyloid deposition and may be correlated to reduction in the size of the corpus callosum, fornix and hippocampus (16). Age-dependent decreases in spontaneous object-recognition performance (12), and deficits in learning a series of spatial locations in the Morris water maze occur from 13 months of age and correlate with amyloid burden (9).

When PDAPP mice were crossed to apolipoprotein E (APOE) knockout mice, there was a dramatic reduction in amyloid plaque density in the cortex and dentate gyrus, and an increase in diffuse amyloid deposits in the hippocampus (21), indicating that apoliprotein-E significantly modifies the phenotype in these mice. While the absence of APOE effected the amount,

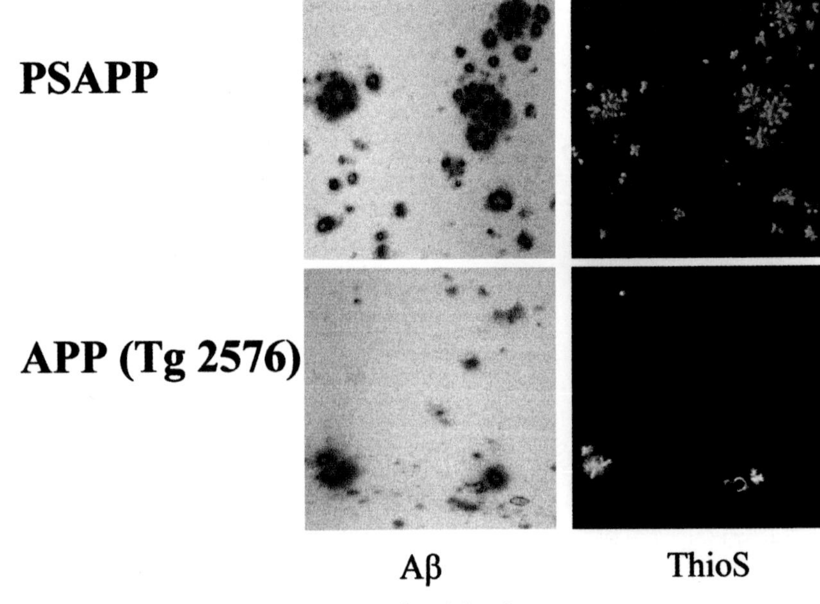

Figure 1. Comparison of pathology in APP (Tg2576) and PSAPP mice. Tg2576 mice have widespread Aβ deposition in the hippocampus, entorhinal and cingluate cortex. A proportion of the senile plaques are thioflavin S-positive. Presenilin-1 accelerates Aβ deposition in Tg2576 mice, and the majority of the Aβ plaques are cored (thioflavin S-positive). Serial sections from age and sex matched Tg2576 and PSAPP mice were immunostained for Aβ (using Bam10 antibody raised against Aβ1-12) and counterstained with thioflavin S.

form and anatomical distribution of Aβ deposits, expression of APP, low density lipoprotein-receptor related protein, and soluble Aβ levels were not affected.

Tg2576 Mice

Probably the most widely studied mutant APP transgenic model is Tg2576 developed by Hsiao and colleagues (20). These mice express the most abundant APP isoform, APP695 with the double mutation K670N, M671L (Swedish mutation) under the control of the hamster prion protein promoter (hPrP). Tg2576 mice had at least 5-fold over-expression of mutant APP over endogenous mouse APP. Both Aβ40 and Aβ42 were elevated and sensitive end-specific ELISA demonstrated a 5-fold increase in Aβ40 and a 14-fold increase in Aβ42 between 2 to 8 months and 11 to 13 months of age. SDS-insoluble Aβ40 and Aβ42 were detected at 6 months of age, when histopathology was minimal. Levels increased exponentially until 10 months of age. The increase in insoluble Aβ was accompanied by a slight decrease in soluble Aβ. Aβ peptides with N-terminal truncation, post-translational modifications and cross-links are found extensively in Aβ deposits in AD brains, but are absent from Tg2576 mice until old age (27).

Amyloid plaques in Tg2576 usually had dense amyloid cores, and were first detected at 9 to 12 months in the frontal, temporal, entorhinal cortex, hippocampus, presubiculum, subiculum and cerebellum in a distribution similar to those described in PDAPP mouse. Only rare isolated plaques can be detected at earlier ages. Increasing amounts of diffuse amyloid deposits were detected in older mice. Astrogliosis, activated microglia and dystrophic neurites were associated with dense amyloid plaques in Tg2576 (13). Phosphorylated tau was detected in dystrophic neurites, but no filamentous tau and no NFTs have been observed (53, 54). A large proportion of plaque-associated dystrophic neurites (74%) were immunoreactive for glycogen synthase kinase 3β (GSK3β) suggesting that GSK3β may be the predominant tau kinase in this location (54). Although Tg2576 mice had no significant neuronal loss, there was localised neuronal and synaptic loss surrounding plaques (53), indicating at least some level of neuronal disruption in the immediate vicinity of fibrillary amyloid deposits (34).

Westerman and colleagues (55) tested a large number of Tg2576 mice in the Morris water maze, eliminating performance-incompetent mice, and identified age-dependent deficits in Tg2576 mice when compared to non-transgenic mice and mice expressing wild-type APP (Tg4569). Spatial reference memory in Tg2576 deteriorated progressively from 6 months of age, coinciding with the appearance of formic acid-extractable, SDS-insoluble Aβ. Memory deficits correlated inversely with insoluble Aβ when the mice were stratified by age, suggesting that a subset of insoluble Aβ, possibly small aggregates, rather than soluble Aβ or fibrillar deposits, may be responsible for the memory decline in these mice (55). Additionally, LTP induction in both hippocampal slices and in the CA1 region of anaesthetised mice was compromised in old Tg2576 mice, but not in wild-type controls or young transgenic animals (8).

The addition of a mutant presenilin-1 (PS1) transgene accelerated pathology in Tg2576 mice (see Figure 1 for comparison of pathology in Tg2576 and PSAPP mice). Not only was Aβ42 selectively increased (by 41%) in the bigenic PSAPP offspring, but also many amyloid deposits developed in the cingulate cortex, followed by the hippocampus and other brain regions (19). Plaques were first observed at 10 weeks (compared to 9 months in Tg2976 mice), and by 6 months deposition was extensive (40). The mice showed reduced spontaneous performance in a Y maze test, before Aβ deposits were widespread. Amyloid plaques disrupted the global neuronal architecture, but no significant neuronal loss was observed (52), suggesting that amyloid deposition alone was not sufficient for neuronal loss. A study of the inflammatory response to amyloidosis revealed activated microglia and astrocytes coincident with amyloid deposition in PSAPP mice. Cyclooxygenase-2 (COX-2) and complement component C1q levels also increased in response to the formation of fibrillar Aβ (39). Swollen cholinergic neurites were detected within cortical plaques in both Tg2576 and PSAPP mice by12 months, but cholinergic cell density and receptor binding remained normal, indicating that the basal forebrain cholinergic system did not degenerate in mice even in the face of very high amyloid plaque burdens (18). Mutant PS transgenes have been shown to accelerate deposition of Aβ in other APP transgenic mice (5, 10).

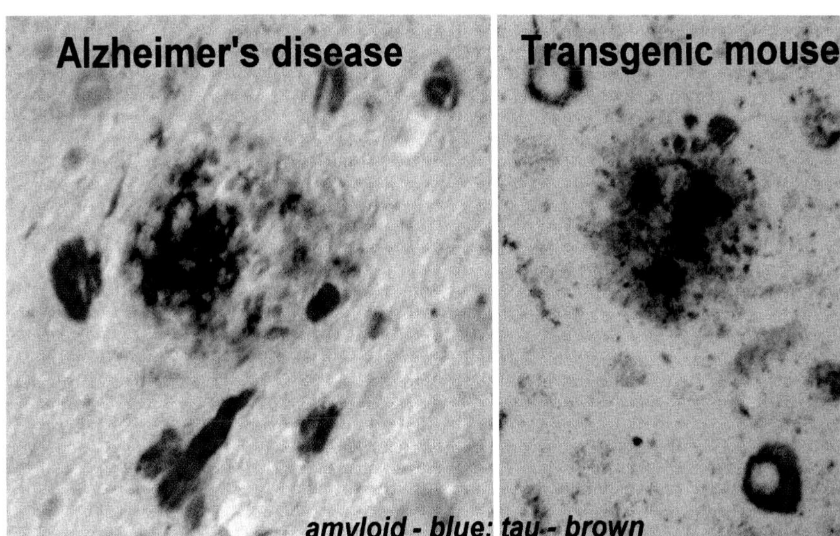

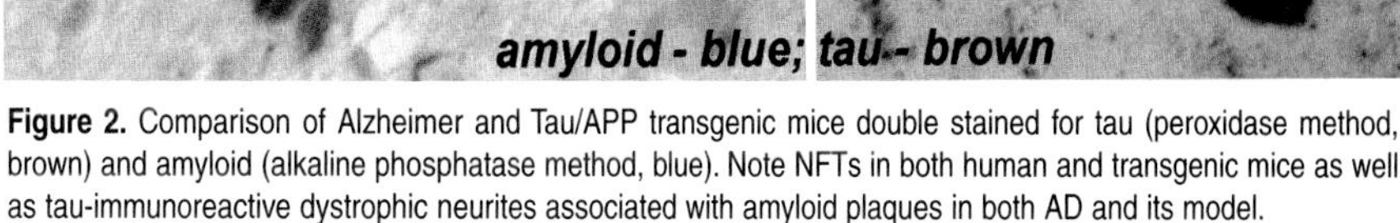

Figure 2. Comparison of Alzheimer and Tau/APP transgenic mice double stained for tau (peroxidase method, brown) and amyloid (alkaline phosphatase method, blue). Note NFTs in both human and transgenic mice as well as tau-immunoreactive dystrophic neurites associated with amyloid plaques in both AD and its model.

APP23 Mice

APP23 mice expressing $hAPPK_{670N, M671L}$ driven by the mouse Thy-1 promoter had 7-fold overexpression of APP. Amyloid deposits were detected at 6 to 12 months of age (50), while the same cDNA directed by the human Thy-1 promoter had no pathology. Transgenic mice with triple APP mutation driven by the Thy-1 promotor, $hAPPK_{670N, M671L+V717I}$ mice (APP22), had amyloid deposits at 18 month with a 2-fold overexpression of mutant APP compared to endogenous APP. No NFTs were identified, but there was increased phospho-tau and hyperphosphorylated tau in dystrophic neurites associated with amyloid plaques. Stereological estimation indicated that the number of CA1 pyramidal neurones was inversely related to plaque burden, with up to 25% neuronal loss noted in mice with high plaque burdens (6). No neuronal loss was detected in the neocortex. In fact, APP23 mice had 14% more neocortical neurones at 8 months compared to 8-month-old wild-type mice or 27-month APP23 mice, suggesting that APP23 mice had more neurones before the development of amyloid plaques, but then lose neurones during ageing and amyloid deposition (2). Aged APP23 mice did not lose cholinergic basal forebrain neurones, but modest decreases in cortical cholinergic enzyme activity have been noted. Coupled with a 30% decrease in cholinergic fibre length (1), the results suggested that the cortical cholinergic deficit in APP23 mice is a local phenomenon. Lesioning of cholinergic neurones projecting to the neocortex actually decreased Aβ levels, strengthening the hypothesis that disruption of the basal forebrain cholinergic system was not responsible for cerebral amyloid deposition in these mice. No behavioural studies have been published to date.

TgCRND8 Mice

In order to maximise Aβ production at a given level of APP expression, TgCRND8 mice were engineered to express APP770 with the Swedish mutation (K670N, M671L) plus the Indiana mutation (V717F) under control of the PrP promoter (10). At 8 to 10 weeks, Aβ42 levels tripled to 298 ng/g brain tissue, while Aβ40 levels only slightly increased, thus increasing the Aβ42/40 ratio. At 26 weeks, Aβ42 levels exceeded 20000 ng/g and Aβ40 levels exceeded 10000 ng/g. Plaques appeared at 3 months and could be detected by both Congo red and thioflavin-S. Plaque burden in the hippocampus and cortex rapidly increased between 3 to 5 months and 8 to 12 months, significantly later than the biochemical increase in Aβ. Dense-cored plaques with associated dystrophic neurites and activated microglia were seen as early as 5 months. Cognitive deficits were also observed by behavioural testing at as young as 11 weeks. The reference memory version of the Morris water maze was used to show that tgCRND8 mice were significantly impaired in acquiring spatial information compared to their non-transgenic littermates. Testing at earlier ages was impractical, as mice were not sexually mature. As seen in other mutant APP mice the addition of mutant PS1 transgene ($PS1_{M146L+L286V}$) accelerated pathology, with lesions detected as early as one month of age.

Other APP Mice

Several other mouse models have been generated, investigating various nuances of APP processing and Aβ deposition. Humanised APP mice with the Swedish mutation had elevated APP processing and increased Aβ, but they failed to develop amyloid deposits (48). TgAPP/Ld/2 mice express $APP695_{V717I}$ and deposit Aβ starting at 12 months of age, but showed behavioural deficits as early as 3 months of age (41). When crossed with PS1 knockout mice, no deposition was seen, but behavioural deficits remained (11). This observation suggests that mutant APP overexpression rather than amyloid deposition might in and of itself contribute to behavioural deficits in transgenic mice.

Conclusion

APP transgenic models develop robust amyloid pathology making them excellent models of amyloidosis and are invaluable to understanding of pathogenesis of AD. These mice have been used successfully to demonstrate the impact of genetic variants such as presenilin mutations and APOE on amyloid deposition, the role of the inflammatory response to brain amyloid and the impact of amyloid deposition on cognitive dysfunction. In addition, APP mice are now widely used to test agents that will reduce Aβ production or hasten amyloid clearance as potential therapies for Alzheimer's disease. They have also been exploited in studies designed to develop biomarkers for AD, particularly in vivo imaging of amyloid

In must be reiterated, however, that current transgenic mice are incomplete models of AD since they generally do not develop overt neuronal loss or NFTs. As a result, considerable work is still required in the development of more authentic transgenic animal models for AD.

The generation of tau transgenic mice is one area where progress has been made. Some tau transgenic mice develop neurofibrillary pathology that is often accompanied by neuronal loss (chapter 3.9). The development of these tau transgenic animals has enabled production of mice with both amyloid plaques and NFTs by cross-breeding mutant APP (Tg2576) and mutant tau P301L (36) mice (Figure 2). Significantly, these tau/APP mice had enhanced neurofibrillary pathology in the limbic system (35), therefore providing evidence that APP dysfunction or Aβ accumulation influences neurofibrillary pathology. These double mutant tau/APP mice are a step closer to a complete model of AD and hopefully herald a new generation of transgenic mice that will develop multiple features of AD pathology.

References

1. Boncristiano S, Calhoun ME, Kelly H, Pfeifer M, Bondolfi L, Stalder M, Phinney AL, Abramowski D, Sturchler-Pierrat C, Enz A, Sommer B, Staufenbiel M, Jucker M (2002) Cholinergic changes in the APP23 transgenic mouse model of cerebral amyloidosis. *J Neurosci* 22: 3234-3243.

2. Bondolfi L, Calhoun M, Ermini MF, Kuhn HG, Wiederhold KH, Walker L, Staufenbiel M, Jucker M (2002) Amyloid-associated neurone loss and gliogenesis in the neocortex of amyloid precursor protein transgenic mice. *J Neurosci* 22: 515-522.

3. Borchelt DR, Davis J, Fischer M, Lee MK, Slunt HH, Ratovitsky T, Regard J, Copeland NG, Jenkins NA, Sisodia SS, Price DL (1996) A vector for expressing foreign genes in the brains and hearts of transgenic mice. *Genet Anal* 13: 159-163.

4. Borchelt DR, Lee MK, Gonzales V, Slunt HH, Ratovitski T, Jenkins NA, Copeland NG, Price DL, Sisodia SS (2002) Accumulation of proteolytic fragments of mutant presenilin 1 and accelerated amyloid deposition are co-regulated in transgenic mice. *Neurobiol Aging* 23: 171-177.

5. Borchelt DR, Ratovitski T, van Lare J, Lee MK, Gonzales V, Jenkins NA, Copeland NG, Price DL, Sisodia SS (1997) Accelerated amyloid deposition in the brains of transgenic mice coexpressing mutant presenilin 1 and amyloid precursor proteins. *Neurone* 19: 939-945.

6. Calhoun ME, Wiederhold KH, Abramowski D, Phinney AL, Probst A, Sturchler-Pierrat C, Staufenbiel M, Sommer B, Jucker M (1998) Neurone loss in APP transgenic mice. *Nature* 395: 755-756.

7. Carlson GA, Borchelt DR, Dake A, Turner S, Danielson V, Coffin JD, Eckman C, Meiners J, Nilsen SP, Younkin SG, Hsiao KK(1997) Genetic modification of the phenotypes produced by amyloid precursor protein overexpression in transgenic mice. *Hum Mol Genet* 6: 1951-1959.

8. Chapman PF, White GL, Jones MW, Cooper-Blacketer D, Marshall VJ, Irizarry M, Younkin L, Good MA, Bliss TV, Hyman BT, Younkin SG, Hsiao KK (1999) Impaired synaptic plasticity and learning in aged amyloid precursor protein transgenic mice. *Nat Neurosci* 2: 271-276.

9. Chen GQ, Chen KS, Knox J, Inglis J, Bernard A, Martin SJ, Justice A, McConlogue L, Games D, Freedman SB, Morris RGM(2000). A learning deficit related to age and beta-amyloid plaques in a mouse model of Alzheimer's disease. *Nature* 408: 975-979.

10. Chishti MA, Yang DS, Janus C, Phinney AL, Horne P, Pearson J, Strome R, Zuker N, Loukides J, French J, Turner S, Lozza G, Grilli M, Kunicki S, Morissette C, Paquette J, Gervais F, Bergeron C, Fraser PE, Carlson GA, George-Hyslop PS, Westaway D (2001). Early-onset amyloid deposition and cognitive deficits in transgenic mice expressing a double mutant form of amyloid precursor protein 695. *J Biol Chem* 276: 21562-21570.

11. Dewachter I, Reverse D, Caluwaerts N, Ris L, Kuiperi C, Van den Haute C, Spittaels K, Umans L, Serneels L, Thiry E, Moechars D, Mercken M, Godaux E, Van Leuven F (2002). Neuronal deficiency of presenilin 1 inhibits amyloid plaque formation and corrects hippocampal long-term potentiation but not a cognitive defect of amyloid precursor protein (V717I) transgenic mice. *J Neurosci* 22: 3445-3453.

12. Dodart JC, Meziane H, Mathis C, Bales KR, Paul SM, Ungerer A (1999) Behavioural disturbances in transgenic mice overexpressing the V717F beta-amyloid precursor protein. *Behav Neurosci* 113: 982-990.

13. Frautschy SA, Yang F, Irrizarry M, Hyman B, Saido TC, Hsiao K, Cole GM (1998) Microglial response to amyloid plaques in APPsw transgenic mice. *Am J Pathol* 152: 307-317.

14. Games D, Adams D, Alessandrini R, Barbour R, Berthelette P, Blackwell C, Carr T, Clemens J, Donaldson T, Gillespie F, et al. (1995) Alzheimer-type neuropathology in transgenic mice overexpressing V717F beta-amyloid precursor protein. *Nature* 373: 523-527.

15. Goate A, Chartier-Harlin MC, Mullan M, Brown J, Crawford F, Fidani L, Giuffra L, Haynes A, Irving N, James L and et al (1991) Segregation of a missense mutation in the amyloid precursor protein gene with familial Alzheimer's disease. *Nature* 349: 704-706.

16. Gonzalez-Lima F, Berndt JD, Valla JE, Games D, Reiman EM(2001) Reduced corpus callosum, fornix and hippocampus in PDAPP transgenic mouse model of Alzheimer's disease. *Neuroreport* 12: 2375-2379.

17. Guenette SY, Tanzi RE (1999). Progress toward valid transgenic mouse models for Alzheimer's disease *Neurobiol Aging* 20: 201-211.

18. Hernandez D, Sugaya K, Qu T, McGowan E, Duff K, McKinney M (2001). Survival and plasticity of basal forebrain cholinergic systems in mice transgenic for presenilin-1 and amyloid precursor protein mutant genes. *Neuroreport* 12: 1377-1384.

19. Holcomb L, Gordon MN, McGowan E, Yu X, Benkovic S, Jantzen P, Wright K, Saad I, Mueller R, Morgan D, Sanders S, Zehr C, O'Campo K, Hardy J, Prada CM, Eckman C, Younkin S, Hsiao K, Duff. K (1998) Accelerated Alzheimer-type phenotype in transgenic mice carrying both mutant amyloid precursor protein and presenilin 1 transgenes. *Nat Med* 4: 97-100.

20. Hsiao K, Chapman P, Nilsen S, Eckman C, Harigaya Y, Younkin S, Yang F, Cole G (1996) Correlative memory deficits, Abeta elevation, and amyloid plaques in transgenic mice. *Science* 274: 99-102.

21. Irizarry MC, Cheung BS, Rebeck GW, Paul SM, Bales KR, Hyman BT (2000) Apolipoprotein E affects the amount, form, and anatomical distribution of amyloid beta-peptide deposition in homozygous APP(V717F) transgenic mice. *Acta Neuropathol (Berl)* 100: 451-458.

22. Irizarry MC, McNamara M, Fedorchak K, Hsiao K, Hyman BT (1997) APPSw transgenic mice develop age-related A beta deposits and neuropil abnormalities, but no neuronal loss in CA1. *J Neuropathol Exp Neurol* 56: 965-973.

23. Irizarry MC, Rebeck GW, Cheung B, Bales K, Paul SM, Holzman D, Hyman BT (2000) Modulation of A beta deposition in APP transgenic mice by an apolipoprotein E null background. *Ann N Y Acad Sci* 920: 171-178.

24. Irizarry MC, Soriano F, McNamara M, Page KJ, Schenk D, Games D, Hyman BT (1997) Abeta deposition is associated with neuropil changes, but not with overt neuronal loss in the human amyloid precursor protein V717F (PDAPP) transgenic mouse. *J Neurosci* 17: 7053-7059.

25. Johnson-Wood K, Lee M, Motter R, Hu K, Gordon G, Barbour R, Khan K, Gordon M, Tan H, Games D, Lieberburg I, Schenk D, Seubert P, McConlogue L (1997) Amyloid precursor protein processing and A beta42 deposition in a transgenic mouse model of Alzheimer disease. *Proc Natl Acad Sci U S A* 94: 1550-1555.

26. Kammesheidt A, Boyce FM, Spanoyannis AF, Cummings BJ, Ortegon M, Cotman C, Vaught JL, Neve RL (1992) Deposition of beta/A4 immunoreactivity and neuronal pathology in transgenic mice expressing the carboxyl-terminal fragment of the Alzheimer amyloid precursor in the brain. *Proc Natl Acad Sci U S A* 89: 10857-10861.

27. Kawarabayashi T, Younkin LH, Saido TC, Shoji M, Ashe KH, Younkin SG(2001) Age-dependent changes in brain, CSF, and plasma amyloid (beta) protein in the Tg2576 transgenic mouse model of Alzheimer's disease. *J Neurosci* 21: 372-381.

28. Kulnane LS, Lamb BT (2001) Neuropathological characterization of mutant amyloid precursor protein yeast artificial chromosome transgenic mice. *Neurobiol Dis* 8: 982-992.

29. Kumar-Singh S, Dewachter I, Moechars D, Lubke U, De Jonghe C, Ceuterick C, Checler F, Naidu A, Cordell B, Cras P, Van Broeckhoven C, Van Leuven F (2000) Behavioural disturbances without amyloid deposits in mice overexpressing human amyloid precursor protein with Flemish (A692G) or Dutch (E693Q) mutation. *Neurobiol Dis* 7: 9-22.

30. LaFerla FM, Tinkle BT, Bieberich CJ, Haudenschild CC, Jay G (1995) The Alzheimer's A beta peptide induces neurodegeneration and apoptotic cell death in transgenic mice. *Nat Genet* 9: 21-30.

31. Lamb BT, Bardel KA, Kulnane LS, Anderson JJ, Holtz G, Wagner SL, Sisodia SS, Hoeger EJ (1999) Amyloid production and deposition in mutant amyloid precursor protein and presenilin-1 yeast artificial chromosome transgenic mice. *Nat Neurosci* 2: 695-697.

32. Lamb BT, Call LM, Slunt HH, Bardel KA, Lawler AM, Eckman CB, Younkin SG, Holtz G, Wagner SL, Price DL, Sisodia SS, Gearhart JD (1997) Altered metabolism of familial Alzheimer's disease-linked amyloid precursor protein variants in yeast artificial chromosome transgenic mice. *Hum Mol Genet* 6: 1535-1541.

33. Lamb BT, Sisodia SS, Lawler AM, Slunt HH, Kitt CA, Kearns WG, Pearson PL, Price DL, Gearhart JD (1993) Introduction and expression of the 400 kilobase amyloid precursor protein gene in transgenic mice. *Nat Genet* 5: 22-30.

34. Le R, Cruz L, Urbanc B, Knowles RB, Hsiao-Ashe K, Duff K, Irizarry MC, Stanley HE, Hyman BT (2001) Plaque-induced abnormalities in neurite geometry in transgenic models of Alzheimer disease: implications for neural system disruption. *J Neuropathol Exp Neurol* 60: 753-758.

35. Lewis J, Dickson DW, Lin WL, Chisholm L, Corral A, Jones G, Yen SH, Sahara N, Skipper L, Yager D, Eckman C, Hardy J, Hutton M, McGowan E (2001) Enhanced neurofibrillary degeneration in transgenic mice expressing mutant tau and APP. *Science* 293: 1487-1491.

36. Lewis J, McGowan E, Rockwood J, Melrose H, Nacharaju P, Van Slegtenhorst M, Gwinn-Hardy K, Murphy MP, Baker M, Yu X, Duff K, Hardy J, Corral A, Lin WL, Yen SH, Dickson DW, Davies P, Hutton M (2000) Neurofibrillary tangles, amyotrophy and progressive motor disturbance in mice expressing mutant (P301L) tau protein. *Nat Genet* 25: 402-405.

37. Malherbe P, Richards JG, Martin JR, Bluethmann H, Maggio J, Huber G (1996) Lack of beta-amyloidosis in transgenic mice expressing low levels of familial Alzheimer's disease missense mutations. *Neurobiol Aging* 17: 205-214.

38. Masliah E, Sisk A, Mallory M, Games D (2001) Neurofibrillary pathology in transgenic mice overexpressing V717F beta-amyloid precursor protein. *J Neuropathol Exp Neurol* 60: 357-368.

39. Matsuoka Y, Picciano M, Malester B, LaFrancois J, Zehr C, Daeschner JM, Olschowka JA, Fonseca MI, O'Banion MK, Tenner AJ, Lemere CA, Duff K (2001) Fibrillar beta-amyloid evokes oxidative damage in a transgenic mouse model of Alzheimer's disease. *Neuroscience* 104: 609-613.

40. McGowan E, Sanders S, Iwatsubo T, Takeuchi A, Saido T, Zehr C, Yu X, Uljon S, Wang R, Mann D, Dickson D, Duff K (1999) Amyloid phenotype characterization of transgenic mice overexpressing both mutant amyloid precursor protein and mutant presenilin1 transgenes. *Neurobiol Dis* 6: 231-244.

41. Moechars D, Dewachter I, Lorent K, Reverse D, Baekelandt V, Naidu A, Tesseur I, Spittaels K, Haute CV, Checler F, Godaux E, Cordell B, Van Leuven F (1999) Early phenotypic changes in transgenic mice that overexpress different mutants of amyloid precursor protein in brain. *J Biol Chem* 274: 6483-6492.

42. Moechars D, Lorent K, Dewachter I, Baekelandt V, De Strooper B, Van Leuven F (1998) Transgenic mice expressing an alpha-secretion mutant of the amyloid precursor protein in the brain develop a progressive CNS disorder. *Behav Brain Res* 95: 55-64.

43. Moechars D, Lorent K, Reverse D, Baekelandt V, Naidu A, Tesseur I, Spittaels K, Haute CV, Checler F, Godaux E, Cordell B, Van Leuven F (1996) Expression in brain of amyloid precursor protein mutated in the alpha-secretase site causes disturbed behavior, neuronal degeneration and premature death in transgenic mice. *EMBO J* 15: 1265-1274.

44. Moechars D, Lorent K, Van Leuven F (1999) Premature death in transgenic mice that overexpress a mutant amyloid precursor protein is preceded by severe neurodegeneration and apoptosis. *Neuroscience* 91: 819-830.

45. Nalbantoglu J, Tirado-Santiago G, Lahsaini A, Poirier J, Goncalves O, Verge G, Momoli F, Welner SA, Massicotte G, Julien JP, Shapiro ML (1997) Impaired learning and LTP in mice expressing the carboxy terminus of the Alzheimer amyloid precursor protein. *Nature* 387: 500-505.

46. Neve RL, Boyce FM, McPhie DL, Greenan J, Oster-Granite ML (1996) Transgenic mice expressing APP-C100 in the brain. *Neurobiol Aging* 17: 191-203.

47. Oster-Granite ML, McPhie DL, Greenan J, Neve RL (1996) Age-dependent neuronal and synaptic degeneration in mice transgenic for the C terminus of the amyloid precursor protein. *J Neurosci* 16: 6732-6741.

48. Reaume AG, Howland DS, Trusko SP, Savage MJ, Lang DM, Greenberg BD, Siman R, Scott RW (1996) Enhanced amyloidogenic processing of the beta-amyloid precursor protein in gene-targeted mice bearing the Swedish familial Alzheimer's disease mutations and a humanized Abeta sequence. *J Biol Chem* 271: 23380-23388.

49. Selkoe DJ (1994) Normal and abnormal biology of the beta-amyloid precursor protein. *Annu Rev Neurosci* 17: 489-517.

50. Sturchler-Pierrat C, Abramowski D, Duke M, Wiederhold KH, Mistl C, Rothacher S, Ledermann B, Burki K, Frey P, Paganetti PA, Waridel C, Calhoun ME, Jucker M, Probst A, Staufenbiel M, Sommer B (1997) Two amyloid precursor protein transgenic mouse models with Alzheimer disease-like pathology. *Proc Natl Acad Sci U S A* 94: 13287-92.

51. Suzuki T, Oishi M, Marshak DR, Czernik AJ, Nairn AC, Greengard P (1994) Cell cycle-dependent regulation of the phosphorylation and metabolism of the Alzheimer amyloid precursor protein. *EMBO J* 13: 1114-1122.

52. Takeuchi A, Irizarry MC, Duff K, Saido TC, Hsiao Ashe K, Hasegawa M, Mann DM, Hyman BT, Iwatsubo T (2000) Age-related amyloid beta deposition in transgenic mice overexpressing both Alzheimer mutant presenilin 1 and amyloid beta precursor protein Swedish mutant is not associated with global neuronal loss. *Am J Pathol* 157: 331-339.

53. Tomidokoro Y, Harigaya Y, Matsubara E, Ikeda M, Kawarabayashi T, Shirao T, Ishiguro K, Okamoto K, Younkin SG, Shoji M (2001) Brain Abeta amyloidosis in APPsw mice induces accumulation of presenilin-1 and tau. *J Pathol* 194: 500-506.

54. Tomidokoro Y, Ishiguro K, Harigaya Y, Matsubara E, Ikeda M, Park JM, Yasutake K, Kawarabayashi T, Okamoto K, Shoji M (2001) Abeta amyloidosis induces the initial stage of tau accumulation in APP(Sw) mice. *Neurosci Lett* 299: 169-172.

55. Westerman MA, Cooper-Blacketer D, Mariash A, Kotilinek L, Kawarabayashi T, Younkin LH, Carlson GA, Younkin SG, Ashe KH (2002) The relationship between Abeta and memory in the Tg2576 mouse model of Alzheimer's disease. *J Neurosci* 22: 1858-1867.

CHAPTER 3

Tauopathies

Chapter Editor: Jean-Jacques Hauw

3.1 Introduction to the Tauopathies 82

3.2 Frontotemporal Dementia and Parkinsonism Linked to Chromosome 17 Associated with *Tau* Gene Mutations (FTDP-17*T*) 86

3.3 Progressive Supranuclear Palsy (PSP) or Steele-Richardson-Olszewski Disease 103

3.4 Corticobasal Degeneration 115

3.5 Pick's Disease 124

3.6 Argyrophilic Grain Disease 132

3.7 Parkinsonism-dementia Complex of Guam 137

3.8 Postencephalitic Parkinsonism 143

3.9 Transgenic Animal Models of Tauopathies 150

Introduction to the Tauopathies

Michel Goedert

AD	Alzheimer's disease
CBD	corticobasal degeneration
MAP	microtubule-associated protein
PiD	Pick's disease
PHF	paired helical filament
PSP	progressive supranuclear palsy

In 1907 Alzheimer described the neuropathological characteristics of the disease that was subsequently named after him. Abundant neuritic plaques and neurofibrillary lesions still constitute the defining neuropathological characteristics of Alzheimer's disease (AD). Although Kidd had described the paired helical filament (PHF) as the major structural component of the neurofibrillary lesions in 1963, the molecular nature of the PHF was only uncovered in the 1980s. By the early 1990s, it was clear that tau is the major, if not the only, component of the PHF and that the latter is made of the 6 brain tau isoforms, each full-length and hyperphosphorylated (for review, see 15). By that time, tau protein-like immunoreactivity had also been described in the pathological deposits of Pick's disease (PiD), progressive supranuclear palsy (PSP) and corticobasal degeneration (CBD) (for review, see 25). In contrast to AD and PiD, the abnormal deposits of PSP and CBD are present in both nerve cells and glial cells. Subsequently, filamentous tau deposits were described in other neurodegenerative diseases (Table 1).

Tau is a microtubule-associated protein (MAP) that binds to microtubules and promotes microtubule assembly. Microtubules are essential cytoskeletal components made of repeating $\alpha\beta$-tubulin heterodimers that are labile unless stabilised by other molecules. Accordingly, most cells express MAPs which stabilise microtubules. Of the neuronal MAPs, tau protein is one of the most abundant. Six tau isoforms are expressed in the adult human brain by alternative mRNA splicing from a single gene (1, 10) (Figure 1). They differ from each other by the presence or absence of 29- or 58-amino acid inserts located in the amino-terminal half and an additional 31-amino acid repeat in the carboxy-terminal half (Figure 1). Inclusion of the latter produces the 3 isoforms with 4 repeats each; the other 3 isoforms have 3 repeats each. The repeats and some adjoining sequences constitute the microtubule-binding domains of tau (8, 24). Similar levels of 3- and 4-repeat tau isoforms are expressed in normal human cerebral cortex (11). This approximately 1:1 ratio is crucial

Diseases in which tau deposits have been described
Alzheimer's disease
Amyotrophic lateral sclerosis/parkinsonism-dementia complex
Argyrophilic grain disease
Autosomal-recessive juvenile parkinsonism
Corticobasal degeneration
Dementia pugilistica
Diffuse neurofibrillary tangles with calcification
Down's syndrome
Familial British dementia
Frontotemporal dementia and parkinsonism linked to chromosome 17
Gerstmann-Sträussler-Scheinker disease
Guadeloupean parkinsonism
Hallervorden-Spatz disease
Myotonic dystrophy
Niemann-Pick disease, type C
Non-Guamanian motor neuron disease with neurofibrillary tangles
Pick's disease
Postencephalitic parkinsonism
Prion protein cerebral amyloid angiopathy
Progressive subcortical gliosis
Progressive supranuclear palsy
Subacute sclerosing panencephalitis
Tangle only dementia

Table 1. Diseases in which tau deposits have been described.

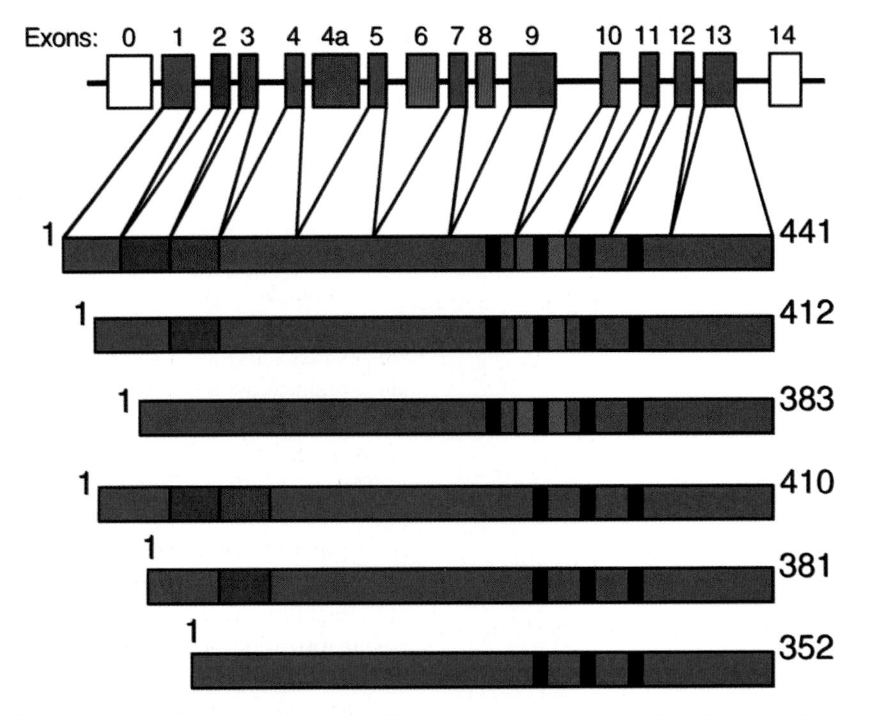

Figure 1. *Schematic representation of the human Tau gene and the 6 tau isoforms (352 to 441 amino acids) that are generated in brain through alternative mRNA splicing.* The human *Tau* gene consists of 16 exons (E) and extends over approximately 100 kb. E0, which forms part of the promoter, and E14 are non-coding (in white). Alternative splicing of E2 (in red), E3 (in green) and E10 (in yellow) gives rise to the six tau isoforms. The constitutively spliced exons (E1, E4, E5, E7, E9, E11, E12, E13) are indicated in blue. E6 and E8 (in violet) are not transcribed in human brain. E4a (in orange) is only expressed in the peripheral nervous system, where its presence gives rise to the tau isoform known as big tau. Black bars indicate the microtubule-binding repeats, with 3 isoforms having 3 repeats each and 3 isoforms having 4 repeats each. The exons and introns are not drawn to scale.

for preventing neurodegeneration and dementia in mid-life (see below).

Tau assembles into filaments through its tandem repeat region, with the amino-terminal half and the carboxy-terminus not participating in the structure of the filament. Following assembly, tau becomes truncated at the amino-terminus. This is necessary for its subsequent ubiquitination (26). Following the death of tangle-bearing cells, the pathological material stays around in the extracellular space, in the form of so-called "ghost tangles" that consist largely of the ubiquitinated repeat region of tau. It thus appears that in AD the ubiquitination of tau filaments is a late, secondary event.

By contrast, the abnormal hyperphosphorylation that characterises PHF-tau at a biochemical level is an early event that appears to precede filament assembly (2). It also renders PHF-tau unable to interact with microtubules (3, 34). Over the years, much effort has gone into the mapping of phosphorylation sites in normal and abnormal tau, and the identification of candidate protein kinases and protein phosphatases. In particular, proline-directed protein kinases and protein phosphatase 2A have been implicated in the phosphorylation and dephosphorylation of tau protein (7, 12, 17, 22).

The abnormal hyperphosphorylation of tau is a feature common to all diseases with tau filaments. The phosphorylated sites are similar, with only minor differences between diseases. However, the pattern of abnormal tau bands varies. Thus, AD is characterised by three major bands of 60, 64 and 68 kDa and a minor band of 74 kDa (16). By contrast, filamentous tau from brains of patients with PSP and CBD lacks the 60-kDa band (9, 23), whereas pathological tau from PiD brain shows major 60- and 64-kDa bands (15). Differences in the tau isoform composition of the pathological filaments explain these patterns of bands. This work revealed that the biochemical composition of tau filaments is not uniform.

It remains to be seen whether the abnormal hyperphosphorylation of tau is either necessary or sufficient for filament assembly. Methods were developed for forming paired helical-like tau filaments from purified full-length protein in vitro (3, 21, 29). They are based on the interaction of non-phosphorylated tau protein with negatively charged substances, such as sulphated glycosaminoglycans and RNA. The characteristics of these filaments closely resemble those of tau filaments from AD brain. However, the precise mechanisms that cause the normally soluble tau protein to assemble into abnormal filaments in brain cells remain to be discovered.

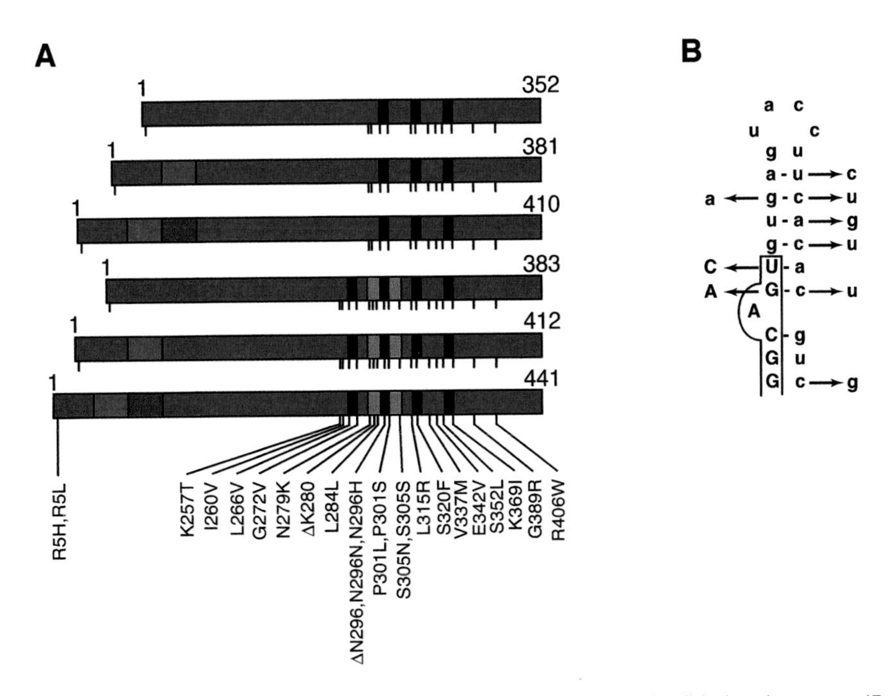

Figure 2. *Mutations in the Tau gene in frontotemporal dementia and parkinsonism linked to chromosome 17 (FTDP-17).* **A.** Schematic diagram of the 6 tau isoforms that are expressed in adult human brain, with mutations in the coding region indicated using the amino acid numbering of the 441 amino acid isoform. Nineteen missense mutations, 2 deletion mutations and 3 silent mutations are shown. **B.** Stem-loop structure in the pre-mRNA at the boundary between E10 and the intron following E10. Nine mutations are shown, 2 of which (S305N anmd S305S) are located in E10. Exon sequences are shown in capital and intron sequences in lower-case letters.

The molecular dissection of the PHF of AD gave quite a complete description of the composition of the filament. It also provided important clues regarding the mechanisms of filament formation. However, it did not provide any direct information as concerning the relevance of filament assembly for the disease process. As a result, tau-positive inclusions were frequently considered to be nothing more than epiphenomena of little or no consequence. What was required was genetic evidence linking dysfunction of tau protein to neurodegeneration and dementia. In 1994. an autosomal-dominantly inherited form of frontotemporal dementia with parkinsonism was linked to chromosome 17q21.2, a region that contains the tau gene (33). This observation was followed by the identification of other forms of frontotemporal dementia that were linked to this region, resulting in the denomination "frontotemporal dementia and parkinsonism linked to chromosome 17" (FTDP-17) for this class of disease. Cases of FTDP-17 were found to exhibit tau-positive inclusions in either nerve cells or in both nerve cells and glial cells. The now widely used term "tauopathy" was introduced because of the sheer abundance of tau inclusions in a family with frontotemporal dementia (31). In 1998, the first mutations in *Tau* in FTDP-17 were reported, with the current total standing at 31 different mutations (Figure 2) (20, 30, 32). The study of FTDP-17 has shown that dysfunction of tau protein is sufficient to cause neurodegeneration and dementia. At a functional level, it has been shown repeatedly that a change in the ratio of 3- to 4-repeat tau isoforms is sufficient to cause disease (20, 32). The finding that many mutations reduce the ability of tau to interact with microtubules suggests that this interaction is crucial for preventing the self-assembly of tau into abnormal filaments (18, 19). Some of these mutations also promote the assembly of tau into filaments (14, 27).

The work on FTDP-17 keeps throwing important light on the pathogenesis of other diseases, since some *Tau* mutations lead to clinical and neuropathological phenotypes similar to those of PSP, CBD and PiD. Moreover, the report (4) of an association between PSP and homozygosity of a common allele at a dinucleotide repeat in the intron following exon 9 of *Tau* (the A0 allele) has been confirmed and extended to CBD (6). Although the precise mechanisms remain to be worked out, the central importance of tau for these diseases is beyond doubt. More unexpected is the reported association between the A0 allele and idiopathic Parkinson's disease (28). It remains to be seen whether tau and α-synuclein are linked in ways that await discovery.

Over the years, much has been learned about the tau inclusions that characterise a surprisingly large number of neurodegenerative diseases. In FTDP-17, the basis underlying disease is a toxic property conferred by the mutations in *Tau*. It is tempting to suggest that a similar toxic property may also be at work in other diseases with tau inclusions. Despite these advances, major questions remain. For example, it is important to know whether the inclusions contribute to pathogenesis or whether they are neutral or even beneficial by-products of the disease process. A related question concerns the molecular events that lead from conformational changes in tau protein to neuronal dysfunction and cell death. Answers to these questions may well lead to the development of effective therapeutic strategies for the tauopathies.

References

1. Andreadis A, Brown MW, Kosik KS (1992) Structure and novel exons of the human tau gene. *Biochemistry* 31: 10626-10633.

2. Braak H, Braak E (1991) Neuropathological stageing of Alzheimer-related changes. *Acta Neuropathol* 82: 239-259.

3. Bramblett GT, Goedert M, Jakes R, Merrick SE, Trojanowski JQ, Lee VMY (1993) Abnormal tau phosphorylation at Ser396 in Alzheimer's disease recapitulates development and contributes to reduced microtubule binding. *Neuron* 19: 1089-1099.

4. Conrad C, Andreadis A, Trojanowski JQ, Dickson DW, Kang D, Chen X, Wiederholt W, Hansen L, Masliah E, Thal LJ, Katzman R, Xia Y, Saitoh T (1997) Genetic evidence for the involvement of tau in progressive supranuclear palsy. *Ann Neurol* 41: 277-281.

5. Delacourte A, Robitaille Y, Sergeant N, Buée L, Hof PR, Wattez A, Laroche-Cholette A, Mathieu J, Chagnon P, Gauvreau D (1996) Specific pathological tau protein variants characterize Pick's disease. *J Neuropathol Exp Neurol* 55: 159-168.

6. Di Maria E, Tabaton M, Vigo T, Abbruzzese G, Bellone E, Donati C, Frasson E, Marchese E, Montagna P, Munoz DG, Pramstaller PP, Zanusso G, Ajmar F, Mandich P (2000) Corticobasal degeneration shares a common genetic background with progressive supranuclear palsy. *Ann Neurol* 47: 374-377.

7. Drewes G, Lichtenberg-Kraag B, Döring F, Mandelkow EM, Biernat J, Dorée M, Mandelkow E (1992) Mitogen-activated protein (MAP) kinase transforms tau protein into an Alzheimer-like state. *EMBO J* 11: 2131-2138.

8. Ennulat DJ, Liem RKH, Hashim GA, Shelanski ML (1989) Two separate 18-amino acid domains of tau promote the polymerization of tubulin. *J Biol Chem* 264: 5327-5330.

9. Flament S, Delacourte A, Verny M, Hauw JJ, Javoy-Agid F (1991) Abnormal tau proteins in progressive supranuclear palsy. Similarities and differences with the neurofibrillary degeneration of the Alzheimer type. *Acta Neuropathol* 81: 591-596.

10. Goedert M, Spillantini MG, Jakes R, Rutherford D, Crowther RA (1989) Multiple isoforms of human microtubule-associated protein tau: sequences and localization in neurofibrillary tangles of Alzheimer's disease. *Neuron* 3: 519-526.

11. Goedert M, Jakes R (1990) Expression of separate isoforms of human tau protein: correlation with the tau pattern in brain and effects on tubulin polymerization. *EMBO J* 9: 4225-4230.

12. Goedert M, Cohen ES, Jakes R, Cohen P (1992) p42 MAP kinase phosphorylation sites in microtubule-associated protein tau are dephosphorylated by protein phosphatase $2A_1$. *FEBS Lett* 312: 95-99.

13. Goedert M, Jakes R, Spillantini MG, Hasegawa M, Smith MJ, Crowther RA (1996) Assembly of microtubule-associated protein tau into Alzheimer-like filaments induced by sulphated glycosaminoglycans. *Nature* 383: 550-553.

14. Goedert M, Jakes R, Crowther RA (1999) Effects of frontotemporal dementia FTDP-17 mutations on heparin-induced assembly of tau filaments. *FEBS Lett* 450: 306-311.

15. Goedert M, Klug A (1999) Tau protein and the paired helical filament of Alzheimer's disease. *Brain Res Bull* 50:469-470.

16. Greenberg SG, Davies P (1990) A preparation of Alzheimer paired helical filaments that displays distinct tau proteins by polyacrylamide gel electrophoresis. *Proc Natl Acad Sci U S A* 87: 5827-5831.

17. Hanger DP, Hughes K, Woodgett JR, Brion JP, Anderton BH (1992) Glycogen synthase kinase-3 induces Alzheimer's disease-like phosphorylation of tau: generation of paired helical filament epitopes and neuronal localization of the kinase. *Neurosci Lett* 147: 58-62.

18. Hasegawa M, Smith MJ, Goedert M (1998) Tau proteins with FTDP-17 mutations have a reduced ability to promote microtubule assembly. *FEBS Lett* 437:207-210.

19. Hong M, Zhukareva V, Vogelsberg-Ragaglia V, Wszolek Z, Reed L, Miller BL, Geschwind DH, Bird TD, McKeel D, Goate A, Morris JC, Wilhelmsen KC, Schellenberg GD, Trojanowski JQ, Lee VMY (1998) Mutation-specific functional impairments in distinct tau isoforms of hereditary FTDP-17. *Science* 282:1914-1917.

20. Hutton M, Lendon CL, Rizzu P, Baker M, Froelich S, Houlden H, Pickering-Brown S, Chakraverty S, Isaacs A, Grover A, Hackett J et al (1998) Association of missense and 5'-splice-site mutations in tau with the inherited dementia FTDP-17. Nature 393: 702-705.

21. Kampers T, Friedhoff P, Biernat J, Mandelkow EM, Mandelkow E (1996) RNA stimulates aggregation of microtubule-associated protein *Tau* into Alzheimer-like paired helical filaments. *FEBS Lett* 399:344-349.

22. Kobayashi S, Ishiguro K, Omori A, Takamatsu M, Atioka M, Imahori K, Uchida T (1993) A cdc-related kinase PSSALRE/cdk5 is homologous with the 30 kDa subunit of tau protein kinase II, a proline-directed protein kinase associated with microtubules. *FEBS Lett* 335: 171-175.

23. Ksiezak-Reding H, Morgan K, Mattiace LA, Davies P, Liu WK, Yen SH, Weidenheim K, Dickson DW (1994) Ultrastructure and biochemical composition of paired helical filaments in corticobasal degeneration. *Am J Pathol* 145: 1496-1508.

24. Lee G, Neve RL, Kosik KS (1989) The microtubule binding domain of tau protein. *Neuron* 2: 1615-1624.

25. Lee VMY, Goedert M, Trojanowski JQ (2001) Neurodegenerative tauopathies. *Annu Rev Neurosci* 24:1121-1159.

26. Morishima-Kawashima M, Hasegawa M, Takio K, Suzuki M, Titani K, Ihara Y (1993) Ubiquitin is conjugated with amino-terminally processed tau in paired helical filaments. *Neuron* 10: 1151-1160.

27. Nacharaju P, Lewis J, Easson C, Yen S, Hackett J, Hutton M, Yen SH (1999) Accelerated filament formation from tau protein with specific FTDP-17 missense mutations. *FEBS Lett* 447: 195-199.

28. Pastor P, Ezquerra M, Munoz E, Marti MJ,, Blesa R, Tolosa E, Oliva R (2000) Significant association

between the tau gene A0/A0 genotype and Parkinson's disease. *Ann Neurol* 47: 242-245.

29. Pérez M, Valpuesta JM, Medina M, Montejo de Garcini E, Avila J (1996) Polymerization of tau into filaments in the presence of heparin: the minimal sequence required for tau-tau interactions. *J Neurochem* 67: 1183-1190.

30. Poorkaj P, Bird TD, Wijsman E, Nemens E, Garruto RM, Anderson L, Andreadis A, Wiederholt WC, Raskind M, Schellenberg GD (1998) Tau is a candidate gene for chromosome 17 frontotemporal dementia. *Ann Neurol* 43: 815-825.

31. Spillantini MG, Goedert M, Crowther RA, Murrell JR, Farlow MJ, Ghetti B (1997) Familial multiple system tauopathy with presenile dementia: a disease with abundant neuronal and glial tau filaments. *Proc Natl Acad Sci U S A* 94: 4113-4118.

32. Spillantini MG, Murrell JR, Goedert M, Farlow MR, Klug A, Ghetti B (1998) Mutation in the tau gene in familial multiple system tauopathy and presenile dementia. *Proc Natl Acad Sci U S A* 95: 7737-7741.

33. Wilhelmsen KC, Lynch T, Pavlou E, Higgins M, Nygaard TG (1994) Localization of disinhibition-dementia-parkinsonism-amyotrophy complex to 17q21-22. *Am J Hum Genet* 55: 1159-1165.

34. Yoshida H, Ihara Y (1993) Tau in paired helical filament is functionally distinct from fetal tau: assembly incompetence of paired helical filament tau. *J Neurochem* 61: 1183-1186.

Frontotemporal Dementia and Parkinsonism Linked to Chromosome 17 Associated with *Tau* Gene Mutations (FTDP-17*T*)

Bernardino Ghetti
Michael L. Hutton
Zbigniew K. Wszolek

AD	Alzheimer's disease
EEG	electroencephalography
EMG	electromyography
FTDP	frontotemporal dementia and parkinsonism
MRI	magnetic resonance imaging
PET	positron emission tomography
PD	Parkinson's disease
PHF	paired-helical filaments
SF	straight filaments

Definition

Frontotemporal dementia and parkinsonism linked to chromosome 17 associated with *Tau* gene mutations (FTDP-17*T*) is a group of genetically-determined, adult-onset, progressive neurodegenerative syndromes, which lead to the accumulation of intracellular deposits of soluble and insoluble hyperphosphorylated tau protein. The clinical phenotypes are characterised by behavioral, cognitive and motor disturbances that may occur in various combinations and in varying degrees of severity. The central element of the neuropathologic phenotypes is tau deposition that occurs either in neurons or in both neurons and glia in multiple areas of the central nervous system with prevalence in the cerebral cortex and some subcortical nuclei.

Synonyms and Historical Annotations

The definition given above represents an evolution of the concept, frontotemporal dementia and parkinsonism linked to chromosome 17, which was developed during the International Consensus Conference in Ann Arbor, Michigan, in 1996 (17). Thirteen families with individuals affected by syndromes linked to chromosome 17q21-22 were presented. These syndromes were characterised clinically by frontotemporal dementia and in some instances parkinsonism. These disorders, some of which had been known for many years, had been given names according to the predominant clinical or pathologic features, such as familial Pick disease, familial progressive subcortical gliosis, familial presenile dementia with tangles, autosomal dominant parkinsonism and dementia with pallido-ponto-nigral degeneration, and multiple system tauopathy with presenile dementia.

The major clinical manifestations of affected individuals included behavioral disturbances, cognitive impairment, and parkinsonism. At the 1996 conference, it was agreed that the name of this new syndrome should reflect these 3 cardinal clinical features and the genetic linkage to chromosome 17 rather than be based on relatively incomplete pathologic observations available at that time; however, it should be noted that a tau abnormality was seen in individuals from 4 of these families.

There is no official synonym for FTDP-17*T*; however, the term "tauopathy" is sometimes used to refer to FTDP-17*T*. The word tauopathy originates from the name of the disease in one of the original 13 families, multiple system tauopathy with presenile dementia, and although it was originally intended to be used for genetically-determined diseases characterised by tau pathology only, this term is used by many investigators to refer to other diseases as well (67).

In view of the facts that: *i)* a linkage to chromosome 17q21-22 was established for the syndrome seen in each of the 13 families presented at the 1996 consensus conference, *ii)* the *Tau* gene had been localised to chromosome 17q21 in 1986, and *iii)* tau pathology was a distinct feature in some of those families, the analysis of the *Tau* gene in the affected subjects and healthy relatives became a priority (4, 17, 25, 39, 42, 47, 51, 77). Several groups carried out this analysis and in 1998 the first point mutations in the *Tau* gene were identified in affected individuals from most of the 13 kindreds (29, 54, 68). It should be noted that 10 of the original 13 families were found to have the syndrome associated with a mutation in the *Tau* gene. To date, the genetic basis for the syndromes in the remaining 3 families is not known. This chapter will deal specifically with disorders associated with *Tau* mutations.

The identification of mutations in *Tau* associated with frontotemporal dementia and parkinsonism linked to chromosome 17 demonstrated that tau dysfunction is sufficient to cause neurodegeneration and focused attention on the role of tau in other neurodegenerative diseases with tau pathology.

Epidemiology

Prevalence and incidence. The prevalence and incidence of FTDP-17*T* are unknown. Currently, approximately 80 families are known to have or have had individuals affected with FTDP-17*T*. These families have been ascertained from the United States, United Kingdom, Japan, The Netherlands, France, Canada, Australia, Italy, Germany, Israel, Ireland, Spain, and Sweden (countries listed according to the number of described families). There are molecular genetic data indicating that some of these families may share a common founder (73). Molecular genetic studies have identified 31 unique *Tau* gene mutations. The 3 most prevalent are P301L, exon 10 5′ +16,

		Mutations not in exon 10					Mutations in exon 10	Exon 10 5' splice-site mutations
		Exon 1	Exon 9	Exon 11	Exon 12	Exon 13		
Clinical features								
Average age at onset	<30						P301S	
	31-40		L266V	S320F		G389R	delN296 S305N	
	41-50		G272V		E342V		N279K P301L	+3 +11 +14 +16
	50<	R5H R5L			V337M K369I	R406W	del280K L284L N296H S305S	+12 +13
Average duration	<5	R5H R5L	L266V			G389R	delK280 delN296 N296H S305N	
	6-10		G272V		E342V K369I		N279K L284L P301L P301S S305S	+11 +12
	11-15			S320F	V337M			+3 +14 +16
	15<					R406W		
First sign	Parkinsonism	R5L					N279K P301L delN296 S305S	+3 +11
	Dementia	R5H		S320F		R406W	L284L delN296	+3 +12
	Personality change		G272V		V337M E342V K369I		P301L N296H S305S S305N	+12 +14 +16
Parkinsonism	Early-prominent						N279K delN296 S305S	+11
	Late-prominent						P301S N296H	+3 +12 +14 +16
	Rare-minimal	R5L	G272V				P301L S305N	
Dementia	Early-prominent		L266V	S320F		R406W	delN296 S305S	+12
	Late-prominent		G272V		V337M K369I		delK280 L284L P301L P301S S305N	+3 +11 +13
	Rare-minimal						N279K	
Personality change	Early-prominent		L266V G272V		V337M K369I	R406W	delK280 L284L P301L P301S S305S S305N	+12 +14 +16
Language difficulties			G272V	S320F		G389R	N279K L284L N296H P301L S305S	+14 +16
Late mutism					V337M	R406W	N279K delK280 N296H P301S S305N	
Eye movement abnormalities							N279K N296H P301S delN296 S305S	+3
Epilepsy							P301S	
Myoclonus					V337M		P301S	+11
Pyramidal signs							N279K P301S S305S	+3 +12
Amyotrophy							P301L	+14

Table 1. (Continued on next page).

and N279K. They account for about 60% of known cases.

Three studies have been carried out in an effort to estimate the prevalence and incidence of mutations in the *Tau* gene in individuals diagnosed with a non-Alzheimer dementia (28, 55, 61). Although *Tau* mutations are uncommon in general, a positive family history of frontotemporal dementia and/or tau pathologic findings increases the likelihood of the presence of a *Tau* gene mutation.

Gender and age distribution. FTDP-17*T* is inherited in an autosomal dominant fashion and therefore has an equal distribution among males and females. The average age at the onset of symptoms is 49 years with a range from 25 to 76 years. The average duration of the clinical course is 8.5 years with a range from 2 to 26 years (59, 80). However, the data on the onset and duration are only available for a limited number of individuals.

Risk factors. There are no known environmental risk factors for FTDP-17*T*. However, FTDP-17*T* phenotypes vary significantly within and between families with the same mutation as well as between families with different mutations (7, 75, 80). Thus, it is plausible to assume that either environmental or other genetic factors partially influence this variability in clinical presentation. As a matter of fact, studies are in progress to determine whether a tau mutation in a H1 or H2 allele may affect the clinical and/or

		Exon 1	Exon 9	Mutations not in exon 10 Exon 11	Exon 12	Exon 13	Mutations in exon 10	Exon 10 5' splice-site mutations
Laboratory findings								
MRI	Frontotemporal atrophy			S320F	K369I	R406W G389R	P301S N296H P301L N279K S305S	+11 +12 +14 +16
	Pontine/ mesencephalic atrophy					N279K		
	Asymmetry				K369I	G389R	N279K P301L N296H	+16
PET	FDG; frontotemporal hypometabolism					G389R	P301S N279K S305S	+14 +16
	6FD; reduced uptake in striatum						N279K	
	RAC; normal						N279K	
SPECT	IMP or PAO; frontotemporal hypometabolism					G389R	P301L	
	IPT (DAT); reduced uptake in striatum						P301S	
	IBZM						P301S	
EEG	Generalized slowness					R406W	P301S G272V N279K P301L	+11 +14
	Epileptiform activity						P301S	
EMG	Denervation change						P301L	+14

Table 1.

References; 1, 4, 6-8, 12-14, 17, 19, 21-25, 28-35, 37, 39-43, 45-46, 50-53, 55-64, 66-73, 77, 79, 81-83

MRI: magnetic resonance imaging, PET: positron emission tomography, FDG: [18F]-fluorodeoxyglucose, 6FD: [18F]-6-fluoro-L-dopa, RAC: [11C]-raclopride, SPECT: single photon emission tomography, IMP: [123I]-isopropyliodoamphetamine, PAO: hexamethyl propylamine oxime, IPT: [123I]-(N)-(3-iodopropen-2-yl)-2beta-carbomethoxy-3beta-(4-chlorophenyl) tropane, DAT; dopamine transporter, IBZM: -[123I]-(S)-2-hydroxy-3-iodo-6-methoxy-[(1-ethyl-2-pyrrolidinyl)methyl] benzamide, EEG: electroencephalography, EMG: electromyography.

pathologic phenotypes (74). Studies of the *Apolipoprotein E* genotype in some families did not provide any evidence that *Apolipoprotein E* influences phenotypic variability (6, 13, 32).

Genetics

FTDP-17*T* is inherited in an autosomal dominant pattern. Linkage analysis in some families established a relationship between the clinical syndrome of frontotemporal dementia and a locus on chromosome 17q21. The *Tau* gene, which is located in that region, has been found to contain mutations associated with FTDP-17. The human *Tau* gene consists of 16 exons; however, only 11 of these exons (Exons 1, 2, 3, 4, 5, 7, 9, 10, 11, 12, and 13) are expressed in the central nervous system (CNS) (Figure 1).

Tau is a microtubule-binding protein that is abundant in neurons and glia; in neurons it is predominantly expressed in axons. A region of the protein tau that is essential for its function is the microtubule-binding domain. Through the binding with tau, microtubules are stabilised and their polymerisation is promoted. The microtubule-binding region, located in the carboxy terminal half of the protein, contains tandem-repeat sequences of 31 or 32 amino acids each, which are encoded by exons 9, 10, 11 and 12. In the adult CNS, the tau protein is present as 6 isoforms resulting from the alternative splicing of exons 2, 3 and 10. The splicing of exon 10 is regulated by a RNA stem loop structure at the boundary between exon 10 and the intron after exon 10. Exons 2 and 3 each encode a 29 amino acid long insert in the amino terminal half, while exon 10 encodes a 31 amino acid long insert in the carboxy terminal half. Thus, 3 isoforms have 3 microtubule binding repeats (3R) and 3 isoforms have 4 microtubule-binding repeats (4R) (36) (Figure 1).

Mutations in the *Tau* gene associated with FTDP-17*T* are either exonic or intronic (Figure 2). The exonic mutations may be missense, deletion, or silent. All but two known exonic mutations occur in exons 9 to 13; these 2 are the R5H and R5L mutations that occur in exon 1. The intronic mutations are clustered in the 5′ splice site of the intron following exon 10. These mutations and some of those located in exon 10 affect the alternative splicing of exon 10 (Figure 3).

Clinical Features

Symptoms and Signs. The onset of FTDP-17*T* is usually insidious. Affected individuals in a fully developed stage of disease present with a constellation of signs, including at least 2 of the 3 cardinal manifestations of FTDP-17*T*: behavioral and personality disturbances, cognitive deficits, and motor dysfunction (most often signs of parkinsonism-plus syndrome).

It should be noted that there is significant clinical phenotypic heterogeneity in individuals with different mutations. In addition, interfamilial and intrafamilial variability of clinical phenotype is often seen among individuals carrying the same mutation. A detailed description of clinical signs as they relate to specific mutations is presented in Table 1.

The behavioral and personality abnormalities include disinhibition, apathy, defective judgment, compulsive behavior, hyper-religiosity, neglect of personal hygiene, alcoholism, illicit drug addiction, verbal and physical aggressiveness, family abuse, and others. The common cognitive disturbances in early stages of the disease are characterised by relative preservation of memory, orientation, and visuospatial function. Progressive speech difficulties with non-fluent aphasia and disorders of executive functions may be initially seen. Later on, progressive deterioration of memory, orientation, and visuospatial functions as well as echolalia, palilalia, and verbal and vocal perseverations are encountered. Finally, progressive dementia and mutism occur. The motor signs are dominated by the occurrence of parkinsonism. The parkinsonism can be the initial manifestation of the disease and as a matter of fact, some FTDP-17*T* patients were misdiagnosed as having Parkinson's disease (PD) or progressive supranuclear palsy (PSP). However, in some families, the parkinsonism occurs late in the course of the illness or not at all. The parkinsonism in FTDP-17*T* is characterised by rather symmetrical bradykinesia, postural instability, rigidity affecting equally

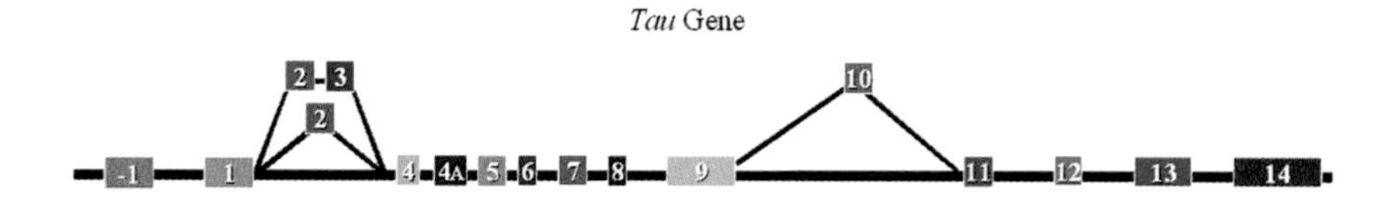

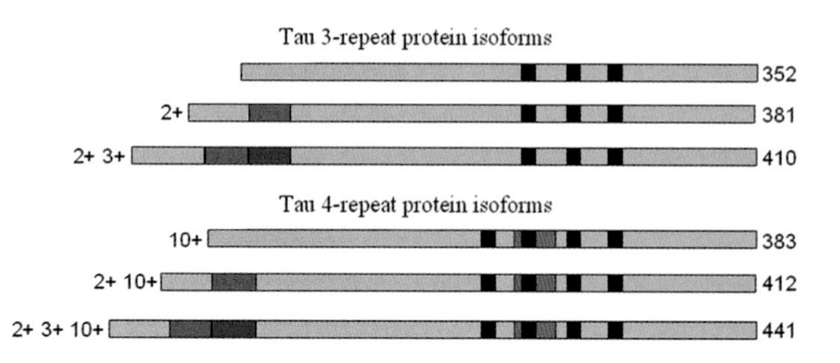

Figure 1. Schematic representation of the human *Tau* gene and the six isoforms generated by alternative mRNA splicing of exons 2, 3 and 10.

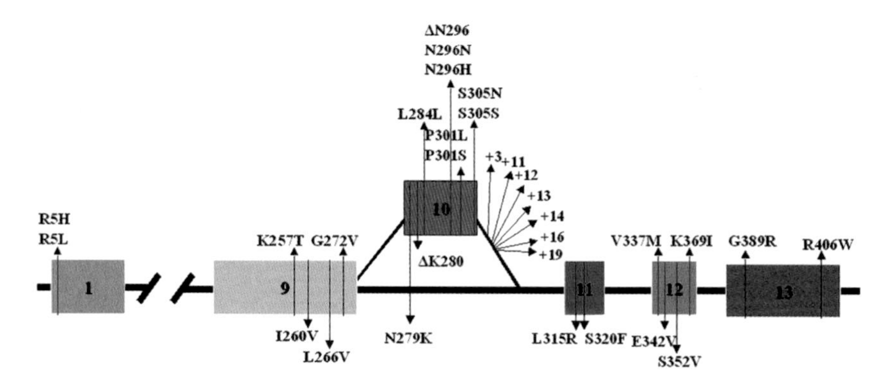

Figure 2. Schematic representation of the exons and intron of the *Tau* gene where mutations have been found.

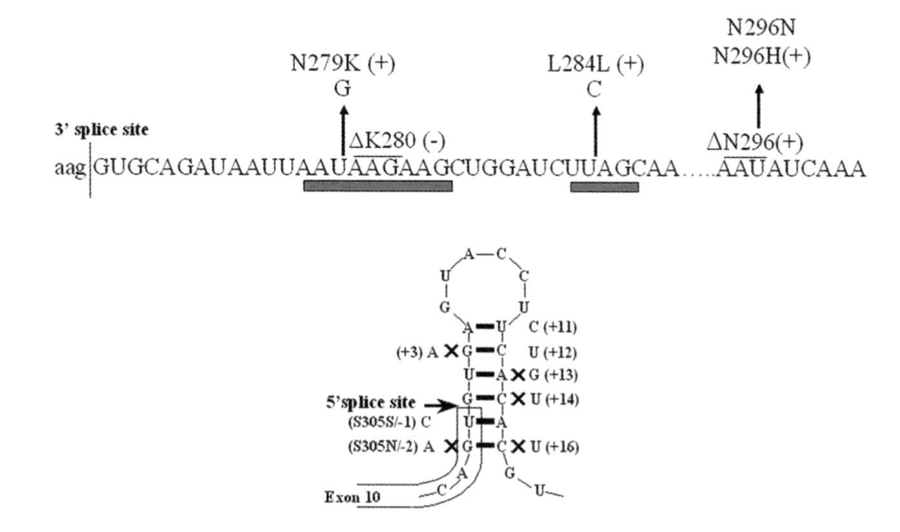

Figure 3. Schematic representation of the mutations in the Tau gene that affect the splicing of exon 10. Three mutations in exon 10 (N279K, ΔK280 and L284L) act on 3 regulatory elements. These elements include an exon splicing enhancer that can either be strengthened (N279K) or be destroyed (ΔK280) resulting in the inclusion or exclusion of exon 10 from tau transcripts. The function of a second regulatory element that is an exon splicing silencer is abolished by mutation L284L resulting in excess exon 10 inclusion. Mutations in the stem loop increase the splicing of exon.

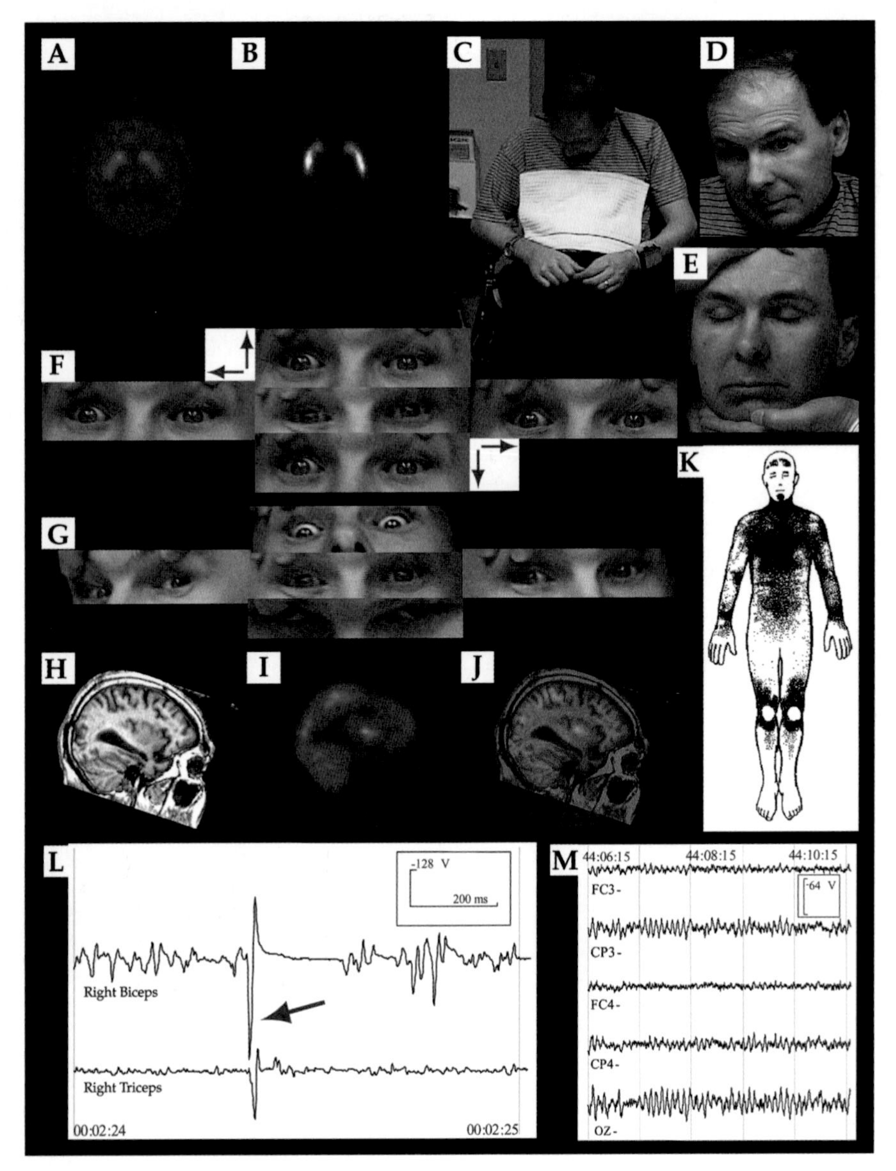

Figure 4. Composite image showing clinical, neuroimaging and neurophysiological features of an affected individual with a N279K mutation. At the age of 41 years, his job performance and motor skills had declined rather rapidly over the period of 6 months. He complained of micrographia. His posture became stooped and his walking was shuffling. On examination he had bradykinesia and asymmetrical rigidity affecting more both right extremities. There was no resting tremor, postural instability or eye movement abnormalities. His cognition was normal but he was somewhat withdrawn. Basic serum and urine laboratory tests, electromyography (EMG), evoked potentials and magnetic resonance imaging (MRI) of the brain were all normal or negative. About a year from the onset of his illness he underwent positron emission tomography (PET) with [18 F]-fluoro-L-dopa (6FD) and [11C]-raclopride (RAC) tracers. The 6FD PET demonstrated reduced FD uptake rate constant throughout the striatum, with the putamen and caudate nucleus affected equally (**A**). RAC PET showed elevated striatal D2-receptor binding also affecting both putamen and caudate nucleus equally (**B**). These abnormalities contrast with that seen in sporadic Parkinson's disease, where the putamen is affected more than the caudate nucleus. He was treated with levodopa/carbidopa and dopamine agonists with only mild initial response. When examined at age 48 years he was wheel chair bounded (**C**) and mute. He had anterocollis (**C**), masked face (**D**) and significantly reduced rate of blinking. His eyes were in fixed mid position (**D**). He had profound eyelid opening apraxia (**E**) to the point that his wife had to help him to open his eyes. He had supranuclear gaze palsy (**F**) with preserved oculocephalic reflexes (**G**). His postural stability was significantly impaired. He was not able to stand without support. Multidisciplinary diagnostic testing including head MRI, 2-deoxy-2-fluoro-[18F]-D-glucose (FDG) PET, EMG, electroencephalography (EEG), autonomic and sleep testing was performed at the time of clinical examination presented above. Head MRI demonstrated severe cortical atrophy in posterior frontal and temporal lobes (**H**). PET showed FDG hypometabolism in the same cortical regions (**I**). Co-registration of MRI and FDG PET studies is shown in J. Autonomic thermoregulatory sweat testing (**K**) demonstrated the anhydrosis predominantly in distal lower and upper extremities with some milder patchy abnormalities in more proximal sites (dark areas indicate normal sweating). EMG multichannel surface recording of the right arm during extension (**L**) showed and EMG discharge that corresponded to a myoclonic jerk. EEG (**M**) demonstrated posterior alpha activity of about 9Hz with occasional theta wave components.
Figure 4 is courtesy of Drs. Caviness (images L and M), Cheshire (image K), Pooley (image J), Tsuboi (images C-G) and Witte (images H and I) from the Mayo Clinic Jacksonville, Florida and Dr. Stoessl (images A and B) from the University of British Clumbia, Vancouver, Canada.

axial and appendicular musculature, usually absence of resting tremor, and poor or no responsiveness to levodopa therapy (Figure 4). Other motor disturbances seen in FTDP-17*T* include dystonia unrelated to medications, supranuclear gaze palsy, upper and lower motor neuron dysfunction, myoclonus, postural and action tremors, eyelid opening and closing apraxia, dysphagia, and dysarthria.

It is still very difficult to carry out precise phenotype/genotype correlations in FTDP-17*T* since the clinical information on some individuals is not detailed enough or not available at all. Nevertheless, some patterns have emerged. There are 2 major groups of clinical phenotypes associated with FTDP-17*T*: dementia-predominant group and parkinsonism-plus-predominant group. The dementia-predominant group is more common and is usually seen in association with exonic mutations that do not affect the splicing of exon 10. The parkinsonism-plus-predominant group is usually seen in association with intronic and exonic mutations that affect exon 10 splicing and lead to an overproduction of four-repeat tau isoforms.

Imaging. Computerised tomography (CT) and magnetic resonance imaging (MRI) of the head frequently reveal some enlargement of the lateral ventricles and atrophy of the frontal, temporal, and parietal lobes (Table 1, Figures 4, 5) (6, 7, 9, 43, 72, 83). In some individuals, the cortical atrophy is asymmetrical (Table 1). MRI T2-weighted images may show accumulation of paramagnetic substances (iron) in mesencephalic nuclei (9).

Functional imaging studies such as single photon emission computerised tomography (SPECT) and positron emission tomography (PET) also demonstrate significant abnormalities (Table 1, Figures 4, 5). PET with 2-deoxy-2-fluoror-[^{18}F]-D-glucose (FDG) often shows reduced frontal-parietal-temporal uptake (Figures 4, 5) similar to patterns seen in sporadic frontotemporal dementia (FTD). PET with [^{18}F]-fluoro-L-dopa(6FD) and [^{11}C]-raclopride tracers reveals uptake abnormalities different than those seen in PD, where the putamen is affected more than the caudate nucleus (49).

Laboratory findings. The routine serum, urine, CSF and other body fluid studies are usually negative. Clinical neurophysiological findings are summarised in Table 1. Electroencephalography (EEG) reveals normal findings early in the disease process and diffuse slowing with clinical progression (78). In sporadic FTD, the slowing of background rhythms usually occurs late in the course of the illness. In individuals with the P301S mutation, EEGs demonstrated the presence of sharp waves, spikes and electrical seizure discharges (64). Nerve conduction studies are normal. Electromyography may show neurogenic patterns related to lower motor neuron dysfunction (39). Evoked potential studies are usually normal. Only limited information is available on the function of the autonomic nervous system (Figure 4) and on the sleep patterns in individuals with FTDP-17*T*. Neuropsychological evaluations are important in determining the severity and extent of cognitive and behavioral dysfunction (6).

Clinical criteria. The International Consensus Conference on FTDP-17 provided useful suggestions based on limited information available at the time of the conference (17). There are no strict criteria regarding the diagnosis of FTDP-17. Nevertheless, FTDP-17 should be considered in the differential diagnosis in the presence of one or more of the following: *i)* an age at onset of the neurological symptoms between the third and fifth decades; *ii)* progressive neuropsychiatric syn-

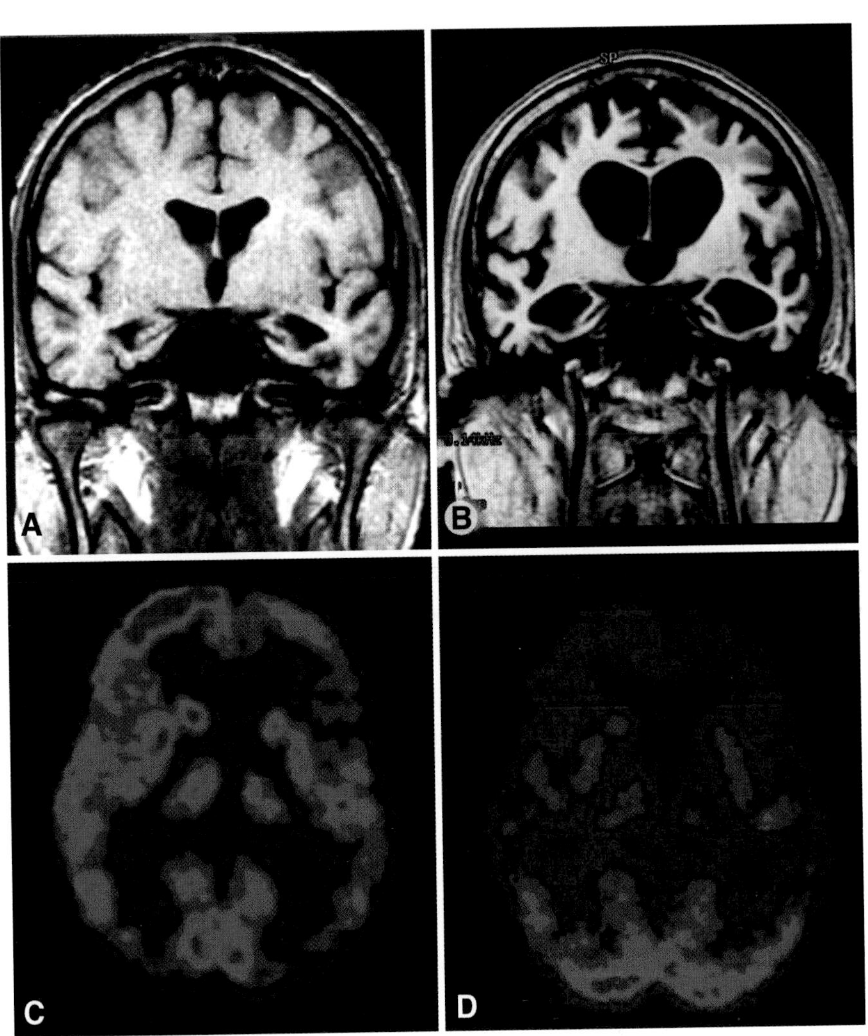

Figure 5. Two MRI scans of the brain of a patient with the G389R mutation illustrate the progression of the cerebral atrophy over a 3-year period. **A.** The first MRI was carried out when the patient was 38-years-old and **B.** the second was obtained when the patient was 41-years-old. **C, D.** Two PET scans of the same individual illustrate the progression of the metabolic alterations over a period of 8 months. **C.** The PET scan, carried out when the patient was 38-years-old, shows hypometabolism of frontal and temporal cortex that is more severe on the left. **D.** The PET scan, carried out when the patient was 39-years-old, shows severe hypometabolism of the frontal and temporal lobes, as well as hypometabolism of thalamic nuclei. Reproduced with permission from the *Journal of Neuropathology and Experimental Neurology.*

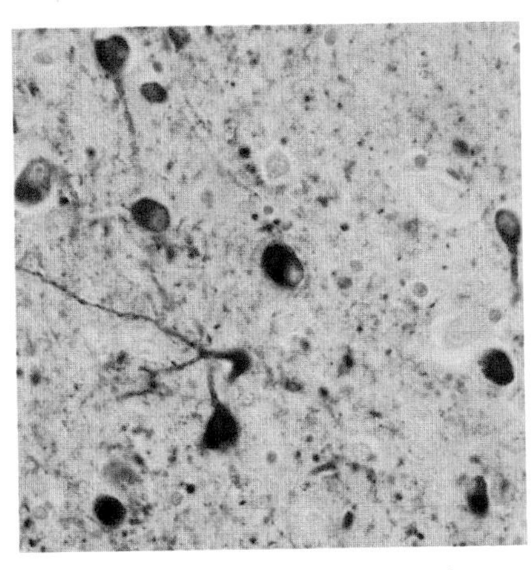

Figure 6. Tau-immunoreactive deposits in the neocortex of an individual with a +3 mutation in the intron following exon 10. Note the tau-immunoreactivity in neuronal perikarya, dendrites and neuropil threads.

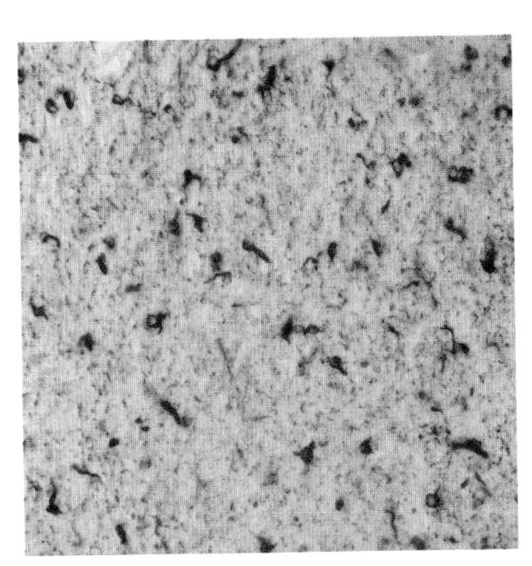

Figure 7. Tau-immunoreactive deposits in the cerebral white matter of an individual with a N279K mutation. Note the tau-immunoreactivity in the perikaryon of oligodendroglial cells and in cell processes.

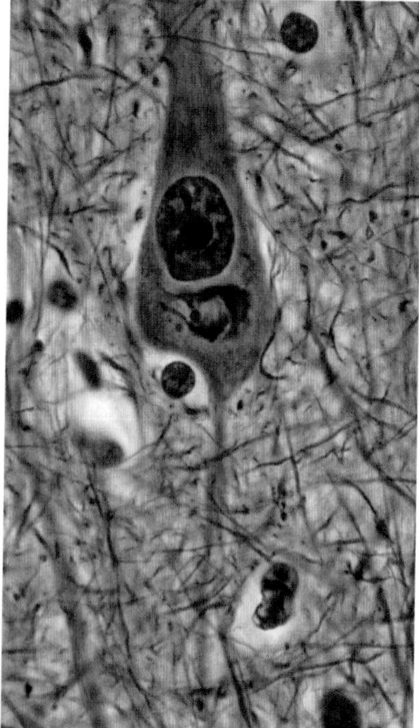

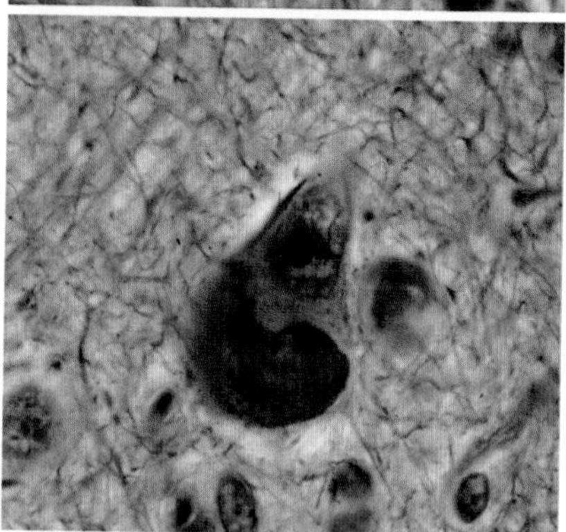

Figure 8. Argentophilic deposit (upper) and neurofibrillary tangle (lower) in neocortical neurons of an individual with a *Tau* mutation. Neurofibrillary tangles similar to those seen in Alzheimer disease are found in individuals with the V337M and R406W.

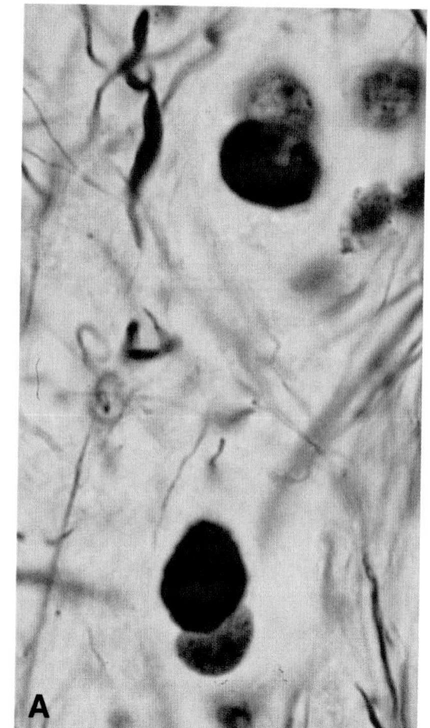

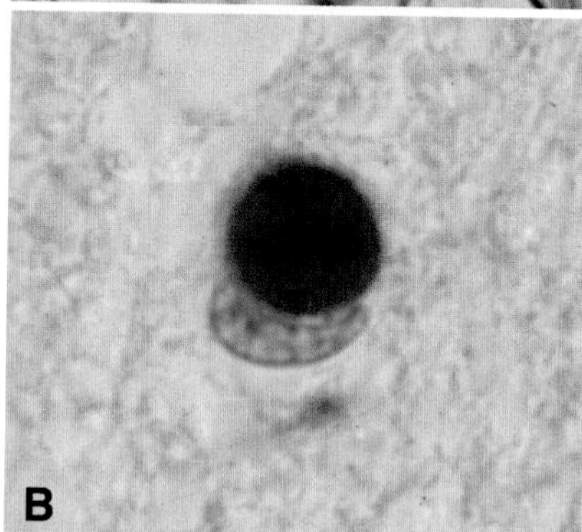

Figure 9. A. Argentophilic and B. tau immunopositive Pick-body-like deposits in the neocortex of an individual with a G389R mutation. Reproduced with permission from the *Journal of Neuropathology and Experimental Neurology.*

drome including personality and behavioral abnormalities and/or frontotemporal dementia; *iii)* parkinsonism-plus syndrome (bradykinesia, rigidity, postural instability, paucity of resting tremor, and poor or no response to dopaminergic therapy), frequently associated with falls and supranuclear gaze palsy and less commonly associated with apraxia, dystonia, and lateralisation; *iv)* progressive speech difficulties from the onset of the illness; *v)* seizure disorder poorly controlled with standard anticonvulsant therapy; and *vi)* positive family history suggestive of autosomal dominant inheritance of a neurodegenerative disorder even if there has been variability in clinical presentations.

Neuropathologic Features

Macroscopy. FTDP-17*T* may have a very long course lasting up to 26 years. The degree of atrophy observed varies with a brain weight ranging from approximately 825 to 1290 grams. The neuropathology of FTDP-17*T* in its early stage has not been described. In the intermediate stage, atrophy of the cerebral hemispheres is mild even though the characteristic histopathological changes in the cortex, subcortical nuclei and white matter are already prominent. There may be mild atrophy of the caudate nucleus and a considerable reduction of the pigmentation of the substantia nigra and locus coeruleus. In the advanced stages, the degree of atrophy varies and may be present throughout the frontal and temporal lobes, caudate nucleus, putamen, globus pallidus, amygdala, hippocampus and ventral hypothalamus. Most often, the superior, middle and inferior frontal gyri as well as the superior, middle and inferior temporal gyri bear the brunt of the disease, the anterior portion of the temporal lobe being particularly vulnerable. The frontal and temporal atrophy may be asymmetric and may be so severe that the gyri have a "knife-edge" appearance. In addition, the orbital, cingulate, and parahippocampal gyri may be involved. The parietal and occipital lobes are less frequently affected. The white matter of the centrum semiovale and of the temporal lobes may be substantially reduced in bulk; the thickness of the corpus callosum is also reduced. The midbrain and pons may be reduced in bulk. The substantia nigra and the locus coeruleus show a marked reduction in pigmentation. In some instances, mild atrophy of the cerebellar cortex as well as discoloration and atrophy of the dentate nucleus may be observed. The lateral ventricles throughout their subdivisions and the third ventricle may be enlarged, often times severely so.

Histopathology and immunohistochemistry. The neuropathologic phenotypes associated with FTDP-17*T* vary substantially not only in morphologic characteristics, but also in severity; however, the neuropathologic hallmark is the presence of tau protein deposits in neurons or in both neurons and glia of the cerebrum, cerebellum, and brain stem (Figures 6, 7). This variability is closely correlated to which *Tau* gene mutation is present. Tau deposits may be abundant in the cerebral cortex, white matter, and some subcortical and brain stem nuclei

(Figures 6, 7). These deposits may also be present in variable amounts in the spinal cord.

Histologically, the cellular pathology of the neuronal perikaryon may resemble that of Alzheimer disease (AD) or Pick disease for the presence of neurofibrillary tangles or Pick bodies (Figures 8, 9). The cellular pathology of glia may resemble that of progressive supranuclear palsy or corticobasal degeneration for the presence of coiled bodies in oligodendroglial cells, tufted astrocytes or astrocytic plaques.

The type of cellular involvement (ie, neurons, astrocytes and oligodendroglia) and the type of neuronal inclusion vary according to the location of the *Tau* gene mutation. Mutations in exons 1 and 10 as well as in the intron following exon 10 are associated with neuronal and glial tau deposition (Figures 10-13). Mutations in exons 9, 11, 12 and 13 lead to deposits of tau filaments predominantly in neurons (Figures 8, 9, 14-17). Three mutations in exon 9, one in exon 11, two in exon 12 and one in exon 13 are associated with the presence of numerous Pick body-like inclusions (Figures 9, 14, 15). Other mutations in exons 12 and 13 lead to the formation of neurofibrillary tangles with paired helical filaments (PHF) and straight filaments (SF) indistinguishable from those seen in AD.

Tau deposits are immunopositive using polyclonal antibodies directed to the amino terminus, microtubule-binding region and carboxy terminus of tau. In addition, phosphorylation-dependent antibodies are used to recognise abnormally phosphorylated sites in tau. According to the longest tau isoform, these sites are threonine 181, 212, 231 and serine 202, 214, 262, 356, 396, 404, 409, 422. An antibody recognising serine 262 and or 356 labels neurofibrillary tangles, but not always Pick bodies. Phosphorylation dependent monoclonal antibody AT8 recognising phosphorylated S202 and T205 is the most sensitive in recognising tau deposits in perikarya and cell processes of neurons and glia (Figures 10-13). Tau deposits are also immunolabeled using anti-ubiquitin antibodies.

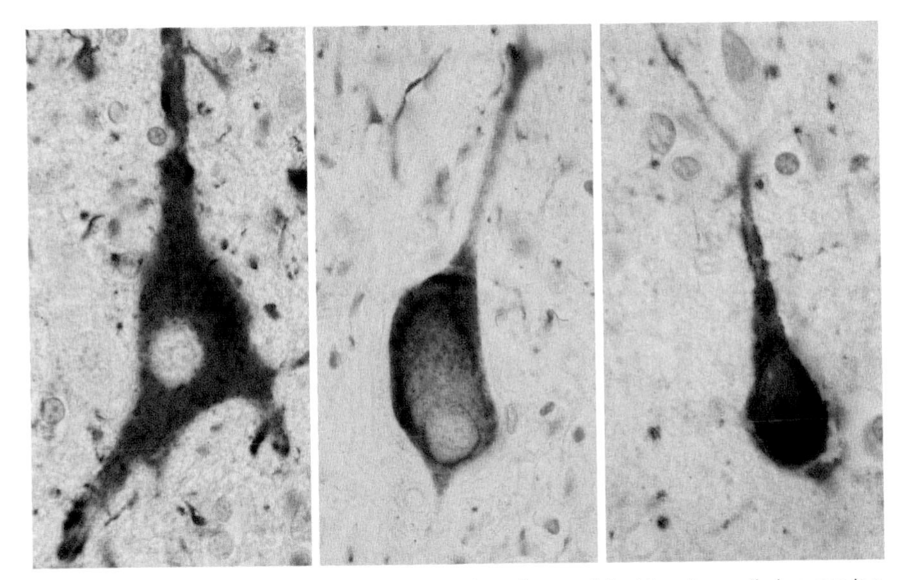

Figure 10. Various types of tau-immunopositive deposits in perikarya and dendrites of neocortical neurons in a patient with the N279K mutation.

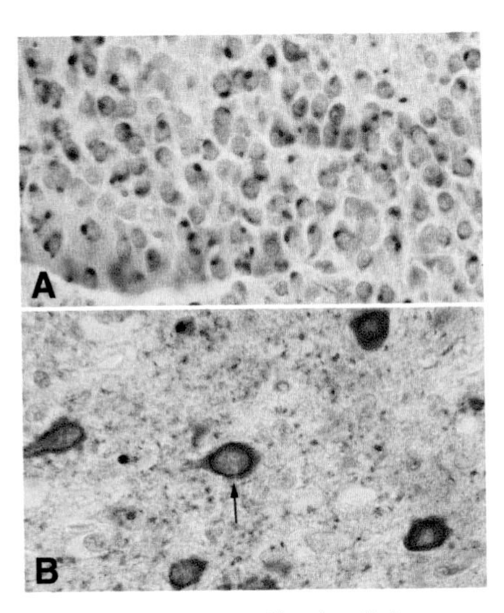

Figure 11. Tau-immunopositive deposits in neurons of the hippocampus in an individual with the P301L mutation. **A.** In the fascia dentata , they are small and round. **B.** In the pyramidal layer, they have the shape of a perinuclear ring.

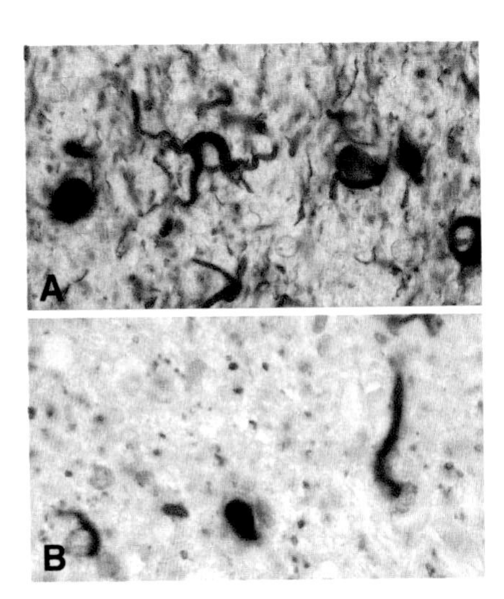

Figure 12. Tau-immunopositive deposits in oligodendroglial cells of the white matter of the centrum semiovale of individuals with **A.** the N279K mutation and **B.** the +3 mutation. Oligodendroglial deposits appear as "coiled bodies" involving the cell perikaryon and extending into the cell processes.

In the following sections, the detailed histopathology for FTDP-17*T* has been organised according to regions of the *Tau* gene affected by a mutation.

Exon 1. Two mutations have been reported at codon 5 of exon 1. They result in the substitution of histidine or leucine for arginine. Although these mutations affect the same residue, the pathologic phenotype associated with each of them differs.

R5H (24). Severe nerve cell loss and gliosis are found in the cortex of the anterior part of the temporal lobe, the hippocampus, parahippocampal gyrus, amygdala and substantia nigra. Neurons contain tau deposits, but neurofibrillary tangles are rare. Prominent tau deposits in oligodendroglial cells and astrocytes are seen throughout the white matter of the frontal and temporal lobes.

R5L (56). Neuronal loss and astrocytosis are seen in the cerebellar dentate nucleus, substantia nigra and locus coeruleus. Neurofibrillary tangles are

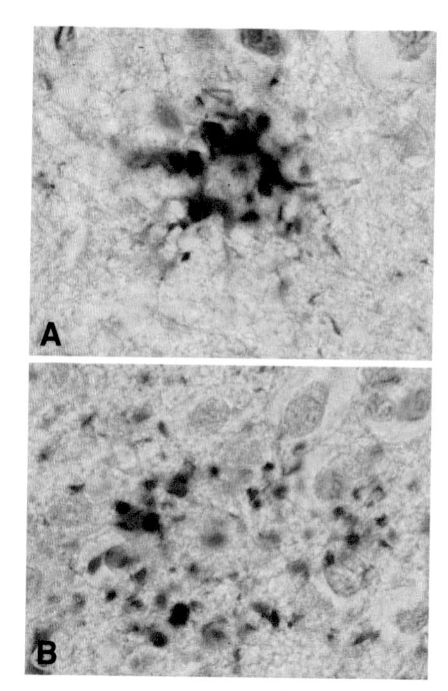

Figure 13. Tau-immunopositive deposits in astrocytes of the cortex of an individual with the P301L mutation. **A.** The tau deposits are present in the cell perikaryon and extend into the proximal segments of the cell processes giving the appearance of a tufted astrocytes. **B.** The tau deposits are present in the cell processes and form a so called "astrocytic" plaque.

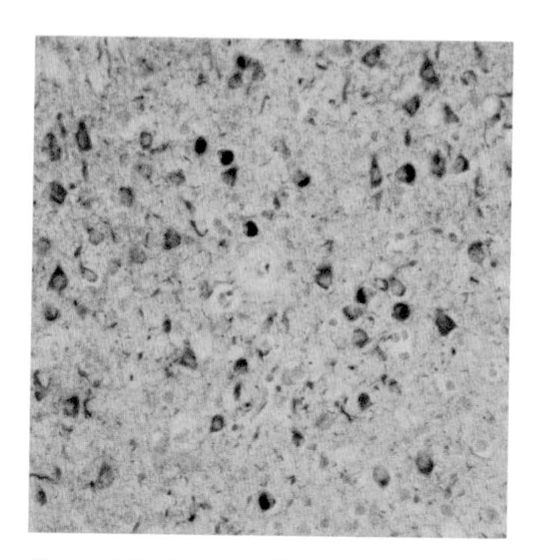

Figure 14. Tau-immunopositive deposits in neurones of the frontal cortex of an individual with the G389R mutation. Numerous perikarya contain round or oval intracytoplasmic tau deposits similar to Pick bodies. Reproduced with permission from the *Journal of Neuropathology and Experimental Neurology.*

most numerous in the putamen, globus pallidus, subthalamic nucleus, thalamus, substantia nigra, locus coeruleus and basis pontis. Tau immunopositive neuropil threads and coiled bodies are most numerous in the periaquaductal gray matter and basis pontis. Tufted astrocytes are numerous in the caudate nucleus, putamen and thalamus.

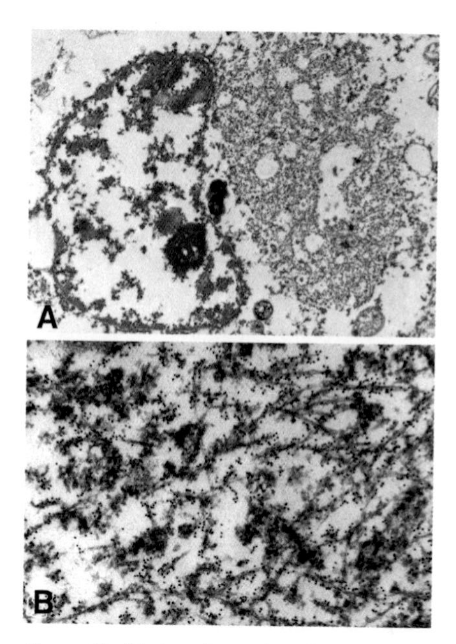

Figure 15. Electronmicrographs of a nerve cell perikaryon from the frontal cortex of an individual with the G389R mutation. **A.** A neurone contains the nucleus and a Pick body-like filamentous deposit. **B.** Tau filaments within the Pick body-like deposit are immunolabeled with a phosphorylation dependent antibody that recognises pSer202/pThr205 (AT8). Reproduced with permission from the *Journal of Neuropathology and Experimental Neurology.*

Exon 9. Four mutations have been reported in exon 9, three of which are associated with a Pick-disease-like neuropathologic phenotype (26, 29, 32a, 52, 60, 80).

K257T, L266V, G272V (22, 26, 32a, 52, 60, 66). Neuronal loss is found in the frontal and temporal cortex as well as in the caudate nucleus, putamen and substantia nigra. Pick body-like inclusions, demonstrated using silver stain and antibodies against tau, may be found in the cortex of the frontal and temporal lobes, striatum, hippocampus and substantia nigra. Ballooned achromatic neurons are numerous in the entorhinal cortex in association with the K257T mutation. Occasionally, glial cells are tau immunopositive.

I260V. At the time of this writing, the associated neuropathology was not published.

*Exon 10.*Ten mutations have been reported in exon 10 (7, 8, 14, 30, 31, 50, 54, 61, 69, 70). The neuropathologic phenotypes have been well documented for the N279K, P301L, and P301S mutations and there are similarities and differences in the cellular pathology of neurons and glia as well as in the topographic distribution of lesions related to tau deposition (1, 7, 12, 33, 39, 45, 58, 66, 81).

N279K (1, 12, 58, 81). Neuronal loss may be severe in the cingulate gyrus, temporal cortex, Ammon's horn, and subiculum. Spongiosis may be present in the superficial layers of the neocortex. Among subcortical nuclei the caudate nucleus, putamen, globus pallidus, amygdala, thalamus, hypothalamus, mammillary bodies, subthalamic nucleus, substantia nigra, locus coeruleus, raphe nuclei, brain stem nuclei (III, V, XII), and inferior olivary nuclei are affected in varying degrees. In the substantia nigra some of the remaining neurons had lost the melanin pigment. Neuronal loss is moderate in the dentate nucleus of the cerebellum and it is associated with grumose plaques. Gliosis is present in both the grey and white matter; however, it is prominent at the junction of the cortex and white matter. Using staining methods for myelin, pallor of the white matter of the frontal and temporal lobes is demonstrated.

Fibrillary changes are found in neurons and glia of the frontal, temporal and parietal cortices and are distributed in various combinations throughout the central nervous system. These changes are most evident in neurons of layers 2 to 6 and in the glial cells of the cortex and white matter junction. A few ballooned neurons are observed in affected cortical areas. Fibrillary changes in neurons are also conspicuous in the midbrain tegmentum, periaqueductal grey matter, substantia nigra and pontine tegmentum.

Strong cytoplasmic immunopositivity is seen in nerve cells and glia using antibodies to tau. Neurons with tau deposits are more numerous than those with fibrillary changes. In the layers II to VI of the frontal and temporal cortices, neuronal perikarya and dendrites show diffuse or punctate tau immunoreactivity; only occasionally round and densely stained inclusions reminiscent of Pick bodies are observed. Among subcortical structures, tau immunopositivity is seen in the globus pallidus, hypothalamus, substantia innominata, and dentate nucleus. Fibrillary tau-immunoreactive inclusion in neurons are infrequent in the neocortex, but numerous in the midbrain, pons and medulla. Rare ballooned neurons show a weak tau immunoreactivity.

Tau immunoreactivity is strong in perikarya and processes of glial cells. Affected glial cells are mostly oligodendroglia, but astrocytes are also involved. The immunoreactivity in glial cells has the appearance of so-called "coiled bodies" and is present in white matter tracts of the cerebrum, cerebellum and brain stem. However, the most intense immunopositivity is seen in glial cells of the lower cortical layers and the subcortical white matter.

P301L and P301S (6, 7, 33, 40, 45). The distribution of neuronal losses and tau-immunoreactive neurons is similar to that seen associated with the N279K mutation; however, the tau pathology in the white matter, subcortical nuclei and brain stem is less severe than that associated with the N279K mutation. The frontal cortex, middle and inferior temporal gyri and parietal cortex are the areas most involved. A feature often reported in association with P301L is the presence of argentophilic tau-immunoreactive perinuclear rings in the neurons of the Ammon's horn, particularly within the CA1 sector and the presence round tau-immunoreactive inclusions in neurons of the fascia dentata (Figure 11). In addition to neurons with tau-immunoreactive deposits, achromatic or ballooned neurons are frequently seen in cortex and some subcortical nuclei associated with the P301L mutation. Both oligodendroglia and astrocytes are affected. Oligodendroglial tau-immunopositive inclusions are in the shape of "coiled bodies." Tufted astrocytes and astrocytic plaque are found in the neocortex. In the white matter, tau-immunopositive oligodendroglial cells are diffusely present, but less numerous than in N279K. In P301S, there is a severe loss of axons with relative sparing of the U fibers.

L284L and N296N (14, 69). These mutations are associated with tau deposition in neurons and glia. In neurons, cytoplasmic granular material and dense bundles of fibrils are immunolabeled by anti-tau antibodies. Tau-immunopositive neurons are present in the neocortex, parahippocampus, hippocampus, and substantia nigra.

N296H (31). In N296H, severe neuronal loss and presence of ballooned neurons is seen in the cerebral cortex along with proliferation of tau-positive astrocytes. Tau-immunopositive deposits (pretangles) are found in neurons of the amygdala, hypothalamus, caudate nucleus, putamen, thalamus, pontine nuclei, inferior olivary nucleus, ocular motor nucleus, hypoglossal nucleus and spinal anterior horn. Tau-immunopositive coiled bodies are present in the subcortical white matter.

ΔK280 and ΔN296 (50,61). The neuropathologic phenotype associated with these mutations has not been characterised.

S305N (30). Neurofibrillary tangles are prominent in the frontal, temporal, insular and post-central cortices. Glial cells containing coiled bodies are seen in the cerebral white matter, basal ganglia and brain stem.

S305S (70). In the S305S mutation, neurofibrillary and glial tangles as well as tufted astrocytes are seen in the cortex, amygdala, periaquaductal gray matter, substantia nigra and oculomotor nuclei. Ballooned neurons are present in the neocortex. Neuronal loss is seen in the cortex, globus pallidus, subthalamus and substantia nigra.

Intron following Exon 10. Seven mutations in the intron following exon 10 (+3, +11, +12, +13, +14, +16, +19) have been reported (15, 21, 29, 41, 68, 70a, 82). Pathologic data are available on all of them except the +19 mutation. The severity of histopathological changes varies from patient to patient; however, there is uniformity in the distribution of lesions. The cortex shows neuronal cell loss and gliosis throughout its thickness. A rarefaction of the neuropil, particularly at the level of the upper 2 layers, and astrogliosis are commonly seen. Among subcortical structures, nerve cell loss and gliosis may be prominent in the caudate nucleus, putamen, globus pallidus, amygdala and hypothalamus. The substantia nigra, locus coeruleus, periaqueductal gray, third and fourth cranial nerve nuclei, reticular nuclei, raphe neurons, and dorsal nucleus of the vagus nerve are all significantly affected by neuronal loss.

Argentophilic tau-immunoreactive inclusions are frequently seen in neurons and oligodendroglia within the neocortex. There is mild neuronal loss in the Ammon's horn and the subiculum. In some patients, large numbers of Hirano bodies may be found in pyramidal neurons of the hippocampus. Neurofibrillary tangles and tau deposits may be seen in the hypothalamus, midbrain nuclei, periaqueductal gray matter, and pontine nuclei. In the cerebellum, there may be a loss of Purkinje cells and neurons of the dentate nucleus. The cerebral white matter shows gliosis and presence of numerous argentophilic tau-immunoreactive inclusions in oligodendroglia, particularly numerous in the frontal and temporal regions. In the spinal cord, axonal swellings and a mild loss of nerve cells are present in the anterior horn and dorsal gray matter. In some instances, a loss of nerve fibers in the propriospinal tract, as well as in ventral and lateral spinothalamic tracts and in the lateral vestibulospinal tract may be observed in myelin preparations (21, 35, 53, 65, 82).

Exon 11. Two mutations have been reported in exon 11 (L315R, S320F).

L315R (76). At the time of this writing, the neuropathology associated with this mutation has not been reported (76).

S320F (62). This mutation in exon 11 of the *Tau* gene is associated with a Pick-disease-like phenotype. Neuronal loss is seen in the temporal cortex, cingulate gyrus, entorhinal cortex and hippocampus. Pick body-like inclusions, demonstrated using antibodies against tau, are numerous in the cortex of the frontal, temporal and parietal lobes, dentate gyrus, amygdala and ventral striatum. A few Pick cells are seen in the temporal cortex. In addi-

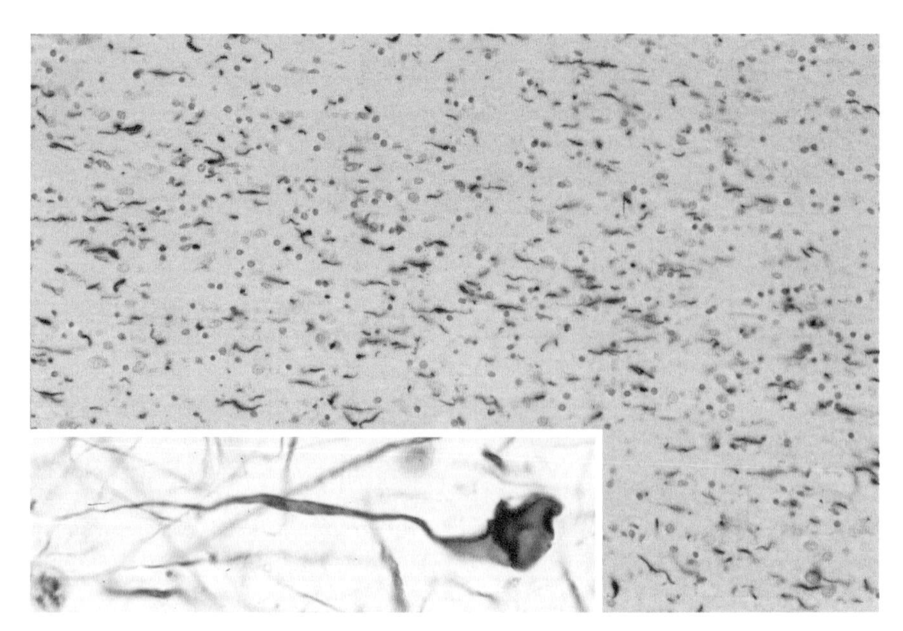

Figure 16. Subcortical white matter of an individual with the G389R mutation. Numerous tau-immunopositive thread-like deposits are seen. Argentophilic axonal segment in the white matter is shown (insert). Reproduced with permission from the *Journal of Neuropathology and Experimental Neurology.*

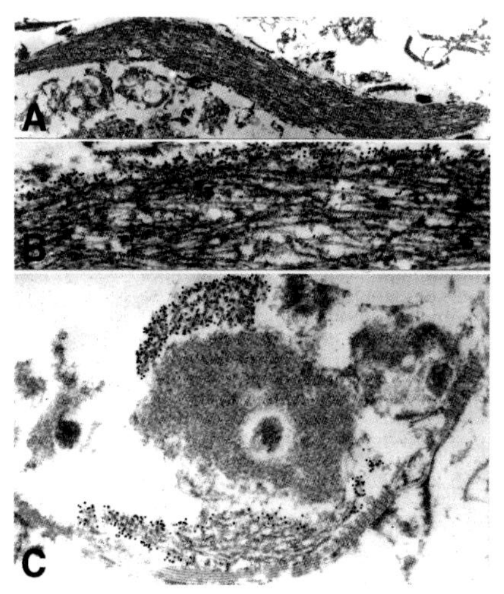

Figure 17. Electronmicrograph of thread-like axonal structures in the white matter of an individual with the G389R mutation. A. The thread-like structure is seen in longitudinal view. B. Straight filaments of the thread-like structure are immunolabeled with monoclonal antibody AT8. C. Electronmicrograph of an axon shows transversally cut filaments labeled with monoclonal antibody AT8. Reproduced with permission from the *Journal of Neuropathology and Experimental Neurology.*

tion, neurons with diffuse tau immunostaining and glial cells containing tau inclusions are seen. The substantia nigra is reportedly not affected (62).

Exon 12. Four mutations have been reported in exon 12 (37, 46, 48, 54).

V337M (54, 65). This mutation is associated with predominantly neuronal pathology. Tau-immunopositive neurofibrillary tangles and neuropil threads are found in the orbital, cingulate and temporal cortices as well as in the subiculum and parahippocampal gyrus. In the cerebral cortex, neurons of layers II, III, IV and V are the most vulnerable. Neuronal loss is variable and its severity may be related to the disease duration. Neuritic plaques are consistently absent. Neuronal loss in the substantia nigra is not described (54, 65, 71).

E342V (37). The histopathology associated with this mutation is characterised by Pick bodies in the dentate fascia and Pick cells that are most abundant in the frontal, insular and temporal cortices, hippocampus, subiculum, claustrum, and nucleus basalis of Meynert. Tufted astrocytes are numerous in the white matter of the frontal lobe (37).

S352V (48). Preliminary neuropathologic information is available on 2 siblings that are homozygous for this mutation. Widespread neurofibrillary tangles are present in brain stem nuclei, a finding similar to that seen in progressive supranuclear palsy (48).

K369I (46). The histopathology associated with this mutation is characterised by severe neuronal loss in the inferior and middle temporal gyri, amygdala, hippocampus, parahippocampal gyrus and caudate nucleus. Tau-immunopositive Pick-body-like inclusions are present in layers II, V and VI of the frontal, temporal, parietal, insular, and cingulate cortices. Pick cells with diffuse tau deposits are also present. No obvious nerve cell loss is present in the substantia nigra. Tufted astrocytes and oligodendroglial cells with coiled bodies are seen. The latter are abundant in the white matter of the internal, external and extreme capsule along with tau-immunopositive focal axonal swellings (46).

Exon 13. There are 2 distinct neuropathologic phenotypes associated with the 2 known mutations in exon 13.

G389R (43, 52). The phenotype associated with the G389R mutation is characterised by severe nerve cell loss and gliosis that are most prominent in the frontal, cingulate, and insular cortices, caudate nucleus, putamen, globus pallidus, amygdala, and substantia nigra. Spongiosis is present in the second cortical layer and in the lower layers of the temporal cortex. Neurons in layers II, V, and VI of the frontal, cingulate, temporal and insular cortices as well as in the fascia dentata, amygdala, raphe and pontine nuclei contain diffusely tau-immunopostive deposits or Pick body-like inclusions (Figures 14, 15). Pick body-like inclusions have not been reported in the substantia nigra. Immunopositivity of glial cell peri-karya is rarely seen. Argentophilic and strongly tau immunoreactive elongated threads and focal axonal swellings ranging between 4 and 40 μm are observed in the cortex, putamen, globus pallidus and thalamus as well as the subcortical white matter of the centrum semiovale (Figures 16, 17), the internal, external, and extreme capsules. In the white matter, a loss of myelin stain is also observed (43, 52).

406W (29, 57, 63). The main features associated with the R406W mutation are neurofibrillary tangles, neuropil threads and neuronal loss in the cortex of the frontal, temporal, parietal, and occipital lobes as well as in the entorhinal cortex, hippocampus, globus pallidus, substantia innominata and amygdala. Neuronal loss in the substantia nigra is not a prominent finding. Neuritic plaques are absent (29, 57, 63).

Electronmicroscopy. Electronmicroscopy of tau filaments has been studied in postmortem fixed tissue and in preparation of dispersed filaments. Morphology of filaments differs according to the *Tau* gene mutation and to which tau isoforms are present in the filaments. The most informative data relevant to our understanding of the biology of tau filaments are obtained from the preparation of dispersed filaments. Using these preparations, tau filaments can be studied by correlating immunoelectronmicroscopy and Western blot analysis.

Fixed tissue. Tau filaments are best identified by immunoelectronmicroscopy. They are strongly immunolabeled with antibody AT8 that recognises the phosphorylated Ser202 and Thr205. According to the *Tau* gene mutation, filaments are present in neurons and glia or in neurons only. In association with mutations in exon 10 and in the intron following exon 10, they are present in both neurons and glia (Figure 18). In association with the N279K mutation, the filaments are arranged into bundles of various thicknesses. They appear as twisted ribbons with a width of 19 to 27 nm and a spacing between crossovers of 130 to 190 nm (12). Filaments associated with mutations in the intron following exon 10 appear as twisted ribbons similar to those seen in association with N279K (Figure 18) (65). Filaments associated with the G389R mutation appear as straight or twisted (Figure 17) (43). The width of the twisted ribbons varies between 8 and 20 nm; however, the periodicity cannot be clearly determined. The SF are 13 nm in width. These filaments are present in both neuronal perikaryon and axons (Figures 15,17). Filaments associated with mutations V337M and R406W are identical to the PHF seen in AD (57, 1).

Dispersed filaments. Dispersed tau filaments are decorated by phosphorylation-independent and phosphorylation-dependent anti-tau antibodies. Their morphology differs according to the *Tau* gene mutation and can be grouped into distinct categories.

Mutations V337M and R406W induce the formation of PHF and SF that are identical to those seen in Alzheimer disease. PHF have a diameter of 8 to 20 nm and a cross over of approximately 80 nm. All 6 tau isoforms are incorporated into the filaments (65).

Mutation G389R induces the formation of 2 classes of filaments. The majority resembling SF of AD, while a minor species is characterised by twisted filaments with a cross over of about 120 nm and a width varying between 6 and 23 nm. The filaments contain the isoforms with 352, 381, 383 and 412 amino acids (43).

Mutation P301L induces the formation of 2 classes of filaments. The majority consists of narrow irregularly twisted ribbons with a maximum width of about 15 nm and a cross over of 130 nm, while a minority consists of SF of 12 nm. The filaments contain the isoforms with 381, 383, and 412 amino acids (66).

Mutations in the intron following exon 10 induce the formation of filaments that appear as irregular twisted-ribbon-like structures with a maximum width of ca. 23 nm and a minimum width of ca. 5 nm at the position of the twist, corresponding to the thickness of the ribbon. The filaments contain the isoforms with four repeats (68).

Biochemistry

The central biochemical questions in FTDP-17*T* revolve around the process by which filaments are formed from the tau protein. In FTDP-17*T*, the tau protein has biochemical characteristics that differ from those of the normal tau protein. These characteristics vary due to the nature and location of the *Tau* gene mutation that is present. A mutation may result in a structurally abnormal protein, an abnormal ratio of tau isoforms produced or both. The

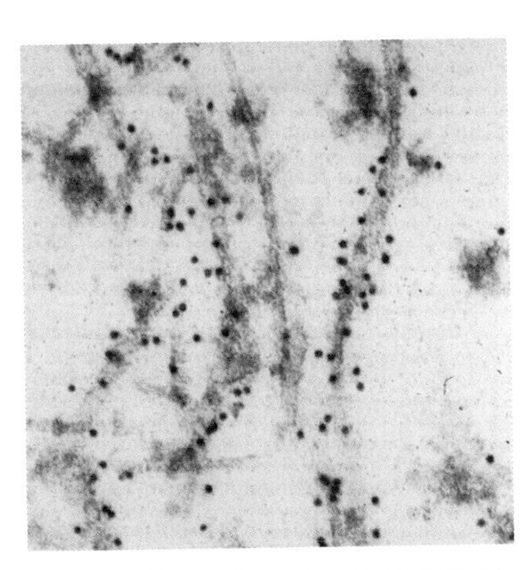

Figure 18. Electronmicrograph of intracytoplasmic tau filaments from a neuronal perikaryon in a patient with the +3 mutation. The tau filaments are decorated with gold particles in a preparation using a phosphorylation dependent monoclonal antibody that recognises pSer396/pSer404 (PHF1).

impact of these abnormalities is that tau becomes hyperphosphorylated and is formed into filaments. The precise order of events related to hyperphosphorylation and filament formation is not clearly understood. Normally, tau is found only in the soluble form; however, in association with FTDP-17*T*, tau may be found in both soluble and insoluble forms. Morphological evidence for the presence of the insoluble form is provided by the facts that some tau deposits are fluorescent using thioflavin S preparations, tau filaments in neurons and glia can be detected by electronmicroscopy, and tau filaments can be visualised following isolation from a sarkosyl insoluble preparation (36).

The protein tau that accumulates in neurons and glia differs according to the *Tau* mutation. Missense mutations in exons 1, 9, 11, 12 and 13 affect structurally all 6 isoforms. Missense and deletion mutations in exon 10 affect structurally only 3 isoforms. Mutations in the stem loop structure of the intron following exon 10 and some mutations in exon 10 affect the splicing of exon 10 thus altering the ratio of the isoforms (36).

Western blot analysis of the tau protein has been used to determine which isoforms are involved in the pathologic process. The 6 human tau isoforms when expressed in bacteria and examined by Western blot analysis form 6 equally spaced bands similar to those observed in Western blots of soluble tau expressed in the normal human brain. Tau in a normal human brain is phosphorylated; however, in FTDP-17*T*, tau becomes hyperphosphorylated predominantly on serine or threonine residues. Hyperphosphorylated tau becomes insoluble and is visualised as 4 or fewer bands depending on the tau mutation (36).

In the soluble tau protein, 4-repeat tau isoforms are more abundant than 3-repeat tau isoforms in association with mutations N279K, L284L, N296N, S305N, S305S, and most mutations in the intron following exon 10. The 6 isoforms are present in equal amounts in association with the other known mutations (36).

Insoluble tau protein shows various patterns suggesting that all or some isoforms may become insoluble depending on the mutation. Grouping, summarising and interpreting these patterns is difficult due to the low number of cases studied and the differences in techniques used by the various laboratories involved. Some patterns are consistently observed. One such pattern is that seen in association with the V337M and R406W mutations. In these cases, the insoluble tau before dephosphorylation is visualised as 4 bands with molecular masses of 60, 64, 68 and 72 kDa; whereas, after dephosphorylation the insoluble tau is visualised as 6 bands corresponding to the 6 isoforms. This pattern is similar to that of insoluble tau in Alzheimer disease. Another commonly seen pattern is that seen in association with mutations that affect the splicing of exon 10 (N279K, L284L, N296N, S305N, S305S, and mutations in the intron following exon 10). The insoluble tau before dephosphorylation is visualised as 3 bands with molecular masses of 64, 68 and 72 kDa; whereas, after dephosphorylation it is visualised as 3 bands corresponding to the 3 isoforms with 383, 412, and 441 amino acids (36, 68).

Individuals with missense (P301L, N279K) or splice site mutations that affect exon 10, and thus 4R isoforms, have tau inclusions consisting predominantly of 4R tau (8, 21, 27, 33, 40, 66, 67). Individuals with missense mutations, outside exon 10, that affect 3R and 4R tau, usually have inclusions composed of all 6 isoforms with tau pathology that is predominantly neuronal in distribution (57, 65, 66). There are exceptions to this pattern most notably the K257T mutation in exon 9 that is associated with Pick disease-like pathology and with insoluble tau deposits that are predominantly composed of 3R tau (60). Pick disease-like pathology has also been observed consistently with a number of *Tau* mutations (K257T, L266V, G272V, G389R, S320F, K369I); however, it is associated with selective 3R tau deposition (K257T) or with the deposition of both 3R and 4R tau (G389R, S320F and K369I) (19, 26, 43, 46, 52, 60, 62, 66).

Differential Diagnosis

Clinically, FTDP-17*T* may mimic several neurodegenerative diseases. The differential diagnosis of FTDP-17*T* includes disorders with initial signs such as behavioral and personality abnormalities, parkinsonism, lower motor neuron dysfunction and cognitive impairment. A neuropathologic study coupled with a molecular genetic analysis of the *Tau* gene are essential steps toward separating FTDP-17*T* from other forms of neurodegenerative diseases associated with tau deposition. The pathologic analysis should include immunohistochemical studies using multiple anti-tau antibodies. In the absence of a positive family history or molecular genetic data, FTDP-17*T* is most frequently confused with Pick disease, progressive supranuclear palsy, and corticobasal degeneration.

Pathogenesis

Mechanism of mutations. Tau is a microtubule-binding protein that is abundant in neurons and glia; in neurons it is predominantly expressed in axons. Tau binds to and stabilises microtubules and promotes microtubule assembly. The majority of the coding region mutations known to date occur within the microtubule-binding region of tau. Most known mutations in non-coding regions affect the splicing of exon 10. The pathogenetic mechanisms operating are related to the altered proportion of tau isoforms or to the ability of tau to bind microtubules and to promote microtubule assembly.

Mutations in *Tau* associated with FTDP-17*T* fall into 2 broad mechanistic groups. One group contains coding mutations (missense and two deletions) that in recombinant protein studies and in transfected cell assays have been shown to disrupt the binding of tau to microtubules (5, 11, 23, 27, 38). In addition, the majority of these mutations have also been shown to accelerate the aggregation of recombinant tau in the presence of polyanions (5, 18, 20, 44). Thus overall these mutations are predicted to both increase the proportion of tau that is unbound to microtubules and available for aggregation and also to directly increase the tendency of the unbound tau to form filaments. This process likely results in the eventual formation of the neurofibrillary tangles and other tau inclusions. It is uncertain if the two mutations reported in exon 1 have mechanistic effects similar to the majority of mutations in exons 9 to 13; however, the R5H mutation has been reported to both disrupt tau-microtubule binding and to increase tau aggregation, in vitro, which is similar to other missense mutations (24).

The second group of *Tau* mutations appears to cause disease by disrupting the alternative splicing of exon 10 and thus the ratio of 4R:3R tau (29, 59, 68). These mutations are a mixture of coding changes, within exon 10 (N279K, ΔK280, L284L, N296N/H, S305S, and S305N) and also intronic mutations close to the 5′ splice site of exon 10 (at positions +3, +11, +12, +13, +14, and +16). All but one of these mutations has been demonstrated to increase the splicing-in of exon 10 and thus the proportion of 4R tau (36, 59). The exception is ΔK280 that, at least in vitro, results in the virtual elimination of exon 10+ mRNA (14). All of these splicing mutations appear to act by disrupting positive or negative cis-acting splice regulatory signals within or just outside exon 10 (15). A group of mutations clustered around the 5′ splice site (S305N, S305S, +3, +11, +12, +13, +14, and +16) likely disrupt a stem-loop structure that is predicted to form over the splice site thus regulating binding of the U1 SnRNP (29). Disruption of this structure by these mutations is predicted to increase U1 SnRNP binding and thus increase exon 10 incorporation and so the production 4R tau. However, these mutations may also act through a direct impact on the strength of the 5′ splice site (S305N, S305S, +3) or through the disruption of an inhibitory splice element located between +11 and +18 (15). Overall, the mechanism of the exon 10 splicing mutations is clear; however, it remains uncertain why the disruption of the 4R:3R tau ratio is sufficient to result in neurodegeneration.

Kinases and tau phosphorylation. In FTDP-17*T*, phosphorylation of tau occurs at sites that are not phosphorylated in a normal tau protein. The abnormally phosphorylated sites are revealed by phosphorylation specific antibodies recognising threonine 181, 212, 231 and serine 202, 214, 262, 356, 396, 404, 409, 422. Mitogen-activated protein kinases (MAPK) phosphorylate the tau protein at many sites in vitro suggesting that they may also be involved in the hyperphosphorylation in vivo. Studies of brain tissue obtained from FTDP-17*T* patients have shown that tau inclusions colocalise with activated kinases of the MAPK family, in particular stress-activated protein kinases (SAPK) (3, 16). These findings are consistent with data obtained in sporadic human diseases associated with tau pathology (eg, AD, PSP, CBD and Pick disease). It remains to be determined whether activation of MAPKs and SAPKs precedes the assembly of tau into filaments.

Neuronal death. The occurrence of neuronal death in the brain of patients affected by FTDP-17*T* may be inferred by the observation of neuronal rarefaction in the brain areas of patients who have died in advanced stages of the disease. Whether glial cell death also occurs as a result of *Tau* gene mutations is not known. The pathway leading from a mutation in the *Tau* gene to cell death is not completely known. It is unlikely that cell death occurs by an apoptotic mechanism. This is supported by the fact that apoptotic profiles, as identified by in situ end labeling, and immunoreactivity of activated caspase 3 have not been found in neurons containing abnormally phosphorylated tau (3). Most likely the effect of most missense mutations is that of reducing the ability of mutant tau to bind to microtubules. This phenomenon results in the destabilisation of microtubules and damage of axoplasmic transport functions. Impairment of the latter is known to have a deleterious effect on the neuronal perikaryon and its processes. In the case of *Tau* gene mutations that affect the ratio of tau isoforms, it is hypothesised that the presence of an excess of specific isoforms may result in tau not bound to microtubules. Unbound tau may become abnormally phosphorylated and susceptible to aggregation into filaments.

Therapy and Future Directions

Currently, a curative treatment for FTDP-17*T* does not exist. However, supportive and symptomatic treatments are available. It is hoped that the development of transgenic mice will provide an opportunity to test therapeutic agents in the near future.

Despite significant progress in the understanding of FTDP-17*T*, there are still many clinical areas that require further exploration. Future research is needed to assess the autonomic nervous system involvement, sleep abnormalities, and eye movement dysfunction. Personality and cognitive deficits await more detailed neuropsychological examinations. Structural and functional imaging has been performed in only some FTDP-17*T* kindreds. PET examinations using newer radiotracers will help demonstrate the nature of the neuronal dysfunction of vulnerable cell populations. There is also a need for the Second International Conference on FTDP-17, which can provide the opportunity to discuss the clinical, molecular genetic, and pathologic progress on this disorder and delineate further research directions.

References

1. Arima K, Kowalska A, Hasegawa M, Mukoyama M, Watanabe R, Kawai M, Takahashi K, Iwatsubo T, Tabira T, Sunohara N (2000) Two brothers with frontotemporal dementia and parkinsonism with an N279K mutation of the tau gene. *Neurology* 54: 1787-1795.

2. Arvanitakis Z, Wszolek ZK (2001) Recent advances in the understanding of tau protein and movement disorders. *Curr Opin Neurol* 14: 491-497.

3. Atzori C, Ghetti B, Piva R, Srinkivasan AN, Zolo P, Delisle MB, Mirra SS, Migheli A (2001) Activation of the JNK/p38 pathway occurs in diseases characterised by tau protein pathology and is related to tau phosphorylation but not to apoptosis. *J Neuropathol Exp Neurol* 60: 1190-1197.

4. Baker M, Kwok JB, Kucera S, Crook R, Farrer M, Houlden H, Isaacs A, Lincoln S, Onstead L, Hardy J, Wittenberg L, Dodd P, Webb S, Hayward N, Tannenberg T, Andreadis A, Hallupp M, Schofield P, Dark F, Hutton M (1997) Localization of frontotemporal dementia with parkinsonism in an Australian kindred to chromosome 17q21-22. *Ann Neurol* 42: 794-798.

5. Barghorn S, Zheng-Fischhofer Q, Ackmann M, Biernat J, von Bergen M, Mandelkow EM Mandelkow E (2000) Structure, microtubule interactions and paired helical filament aggregation by tau mutants of frontotemporal dementias. *Biochemistry* 39: 11714-11721.

6. Bird TD, Nochlin D, Poorkaj P, Cherrier M, Kaye J, Payami H, Peskind E, Lampe TH, Nemens E, Boyer PJ, Schellenberg GD (1999) A clinical pathological comparison of three families with frontotemporal dementia and identical mutations in the tau gene (P301L). *Brain* 122: 741-756.

7. Bugiani O, Murrell JR, Giaccone G, Hasegawa M, Ghigo G, Tabaton M, Morbin M, Primavera A, Carella F, Solaro C et al (1999) Frontotemporal dementia and corticobasal degeneration in a family with a P301S mutation in tau. *J Neuropathol Exp Neurol* 58: 667-677.

8. Clark LN, Poorkaj P, Wszolek Z, Geschwind DH, Nasreddine ZS, Miller B, Li D, Payami H, Awert F, Markopoulou K et al (1998) Pathogenic implications of mutations in the tau gene in pallido-ponto-nigral degeneration and related neurodegenerative disorders linked to chromosome 17. *Proc Natl Acad Sci U S A* 95: 13103-13107.

9. Cordes M, Wszolek ZK, Calne DB, Rodnitzky RL, Pfeiffer RF (1992) Magnetic resonance imaging studies in rapidly progressive autosomal dominant parkinsonism and dementia with pallido-ponto-nigral degeneration. *Neurodegeneration* 1: 217-224.

10. Crowther RA, Goedert M (2000) Abnormal tau-containing filaments in neurodegenerative diseases. *J Struct Biol* 130: 271-279.

11. Dayanandan R, Van Slegtenhorst M, Mack TG, Ko L, Yen SH, Leroy K, Brion JP, Anderton BH, Hutton M, Lovestone S (1999) Mutations in tau reduce its microtubule-binding properties in intact living cells. *FEBS Lett* 446: 228-232.

12. Delisle MB, Murrell JR, Richardson R, Trofatter JA, Rascol O, Soulages X, Mohr M, Calvas P, Ghetti B (1999) A mutation at codon 279 (N279K) in exon 10 of the Tau gene causes a tauopathy with dementia and supranuclear palsy. *Acta Neuropathol (Berl)* 98: 62-77.

13. Dumanchin C, Camuzat A, Campion D, Verpillat P, Hannequin D, Dubois B, Saugier-Veber P, Martin C, Penet C, Charbonnier F et al (1998) Segregation of a missense mutation in the microtubule-associated protein tau gene with familial frontotemporal dementia and parkinsonism. *Hum Mol Genet* 7: 1825-1829.

14. D'Souza I, Poorkaj P, Hong M, Nochlin D, Lee VM, Bird TD, Schellenberg GD (1999) Missense and silent tau gene mutations cause frontotemporal dementia with parkinsonism-chromosome 17 type, by affecting multiple alternative RNA splicing regulatory elements. *Proc Natl Acad Sci U S A* 96: 5598-5603.

15. D'Souza I, Schellenberg GD (2002) Tau Exon 10 expression involves a bipartite intron 10 regulatory sequence and weak 5′ and 3′ splice sites. *J Biol Chem* 277: 26587-26599.

16. Ferrer I, Pastor P, Rey MJ, Munoz E, Puig B, Pastor E, Oliva R, Tolosa E (2003) Tau phosphorylation and kinase activation in familial tauopathy linked to ΔN296 mutation. *Neuropathol Appl Neurobiol* 29: 23-34.

17. Foster NL, Wilhelmsen K, Sima AA, Jones MZ, D'Amato CJ, Gilman S (1997) Frontotemporal dementia and parkinsonism linked to chromosome 17: a consensus conference. Conference Participants. *Ann Neurol* 41: 706-715.

18. Gamblin TC, King ME, Dawson H, Vitek MP, Kuret J, Berry RW, Binder LI (2000) In vitro polymerization of tau protein monitored by laser light scattering: method and application to the study of FTDP-17 mutants. *Biochemistry* 39: 6136-6144.

19. Ghetti B, Murrell JR, Zolo P, Spillantini MG, Goedert M (2000) Progress in hereditary tauopathies: a mutation in the Tau gene (G389R) causes a Pick disease-like syndrome. Ann N Y Acad Sci 920: 52-62.

20. Goedert M, Jakes R, Crowther RA (1999) Effects of frontotemporal dementia FTDP-17 mutations on heparin-induced assembly of tau filaments. *FEBS Lett* 450: 306-311.

21. Goedert M, Spillantini MG, Crowther RA, Chen SG, Parchi P, Tabaton M, Lanska DJ, Markesbery WR, Wilhelmsen KC, Dickson DW, Petersen RB, Gambetti P (1999) Tau gene mutation in familial progressive subcortical gliosis. *Nat Med* 5: 454-457.

22. Groen JJ, Endtz LJ (1982) Hereditary Pick's disease: second re-examination of a large family and discussion of other hereditary cases, with particular reference to electroencephalography and computerized tomography. *Brain* 105: 443-459.

23. Hasegawa M, Smith MJ, Goedert M (1998) Tau proteins with FTDP-17 mutations have a reduced ability to promote microtubule assembly. *FEBS Lett* 437: 207-210.

24. Hayashi S, Toyoshima Y, Hasegawa M, Umeda Y, Wakabayashi K, Tokiguchi S, Iwatsubo T, Takahashi H (2002) Late-onset frontotemporal dementia with a novel exon 1 (Arg5His) tau gene mutation. *Ann Neurol* 51: 525-530.

25. Heutink P, Stevens M, Rizzu P, Bakker E, Kros JM, Tibben A, Niermeijer MF, van Duijn CM, Oostra BA, van Swieten JC (1997) Hereditary frontotemporal dementia is linked to chromosome 17q21-q22: a genetic and clinicopathological study of three Dutch families. *Ann Neurol* 41: 150-159.

26. Hogg M, Baker M, Hutton ML, Gruijic ZM, Demirci S, Sweet AP, Herzog LL, Weintraub S, Mesulam MM et al (2002) A novel tau mutation L266V produces a tauopathy clinically and pathologically consistent with Pick's disease. *Neurobiol Aging* 23: S459.

27. Hong M, Zhukareva V, Vogelsberg-Ragaglia V, Wszolek Z, Reed L, Miller BI, Geschwind DH, Bird TD, McKeel D, Goate A et al (1998) Mutation-specific functional impairments in distinct tau isoforms of hereditary FTDP-17. *Science* 282: 1914-1917.

28. Houlden H, Baker M, Adamson J, Grover A, Waring S, Dickson D, Lynch T, Boeve B, Petersen RC, Pickering-Brown S et al (1999) Frequency of tau mutations in three series of non-Alzheimer's degenerative dementia. *Ann Neurol* 46: 243-248.

29. Hutton M, Lendon CL, Rizzu P, Baker M, Froelich S, Houlden H, Pickering-Brown S, Chakraverty S, Isaacs A, Grover A, Hackett J et al (1998) Association of missense and 5′-splice-site mutations in tau with the inherited dementia FTDP-17. *Nature* 393: 702-705.

30. Iijima M, Tabira T, Poorkaj P, Schellenberg GD, Trojanowski JQ, Lee VM, Schmidt ML, Takahashi K, Nabika T, Matsumoto T, Yamashita Y, Yoshioka S, Ishino H (1999) A distinct familial presenile dementia with a novel missense mutation in the tau gene. *Neuroreport* 10: 497-501.

31. Iseki E, Matsumura T, Marui W, Hino H, Odawara T, Sugiyama N, Suzuki K, Sawada H, Arai T, Kosaka K (2001) Familial frontotemporal dementia and parkinsonism with a novel N296H mutation in exon 10 of the tau gene and a widespread tau accumulation in the glial cells. *Acta Neuropathol (Berl)* 102: 285-292.

32. Janssen JC, Warrington EK, Morris HR, Lantos P, Brown J, Revesz T, Wood N, Khan MN, Cipolotti L, Fox NC, Rossor MN (2002) Clinical features of frontotemporal dementia due to the intronic tau 10(+16) mutation. *Neurology* 58: 1161-1168.

32a. Kobayashi T, Ota S, Tanaka K, Ito Y, Hasegawa M, Umeda Y, Moroi Y, Takanashi M, Yasuhara M, Anno M, Mizuno Y, Mori H (2003) A novel L266V mutation of the tau gene causes frontotemporal dementia with a unique tau pathology. *Ann Neurol* 53: 133-137.

33. Kodama K, Okada S, Iseki E, Kowalska A, Tabira T, Hosoi N, Yamanouchi N, Noda S, Komatsu N, Nakazato M et al (2000) Familial frontotemporal dementia with a P301L tau mutation in Japan. *J Neurol Sci* 176: 57-64.

34. Lanska DJ, Currier RD, Cohen M, Gambetti P, Smith EE, Bebin J, Jackson JF, Whitehouse PJ, Markesbery WR (1994) Familial progressive subcortical gliosis. *Neurology* 44: 1633-1643.

35. Lantos PL, Cairns NJ, Khan MN, King A, Revesz T, Janssen JC, Morris H, Rossor MN (2002) Neuropathologic variation in frontotemporal dementia due to the intronic tau 10 (+16) mutation. *Neurology* 58: 1169-1175.

36. Lee VMY, Goedert M, Trojanowski JQ (2001) Neurodegenerative tauopathies. *Annu Rev Neurosci* 24: 1121-1159.

37. Lippa CF, Zhukareva V, Kawarai T, Uryu K, Shafiq M, Nee LE, Grafman J, Liang Y, St George-Hyslop PH, Trojanowski JQ, Lee VM (2000) Frontotemporal dementia with novel tau pathology and a Glu342Val tau mutation. *Ann Neurol* 48: 850-858.

38. Lu M, Kosik KS (2001) Competition for microtubule-binding with dual expression of tau missense and splice isoforms. *Mol Biol Cell* 12: 171-184.

39. Lynch T, Sano M, Marder KS, Bell KL, Foster NL, Defendini RF, Sima AA, Keohane C, Nygaard TG, Fahn S et al (1994) Clinical characteristics of a family with chromosome 17-linked disinhibition-dementia-parkinsonism-amyotrophy complex. *Neurology* 44: 1878-1884.

40. Mirra SS, Murrell JR, Gearing M, Spillantini MG, Goedert M, Crowther RA, Levey AI, Jones R, Green J, Shoffner JM et al (1999) Tau pathology in a family with dementia and a P301L mutation in tau. *J Neuropathol Exp Neurol* 58: 335-345.

41. Miyamoto K, Kowalska A, Hasegawa M, Tabira T, Takahashi K, Araki W, Akiguchi I, Ikemoto A (2001) Familial frontotemporal dementia and parkinsonism with a novel mutation at an intron 10+11-splice site in the tau gene. *Ann Neurol* 50: 117-120.

42. Murrell JR, Koller D, Foroud T, Goedert M, Spillantini MG, Edenberg HJ, Farlow MR, Ghetti B (1997) Familial multiple-system tauopathy with presenile dementia is localized to chromosome 17. *Am J Hum Genet* 61: 1131-1138.

43. Murrell JR, Spillantini MG, Zolo P, Guazzelli M, Smith MJ, Hasegawa M, Redi F, Crowther RA, Pietrini P, Ghetti B, Goedert M (1999) Tau gene mutation G389R causes a tauopathy with abundant Pick body-like inclusions and axonal deposits. *J Neuropathol Exp Neurol* 58: 1207-1226.

44. Nacharaju P, Lewis J, Easson C, Yen S, Hackett J, Hutton M, Yen, SH (1999) Accelerated filament formation from tau protein with specific FTDP-17 missense mutations. *FEBS Lett* 447: 195-199.

45. Nasreddine ZS, Loginov M, Clark LN, Lamarche J, Miller BL, Lamontagne A, Zhukareva V, Lee VM, Wilhelmsen KC, Geschwind DH (1999) From genotype to phenotype: a clinical, pathological, and biochemical investigation of frontotemporal dementia and parkinsonism (FTDP-17) caused by the P301L tau mutation. *Ann Neurol* 45: 704-715.

46. Neumann M, Schulz-Schaeffer W, Crowther RA, Smith MJ, Spillantini MG, Goedert M, Kretzschmar HA (2001) Pick's disease associated with the novel Tau gene mutation K369I. *Ann Neurol* 50: 503-513.

47. Neve RL, Harris P, Kosik KS, Kurnit DM, Donlon TA (1986) Identification of cDNA clones for the human microtubule-associated protein tau and chromosomal localization of the genes for tau and microtubule-associated protein 2. *Brain Res* 387: 271-280.

48. Nicholl DJ, Greenstone MA, Rizzu P, Clarke CE, Crooks D, Heutink P (2002) A Yorkshire kindred with young onset atypical PSP and central hypoventilation due to a novel homozygous S352L tau mutation. *Movement Disorders* 17: S30.

49. Pal PK, Wszolek ZK, Kishore A, de la Fuente-Fernandez R, Sossi V, Uitti RJ, Dobko T, Stoessl AJ (2001) Positron emission tomography in pallido-ponto-nigral degeneration (PPND) family (frontotemporal dementia with parkinsonism linked to chromosome 17 and point mutation in tau gene). *Parkinsonism Relat Disord* 7: 81-88.

50. Pastor P, Pastor E, Carnero C, Vela R, Garcia T, Amer G, Tolosa E, Oliva R (2001) Familial atypical progressive supranuclear palsy associated with homozigosity for the delN296 mutation in the tau gene. *Ann Neurol* 49: 263-267.

51. Petersen RB, Tabaton M, Chen SG, Monari L, Richardson SL, Lynch T, Manetto V, Lanska DJ, Markesbery WR, Currier RD et al (1995) Familial progressive subcortical gliosis: presence of prions and linkage to chromosome 17. *Neurology* 45: 1062-1067.

52. Pickering-Brown S, Baker M, Yen SH, Liu WK, Hasegawa M, Cairns N, Lantos PL, Rossor M, Iwatsubo T, Davies Y, Allsop D, Furlong R, Owen F, Hardy J, Mann D, Hutton M (2000) Pick's disease is associated with mutations in the tau gene. *Ann Neurol* 48: 859-867.

53. Pickering-Brown SM, Richardson AM, Snowden JS, McDonagh AM, Burns A, Braude W, Baker M, Liu WK, Yen SH, Hardy J et al (2002) Inherited frontotemporal dementia in nine British families associated with intronic mutations in the tau gene. *Brain* 125: 732-751.

54. Poorkaj P, Bird TD, Wijsman E, Nemens E, Garruto RM, Anderson L, Andreadis A, Wiederholt WC, Raskind M, Schellenberg GD (1998). Tau is a candidate gene for chromosome 17 frontotemporal dementia. *Ann Neurol* 43: 815-825.

55. Poorkaj P, Grossman M, Steinbart E, Payami H, Sadovnick A, Nochlin D, Tabira T, Trojanowski JQ, Borson S, Galasko D, Reich S, Quinn B, Schellenberg G, Bird TD (2001) Frequency of tau gene mutations in familial and sporadic cases of non-Alzheimer dementia. *Arch Neurol* 58: 383-387.

56. Poorkaj P, Muma NA, Zhukareva V, Cochran EJ, Shannon KM, Hurtig H, Koller WC, Bird TD, Trojanowski JQ, Lee VM, Schellenberg GD (2002) An R5L tau mutation in a subject with a progressive supranuclear palsy phenotype. *Ann Neurol* 52: 511-516.

57. Reed LA, Grabowski TJ, Schmidt ML, Morris JC, Goate A, Solodkin A, Van Hoesen GW, Schelper RL, Talbot CJ, Wragg MA, Trojanowski JQ (1997) Autosomal dominant dementia with widespread neurofibrillary tangles. *Ann Neurol* 42: 564-572.

58. Reed LA, Schmidt ML, Wszolek ZK, Balin BJ, Soontornniyomkij V, Lee VM, Trojanowski JQ, Schelper RL (1998) The neuropathology of a chromosome 17-linked autosomal dominant parkinsonism and dementia ("pallido-ponto-nigral degeneration"). *J Neuropathol Exp Neurol* 57: 588-601.

59. Reed LA, Wszolek ZK, Hutton M (2001) Phenotipic correlations in FTDP-17. *Neurobiol Aging* 22: 89-107.

60. Rizzini C, Goedert M, Hodges JR, Smith MJ, Jakes R, Hills R, Xuereb JH, Crowther RA, Spillantini MG (2000) Tau gene mutation K257T causes a tauopathy similar to Pick's disease. *J Neuropathol Exp Neurol* 59: 990-1001.

61. Rizzu P, Van Swieten JC, Joosse M, Hasegawa M, Stevens M, Tibben A, Niermeijer MF, Hillebrand M, Ravid R, Oostra BA et al (1999) High prevalence of mutations in the microtubule-associated protein tau in a population study of frontotemporal dementia in the Netherlands. *Am J Hum Genet* 64: 414-421.

62. Rosso SM, van Herpen E, Deelen W, Kamphorst W, Severijnen LA, Willemsen R, Ravid R, Niermeijer MF, Dooijes D, Smith MJ et al (2002) A novel tau mutation, S320F, causes a tauopathy with inclusions similar to those in Pick's disease. *Ann Neurol* 51: 373-376.

63. Saito Y, Geyer A, Sasaki R, Kuzuhara S, Nanba E, Miyasaka T, Suzuki K, Murayama S (2002) Early-onset, rapidly progressive familial tauopathy with R406W mutation. *Neurology* 58: 811-813.

64. Sperfeld AD, Collatz MB, Baier H, Palmbach M, Storch A, Schwarz J, Tatsch K, Reske S, Joosse M, Heutink P, Ludolph AC (1999) FTDP-17: an early-onset phenotype with parkinsonism and epileptic seizures caused by a novel mutation. *Ann Neurol* 46: 708-715.

65. Spillantini MG, Bird TD, Ghetti B (1998) Frontotemporal dementia and parkinsonism linked to chromosome 17: a new group of tauopathies. *Brain Pathol* 8: 387-402.

66. Spillantini MG, Crowther RA, Kamphorst W, Heutink P, van Swieten JC (1998) Tau pathology in two Dutch families with mutations in the microtubule-binding region of tau. *Am J Pathol* 153: 1359-1363.

67. Spillantini MG, Goedert M, Crowther RA, Murrell JR, Farlow MR, Ghetti B (1997) Familial multiple system tauopathy with presenile dementia: a disease with abundant neuronal and glial tau filaments. *Proc Natl Acad Sci U S A* 94: 4113-4118.

68. Spillantini MG, Murrell JR, Goedert M, Farlow MR, Klug A, Ghetti B (1998) Mutation in the tau gene in familial multiple system tauopathy with presenile dementia. *Proc Natl Acad Sci U S A* 95: 7737-7741.

69. Spillantini MG, Yoshida H, Rizzini C, Lantos PL, Khan N, Rossor MN, Goedert M, Brown J (2000) A novel tau mutation (N296N) in familial dementia with swollen achromatic neurons and corticobasal inclusion bodies. *Ann Neurol* 48: 939-943.

70. Stanford PM, Halliday GM, Brooks WS, Kwok JB, Storey CE, Creasey H, Morris JG, Fulham MJ, Schofield PR (2000) Progressive supranuclear palsy pathology caused by a novel silent mutation in exon 10 of the tau gene: expansion of the disease phenotype caused by tau gene mutations. *Brain* 123: 880-893.

70a. Stanford PM, Shepherd CE, Halliday GM, Brooks WS, Schofield PW, Brodaty H, Martins RN, Kwok JBJ, Schofield PR. (2003) Mutations in the tau gene cause an increase in three repeat tau and frontotemporal dementia. *Brain* in press.

71. Sumi SM, Bird TD, Nochlin D, Raskind MA (1992) Familial presenile dementia with psychosis associated with cortical neurofibrillary tangles and degeneration of the amygdala. *Neurology* 42: 120-127.

72. Tanaka R, Kobayashi T, Motoi Y, Anno M, Mizuno Y, Mori H (2000) A case of frontotemporal dementia with tau P301L mutation in the Far East. *J Neurol* 247: 705-707.

73. Tsuboi Y, Baker M, Hutton ML, Uitti RJ, Rascol O, Delisle MB, Soulages X, Murrell JR, Ghetti B, Yasuda M, Komure O, Kuno S, Arima K, Sunohara N, Kobayashi T, Mizuno Y, Wszolek ZK (2002) Clinical and genetic studies of families with the tau N279K mutation (FTDP-17). *Neurology* 59: 1791-1793.

74. Tsuboi Y, Baker M, Hutton M, Uitti RJ, Yasuda M, Bugiani O, Ghetti B, Wszolek ZK (2002) Tau haplotype and clinical features of FTDP-17 families with P301S tau mutation. *Movement Disorder* 17: 1107.

75. Tsuboi Y, Uitti RJ, Wszolek ZK (2002) Differences in clinical presentation among branches of pallido-ponto-nigral degeneration family (FTDP-17, N279K mutation on the tau gene). *J Investigative Medicine* 50: 164A.

76. van Herpen E, Rosso SM, Severijnen LA, Niermeijer MF, Heutink P, van Swieten JC, Ravid R, Smith MJ, Goedert M (2002) Characterization of two novel mutations in exon 11 of the tau gene. *Neurobiol Aging* 23: S459.

77. Wilhelmsen KC, Lynch T, Pavlou E, Higgins M, Nygaard TG (1994) Localization of disinhibition-dementia-parkinsonism-amyotrophy complex to 17q21-22. *Am J Hum Genet* 55: 1159-1165.

78. Wszolek ZK, Lagerlund TD, Steg RF, McManis PG (1998) Clinical neurophysiologic findings in patients with rapidly progressive familial parkinsonism and dementia with pallido-ponto-nigral degeneration. *Electroenceph Clin Neurophysiol* 107: 213-222.

79. Wszolek ZK, Pfeiffer RF, Bhatt MH, Schelper RL, Cordes M, Snow BJ, Rodnitzky RL, Wolters EC, Arwert F, Calne DB (1992) Rapidly progressive autosomal dominant parkinsonism and dementia with pallido-ponto-nigral degeneration. *Ann Neurol* 32: 312-320.

80. Wszolek ZK, Tsuboi Y, Farrer M, Uitti RJ, Hutton ML (2003) Hereditary tauopathies and parkinsonism. *Adv Neurol* 91: 153-163.

81. Yasuda M, Kawamata T, Komure O, Kuno S, D'Souza I, Poorkaj P, Kawai J, Tanimukai S, Yamamoto Y, Hasegawa H, Sasahara M, Hazama F, Schellenberg GD, Tanaka C (1999) A mutation in the microtubule-associated protein tau in pallido-nigro-luysian degeneration. *Neurology* 53: 864-868.

82. Yasuda M, Takamatsu J, D'Souza I, Crowther RA, Kawamata T, Hasegawa M, Hasegawa H, Spillantini MG, Tanimukai S, Poorkaj P, Varani L, Varani G, Iwatsubo T, Goedert M, Schellenberg DG, Tanaka C (2000) A novel mutation at position +12 in the intron following exon 10 of the tau gene in familial frontotemporal dementia (FTD-Kumamoto). *Ann Neurol* 47: 422-429.

83. Yasuda M, Yokoyama K, Nakayasu T, Nishimura Y, Matsui M, Yokoyama T, Miyoshi K, Tanaka C (2000) A Japanese patient with frontotemporal dementia and parkinsonism by a tau P301S mutation. *Neurology* 55: 1224-1227.

Progressive Supranuclear Palsy (PSP) or Steele-Richardson-Olszewski Disease

Jean-Jacques Hauw
Yves Agid

A	amygdala
BNM	basal nucleus of Meynert
CN	caudate nucleus
CoS	superior colliculus
CS	cortico-spinal tract
DN	dentate nucleus
GCM	griseum centrale mesencephali and metencephali
IO	inferior olive
IRZ	intermediate reticular zone
LC	locus coeruleus
NCS	nucleus centralis superior
NP	pons nuclei
Npp	pedunculo pontine nucleus
NR	red nucleus
NTF	neurofibrillary tangle
Pa	pallidum
PHF	paired helical filament
PSP	progressive supranuclear palsy
Pu	putamen
SN	substantia nigra
ST	subthalamic nucleus
TANC	tangle-associated neuritic cluster

Definition

Progressive supranuclear palsy (PSP) can be defined as a multisystem degeneration of middle and late age characterised clinically by parkinsonism associated with other symptoms and signs (usually including supranuclear ophthalmoplegia), and pathologically by tau-associated lesions in selective regions of the basal ganglia, brain stem, cerebellum and cerebral cortex. PSP is one of the neurodegenerative tauopathies (58).

Synonyms and Historical Annotations

John C. Steele, J. Clifford Richardson and Jerzy Olszewski in Toronto, Canada, 1964, described PSP as a "heterogeneous degeneration involving the brain stem, basal ganglia and cerebellum with vertical gaze and pseudobulbar palsy, nuchal dystonia and dementia" (101). Their paper was accepted as the seminal description of a clinicopathological entity. PSP is also named Steele, Richardson and Olszewski syndrome, in spite of the fact that a few similar cases had been published earlier, one of which with clinico-neuropathological examination (16).

Epidemiology

Prevalence and incidence. The prevalence of PSP has been underestimated. Using passive referral evaluation, Nath et al found a prevalence in the United Kingdom of 1 per 1000000 (80). With an active multiple source case ascertainment, the crude and age-adjusted prevalence in northern England is of 3.1 (95% CI 2.4-3.8) and 2.4 (1.9-3.0) per 100000, respectively (80). Screening the records of 15 general practices in London, United Kingdom, Schrag et al evaluated the age-adjusted prevalence to 6.4 per 100000 (94). The annual incidence rate for ages 50 to 99 years was 5.3, and increased from 1.7 at 50 to 59 years to 14.7 at 80 to 99 years in Olmsted County, Minn, during the years 1976 to 1990. Median survival time from symptom onset was 5.3 years in this study (11).

Sex and age distribution. PSP is a disease of middle and late age (median age at onset: 65-69 years) (80). In a large clinically diagnosed series 61.8% of the deceased sample were men (92).

Risk factors. Advanced age can be considered the only risk factor for PSP. Possible aetiological influences, both environmental and genetic, have been suggested, but none has been established. An association between a history of hypertension and PSP has been reported. This may be connected to the high prevalence of lacunes described in PSP. Consumption of herbal tea and tropical fruit from the Annonaceae family (that contain neurotoxic benzyltetrahydroisoquinoline alkaloids) in the French West Indies may be more frequent in PSP and atypical parkinsonism than in Parkinson's disease (14). No relationship between PSP and smoking could be established (109).

Genetics

PSP is a sporadic disease although a few familial cases with a PSP-like phenotype have been reported, some of which have been validated by a neuropathological study (31, 90). Autosomal recessive and dominant transmission with incomplete penetrance have been suggested (88, 90). Several mutations of the tau gene have been identified in rare familial cases (90) including a silent mutation in exon 10 of the tau gene (100). The diagnosis of these cases is debated, some authors believing that they should be classified as FTDP-17 (115). Several polymorphisms in the tau gene have been reported. The first was a dinucleotide repeat polymorphism in intron 9, for which several studies demonstrated an increased frequency of the A0 allele and of the A0/A0 genotype in PSP patients (17). In the Caucasian, but not Asian populations, the homozygous tau allele A0 is over-represented in PSP patients compared with controls and Alzheimer's disease affected patients (17, 77). It was subsequently demonstrated that this polymorphism is associated with at least 9 others which cover the 100 Kb tau gene and constitute 2 haplotypes in complete linkage dysequilibrium: H1 including the A0, A1 and A2 alleles and H2 with the A3 and A4 alleles (6). Most cases of PSP are associated with the H1 haplotype and H1/H1 genotype (6, 44, 77, 78); however, the H1 haplotype is also present in 60% of the normal Caucasian and 100% of the Japanese populations. It is not known which allele of the H1 haplotype represents the risk factor for PSP or if this haplotype is simply in linkage disequilibrium with another still unknown variant of the tau, or a tightly-linked gene responsible for the biological effect. Recently,

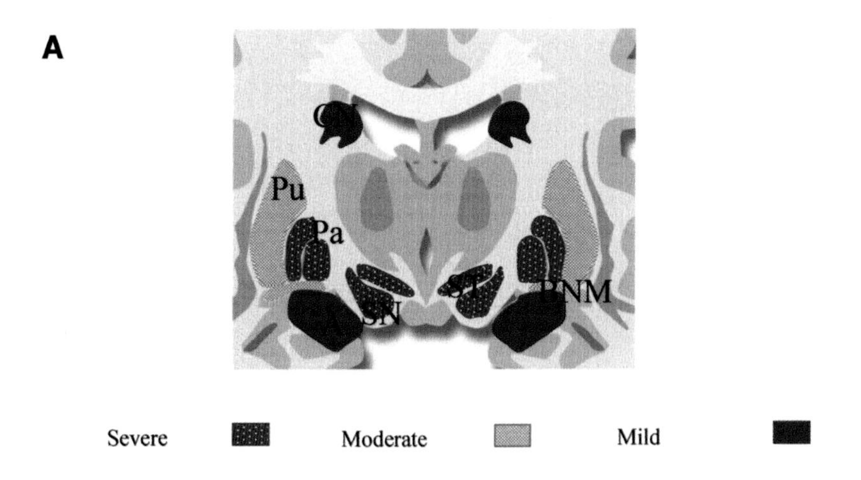

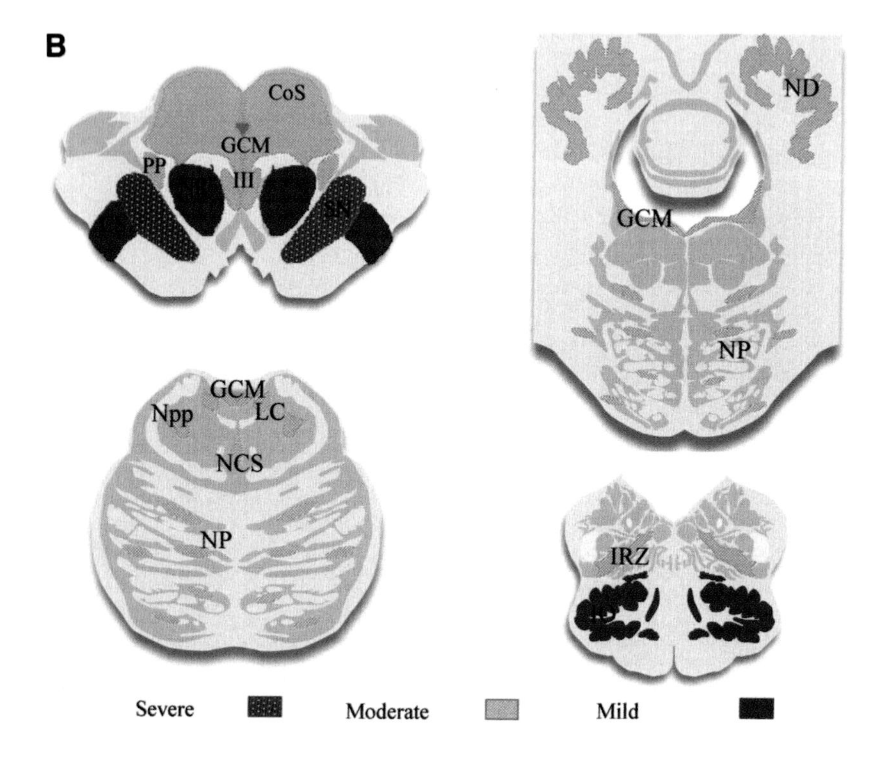

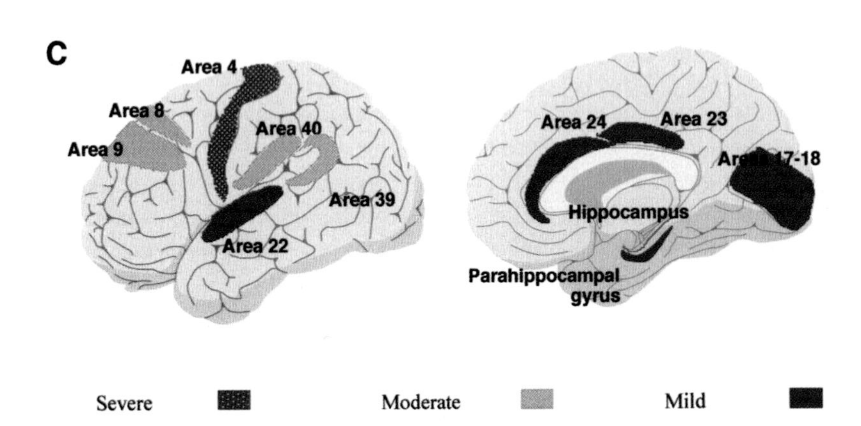

Figure 1. Schematic distribution of tau-associated lesions. **A.** Basal ganglia, **B.** Brain stem, **C.** Cerebral cortex.

an extended 5′-tau haplotype, HapA, has shown a high sensitivity (98%) and a moderate specificity (67%) as a marker for PSP (39). A recent study found an earlier age of onset in patients with the tau protein A0/A0 genotype (75). Another team, on the contrary, found that H1/H1genotype or A0/A0 genotype, independently or in conjunction with selected environmental risk factors (history of hypertension, thyroid condition, diabetes, smoking and alcohol abuse) did not influence the age at onset, severity, or survival in patients with PSP (64). No effect of α-synuclein, synphilin, or APOE genotypes on the development of PSP have been demonstrated (40, 78).

Clinical Features

A few reviews on PSP have been published recently (61, 88). Detailed descriptions can be found in early comprehensive reports (15, 62).

Symptoms and signs. The onset is insidious. Falls and postural instability are the most common presenting features. Symmetric axial rigidity with abnormal posturing of the neck (retrocolis), bradykinesia, slow and unsteady gait, impaired eye movements (particularly downward gaze supranuclear palsy, but later involvement in all directions), pseudobulbar palsy, frontal lobe-type symptoms and dementia, are usually the main signs, but these are neither specific nor found in all patients. PSP symptoms do not respond or respond poorly and transiently to levodopa therapy (66, 92, 111). In a series of 24 patients with the clinicopathological diagnosis of PSP fulfilling the NINDS neuropathologic criteria (37), survival was 6.6±0.6 years.

PSP can be classified as "Parkinson plus" together with multisystem atrophy, corticobasal degeneration and a few rare disorders (see Differential Diagnosis) because examination shows signs that are not seen in

Parkinson's disease. The main differential diagnosis being corticobasal degeneration and FTDP-17, the clinical features that can help to distinguish these diseases from PSP, such as apraxia (87) impaired executive functions (97) and neuropsychiatric symptoms (1), have been recently more specifically studied. When vertical supranuclear gaze palsy is lacking in PSP patients, or when corticobasal degeneration patients present with early severe frontal dementia (8) and bilateral parkinsonism, these disorders are generally misdiagnosed (66). The symptoms and signs in kindred classified as frontotemporal dementia and parkinsonism linked to chromosome 17 (FTDP-17) (115) or PSP (99) may overlap, the more so since there are wide phenotypic variations in the same family: Parkinsonism, eye movement abnormalities, including supranuclear gaze palsies, frontotemporal dementia, dystonia may occur in FTDP-17.

Imaging. Imaging studies help exclude other diagnoses such as CBD, MSA, multi-infarct dementia, hydrocephalus, and tumours. In addition, measuring the anteroposterior diameters in the midline sagittal T1-weighted image in MRI may support the diagnosis. PSP patients have a small rostral midbrain tegmentum contrasting with a normal pons (5, 95, 114). Proton density-weighted MRI (83) and magnetisation transfer measurement (35) have been proposed to better characterise parkinsonism cases but the specificity of the findings is not ascertained.

Functional imaging studies such as SPECT and PET show bilateral frontal hypoactivity in PSP. Cerebral blood flow reductions are less extensive and asymmetric in PSP than in corticobasal degeneration (84). Imaging of dopaminergic transporters with [^{123}I]beta-CIT SPECT or [^{18}F]DOPA PET visualise and quantify the nigrostriatal dopaminergic lesions. D2 receptor imaging can help to differentiate PSP from Parkinson disease (12).

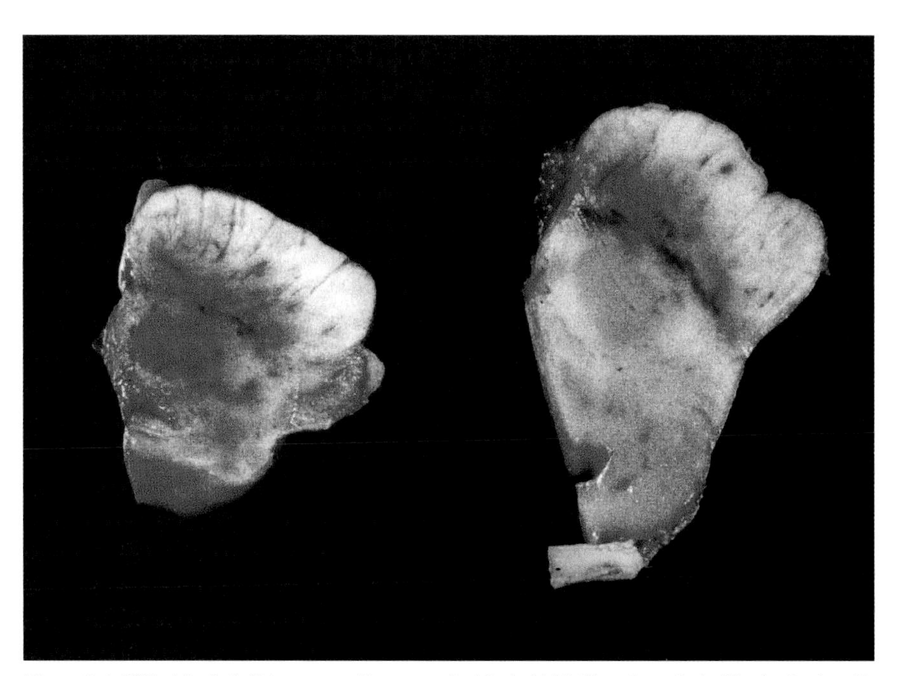

Figure 2. A PSP midbrain (left) is compared to a normal midbrain (right). There is marked midbrain atrophy with discoloration of substantia nigra, Courtesy of Pr Catherine Bergeron.

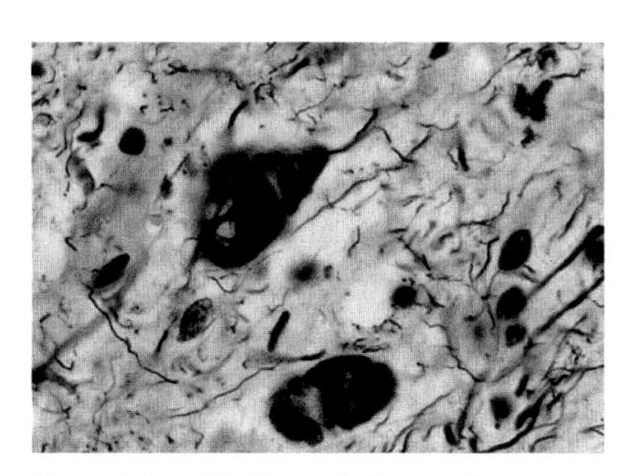

Figure 3. Two globoid neurofibrillary tangles are seen in the cytoplasm of large neurons in the subthalamic nucleus. Bodian stain combined with luxol fast blue. ×500.

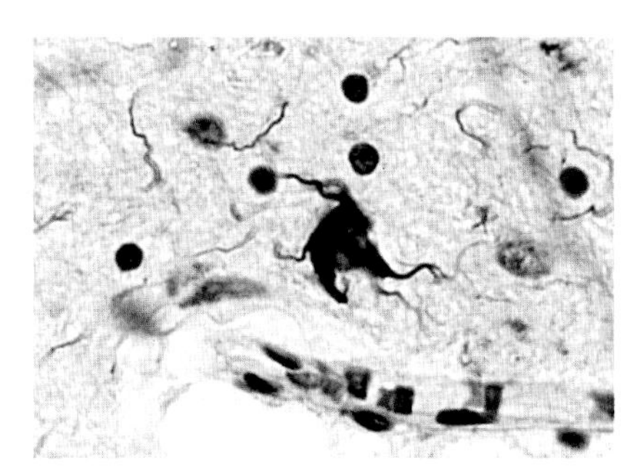

Figure 4. A small cell is stained by Gallias technique in the external pallidum. The cell body and the main cell processes are demonstrated. The exact nature of such cells, neuronal or glial, is sometimes difficult to ascertain without combined immunohistochemistry. ×500.

Laboratory findings. Electrooculographic recordings show hypometric horizontal voluntary saccades of variable latency that can help differentiate PSP from other parkinsonian disorders (72, 89). Absent or delayed auditory startle response and absent orbicularis oculi response on median nerve stimulation seem to be specific for PSP (108, 112). Other research tools include evoked potentials (visual, auditory, P300) and polysomnography that are abnormal. Tau protein level in cerebrospinal fluid is significantly higher in early PSP than in early corticobasal degeneration (107).

Clinical criteria. NINDS-SPSP criteria (63) have been evaluated retrospectively in a pathologically confirmed series of 83 patients. Specificity, sensitivity and predictive value were found superior to those in existing PSP diagnostic criteria. Interrater diagnostic agreement is near-perfect (0.91) (69).

Macroscopy

Brain weight, usually slightly decreased, remains within normal range. Gross examination may be normal, but in most cases there is midbrain atrophy predominating on the superior colliculi, dilatation of the aqueduct of Sylvius, and discoloration of the substantia nigra. Other possible changes include atrophy of the pallidum, thalamus, subthalamic nucleus

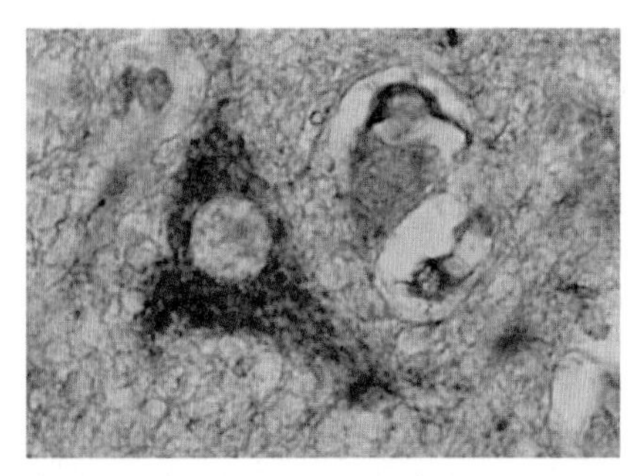

Figure 5. Granular anti-tau cytoplasmic labelling in a pretangle neuron of the motor cortex. A tau positive coiled body is seen close to another neuron. ×500.

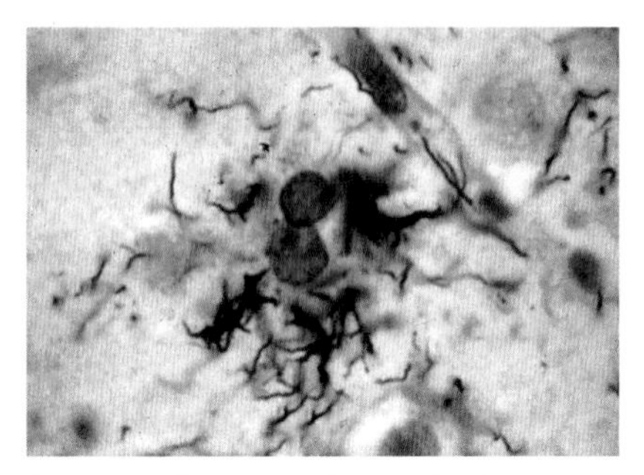

Figure 6. Tuft astrocyte showing the characteristic paired nuclei surrounded by densely packed fibres of varying diameters. Gallias technique. ×500.

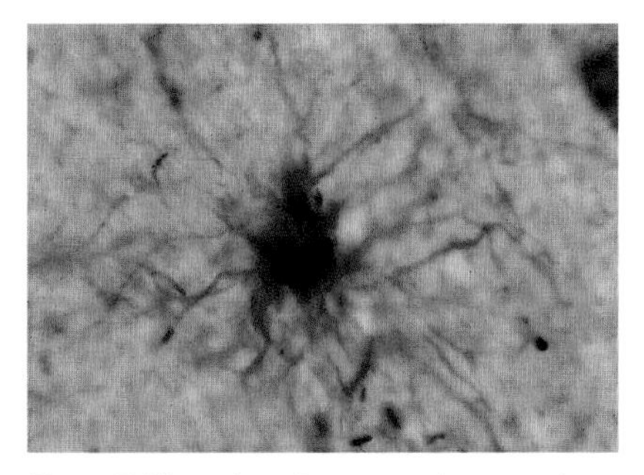

Figure 7. Thorn-shaped astrocytes have prominent argyrophilic and tau positive cytoplasm and a few thick processes. They are usually located in the subpial and subependymal regions. Double immunostaining with anti-tau (purple) and anti GFAP (yellow) antibodies. ×500. Reproduced with permission from 47.

and superior cerebellar peduncle; dilatation of the third and fourth ventricles; and loss of neuromelanin pigment of the locus ceruleus. None of these findings is specific. Mild atrophy of the cerebral cortex, either generalised or predominating in the posterior frontal, precentral and postcentral gyri, rarely with a "knife-edge appearance" has been documented. Asymmetric atrophy is not a feature of PSP. (For review, see 21, 37, 70), and for early reports see (53, 110). Image

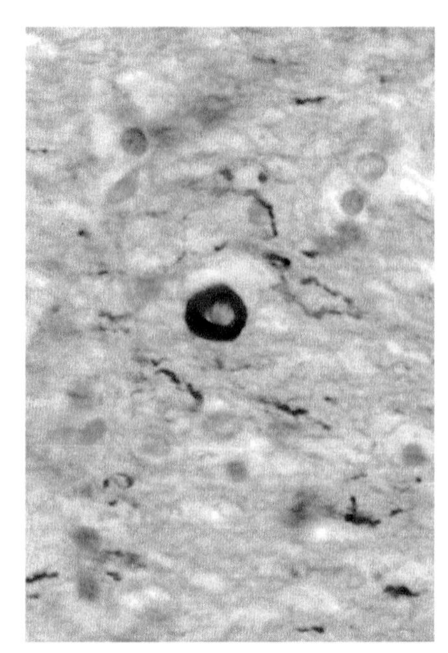

Figure 8. Coiled body adn neuropil threads in the pallidum. Tau immunohistochemistry. ×500.

analysis of fixed sections has confirmed the reduction in the cross-sectional areas of the putamen and globus pallidus; lateral and medial thalamus; tegmentum (midbrain and upper pons); basis pontis; and frontal cortex (73, 85). This was associated with a 25% reduction in the thickness of the corpus callosum (73). Greater frontal lobe atrophy tends to be correlated with clinical dementia (18).

Histopathology

The distinctive changes are neurofibrillary tangles (NFTs), neuroglial pathology (mainly tufted astrocytes), and neuropil threads associated with fibrillary astrogliosis and neuronal loss in selective areas (24, 37). The microscopical lesions are illustrated in Figures 3 to 8. The distribution of the lesions is presented in Figure 1.

Neurofibrillary tangles. Numerous NFTs in the basal ganglia and brain stem are the most helpful markers. Routine techniques (H&E, Klüver and Barrera, Congo red or thioflavin) are not useful. Silver stains used in diagnostic neuropathology such as Bodian's stain and modified Bielschowsky's stain are less sensitive that Gallyas-Braak's technique in showing NFT and other tau-related lesions. Tau immunohistochemistry, however, is as sensitive and more specific than any other method (23, 43). NFTs are mainly of the globose type in the brain stem, in the basal nucleus of Meynert and in subthalamic nucleus. Globose NFTs are characterised by skeins of argyrophilic fibrils that whirl together to make up rounded intracytoplasmic inclusions, sometimes reaching the diameter of the large neurons. In other regions (subthalamus, pallidum and cerebral cortex), NFT are more frequently flame-shaped or curvilinear. Looped forms, extending from the cell body to the main cell processes or from one dendrite to another, can be seen in small neurones, particularly in cortical layers V or VI and in the basal ganglia. These small tangles can be easily overlooked and have to be distinguished from neuroglial inclusions. NFTs have been subdivided into mature and immature according to the intensity of staining properties with anti-tau antibodies (59). In addition, numerous tangle-free neurones exhibit diffuse or granular anti-tau cytoplasmic labeling and are named "pre-tangle" neurons (53). Abnormal tau accumulation seems thus to precede genuine tangles. Ghost tangles (extracellular NFTs) are found in the hippocampus and the parahippocampal cortex, sometimes within tangle-associated neuritic clusters (TANCs) in cases with concurrent Alzheimer-type pathology (3).

In typical cases of PSP, numerous NFTs are seen in the following structures: striatum, pallidum, subthalamic nucleus, nucleus basalis of Meynert, brain stem (including colliculi, tegmentum, periaqueductal grey, red nucleus, basis pontis) and dentate nucleus. The oculomotor complex, the nucleus of the trochlear nerve and the inferior olive are also frequently affected (19, 37). The distribution of the lesions differs from case to case. A review of pathologically confirmed PSP cases selected following the NINDS criteria of typical PSP (38, 67) showed that NFTs were numerous in more than 80% of cases in the pallidum, subthalamic nucleus and substantia nigra. Some NFTs (and neuropil threads, when mentioned) were always observed in these regions. NFT were numerous in more than 50% of the cases in the periaqueductal grey matter, locus ceruleus, basal nucleus of Meynert, central pontine nuclei and dentate nucleus. They were occasional or absent in at least 50% of cases in the claustrum, putamen, caudate and olivary complex. The density of lesions was quite variable in the superior colliculus, the oculomotor complex, the pedunculopontine nucleus and the central pontine nucleus. They were usually absent, or rare, in the thalamus, red nucleus, and cuneiform or subcuneiform nuclei (110). In the cerebellum, mossy fibre exhibit tau-positive excrescences (2), but the cortex is spared. NFTs and tau-positive neurones are also seen in the spinal cord, where they can be found in the anterior, posterior and lateral horns (101). They are more frequent at the cervical level (55) and in Onuf's nucleus (93) They can be found in spinal ganglia (81).

The specificity of NFTs and tau-positive neurones in the cortex of PSP brains is now established, but it should be emphasised that isocortical NFTs are less numerous in PSP than in cortico-basal degeneration or Alzheimer's disease. They are mainly found in layers V and VI in small and large neurones, such as Betz cells (110). It is more difficult to distinguish PSP from age-associated lesions in the allocortex because the changes are virtually confined to the transentorhinal region selectively affected in ageing. However, NFTs can be seen in the granule layer of the dentate gyrus, which is usually spared in Alzheimer's disease (24, 37). As a whole, tau-positive inclusions are found in the following rank order: areas 4, 39, 8, subiculum, areas 40, 9, 23, 24, 22, parahippocampal gyrus, and finally areas 17-18, the occipital cortex being usually completely spared (110).

Neuropil threads. These short, tortuous, irregularly intermingled processes are of neuronal and oligodendroglial origin, astrocytic threads being still debated. Best recognised with Gallyas-Braak silver stain and tau immunohistochemistry, neuropil threads lack spindle-shaped thickenings, which characterise argyrophilic grains. They are seen in both grey and white matters (where they are also called white matter or interfascicular threads), in various subcortical regions: the pallidum, nucleus subthalamicus and substantia nigra, the medullary laminae of the pallidum, the striatofugal fibres to the pallidum, ansa lenticularis, fasciculus lenticularis, the corticospinal fibres. They are also seen in the cerebral cortex, constantly in the frontal regions (even in cases where NFT are lacking in the same area), especially in the precentral gyrus, and predominate in the subcortical white matter (23, 34, 37, 56, 86); however, they remain less frequent in the cerebral cortex of PSP than in corticobasal degeneration and Alzheimer's disease (1.12% in PSP, compared to 6.8% in Alzheimer disease and 0.3% in Parkinson disease) (20). In grey matter, they are seen in increasing numbers in the cortex, basal ganglia and the brainstem. On the contrary, similar densities are seen in cortical, basal ganglia and brain stem white matter (27).

Tau-positive glial fibrillary tangles. The most significant are the tufted astrocytes (synonyms: "tufts of abnormal fibers," "star-like tufts," "astrocytic tufts," or "glial fibrillary tangles") shown by silver stains (especially Gallyas-Braak technique) and tau immunohistochemistry (9, 45, 46, 106). These densely packed fibres of varying diameters, sometimes larger in the centre of the tuft, may be followed to adjacent tau positive protoplasmic astrocytes that may be binucleated. Immunostaining with anti-GFAP is negative or faintly positive, but anti-CD (43) is positive. Tuft astrocytes are seen almost exclusively in PSP, especially in the striatum, the medial thalamus, subthalamic nucleus and the frontal cortex (particularly in precentral gyri). They are rare or absent in corticobasal degeneration. Thorn-shaped astrocytes (47) (synonym: "thorn like cytoplasmic profiles with radial processes" [34]) are fibrillary astrocytes, especially seen in subpial and subependymal regions. They have a few short processes and a small eccentric nucleus, and exhibit the same histochemical properties as tuft astrocytes. These non-specific lesions are found in a wide range of cytoskeletal disorders, including corticobasal degeneration, and may be found in control cases. Other astrocytic lesions, such as astrocytic plaques, are not characteristic of PSP, and are indicative of corticobasal degeneration.

Coiled bodies (synonyms: "oligodendroglia microtubular masses" [116]) are oligodendroglial inclusions. These intra-cytoplasmic tau-positive profiles adjoin or surround the nucleus of oligodendrocytes. They have coil-like, or coma-like shapes, and can adopt more complicated shapes (spine-like or branched) (34, 46, 56). They are easily differentiated from the cap-shaped glial cytoplasmic inclusions characteristic of multisystem atrophy. They are frequently found in the cortex and adjacent white matter, subthalamic nucleus, pallidum, thalamus (lateral nuclei), substantia nigra, tegmentum pontis, and red nucleus. Coiled bodies are not specific for PSP and can also be found in corticobasal degeneration and argyrophilic grain disease. They are, on average, more numerous and more diffuse than astroglial lesions (56, 116).

Neuronal loss and gliosis. Neuronal loss and gliosis are most severe in areas containing NFTs and glial tau pathology, but exceptions are possible. A selective decrease in the density of large neurones has been reported in the head of the caudate nucleus, the putamen and the nucleus accumbens. In the substantia nigra, the nonpigmented neurones are particularly depleted in the ventral part and relative preservation of the pigmented neurones is observed in the medial part (86). Data concerning the locus ceruleus and the cerebral cortex are controversial (37). A decrease in synaptophysin concentrations was recently described in frontal, temporal, and parietal lobes, and in the cerebellum (10).

Reactive astrogliosis is usually linked to neuronal loss. Interestingly, the astrocytic tau pathology is not always associated with a large number of reactive GFAP-positive astrocytes (104). Microglial activation, neuronophagia and perivascular cuffs of lymphoid cells are not prominent on routine stains. The microglial burden is linked to immunoreactivity for TGF-beta type 1 and II receptors (60). It correlates with the tau burden in most areas, but not in the brainstem, which suggests that brainstem pathology in PSP is not exclusively due to tau pathology (49).

Other non-specific markers include ballooned neurones (also named "achromatic neurones," "swollen neurones," or "Pick cells"). Although rare, and even absent in some cases (19, 76), they have been reported in tegmental nuclei, amygdala and cerebral cortex. They are found mainly in the limbic system, including the parahippocampus gyrus (41), usually in the entorhinal and transentorhinal cortex (71). A high number is indicative of other diagnoses, such as corticobasal degeneration, Pick disease or argyrophilic grain disease (25, 103). Pigment accumulation and spheroid degeneration of the pallidonigral system are non-specific findings. Grumose (foamy) spheroid bodies are associated with aberrant sprouting of axons in the degenerated pars reticulata of substantia nigra (79). Grumose degeneration occurs in the dentate nuclei. Small eosinophilic and argyrophilic granular structures, consisting of clusters of degenerating axon terminals, surround large neurones, some of which are swollen and achromatic. This non-specific change may be related to the degeneration of the dentatorubrothalamic tract as well as the cerebellar hemispheric white matter (51). Hypertrophy of the olivary nuclei may occur, presumably as a consequence of lesions of the central tegmental tracts (33). Granulovacuolar degeneration, although mentioned in the original descriptions, is uncommon and non-specific

White matter degeneration. Some white matter pallor and atrophy, which remains usually moderate and is mainly due to neuronal or axonal degeneration, and tau-positive bundles of fibers, are seen in the most affected areas (posterior internal capsule and cerebral peduncle, superior cerebellar peduncle). Primary demyelination related to oligodendroglial tau pathology cannot be dismissed.

Neuropathological subgroups. Atypical cases (38) are variants in which the severity or distribution of lesions deviates from the typical pattern described by Steele et al (101). No specific symptoms or signs appear to characterise these cases (19, 65, 67). In typical PSP, two main subgroups of patients may be found, one of which is characterised by predominant pallidoluysonigral lesions, the other by more severe cortical lesions, in the absence of the characteristics of corticobasal degeneration (111). The H1 haplotype has no effect on the pathological phenotype of PSP (68). In combined cases of PSP, other neurologic disorders exist concomitantly with typical PSP. For example, concomitant Alzheimer's disease and the presence of Lewy or Pick bodies have been described (27, 30, 37, 53, 70).

Neuropathologic criteria. As already mentioned, neuropathological criteria have been established and validated (38, 67). They are based on the distribution of tau associated lesions and exclusion of other degenerative disorders associated with parkinsonism and dementia (see below). Lastly, it may be mentioned that rare cases do not fall in existing criteria, and that their classification may be difficult (8, 24).

Immunohistochemistry and ultrastructural findings. *Immunohistochemistry of NFT and other tau-associated lesions.* NFT and other cytoskeletal lesions are labeled by most anti-paired helical filament (PHF) and by anti-tau antibodies, with the exception of antibodies directed against 3 repeat tau 55 kD. They bear phosphorylated epitopes (37, 53, 56, 70).

The immunoreactivities are different in PSP and Alzheimer's disease: NFT share a number of epitopes in both diseases, but they react differently to some antibodies. Alz50, a monoclonal antibody that recognises A68, an epitope of the N-terminal region of abnormal tau in Alzheimer brain, stains two major bands on Western blots in PSP brain, and three major bands in Alzheimer's disease. Fewer tangles are labeled by Alz50 immunohistochemistry in PSP than in Alzheimer's disease. An antibody against the alternatively spliced tau exon 3 (one of two N-terminal exons) recognises the lesions in PSP and Alzheimer's disease, but not in corticobasal degeneration (26). The antibodies anti exon 10 (the alternative expression of which leads to formation of three- or four-repeat tau isoforms) do not label NFT and tau-positive glial inclusions, but pretreatment with formic acid exposes the epitope. This is consistent with the hypothesis that PSP inclusions contain four-repeat tau (50). A small number of NFTs in PSP are labeled by an anti-ubiquitin monoclonal antibody (53), and some, especially compact globose tangles, by UBB+1, an aberrant form of ubiquitin derived from the ubiquitin-B gene (28). However, most NFTs and tau-positive glial cells (34) are not stained by polyclonal antibodies against ubiquitin. This is in sharp contrast with the results obtained in Alzheimer's disease, and indicate that ubiquitination is a later -and rarer- phenomenon in PSP than in Alzheimer disease.

At present, tau is the only known constituent of PSP tangles. Phosphorylated epitopes of high- and middle-molecular weight neurofilament proteins are lacking in PSP, whereas they are present in subcortical NFT of Alzheimer's disease cases (53).

Electron microscopy of NFTs and other tau-associated lesions. There are several reviews on the electron microscopy of NFTs and other tau-associated lesions (43, 45, 53, 56). NFTs are principally made of clusters of straight 12 to 20 nm filaments with circular profiles on cross section. They differ from the PHF seen in Alzheimer disease, ageing, and a number of other diseases (43, 48). Some PHF, however, may also be seen in PSP, and straight filaments contiguous with PHF may contribute to the same tangle. This has also been reported in Alzheimer disease (42, 53). By immunoelectron microscopy, the anti-tau immunoreactivity is usually associated with 12 to 20 nm straight filaments (Figure 9). Antibodies directed against PHF and sometimes ubiquitin can decorate these filaments. Anti-tau and anti-PHF also label some amorphous material. Alz50 labels short straight filaments, which could be early lesions (53). Cortical NFT in PSP may be made either of straight filaments or of PHF (53). It may be added that in the dentate granule cells of patients with Alzheimer's disease, Lewy body disease and PSP, NFT consist of straight tubular structures about 18 to 25 nm in diameter (113). Tangle-associated neuritic clusters (TANCs) are made of numerous reactive or degenerative axon terminals surrounding extracellular tubules, without amyloid. Some axons contain 13- to 15-nm-thick straight tubules that show tau immunoreactivity (3). Thorn-shaped astrocytes are made of bundles of 15-nm straight tubules and amorphous material co-existing with densely packed glial fibrils. Electron microscopy of tufted astrocytes shows fibres, 20 to 25 nm in diameter. In Gallyas-Braak-stained sections, amorphous structures and rare tubular structures are also seen. Argyrophilic threads consist in a meshwork or bundles of fibrils and in amorphous tau-immunoreactive structures. Interfascicular threads seen in the processes of oligodendrocytes, are found in the outer and inner loops of myelin, and are made of 13 to 15 nm tubules (4, 45, 56).

Biochemistry

Tau phosphorylation. Filamentous neuronal and glial tau inclusions associated with PSP are made of abnormally phosphorylated tau (22, 43, 58, 98). Six human brain tau isoforms result from alternative splicing of the tau gene located on chromosome 17. These isoforms have either 3 (3R tau) or four (4R tau) MT-binding repeats (consecutive imperfect motifs of 31 or 32 amino acids in the carboxy-terminal half of the protein). The repeat domain, which is expressed in 4R tau, is coded by exon 10. In PSP, analysis of Western blot banding patterns of filamentous (insoluble) tau from affected regions, following resolution by sodium dodecyl sulphate-polyacrylamide gel electrophoresis and immunoblotting with phosphorylation-independent anti-tau antibodies, shows 2 prominent bands of 68 and 64 kDa (a minor 72-kDa band is variably detected). These bands are made of hyperphosphorylated 4R-tau isoforms. The soluble fraction contains all 6 isoforms of tau (58, 96, 98). Similar results are found in cases of corticobasal degeneration and FTDP-17 with the P301L mutation. In contrast, in Alzheimer's disease and some FTDP-17 mutations that do not affect splicing (V337M and R406W), 3 major bands of 68, 64, and 60 kDa (and a minor variably detected band of 72 kDa) are seen. When dephosphorylated, they resolve into the 6 bands normal tau. In Pick's disease and some FTDP-17 mutations (K257T, G389R) that do not affect splicing, predominantly soluble 3R tau is expressed in the brain (13, 58, 98). The H1 haplotype does not influence the biochemical phenotype of PSP (68).

Neurotransmitters (37, 52, 91). The nigrostriatal dopaminergic pathway is dramatically affected, as shown by the 90% reduction in dopamine and tyrosine hydroxylase levels in the putamen and the caudate nucleus, and the loss of dopaminergic neurons in the substantia nigra. In contrast to Parkinson's disease, the meso-cortico-limbic dopaminergic projections from the

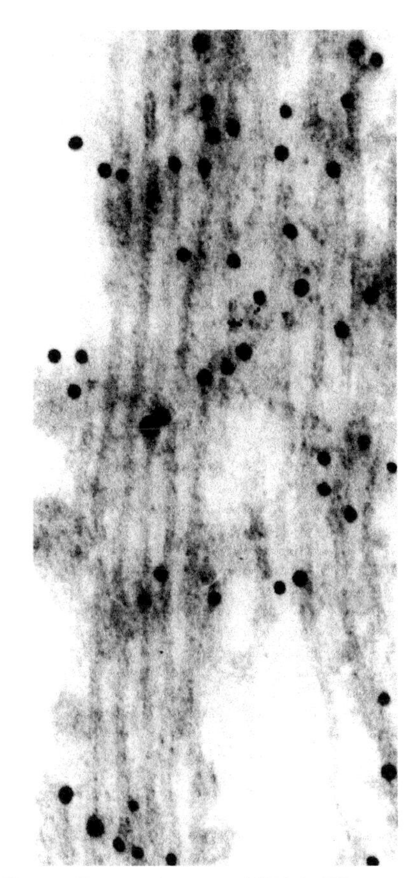

Figure 9. Electron microscopy of NFTs in PSP, consisting of straight filaments labelled by polyclonal anti-tau. ×55000 (from 53, with permission).

ventro-tegmental area to the nucleus accumbens and the cerebral cortex are relatively preserved. Whereas the density of dopaminergic D1 receptors is unaltered in the caudate nucleus and putamen, the number of D2 receptors is decreased by 30 to 50% in the same nuclei. This is likely due to the loss of dopaminoceptive neurones, and may explain, at least in part, the limited response of patients to levodopa treatment.

In contrast to Parkinson's disease, most cholinergic neuronal systems are markedly affected in PSP cases as suggested by a 40 to 80 % reduction in the choline-acetyl-transferase activity in the hippocampus, striatum, globus pallidus, substantia innominata; as well as loss of cholinergic neurons in the striatum and various nuclei of the brain stem (including the superior colliculus, the Edinger-Westphal nucleus, the interstitial nucleus of Cajal, the rostral interstitial nucleus of the medial longitudinal faciculus, the nucleus tegmenti

Distribution of lesions *	PSP type A (classical)	PSP type B* (pallidoluysonigral)
Striatum, Pallidum, Subthalamic nucleus	+++	+++
Substantia nigra, Oculomotor complex, IV nucleus	++/+++	++/+++
Inferior olives, Dentate nucleus	+/++	+/++
Basis pontis	+/++	+/++
Hippocampus and Entorhinal cortex	-/++	-/+
Prefrontal and Precentral cortex	++	-/+
Associative cortex	-/+	-/+

Table 1. Schematic distribution of tau-associated lesions in PSP (modified from [105]).
* There is often severe involvement of the basal nucleus of Meynert and of the pedunculopontine and superior centralis nuclei. The severity of the changes may vary as a function of the age of the disease.

pedunculopontis, the laterodorsal tegmental nucleus, the nucleus pontis centralis caudalis).

Cell counting of neuronal cell bodies, and measurement of the concentration of neurotransmitters show the relative integrity of the coeruleo-cortical noradrenergic system and the raphe-telencephalic serotoninergic neurons. The concentrations of many peptide neurotransmitters (methionine-enkephalin, leucine-enkephalin, substance P, cholecystokinin (9)) are not different from controls in PSP patients. Unexpectedly, there is a 40 to 60% reduction of glutamic-acid-decarboxylase, the synthetic enzyme for GABA, in the putamen, external pallidum, subthalamic nucleus and hippocampus.

Differential Diagnosis

The differential diagnosis of PSP includes disorders characterised by parkinsonism and other movement disorders, by cognitive changes, or both. Other tauopathies, such as Alzheimer disease, dementia pugilistica, Parkinson-Dementia complex of Guam, and especially corticobasal degeneration, post-encephalitic parkinsonism and FTDP-17 are the most difficult to distinguish from PSP. Neurofibrillary tangles are non-specific lesions indicating only the presence of abnormally phosphorylated and fibrillary tau proteins. They have been seen in association with a large number of disorders, in infants as young as 16-month-old (7) and they are nearly constant in centenarians, whatever the mental status (36). They can be seen in reaction to a number of chronic cell injuries, including hypoxia-ischemia (74).

The following main difficulties can arise:

i) Corticobasal degeneration and FTDP. Some cases of these diseases are very close to PSP. The distribution of NFTs and the absence of other lesions such as asymmetric focal cortical atrophy and severe white matter pathology, ballooned neurones and astrocytic plaques dismisses the diagnosis of corticobasal degeneration (23); however, some corticobasal cases may be difficult to distinguish from cases of PSP with severe cortical lesions. Similarly, distinguishing some cases of FTDP 17 from PSP (especially when the density of lesions is low or their distribution atypical) can be difficult.

ii) Alzheimer's disease. The diagnosis of Alzheimer's disease and of Alzheimer's type pathology in patients without a definite history of dementia relies on the presence of allocortical, and especially isocortical, neurofibrillary tangles and of isocortical neuritic plaques in sufficient number (depending on the age of the patient). Distinguishing Alzheimer's disease from PSP may be difficult because NFTs can be numerous in the basal ganglia and in the brain stem in some cases of Alzheimer's disease. Conversely, Alzheimer's type pathology can be seen in aged PSP patients. The use of the criteria proposed by a working group at the National Institute on Aging, and Reagan Institute allows an operational diagnosis of Alzheimer's disease.

iii) Postencephalitic parkinsonism and parkinsonism-dementia complex of Guam. The diagnosis of these rare disorders heavily depends on clinical information (67) The distribution of lesions and the tauopathy in parkinsonism-dementia complex of Guam are very close to that of Alzheimer's disease.

iv) Combined pathologies. It is debated if the presence of Lewy bodies should exclude a diagnosis of typical PSP (38) for two reasons: i) Whether Lewy bodies found with an increasing prevalence in oldest individuals is related to "normal ageing" or to "incipiens" Parkinson disease is a matter of opinion. ii) Lewy bodies have been seen in a number of PSP cases (30). Whether this is more than a chance association remains to be proven by the study of larger series.

Animal and Experimental Models

Abnormal neuronal and glial argyrophilic fibrillary structures have been described in the brain of an aged albino cynomolgus monkey (54). Transgenic models of human tauopathies (32, 117) provide animal models for neuro- and glial- fibrillary lesion formation. Stably transfected human neuroblastoma with either 3R- or 4R-tau isoforms have also been established (72).

Pathogenesis

Phosphatases and kinases that regulate tau phosphorylation. The involvement of various pathways of tau phosphorylation and dephosphorylation in vitro, and in various tauopathies, including PSP, has been extensively studied. Recent data have implicated protein kinases GSK-3β, cdk5, ERK1, ERK2 and phosphatases PP1, PP2A, PP2B, and PP2C in the in vivo regulation of tau phosphorylation (13, 29, 58). Further studies are needed to define the specific role of individual kinases and phosphatases in PSP.

Neuronal death. It has been suggested that p53- or CD95-associated apoptosis may be a mechanism of cell loss in PSP (22). Double-labelling immunohistochemistry to Bcl-2 and Bax and to tau protein suggests that Bcl-2 and Bax are probably not implicated in neurofibrillary tangle formation in PSP (105). A strong inducible NOS-like immunoreactivity was detected in tuft astrocytes but was not found in coiled bodies containing oligodendrocytes, in microglia or in neurones with neurofibrillary tangles (57). Antioxidant enzyme activities were elevated in PSP transmitochondrial cytoplasmic hybrid cell lines expressing mitochondrial genes from patients with PSP. These data suggest that mtDNA aberration occurs in PSP (102). Unlike in AD, lipid peroxidation is selectively associated with NFT formation in PSP. The intraneuronal accumulation of toxic aldehydes may contribute to hamper tau degradation, leading to its aggregation in the PSP specific abnormal filaments (82).

Distribution and progression of lesions. The brunt of the lesions is on the pallidum, the substantia nigra and the subthalamic nucleus, suggesting that the pathological process starts there. Neither anterograde nor retrograde spread can explain easily the distribution of other subcortical or cortical lesions. Another still unexplained mechanism is needed to explain the selective vulnerability of some neuronal networks and of the glial cells in PSP (110).

Therapy and Future Directions

Although a number of therapeutic trials have been conducted, the disease remains progressive, and by in large untreatable. A better knowledge of the genetics and tauopathy of PSP and of the mechanism of neuronal degeneration and death is required.

References

1. Aarsland D, Litvan I, Larsen JP (2001) Neuropsychiatric symptoms of patients with progressive supranuclear palsy and Parkinson's disease. *J Neuropsychiatry Clin Neurosci* 13: 42-49.

2. Arai K, Braak E, de Vos RA, Jansen Steur EN, Braak H (1999) Mossy fiber involvement in progressive supranuclear palsy. *Acta Neuropathol (Berl)* 98: 341-344.

3. Arima K, Nakamura M, Sunohara N, Nishio T, Ogawa M, Hirai S, Kawai M, Ikeda K (1999) Immunohistochemical and ultrastructural characterization of neuritic clusters around ghost tangles in the hippocampal formation in progressive supranuclear palsy brains. *Acta Neuropathol (Berl)* 97: 565-576.

4. Arima K, Nakamura M, Sunohara N, Ogawa M, Anno M, Izumiyama Y, Hirai S, Ikeda K (1997) Ultrastructural characterization of the tau-immunoreactive tubules in the oligodendroglial perikarya and their inner loop processes in progressive supranuclear palsy. *Acta Neuropathol (Berl)* 93: 558-566.

5. Asato R, Akiguchi I, Masunaga S, Hashimoto N (2000) Magnetic resonance imaging distinguishes progressive supranuclear palsy from multiple system atrophy. *J Neural Transm* 107: 1427-1436

6. Baker M, Litvan I, Houlden H, Adamson J, Dickson D, Perez-Tur J, Hardy J, Lynch T, Bigio E, Hutton M (1999) Association of an extended haplotype in the tau gene with progressive supranuclear palsy. *Hum Mol Genet* 8: 711-715.

7. Bancher C, Jellinger KA, Zwiauer K (1996) Neurofibrillary tangles in the brain of a 16 month old infant. *J Neurol Neurosurg Psychiatry* 60: 231.

8. Bergeron C, Davis A, Lang AE (1998) Corticobasal ganglionic degeneration and progressive supranuclear palsy presenting with cognitive decline. *Brain Pathol* 8: 355-365.

9. Bergeron C, Pollanen MS, Weyer L, Lang AE (1997) Cortical degeneration in progressive supranuclear palsy. A comparison with cortical-basal ganglionic degeneration. *J Neuropathol Exp Neurol* 56: 726-734.

10. Bigio EH, Vono MB, Satumtira S, Adamson J, Sontag E, Hynan LS, White CL, 3rd, Baker M, Hutton M (2001) Cortical synapse loss in progressive supranuclear palsy. *J Neuropathol Exp Neurol* 60: 403-410.

11. Bower JH, Maraganore DM, McDonnell SK, Rocca WA (1997) Incidence of progressive supranuclear palsy and multiple system atrophy in Olmsted County, Minnesota, 1976 to 1990. *Neurology* 49: 1284-1288.

12. Brucke T, Djamshidian S, Bencsits G, Pirker W, Asenbaum S, Podreka I (2000) SPECT and PET imaging of the dopaminergic system in Parkinson's disease. *J Neurol* 247 Suppl 4: IV/2-7.

13. Buee L, Bussiere T, Buee-Scherrer V, Delacourte A, Hof PR (2000) Tau protein isoforms, phosphorylation and role in neurodegenerative disorders. *Brain Res Brain Res Rev* 33: 95-130.

14. Caparros-Lefebvre D, Elbaz A (1999) Possible relation of atypical parkinsonism in the French West Indies with consumption of tropical plants: a case-control study. Caribbean Parkinsonism Study Group. *Lancet* 354: 281-286.

15. Cardoso F, Jankovic J (1994) Progressive supranuclear palsy. In *Neurodegenerative diseases*, DB Calne (eds). WB Saunders: Philadelphia. pp. 769-786

16. Chavany A, Van Bogaert L, Godlewski S (1951) Un syndrome de rigidité à prédominance axiale avec perturbation des automatismes oculo-palpébraux d'origine encéphalitique. *Presse Méd (Paris)* 45: 956-962

17. Conrad C, Amano N, Andreadis A, Xia Y, Namekataf K, Oyama F, Ikeda K, Wakabayashi K, Takahashi H, Thal LJ, Katzman R, Shackelford DA, Matsushita M, Masliah E, Sawa A (1998) Differences in a dinucleotide repeat polymorphism in the tau gene between Caucasian and Japanese populations: implication for progressive supranuclear palsy. *Neurosci Lett* 250: 135-137.

18. Cordato NJ, Halliday GM, Harding AJ, Hely MA, Morris JG (2000) Regional brain atrophy in progressive supranuclear palsy and Lewy body disease. *Ann Neurol* 47: 718-728.

19. Daniel SE, de Bruin VM, Lees AJ (1995) The clinical and pathological spectrum of Steele-Richardson-Olszewski syndrome (progressive supranuclear palsy): a reappraisal. *Brain* 118: 759-770.

20. Davis DG, Wang HZ, Markesbery WR (1992) Image analysis of neuropil threads in Alzheimer's, Pick's, diffuse Lewy body disease and in progressive supranuclear palsy. *J Neuropathol Exp Neurol* 51: 594-600.

21. De Armond S, Dickson D, DeArmond B (1997) Degenerative diseases of the central nervous system. In *Textbook of Neuropathology*, R Davis, D Robertson (eds). Williams & Wilkins: Baltimore. pp. 1063-1178

22. Delacourte A, Buee L (2000) Tau pathology: a marker of neurodegenerative disorders. *Curr Opin Neurol* 13: 371-376.

23. Dickson D, Liu W-K, Ksiezak-Reding H, Yen S-H (2000) Neuropathologic and molecular considerations. In *Advances in Neurology, Vol 42 Corticobasal degeneration and related disorders*, I Litvan, C Goetz, AE Lang (eds). Lippingott William & Wilkins: Philadelphia. pp. 9-27

24. Dickson DW (1999) Neuropathologic differentiation of progressive supranuclear palsy and corticobasal degeneration. *J Neurol* 246 Suppl 2: II6-15.

25. Feany MB, Dickson DW (1995) Widespread cytoskeletal pathology characterizes cortico-basal degeneration. *Am J Pathol* 90: 37-43

26. Feany MB, Ksiezak-Reding H, Liu WK, Vincent I, Yen SH, Dickson DW (1995) Epitope expression and hyperphosphorylation of tau protein in corticobasal degeneration: differentiation from progressive supranuclear palsy. *Acta Neuropathol* 90: 37-43

27. Feany MB, Mattiace LA, Dickson DW (1996) Neuropathologic overlap of progressive supranuclear palsy, Pick's disease and corticobasal degeneration. *J Neuropathol Exp Neurol* 55: 53-67.

28. Fergusson J, Landon M, Lowe J, Ward L, van Leeuwen FW, Mayer RJ (2000) Neurofibrillary tangles in progressive supranuclear palsy brains exhibit immunoreactivity to frameshift mutant ubiquitin-B protein. *Neurosci Lett* 279: 69-72.

29. Ferrer I, Blanco R, Carmona M, Ribera R, Goutan E, Puig B, Rey MJ, Cardozo A, Vinals F, Ribalta T (2001) Phosphorylated map kinase (ERK1, ERK2) expression is associated with early tau deposition in neurones and glial cells, but not with increased nuclear DNA vulnerability and cell death, in Alzheimer disease, Pick's disease, progressive supranuclear palsy and corticobasal degeneration. *Brain Pathol* 11: 144-158.

30. Gearing M, Olson DA, Watts RL, Mirra SS (1994) Progressive supranuclear palsy: neuropathologic and clinical heterogeneity. *Neurology* 44: 1015-1024.

31. Golbe LI, Dennis NJ, Dickson W (1995) Familial autopsy-proven progressive supranuclear palsy. *Neurology* 45: A255

32. Gotz J, Tolnay M, Barmettler R, Ferrari A, Burki K, Goedert M, Probst A, Nitsch RM (2001) Human tau transgenic mice. Towards an animal model for neuro- and glialfibrillary lesion formation. *Adv Exp Med Biol* 487: 71-83

33. Hanihara T, Amano N, Takahashi T, Itoh Y, Yagishita S (1998) Hypertrophy of the inferior olivary nucleus in patients with progressive supranuclear palsy. *Eur Neurol* 39: 97-102

34. Hanihara T, Amano N, Takahashi T, Nagatomo H, Yagashita S (1995) Distribution of tangles and threads in the cerebral cortex in progressive supranuclear palsy. *Neuropathol Appl Neurobiol* 21: 319-326.

35. Hanyu H, Asano T, Sakurai H, Takasaki M, Shindo H, Abe K (2001) Magnetisation transfer measurements of the subcortical grey and white matter in Parkinson's disease with and without dementia and in progressive supranuclear palsy. *Neuroradiology* 43: 542-546.

36. Hauw J-J, Duyckaerts C (2001) Alzheimer's disease. In *Pathology of the aging human nervous system*, S Duckett, JC de la Torre (eds). Oxford University Press: Oxford. pp. 207-263

37. Hauw J-J, Verny M, Ruberg M, Duyckaerts C (1998) The neuropathology of progressive supranuclear palsy (PSP) or Steele-Richardson-Olszewski disease. In *The neuropathology of dementing disorders*, W Markesbery (eds). Edward Arnold: London. pp. 193-218

38. Hauw JJ, Daniel SE, Dickson D, Horoupian DS, Jellinger K, Lantos PL, McKee A, Tabaton M, Litvan I (1994) Preliminary NINDS neuropathologic criteria for Steele-Richardson- Olszewski syndrome (progressive supranuclear palsy). *Neurology* 44: 2015-2019.

39. Higgins JJ, Golbe LI, De Biase A, Jankovic J, Factor SA, Adler RL (2000) An extended 5′-tau susceptibility haplotype in progressive supranuclear palsy. *Neurology* 55: 1364-1367.

40. Higgins JJ, Litvan I, Pho LT, Li W, Nee LE (1998) Progressive supranuclear gaze palsy is in linkage disequilibrium with the tau and not the alpha-synuclein gene. *Neurology* 50: 270-273.

41. Higuchi Y, Iwaki T, Tateishi J (1995) Neurodegeneration in the limbic and paralimbic system in progressive supranuclear palsy. *Neuropathol Appl Neurobiol* 21: 246-254.

42. Hirano A, Llena JF (1994) Structures of neurons in the aging nervous system. In *Neurodegenerative diseases*, DB Calne (eds). WB Saunders: Philadelphia. pp. 3-14

43. Hong M, Trojanowski J, Lee V (2000) Neurofibrillary lesions are the common pathology of Alzheimer's disease and other neurodegenerative tauopathies. In *Neurodegenerative dementias*, C Clark, J Trojanowski (eds). McGraw-Hill: New York. pp. 161-175

44. Houlden H, Baker M, Morris HR, MacDonald N, Pickering-Brown S, Adamson J, Lees AJ, Rossor MN, Quinn NP, Kertesz A, Khan MN, Hardy J, Lantos PL, St George-Hyslop P, Munoz DG, Mann D, Lang AE, Bergeron C, Bigio EH, Litvan I, Bhatia KP, Dickson D, Wood NW, Hutton M (2001) Corticobasal degeneration and progressive supranuclear palsy share a common tau haplotype. *Neurology* 56: 1702-1706.

45. Ikeda K, Akiyama H, Arai T, Nishimura T (1998) Glial tau pathology in neurodegenerative diseases: their nature and comparison with neuronal tangles. *Neurobiol Aging* 19: S85-91.

46. Ikeda K, Akiyama H, Haga C, Kondo H, Arima K, Oda T (1994) Argyrophilic thread-like structure in corticobasal degeneration and supranuclear palsy. *Neurosci Lett* 174: 157-159.

47. Ikeda K, Akiyama H, Kondo H, Haga C, Tanno E, Tokuda T, Ikeda S (1995) Thorn-shaped astrocytes: possibly secondarily induced tau-positive glial fibrillary tangles. *Acta Neuropathol* 90: 620-625

48. Iqbal K, Alonso AD, Gondal JA, Gong CX, Haque N, Khatoon S, Sengupta A, Wang JZ, Grundke-Iqbal I (2000) Mechanism of neurofibrillary degeneration and pharmacologic therapeutic approach. *J Neural Transm* Suppl 59: 213-222

49. Ishizawa K, Dickson DW (2001) Microglial activation parallels system degeneration in progressive supranuclear palsy and corticobasal degeneration. *J Neuropathol Exp Neurol* 60: 647-657.

50. Ishizawa K, Ksiezak-Reding H, Davies P, Delacourte A, Tiseo P, Yen SH, Dickson DW (2000) A double-labeling immunohistochemical study of tau exon 10 in Alzheimer's disease, progressive supranuclear palsy and Pick's disease. *Acta Neuropathol (Berl)* 100: 235-244.

51. Ishizawa K, Lin WL, Tiseo P, Honer WG, Davies P, Dickson DW (2000) A qualitative and quantitative study of grumose degeneration in progressive supranuclear palsy. *J Neuropathol Exp Neurol* 59: 513-524.

52. Javoy-Agid F (1994) Cholinergic and peptidergic systems in PSP. *J Neural Transm* Suppl 42: 205-218

53. Jellinger KA, Bancher C (1992) Neuropathology. In *Progressive Supranuclear Palsy, Clinical and Research Approaches*, I Litvan, Y Agid (eds). Oxford University Press: New-York. pp. 44-88

54. Kiatipattanasakul W, Nakayama H, Yongsiri S, Chotiapisitkul S, Nakamura S, Kojima H, Doi K (2000) Abnormal neuronal and glial argyrophilic fibrillary structures in the brain of an aged albino cynomolgus monkey (Macaca fascicularis). *Acta Neuropathol (Berl)* 100: 580-586.

55. Kikuchi H, Doh-ura K, Kira J, Iwaki T (1999) Preferential neurodegeneration in the cervical spinal cord of progressive supranuclear palsy. *Acta Neuropathol (Berl)* 97: 577-584.

56. Komori T (1999) Tau-positive glial inclusions in progressive supranuclear palsy, corticobasal degeneration and Pick's disease. *Brain Pathol* 9: 663-679.

57. Komori T, Shibata N, Kobayashi M, Sasaki S, Iwata M (1998) Inducible nitric oxide synthase (iNOS)-like immunoreactivity in argyrophilic, tau-positive astrocytes in progressive supranuclear palsy. *Acta Neuropathol (Berl)* 95: 338-344.

58. Lee VM, Goedert M, Trojanowski JQ (2001) Neurodegenerative tauopathies. *Annu Rev Neurosci* 24: 1121-1159

59. Li F, Iseki E, Odawara T, Kosaka K, Yagishita S, Amano N (1998) Regional quantitative analysis of tau-positive neurons in progressive supranuclear palsy: comparison with Alzheimer's disease. *J Neurol Sci* 159: 73-81.

60. Lippa CF, Flanders KC, Kim ES, Croul S (1998) TGF-beta receptors-I and -II immunoexpression in Alzheimer's disease: a comparison with aging and progressive supranuclear palsy. *Neurobiol Aging* 19: 527-533.

61. Litvan I (2001) Diagnosis and management of progressive supranuclear palsy. *Semin Neurol* 21: 41-48

62. Litvan I, Agid Y (1993) *Progressive supranuclear palsy: clinical and research approaches.* Oxford University Press: Oxford.

63. Litvan I, Agid Y, Calne D, Campbell G, Dubois B, Duvoisin RC, Goetz CG, Golbe LI, Grafman J, Growdon JH, Hallett M, Jankovic J, Quinn NP, Tolosa E, Zee DS (1996) Clinical research criteria for the diagnosis of progressive supranuclear palsy (Steele-Richardson-Olszewski syndrome): report of the NINDS-SPSP international workshop. *Neurology* 47: 1-9.

64. Litvan I, Baker M, Hutton M (2001) Tau genotype: no effect on onset, symptom severity, or survival in progressive supranuclear palsy. *Neurology* 57: 138-140.

65. Litvan I, DeLeo JM, Hauw JJ, Daniel SE, Jellinger K, McKee A, Dickson D, Horoupian DS, Lantos PL, Tabaton M (1996) What can artificial neural networks teach us about neurodegenerative disorders with extrapyramidal features? *Brain* 119: 831-839.

66. Litvan I, Grimes DA, Lang AE, Jankovic J, McKee A, Verny M, Jellinger K, Chaudhuri KR, Pearce RK (1999) Clinical features differentiating patients with postmortem confirmed progressive supranuclear palsy and corticobasal degeneration. *J Neurol* 246 Suppl 2: II1-5.

67. Litvan I, Hauw JJ, Bartko JJ, Lantos PL, Daniel SE, Horoupian DS, McKee A, Dickson D, Bancher C, Tabaton M, Jellinger K, Anderson DW (1996) Validity and reliability of the preliminary NINDS neuropathologic criteria for progressive supranuclear palsy and related disorders. *J Neuropathol Exp Neurol* 55: 97-105.

68. Liu WK, Le TV, Adamson J, Baker M, Cookson N, Hardy J, Hutton M, Yen SH, Dickson DW (2001) Relationship of the extended tau haplotype to tau biochemistry and neuropathology in progressive supranuclear palsy. *Ann Neurol* 50: 494-502.

69. Lopez OL, Litvan I, Catt KE, Stowe R, Klunk W, Kaufer DI, Becker JT, DeKosky ST (1999) Accuracy of four clinical diagnostic criteria for the diagnosis of neurodegenerative dementias. *Neurology* 53: 1292-1299.

70. Lowe J, Lennox G, Leigh P (1997) Disorders of movement and system degeneration. In *Greenfield's*

Neuropathology, D Graham, P Lantos (eds). 2 Arnold: London. pp. 280-366

71. Mackenzie IR, Hudson LP (1995) Achromatic neurons in the cortex of progressive supranuclear palsy. *Acta Neuropathol* 90: 615-619

72. Mailliot C, Bussiere T, Hamdane M, Sergeant N, Caillet ML, Delacourte A, Buee L (2000) Pathological tau phenotypes. The weight of mutations, polymorphisms, and differential neuronal vulnerabilities. *Ann N Y Acad Sci* 920: 107-114

73. Mann DM, Oliver R, Snowden JS (1993) The topographic distribution of brain atrophy in Huntington's disease and progressive supranuclear palsy. *Acta Neuropathol* 85: 553-559

74. Mokhtari K, Uchihara T, Clemenceau S, Baulac M, Duyckaerts C, Hauw JJ (1998) Atypical neuronal inclusion bodies in meningioangiomatosis. *Acta Neuropathol (Berl)* 96: 91-96.

75. Molinuevo JL, Valldeoriola F, Alegret M, Oliva R, Tolosa E (2000) Progressive supranuclear palsy: earlier age of onset in patients with the tau protein A0/A0 genotype. *J Neurol* 247: 206-208.

76. Mori H, Oda M, Mizuno Y (1996) Cortical ballooned neurons in progressive supranuclear palsy. *Neurosci Lett* 209: 109-112.

77. Morris HR, Lees AJ, Wood NW (1999) Neurofibrillary tangle parkinsonian disorders--tau pathology and tau genetics. *Mov Disord* 14: 731-736.

78. Morris HR, Vaughan JR, Datta SR, Bandopadhyay R, Rohan De Silva HA, Schrag A, Cairns NJ, Burn D, Nath U, Lantos PL, Daniel S, Lees AJ, Quinn NP, Wood NW (2000) Multiple system atrophy/progressive supranuclear palsy: alpha- Synuclein, synphilin, tau, and APOE. *Neurology* 55: 1918-1920.

79. Nagao M, Kato S, Oda M, Hirai S (1998) Expression of phosphotyrosine and SNAP-25 immunoreactivity in grumose (foamy) spheroid bodies suggests axonal regeneration. *Acta Neuropathol (Berl)* 96: 388-394.

80. Nath U, Ben-Shlomo Y, Thomson RG, Morris HR, Wood NW, Lees AJ, Burn DJ (2001) The prevalence of progressive supranuclear palsy (Steele-Richardson- Olszewski syndrome) in the UK. *Brain* 124: 1438-1449.

81. Nishimura M, Namba Y, Ikeda K, Akiguchi I, Oda M (1993) Neurofibrillary tangles in the neurons of spinal dorsal root ganglia of patients with progressive supranuclear palsy. *Acta Neuropathol* 85: 453-457

82. Odetti P, Garibaldi S, Norese R, Angelini G, Marinelli L, Valentini S, Menini S, Traverso N, Zaccheo D, Siedlak S, Perry G, Smith MA, Tabaton M (2000) Lipoperoxidation is selectively involved in progressive supranuclear palsy. *J Neuropathol Exp Neurol* 59: 393-397.

83. Oka M, Katayama S, Imon Y, Ohshita T, Mimori Y, Nakamura S (2001) Abnormal signals on proton density-weighted MRI of the superior cerebellar peduncle in progressive supranuclear palsy. *Acta Neurol Scand* 104: 1-5.

84. Okuda B, Tachibana H, Kawabata K, Takeda M, Sugita M (2000) Cerebral blood flow in corticobasal degeneration and progressive supranuclear palsy. *Alzheimer Dis Assoc Disord* 14: 46-52.

85. Oyanagi K, Makifuchi T, Ohtoh T, Ikuta F, Chen KM, Chase TN, Gajdusek DC (1994) Topographic investigation of brain atrophy in parkinsonism-dementia complex of Guam: a comparison with Alzheimer's disease and progressive supranuclear palsy. *Neurodegeneration* 3: 301-304.

86. Oyanagi K, Tsuchiya K, Yamazaki M, Ikeda K (2001) Substantia nigra in progressive supranuclear palsy, corticobasal degeneration, and parkinsonism-dementia complex of Guam: specific pathological features. *J Neuropathol Exp Neurol* 60: 393-402.

87. Pharr V, Uttl B, Stark M, Litvan I, Fantie B, Grafman J (2001) Comparison of apraxia in corticobasal degeneration and progressive supranuclear palsy. *Neurology* 56: 957-963.

88. Rehman HU (2000) Progressive supranuclear palsy. *Postgrad Med J* 76: 333-336.

89. Rivaud-Pechoux S, Vidailhet M, Gallouedec G, Litvan I, Gaymard B, Pierrot-Deseilligny C (2000) Longitudinal ocular motor study in corticobasal degeneration and progressive supranuclear palsy. *Neurology* 54: 1029-1032.

90. Rojo A, Pernaute RS, Fontan A, Ruiz PG, Honnorat J, Lynch T, Chin S, Gonzalo I, Rabano A, Martinez A, Daniel S, Pramstaller P, Morris H, Wood N, Lees A, Tabernero C, Nyggard T, Jackson AC, Hanson A, de Yebenes JG, Pramsteller P (1999) Clinical genetics of familial progressive supranuclear palsy. *Brain* 122: 1233-1245.

91. Ruberg M, Hirsch E, Javoy-Agid F (1992) Neurochemistry. In *Progressive supranuclear palsy. Clinical and research approaches*, I Litvan, Y Agid (eds). Oxford University Press: New York. pp. 89-109

92. Santacruz P, Uttl B, Litvan I, Grafman J (1998) Progressive supranuclear palsy: a survey of the disease course. *Neurology* 50: 1637-1647.

93. Scaravilli T, Pramstaller PP, Salerno A, Egarter-Vigl E, Giometto B, Vitaliani R, An SF, Revesz T (2000) Neuronal loss in Onuf's nucleus in three patients with progressive supranuclear palsy. *Ann Neurol* 48: 97-101.

94. Schrag A, Ben-Shlomo Y, Quinn NP (1999) Prevalence of progressive supranuclear palsy and multiple system atrophy: a cross-sectional study. *Lancet* 354: 1771-1775.

95. Schrag A, Good CD, Miszkiel K, Morris HR, Mathias CJ, Lees AJ, Quinn NP (2000) Differentiation of atypical parkinsonian syndromes with routine MRI. *Neurology* 54: 697-702.

96. Sergeant N, Wattez A, Delacourte A (1999) Neurofibrillary degeneration in progressive supranuclear palsy and corticobasal degeneration: tau pathologies with exclusively "exon 10" isoforms. *J Neurochem* 72: 1243-1249.

97. Soliveri P, Monza D, Paridi D, Carella F, Genitrini S, Testa D, Girotti F (2000) Neuropsychological follow up in patients with Parkinson's disease, striatonigral degeneration-type multisystem atrophy, and progressive supranuclear palsy. *J Neurol Neurosurg Psychiatry* 69: 313-318.

98. Spillantini MG, Goedert M (1998) Tau protein pathology in neurodegenerative diseases. *Trends Neurosci* 21: 428-433.

99. Stanford P, Haliday G, Brooks W, Kwok J, Schofield P (2001) Progressive supranuclear palsy pathology,frontotemporal dementia with parkinsonism linked to chromosome 17 and familial tauopathies. *Brain* 124: 1670-1675

100. Stanford PM, Halliday GM, Brooks WS, Kwok JB, Storey CE, Creasey H, Morris JG, Fulham MJ, Schofield PR (2000) Progressive supranuclear palsy pathology caused by a novel silent mutation in exon 10 of the tau gene: expansion of the disease phenotype caused by tau gene mutations. *Brain* 123: 880-893.

101. Steele JC, Richardson JC, Olszewski J (1964) Progressive supranuclear palsy; a heterogeneous degeneration involving the brain stem, basal ganglia and cerebellum with vertical gaze and pseudobulbar palsy, nuchal dystonia and dementia. *Arch Neurol* 10: 333-359

102. Swerdlow RH, Golbe LI, Parks JK, Cassarino DS, Binder DR, Grawey AE, Litvan I, Bennett JP, Jr., Wooten GF, Parker WD (2000) Mitochondrial dysfunction in cybrid lines expressing mitochondrial genes from patients with progressive supranuclear palsy. *J Neurochem* 75: 1681-1684.

103. Togo T, Dickson D (2002) Balloned neurons in PSP are usually due to concurrent argyrophilic grain disease. *Acta Neuropathol* 104: 53-56.

104. Togo T, Dickson DW (2002) Tau accumulation in astrocytes in progressive supranuclear palsy is a degenerative rather than a reactive process. *Acta Neuropathol* 104: 398-402.

105. Tortosa A, Blanco R, Ferrer I (1998) Bcl-2 and Bax protein expression in neurofibrillary tangles in progressive supranuclear palsy. *Neuroreport* 9: 1049-1052.

106. Uchihara T, Mitani K, Mori H, Kondo H, Yamada M, Ikeda K (1994) Abnormal cytoskeletal pathology peculiar to corticobasal degeneration is different from that of Alzheimer's disease or progressive supranuclear palsy. *Acta Neuropathol* 88: 379-383

107. Urakami K, Wada K, Arai H, Sasaki H, Kanai M, Shoji M, Ishizu H, Kashihara K, Yamamoto M, Tsuchiya-Ikemoto K et al (2001) Diagnostic significance of tau protein in cerebrospinal fluid from patients with corticobasal degeneration or progressive supranuclear palsy. *J Neurol Sci* 183: 95-98.

108. Valls-Sole J, Valldeoriola F, Tolosa E, Marti MJ (1997) Distinctive abnormalities of facial reflexes in patients with progressive supranuclear palsy. *Brain* 120: 1877-1883.

109. Vanacore N, Bonifati V, Fabbrini G, Colosimo C, Marconi R, Nicholl D, Bonuccelli U, Stocchi F, Lamberti P, Volpe G, De Michele G, Iavarone I, Bennett P, Vieregge P, Meco G (2000) Smoking habits in multiple system atrophy and progressive supranuclear palsy. European Study Group on Atypical Parkinsonisms. *Neurology* 54: 114-119.

110. Verny M, Duyckaerts C, Agid Y, Hauw JJ (1996) The significance of cortical pathology in progressive supranuclear palsy. Clinico-pathological data in 10 cases. *Brain* 119: 1123-1136.

111. Verny M, Jellinger KA, Hauw JJ, Bancher C, Litvan I, Agid Y (1996) Progressive supranuclear palsy: a clinicopathological study of 21 cases. *Acta Neuropathol* 91: 427-431

112. Vidailhet M, Rothwell JC, Thompson PD, Lees AJ, Marsden CD (1992) The auditory startle response in the Steele-Richardson-Olszewski syndrome and Parkinson's disease. *Brain* 115: 1181-1192.

113. Wakabayashi K, Hansen LA, Vincent I, Mallory M, Masliah E (1997) Neurofibrillary tangles in the dentate granule cells of patients with Alzheimer's disease, Lewy body disease and progressive supranuclear palsy. *Acta Neuropathol (Berl)* 93: 7-12.

114. Warmuth-Metz M, Naumann M, Csoti I, Solymosi L (2001) Measurement of the midbrain diameter on routine magnetic resonance imaging: a simple and accurate method of differentiating between Parkinson disease and progressive supranuclear palsy. *Arch Neurol* 58: 1076-1079.

115. Wszolek ZK, Tsuboi Y, Uitti RJ, Reed L, Hutton ML, Dickson DW (2001) Progressive supranuclear palsy as a disease phenotype caused by the S305S tau gene mutation. *Brain* 124: 1666-1670.

116. Yamada T, Calne DB, Akiyama H, McGeer EG, McGeer PL (1993) Further observations on Tau-positive glia in the brains with progressive supranuclear palsy. *Acta Neuropathol* 85: 308-315

117. Yen SH, Hutton M, DeTure M, Ko LW, Nacharaju P (1999) Fibrillogenesis of tau: insights from tau missense mutations in FTDP-17. *Brain Pathol* 9: 695-705.

Corticobasal Degeneration

Dennis Dickson
Irene Litvan

AD	Alzheimer's disease
BN	balooned neuron
CBD	corticobasal degeneration
NFT	neurofibrillary tangle
PiD	Pick's disease
PSP	progressive supranuclear palsy

Definition

Corticobasal degeneration (CBD) was initially characterised as asymmetric akinetic-rigid parkinsonism, but more recently pathologically confirmed cases of CBD have presented with primary aphasia, dementia, visual inattention or rapidly progressive mutism. The salient histologic features are focal cortical degeneration with widespread tau pathology in neurones and glia in cortical and subcortical grey and white matter.

Synonyms and Historical Annotations

CBD was first reported by Rebeiz and co-workers (53), who referred to the disorder as "corticodentatonigral degeneration with neuronal achromasia." Subsequent reports referred to the disorder as corticonigral degeneration (4, 20, 38, 52, 66), and Gibb and coworkers coined the term "corticobasal degeneration" (CBD) (26). Some groups have also used the term "corticobasal ganglionic degeneration" (5-7). All names emphasise the predominant distribution of pathology to cortex and deep grey matter structures. The advantage of the term corticobasal over the others is that it is the most generic and encompasses degenerative changes in deep grey matter areas other than the basal ganglia, substantia nigra and cerebellar dentate.

Epidemiology

Incidence and prevalence. True prevalence rates of CBD are difficult to estimate since clinical and pathologic criteria for diagnosis of CBD are undergoing reappraisal.The range of clinical presentations for CBD is expanding, based upon recent clinicopathologic studies (36). Original descriptions of CBD emphasized a syndrome of progressive asymmetrical apraxia and rigidity (26, 55) but more recent reports have indicated that individuals with postmortem findings of CBD may also present with focal cortical syndromes, such as frontal dementia and progressive aphasia (4-6, 26, 30, 36, 52). Using assumptions about the presenting features of CBD and its frequency among parkinsonian disorders, a calculated estimate of the incidence of CBD is less than 1 per 100000 per year, which compares with 12 per 100000 for Parkinson's disease (39).

Sex and age distribution. There is no clear sex or ethnic preponderance for CBD. In a large postmortem confirmed clinicopathologic series, the male to female ratio was approximately equal and the average age of onset was 63±7.7 years with an average disease duration of 7.9±2.6 years (67).

Risk factors. There are no known risk factors, but genetic factors in the form of variants in the tau gene may play a role in some cases.

Genetics

Almost all reported cases of CBD have been sporadic, but there are rare familial reports of CBD (12). Whether these are actual cases of CBD or frontotemporal dementia and parkinsonism linked to chromosome 17 (FTDP-17) remains to be determined by evaluation of these purported familial CBD cases for tau mutations. FTDP-17 has a number of clinical and pathologic features in common with CBD (14). In particular, familial multi-system tauopathy (59, 60) and familial pallido-ponto-nigral degeneration (54) have many histological, ultrastructural and biochemical similarities to CBD. Similarly, as described in detail in chapter 3.2 on PSP there are many similarities to CBD. It remains to be demonstrated that the polymorphisms described in PSP are relevant for CBD, but two recent studies have shown that CBD shares the same genetic background as PSP (18, 29).

Clinical Features

Signs and symptoms. CBD is a focal cortical degenerative disorder, and the clinical phenotype is a function of the location of the dominant cortical pathology. Phenotype at presentation seems to predict prognosis. Patients with a lateralized presentation live longer than those with a bilateral/dementia presentation (dementia, bilateral parkinsonism) (39). The usual clinical presentation corresponds to damage to the dorsal peri-Rolandic, superior frontal and superior parietal cortices, whereas cases with aphasia show pathology in the peri-Sylvian region (30, 44). The clinical syndrome of progressive asymmetrical apraxia and rigidity, while typical of CBD, can be due to other pathologic disorders (9, 28).

The initial signs of typical cases of CBD are unilateral or asymmetrical apraxia, rigidity and dystonia.This may be associated with myoclonic jerks, grasp reflex, cortical sensory signs and the alien limb phenomenon.The affected hand may develop dystonic flexion contractures late in the disease. Cognitive impairment is not universal in CBD. Dementia in CBD most often has features of a frontal lobe dementia marked by personality change, disorder of conduct, impaired attention and distractibility. Frontal lobe signs, including grasp reflex, forced groping, utilization behaviour and inter-manual conflict, characteristically are unilateral at onset and markedly asymmetric.

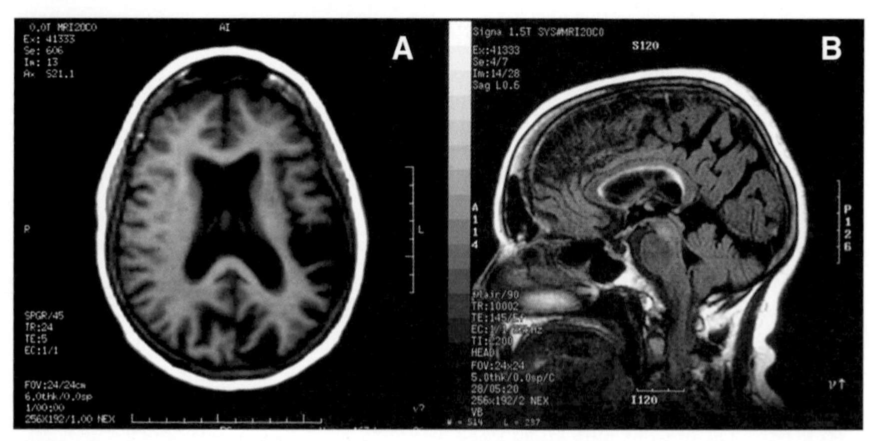

Figure 1. A. Horizontal MRI of CBD shows asymmetrical atrophy (enlarged sulcal spaces and narrow gyri) affecting the left parietal and occipital lobe with asymmetrical enlargement of the lateral ventricle. **B.** Sagittal MRI of CBD shows superior frontal atrophy and increased signal in a thinned corpus callosum.

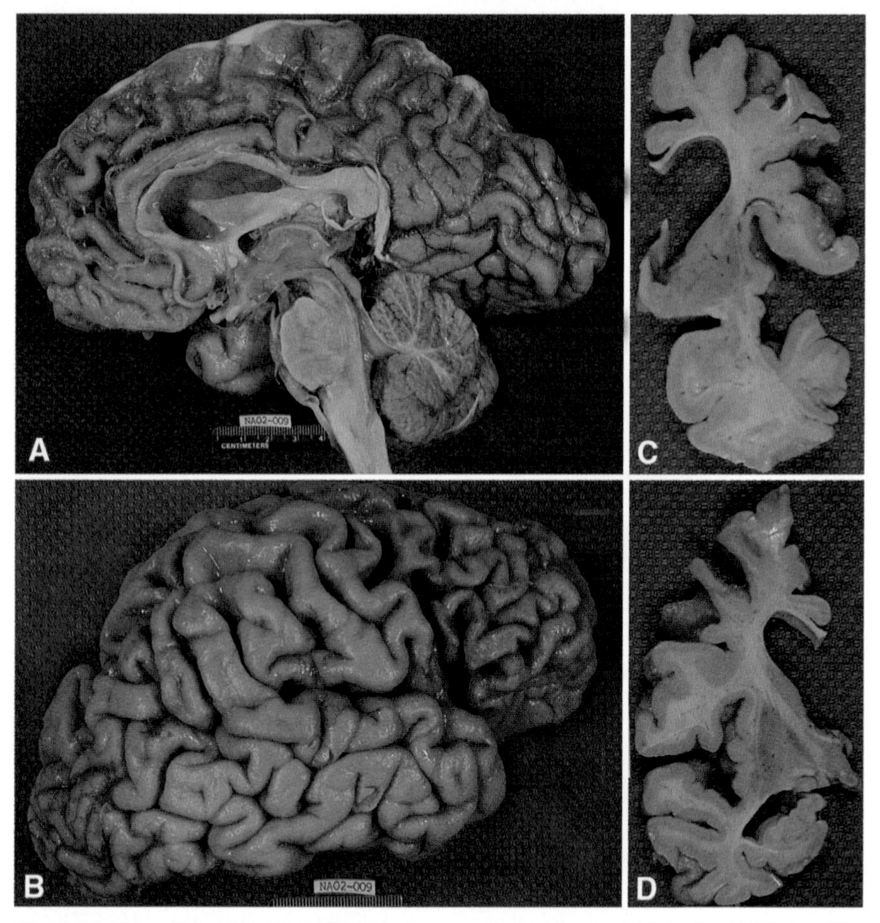

Figure 2. A. Mid-sagittal section of fixed CBD brain shows superior frontal and parietal atrophy with thinning of the corpus callosum. **B.** The convexity view shows frontal atrophy most marked in the premotor cortex. Note preservation of temporal, occipital and inferior parietal lobes. **C.** Coronal section at the level of the nucleus accumbens show enlargement of the frontal horn of the lateral ventricle, thinning of the corpus callosum and slight flattening of the head of the caudate nucleus. **D.** Coronal section at the level of the mammillary body shows atrophy of the dorsal aspects of the frontal lobe (also visible in **C**) with sparing of the inferior frontal and temporal lobe, including the hippocampus.

The alien limb phenomenon, which includes involuntary movement, such as elevation of the arm or leg in the air, but also the feeling of not owning a limb (22) is often emphasised in CBD, but it is neither specific to CBD nor found in all cases. Cortical sensory deficits due to parietal lobe involvement and characterised by hemineglect, agraphesthesia and astereognosis are frequent in CBD .

Imaging. Structural imaging may be helpful in CBD, where magnetic resonance imaging may show asymmetrical atrophy of the superior parietal lobule variably extending into frontal regions, with less prominent atrophy elsewhere (58). Structural changes become more obvious as the disease progresses. Asymmetrical cortical atrophy may be subtle or absent in initial stages (Figure 1). Asymmetrical cortical atrophy is not specific, since Pick's disease, nonspecific frontotemporal dementia, primary progressive aphasia and some individuals with FTDP-17 may have asymmetrical cortical atrophy. MRI scans in CBD may show hyperintense signals in white matter in regions of brain atrophy and sometimes atrophy of and increased signal in the corpus callosum (21, 69) (Figure 1).

Functional imaging is often informative. The hallmark finding is asymmetrical hypometabolism in superior frontal and parietal lobes (8, 56). Hypometabolism is sometimes also detected in caudate, putamen or thalamus. PET scans assessing dopa-mine metabolism with $[^{18}F]$-DOPA may show reduction of striatal and medial frontal uptake (56). Striatal uptake is usually most severely impaired contralateral to the clinically most affected limbs.

Laboratory findings. No specific laboratory tests are available for CBD. Measurements of CSF tau have produced conflicting results. While initial studies failed to find increases of tau in CSF in CBD (2), more recent studies with larger sample sizes have shown increases over controls and even PSP (45, 64). Use of assays for hyperphosphorylated tau and for specific isoforms of tau, namely 4R tau, have yet to be published, but hold promise for more specific assays with greater differential diagnostic value.

Macroscopy

On external examination, the brain usually shows narrowing of cortical gyri that is most marked in parasagittal regions. (Figure 2). The superior frontal gyrus is often more affected than middle and inferior frontal gyri in cases with a typical progressive asymmetrical rigidity and apraxia syndrome. The pre- and post-central regions are also affected to varying degrees. Postmortem volumetric studies confirm the selective atrophy of the precentral gyrus (17). The temporal and occipital lobes are usually spared. In cases presenting with dementia or progressive aphasia the distribution of the atrophy is often more generalised and involves the inferior frontal and temporal lobes, as well. The atrophy is often asymmetric, but the side-to-side differences can be subtle.

On sectioning the brain, cortical atrophy is often obvious in the dorsal half of the frontal lobe, with sometimes striking preservation of the frontal opercular region and the temporal lobe (Figure 2). The cingulate gyrus is not consistently affected. The brainstem and cerebellum are not consistently reduced in size.

The cerebral white matter in affected areas is often attenuated and may have a grey and gelatinous consistency in severe cases. The anterior corpus callosum is sometimes thinned. The anterior limb of the internal capsule may show attenuation, as well, but other white matter tracts, such as the optic tract, anterior commissure and fornix, are preserved.

There may be flattening of the head of the caudate, and in many cases the thalamus is smaller than expected. In some cases there is a rust-like color of the globus pallidus, red nucleus and pars reticularis of the substantia nigra. Transverse sections of the brainstem invariably show loss of neuromelanin pigment in the substantia nigra, usually atrophy of the midbrain tegmentum and dilation of the aqueduct. The neuromelanin pigment in the locus ceruleus may be preserved.The cerebral peduncles may show attenuation of the medial third. It is unusual to detect gross atrophy of the pons and medulla, and significant degeneration of the cerebellar dentate nucleus.

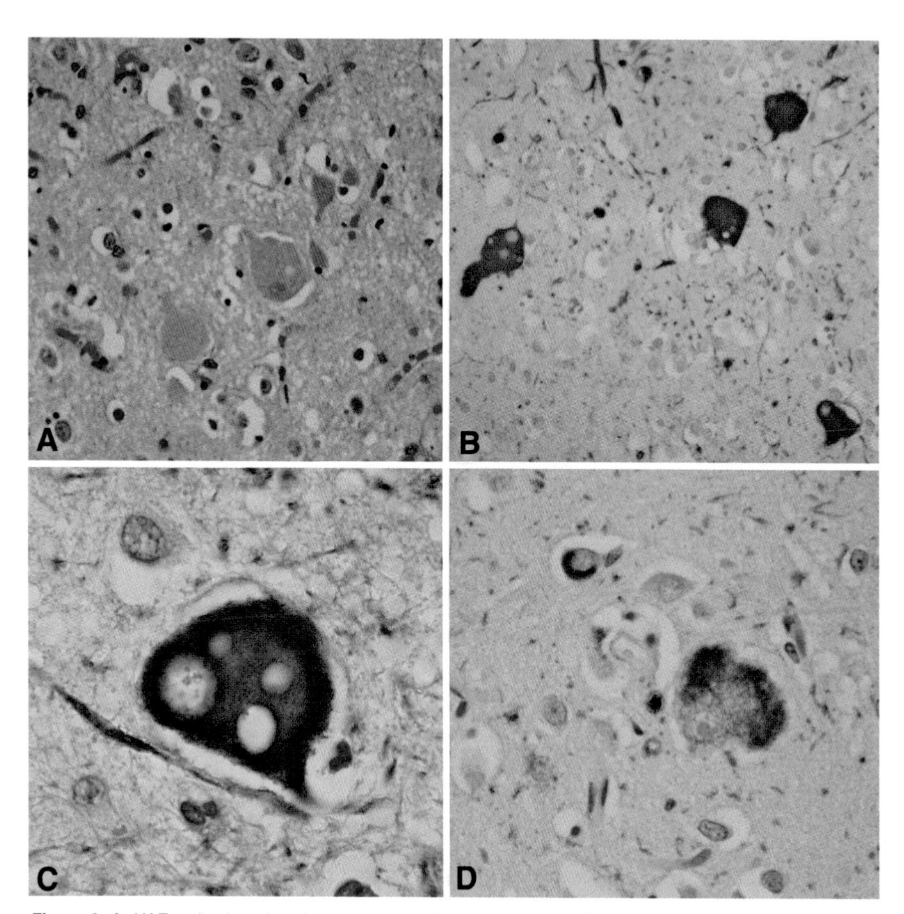

Figure 3. A. H&E stained section shows several ballooned neurons. **B.** Neurofilament immunostaining demonstrates ballooned neurons selectively and show enlargement of proximal processes of some ballooned neurons. **C.** Higher magnification of neurofilament stained ballooned neurons shows vacuolation of cytoplasm. **D.** Phospho-tau immunoreactivity of the ballooned neuron is limited to the periphery of the cytoplasm. Note the ring-shaped inclusion in an adjacent small neuron.

Histopathology

In affected cortical areas the cortical ribbon is usually thinner than expected and rarefied due to neuronal loss and gliosis. Superficial spongiosis is a common finding in atrophic cortical regions. There is also astrocytic gliosis that is prominent in the superficial cortical layers and at the grey-white junction. The cerebral white matter shows mild loss of myelin and gliosis that follows the topographic distribution of the cortical atrophy. Most cases do not have senile plaques or neurofibrillary tangles (NFT).

In affected areas swollen cortical neurones are scattered in third, fifth and sixth cortical layers. These swollen neurones are the histological hallmark of CBD (Figure 3) and have been likened to "chromatolysis" (15). Given that there is no direct evidence to support the hypothesis that axonal damage is the cause of swollen cortical neurones in CBD, many authors have preferred to use more descriptive terms such as "achromatic neurones" or "ballooned neurones" (BN) (20, 40, 46, 48, 49, 57). The latter term has gained wide acceptance and has largely replaced the term "achromasia" and "chromatolysis." In PiD swollen neurones analogous to BN are sometimes referred to as "Pick cells" (16, 19).

The most common locations for BN are anterior cingulate gyrus, amygdala, insular cortex and claustrum, but this limbic and paralimbic distribution should not be considered specific. It is not uncommon to find BN limited to the limbic and paralimbic gray matter in a host of other disorders, most notably Braak's argyrophilic grain disease (63), which can occur in conjunc-

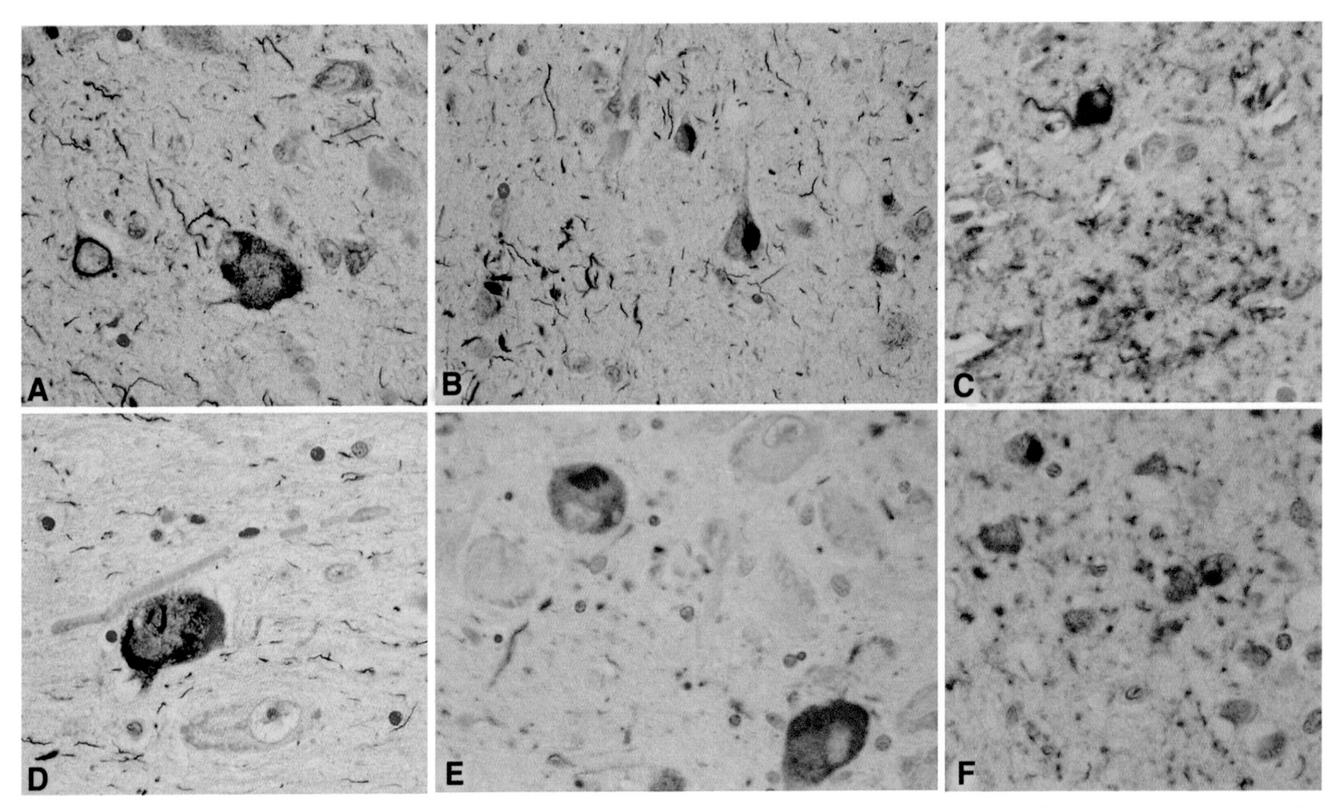

Figure 4. Heterogeneity of neuronal inclusions **A.** A perinuclear rim of tau immunoreactivity. Note also threads and a partially stained ballooned neuron. **B.** A small tangle-like inclusion and a round Pick body-like inclusion. Note threads and an astrocytic plaque (lower left). **C.** A small neuron with an inclusion that diffusely fills the cytoplasm. Note also threads and an astrocytic plaque (lower center). **D.** A large neuron with several discrete fibrils. **E.** Large neurons in the basal nucleus with irregular clumps of fibrils or diffuse granular cytoplasmic immunoreactivity. **F.** Several small Pick body-like inclusions in the dentate fascia.

tion with PSP (62). Of much more diagnostic significance is the presence of BN in convexity cortical areas, such as the superior frontal gyrus. On routine histological stains BN are eosinophilic to amphophilic, often vacuolated and have swelling of proximal dendrites. They may be weakly argyrophilic and negative with thioflavin S fluorescence microscopy. Some BN may have granulovacuolar bodies. They are strongly immunoreactive for phosphorylated neurofilaments (20, 57) (Figure 3) and for alpha B-crystallin (40, 49), but have inconsistent immunoreactivity for ubiquitin (23, 27). Focal tau immunoreactivity is also sometimes detected in BN, most often at the cell margins.

In addition to BN, scattered neurones in atrophic cortical areas have tau immunoreactivity. The tau-immunoreactive neuronal lesions are structurally pleomorphic. In some neurones the immunoreactivity is densely packed into a small inclusion body somewhat reminiscent of Pick bodies or small NFT (Figure 4). In other neurones the filamentous inclusions are more dispersed and disorderly or even granular, consistent with a so-called "pre-tangle" (10). Neurofibrillary lesions in brainstem monoaminergic nuclei, such as the locus ceruleus and substantia nigra, are common and resemble globose NFT, but have also been referred to as "corticobasal bodies" (26) (Figure 5).

The neuropil of both grey and white matter invariably contains many tau-immunoreactive cell processes (Figure 6). The predominance of tau-immunoreactivity in cell processes is an important attribute of CBD and a useful feature in differentiating it from other disorders. In other disorders with which CBD can be confused, tau-related pathology is more often located in cell bodies (eg, NFT and Pick bodies) and the proximal cell processes of neurones and glia. Accompanying white matter thread-like lesions are tau-positive argyrophilic inclusions in oligodendroglia, which are referred to as "oligodendroglia microtubular masses" (68) or "coiled bodies" (11).

In grey matter characteristic tau-immunoreactive astrocytic lesions are found in CBD (Figure 7). These lesions appear as annular clusters of grain-like processes, which may be suggestive of a neuritic plaque. In contrast to neuritic plaques, there is no amyloid, and the tau immunoreactivity is not within dystrophic neuronal processes, but rather processes of astrocytes. These lesions are called "astrocytic plaques" (23).

Neuroanatomical distribution of lesions. The brunt of the cortical pathology is in the superior frontal gyrus, superior parietal lobule and parasagittal pre- and post-central gyri. In most cases the hippocampus and parahippocampus show normal neuronal content and organisation without gliosis. Although a few pyramidal neurones may contain NFT and granulovacuolar degeneration, this is usually not greater than expected for the age of the individual. Tau-immunoreactive grains may be detected in some cases. The caudate nucleus and putamen invariably have tau-immunoreactive lesions, and these often have a predilection for the striatal fiber bundles. Scattered neurones may have NFT, but pretangles are more numerous, and there may be astrocytic plaques in the striatum. The globus pallidus and inner putamen show nerve cell depletion with gliosis and occasional NFT. There may be granular axonal spheroids and hemosiderin-like pigmentary degeneration in the globus pallidus and pars reticularis of the substantia nigra. The basal nucleus of Meynert is usually well populated, but may have NFT and more often pretangles.

The red nucleus and subthalamic nucleus may have mild neuronal loss, gliosis and tau-immunoreactive neurofibrillary lesions. Thalamic nuclei may also be affected, particularly the ventrolateral nucleus. The substantia nigra usually has moderate to marked neuronal loss with extraneuronal neuromelanin in phagocytes. Residual neurones often contain NFT. Pretangles and threads are also numerous in the substantia nigra and may help differentiate CBD from PSP (51). The locus ceruleus, raphe nuclei and tegmental grey have similar neurofibrillary lesions. There is mild or no neuronal depletion and gliosis of the cerebellar dentate nucleus. The cerebellar cortex is relatively unaffected, but scattered Purkinje cell axonal torpedoes and mild Bergmann gliosis are not uncommon.

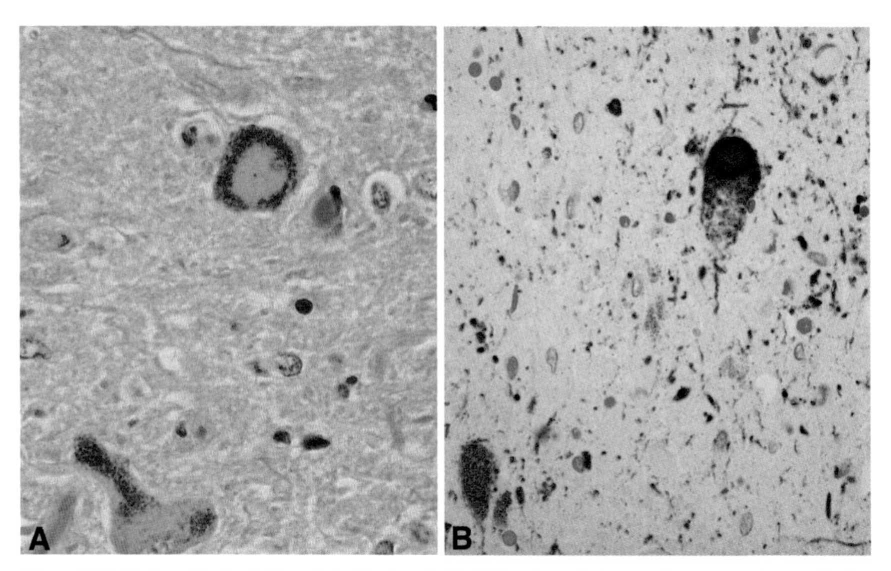

Figure 5. Corticobasal bodies in the substantia nigra. **A.** On H&E a pigmented neuron has an round area with pigment displacement. **B.** On tau immunostaining the round area is positive and similar to a globose NFT. Note also many grain-like and thread-like processes in the neuropil.

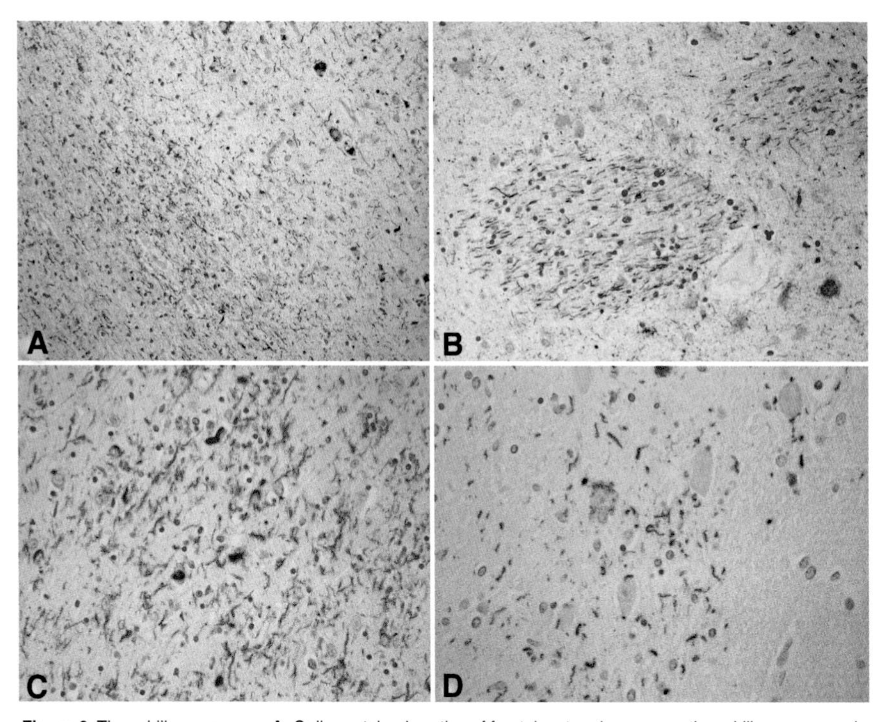

Figure 6. Thread-like processes. **A.** Gallyas stained section of frontal cortex shows many thread-like processes in gray and white matter, with densest accumulation at the gray-white junction. **B.** Threads in the basal ganglia are prominent in the pencil fibers, but also present in gray matter of the striatum (Gallyas stain). **C.** Tau immunostain shows many thread-like processes in the internal capsule, as well as some ring-like inclusions in small glial cells (so-called coiled bodies). **D.** In the pontine nuclei there are also sparse thread-like lesions as well as diffuse cytoplasmic immunoreactivity (pre-tangles).

Immunohistochemistry and Ultrastructural Findings

There are only a limited number of published reports on the fine structural alterations in CBD (47, 61, 65), with much of the research focussed on morphology of isolated filaments (34, 35), where the cell of origin is not known. Given that abnormal cytoskeletal lesions are found in neurones and glia in CBD, additional descriptive studies are warranted.

Ultrastructurally, the cytoplasm of cortical neurones with ballooning degeneration usually contains a disorderly array of filaments about 10 nm in diameter, interspersed with other cytoplasmic elements (15). In contrast, the filaments in tau-positive lesions tend to have a wider diameter (20-24 nm) and paired helical filament-like structure. These wider filaments are also the predominant and most characteristic finding in isolated filament preparations. They have been referred to as "twisted tubules" or "twisted ribbons." While they appear somewhat similar to paired helical filaments of AD, they

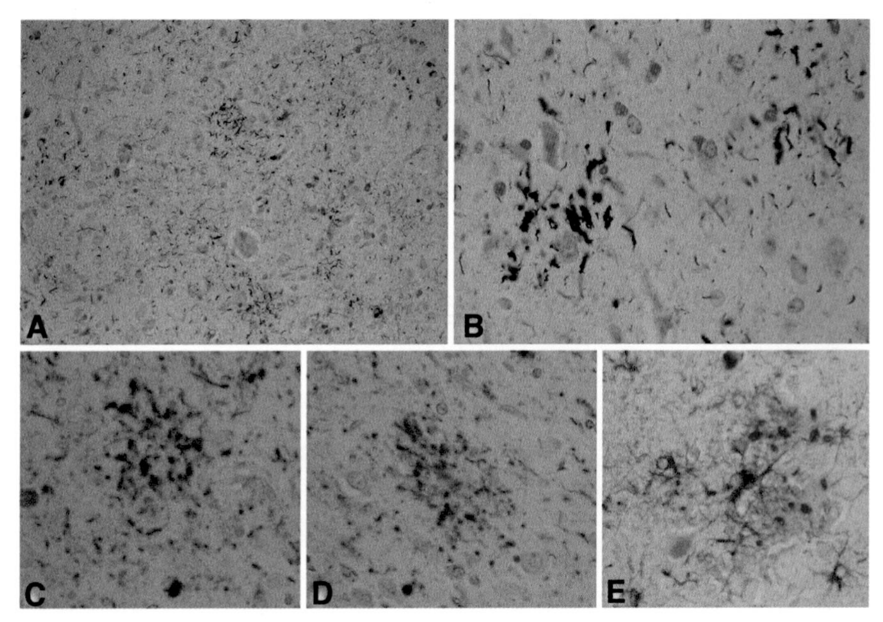

Figure 7. A. Several astrocytic plaques are apparent in frontal cortex with Gallyas stain. Note also the numerous thread-like lesions. **B.** At higher magnification the astrocytic plaque is composed of an annular array of short stubby processes with irregular thickness and fuzzy outlines. **C.** and **D.** Tau immunostaining shows astrocytic plaques that sometimes have no obvious central cell (**C**) or have a central cell consistent with an astrocyte (**D**). Double immunostaining for tau (blue) and GFAP (brown) (**E**) shows an astrocyte in the center of an astrocytic plaque.

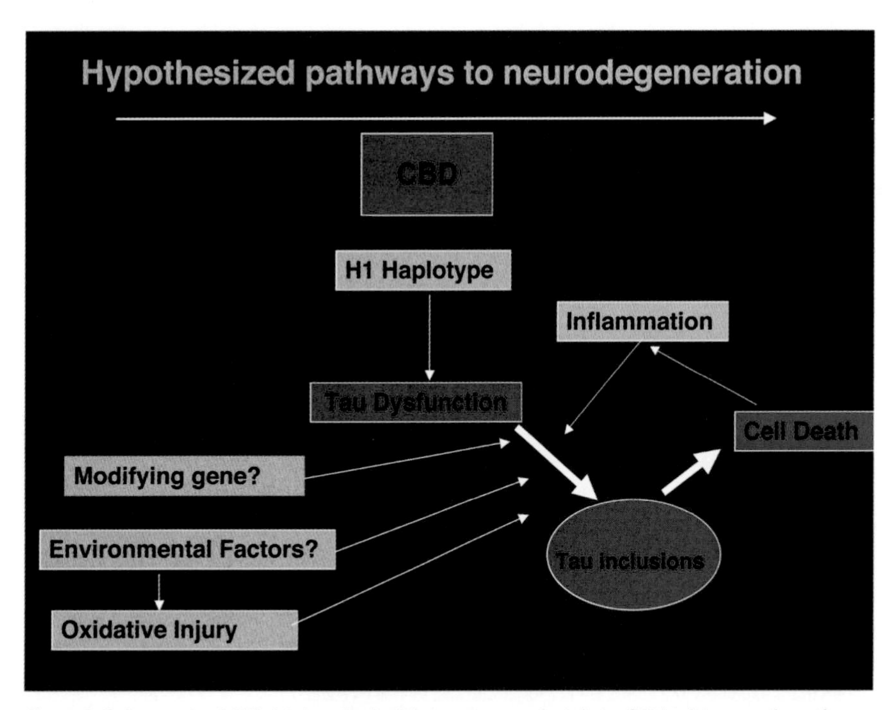

Figure 8. Pathogenesis of CBD. It is hypothesized that sequence variants in tau [H1 haplotype or other polymorphism(s)] predispose to the selective deposition of insoluble 4-R tau. Certain unknown environmental risk factors (eg, pesticides) may trigger the development of the disease in susceptible individuals. The environmental trigger may be mediated through an increase in free radicals and lipoperoxidation, which initiate and maintain a cascade of events that eventually leads to neurodegeneration of certain population of cells in mid to late in life. Finally, it is proposed that neurodegeneration triggers an inflammatory response, which in turn promotes further neurodegeneration through the release of cytokines or other toxic factors. The eventual development of the different CBD phenotypes may be the consequence of exposure to certain environmental upon a specific background.

have several differences. The twisted ribbons of CBD are wider, have a longer periodicity of the twists, less mass per unit length and greater instability as assessed by increased tendency to dissociate into protofilaments (35). They are also less phosphorylated and less ubiquitinated than filaments in AD (70). Fine structural analysis of grain-like lesions has not been reported in CBD, but these lesions have been described in other disorders, where they appear to be composed of 15 to 18 nm diameter straight filaments and granular material (31). Ultrastructural analysis of neuropil threads and thread-like structures in CBD is complicated by the fact that they undoubtedly have multiple cellular origins, including neurones, astrocytes and oligodendroglia. Threads in CBD contain 15 to 18 nm diameter straight filaments or 20 to 24 nm diameter twisted filaments (50). Ultrastructural studies of astrocytic plaques have yet to be reported. The proximal cell bodies of astrocytes in CBD cortex contain accumulations of intermediate-sized (18-20 nm diameter) straight filaments (23).

Biochemistry

There are very few studies of postmortem neurochemical changes in CBD. In one of the first studies, Clark and coworkers showed that cortical choline acetyl transferase, a marker for cholinergic neurones, was not decreased (15), which demonstrated a significant difference between CBD and AD. Given the marked loss of pigmented neurones in the pars compacta of the substantia nigra, a population of neurones known to be the major dopaminergic innervation of the basal ganglia, it is not surprising that decreases in dopamine in the basal ganglia have been found in postmortem studies of CBD (43). Other neurotransmitter abnormalities have not been documented in CBD. It is unknown, for example, if the involvement of cortical neurons has any selectivity with respect to neurotransmitter.

By far most of the biochemical studies that have been conducted on CBD have focussed on cytoskeletal proteins, especially tau protein (3, 13, 41). Tau protein is a microtubule-associated protein that promotes tubulin polymerization and stabilization of microtubules. It undergoes extensive post-translational modification, in-

	CBD	PSP	Pick's disease
		GROSS FINDINGS	
Cortical atrophy	Mild to moderate, focal (often asymmetric, superior frontoparietal or parasagittal)	Mild (usually symmetric, frontal, parasagittal or paracentral)	Marked, lobar (often asymmetric, frontotemporal & limbic lobe; paracentral spared)
White matter pathology	Frontal (corticostriate fibers in anterior internal capsule & corticobulbar fibers in cerebral peduncle)	Central & cerebellar outflow (corticospinal in posterior internal capsule & cerebral peduncle; superior cerebellar peduncle)	Frontotemporal (Papez circuit; anterior commissure; corticostriatal fibers in anterior internal capsule)
Basal ganglia	Caudate atrophy Pallidonigral pigment-spheroid degeneration	Pallidonigral pigment-spheroid degeneration; subthalamic nucleus atrophy	Caudate atrophy
		MICROSCOPIC FINDINGS	
Cortical changes	Superficial laminar spongiosis	Minimal cortical changes	Severe status spongiosis
Ballooned neurons	Present in affected cortical areas	Rare (or none)	Present in affected cortical areas, especially limbic lobe
Neuronal tau-pathology	Corticobasal bodies (ie, globose NFT) and other neurofibrillary lesions Cortex Basal ganglia Thalamus Substantia nigra Locus ceruleus	NFT and pre-tangles Basal ganglia Subthalamic nucleus Substantia nigra Oculomotor nuclei Raphe nuclei Locus ceruleus Pontine nuclei Tegmental gray Inferior olive Cerebellar dentate	Pick bodies Cortex Dentate fascia Amygdala External pallidum Substantia nigra Locus ceruleus Pontine nuclei
Neuropil threads	Usually numerous Cerebral cortex Cerebral white matter Internal capsule Pencil fibers in striatum Thalamic fasciculus Cerebral peduncle (corticobulbar) Tegmental fibers Pontine base Inferior olive Cerebellar dentate nucleus	Usually sparse in telencephalon, but may be dense in diencephalon Basal ganglia Internal capsule Thalamic fasciculus (often numerous) Cerebral peduncle (corticospinal)	Variable amount Cortex Limbic lobe
Astrocytic tau pathology	Many astrocytic plaques Cortex	Many tufted astrocytes Motor cortex Corpus striatum	Variable number of thorn-shaped Astrocytes Cortex
Oligodendroglial tau pathology (coiled bodies)	Numerous Cerebral white matter Basal ganglia fibers Internal capsule Thalamic fasciculus	Many Central white matter Basal ganglia fibers Thalamic fasciculus	Variable Cerebral white matter

Table 1. Neuropathologic differential diagnosis of corticobasal degeneration (CBD), progressive supranuclear palsy (PSP) and Pick's disease (PD).

cluding phosphorylation, which controls its functional state (42). Phosphorylated tau is less efficient in promoting tubulin polymerization. The tau gene, located on chromosome 17, has 15 exons, 3 of which are alternatively spliced (1). In the carboxyl-terminal half of the molecule are 4 conserved 30-amino acid tandem repeats that are essential for interaction of tau with microtubules. One of the repeat domains is the product of exon 10 and is alternatively spliced, generating 2 families of tau splice forms—4 repeat tau (4R tau) and 3 repeat tau (3R tau). Western blots of normal brain tissue homogenates show 6 bands in a range of 50 to 62 kDa composed of 3R and 4R tau. Homogenates of detergent soluble tau protein from CBD migrates at a higher molecular weight due to increased phosphorylation. In addition the immunoblotting pattern is reduced to 2 major bands at about 64 and 68 kDa (44, 65) due to preferential accumulation of 4R tau.

Differential Diagnosis

The major neuropathological differential diagnosis of CBD is limited to those disorders associated with cortical and deep gray matter pathology associated with tau-immunoreactive inclusions in neurons and glia (24, 25). The major disorders in this category are PSP, Pick's disease and FTDP-17.

Table 1 summarizes neuropathologic and molecular features that are useful to consider in differential diagnosis. FTDP-17 can be differentiated from CBD by clinical history since it is an autosomal dominant disorder and CBD is sporadic.

Experimental Models

There are no animal models for CBD, but transgenic mice with tau mutations (37) have some features in common with CBD (chapter 3.9). None of the transgenic models have shown any evidence for focal cortical pathology, however, which remains a unique feature of the human disease.

Pathogenesis

Little is known about the pathogenesis of CBD. The interaction of environmental factors and a genetic predisposition conferred by specific polymorphic variants in the tau gene are likely to be involved. Neuroinflammation is involved in the pathology of CBD, at least as reflected by class II major histocompatibility antigen immunoreactivity in reactive microglia (32) but there is little to suggest that neuroinflammatory processes are anything but secondary to the neurodegeneration (Figure 8).

Future Directions and Therapy

Given the prominent tau pathology in CBD, efforts to interrupt tau fibrillogenesis would seem to offer hope for possible future therapies. Additional clinical pathological studies are warranted to improve antemortem clinical recognition of CBD. Development of viable biomarkers for the disease, such as neuroimaging methods or CSF tau assays, would seem to be a critical clinical need.

References

1. Andreadis A, Brown WM, Kosik KS (1992) Structure and novel exons of the human tau gene. *Biochemistry* 31: 10626-10633.

2. Arai H, Morikawa Y, Higuchi M, Matsui T, Clark CM, Miura M, Machida N, Lee VM, Trojanowski JQ, Sasaki H (1997) Cerebrospinal fluid tau levels in neurodegenerative diseases with distinct tau-related pathology. *Biochem Biophys Res Commun* 236: 262-264.

3. Arai T, Ikeda K, Akiyama H, Shikamoto Y, Tsuchiya K, Yagishita S, Beach T, Rogers J, Schwab C, McGeer PL (2001) Distinct isoforms of tau aggregated in neurons and glial cells in brains of patients with Pick's disease, corticobasal degeneration and progressive supranuclear palsy. *Acta Neuropathol (Berl)* 101: 167-173.

4. Arima K, Uesugi H, Fujita I, Sakurai Y, Oyanagi S, Andoh S, Izumiyama Y, Inose T (1994) Corticonigral degeneration with neuronal achromasia presenting with primary progressive aphasia: ultrastructural and immunocytochemical studies. *J Neurol Sci* 127: 186-197.

5. Bergeron C, Davis A, Lang AE (1998) Corticobasal ganglionic degeneration and progressive supranuclear palsy presenting with cognitive decline. *Brain Pathol* 8: 355-365.

6. Bergeron C, Pollanen MS, Weyer L, Black SE, Lang AE (1996) Unusual clinical presentations of cortical-basal ganglionic degeneration. *Ann Neurol* 40: 893-900.

7. Bergeron C, Pollanen MS, Weyer L, Lang AE (1997) Cortical degeneration in progressive supranuclear palsy. A comparison with cortical-basal ganglionic degeneration. *J Neuropathol Exp Neurol* 56: 726-734.

8. Blin J, Vidailhet MJ, Pillon B, Dubois B, Feve JR, Agid Y (1992) Corticobasal degeneration: decreased and asymmetrical glucose consumption as studied with PET. *Mov Disord* 7: 348-354.

9. Boeve BF, Maraganore DM, Parisi JE, Ahlskog JE, Graff-Radford N, Caselli RJ, Dickson DW, Kokmen E, Petersen RC (1999) Pathologic heterogeneity in clinically diagnosed corticobasal degeneration. *Neurology* 53: 795-800.

10. Braak E, Braak H, Mandelkow EM (1994) A sequence of cytoskeleton changes related to the formation of neurofibrillary tangles and neuropil threads. *Acta Neuropathol* 87: 554-567

11. Braak H, Braak E (1989) Cortical and subcortical argyrophilic grains characterize a disease associated with adult onset dementia. *Neuropathol Appl Neurobiol* 15: 13-26.

12. Brown J, Lantos PL, Roques P, Fidani L, Rossor MN (1996) Familial dementia with swollen achromatic neurons and corticobasal inclusion bodies: a clinical and pathological study. *J Neurol Sci* 135: 21-30.

13. Buee Scherrer V, Hof PR, Buee L, Leveugle B, Vermersch P, Perl DP, Olanow CW, Delacourte A (1996) Hyperphosphorylated tau proteins differentiate corticobasal degeneration and Pick's disease. *Acta Neuropathol* 91: 351-359

14. Bugiani O, Murrell JR, Giaccone G, Hasegawa M, Ghigo G, Tabaton M, Morbin M, Primavera A, Carella F, Solaro C, Grisoli M, Savoiardo M, Spillantini MG, Tagliavini F, Goedert M, Ghetti B (1999) Frontotemporal dementia and corticobasal degeneration in a family with a P301S mutation in tau. *J Neuropathol Exp Neurol* 58: 667-677.

15. Clark AW, Manz HJ, White CL, 3rd, Lehmann J, Miller D, Coyle JT (1986) Cortical degeneration with swollen chromatolytic neurons: its relationship to Pick's disease. *J Neuropathol Exp Neurol* 45: 268-284.

16. Constantinidis J, Richard J, Tissot R (1974) Pick's disease. Histological and clinical correlations. *Eur Neurol* 11: 208-217

17. Cordato NJ, Halliday GM, McCann H, Davies L, Williamson P, Fulham M, Morris JG (2001) Corticobasal syndrome with tau pathology. *Mov Disord* 16: 656-667.

18. Di Maria E, Tabaton M, Vigo T, Abbruzzese G, Bellone E, Donati C, Frasson E, Marchese R, Montagna P, Munoz DG, Pramstaller PP, Zanusso G, Ajmar F, Mandich P (2000) Corticobasal degeneration shares a common genetic background with progressive supranuclear palsy. *Ann Neurol* 47: 374-377.

19. Dickson DW (1998) Pick's disease: a modern approach. *Brain Pathol* 8: 339-354.

20. Dickson DW, Yen SH, Suzuki KI, Davies P, Garcia JH, Hirano A (1986) Ballooned neurons in select neurodegenerative diseases contain phosphorylated neurofilament epitopes. *Acta Neuropathol* 71: 216-223

21. Doi T, Iwasa K, Makifuchi T, Takamori M (1999) White matter hyperintensities on MRI in a patient with corticobasal degeneration. *Acta Neurol Scand* 99: 199-201.

22. Doody RS, Jankovic J (1992) The alien hand and related signs. *J Neurol Neurosurg Psychiatry* 55: 806-810.

23. Feany MB, Dickson DW (1995) Widespread cytoskeletal pathology characterizes corticobasal degeneration. *Am J Pathol* 146: 1388-1396.

24. Feany MB, Dickson DW (1996) Neurodegenerative disorders with extensive tau pathology: a comparative study and review. *Ann Neurol* 40: 139-148.

25. Feany MB, Mattiace LA, Dickson DW (1996) Neuropathologic overlap of progressive supranuclear palsy, Pick's disease and corticobasal degeneration. *J Neuropathol Exp Neurol* 55: 53-67.

26. Gibb WR, Luthert PJ, Marsden CD (1989) Corticobasal degeneration. *Brain* 112: 1171-1192.

27. Halliday GM, Davies L, McRitchie DA, Cartwright H, Pamphlett R, Morris JG (1995) Ubiquitin-positive achromatic neurons in corticobasal degeneration. *Acta Neuropathol* 90: 68-75

28. Horoupian DS, Wasserstein PH (1999) Alzheimer's disease pathology in motor cortex in dementia with Lewy bodies clinically mimicking corticobasal degeneration. *Acta Neuropathol (Berl)* 98: 317-322.

29. Houlden H, Baker M, Morris HR, MacDonald N, Pickering-Brown S, Adamson J, Lees AJ, Rossor MN, Quinn NP, Kertesz A et al (2001) Corticobasal degeneration and progressive supranuclear palsy share a common tau haplotype. *Neurology* 56: 1702-1706.

30. Ikeda K, Akiyama H, Iritani S, Kase K, Arai T, Niizato K, Kuroki N, Kosaka K (1996) Corticobasal degeneration with primary progressive aphasia and accentuated cortical lesion in superior temporal gyrus: case report and review. *Acta Neuropathol (Berl)* 92: 534-539.

31. Ikeda K, Akiyama H, Kondo H, Haga C (1995) A study of dementia with argyrophilic grains. Possible cytoskeletal abnormality in dendrospinal portion of

neurons and oligodendroglia. *Acta Neuropathol* 89: 409-414

32. Ishizawa K, Dickson DW (2001) Microglial activation parallels system degeneration in progressive supranuclear palsy and corticobasal degeneration. *J Neuropathol Exp Neurol* 60: 647-657.

33. Komori T, Arai N, Oda M, Nakayama H, Mori H, Yagishita S, Takahashi T, Amano N, Murayama S et al (1998) Astrocytic plaques and tufts of abnormal fibers do not coexist in corticobasal degeneration and progressive supranuclear palsy. *Acta Neuropathol (Berl)* 96: 401-408.

34. Ksiezak-Reding H, Morgan K, Mattiace LA, Davies P, Liu WK, Yen SH, Weidenheim K, Dickson DW (1994) Ultrastructure and biochemical composition of paired helical filaments in corticobasal degeneration. *Am J Pathol* 145: 1496-1508.

35. Ksiezak-Reding H, Tracz E, Yang LS, Dickson DW, Simon M, Wall JS (1996) Ultrastructural instability of paired helical filaments from corticobasal degeneration as examined by scanning transmission electron microscopy. *Am J Pathol* 149: 639-651.

36. Lang AE, Bergeron C, Pollanen MS, Ashby P (1994) Parietal Pick's disease mimicking cortical-basal ganglionic degeneration. *Neurology* 44: 1436-1440.

37. Lewis J, McGowan E, Rockwood J, Melrose H, Nacharaju P, Van Slegtenhorst M, Gwinn-Hardy K, Paul Murphy M et al (2000) Neurofibrillary tangles, amyotrophy and progressive motor disturbance in mice expressing mutant (P301L) tau protein. Nat Genet 25: 402-405.

38. Lippa CF, Smith TW, Fontneau N (1990) Corticonigral degeneration with neuronal achromasia. A clinicopathologic study of two cases. *J Neurol Sci* 98: 301-310.

39. Litvan I, Grimes DA, Lang AE (2000) Phenotypes and prognosis: clinicopathologic studies of corticobasal degeneration. *Adv Neurol* 82: 183-196

40. Lowe J, Errington DR, Lennox G, Pike I, Spendlove I, Landon M, Mayer RJ (1992) Ballooned neurons in several neurodegenerative diseases and stroke contain alpha B crystallin. *Neuropathol Appl Neurobiol* 18: 341-350.

41. Mailliot C, Sergeant N, Bussiére T, Caillet-Boudin ML, Delacourte A, Buée L (1998) Phosphorylation of specific sets of tau isoforms reflects different neurofibrillary degeneration processes. *FEBS Lett* 433: 201-204.

42. Mandelkow EM, Biernat J, Drewes G, Steiner B, Lichtenberg-Kraag B, Wille H, Gustke N, Mandelkow E (1993) Microtubule-associated protein tau, paired helical filaments, and phosphorylation. *Ann N Y Acad Sci* 695: 209-216.

43. Marshall EF, Perry RH, Perry EK, Piggott MA, Thompson P, Jaros E, Burn DJ (1997) Striatal dopaminergic loss without parkinsonism in a case of corticobasal degeneration. *Acta Neurol Scand* 95: 287-292.

44. Mimura M, Oda T, Tsuchiya K, Kato M, Ikeda K, Hori K, Kashima H (2001) Corticobasal degeneration presenting with nonfluent primary progressive aphasia: a clinicopathological study. *J Neurol Sci* 183: 19-26.

45. Mitani K, Furiya Y, Uchihara T, Ishii K, Yamanouchi H, Mizusawa H, Mori H (1998) Increased CSF tau protein in corticobasal degeneration. *J Neurol* 245: 44-46.

46. Mizutani T, Inose T, Nakajima S, Kakimi S, Uchigata M, Ikeda K, Gambetti P, Takasu T (1998) Familial parkinsonism and dementia with ballooned neurons, argyrophilic neuronal inclusions, atypical neurofibrillary tangles, tau-negative astrocytic fibrillary tangles, and Lewy bodies. *Acta Neuropathol (Berl)* 95: 15-27.

47. Mori H, Nishimura M, Namba Y, Oda M (1994) Corticobasal degeneration: a disease with widespread appearance of abnormal tau and neurofibrillary tangles, and its relation to progressive supranuclear palsy. *Acta Neuropathol* 88: 113-121

48. Mori H, Oda M (1997) Ballooned neurons in corticobasal degeneration and progressive supranuclear palsy. *Neuropathology* 17: 248-252

49. Mori H, Oda M, Mizuno Y (1996) Cortical ballooned neurons in progressive supranuclear palsy. *Neurosci Lett* 209: 109-112.

50. Nishimura T, Ikeda K, Akiyama H, Kondo H, Kato M, Li F, Iseki E, Kosaka K (1995) Immunohistochemical investigation of tau-positive structures in the cerebral cortex of patients with progressive supranuclear palsy. *Neurosci Lett* 201: 123-126.

51. Oyanagi K, Tsuchiya K, Yamazaki M, Ikeda K (2001) Substantia nigra in progressive supranuclear palsy, corticobasal degeneration, and parkinsonism-dementia complex of Guam: specific pathological features. *J Neuropathol Exp Neurol* 60: 393-402.

52. Paulus W, Selim M (1990) Corticonigral degeneration with neuronal achromasia and basal neurofibrillary tangles. *Acta Neuropathol* 81: 89-94

53. Rebeiz JJ, Kolodny EH, Richardson EP, Jr. (1967) Corticodentatonigral degeneration with neuronal achromasia: a progressive disorder of late adult life. *Trans Am Neurol Assoc* 92: 23-26

54. Reed LA, Schmidt ML, Wszolek ZK, Balin BJ, Soontornniyomkij V, Lee VM, Trojanowski JQ, Schelper RL (1998) The neuropathology of a chromosome 17-linked autosomal dominant parkinsonism and dementia ("pallido-ponto-nigral degeneration"). *J Neuropathol Exp Neurol* 57: 588-601.

55. Riley DE, Lang AE, Lewis A, Resch L, Ashby P, Hornykiewicz O, Black S (1990) Cortical-basal ganglionic degeneration. *Neurology* 40: 1203-1212.

56. Sawle GV, Brooks DJ, Marsden CD, Frackowiak RS (1991) Corticobasal degeneration. A unique pattern of regional cortical oxygen hypometabolism and striatal fluorodopa uptake demonstrated by positron emission tomography. *Brain* 114: 541-556.

57. Smith TW, Lippa CF, de Girolami U (1992) Immunocytochemical study of ballooned neurons in cortical degeneration with neuronal achromasia. *Clin Neuropathol* 11: 28-35.

58. Soliveri P, Monza D, Paridi D, Radice D, Grisoli M, Testa D, Savoiardo M, Girotti F (1999) Cognitive and magnetic resonance imaging aspects of corticobasal degeneration and progressive supranuclear palsy. *Neurology* 53: 502-507.

59. Spillantini MG, Goedert M (1998) Tau protein pathology in neurodegenerative diseases. *Trends Neurosci* 21: 428-433.

60. Spillantini MG, Murrell JR, Goedert M, Farlow MR, Klug A, Ghetti B (1998) Mutation in the tau gene in familial multiple system tauopathy with presenile dementia. *Proc Natl Acad Sci U S A* 95: 7737-7741.

61. Takahashi T, Amano N, Hanihara T, Nagatomo H, Yagishita S, Itoh Y, Yamaoka K, Toda H, Tanabe T (1996) Corticobasal degeneration: widespread argentophilic threads and glia in addition to neurofibrillary tangles. Similarities of cytoskeletal abnormalities in corticobasal degeneration and progressive supranuclear palsy. *J Neurol Sci* 138: 66-77.

62. Togo T, Dickson DW (2002) Ballooned neurons in progressive supranuclear palsy are usually due to concurrent argyrophilic grain disease. *Acta Neuropathol* 104: 53-56.

63. Tolnay M, Probst A (1998) Ballooned neurons expressing alphaB-crystallin as a constant feature of the amygdala in argyrophilic grain disease. *Neurosci Lett* 246: 165-168.

64. Urakami K, Wada K, Arai H, Sasaki H, Kanai M, Shoji M, Ishizu H, Kashihara K, Yamamoto M, Tsuchiya-Ikemoto K et al (2001) Diagnostic significance of tau protein in cerebrospinal fluid from patients with corticobasal degeneration or progressive supranuclear palsy. *J Neurol Sci* 183: 95-98.

65. Wakabayashi K, Oyanagi K, Makifuchi T, Ikuta F, Homma A, Homma Y, Horikawa Y, Tokiguchi S (1994) Corticobasal degeneration: etiopathological significance of the cytoskeletal alterations. *Acta Neuropathol* 87: 545-553

66. Wang LN, Kowall NW, Richardson EP, Jr. (1991) Phosphorylated neurofilament epitopes in the achromasic neurons of corticonigral degeneration. *Chin Med J (Engl)* 104: 1011-1017.

67. Wenning GK, Litvan I, Jankovic J, Granata R, Mangone CA, McKee A, Poewe W, Jellinger K, Ray Chaudhuri K, D'Olhaberriague L, Pearce RK (1998) Natural history and survival of 14 patients with corticobasal degeneration confirmed at postmortem examination. *J Neurol Neurosurg Psychiatry* 64: 184-189.

68. Yamada T, McGeer PL (1995) Oligodendroglial microtubular masses: an abnormality observed in some human neurodegenerative diseases. *Neurosci Lett* 120: 163-166

69. Yamauchi H, Fukuyama H, Nagahama Y, Katsumi Y, Dong Y, Hayashi T, Konishi J, Kimura J (1998) Atrophy of the corpus callosum, cortical hypometabolism, and cognitive impairment in corticobasal degeneration. *Arch Neurol* 55: 609-614.

70. Yang L, Ksiezak-Reding H (1998) Ubiquitin immunoreactivity of paired helical filaments differs in Alzheimer's disease and corticobasal degeneration. *Acta Neuropathol (Berl)* 96: 520-526.

Pick's Disease

Catherine Bergeron
Huw R. Morris
Martin Rossor

CBD	corticobasal degeneration
FTDP	frontotemporal dementia and Parkinsonism
PSP	progressive supranuclear palsy

Definition

Pick's disease is a neurodegenerative disorder characterised by severe circumscribed lobar atrophy, marked neuronal loss and gliosis, swollen neurons, and Pick bodies (16, 34, 40, 43, 55).

Synonyms and Historical Annotations

Pick's disease is named after the neuropsychiatrist Arnold Pick (1851-1924). His original publication (63) was confined to macroscopic findings. The histological observations, including the description of swollen neurons and the discovery of Pick bodies, were contributed by Alois Alzheimer nearly 20 years later (1). A few years later, the terms Pick's atrophy and Pick's disease were used to refer to cases of circumscribed lobar atrophy with no neurofibrillary tangles or neuritic plaques, independent of the presence of Pick bodies (23, 61). About 50 years later, Tissot et al revisited the issue and subdivided Pick's disease into 3 subgroups (13, 78): Pick's disease type A (neuronal loss and gliosis, Pick bodies and swollen neurons), type B (neuronal loss and gliosis with swollen neurons), or type C (neuronal loss and gliosis). The term Pick's disease was subsequently commonly used for all disorders characterised by neuronal loss and gliosis, independent of the presence or absence of swollen neurons and Pick bodies. The recent widespread use of immunohistochemistry for the study of neurodegenerative diseases has resulted in a new classification in which Pick's disease is a distinctive and specific pathological entity as defined above.

Epidemiology

Incidence and prevalence. There are no reliable data on the epidemiology of Pick's Disease. The clinical features are those of frontotemporal degeneration (59). Using clinical criteria, patients with frontotemporal degeneration form the second or third commonest cause of dementia. It appears to be commoner in the younger age group, although this may reflect difficulties of diagnosis in the older age group and the tendency to diagnose Alzheimer's disease. A community-based series of young onset dementia, that is, those below the age of 65 years, found that 10% of patients fulfilled the criteria for frontotemporal degeneration (32).

Sex and age distribution. Both sexes are affected. A retrospective analysis of 50 cases of neuropathologically diagnosed cases of Pick's disease based on the presence of Pick bodies revealed a male preponderance. The age range is wide although it appears uncommon above the age of 70 years; this may reflect lack of diagnosis in older patients (77). Young cases have been reported, for example, onset at the age of 27 years (41).

Risk factors. Unknown.

Genetics

Unlike progressive supranuclear palsy (PSP) and corticobasal degeneration (CBD), sporadic Pick's disease is not related to common tau gene haplotypes (72). The sporadic 4-repeat tau deposition disorders, PSP and CBD, are associated with the tau H1 haplotype whereas Pick's disease, a 3-repeat tau disorder, is not related to either tau H1 or H2 haplotypes. Familial Pick's disease is a controversial entity. Initially it was thought that familial Pick's disease was common; however, it appears that many of the kindreds described as having familial Pick's disease in fact have frontotemporal dementia linked to chromosome 17 (FTDP-17), with pathological features that are different to classical Pick's disease (22). The majority of FTDP-17 kindreds, in which neurodegeneration is due to mutations in tau, are different from Pick's disease. However, some kindreds have closer similarities to Pick's disease and may be regarded as familial forms of Pick's disease.

The exon 13 tau mutation G389R leads to frontotemporal dementia with the formation of Pick-like bodies (58). However, these tau inclusions are immunoreactive with tau antibody 12-E8 indicating that they have a different biochemical composition to most cases of sporadic Pick's disease (58). Tau in G389R FTDP-17 forms a doublet of bands similarly to Pick's disease, but this seems to be composed of both 3-repeat and 4-repeat tau. Clinically, G389R mutation individuals have a relatively young age at onset and may not have a definite family history (58, 64). The exon 9 tau mutation K257T also leads to dementia with the formation of Pick-like bodies which are not immunoreactive with 12E8, indicating that these are biochemically more similar to Pick's disease Pick bodies (70). The tau in K257T dementia is predominantly three repeat tau, like Pick's disease. In vitro analysis of the FTDP-17 mutation ΔK280 indicates that it leads to an overexpression of 3-repeat tau and thus would be predicted to lead to a Pick's disease like profile (71). This mutation has not been identified in pathologically confirmed individuals. Finally, an exon 12 K369I mutation has been identified in a single 52-year-old patient (60). The neuropathological features of this case are identical to those of classical Pick's disease including the lack of staining with

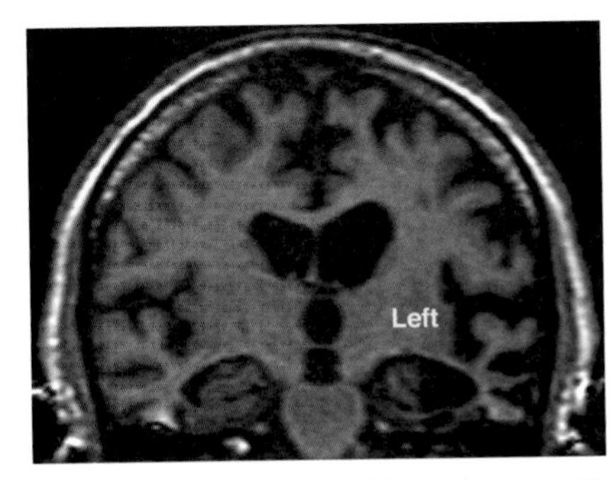

Figure 1. Coronal MRI of a 61-year-old male with Pick's disease showing severe focal atrophy of the left temporal lobe.

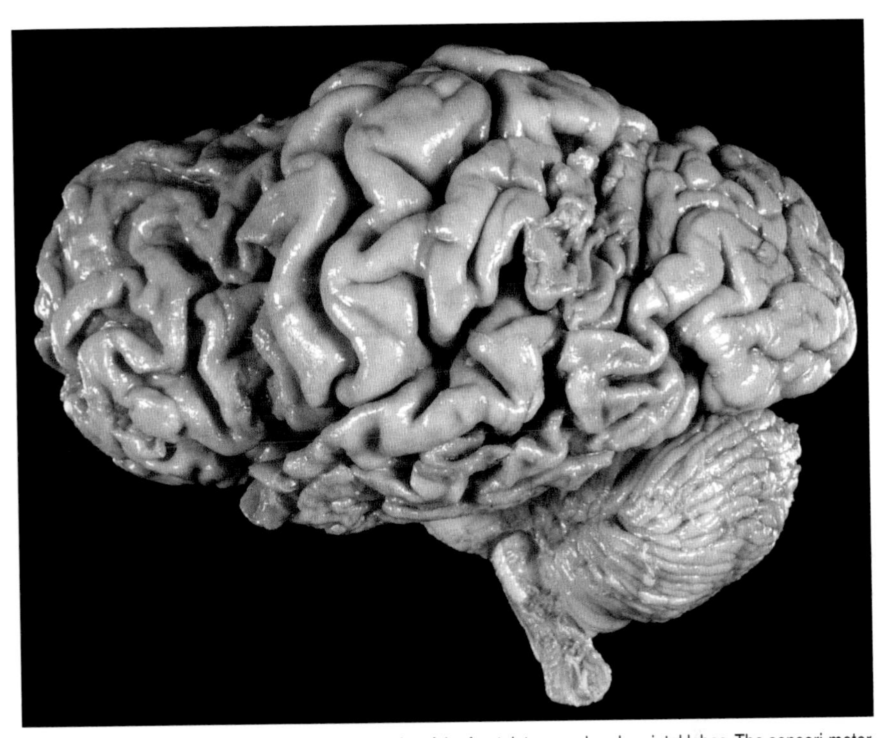
Figure 2. Severe circumscribed "knife-edge" atrophy of the frontal, temporal and parietal lobes. The sensori-motor cortex and the posterior two thirds of the superior temporal gyrus are preserved, as is the occipital lobe. The brain stem and cerebellum are unremarkable.

12E8. This mutation is associated with both 3-repeat and 4-repeat tau. Although some cases of FTDP-17 are undoubtedly very similar to Pick's disease the majority of cases of Pick's disease that have been studied are sporadic and not caused by tau mutations, and genetic risk factors predisposing to sporadic Pick's disease have not yet been identified.

Clinical Features

Signs and symptoms. The clinical features reflect the topographical distribution of the pathology and thus include impairments of behaviour, speech production and language. In general, the abnormalities are confined to higher cortical functions although extrapyramidal and pyramidal symptoms can sometimes be observed, presumably reflecting the involvement of the basal ganglia and pyramidal tracts. The majority of clinical descriptions of Pick's disease have either lacked neuropathology or have relied on the macroscopic features, that is, those of fronto-temporal lobar atrophy, rather than a specific histology. They often followed the earlier classification of Constantinidis et al (13) and as such subsumed a number of different nosological entities.

In general 3 prototypic clinical syndromes are associated with frontotemporal degeneration: a behavioural syndrome referred to as fronto-temporal dementia, progressive non-fluent aphasia and semantic dementia (59). The behavioural presentation reflects the predominant involvement of the frontal lobe and can range from a dysexecutive syndrome to prominent, and distressing, social disinhibition. A behavioural syndrome can also arise from temporal lobe involvement; for example, the striking atrophy of the amygdala which is sometimes observed is commonly associated with the inability to recognise and distinguish facial expressions. This will often result in patients appearing insensitive and lacking empathy. The non-fluent aphasia patients have a prominent speech production deficit which will often progress to mutism. The term semantic dementia draws upon the distinction between episodic memory and semantic memory. Episodic memory provides our recollection of day to day personal events and is dependent upon hippocampal function. Many patients with Pick's disease will have well preserved episodic memory. By contrast, semantic memory informs our meaning of stimuli and encompasses both verbal and visual domains. Patients with semantic verbal impairment lose their comprehension of language, but within the constraints of a limited vocabulary their speech is fluent, in striking contrast the non-fluent progressive aphasia. Verbal semantic memory impairment was originally referred to as transcortical sensory aphasia. Semantic memory impairment can involve the visual domain and indeed patients often progress to an associative visual agnosia. The clinical progression of Pick's disease is variable; some cases can extend over 15 to 20 years.

Imaging. Imaging reflects the fronto-temporal lobar atrophy. This can be seen on functional imaging with both PET and SPECT. The changes are less evident with CT but are often striking with MRI. In the early stages of the disease there can be a striking asymmetry more commonly on the left (Figure 1).

Laboratory findings. Neurological investigations are usually normal in Pick's disease. Examination of the cerebrospinal fluid is routinely normal although there is an excess of tau and S100β (28, 29). The EEG in Pick's disease tends to be normal particularly by comparison with Alzheimer's disease (44).

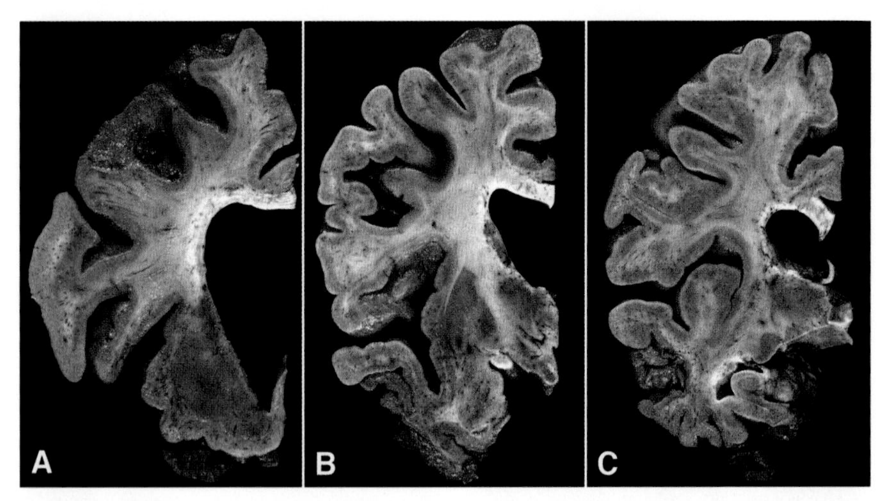

Figure 3. A. The head of the caudate nucleus is flattened and the anterior horn of the lateral ventricle is dilated. The bulk of the centrum semiovale is decreased. **B.** The amygdala and entorhinal cortex are severely atrophic. **C.** The hippocampus is occasionally spared.

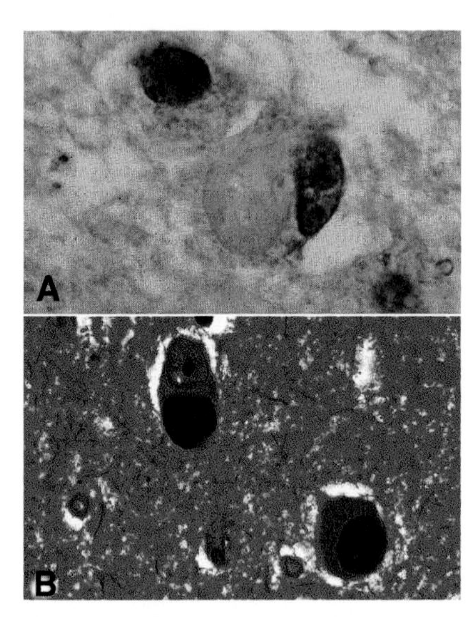

Figure 4. The Pick body is a basophilic, round, well demarcated, fibrillary inclusion. **A.** It is argentophilic on silver stains such as the Bielschowsky and Bodian preparations (**B**), but fails to stain with the Gallyas method. **A.** H&E ×1000. **B.** Bielschowsky stain, ×1000.

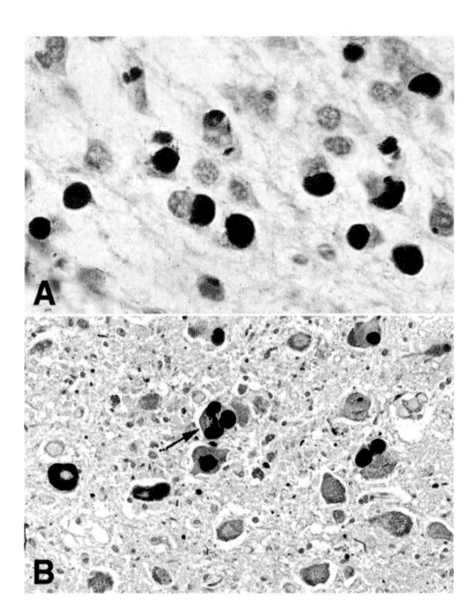

Figure 5. A. Pick bodies are consistently found in large numbers in the dentate fascia of the hippocampus. **B.** Although usually single, multiple Pick bodies can be seen within a neuron, particularly in the locus coeruleus . AT8 ×400.

Macroscopy

The gross appearance of the brain in Pick's disease is remarkably consistent from case to case and is well documented in Tissot's original monograph and in more recent publications (16, 78). Cortical atrophy is severe and exhibits a "knife-edge" or "dried walnut" appearance; it is sharply circumscribed and frequently asymmetrical. The atrophy involves the frontal and temporal lobes and may extend to the parietal lobe. The pre-central gyrus and the posterior two-thirds of the superior temporal gyrus are consistently relatively preserved (Figure 2). The head of the caudate nucleus is usually flattened and the anterior horn of the lateral ventricle is dilated; the white matter underlying the affected cortex is decreased in bulk, granular and rubbery. In cases with severe frontal involvement, the corpus callosum is thin. The atrophy also involves the limbic structures (amygdala, entorhinal cortex and cingulate gyrus); the hippocampus is often relatively preserved (Figure 3). Ventricular dilatation is always present and often severe (Figure 3). The substantia nigra is usually well pigmented or mildly depigmented. The cerebellum and brain stem are unremarkable.

Histopathology

The histopathological changes are illustrated in Figures 4 to 10. The affected cortex shows severe pancortical gliosis (Figure 6). In the less severely involved regions at the periphery of the gross circumscribed atrophy, there is milder loss, often with microvacuolation of the superficial cortical layers. Morphometric studies have shown that both large and small neurons are lost (31). The subcortical white matter shows severe atrophy and gliosis in keeping with the degree of cortical atrophy. Neuronal loss and gliosis is frequent in the caudate nucleus (60% of cases) and thalamus (60%) and consistently absent in the pallidum (78, 80). In the amygdala, the basolateral group is more severely involved than the corticomedial group (80). Neuronal loss has also been reported in the nucleus basalis (83). Uchihara et al (82) performed a morphometric study of the substantia nigra in 13 cases of Pick's disease and reported a loss of 38 to 50% of pigmented nigral neurons. On closer examination, however, 11 of their cases showed no Pick bodies or swollen neurons and most likely represent frontotemporal degeneration. Kosaka et al (49) studied striatopallidonigral degeneration in 41 cases of Pick's disease. As in Uchihara's study their series included a majority of cases without Pick bodies. However, they subdivided their cases in three groups according to the severity of the degeneration. Group I consisted of 5 cases with severe nigral degeneration, one with moderate loss and 2 with mild loss, none of which had Pick bodies. Group II included 8 cases in which the nigra was examined. Half these cases showed moderate nigral loss and the other half only mild loss. The incidence of Pick bodies in this group is 11.1% or one case. Group III included 6 cases with mild nigral loss and 5 with a normal substantia nigra. The incidence of Pick bodies in this group is higher at 33%. All 9 cases in Group IV where the incidence of Pick bodies is

55% showed no nigral changes. In conclusion, Kosaka's data indicates that Pick's disease usually shows no or only mild nigral loss (49), as reported by Tissot (78). Pale basophilic inclusions similar to those seen in CBD are often found in the substantia nigra (24) (Figure 7).

Pick bodies are spherical cytoplasmic inclusions (Figure 4), but oblong, falciform and irregular forms can also occur; they are well demarcated, amorphous and slightly basophilic on hematoxylin-eosin stain. They are argentophilic with Bielschowsky and Bodian silver stains (Figure 4) but fail to react with the Gallyas stain (67). The Pick bodies vary in size depending on the neuronal volume. They are usually single but multiple Pick bodies can be seen in a single cell, particularly in the locus ceruleus (21) (Figure 5). They are abundant in the dentate gyrus of the hippocampus (Figure 5), induseum griseum, amygdala and septal nuclei; they are also common in the cerebral cortex where they are found mostly in layers II and III and in some cases, in layer VI (5, 35, 78). Other sites include the caudate, putamen, hypothalamus, thalamus, pallidum, claustrum, anterior olfactory nucleus, tectum and central grey of the midbrain, red nucleus, substantia nigra, reticular formation, locus ceruleus, pontine nuclei, dorsal vagal nuclei and anterior horn of the uppermost cervical cord (3, 21, 88, 89). Their distribution in the hippocampus is stereotyped: they are frequent in CA1 and much less common in CA2-4 and presubiculum (7, 78). Pick bodies are not uniformly or randomly distributed in cortex and dentate gyrus but occur in large clusters (4, 6). Swollen neurons are consistently observed in affected areas and are seen in largest numbers in the regions at the periphery of the severe cortical atrophy (Figure 7). Small numbers of neurofibrillary tangles are also often found in limbic and neocortical areas; in contrast with Alzheimer's diseases where tangles predominate in cortical infragranular layers, in Pick's disease the tangles are preferentially located in layers II and III (4, 5, 35, 42).

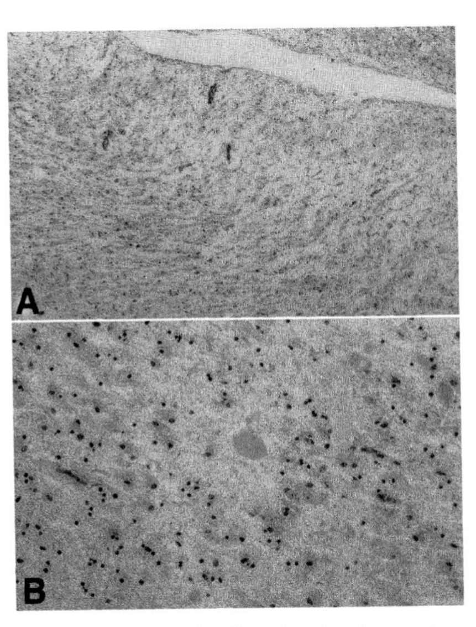

Figure 6. The severely affected cortex shows extensive neuronal loss with complete effacement of the cortical cytoarchitecture and status spongiosus. H&E ×25 (**A**) and ×100 (**B**).

Immunohistochemistry and Ultrastructural Findings

Pick bodies stain uniformly with antibodies to phosphorylated neurofilaments, tubulin, MAP-2, Alzheimer's paired helical filaments, tau and ubiquitin (21, 51, 57, 62, 66, 68, 84). Pick bodies stain with most tau antibodies with the exception of 12E8 which recognises a phosphorylated site at Ser 262 (67). At the ultrastructural level they appear as poorly demarcated accumulations of filamentous material with interspersed osmiophilic granular and vesicular structures (Figure 8). There is no limiting membrane at the periphery of the inclusion. The appearance of the filaments is heterogeneous: straight 12 to 18 nm filaments devoid of sidearms arranged randomly or occasionally forming small bundles, or thicker 25 nm filaments with 12 nm constrictions at long-period intervals (46, 69, 73, 79, 85). A recent ultrastructural study of purified Pick body filaments confirmed the presence of straight filaments 10 nm in diameter along with some paired helical filaments with periodicities of 90 or 145 nm (47). Swollen neurons stain with antibodies for phosphorylated neurofilaments, MAP-2, tubulin and ubiquitin (17, 45, 52, 57, 66, 75).

Tau immunohistochemistry has revealed additional cytoskeletal changes in Pick's disease including neuritic profiles and astrocytic and oligodendroglial inclusions (20, 86). The tau positive neuritic profiles of Pick's disease differ from the neuropil threads of Alzheimer's disease: they are thinner, more regular in diameter and are negative with Gallyas stains (Figure 10) (67). In addition, unlike the Alzheimer's threads, the profiles of Pick's disease cannot be traced back to neuronal perikarya with Pick bodies but are most likely axonal in nature (67). Tau positive glia are a feature of Pick's disease (20, 39, 48, 86, 87), including thorn-shaped astrocytes and coiled bodies. More specific to Pick's disease are small circular inclusions

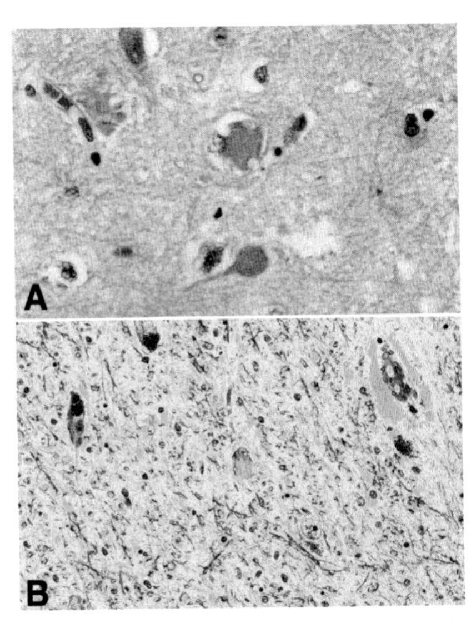

Figure 7. Balloned neurons are usually seen frequently and may be easier to find in the better preserved cortex (**A**). The substantia nigra often shows basophilic inclusions reminiscent of corticobasal bodies or neurofibrillary tangles (**B**). H&E ×600 (**A**), ×400 (**B**).

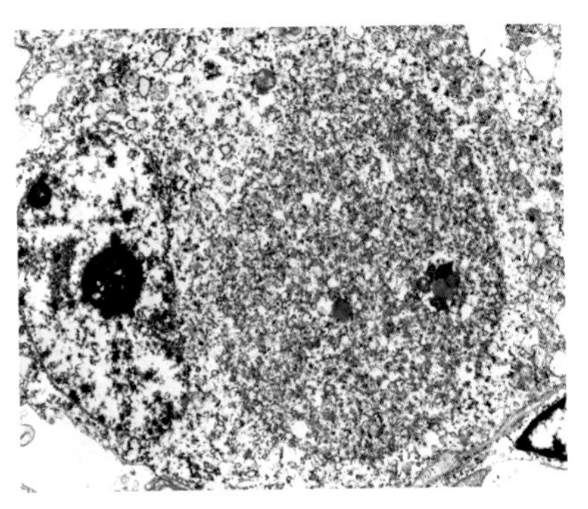

Figure 8. At the ultrastructural level Pick bodies appear as poorly demarcated accumulations of filamentous material with interspersed osmiophilic granular and vesicular structures.

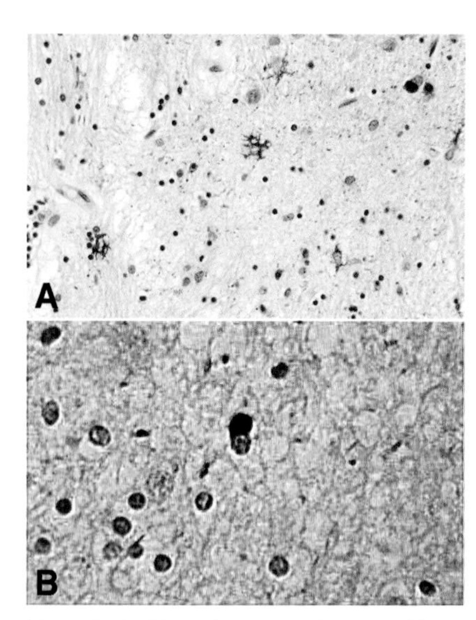

Figure 9. Ramified astrocytes can be seen with tau stains (**A**) as well as small spherical inclusions in white matter oligodendroglial cells (**B**) AT8 tau, putamen ×400 (**A**), frontal lobe white matter ×400 (**B**)

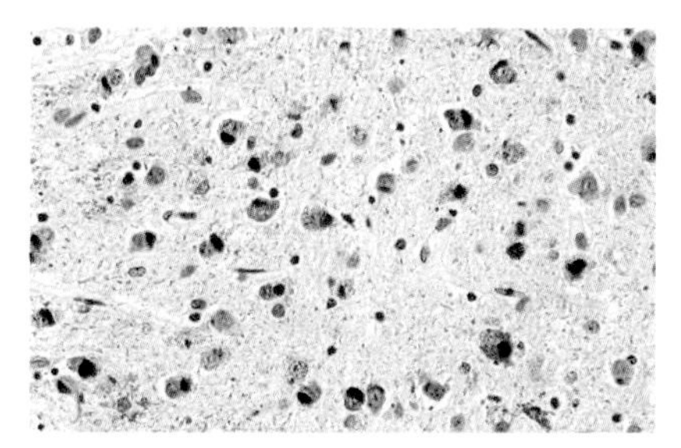

Figure 10. Neuronal threads are present in affected areas. They are thin and delicate and fail to stain with Gallyas stains. Putamen, AT8 tau, ×400.

occasionally found in the subcortical white matter and ramified astrocytes (Figure 9). These tau positive astrocytes differ from the better known tufted astrocytes in that tau immunodeposits occupy a greater area of the glial cytoplasm with scantier and shorter ramifications in the astrocytic processes. Interestingly, as in the case of the Pick body, both types of glial inclusions fail to stain with the Gallyas stain (48).

Biochemistry

As described, Pick's disease is characterised by the deposition of tau protein in Pick bodies and glial inclusions. The use of a range of tau antibodies in immunohistochemistry and immunoelectrophoresis has allowed a biochemical description of Pick's disease and a comparison with other tauopathies. As in Alzheimer's disease tau in Pick's disease is abnormally hyperphosphorylated and recognised by phosphorylation dependant antibodies such as AT8 (67). It differs from Alzheimer's disease in the absence of phosphorylation of the exon 9 tau residue Ser262 (67). This hyperphosphorylated residue is recognised by antibody 12E8, and so Pick bodies, unlike neurofibrillary tangles and tau inclusions in Alzheimer's disease, PSP and CBD are 12E8 negative (8). Immunoelectrophoresis demonstrates that tau in Pick's disease forms a doublet of hyperphosphorylated bands at 55 and 64 kDa, in contrast to Alzheimer's disease tau which forms a major triplet of bands at 55, 64 and 69 kDa with a minor band at 72 kDa (11, 14). The use of dephosphorylation analysis and more recently the use of tau exon 10 specific antibodies indicates that the different hyperphosphorylated bands seen on Western blotting reflect the presence of different tau protein isoforms (15, 27). In general, Pick's disease tau protein does not stain with exon 10 specific antibodies, either in Western blots or immunohistochemistry (2, 15, 37). This indicates that the abnormal hyperphosphorylated tau in Pick's disease in composed primarily of 3-repeat tau, which does not contain tau exon 10. A more recent study using purified Pick bodies rather than brain homogenates has demonstrated conclusively the while most of the tau in Pick's disease consists of 3-repeat tau, a significant amount of 4-repeat tau is also present (47). This surprising finding was also confirmed immunohistochemically using exon 10 specific antibodies; 4-repeat tau is detected in virtually all dentate fascia Pick bodies after formic acid treatment (37). Exon 10 specific antibodies also detected 4-repeat tau in some thorn shaped astrocytes (2). Neurochemistry studies have shown no changes in cholinergic markers, but alterations in serotonergic function and monoamine oxidases (53).

Differential Diagnosis of Pick's Disease

Cortical neuronal loss and gliosis, swollen neurons and Pick bodies are features of both CBD and Pick's disease. Important distinctions exist between the 2 conditions, however. The characteristic "knife-edge" lobar atrophy of Pick's disease is only rarely seen in CBD. Similarly the degree of neuronal loss and gliosis in the neocortex only rarely reaches the severity of that seen in Pick's disease with complete loss of the cortical cytoarchitecture. Finally, although Pick bodies can be seen in CBD their numbers are far fewer than in Pick's disease and they are usually absent in the hippocampus of CBD cases, in contrast to the massive numbers seen in this region in Pick's disease (9). Furthermore, the staining properties of "Pick bodies" in the 2 conditions are different: true Pick bodies in Pick disease are Gallyas negative, while in CBD they are readily detected by this method. Conversely, Pick bodies are readily stained with Bodian and Bielschowsky stains while the Pick-like inclusions of CBD stain poorly or not at all. The 2 inclusions can be further differentiated immunohistochemically: the anti-tau antibody 12E8 which detects phosphorylation at Ser262/356 stains the inclusions in CBD but not Pick bodies (8). In addition the nature and relative distribution of the tau immunodeposits further allows the distinction between Pick's disease and CBD (9, 19, 20).

Frontotemporal degeneration also shares some features with Pick's disease, namely the neuronal loss and gliosis, which can be severe, and the occasional presence of swollen neurons (40). The absence of tau immunoreactivity or Pick bodies readily differentiate this condition form Pick's disease. Rare cases of concomitant Pick's disease and Alzheimer's disease have been reported (10, 65, 74). One should exercise great caution when making this diagnosis. Pick-like bodies are frequently found in the dentate fascia of cases of severe Alzheimer's disease, often in large numbers (18), and scattered swollen neurons also occur in AD (12). These two features in isolation should therefore not be taken as evidence of concomitant Pick's and AD. Finally, neocortical tangles are also found in Pick's disease but in contrast to AD, they predominate in small neurons of the superficial cortical layers (35). In 1984, Munoz and Ludwin coined the term "generalised variant of Pick's disease" (56). The term refers to a disease characterised by severe subcortical involvement and neuronal inclusions, which are unique in their nature and distribution. The inclusions are variably basophilic or eosinophilic, poorly argentophilic and contain variable amounts of RNA. They fail to stain with tau, ubiquitin, neurofilament, αB-crystallin and α-synuclein (81). Their ultrastructure differs from that of Pick bodies and consists of filaments coated along most of their length by granular and fuzzy material. Finally, they are only rarely seen in neocortex, they are absent in hippocampus and are easily found in subcortical structures and anterior horn cells. Of interest, the inclusions are similar to those seen in some cases of sporadic ALS, both juvenile (54) and adult onset (38). Similar cases with prominent extrapyramidal symptoms have also recently been described (81). This disorder is clearly different from Pick's disease and the term "basophilic inclusion body disease" is preferred to that of "generalised variant of Pick's disease."

Experimental Models

Transgenic mice overexpressing the shortest human tau protein have been generated (36, 50). The mice develop spherical argentophilic inclusions in the cytoplasm and proximal axon of neurons in the brain and spinal cord. These filamentous inclusions are composed of 3-repeat tau, which is hyperphosphorylated and becomes insoluble as the disease progresses. The inclusions are accompanied by severe neuronal loss and gliosis. Axonal degenerations is extensive. The mice also show decreased numbers of microtubules and reduced fast axonal transport. The authors suggest that tau overexpression results in a toxic gain of function of the excess tau protein that cannot bind microtubules. Excess tau then aggregates in the neuronal cytoplasm, blocks axonal transport and leads to neuronal death. In another model, the shortest form of human tau was overexpressed in the anterior bulbar cells of the lamprey (30). Tau filaments formed rapidly and aggregated with microtubules and membrane bounded organelles. The affected neurons showed membrane degeneration and synapse loss.

Pathogenesis

The pathogenesis of Pick's disease remains obscure. The recent discovery of genetic forms of Pick's disease, however, points to a possible defect in tau expression or metabolism (58, 60, 64, 70, 76). Tau mutant proteins found in Pick's disease have been shown to severely decrease the ability of tau to promote microtubule assembly (33, 58, 60, 64, 70), and to stimulate the heparin-induced filament assembly of recombinant tau (26). The mutant tau protein is also abnormally susceptible to calpain digestion (64). How a possible alteration in tau metabolism can lead to cell death is still unknown, but the experimental models suggest that the accumulation of tau filaments may lead to defective microtubule function and axonal transport or exert a direct toxic effect on the neuron. The mechanism of neuronal death was recently examined in Pick's disease; extensive DNA fragmentation is present in both neurons and glia, independent of inclusion formation, suggesting the activation of cell death and repair mechanisms (25).

Future Directions and Therapy

Unlike Alzheimer's disease and Lewy body disease where modulation of the cholinergic system may help patients, there is no effective therapy available for Pick's disease. The generation of animal models of tauopathies will allow our further understanding of tau metabolism and filament formation and will allow the screening of potential new therapies.

References

1. Alzheimer A (1911) Über einenartige Krankheitsfälle des späteren alters. *Z Gemsamte Neurol Psychiate* 4: 356-385.

2. Arai T, Ikeda K, Akiyama H, Shikamoto Y, Tsuchiya K, Yagishita S, Beach T, Rogers J, Schwab C, McGeer PL (2001) Distinct isoform of tau aggregated in neurons and glial cells in brains of patients with Pick's disease, corticobasal degeneration and progressive supranuclear palsy. *Acta Neuropathol* 101: 167-173.

3. Arima K,Akashi T (1990) Involvement of the locus coeruleus in Pick's disease with or without Pick body formation. *Acta Neuropathol* 79: 629-633.

4. Armstrong R, Cairns N,Lantos P (1999) Laminar distribution of Pick bodies, Pick cells and Alzheimer disease pathology in the frontal and temporal cortex in Pick's disease. *Neuropath Appl Neurobiol* 25: 266-271.

5. Armstrong R, Cairns N,Lantos P (1999) Quantification of pathological lesions in the frontal and temporal lobe of ten patients diagnosed with Pick's disease. *Acta Neuropathol* 97: 456-462.

6. Armstrong R, Cairns N,Lantos P (2000) Clustering of Pick bodies in the dentate gyrus in Pick's disease. *Neuropathol* 20: 170-175.

7. Ball M (1979) Topography of Pick inclusion bodies in hippocampi of demented patients. *J Neuropathol Exp Neurol* 38: 614-620.

8. Bell K, Cairns N, Lantos P,Rossor M (2000) Immunohistochemistry distinguishes between Pick's disease and corticobasal degeneration. *J Neurol Neurosurg Psychiatry* 69: 835-836.

9. Bergeron C, Davis A, Lang AE (1998) Corticobasal ganglionic degeneration and progressive supranuclear palsy presenting with cognitive decline. *Brain Pathol* 8: 355-365.

10. Berlin L (1949) Presenile sclerosis (Alzheimer's disease) with features resembling Pick's disease. *Arch Neurol Psychiatry* 61: 369-384.

11. Buée-Scherrer V, Hof P, Buée L, Leveugle B, Vermersch P, Perl D, Olanow C,Delacourte A (1996) Hyperphosphorylated tau proteins differentiate corticobasal degeneration and Pick's disease. *Acta Neuropathol* 91: 351-359.

12. Clark AW, Manz HJ, White III CL, Lehmann J, Miller D,Coyle JT (1986) Cortical degeneration with swollen chromatolytic neurons: its relationship to Pick's disease. *J Neuropathol Exp Neurol* 45: 268-284.

13. Constantinidis J, Richard J,Tissot R (1974) Pick's disease: histological and clinical correlations. *Eur J Neurol* 11: 208-217.

14. Delacourte A, Robitaille Y, Sergeant N, Buée L, Hof PR, Wattez A, Laroche-Cholette A, Mathieu J, Chagnon P,Gauvreau D (1996) Specific pathological tau protein variants characterize Pick's disease. *J Neuropathol Exp Neurol* 55: 159-168.

15. Delacourte A, Sergeant N, Wattez A, Gauvreau D,Robitaille Y (1998) Vulnerable neuronal subsets in Alzheimer's and Pick's disease are distinguished by their t isoform distribution and phosphorylation. *Ann Neurol* 43: 193-204.

16. Dickson D (1998) Pick's disease: a modern approach. *Brain Pathol* 8: 339-354.

17. Dickson D, Yen S, Suzuki K, Davies P, Garcia J,Hirano A (1986) Balooned neurons in select neurodegenerative diseases contain phosphorylated neurofilament epitopes. *Acta Neuropathol* 71: 216-223.

18. Dickson D, Yen S-H, Horoupian D (1986) Pick body-like inclusions in the dentate fascia of the hippocampus in Alzheimer's disease. *Acta Neuropathol* 71: 38-45.

19. Feany MB,Dickson DW (1995) Widespread cytoskeletal pathology characterizes corticobasal degeneration. *Am J Pathol* 146: 1388-1396.

20. Feany MB, Mattiace LA,Dickson DW (1996) Neuropathologic overlap of progressive supranuclear palsy, Pick's disease and corticobasal degeneration. *J Neuropathol Exp Neurol* 55: 53-67.

21. Forno L, Eng L,Selkoe D (1989) Pick bodies in the locus ceruleus. *Acta Neuropathol* 79: 10-17.

22. Foster N, Wilhelmsen K, Sima AA, Jones MZ, D'Amato CJ,Gilman S (1997) Frontotemporal dementia and Parkinsonism linked to chromosome 17: a consensus conference. *Ann Neurol* 41: 706-715.

23. Gans A (1923) Betrachtungen über Art und Ausbreitung des krankhaften Prozesses in einem Fall von Pickscher Krankheit des Stirnhirns. *Z Neur* 80: 10.

24. Gibb WRG, Luthert PJ,Marsden CD (1989) Corticobasal degeneration. *Brain* 112: 1171-1192.

25. Gleckman A, Jiang Z, Liu Y,Smith T (1999) Neuronal and glial DNA fragmentation in Pick's disease. *Acta Neuropathol* 98: 55-61.

26. Goedert M, Jakes R,Crowther A (1999) Effects of frontotemporal dementia FTDP-17 mutations on heparin-induced assembly of tau filaments. *FEBS Lett* 450: 306-311.

27. Goedert M, Spillantini MG, Cairns N,Crowther A (1992) Tau proteins of Alzheimer paired helical filaments: abnormal phosphorylation of all six brain isoforms. *Neuron* 8: 159-168.

28. Green AJ, Harvey RJ, Thompson EJ,Rossor MN (1997) Increased S100beta in the cerebrospinal fluid of patients with frontotemporal dementia. *Neurosci Lett* 235: 5-8.

29. Green AJ, Harvey RJ, Thompson EJ,Rossor MN (1999) Increased tau in the cerebrospinal fluid of patients with frontotemporal dementia and Alzheimer's disease. *Neurosci Lett* 259: 133-135.

30. Hall GF, Chu B, Lee G,Yao J (2000) Human tau filaments induce microtubule and synapse loss in an in vivo model of neurofibrillary degenerative disease. *J Cell Sci* 113: 1373-1387.

31. Hansen LA, De Teresa R, Tobias H, Alvord M,Terry RD (1988) Neocortical morphometry and cholinergic neurochemistry in Pick's disease. *Am J Pathol* 131: 507-518.

32. Harvey RJ, Rossor MN, Skelton-Robinson M (1998) Young onset dementia: epidemiology,clinical symptoms, family burden and outcome. Dementia Research Group, Imperial College School of Medicine.

33. Hasegawa M, Smith MJ,Goedert M (1998) Tau proteins with FTDP-17 mutations have a reduced ability to promote microtubule assembly. *FEBS Lett* 437: 207-210.

34. Hauw J, Duyckaerts C, Seilhean D, Camilleri S, Sazdovitch V, Rancurel G (1996) The neuropathologic diagnostic criteria of frontal lobe dementia revisited. A study of ten consecutive cases. *J Neural Transm* (Suppl) 47: 47-59.

35. Hof P, Bouras C, Perl D,Morrisson J (1994) Quantitative neuropathologic analysis of Pick's disease cases: cortical distribution of Pick bodies and coexistence with Alzheimer's disease. *Acta Neuropathol* 87: 115-124.

36. Ishihara T, Hong M, Zhang B, Nakagawa Y, Lee MK, Trojanowski JQ, Lee VM-Y (1999) Age-dependent emergence and progression of a tauopathy in transgenic mice overexpressing the shortest human tau isoform. *Neuron* 24: 751-762.

37. Ishizawa K, Ksiezak-Reding H, Davies P, Delacourte A, Tiseo P, Yen S-H, Dickson D (2000) A double -labeling immunohistochemical study of tau exon 10 in Alzheimer's disease, progressive supranuclear palsy and Pick's disease. *Acta Neuropathol* 100: 235-244.

38. Ito H, Kusaka H, Matsumoto S (1995) Topographic involvement of the striatal efferents in basal ganglia of patients with adult-onset motor neuron disease with basophilic inclusions. *Acta Neuropathol* 89: 513-518.

39. Iwatsubo T, Hasegawa M, Ihara Y (1994) Neuronal and glial tau-positive inclusions in diverse neurologic diseases share common phosphorylation characteristics. *Acta Neuropathol* 88: 129-136.

40. Jackson M, Lowe J (1996) The new neuropathology of degenerative frontotemporal dementias. *Acta Neuropathol* 91: 127-134.

41. Jacob J, Revesz T, Thom M,Rossor MN (1999) A case of sporadic Pick disease with onset at 27 years. *Arch Neurol* 56: 1289-1291.

42. Jellinger K (1994) Quantitative neuropathologic analysis of Pick's disease. *Acta Neuropathol* 87: 223-224.

43. Jellinger K (1996) Structural basis of dementia in neurodegenerative disorders. *J Neural Transm* (Suppl) 47: 1-29.

44. Johannesson G, Brun A, Gustafson I, Ingvar DH (1977) EEG in presenile dementia related to cerebral blood flow and autopsy findings. *Acta Neurol Scand* 56: 89-103.

45. Kato S, Hirano A, Umahara T, Kato M, Herz F, Ohama E (1992) Comparative immunohistochemical study on the expression of αB crystallin, ubiquitin and stress-response protein 27 in balooned neurons in various disorders. *Neuropath Appl Neurobiol* 18: 335-340.

46. Kato S, Nakamura H (1990) Presence of two different fibril subtypes in the Pick body: an immunoelectron microscopic study. *Acta Neuropathol* 81: 125-129.

47. King ME, Ghoshal N, Wall JS, Binder L, Ksiezak-reding H (2001) Structural analysis of Pick's disease-derived and in vitro-assembled tau filaments. *Am J Pathol* 158: 1481-1490.

48. Komori T (1999) Tau-positive glial inclusions in progressive supranuclear palsy, corticobasal degeneration and Pick's disease. *Brain Pathol* 9: 663-679.

49. Kosaka K, Ikeda K, Kobayashi K, Mehraein P (1991) Striatopallidonigral degeneration in Pick's disease: a clinicopathological study of 41 cases. *J Neurol* 238: 151-160.

50. Lee VM-Y, Trojanowski JQ (2001) Transgenic mouse models of tauopathies : prospects for animal models of Pick's disease. *Neurology* 56: S26-S30.

51. Love S, Saitoh T, Quijada S, Cole G,Terry R (1988) ALz-50, ubiquitin and tau immunoreactivity of neurofibrillary tangles, Pick bodies and Lewy bodies. *J Neuropathol Exp Neurol* 47: 393-405.

52. Lowe J, Errington DR, Lennox G, Pike I, Spendlove I, Landon M, Mayer RJ (1992) Balooned neurons in several neurodegenerative diseases and stroke contain αB crystallin. *Neuropath Appl Neurobiol* 18: 341-350.

53. Markesberry WR (1998) Pick's disease, in *Neuropathology of dementing disorders*, Markesberry WR (eds). Arnold: London. pp. 145.

54. Matsumoto S, Kusaka H, Murakami N, Hashizume Y, Okazaki H, Hirano A (1992) Basophilic inclusions in sporadic juvenile amyotrophic lateral sclerosis: an immunocytochemical and ultrastructural study. *Acta Neuropathol* 83: 579-583.

55. McKhann GM, Albert MS, Grossman M, Miller B, Dickson DW, Trojanowski JQ (2001) Clinical and pathological diagnosis of frontotemporal dementia: Report of Workgroup on frontotemporal dementia and Pick's disease. *Arch Neurol* in press

56. Munoz-Garcia D, Ludwin S (1984) Classic and generalized variants of Pick's disease: a clinicopathological, ultrastructural, and immunocytochemical comparative study. *Ann Neurol* 16: 467-480.

57. Murayama S, Mori H, Ihara Y, Tomonaga M (1990) Immunocytochemical and ultrastructural studies of Pick's disease. *Ann Neurol* 27: 394-405.

58. Murrell JR, Spillantini MG, Zolo p, Guazelli M, Smith MJ, Hasegawa M, Redi F, Crowther A, Pietrini P, Ghetti B, Goedert M (1999) Tau gene mutation G389R causes a tauopathy with abundant Pick body-like inclusions and axonal deposits. *J Neuropathol Exp Neurol* 58: 1207-1226.

59. Neary D, Snowden JS, Gustafson L, Passant U, Stuss D, Black S, Freedman M, Kertesz A, Robert PH, Albert M, Boone K, Miller BL, Cummings J, Benson DF (1998) Frontotemporal lobar degeneration: a consensus on clinical diagnostic criteria. *Neurology* 51: 1546-1554.

60. Neumann M, Schulz-Schaeffer WJ, Crowther A, Smith MJ, Spillantini MG, Goedert M, Kretzschmar HA (2001) Pick's disease associated with the novel tau gene mutation K369I. *Ann Neurol* 50: 503-513.

61. Onari K, Spatz H (1926) Anatomische Beiträge zur Lehre von der Pickschen umschriebenen Grosshirnrindenatrophie. (Picksche Krankheit). *Z Neur* 101: 470-511.

62. Perry G, Stewart D, Friedman R, Manetto V, Autilio-Gambetti L, Gambetti P (1987) Filaments of Pick's bodies contain altered cytoskeletal elements. *Am J Pathol* 127: 559-568.

63. Pick A (1892) Ueber die Beziehungen der senilen Hirnatrophie zur Aphasie. *Prager Med Wochenschr* 17: 165-167.

64. Pickering-Brown S, Baker M, Yen S-H, Liu W-K, Hasegawa M, Cairns N, Lantos PL, Rossor M, Iwatsuboto T, Davies Y, Allsop D, Furlong R, Owen F, Hardy J, Mann D, Hutton M (2000) Pick's disease is associated with mutations in the tau gene. *Ann Neurol* 48: 859-867.

65. Pogacar S, Rubio A (1982) Morphological features of Pick's and atypical Alzheimer's disease in Down's syndrome. *Acta Neuropathol* 1982: 249-254.

66. Probst A, Anderton B, Ulrich J, Kohler R, Kahn J, Heitz P (1983) Pick's disease: an immunocytochemical study of neuronal changes. Monoclonal antibodies show that Pick bodies share antigenic determinants with neurofibrillary tangles and neurofilaments. *Acta Neuropathol* 60: 175-182.

67. Probst A, Tolnay M, Langui D, Goedert M, Spillantini M (1996) Pick's disease: hyperphosphorylated tau protein segregates to the somatoaxonal compartment. *Acta Neuropathol* 92: 588-596.

68. Rasool C, Selkoe D (1985) Sharing of specific antigens by degenerating neurons in Pick's disease and Alzheimer's disease. *N Engl J Med* 312: 700-705.

69. Rewcastle N, Ball M (1968) Electron microscopic structure of the "inclusion bodies" in Pick's disease. *Neurology* 18: 1205-1213.

70. Rizzini C, Goedert M, Hodges JR, Smith MJ, Jakes R, Hills R, Xuereb JH, Crowther A, Spillantini MG (2000) Tau gene mutation K257T causes a tauopathy similar to Pick's disease. *J Neuropathol Exp Neurol* 59: 990-1001.

71. Rizzu P, van Swieten JC, Joose M, Hasegawa M, Stevens M, Tibben A, Niermeijer MF, Hillebrand M, Ravid R, Oostra BA, Goedert M, van Duijn CM, Heutink P (1999) High prevalence of mutations in the microtubule-associated protein tau in a population study of frontotemporal dementia in the Netherlands. *Am J Hum Genet* 64: 414-421.

72. Russ C, Lovestone S, Baker M, Pickering-Brown S, Andersen P, Furlong R, Mann D, Powell JF (2001) The extended haplotype of the microtubule associated protein tau gene is not associated with Pick's disease. *Neurosci Lett* 299: 156-158.

73. Schochet SJ, Lampert P, Lindenberg R (1968) Fine structure of Pick and Hirano bodies in a case of Pick's disease. *Acta Neuropathol* 11: 330-337.

74. Smith D, Lantos P (1983) A case of combined Pick's disease and Alzheimer's disease. *J Neurol Neurosurg Psychiatry* 46: 675-677.

75. Smith T, Lippa C,de Girolami U (1992) Immunocytochemical study of ballooned neurons in cortical degeneration with neuronal achromasia. *Clin Neuropathol* 11: 28-35.

76. Spillantini MG, Crowther A, Kamphorst W, Heutink P, van Swieten J (1998) Tau pathology in two Dutch families with mutations in the microtubule -binding region of tau. *Am J Pathol* 153: 1359.

77. The European Concerted Action on Pick's disease (ECAPD) Consortium (1998) Provisional clinical and neuroradiological criteria for the diagnosis of Pick's disease. *Eur J Neurol* .

78. Tissot R, Constantinidis J, Richard J, *La maladie de Pick*. 1975, Paris: Masson et Cie.

79. Towfighi J (1972) Early Pick's disease. *Acta Neuropathol* 21: 224-231.

80. Tsuchiya K, Arima K, Fukui T, Kuroiwa T, Haga C, Iritiani S, Hirai S, Nakano I, Takemura T, Masaaki M, Ikeda K (1999) Distribution of basal ganglia lesions in Pick's disease with Pick bodies: a topographic neuropathological study of eight autopsy cases. *Neuropathol* 19: 370-379.

81. Tsuchiya K, Ishizu H, Nakano I, Kita Y, Sawabe M, Haga C, Kuyama K, Nishinaka T, Oyanagi K, Ikeda K,S K (2001) Distribution of basal ganglia lesions in generalized variant of Pick's disease: a clinicopathological study of four autopsy cases. *Acta Neuropathol* 102: 441-448.

82. Uchihara T, Tsuchiya K, Kosaka K (1990) Selective loss of nigral neurons in Pick's disease: a morphometric study. *Acta Neuropathol* 81: 155-161.

83. Uhl GR, Hilt DC, Hedreen JC, Whitehouse PJ, Price DL (1983) Pick's disease (lobar sclerosis): depletion of neurons in the nucleus basalis of Meynert. *Neurology* 33: 1470-1473.

84. Ulrich J, Haugh M, Anderton B, Probst A, Lautenschlager C, His B (1987) Alzheimer dementia and Pick's disease: neurofibrillary tangles and Pick bodies are associated with identical phosphorylated neurofilament epitopes. *Acta Neuropathol* 73: 240-246.

85. Wisniewski HM, Coblentz JM, Terry RD (1972) Pick's disease. A clinical and ultrastructural study. *Arch Neurol* 26: 97-108.

86. Yamazaki M, Nakano I, Imazu O, Kaieda R, Terashi A (1994) Astrocytic straight tubules in the brain of a patient with Pick's disease. *Acta Neuropathol* 88: 587-591.

87. Yasuhara O, Matsuo A, Tooyama I, Kimura H, McGeer EG, McGeer PL (1995) Pick's disease immunohistochemistry: new alterations and Alzheimer's disease comparisons. *Acta Neuropathol* 89: 322-330.

88. Yoshimura N (1988) Olfactory bulb involvement in Pick's disease. *Acta Neuropathol* 77: 202-205.

89. Yoshimura N (1989) Topography of Pick body distribution in Pick's disease: a contribution to understanding the relationship between Pick's and Alzheimer's diseases. *Clin Neuropathol* 8: 1-6.

Argyrophilic Grain Disease

Markus Tolnay
Estifanos Ghebremedhin
Alphonse Probst
Heiko Braak

Aβ	amyloid β
AD	Alzheimer's disease
AgD	argyrophilic grain disease
ArG	argyrophilic grain
BN	ballooned neuron
NFL	neurofibrillary lesion
PB	Pick body

Definition

Argyrophilic grain disease (AgD) is a late-onset dementia morphologically characterised by the presence of abundant spindle-shaped argyrophilic grains (ArGs) in neuronal processes and coiled bodies in oligodendrocytes. Both of these filamentous lesions consist of the microtubule-associated protein tau in an abnormally and hyperphosphorylated state. Since only a fraction of the emerging abnormal intracellular deposits consists of argyrophilic fibrils the bulk of the pathology associated with AgD only can be assessed by using immunoreactions for abnormally phosphorylated tau protein. At the present time, there are no reliable clinical features that permit diagnosis of AgD. Therefore, AgD only can be identified by means of postmortem neuropathological analysis.

Synonyms and Historical Annotations.

Argyrophilic grains originally were described in the late eighties by Braak and Braak in cases of adult onset dementia with no or only sparse pathological Alzheimer-related changes (4, 5). Subsequently, the term "argyrophilic grain disease" was introduced. Alternative designations include dementia with grains, dementia with argyrophilic grains, and argyrophilic grain dementia.

Epidemiology

Incidence and prevalence. Since AgD represents a relatively new disorder and neither uniform neuropathological nor clinical criteria have been applied yet to their definition, reliable epidemiological data are not available. It became apparent from several consecutive and non-consecutive autopsy studies, however, that AgD might account for approximately 5% of all dementia cases (8, 21, 30). Moreover, a recent study suggests that AgD is the second most common cause of degenerative dementia in Japan, after Alzheimer's disease (AD).

Gender and age distribution. AgD shows a significant correlation with advancing age, and the mean age of affected patients has been reported to be roughly 80 years (8, 16, 30). There is no overt difference in gender distribution.

Risk factors. Presently, advanced age can be considered the only risk factor for AgD.

Genetics

No hereditary form of AgD has been reported to date, and no causative gene is known (eg, there is no reported mutation or polymorphism on the tau gene). Recently, the apolipoprotein E (ApoE) genotypes were analysed in AgD (12, 21, 25). In most studies a low ApoE e4 allele frequency was found, which significantly differed from the e4 allele frequencies in AD, but not from age-matched control subjects. In one of these studies, a significantly higher incidence of the ApoE e2 allele was reported in AgD cases than in AD and age-matched controls (12). Further studies have to confirm whether AgD is indeed associated with polymorphisms in alpha-2 macroglobulin and low-density lipoprotein receptor-related protein genes as suggested by Ghebremedhin and coworkers (13).

Clinical Features

Currently, very little is known about the clinical aspects of AgD patients, especially the early symptoms. However, recent studies (3, 15) suggest that cognitive impairment does not constitute an early event in AgD patients. Instead, in contrast to what is generally observed in AD patients, it seems likely that in AgD behavioural disturbances (eg, paroxysmal agitation and violence, inappropriate social conduct, personality changes, aggressiveness, restlessness, loss of personal awareness) precede memory failure and cognitive decline. Nonetheless, in late stages of the disease process, when dementia already is present, AgD may become clinically indistinguishable from AD. Based upon retrospective clinicopathological studies, it also has become apparent that the presence of ArGs in human brain is not necessarily associated with cognitive decline (23, 24).

Macroscopy

Upon gross examination, the majority of AgD brains appear virtually unchanged or show only mild, diffuse or frontotemporal cortical atrophy. In particular, there is no marked atrophy of the hippocampus and/or the amygdaloid complex, and the temporal portion of the lateral ventricles is not enlarged (8, 30). However, AgD cases exhibiting prominent atrophy of the medial temporal lobes and the ambient gyrus have also been described (19, 32)

Histopathology

Argyrophilic grains (ArGs). ArGs constitute the most important histopathological hallmark of AgD. They can best be detected in routine paraffin-embedded tissue by the use of conventional silver methods (eg, Bielschowsky or Bodian stain) but are more easily recognized in tissue sections processed with the Gallyas silver iodide technique (Figure 1A, B). In such sections, the tiny ArGs stand out clearly against their background. ArGs are spindle- or comma-shaped structures with a long axis extending up to 9 μm and a diameter reaching 4 μm. Variations in shape include straight or kinked rod- or drumstick-like structures, often with tiny excrescences along the surface (Figure 1B). ArGs are found in both cortical and subcortical structures. Among cortical areas, the transentorhinal and entorhinal cortices are most susceptible to the development of ArGs. The brunt of the ArG pathology occurs in the upper pre-β layer, although scattered ArGs also are present within the deep pri-α layer and the cellular islands of layer pre-α. From the amygdala and temporal allocortex, ArGs typically spread out into layer III of the temporal neocortex. ArGs are sparse in the anterobasal portions of the insula as well as in the temporopolar and frontoorbital neocortex, and they are almost absent in other neocortical regions. ArGs are abundantly present in the external and internal pyramidal layers of the first Ammon's horn sector (CA1) (Figure 1A). The prosubiculum usually exhibits the highest ArG density in the hippocampal region, whereas the subiculum proper contains only a small number of lesions. A few ArGs may be found in sectors CA2-4 and the parasubiculum. At the subcortical level, ArGs are densely distributed throughout the basolateral nuclei of the amygdaloid complex. High densities of ArGs also are present in the hypothalamic lateral tuberal nucleus, whereas the adjoining hypothalamic nuclei and the entire thalamus appear nearly devoid of lesions (20). On rare occasions, ArGs may be found in basal portions of the claustrum but the striatum and the magnocellular nuclei of the basal forebrain remain consistently free of grains (8, 30). Occasionally, a few grains may be found in the lower brain stem.

As mentioned earlier, ArGs in human brain are not necessarily associated with cognitive decline. In a recent study, the distribution and density of ArGs were carefully assessed in well-documented demented and nondemented AgD subjects (24). A significantly more widespread rostrocaudal extension of ArG changes was encountered in the limbic area (eg, sector CA1 of the hippocampus, entorhinal and transentorhinal cortex, parahippocampal cortex) of subjects with documented cognitive decline than in that of cognitively unimpaired subjects suggesting that early (subclinical) changes in AgD might begin in the rostral hippocampus and/or in the most anterior entorhinal cortex and amygdaloid complex (22). A more recent study further suggests that the selective severe involvement of the ambient gyrus might explain some of the clinical manifestations in AgD patients (19).

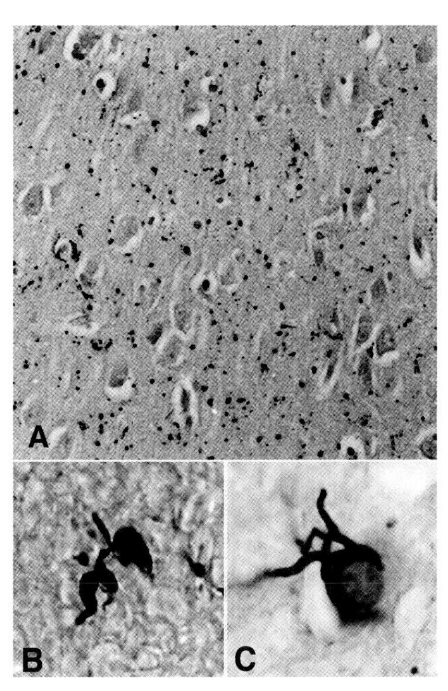

Figure 1. Gallays staining. **A.** Argyrophilic grains (ArGs) in the intercellular grey matter of the hippocampus (sector CA1). Note the complete absence of neurofibrillary changes and neuropil threads in this area of the cortex. **B.** ArGs sometimes show saccular or filiform protrusions. **C.** Subcortical white matter, hippocampus region. A coiled body surrounding the cell nucleus of an oligodendrocyte.

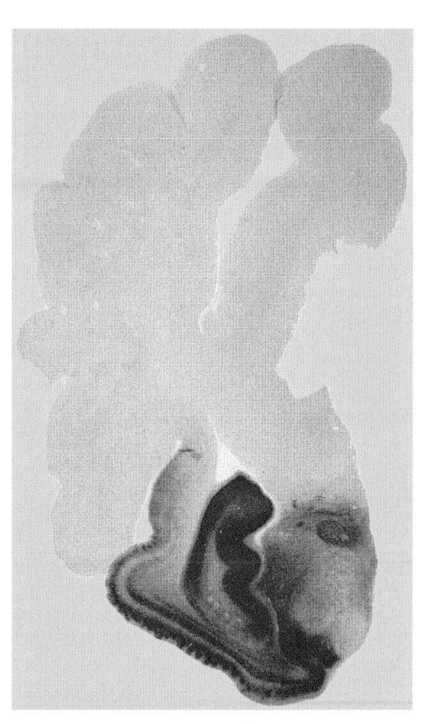

Figure 2. Typical distribution pattern of the pathology related to argyrophilic grain disease. Note that all of the lesions are almost exclusively concentrated on the anteromedial portion of the temporal lobe. The neocortex here is devoid of pathology. 100 μm thick polyethylene glycol (PEG) embedded section. AT8 immunostaining.

Coiled bodies. Coiled bodies are conspicuous, curvaceous, whip-like, and often, branching oligodendroglial inclusions, located in the vicinity of the cell nucleus (Figure 1C). Like ArGs, they easily can be detected with appropriate silver stains. Coiled bodies can be found in varying amounts in other degenerative disorders of the central nervous system and, therefore, are considered a non-specifc finding (9). In AgD, however, coiled bodies represent a consistent finding in the white matter close to cortical areas and subcortical nuclei rich in ArGs, and coiled bodies also may be encountered in deep layers of involved cortical regions. Accordingly, in addition to ArGs, coiled bodies should be considered as one of the essential histopathological hallmarks of AgD.

Changes of the Alzheimer-type. One of the reasons why AgD still is called into question as a distinct disease entity is the observation that most of the reported AgD cases show associated changes of the AD-type, eg, neurofibrillary lesions (NFLs). AgD, therefore, has been regarded as a variant of AD. Closer inspection, however, reveals notable differences between AD-type changes in AgD and AD, which strongly argue against the for-

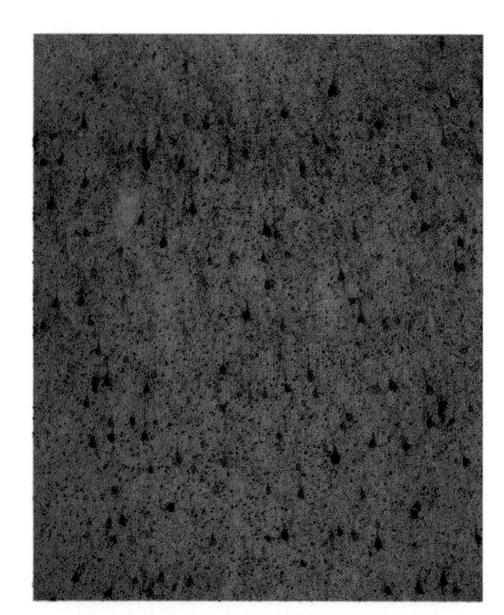

Figure 3. Transentorhinal region. Note the dense distribution pattern of the tiny ArGs throughout the external cortical layers. In addition there are numerous pretangle neurons. 100 μm thick PEG embedded section. AT8 immunostaining.

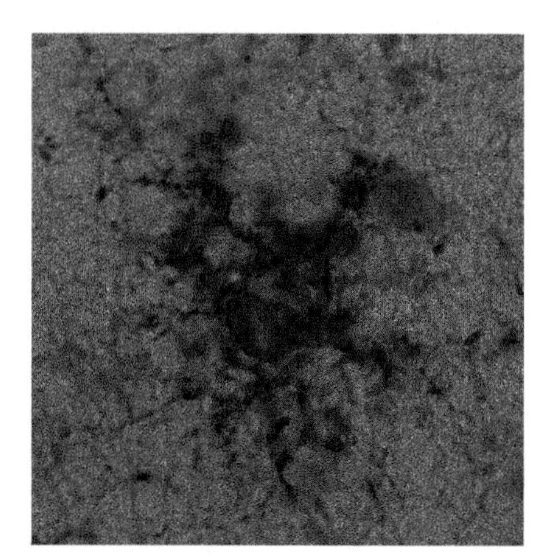

Figure 5. AT8-stained, non-argyrophilic, highly branched astrocyte in the amygdala of an AgD case.

mer hypothesis. Large series of AgD cases (8, 27) have revealed NFLs corresponding to early (entorhinal and limbic) Braak stages, which generally are not associated with cognitive decline (6). Moreover, when using appropriate silver staining techniques and/or Aβ immunohistochemistry, senile plaques (mainly in the form of diffuse Aβ-deposits) are found in only about two-thirds of AgD cases, whereas senile plaques are completely lacking in the remaining cases (8, 29).

Ballooned neurons. Ballooned neurons (BNs) are a frequent feature of amygdaloid nuclei in patients with AgD (Figure 4) (26). Moderate numbers of cortical BNs also have been encountered in layers V and VI of basal temporal neocortical areas (8, 17, 21, 26).

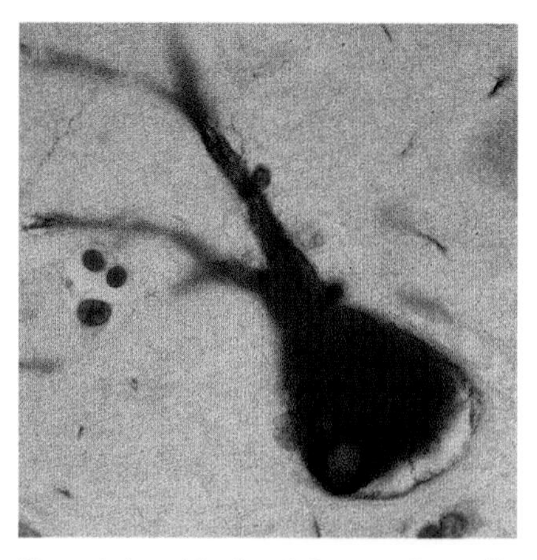

Figure 4. Amygdala of an AgD case. αB-crystallin immunoreactive ballooned cell.

Other findings. In some AgD cases, a prominent superficial laminar spongiosis in cortical areas rich in ArGs has been reported (17). In addition, extensive cortical and subcortical gliosis can be found in rare instances of AgD (32, 33). Nevertheless, based on the authors' own experience involving numerous AgD cases, it seems likely that both features—cortical spongiosis and subcortical gliosis—represent atypical findings and therefore are not essential to the diagnosis of AgD.

Immunohistochemistry and Ultrastructural Findings

Several studies have confirmed that the main protein constituent of both ArGs and coiled bodies is the abnormally and hyperphosphorylated tau protein (Figures 2, 3) (16). Furthermore, it has been shown that the tau protein in ArGs and coiled bodies shares a high number of phosphorylated sites with the NFLs of AD (23). Earler immunohistochemical studies failed to stain ArGs and coiled bodies with antibodies directed against phosphorylated Ser262 (23), and AgD changes therefore shared this particular tau antigenic property with Pick bodies (Pbs) in Pick's disease (10, 18). Recent immunohistochemical and biochemical studies, however, strongly suggest that Ser262 is indeed phosphorylated in both Pbs and ArGs (11, 31).

The bulk of pathological changes in AgD only becomes visible by using tau immunohistochemistry (eg, antibody AT8) (Figures 2, 3). Thus, an additional striking feature in AgD cases consists of a widespread hyperphosphorylation of the tau protein in the somatodendritic domain of limbic neurons (8, 20, 23) (Figure 3). Furthermore, it has been shown that the majority of the afflicted nerve cells are projection neurons (eg, the projection cells of the transentorhinal and entorhinal layers pre-α and pri-α, the principal cells of the lateral tuberal nucleus, the projection cells in both the central nucleus and the basolateral nuclei of the amygdala, the pyramidal cells in sector CA1, the hilar mossy cells as well as granule cells of the fascia dentata [8]). The intraneuronal distribution of the hyperphosphorylated tau in AgD very much resembles that of the pretangle neurons in AD (1, 7). By using combined AT8/Gallyas staining, it could be shown recently that a substantial subset of ArGs is formed within dendrites and dendritic side branches but not in perikarya of neurons containing the hyperphosphorylated tau protein (27), a finding that corroborates previous studies suggesting a dendritic origin for ArGs (14, 20). Ballooned cells in AgD also stain for tau but are best visualised with antibodies against neurofilament or αB-crystallin (Figure 4) (26). Approximately 50% of ArGs and a subset of coiled bodies are stained with antibodies against ubiquitin. However, these lesions do not stain with antibodies for α-synuclein, β-amyloid, αB-crystallin, neurofilament, or GFAP.

In addition to coiled bodies, glial tau pathology in AgD also is present in astrocytes. Recently, non-argyrophilic astrocytes expressing hyperphosphorylated tau epitopes were reported as constant features in anterior limbic structures, such as the amygdala and anterior entorhinal cortex in AgD cases (Figure 5) (2).

Ultrastructurally, ArGs consist of aggregates of straight filaments with diameters of 9 to 18 nm and bundles of smooth tubules with diameters of 25 nm. AD paired helical filaments are absent. Coiled bodies are made up of straight filaments with diameters of 10 to 13 nm or tubular structures (16).

Biochemistry

Using antibodies specific to 3R and 4R tau as well as biochemistry, it has recently been shown that AgD is a tauopathy with preferential accumulation of 4R tau within grains (22, 31, 34). While not statistically significant AgD cases also had increased frequency of tau H1 haplotye similar to other 4R tauopathies, namely PSP and CBD (22).

Differential Diagnosis

ArGs can easily be distinguished from the NFLs of AD. They are much smaller than neurofibrillary tangles and are never seen in neuronal cell perikarya. Extracellular "ghost" tangles are larger, and they show much less argyrophilia than ArGs (1, 7). Neuropil threads are slender filiform structures without spindle-shaped thickenings and are more varied in size and shape than the sturdy ArGs, which exhibit little variation. Although ArGs are distributed evenly throughout the neuropil, clusters of grains may be observed in some cases, which—at first glance—may resemble AD neuritic plaques (NPs) or astrocytic plaques as seen in corticobasal degeneration (28). Dystrophic neurites of NPs, however, vary greatly in size and shape compared with the much more uniform ArGs, and the diameters of both NPs and astrocytic plaques generally exceed those of ArGs clusters. Moreover, Aβ-deposits are not encountered in clustered ArGs. ArGs also can be easily distinguished from tufted astrocytes of PSP (28). PBs of Pick's disease are much larger than ArGs and are found exclusively in neuronal cell perikarya. Furthermore, PBs, although argyrophilic, are not stained with the Gallyas silver iodide technique (18). Co-occurring ArGs have been reported in a variety of neurodegenerative disorders, among them Pick's disease, progressive supranuclear palsy, corticobasal degeneration, Parkinson's disease, dementia with Lewy bodies, tangle-predominant form of senile dementia, Creutzfeldt-Jakob disease and multiple system atrophy (30). As such, it has been suggested that AgD does not represent a separate disease entity, and some authors have proposed that AgD be classified as a variant of the lobar atrophy complex (Pick's complex) (15) or PSP (17). However, in all these disorders ArGs are an inconsistent feature and are only found in a subset of cases. Moreover, although not regularly present, ArGs constitute a frequent finding in brains of old and very old subjects, and it is therefore not surprising that some ArGs occur as incidental features in various neurodegenerative disorders in old age.

1. Core lesions of AgD

Essential for diagnosis

a) Argyrophilic grains

Consistent features but not essential for diagnosis

b) Coiled bodies

c) Non-argyrophilic limbic projection neurons containing hyperphosphorylated tau protein in all cell compartments

2. AgD-associated lesions—frequent findings but not essential for diagnosis

a) Ballooned neurons (frequent finding in amygdala and layers V and VI of basal temporal neocortical areas)

b) Non-argyrophilic tau immunoreactive astrocytes (frequent finding in amygdala and entorhinal and transen torhinal cortex)

c) Associated lesions of the Alzheimer-type

- Neurofibrillary lesions corresponding to Braak stages I-III (frequent finding)
- Some senile plaques, mainly of the diffuse type (two-thirds of cases)

AgD-associated lesions—infrequent findings

a) Superficial laminar spongiosis (layers II-III of basal temporal neocortical areas)

b) Cortical and subcortical gliosis (entorhinal and transentorhinal cortex, posterior parahippocampal cortex)

Table 1. Argyrophilic grain disease: neuropathological features.

Experimental Models

There are no animal models currently in existence for AgD.

Future Directions

Since the first reports by Braak and Braak more than 10 years ago (4, 5), AgD in the meantime constitutes a morphologically well-defined disease entity (Table 1). Nonetheless, more work needs to be done to establish AgD within the large and heterogeneous group of tauopathies, eg, to define it's possible relationship to other 4R tauopathies, namely PSP and CBD. Presently, the diagnosis "argyrophilic grain disease" still is based exclusively on postmortem examination. Accordingly it is crucial to develop diagnostic criteria, which will permit a clinical diagnosis of AgD.

References

1. Bancher C, Brunner C, Lassmann H, Budka H, Jellinger K, Wiche G, Seitelberger F, Grundke-Iqbal I, Wiesniewski HM (1989) Accumulation of abnormally phosphorylated tau precedes the formation of neurofibrillary tangles in Alzheimer's disease. Brain Res 477: 90-99.

2. Botez G, Probst A, Ipsen S, Tolnay M (1999) Astrocytes expressing hyperphosphorylated tau protein without glial fibrillary tangles in argyrophilic grain disease. Acta Neuropathol 98: 251-256.

3. Botez G, Schultz C, Ghebremedhin E, Bohl J, Braak E, Braak H (2000) Clinical aspects of argyrophilic grain disease. Nervenarzt 71: 38-43.

4. Braak H, Braak E (1987) Argyrophilic grains: characteristic pathology of cerebral cortex in cases of adult onset dementia without Alzheimer changes. Neurosci Lett 76: 124-127.

5. Braak H, Braak E (1989) Cortical and subcortical argyrophilic grains characterize a disease associated with adult onset dementia. Neuropathol Appl Neurobiol 15: 13-26.

6. Braak H, Braak E (1991) Neuropathological stageing of Alzheimer-related changes. Acta Neuropathol 82: 239-259.

7. Braak E, Braak H, Mandelkow EM (1994) A sequence of cytoskeleton changes related to the formation of neurofibrillary tangles and neuropil threads. Acta Neuropathol 87: 554-567.

8. Braak H, Braak E (1998) Argyrophilic grain disease: frequency of occurrence in different age categories and neuropathological diagnostic criteria. J Neural Transm 105: 801-819.

9. Chin SS-M, Goldman EJ (1996) Glial inclusions in CNS degenerative diseases. J Neuropathol Exp Neurol 55: 499-508.

10. Delacourte A, Sergeant N, Wattez A, Gauvreau D, Robitaille Y (1998) Vulnerable neuronal subsets in Alzheimer's and Pick's disease are distinguished by their tau isoform distribution and phosphorylation. Ann Neurol 43: 193-204.

11. Ferrer I, Barrachina M, Puig B (2002) Anti-tau phospho-specific Ser(262) antibody recognizes a variety of abnormal hyper-phosphorylated tau deposits in tauopathies including Pick bodies and argyrophilic grains. *Acta Neuropathol* 104: 658-664.

12. Ghebremedhin E, Schultz C, Botez G, Rüb U, Sassin I, Braak E, Braak H (1998) Argyrophilic grain disease is associated with apolipoprotein E e2 allele. Acta Neuropathol 96: 222-224.

13. Ghebremedhin E, Schultz C, Thal DR, Del Tredici K, Rueb U, Braak H (2002) Genetic association of argyrophilic grain disease with polymorphisms in alpha-2 macroglobulin and low-density lipoprotein receptor-related protein genes. *Neuropath Appl Neuro* 28: 308-313.

14. Ikeda K, Akiyama H, Kondo H, Haga C (1995) A study of dementia with argyrophilic grains. Possible cytoskeletal abnormality in dendrospinal portion of neurons and oligodendroglia. Acta Neuropathol 89: 409-414.

15. Ikeda K, Akiyama H, Arai T, Matsushita M, Tsuchiya K, Miyazaki H (2000) Clinical aspects of argyrophilic grain disease. Clin Neuropathol 19: 278-284.

16. Jellinger K (1998) Dementia with grains (argyrophilic grain disease). Brain Pathol 8: 377-386.

17. Martinez-Lage P, Munoz DG (1997) Prevalence and disease association of argyrophilic grains of Braak. J Neuropathol Exp Neurol 56: 157-164.

18. Probst A, Tolnay M, Langui D, Goedert M, Spillantini MG (1996) Pick's disease: hyperphosphorylated tau protein segregate to the somatoaxonal compartment. Acta Neuropathol 92: 588-596.

19. Saito Y, Nakahara K, Yamanouchi H, Murayama S (2002) Severe involvement of ambient gyrus in dementia with grains. *J Neuropathol Exp Neurol* 61: 789-796.

20. Schultz C, Koppers D, Sassin I, Braak E, Braak H (1998) Cytoskeletal alterations in the human tuberal hypothalamus related to argyrophilic grain disease. Acta Neuropathol 96: 596-602.

21. Togo T, Cookson N, Dickson DW (2002) Argyrophilic grain disease: Neuropathology, frequency in a dementia brain bank and lack of relationship with apolipoprotein E. Brain Pathology 12:45-52.

22. Togo T, Sahara N, Yen S-H, Cookson N, Ishizawa T, Hutton M, de Silva R, Lees A, Dickson DW. Argyrophilic grain disease is a sporadic 4-repeat tauopathy. J Neuropathol Exp Neuro 2002:(in press)

23. Tolnay M, Spillantini MG, Goedert M, Ulrich J, Langui D, Probst A (1997) Argyrophilic grain disease: widespread hyperphosphorylation of tau protein in limbic neurons. Acta Neuropathol 93: 477-484.

24. Tolnay M, Schwietert M, Monsch AU, Staehelin HB, Langui D, Probst A (1997) Argyrophilic grain disease: distribution of grains in patients with and without dementia. Acta Neuropathol 94: 353-358.

25. Tolnay M, Probst A, Monsch AU, Staehelin HB, Egensperger R (1998) Apolipoprotein E allele frequencies in argyrophilic grain disease. Acta Neuropathol 96: 225-227.

26. Tolnay M, Probst A (1998) Ballooned neurons expressing αB-crystallin as a constant feature of the amygdala in argyrophilic grain disease. Neurosci Lett 246: 165-168.

27. Tolnay M, Mistl C, Ipsen S, Probst A (1998) Argyrophilic grains of Braak: occurrence in dendrites of neurons containing hyperphosphorylated tau protein. Neuropathol Appl Neurobiol 24: 53-59.

28. Tolnay M, Probst A (1999) Review: Tau protein pathology in Alzheimer's disease and related disorders. Neuropathol Appl Neurobiol 25: 171-187.

29. Tolnay M, Calhoun M, Pham HC, Egensperger R, Probst A (1999) Low amyloid (Aβ) plaque load and relative predominance of diffuse plaques distinguish argyrophilic grain disease from Alzheimer's disease. Neuropathol Appl Neurobiol 25: 295-305.

30. Tolnay M, Monsch AU, Probst A (2001) Argyrophilic grain disease: a frequent dementing disorder in aged patients. Adv Exp Med Biol 487: 39-58.

31. Tolnay M, Sergeant N, Ghestern A, Chalbot S, De Vos RAI, Jansen Steur EN, Probst A, Delacourte A (2002) Argyrophilic grain disease and Alzheimer's disease are distinguished by their different distribution of tau protein isoforms. *Acta Neuropathol* 104: 425-434.

32. Tsuchiya K, Mitani K, Arai T, Yamada S, Komiya T, Esaki Y, Haga C, Yamanouchi H, Ikeda K (2001) Argyrophilic grain disease mimicking temporal Pick's disease: a clinical, radiological, and pathological study of an autopsy case with a clinical course of 15 years. Acta Neuropathol 102: 195-199.

33. Yamada T, McGeer PL, McGeer EG (1992) Some immunohistochemical features of argyrophilic grain dementia with normal cortical choline acetyltransferase levels but extensive subcortical pathology and markedly reduced dopamine. J Geriatr Psychiatry Neurol 5: 3-13.

34. Zhukareva V, Shah K, Uryu K, Braak H, Del Tredici K, Sundarraj S, Clark C, Trojanowski JQ, Lee VM (2002) Biochemical analysis of tau proteins in argyrophilic grain disease, Alzheimer's disease, and Pick's disease: a comparative study. *Am J Pathol* 161: 1135-1141.

Parkinsonism-dementia Complex of Guam

Kiyomitsu Oyanagi

AD	Alzheimer's disease
ALS	amyotrophic lateral sclerosis
CBD	corticobasal degeneration
Guam PDC	Parkinsonism-dementia complex of Guam
NFT	neurofibrillary tangle
PDC	Parkinson-dementia complex
PEP	postencephalitic Parkinsonism
PHF	paired helical filament
PSP	progressive supranuclear palsy
SF	straight filament

Definition

Parkinsonism-dementia complex of Guam (Guam PDC) is a disease occurring in the Chamorro people of Guam first characterised in clinicopathological studies by Hirano et al (18). Its neuropathological hallmarks are widespread neurofibrillary tangles (NFTs) and neuronal loss, which exhibit a characteristic distribution in cortical and subcortical regions. The NFTs have ultrastructural and biochemical properties similar to those in Alzheimer's disease (AD). Unlike AD, there are only a few neuropil threads and senile plaques (18, 44, 61) and recent studies have also demonstrated distinct tau- and Gallyas-positive astrocytic inclusions not found in AD (39).

Synonyms and Historical Annotations

Before the discovery of PDC, a high incidence of amyotrophic lateral sclerosis (ALS) was observed on Guam (27). Malamud (30) and Hirano (19) proposed that ALS of Guam and Guam PDC were a single disease entity, and that Guam ALS was a disease different from typical sporadic ALS. Guam ALS was considered distinct because: *i)* the topographic distribution of NFTs and neuronal loss in ALS was similar to Guam PDC, *ii)* patients with combined PDC and ALS (PDC-ALS) were recognised, and *iii)* ALS as well as PDC patients were sometimes admixed within a kindred. Recently, however, it has become clear that NFTs are prevalent in the normal population of Guam (4) and that NFTs in the setting of Guam ALS are merely a background phenomenon (41). The current evidence suggests that the mechanism of neuronal degeneration in Guam ALS is similar to typical ALS (41, 44, 60). Guam PDC, on the other hand, is a distinctive disease process and the focus of this chapter. For more information about ALS, please see chapter 8. 2.

Epidemiology

The maximum annual incidence rate of Guam PDC from 1955 to 1965 (Figure 1) was reported to be about 60 per 100000 for men; and about 20 per 100000 for women (15, 49). The mortality rate of PDC in Chamorro people on Saipan, a northern island of Guam, whose genotypic composition is similar to Guam Chamorro, was strikingly low suggesting an environmental risk factor (63). Filipino migrants to Guam are susceptible to the disease further supporting an environmental over genetic etiology (13). The increased risk to spouses of affected indiviudals in a longitudinal case-control study also strongly implicated environmental factors (47). Since 1965, the incidence rate of Guam PDC has been decreasing, especially in men, but has remained at about 10 to 25 per 100000 when last estimated for the period of 1980 to 1990 (59). These findings suggest that environmental factors in combination with possible genetic risk factors may predispose to Guam PDC and account for the decreasing incidence in recent years. Similarly, the incidence rate for ALS has markedly decreased in recent years and is now similar to the rate in the rest of the world, namely about 3 to 5 per 100000 (Chen K-M, personal communication).

Genetics

A definitive genetic cause for Guam PDC has not been identified (45); however, a number of candidate genes have been studied. The G-to-C polymorphism in exon 9 of the CYP2D6 gene, which is linked to slower metabolism of exogenous toxins, was reported to be higher in Chamorro control subjects and PDC patients than that in Caucasian controls (9). The apolipoprotein E $\epsilon4$ allele frequency,

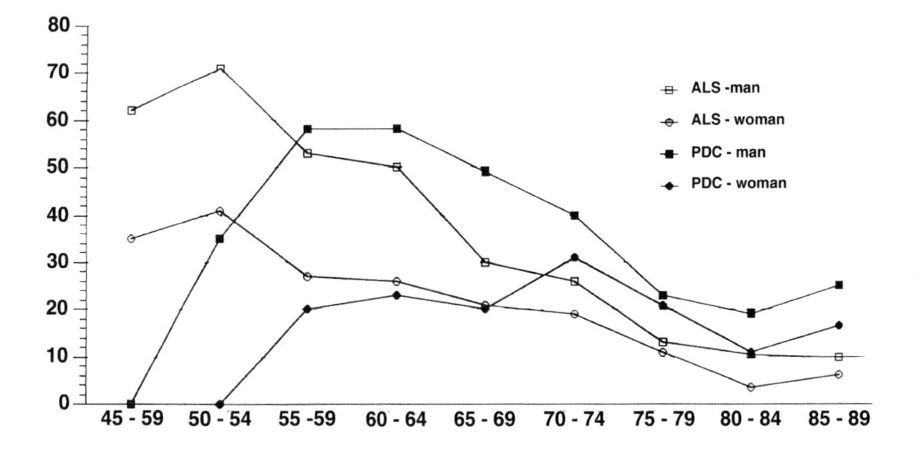

Figure 1. Five-year average annual incidence rates for ALS and PDC per 100000 population (1945-1989). Age adjusted to the 1960 Guam population. Adapted from Ralph Garruto et al (1995). Cited with permission from K Tashiro et al (1995).

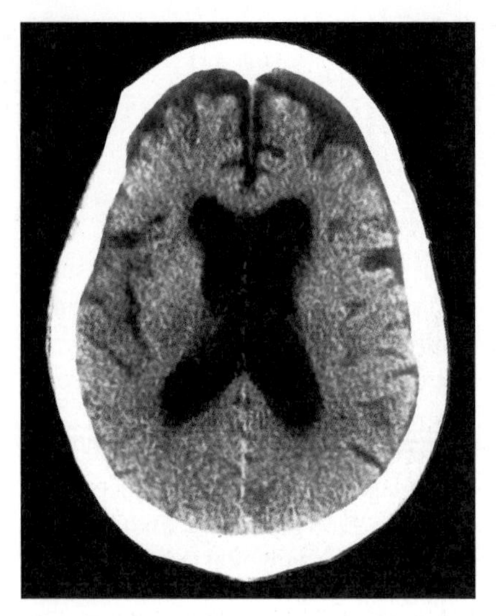

Figure 2. A brain CT of a 71-year-old male patient with PDC. By courtesy of Dr K-M Chen.

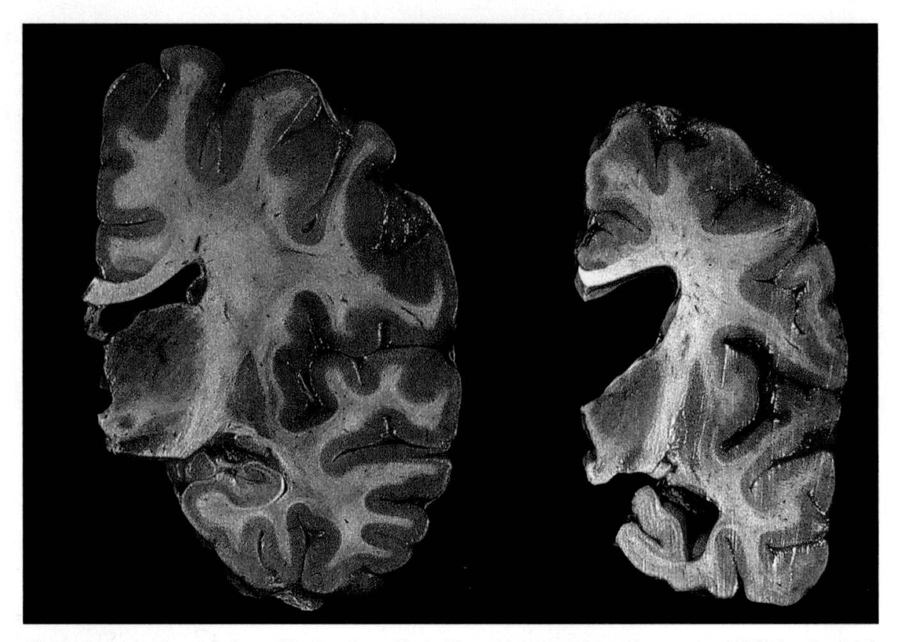

Figure 3. Coronally cut surface of brains of a patient with parkinsonism-dementia complex (PDC) (on the right) and of an age-matched non-PDC non-amyotrophic lateral sclerosis (ALS) subject (on the left). From Oyanagi et al (1999), Steinkopff Verlag with permission.

which is a risk factor for AD, was not increased in PDC, but both Chamorro controls and PDC patients had considerably lower ϵ2 allele frequencies than Caucasian controls (6, 9). The percentage of subjects that were homozygous for TAU A_0, a dinucleotide repeat polymorphism in the TAU gene, was somewhat higher in Chamorro controls and PDC patients than Caucasian controls (10). No mutations have been detected in the TAU gene in PDC (45, 48), but association studies implicate TAU as a susceptibility factor or a disease-modifying factor (48).

Clinical Features

Guam PDC is characterised by extrapyramidal symptoms (rigidity, tremors and bradykinesia) and dementia in the fifth to sixth decade of life, and progression to a vegetative state with pelvicrural flexion contractures within 4 to 6 years. In addition to marked akinetic-rigid state that can lead to limb deformities (36), oculomotor signs have been observed in some patients (8). Pigmentary retinal lesions have been reported (11) and have been histologically characterised (7) but are not specific to PDC and are found in unaffected Chamorro (7). Similar to idiopathic Parkinson's disease, olfactory dysfunction is common in PDC (3, 12), which probably correlates with severe pathology in olfactory related brain structures. Autonomic dysfunction is also frequent (29). More than half the cases of PDC have clinical evidence of diabetes mellitus, but diabetes is also common in unaffected Chamorro (1). Only a limited number of imaging studies have been reported in PDC, but ^{18}F-DOPA PET scans show decreased uptake in the basal ganglia due to degeneration of dopaminergic input similar to Parkinson's disease (57). Figure 2 shows the CT changes seen in one case with PDC.

Macroscopy

The average brain weight of Guam PDC patients is about 1070 g (44) The cerebrum has diffuse atrophy accentuated in the frontal and temporal lobes. The thickness of the cerebral cortex is generally reduced, especially in the hippocampus and parahippocampal gyrus (Figure 3). The basal ganglia and thalamus show moderate atrophy, and the white matter of the cerebrum and brainstem are diffusely atrophic. The midbrain and pons atrophy parallels that of the cerebrum. The substantia nigra and locus coeruleus have loss of neuromelanin pigmentation. The volume of the superior colliculus, cerebellum and medulla oblongata are preserved (42, 44).

Histopathology and Distribution of Lesions

Cerebral cortex and white matter. The topographic distribution of brain atrophy roughly coincides with that of neuronal loss and NFTs (18, 41, 42). Complete loss of neurons is seen in Sommer's sector, and severe to moderate loss is observed in the temporal, insular and frontal cortices. Many NFTs are observed in Sommer's sector, parahippocampal gyrus, temporal neocortex, and frontal cortex. The NFTs are predominantly distributed in the superficial layers in the cerebral cortex (20) and are immunopositive for tau (Figure 4) (44), Aβ (22), and Apo E (6, 53). Many granulovacuolar bodies and Hirano bodies are detected in Ammon's horn (17). Although a few cases may have relatively large numbers of senile plaques, most cases have no or only a few senile plaques (18, 44, 50). Neuropil threads (curly fibers) are absent or sparse (61) (Figure 4). The cerebral white matter has severe atrophy, but myelin pallor and tau-positive thread-like structures are not present in most cases.

Basal ganglia and thalamus. The large neurons in the neostriatum are decreased to 40% of control levels, while the loss is only 10% of control levels in the nucleus accumbens (40). The neurons in the basal nucleus of Meynert are also decreased (32, 37). Many of the residual large neurons in the neostriatum contain NFTs (40). The globus pallidus has moderate neuronal loss and some NFTs. Many α-synuclein positive neuronal inclusions (Lewy bodies) and Lewy neurites are observed in the amygdaloid nucleus; synuclein immunoreactive inclusions frequently coexist in neurons with tau-positive pretangles and NFTs (62) (Figure 6). The thalamus, particularly the lateral nucleus, has moderate neuronal loss and NFTs, while neuronal loss and NFTs are much less in the medial nucleus. Marked neuronal loss and many NFTs are evident in the hypothalamus. The subthalamic nucleus has only slight neuronal loss and a few NFTs (44).

Brain stem. The substantia nigra has very severe neuronal loss and many NFTs affecting not only pigmented, but also nonpigmented neurons (16, 43). Similar changes are noted in the ventral tegmental area. Lewy bodies are rarely detected in the substantia nigra. The locus coeruleus and superior central nucleus have marked neuronal loss and many NFTs. The pedunculopontine and pontine nuclei have NFTs, but relatively mild neuronal loss. The superior colliculus has a few NFTs, but the large neurons in the deeper layer are preserved (44).

Cerebellum and spinal cord. The Purkinje and granule cell layers are preserved. Although a few NFTs are observed in the dentate nucleus, no neuronal loss is usually evident and grumose degeneration is not usually present (44). The cerebellar and spinal white matter is usually free of significant pathology. Anterior horn cells are pyknotic, but usually not reduced in number. A few NFTs are observed in the intermediate zone and posterior horn, and occasionally in the anterior horn (25, 41, 51).

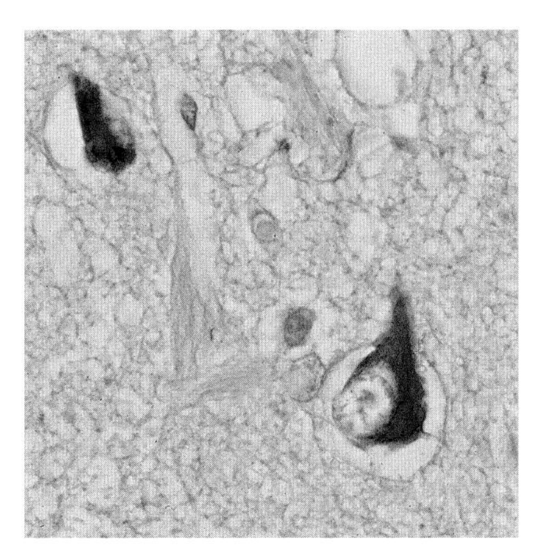

Figure 4. A number of neurons in the cerebral cortex in PDC showed robust immunohistochemical staining for human tau protein. The extracellular ghost tangles were negative for the staining. Cited from Oyanagi et al (1999), Steinkopff Verlag with permission.

Glial inclusions. Tau-immunopositive and Gallyas-positive glial inclusions are observed in PDC. Astrocytes in amygdala, motor cortex, and inferior olivary nucleus have granular hazy inclusions (Figure 7) (39, 44). Crescent or coiled shaped inclusions are present in the oligodendroglia of the anterior nucleus of the thalamus, motor cortex, midbrain tegmentum, and medullary pyramids (39, 44).

Immunohistochemistry and Ultrastructural Findings

Like NFTs in AD, NFTs of Guam PDC are immunoreactive for tau (Figure 4) and ubiquitin (6, 23, 33, 44, 52). In areas with severe pathology (eg, hippocampus) many of the NFTs are extracellular and have additional immunoreactivity, including apolipoprotein-E, amyloid P component, Aβ40, and complement factor C4d (53-55). The extracellular NFT are also frequently associated with neuritic clusters (56) and a prominent microglial and astrocytic reaction (53, 55). Based upon immunohistochemical studies of NFTs with tau and amyloid P component antibodies and neuronal counts, it is estimated that the majority of neurons that die in the hippocampus in PDC go through a NFT stage.

At the ultrastructural level NFTs in cerebrum and spinal cord are mostly composed of paired helical filaments (PHFs) and some straight filaments (SFs) similar to NFTs in AD (Figure 5) (17, 25, 40, 41, 44). NFTs in the spinal cord of PDC and PDC-ALS patients were mostly composed of SFs (41).

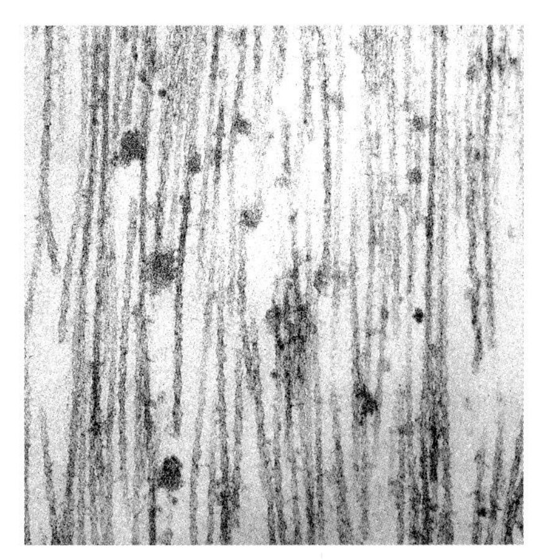

Figure 5. Electron micrograph of neurofibrillary tangles (NFTs) in a neuron in the subiculum of a PDC patient. The NFTs are composed mainly of 11- to 25-nm-wide paired helical filaments (PHFs) with a periodicity of 63 to 87 nm. Uranyl acetate-lead citrate.

Biochemistry

Brain homogenates subjected to western blot studies show that abnormal tau protein in Guam PDC is composed of a major tau triplet, with molecular weights of 68, 64, and 55 kDa with and a minor variant at 74 kDa (5, 34) consistent with a mixture of 3 repeat (3R) and 4 repeat (4R) tau. This is the same pattern as in AD and is different from the 4R in progressive supranuclear palsy (PSP). Examination of antibodies specific to multiple phospho-epitopes in tau showed great similarity between AD and Guam PDC. Western blots of spinal cord samples revealed similar tau abnormalities (51).

Analysis of choline acetyl transferase levels in postmortem tissue shows deficits comparable to those found in AD (31), which correlate with evidence of neuronal loss in the basal nucleus of Meynert.

Using x-ray microprobe or laser microprobe methods to study NFTs in Guam PDC reveals high concentrations of aluminum (Al), calcium (Ca) and iron (Fe) (15, 24, 46) with Al levels higher than in AD (46).

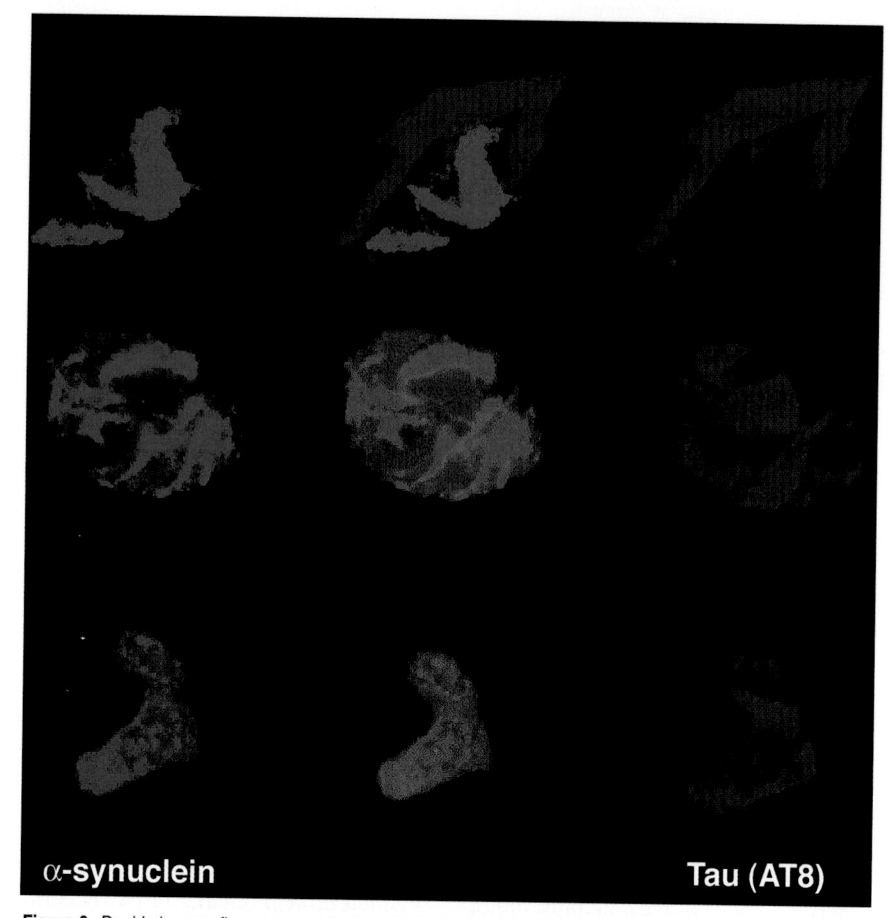

Figure 6. Double immunofluorescence labeling with AT8 (Alexa 594: red) and α-synuclein #17 (Alexa 488: green) showed that many α-synuclein-positive inclusions coexisted with NFTs in the same neurons in the amygdaloid nucleus of a patient with Guam PDC. *i)* α-synuclein-positive inclusions were intermingled with NFTs; *ii)* α-synuclein-positive inclusions were covered by a thin, tau-positive layer; and *iii)* a small number of pretangles/NFTs were encapsulated by an α-synuclein-positive thin shell.

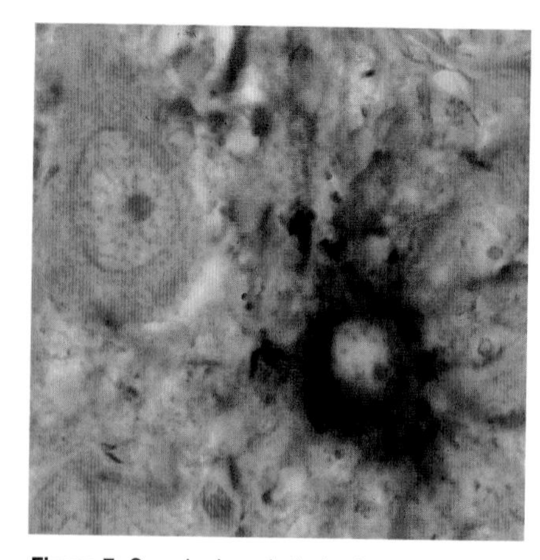

Figure 7. Granular hazy inclusion in an astrocyte in the motor cortex of a patient with PDC. Double staining involving Gallyas preparation (black) and glial fibrillary acidic protein immunostaining (brown).

Differential Diagnosis

Disorders of the elderly exhibiting dementia and movement disorders with widespread NFTs and glial tangles composed of abnormally phosphorylated tau proteins are in the differential diagnosis given the clinical history. Guam PDC has not been described in western societies, but cases of PDC on Kii Peninsula in Japan have many similarities (28). The major differential includes progressive supranuclear palsy (PSP), corticobasal degeneration (CBD), postencephalitic Parkinsonism (PEP), frontotemporal dementia and Parkinsonism linked to chromosome 17 (FTDP-17).

The predominance of NFTs with relatively few neuropil threads and glial tangles in Guam PDC are different from the widespread occurrence of numerous threads and glial tangles in the gray and white matter in PSP, CBD and FTDP-17. The minimal neuronal loss in the subthalamic nucleus, absence of grumose degeneration in the cerebellar dentate nucleus and rare tufted-astrocytes help to differentiate Guam PDC from PSP. The absence of astrocytic plaques and ballooned neurons, and the relatively small number of pretangles and foamy axonal spheroids help differentiate Guam PDC from CBD (26, 43). Thorn-shaped tau-positive astrocytes have been reported to be restricted to within the third ventricle wall and around the cerebral aqueduct in PEP, but these lesions can also be found in non-tauopathies and lack specificity (21). In contrast, the granular hazy astrocytic inclusions have been exclusively reported in Guam PDC.

Pathogenesis

Despite decades of research, the etiology and pathogenesis of Guam PDC remains unknown. Environmental factor(s), such as low Mg and Ca and high Al intake (64), and some plant neurotoxins (from cycad flour) (58), and a certain genetic predisposition (48) have been proposed. When PDC and controls are carefully screened for metabolic and disorders of mineral metabolism, there has been no compelling evidence to support the calcium/heavy metal hypothesis (2).

Experimental Models

Based on the possible pathogenesis proposed, experimental studies focusing on low Mg and Ca and high Al and on plant neurotoxins have been explored; however, no animal model completely recapiltulates Guam PDC. Repeated oral administration of α-amino-β-methylaminopropionic acid (L-BMAA), the proposed toxic factor within cycad flour, to macaques produces chromatolysis of Betz cells, simple atrophy of spinal anterior horn cells and neuritic swelling in the substantia nigra (58). A low-Ca, high-Al diet in monkeys induces neurofibrillary pathology characterised by accumulation of phosphorylated neurofilaments in anterior horn cells (14). Loss of dopaminergic neurons in the substantia nigra is observed in rats with long duration exposure of low Mg intake over two generations (38).

Future Directions and Therapy

Extensive long-range studies on Guam PDC have led to the idea of exogenous cause(s) of the disease possibly in combination with some aspects of the genetic background. Further studies on Guam PDC are needed to determine causative factors and the pathogenetic mechanisms of neurodegeneration, which will provide rational therapeutic strategies for the tauopathies.

References

1. Ahlskog JE, Petersen RC, Waring SC, Esteban-Santillan C, Craig UK, Maraganore DM, Lennon VA, Kurland LT (1997) Guamanian neurodegenerative disease: are diabetes mellitus and altered humoral immunity clues to pathogenesis? *Neurology* 48: 1356-1362.

2. Ahlskog JE, Waring SC, Kurland LT, Petersen RC, Moyer TP, Harmsen WS, Maraganore DM, O'Brien PC, Esteban-Santillan C, Bush V (1995) Guamanian neurodegenerative disease: investigation of the calcium metabolism/heavy metal hypothesis. *Neurology* 45: 1340-1344.

3. Ahlskog JE, Waring SC, Petersen RC, Esteban-Santillan C, Craig UK, O'Brien PC, Plevak MF, Kurland LT (1998) Olfactory dysfunction in Guamanian ALS, parkinsonism, and dementia. *Neurology* 51: 1672-1677.

4. Anderson FH, Richardson EP, Jr., Okazaki H, Brody JA (1979) Neurofibrillary degeneration on Guam: frequency in Chamorros and non Chamorros with no known neurological disease. *Brain* 102: 65-77.

5. Buée L, Delacourte A (1999) Comparative biochemistry of tau in progressive supranuclear palsy, corticobasal degeneration, FTDP-17 and Pick's disease. *Brain Pathol* 9: 681-693.

6. Buée L, Perez-Tur J, Leveugle B, Buée-Scherrer V, Mufson EJ, Loerzel AJ, Chartier-Harlin MC, Perl DP, Delacourte A, Hof PR (1996) Apolipoprotein E in Guamanian amyotrophic lateral sclerosis/parkinsonism-dementia complex: genotype analysis and relationships to neuropathological changes. *Acta Neuropathol* 91: 247-253

7. Campbell RJ, Steele JC, Cox TA, Loerzel AJ, Belli M, Belli DD, Kurland LT (1993) Pathologic findings in the retinal pigment epitheliopathy associated with the amyotrophic lateral sclerosis/parkinsonism-dementia complex of Guam. *Ophthalmology* 100: 37-42.

8. Chen KM, Chase TN (1985) Parkinsonism-dementia. *Handb Clin Neurol* 49: 167-183.

9. Chen X, Xia Y, Gresham LS, Molgaard CA, Thomas RG, Galasko D, Wiederholt WC, Saitoh T (1996) ApoE and CYP2D6 polymorphism with and without parkinsonism-dementia complex in the people of Chamorro, Guam. *Neurology* 47: 779-784.

10. Conrad C, Andreadis A, Trojanowski JQ, Dickson DW, Kang D, Chen X, Wiederholt W, Hansen L, Masliah E, Thal LJ, Katzman R, Xia Y, Saitoh T (1997) Genetic evidence for the involvement of tau in progressive supranuclear palsy. *Ann Neurol* 41: 277-281.

11. Cox TA, McDarby JV, Lavine L, Steele JC, Calne DB (1989) A retinopathy on Guam with high prevalence in Lytico-Bodig. *Ophthalmology* 96: 1731-1735.

12. Doty RL, Perl DP, Steele JC, Chen KM, Pierce JD, Jr., Reyes P, Kurland LT (1991) Odor identification deficit of the parkinsonism-dementia complex of Guam: equivalence to that of Alzheimer's and idiopathic Parkinson's disease. *Neurology* 41: 77-80; discussion 80-71.

13. Garruto RM, Gajdusek DC, Chen KM (1981) Amyotrophic lateral sclerosis and parkinsonism-dementia among Filipino migrants to Guam. *Ann Neurol* 10: 341-350.

14. Garruto RM, Shankar SK, Yanagihara R, Salazar AM, Amyx HL, Gajdusek DC (1989) Low-calcium, high-aluminum diet-induced motor neuron pathology in cynomolgus monkeys. *Acta Neuropathol* 78: 210-219

15. Garruto RM, Yanagihara R, Gajdusek DC (1985) Disappearance of high-incidence amyotrophic lateral sclerosis and parkinsonism-dementia on Guam. *Neurology* 35: 193-198.

16. Goto S, Hirano A, Matsumoto S (1990) Immunohistochemical study of the striatal efferents and nigral dopaminergic neurons in parkinsonism-dementia complex on Guam in comparison with those in Parkinson's and Alzheimer's diseases. *Ann Neurol* 27: 520-527.

17. Hirano A, Dembitzer HM, Kurland LT, Zimmerman HM (1968) The fine structure of some intraganglionic alterations. Neurofibrillary tangles, granulovacuolar bodies and "rod-like" structures as seen in Guam amyotrophic lateral sclerosis and parkinsonism-dementia complex. *J Neuropathol Exp Neurol* 27: 167-182.

18. Hirano A, Kurland LT, Krooth RS, Lessell S (1961) Parkinsonism-dementia complex, an endemic disease on Guam. II Pathological features. *Brain* 84: 622-631

19. Hirano A, Malamud N, Elizan TS, Kurland LT (1966) Amyotrophic lateral sclerosis and Parkinsonism-dementia complex on Guam. Further pathologic studies. *Arch Neurol* 15: 35-51.

20. Hof PR, Perl DP, Loerzel AJ, Morrison JH (1991) Neurofibrillary tangle distribution in the cerebral cortex of parkinsonism-dementia cases from Guam: differences with Alzheimer's disease. *Brain Res* 564: 306-313.

21. Ikeda K, Akiyama H, Kondo H, Haga C, Tanno E, Tokuda T, Ikeda S (1995) Thorn-shaped astrocytes: possibly secondarily induced tau-positive glial fibrillary tangles. *Acta Neuropathol* 90: 620-625.

22. Ito H, Hirano H, Yen SH, Kato S (1991) Demonstration of beta amyloid protein-containing neurofibrillary tangles in parkinsonism-dementia complex on Guam. *Neuropathol Appl Neurobiol* 17: 365-373.

23. Joachim CL, Morris JH, Kosik KS, Selkoe DJ (1987) Tau antisera recognize neurofibrillary tangles in a range of neurodegenerative disorders. *Ann Neurol* 22: 514-520.

24. Kasarskis EJ, Tandon L, Lovell MA, Ehmann WD (1995) Aluminum, calcium, and iron in the spinal cord of patients with sporadic amyotrophic lateral sclerosis using laser microprobe mass spectroscopy: a preliminary study. *J Neurol Sci* 130: 203-208.

25. Kato S, Hirano A, Llena JF, Ito H, Yen SH (1992) Ultrastructural identification of neurofibrillary tangles in the spinal cords in Guamanian amyotrophic lateral sclerosis and parkinsonism- dementia complex on Guam. *Acta Neuropathol* 83: 277-282

26. Komori T (1999) Tau-positive glial inclusions in progressive supranuclear palsy, corticobasal degeneration and Pick's disease. *Brain Pathol* 9: 663-679.

27. Kurland LT, Mulder DW (1954) Epidemiologic investigations of amyotrophic lateral sclerosis. Part 1. Preliminary report on geographic distribution, with special reference to the Mariana Islands, including clinical and pathological observations. *Neurology* 4: 355-378, 438-448.

28. Kuzuhara S, Kokubo Y, Sasaki R, Narita Y, Yabana T, Hasegawa M, Iwatsubo T (2001) Familial amyotrophic lateral sclerosis and parkinsonism-dementia complex of the Kii Peninsula of Japan: clinical and neuropathological study and tau analysis. *Ann Neurol* 49: 501-511.

29. Low PA, Ahlskog JE, Petersen RC, Waring SC, Esteban-Santillan C, Kurland LT (1997) Autonomic failure in Guamanian neurodegenerative disease. *Neurology* 49: 1031-1034.

30. Malamud N, Hirano A, Kurland LT (1961) Pathoanatomic changes in amytrophic lateral sclerosis on Guam. *Arch Neurol* 5: 301-311

31. Masliah E, Alford M, Galasko D, Salmon D, Hansen LA, Good PF, Perl DP, Thal L (2001) Cholinergic deficits in the brains of patients with parkinsonism- dementia complex of Guam. *Neuroreport* 12: 3901-3903.

32. Masullo C, Pocchiari M, Mariotti P, Macchi G, Garruto RM, Gibbs CJ, Jr., Yanagihara R, Gajdusek DC (1989) The nucleus basalis of Meynert in parkinsonism-dementia of Guam: a morphometric study. *Neuropathol Appl Neurobiol* 15: 193-206.

33. Matsumoto S, Hirano A, Goto S (1990) Spinal cord neurofibrillary tangles of Guamanian amyotrophic lateral sclerosis and parkinsonism-dementia complex: an immunohistochemical study. *Neurology* 40: 975-979.

34. Mawal-Dewan M, Schmidt ML, Balin B, Perl DP, Lee VM, Trojanowski JQ (1996) Identification of phosphorylation sites in PHF-TAU from patients with Guam amyotrophic lateral sclerosis/parkinsonism-dementia complex. *J Neuropathol Exp Neurol* 55: 1051-1059.

35. Morris HR, Al-Sarraj S, Schwab C, Gwinn-Hardy K, Perez-Tur J, Wood NW, Hardy J, Lees AJ, McGeer PL, Daniel SE, Steele JC (2001) A clinical and pathological study of motor neurone disease on Guam. *Brain* 124: 2215-2222.

36. Murakami N (1999) Parkinsonism-dementia complex on Guam - overview of clinical aspects. *J Neurol* 246 Suppl 2: II16-18.

37. Nakano I, Hirano A (1983) Neuron loss in the nucleus basalis of Meynert in parkinsonism-dementia complex of Guam. *Ann Neurol* 13: 87-91.

38. Oyanagi K, Kawakami E, Kikuchi K, Ohara K, Ogata K, Wada M, Kihira T, Yasui M (2002) Degeneration of substantia nigra in magnesium deficiency in rats for two generations. *J Neuropathol Exp Neurol* 61: 461.

39. Oyanagi K, Makifuchi T, Ohtoh T, Chen KM, Gajdusek DC, Chase TN (1997) Distinct pathological features of the gallyas- and tau-positive glia in the Parkinsonism-dementia complex and amyotrophic lateral sclerosis of Guam. *J Neuropathol Exp Neurol* 56: 308-316.

40. Oyanagi K, Makifuchi T, Ohtoh T, Chen KM, Gajdusek DC, Chase TN, Ikuta F (1994) The neostriatum and nucleus accumbens in parkinsonism-dementia complex of Guam: a pathological comparison with Alzheimer's disease and progressive supranuclear palsy. *Acta Neuropathol* 88: 122-128.

41. Oyanagi K, Makifuchi T, Ohtoh T, Chen KM, van der Schaaf T, Gajdusek DC, Chase TN, Ikuta F (1994) Amyotrophic lateral sclerosis of Guam: the nature of the neuropathological findings. *Acta Neuropathol* 88: 405-412.

42. Oyanagi K, Makifuchi T, Ohtoh T, Ikuta F, Chen KM, Chase TN, Gajdusek DC (1994) Topographic investigation of brain atrophy in parkinsonism-dementia complex of Guam: a comparison with Alzheimer's disease and progressive supranuclear palsy. *Neurodegeneration* 3: 301-304.

43. Oyanagi K, Tsuchiya K, Yamazaki M, Ikeda K (2001) Substantia nigra in progressive supranuclear palsy, corticobasal degeneration, and parkinsonism-dementia complex of Guam: specific pathological features. *J Neuropathol Exp Neurol* 60: 393-402.

44. Oyanagi K, Wada M (1999) Neuropathology of parkinsonism-dementia complex and amyotrophic lateral sclerosis of Guam: an update. *J Neurol* 246 Suppl 2: II19-27.

45. Perez-Tur J, Buee L, Morris HR, Waring SC, Onstead L, Wavrant-De Vrieze F, Crook R, Buee-Scherrer V, Hof PR, Petersen RC, McGeer PL, Delacourte A, Hutton M, Siddique T, Ahlskog JE, Hardy J, Steele JC (1999) Neurodegenerative diseases of Guam: analysis of TAU. *Neurology* 53: 411-413.

46. Perl DP, Gajdusek DC, Garruto RM, Yanagihara RT, Gibbs CJ (1982) Intraneuronal aluminum accumulation in amyotrophic lateral sclerosis and Parkinsonism-dementia of Guam. *Science* 217: 1053-1055.

47. Plato CC, Garruto RM, Fox KM, Gajdusek DC (1986) Amyotrophic lateral sclerosis and parkinsonism-dementia on Guam: a 25- year prospective case-control study. *Am J Epidemiol* 124: 643-656.

48. Poorkaj P, Tsuang D, Wijsman E, Steinbart E, Garruto RM, Craig UK, Chapman NH, Anderson L, Bird TD, Plato CC, Perl DP, Weiderholt W, Galasko D, Schellenberg GD (2001) TAU as a susceptibility gene for amyotropic lateral sclerosis- parkinsonism dementia complex of Guam. *Arch Neurol* 58: 1871-1878.

49. Reed DM, Brody JA (1975) Amyotrophic lateral sclerosis and parkinsonism-dementia on Guam, 1945- 1972. I. Descriptive epidemiology. *Am J Epidemiol* 101: 287-301.

50. Schmidt ML, Lee VM, Saido T, Perl D, Schuck T, Iwatsubo T, Trojanowski JQ (1998) Amyloid plaques in Guam amyotrophic lateral sclerosis/parkinsonism-dementia complex contain species of A beta similar to those found in the amyloid plaques of Alzheimer's disease and pathological aging. *Acta Neuropathol (Berl)* 95: 117-122.

51. Schmidt ML, Zhukareva V, Perl DP, Sheridan SK, Schuck T, Lee VM, Trojanowski JQ (2001) Spinal cord neurofibrillary pathology in Alzheimer disease and Guam Parkinsonism-dementia complex. *J Neuropathol Exp Neurol* 60: 1075-1086.

52. Schwab C, Steele JC, Akiyama H, McGeer EG, McGeer PL (1995) Relationship of amyloid beta/A4 protein to the neurofibrillary tangles in Guamanian parkinsonism-dementia. *Acta Neuropathol* 90: 287-298.

53. Schwab C, Steele JC, Akiyama H, McGeer PL (1996) Distinct distribution of apolipoprotein E and beta-amyloid immunoreactivity in the hippocampus of Parkinson dementia complex of Guam. *Acta Neuropathol (Berl)* 92: 378-385.

54. Schwab C, Steele JC, McGeer EG, McGeer PL (1997) Amyloid P immunoreactivity precedes C4d deposition on extracellular neurofibrillary tangles. *Acta Neuropathol (Berl)* 93: 87-92.

55. Schwab C, Steele JC, McGeer PL (1996) Neurofibrillary tangles of Guam parkinson-dementia are associated with reactive microglia and complement proteins. *Brain Res* 707: 196-205.

56. Schwab C, Steele JC, McGeer PL (1997) Dystrophic neurites are associated with early stage extracellular neurofibrillary tangles in the parkinsonism-dementia complex of Guam. *Acta Neuropathol (Berl)* 94: 486-492.

57. Snow BJ, Peppard RF, Guttman M, Okada J, Martin WR, Steele J, Eisen A, Carr G, Schoenberg B, Calne D (1990) Positron emission tomographic scanning demonstrates a presynaptic dopaminergic lesion in Lytico-Bodig. The amyotrophic lateral sclerosis-parkinsonism-dementia complex of Guam. *Arch Neurol* 47: 870-874.

58. Spencer PS, Nunn PB, Hugon J, Ludolph AC, Ross SM, Roy DN, Robertson RC (1987) Guam amyotrophic lateral sclerosis-parkinsonism-dementia linked to a plant excitant neurotoxin. *Science* 237: 517-522.

59. Tashiro K, Okumura H, Moriwaka F, Chen K-M, Kurland LT (1995) Recent epidemiologic study of amyotrophic lateral sclerosis (ALS) and parkinsonism-dementia complex (PDC) in Guam island. *Annual report of the research committee of CNS degenerative diseases, the Ministry of Health and Welfare of Japan*: 174-176.

60. Wada M, Uchihara T, Nakamura A, Oyanagi K (1999) Bunina bodies in amyotrophic lateral sclerosis on Guam: a histochemical, immunohistochemical and ultrastructural investigation. *Acta Neuropathol (Berl)* 98: 150-156.

61. Wakayama I, Kihira T, Yoshida S, Garruto RM (1993) Rare neuropil threads in amyotrophic lateral sclerosis and parkinsonism- dementia on Guam and in the Kii Peninsula of Japan. *Dementia* 4: 75-80.

62. Yamazaki M, Arai Y, Baba M, Iwatsubo T, Mori O, Katayama Y, Oyanagi K (2000) Alpha-synuclein inclusions in amygdala in the brains of patients with the parkinsonism-dementia complex of Guam. *J Neuropathol Exp Neurol* 59: 585-591.

63. Yanagihara RT, Garruto RM, Gajdusek DC (1983) Epidemiological surveillance of amyotrophic lateral sclerosis and parkinsonism-dementia in the Commonwealth of the Northern Mariana Islands. *Ann Neurol* 13: 79-86.

64. Yase Y (1978) ALS in the Kii peninsula: one possible etiological hypothesis. In *Amyotrophic Lateral Sclerosis*, T. Tsubaki, Y Toyokura (eds.), University of Tokyo Press: Tokyo. pp. 307-318.

Postencephalitic Parkinsonism

James M. Henry
Kurt A. Jellinger

This chapter is dedicated to Dr Kenneth M. Earle, Chairman Department of Neuropathology, Armed Forces Institute of Pathology, 1962-1982.

AD	Alzheimer's disease
AFIP	American Forces Institute of Pathology
ALS-PDC	amyotrophic lateral sclerosis-parkinsonism/dementia complex of Guam
APP	amyloid precursor protein
CBD	corticobasal degeneration
EL	encephalitis lethargica
GFT	glial fibrillary tangle
IPD	idiopathic Parkinson's disease
LB	Lewy body
LBI	Ludwig Boltzman Institute
LC	locus coeruleus
NFT	neurofibrillary tangle
PCR	polymerase chain reaction
PEP	postencephalitic parkinsonism
PHF	paired helical filament
pNFP	phosphorylated neurofilament protein
PSP	progressive supranuclear palsy
SN	substantia nigra
ST	straight tubule

Definition

Postencephalitic parkinsonism (PEP) is a progressive neurodegenerative disease with clinical features referable mainly to the extrapyramidal and oculomotor systems. It represents a chronic complication of *encephalitis lethargica* (EL), and clinically resembles idiopathic Parkinson's disease (IPD), with which it may be confused. It shares histopathological features with other tauopathies and is characterised by tau-positive neurofibrillary tangles (NFTs) that have biochemical and ultrastructure features similar to Alzheimer disease (AD).

Synonyms and Historical Background

EL and PEP emerged mysteriously during and after the First World War, only to wane and disappear in subsequent decades, with the exception of occasional case reports of sporadic PEP (34, 41). Constantin von Economo, a Viennese neurologist, first described a hitherto unknown variant of acute encephalitis, originally designated by him as *encephalitis lethargica* and subsequently titled as *von Economo's encephalitis, von Economo's disease* or *sleep sickness* (9, 48). PEP refers to the most frequent chronic complication of acute EL. Von Economo's original description comprised 6 clinical cases observed in Vienna during the winter of 1915 to 1916, including 2 autopsies (9-11). The disease subsequently spread throughout Europe and North America in epidemic and pandemic proportions, subsiding in 1924 to 1925, and disappeared from the medical scene as mysteriously as it had emerged.

The neurological manifestations of acute EL were polymorphic, thus leading von Economo to classify the protean symptom complex into 3 clinical categories: the *somnolent-ophthalmoplegic form*, characterised by profound lethargy (*sleep sickness*) and ophthalmoplegia; the *hyperkinetic form*, reflecting intense restlessness, a frenzied mental state, choreiform movements, inverted sleep patterns, and ophthalmoplegia; and the *amyostatic-akinetic variant* with external ophthalmoplegia, bradykinesia, and rigidity, resembling an acute form of parkinsonism (10, 11). The mortality rate for acute EL often approached 40% and residual morbidity, in the form of chronic complications, was common. About one-third of patients died in the acute phase, one third survived with chronic disability, and one-third recovered, many of whom developed PEP following a latency of months to years (17). Repeated pandemics of a particularly virulent and lethal strain of influenza virus occurred contemporaneously, although not simultaneously, with acute EL during and after the First World War. Von Economo recognised the relatively noninfectious and nontransmissible nature of EL, in contrast to the highly infectious character of influenza, and denied an aetiological relationship between the 2 diseases, stating the EL represented a unique, new disease, distinct from influenza. His hypothesis was ignored by subsequent neuroscientists who, no longer familiar with the clinical aspects of EL, postulated aetiological commonality (6, 12, 13, 26, 40, 45). As epidemic EL disappeared by 1925, cases of chronic PEP flooded the clinical scene until the late 1930s, mimicking IPD. Although PEP, like EL, was associated with mortality rates approaching 40%, residual survivors often survived into old age (5, 17, 44, 48). Although sporadic cases of PEP are occasionally reported, they should be viewed with circumspection, particularly in the absence of a prior history of EL, due to clinico-pathological overlap phenomena with other tauopathies (17, 21, 22, 30, 31, 48).

Epidemiology

Incidence and prevalence. Morbidity and mortality statistics for EL and PEP were maintained only in England and the United States (39). The onset of EL in England was reported in 1918, with annual recurrences, resulting in a peak of 1470 cases in 1921, followed by recession and ultimate disappearance of the disease in 1925. The total number of acute EL cases in England was about 5500 from 1919 to 1924, in association with a mortality rate of about 40%. Although accurate statistics were not available for other European countries, the total number of EL cases throughout Europe during this period is estimated at approximately

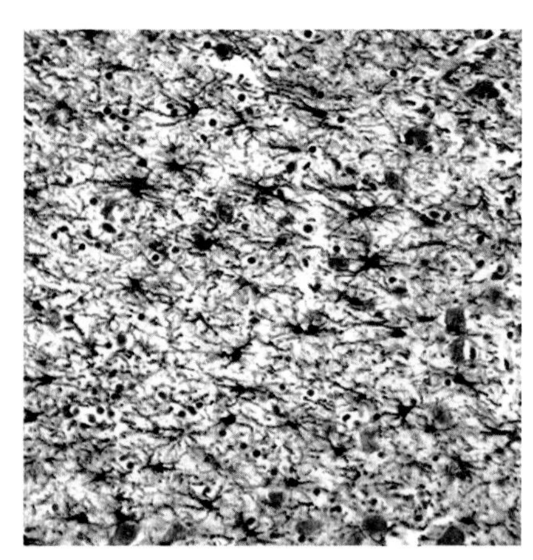

Figure 1. Diffuse reactive astrogliosis in colliculi. ×200

100 000. Acute EL made its initial US debut in New York, in autumn of 1918, and spread rapidly westward, peaking in 1922 and disappearing by 1924. The total number of cases is estimated at 25 000 to 40 000, contingent on the accuracy of the clinical diagnosis, with a mortality rate of 30 to 40%.

After the disappearance of EL, chronic cases of PEP continued to soar from 1925 to 1938, representing almost 50% of all cases or parkinsonism diagnosed at that time. The high mortality rate of about 40% resulted in approximately 15 000 PEP-related deaths from 1925 to 1938. Later on, the incidence of PEP in the literature was considered to range from 4% to 30% with a means of 13% of all cases of parkinsonism, while in recent autopsy series, its incidence dropped from 6% (1957-1970) to zero in the last decade (32).

Sex and age distribution. No gender bias was noted. Acute EL and chronic PEP involved a much younger population than IPD, ranging from 20 to 40 years of age, in addition to childhood cases.

Risk factors. With the exception of pandemic influenza as a positive risk factor, the aetiology of EL and PEP remains undetermined and definite risk factors cannot be ascertained.

Genetics

There is no known genetic factor associated with EL or PEP, which resembles an infectious disease with a low degree of interpersonal transmissibility, analogous to the epidemiological profile of an arbovirus disease.

Clinical Features

Signs and symptoms. The clinical features of PEP presenting with bradykinesia, rigidity, hypomimia, postural instability, gait disturbances with falls, and sialorhoea. Although similar to IPD, PEP shows significant differential parameters: *i)* onset of symptoms in a younger age group, including children and adults aged 25 to 40 years; *ii)* rare occurrence of the characteristic resting tremor of IPD; *iii)* progression of the disease in discontinuous spurts; *iv)* ophthalmoplegia and oculogyric crises; and *v)* a prior history of acute EL (38, 40-48). Patients may variably respond to levodopa therapy (17, 48). Elderly PEP patients may continue to suffer from progressive deterioration of motor function with dysphagia, incontinence, levodopa-induced psychoses and depression, rare pyramidal signs, dystonia, and cognitive deterioration (17, 27, 48).

Imaging. MRI studies in EL have shown bilateral hyperintense lesions of the substantia nigra (SN) (47), and may have atrophy of the SN, corresponding to the gross morphological findings in PEP. Recent PET studies revealed a bilateral reduction of ^{18}F-DOPA in the striatum with striatal glucose hypermetabolism, different from the findings in IPD (5, 18).

Laboratory findings. There are no specific or diagnostic laboratory findings or disease markers but some patients with suspected PEP have oligoclonal IgG bands in CSF (18).

Macroscopy

The gross pathological findings of acute EL are nonspecific, including oedema, hyperaemia, and occasional petechial haemorrhages. In PEP, the brain shows depigmentation and atrophy of the pigmented brainstem nuclei, particularly the SN and, to a lesser degree, the locus coeruleus (LC). The degree of depigmentation in the SN is more severe than in IPD (2, 19).

Histopathology

The microscopical appearance of acute and subacute EL shows leptomeningeal and parenchymal perivascular lympho-plasmocytic infiltrates, with scattered foci of acute neuronal injury manifested by neuronophagia in the absence of inclusions of demonstrable organisms, most severely involving the brainstem (2, 4, 9, 34, 39).

Although originally considered as a focal disease, due to the prominent and severe degeneration of the SN, PEP is now considered a multisystem tauopathy with widespread neuronal loss and neurodegeneration with widespread occurrence of tau-related lesions in neurons and glia. It thus shares histopathological features with other tauopathies, including progressive supranuclear palsy (PSP), amyotrophic lateral sclerosis-parkinsonism/dementia complex of Guam (ALS-PDC), and corticobasal degeneration (CBD).

There is marked neuronal loss and gliosis throughout the brainstem, particularly in the SN and to a lesser degree in the LC (Figure 1). No Lewy bodies (LB) are detected, but there are prominent globose NFTs in residual neurones of the SN, LC and other non-pigmented brainstem nuclei (4, 10, 11, 19, 20, 22, 32, 46, 48). Severe neuronal loss, averaging over 90% of pigmented cells in the SN, involves all parts of the pars compacta with no prevalence for the ventral tier as in IPD (31, 32). There is severe involvement of various nuclei, including the oculomotor nuclear complex, the colliculi, the midbrain raphe, the pontine tegmentum, the reticular formation, the subthalamic nucleus, amygdaloid complex and the basal nucleus of Meynert. Less severe involvement of the striopallidum, thalamus, hypothalamus, periaqueductal grey matter, ventral tegmentum, pontine base and vestibular nuclei and cerebellar dentate nucleus (Figure 2). Cortical pathology is common, with NFTs mainly in the hippocampus as well as entorhinal, temporal, frontal and insular cortices. There is relative preservation of the precentral, cingulate and parietal cortices. Within affected cortices, the prominent neurofibrillary degeneration in cortical layers II and III differs from AD, which is usually more prominent in infragranular layers (24). Involvement of the spinal cord has been described, while the cerebellum, inferior olives, and the hypoglossal and arcuate nuclei are relatively spared (17, 19, 24, 32, 45, 46). The distribution of lesions shows some similarities with PSP (17, 23, 48).

Immunohistochemistry and Ultrastructural Findings

The immunohistochemical characteristics are presented in Figures 3 to 7. The NFTs in PEP are immunoreactive for tau protein similar to AD and Guam ALS-PDC. They also show variable immunoreactivity for ubiquitin, phosphorylated neurofilament protein (pNFP), alpha-B crystallin, and amyloid precursor protein (APP) (22, 31, 42). An examination of the archival material of the AFIP and the LBI using modern immunohistochemical methods revealed diffuse dissemination of tau-immunoreactive NFTs and less frequent neuropil threads throughout the grey matter of the brainstem, with prominent involvement of the oculomotor complex, where virtually all of the remaining neurons were affected (Figure 4). Round, tau-positive and argyrophilic intraneuronal inclusions resembling Pick bodies were rarely observed in collicular neurons. LBs were not detected with ubiquitin and α-synuclein immunostains (31, 33, 48). Neurofilament immunostaining revealed diffuse neuritic pathology throughout the brainstem, manifested by fragmented and swollen neuronal processes and formation of axonal bodies, particularly evident in cross-sections of fiber tracts (Figure 6). Tau- and ubiquitin-immunoreactive crescentic, semilunar or navicular-shaped inclusions were detected within the cytoplasm of astrocytes throughout the

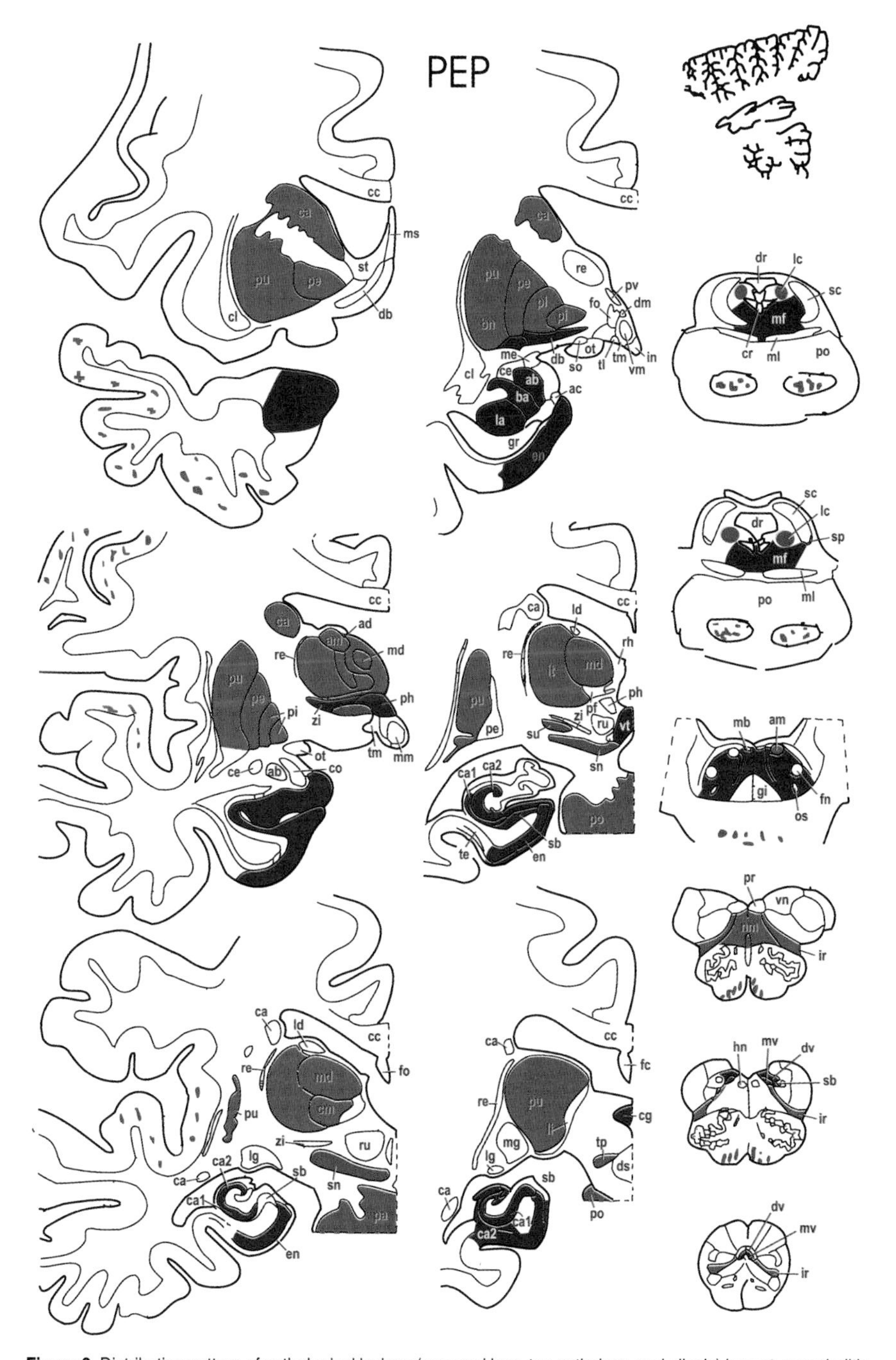

Figure 2. Distribution pattern of pathological lesions (neuronal loss, tau-pathology, and gliosis) in post-encephalitic Parkinsonism. Green = severe, red = moderate, yellow = mild lesions.

brainstem (Figure 7). Similar to glial fibrillary tangles (GFTs), although barely visible with Bodian and Bielschowsky stains, they are optimally illustrated with the Gallyas-Braak silver impregnation method. These GFTs differ from synuclein-immunoreactive glial cytoplasmic inclusions of multiple system atrophy (36). There were occasional tau-positive lesions resembling astrocytic plaques of CBD (8, 14, 29, 36) (Figure 7).

Ultrastructurally NFT in PEP are composed of 22 nm paired helical filaments (PHF) and occasional 15 nm straight tubules (ST), similar to paired helical filaments of AD. They differ histochemically and ultrastructurally from neuronal lesions in PSP, CBD and Pick's disease (3, 8, 14, 22, 28, 29, 31). Astrocytic lesions that were tau-positive and variably immunoreactive for ubiquitin are composed of 15 nm

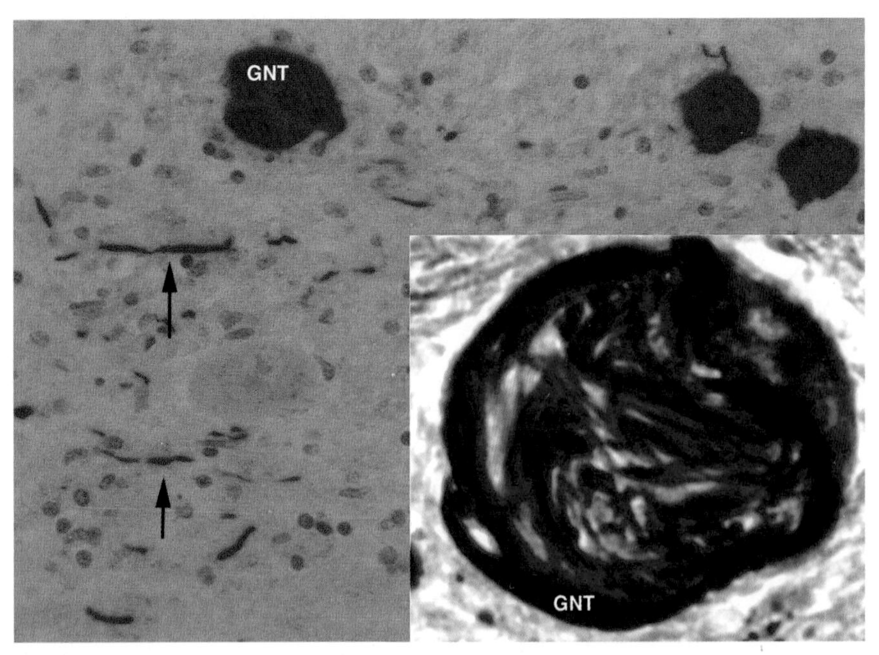

Figure 3. Globose neurofibrillary tangles (GNT) and neuropil threads (arrows) in medial substantia nigra zona compacta with diffuse astrogliosis. AT-8 antibody. ×350, inset Bodian ×600.

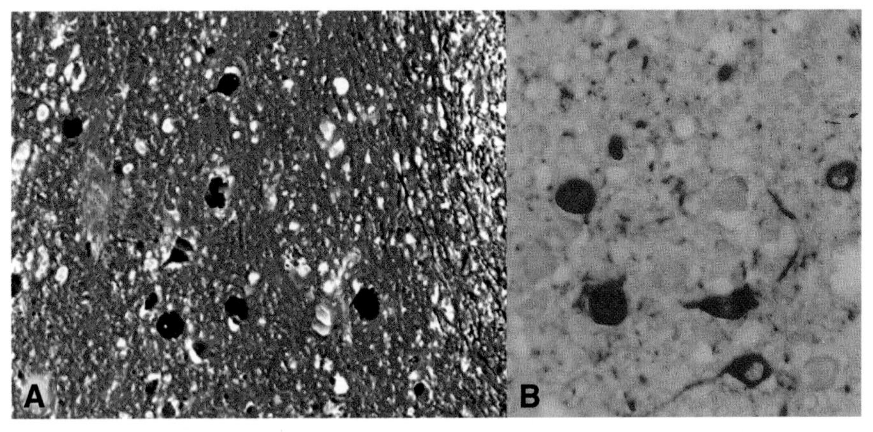

Figure 4. A. Oculomotor nucleus with multiple globose NFTs. Bielschowsky ×96. **B.** Westphal-Edlinger nucleus with multiple globose NFTs and neuropil threads. AT-8 ×200.

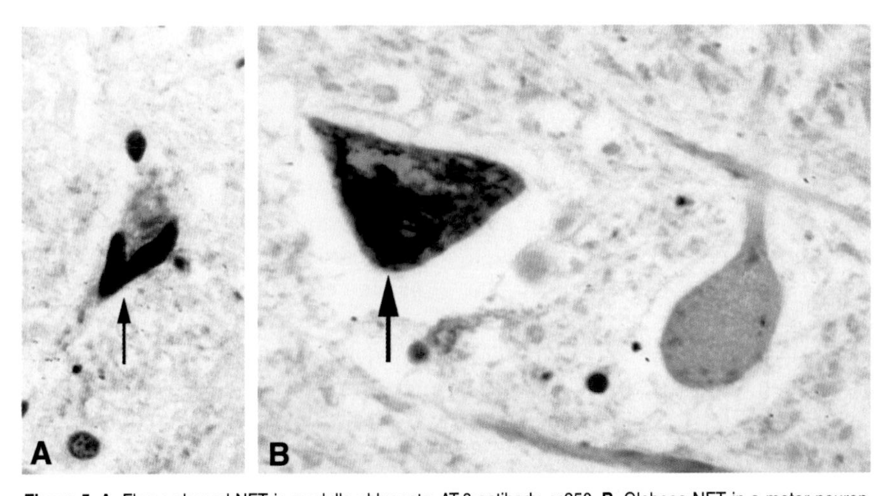

Figure 5. A. Flame-shaped NFT in medulla oblongata. AT-8 antibody, ×250. **B.** Globose NFT in a motor neuron (arrow) of cervical spinal cord. AT-8 ×640.

straight tubules and intermediate filaments (7, 22, 29, 37).

Biochemistry

The biochemistry of tau protein in PEP is essentially the same as in AD. Western blots of brain homogenates show hyperphosphorylated tau protein with three prominent bands at 55, 64 and 68 kDa. This "tau triplet" differs from 68- and 64-kDa "tau doublet" of PSP and CBD and from the 64- and 55-kDa tau doublet of Pick's disease (3, 8, 37).

The severe loss of dopaminergic neurones in the SN causes a massive depletion of dopamine in the striatum, which is more severe than in IPD. Dopamine concentrations in the putamen are reduced to 0.6% to 6% of controls and to 1.5% to 6% of controls in the caudate nucleus; in comparison dopamine concentrations are 10% to 30% of controls in IPD. There are similar, but less severe reductions of homovanillic acid (HVA) the major metabolite of dopamine (1).

Differential Diagnosis

Overlap of PEP is evident at clinical, light microscopical, immunohistochemical, and ultrastructural levels with other tauopathies, in particular with PSP and CBD, based on the lack of specificity of several parameters (15, 17, 31, 37). Both PEP and PSP share some clinical and histopathological features that often do not allow a clear distinction between these disorders. Gaze palsies with a vertical component and eyelid abnormalities, in addition to bradykinesia, rigidity, and gait disorders are prominent clinical features in both PEP and PSP which are related to similar , but not identical distribution patterns of morphological lesions (16, 17, 21, 25, 30, 31, 45, 48). In particular, the presence of NFTs in the SN and in cholinergic subcortical centers of eye movement, including the dorsal central grey nucleus, nucleus centralis pontis oralis, nucleus dorsal raphe interpositus, and the oculomotor complex (nucleus interstitialis of Cajal) may be responsible for the clinical signs of oculogyric crises, ble-

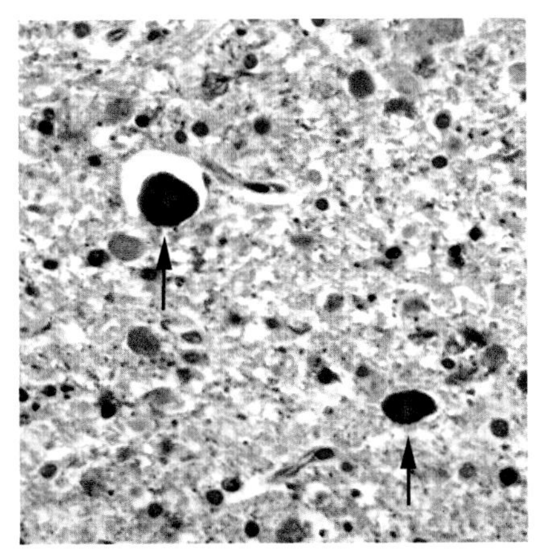

Figure 6. Swollen axonal spheroids (arrows) in brainstem. Ubiquitin ×600.

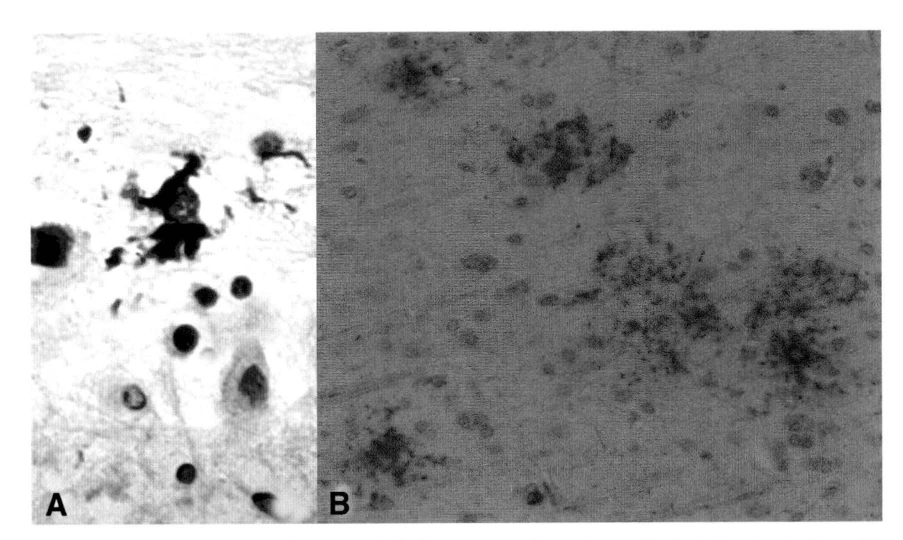

Figure 7. A. Glial fibrillary tangle in astrocyte in brainstem presenting as tau-positive inclusions in cytoplasm, AT-8 ×300. B. Tufted astrocytes and astrocytic plaques in white matter. AT-8 ×320.

pharospasm, and gaze palsy, and eye lid apraxia (21, 31, 48).

Globose NFTs are seen in other tauopathies, including PSP, Guam ALS-PD and CBD (8, 14-17, 25, 35). Although their anatomical distribution in PEP differs from these disorders (8, 23, 24, 28, 30, 31, 37, 45, 48) it does not appear possible to differentiate these disorders solely on the morphological appearance of neuronal tau pathology (15, 17, 30, 31, 48).

There are a number of distinctive differences between PEP and PSP. Clinically, PEP has a younger age onset, longer duration, and often a history of encephalitis, with bradykinesia, rigidity, resting tremor, and oculogyric crises as presenting symptoms. In contrast PSP is associated with postural instability, gait disorders, falls, and bradykinesia as presenting symptoms with later akinesia-rigidity and vertical gaze palsy. PEP is partially levodopa-responsive, while PSP is usually levodopa non-responsive. Neuropathologically, there are subtle differences in the anatomical distribution of neuronal depletion and NFTs, with only rare involvement of the red nucleus, cranial nerve nuclei IV and XII, pontine basis, inferior olives, dentate nuclei, striatum, and globus pallidus in PEP, while these nuclei are consistently affected in PSP. Cortical involvement in PEP differs from that in PSP, with comparative preservation of the precentral, cingulate, and parietal areas. In contrast to PSP there is very little tau pathology in the white matter and fewer positive astrocytes and oligodendroglia in white matter in PEP (24, 30). Biochemical and ultrastructural differences that differentiate PEP from PSP include PHF and triplet tau in PEP, while PSP has straight filaments and doublet tau.

Experimental Models

No experimental models for EL and PEP are available.

Pathogenesis

In the absence of a known aetiology of EL and its chronic complication, PEP, the elucidation of pathogenesis remains enigmatic. Hallervorden and others hypothesised that initial neuronal damage during the acute phase of EL may predispose surviving neurons to subsequent progressive degeneration, a form of "infectious abiotrophy" (20, 17). Although the specific mechanism of neuronal degeneration was unknown, the presence of globose NFTs was considered a structural manifestation of this injury. It remains undetermined whether NFTs or other inclusions in the tauopathies are causes of neuronal loss or merely a nonspecific secondary manifestation of neuronal injury due to other precipitating factors.

The association of diffuse neurofibrillary degeneration and neuritic injury as well as glial pathology in PEP in structural compartments of the brain stem that also bear the brunt of pathology in acute EL suggests a causal relationship; however, the relationship of influenza virus as the aetiologcal factor for PEP is uncertain. Recent studies using polymerase chain reaction (PCR) methodology that was successfully used to characterise the H1N1 influenza virus responsible for the influenza pandemics during and after the First World War failed to identify this virus in archival cases of either EL or PEP (39, 45). The inability to demonstrate the influenza virus in this material represents an additional step in validating von Economo's original hypothesis that acute EL was a noninfectious disease entity *sui generis*, distinct from any known complication of influenza. There is no evidence to suggest that the wild-type influenza virus, a primary resident of the respiratory tract, is capable of spontaneously developing pantropic or neurotropic features enabling it to infect the CNS.

The race between 2 teams of medical investigators to identify and characterise the influenza virus during 1918 to 1921 reads like a medical detective story and contributed to our understanding of the influenza pandemic that occurred contemporaneously with EL (35, 45); however, the relationship between influenza and EL remain enigmatic.

Future Directions and Therapy

In the absence of a known aetiological agent and the lack of contemporary disease entities due to the extinction of both EL and PEP from the contemporary scene, progress in solving the problems of pathogenesis of PEP is limited. Repository archival material represents the only source for modern investigation, but current research has failed to identify a causative or transmissible agent. It may be reasonably concluded that in reference to PEP and its relationship to other tauopathies, we are learning more and more about less and less.

References

1. Bernheimer H, Birkmayer W, Hornykiewicz O, Jellinger K, Seitelberger F (1973) Brain dopamine and the syndromes of Parkinson and Huntington. Clinical, morphological and neurochemical correlations. *J Neurol Sci* 20: 415-455.

2. Boyd W (1921) Epidemic encephalitis. *Ann Med* 1: 195-221

3. Buee-Scherrer V, Buee L, Leveugle B, Perl DP, Vermersch P, Hof PR, Delacourte A (1997) Pathological tau proteins in postencephalitic parkinsonism: comparison with Alzheimer's disease and other neurodegenerative disorders. *Ann Neurol* 42: 356-359.

4. Buzzard EF, Greenfield JG (1919) Lethargie encephalitis: its sequelae and morbid anatomy. *Brain* 42: 305-338

5. Caparros-Lefebvre D, Cabaret M, Godefroy O, Steinling M, Remy P, Samson Y, Petit H (1998) PET study and neuropsychological assessment of a long-lasting post-encephalitic parkinsonism. *J Neural Transm* 105: 489-495

6. Casals J, Elizan TS, Yahr MD (1998) Postencephalitic parkinsonism—a review. *J Neural Transm* 105: 645-676

7. Chin SS, Goldman JE (1996) Glial inclusions in CNS degenerative diseases. *J Neuropathol Exp Neurol* 55: 499-508.

8. Dickson DW (2001) Progressive supranuclear palsy and corticobasal degeneration. In *Functional Neurobiology of Aging*, RH RR., L Mobbs (eds). Academic Press: pp. 155-171

9. Economo Von C (1917) Encephalitis lethargica. *Wien Klin Wochenschr* 30: 581-583

10. Economo Von C (1929) Die Encephalitis lethargica, ihre Nachkrankheiten und ihre Behandlung. Urban & Schwarzenberg: Berlin-Wien.

11. Economo Von C (1931) *Encephalitis lethargica: Its Sequelae and Treatment.* Oxford University Press: London.

12. Elizan TS, Casals J (1991) Astrogliosis in von Economo's and postencephalitic Parkinson's diseases supports probable viral etiology. *J Neurol Sci* 105: 131-134.

13. Elizan TS, Casals J, Swash M (1989) No viral antigens detected in brain tissue from a case of acute encephalitis lethargica and another case of postencephalitic parkinsonism. *J Neurol Neurosurg Psychiatry* 52: 800-801.

14. Feany MB, Dickson DW (1995) Widespread cytoskeletal pathology characterizes corticobasal degeneration. *Am J Pathol* 146: 1388-1396.

15. Feany MB, Mattiace LA, Dickson DW (1996) Neuropathologic overlap of progressive supranuclear palsy, Pick's disease and corticobasal degeneration. *J Neuropathol Exp Neurol* 55: 53-67.

16. Gearing M, Olson DA, Watts RL, Mirra SS (1994) Progressive supranuclear palsy: neuropathologic and clinical heterogeneity. *Neurology* 44: 1015-1024.

17. Geddes JF, Hughes AJ, Lees AJ, Daniel SE (1993) Pathological overlap in cases of parkinsonism associated with neurofibrillary tangles. A study of recent cases of postencephalitic parkinsonism and comparison with progressive supranuclear palsy and Guamanian parkinsonism-dementia complex. *Brain* 116: 281-302.

18. Ghaemi M, Rudolf J, Schmulling S, Bamborschke S, Heiss WD (2000) FDG- and Dopa-PET in postencephalitic parkinsonism. *J Neural Transm* 107: 1289-1295

19. Greenfield JG, Bosanquet FD (1953) The brainstem lesions in parkinsonism. *J Neurosurg Psychiatry* 16: 213-226

20. Hallervorden J (1935) Anatomische Untersuchungen zur Pathogenese des postencephalitischen Parkinsonismus. *Dtsch Z Nervenheilk* 136: 68-77

21. Halliday GM, Hardman CD, Cordato NJ, Hely MA, Morris JG (2000) A role for the substantia nigra pars reticulata in the gaze palsy of progressive supranuclear palsy. *Brain* 123: 724-732.

22. Haraguchi T, Ishizu H, Terada S, Takehisa Y, Tanabe Y, Nishinaka T, Kawai K, Kuroda S, Komoto Y, Namba M (2000) An autopsy case of postencephalitic parkinsonism of von Economo type: some new observations concerning neurofibrillary tangles and astrocytic tangles. *Neuropathology* 20: 143-148.

23. Hauw JJ, Daniel SE, Dickson D, Horoupian DS, Jellinger K, Lantos PL, McKee A, Tabaton M, Litvan I (1994) Preliminary NINDS neuropathologic criteria for Steele-Richardson-Olszewski syndrome (progressive supranuclear palsy). *Neurology* 44: 2015-2019.

24. Hof PR, Charpiot A, Delacourte A, Buee L, Purohit D, Perl DP, Bouras C (1992) Distribution of neurofibrillary tangles and senile plaques in the cerebral cortex in postencephalitic parkinsonism. *Neurosci Lett* 139: 10-14.

25. Horoupian DS, Chu PL (1994) Unusual case of corticobasal degeneration with tau/Gallyas-positive neuronal and glial tangles. *Acta Neuropathol* 88: 592-598

26. Howard RS, Lees AJ (1987) Encephalitis lethargica. A report of four recent cases. *Brain* 110: 19-33.

27. Hudson AJ (1981) Amyotrophic lateral sclerosis and its association with dementia, parkinsonism and other neurological disorders: a review. *Brain* 104: 217-247.

28. Ikeda K, Akiyama H, Kondo H (1993) Anti-tau-positive glial fibrillary tangles in the brain of postencephalitic parkinsonism of Economo type. *Neurosci Lett* 162: 176-178.

29. Ikeda K, Akiyama H, Kondo H, Haga C, Tanno E, Tokuda T, Ikeda S (1995) Thorn-shaped astrocytes: possibly secondarily induced tau-positive glial fibrillary tangles. *Acta Neuropathol* 90: 620-625

30. Ishii T, Nakamura Y (1981) Distribution and ultrastructure of Alzheimer's neurofibrillary tangles in postencephalitic Parkinsonism of Economo type. *Acta Neuropathol* 55: 59-62

31. Jellinger KA (1999) Movement disorders with tau protein cytoskeletal pathology. *Adv Neurol* 80: 303-311

32. Jellinger KA (2001) The pathology of Parkinson's disease. *Adv Neurol* 86: 55-72

33. Josephs KA, Parisi JE, Dickson DW (2002) Alpha-synuclein studies are negative in postencephalitic parkinsonism of von Economo. *Neurology* 59: 645-646.

34. Kiley M, Esiri MM (2000) A contemporary case of encephalitis lethargica. *Clin Neuropathol* 20: 2-7

35. Kolata G (1999) *Flu: The Story of the Great Influenza Pandemic of 1918 and the Search for the Virus that Caused it.* Farrar, Straus and Giroux: New York.

36. Lantos PL (1998) The definition of multiple system atrophy: a review of recent developments. *J Neuropathol Exp Neurol* 57: 1099-1111.

37. Litvan I, Goetz CG, Lang AE (2000) Corticobasal degeneration and related disorders. *Adv Neurol* 82

38. Litvan II, Jankovic J, Goetz CG, Wenning GK, Sastry N, Jellinger K, McKee A, Lai EC, Brandel JP, Verny M, Ray-Chaudhuri K, Pearce RK, Bartko JJ, Agid Y (1998) Accuracy of the clinical diagnosis of postencephalitic parkinsonism: a clinicopathologic study. *Eur J Neurol* 5: 451-457.

39. McCall S, Henry JM, Reid AH, Taubenberger JK (2001) Influenza RNA not detected in archival brain tissue from acute encephphalitic lethargica cases of postencephalitic parkinsonism. *J Neuropathol Exp Neurol* 60: 606-704

40. Ravenholt RT, Foege WH (1982) 1918 influenza, encephalitis lethargica, parkinsonism. *Lancet* 2: 860-864.

41. Reid AH, McCall S, Henry JM, Taubenberger JK (2001) Experimenting on the past: the enigma of von Economo's encephalitis lethargica. *J Neuropathol Exp Neurol* 60: 663-670.

42. Tabaton M, Perry G, Autilio-Gambetti L, Manetto V, Gambetti P (1988) Influence of neuronal location on antigenic properties of neurofibrillary tangles. *Ann Neurol* 23: 604-610.

43. Tabaton M, Whitehouse PJ, Perry G, Davies P, Autilio-Gambetti L, Gambetti P (1988) Alz 50 recognizes abnormal filaments in Alzheimer's disease and progressive supranuclear palsy. *Ann Neurol* 24: 407-413.

44. Takahashi M, Yamada T, Nakajima S, Nakajima K, Yamamoto T, Okada H (1995) The substantia nigra is a major target for neurovirulent influenza A virus. *J Exp Med* 181: 2161-2169.

45. Taubenberger JK, Reid AH, Krafft AE, Bijwaard KE, Fanning TG (1997) Initial genetic characterization of the 1918 "Spanish" influenza virus. *Science* 275: 1793-1796.

46. Torvik A, Meen D (1966) Distribution of the brain stem lesions in postencephalitic Parkinsonism. *Acta Neurol Scand* 42: 415-425

47. Verschueren H, Crols R (2001) Bilateral substantia nigra lesions on magnetic resonance imaging in a patient with encephalitis lethargica. *J Neurol Neurosurg Psychiatry* 71: 275.

48. Wenning GK, Jellinger K, Litvan I (1997) Supranuclear gaze palsy and eyelid apraxia in postencephalitic parkinsonism. *J Neural Transm* 104: 845-865

49. Wilkins RH, Brody IA (1968) Encephalitis lethargica. *Arch Neurol* 18: 324.

Transgenic Animal Models of Tauopathies

Jada Lewis
Dennis W. Dickson

BS	brain stem
AD	Alzheimer's disease
FTDP	frontal lobe dementia and parkinsonism
GFAP	glial fbrillary acidic protein
NFT	neurofibrillary tangle
PAC	P1 artificial chromosome
SC	spinal cord
tau-ir	tau-immunoreactivity

Introduction

The discovery of mutations in the tau gene in frontotemporal dementia and parkinsonism linked to chromosome 17 (FTDP-17) (5, 12, 23, 27) has demonstrated that tau dysfunction can result in neurodegeneration and has allowed researchers to generate transgenic models of the human tauopathies (25) (Table 1). Transgenic models permit studies on the mechanisms of formation of filamentous tau lesions in neurons and glia as well as their role in neurodegeneration. They also serve as models to develop treatments for tauopathies.

The tau gene is subject to alternative splicing of three exons, which generates 6 tau isoforms (7, 8). Additional heterogeneity is derived from post-translational modifications of tau. Two exons in the amino-half of the molecule (exon 2 and exon 3) and one exon in the microtubule-binding domain (exon 10) are alternatively spliced (17). Exon 2 is included (1N) or excluded (0N), while exon 3 is always co-expressed with exon 2 (2N). Exon 10 contains a conserved repeat domain that is also present in exons 9, 11 and 12. Inclusion of exon 10 generates tau with 4 repeats (4R), while exclusion generates tau with 3 repeats (3R). The various splice combinations of tau are thus abbreviated as follows: 0N3R, 0N4R, 1N3R, 1N4R, 2N3R and 2N4R. Adult brain has all 6 isoforms, while fetal tau is composed of 3R tau (16).

Transgenic Mice Expressing Wild-type Tau Transgenes

Two tau transgenic models have been reported that overexpress the longest isoform of wild-type 4R tau (2N4R). These mice expressed the transgene up to 10-fold over the level of endogenous tau and displayed somatodendritic localisation of tau in neurons reminiscent of the "pre-tan-

Promoter	Isoform	Tau mutation	Mouse strain	Major pathologic findings	Tau antibodies used	Ref
mouse prion	0N3R	Wild-type	B6/D2	tau-ir axonal spheroids; rare NFTs in old mice	AT8, 12E8, AT270, PHF1, PHF6, T3P	13, 14
Tα1-tubulin	(0N,1N,2N)3R	Wild-type	B6/SJL	tau-ir fibrillary inclusions in glia; oligodendroglial loss with age	AT8, AT270, PHF1, PHF6, T3P	11
PAC (mouse tau)	(0N,1N,2N)3R > (0N,1N,2N)4R	Wild-type	B6/D2/SW	tau-ir pretangles & dendritic processes	MC-1	6
mouse thy-1	2N4R	Wild-type	B6/D2	axonopathy; dystrophic neurites; gliosis in brain & SC	AT8, AT180, PHF1	24
mouse thy-1	2N4R	Wild-type	FVB/N	tau-ir pretangles; axonopathy; dystrophic neurites; gliosis in brain & SC	AT8, ALZ50, PHF1, AT180, AT270, MC1	28
mouse prion	0N4R	P301L	B6/D2/SW	neuronal loss, gliosis & NFT in limbic cortex, BS & SC; tau-ir glial inclusions	AT8, ALZ50, PHF1, AT180, AT100, CP3, CP9, CP13, MC1	18
mouse thy-1	2N4R	P301L	B6/D2	tau-ir pretangles and NFT in cortex, BS & SC	AT8, AD199, AT180, MC1, TG3	9
mouse thy-1	0N4R	P301S	B6/CBA	neuronal loss, gliosis & NFT in limbic cortex, BS & SC	AT8, ALZ50, PHF1, AT180, 12E8, AT100, AP422, CP3, PG5	2
mouse prion-tTA/tetOp-tau	2N4R	G272V	B6/D2	tau-ir pretangles; tau-ir & filamentous inclusions in oligodendroglia	AT8, 12E8, AD2, TG3	10
PDGFβ	2N4R	V337M	B6/SJL	tau-ir pretangles	AT8, ALZ50, PS199	30, 31
CamKII	2N4R	R406W	B6/SJL	tau-ir pretangles & a few NFT in old mice	ALZ50, AT180, PS199, PS404	32
mouse thy-1	2N4R	G272V, P301L, R406W	B6/CBA	dystrophic neurites; tau-ir pretangles; increased lysosomal bodies	AT8, AT180	19

Table 1. Tau models.

gle" state observed in human tauopathies including Alzheimer's disease (24, 28). The 2N4R animals also showed motor disturbances in tasks involving balancing on a rod and clinging from an inverted grid. This observation was consistent with the presence of prominent axonopathy characterised by swollen axons with neurofilament, tubulin, mitochondria, and vesicles in the brains and spinal cords of these mice. Dystrophic neurites that stained with antibodies recognising hyperphosphorylated and conformational- tau epitopes (eg, Alz50) were also identified. Astrogliosis, demonstrated by glial fibrillary acidic protein (GFAP) immunoreactivity, was also observed in the cortex and spinal cord. Wild-type 4R tau transgenic mice did not, however, develop filamentous tau inclusions characteristic of neurofibrillary tangles (NFTs) and neuronal loss was not observed.

To examine the role of tau hyperphosphorylation in disease pathogenesis 2N4R wild-type tau animals were crossed with mice overexpressing glycogen synthase 3 beta (GSK3β), a possible tau protein kinase (29). These mice displayed a 2-fold increase in GSK3β activity and tau phosphorylation that surprisingly did not lead to NFTs, but instead resulted in rescue of axonopathy and motor deficits observed in the wild-type tau 2N4R transgenic mice. This observation indicates that tau hyperphosphorylation does not inevitably result in abnormal tau aggregation, although clearly GSK3β and tau hyperphosphorylation could still play a role in the pathogenesis of tauopathies.

The adult mouse brain predominantly expresses 4R tau isoforms. Therefore, Ishihara and coworkers generated transgenic mice that over express the shortest tau isoform (0N3R) to test the hypothesis that absence of 3R tau inhibits the development of neurofibrillary pathology (13). Five to 10-fold overexpression of the 0N3R wild-type transgene resulted in axonal spheroids in the spinal cord from one month of age that were immunopositive for multiple phospho-dependent tau antibodies. The spheroids also stained for neurofilament. The spinal cord inclusions in the 3R mice were argyrophilic with the Gallyas stain, but negative for thioflavin S. Binding of thioflavin S and other "congophilic" dyes to the neurofibrillary pathology in AD and other tauopathies is consistent with the presence of tau filaments with a β-sheet structure. It was therefore interesting that after 2 years of age, occasional (1-2 NFTs per mouse brain section) NFTs were observed in the hippocampus of these mice. These inclusions consisted of straight tau filaments of 10 to 20 nm diameter that did not stain with neurofilament antibodies. Additionally, insoluble tau accumulated in the brains and spinal cords of these tau mice with age. Because the NFTs were sparse and required up to two years to develop, it has been suggested that these mice represent a model of normal aging (14). It will be interesting to determine whether modifying factors can be identified that accelerate the development of neurofibrillary pathology in these mice.

In another approach to modeling tauopathy Duff and coworkers (6) created mice that expressed a P1-derived artificial chromosome (PAC) transgene containing the entire human tau gene. These mice produce all six human tau isoforms with a 3.7-fold increase total tau levels. Interestingly, in the mouse brain, splicing of the Human genomic tau transgene is altered to favor the production of exon 10-negative mRNA and 3R tau. In these mice neuronal processes and synaptic terminals were positive for human tau. With the exception of immunoreactivity with certain conformation-specific tau antibodies (eg, MC-1), these mice lacked evidence of abnormal tau pathology or behavioral changes up to 8 months of age. It is uncertain why these mice, despite relatively high tau expression levels, develop little overt pathology. One possibility is that the pattern of expression of the tau promoter is diffuse when compared with the heterologous promoters used in tau cDNA transgenic mice, preventing the accumulation of tau in specific brain regions. Alternatively, the high proportion of 3R tau generated by this transgene may be linked to the lack of pathology. Several laboratories are currently generating genomic (PAC) tau mice with FTDP-17 mutations.

Higuchi and coworkers generated transgenic mice using the Tα1-tubulin promoter to obtain 3R tau expression (11), but instead of a cDNA with 0N3R tau, they used a minigene construct that permitted expression of three human tau isoforms (0N3R, 1N3R and 2N3R). Hyperphosphorylated tau accumulated in glia and insoluble tau, extracted in formic acid, accumulated in spinal cord and cerebellum by 12 months. At 24 months of age the glial inclusions were argyrophilic and immunoelectron microscopy showed tau immunoreactive fibrils within oligodendrocyte inclusions. There was also an age-related decrease in oligodendrocytes in spinal cord.

Transgenic Mice Expressing FTDP-17-associated P301L Mutant Tau Transgenes

Overexpression of wild-type tau transgenes has had only limited success in modeling the pathology observed in the human tauopathies. As a result, several groups have generated mice that express human tau containing FTDP-17-associated mutations in an attempt to accelerate the development of neurofibrillary inclusions and other tau-related pathology.

Lewis and coworkers (18) reported a tau (P301L) transgenic mouse that expresses at about 1- to 2-fold above endogenous levels the shortest 4R tau isoform (0N4R) with the P301L mutation in exon 10. Hemizygous and homozygous animals developed motor and behavioral deficits, initially presenting with hind-limb dysfunction starting at 7 and 4.5 months, respectively. Dystonic posturing and immobility developed within 1 to 2 months of the initial symptoms. Additional features of the phenotype included docility, reduced weight, decreased vocalisation and eye irritations.

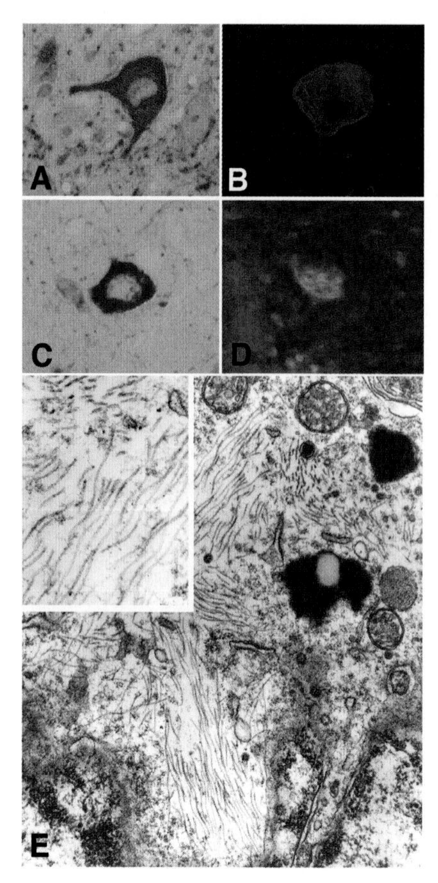

Figure 1. *Neurofibrillary tangles in transgenic (P301L) mouse.* **A.** Tau immunoreactivity, **B.** Congo-red fluorescence, **C.** Argyrophilia with Gallyas stain, **D.** Thioflavin-S fluorescence, **E.** Filamentous cytoplasmic aggregates (about 20-nm thick, wavy and straight or slightly twisted—see inset) at electron microscopy. (EM courtesy of Dr. Wen-lang Lin, Mayo Clinic Jacksonville).

The P301L tau mice developed NFTs composed of 15- to 20-nm diameter straight and wavy tau filaments that were concentrated in the spinal cord, brain stem and basal telencephalon (Figure 1). Occasional NFTs (1-2 per section) were observed in the cortex and hippocampus. Pretangles had a much wider brain distribution. The NFTs contained hyperphosphorylated tau, were congophilic and were positive with silver stains. Additionally, NFTs were negative for neurofilament and some were positive for ubiquitin. In addition to NFT, argyrophilic oligodendroglial inclusions were also detected in the spinal cord, and the glial inclusions were composed of tau-immunoreactive fibrils with electron microscopy (20). Tau-immunoreactive astrocytes were also detected, but they did not have argyrophilia and ultrastructural studies showed dispersed tau fibrils (20). Consistent with the neuropathology, the mice accumulated hyperphosphorylated tau that was insoluble after sarkosyl extraction of brain tissue including a prominent hyperphosphorylated 64 kD species that co-migrated with pathologic tau from FTDP-17 and AD patients. Associated with the neurofibrillary pathology, the P301L animals demonstrated almost 50% neuronal loss in the spinal cord (neuronal counts in other brain regions were not reported), which likely explains much of the motor dysfunction in these mice.

A second P301L tau transgenic mouse expressing the longest 4R tau isoform (2N4R) under the mouse Thy-1 promoter was described by Götz and coworkers (9). Pre-tangles and some thioflavin-S-positive neurofibrillary-like structures were identified in the cortex, brain stem, and spinal cord of 8 month-old P301L animals. Tau filaments with straight and twisted ribbon morphologies were observed in brain extracts. Additionally, astrocytosis and neuronal apoptosis, as demonstrated with terminal transferase-mediated dUTP nick end labeling (TUNEL), accompanied the tau pathology.

Transgenic Mice Expressing Other FTDP-17-associated Mutant Tau Transgenes

Similar to Christi and colleagues approach to modeling accelerated amyloid pathology in transgenic mice (4), Lim and coworkers generated transgenic mice expressing 4R2N human tau containing three different FTDP-17 mutations under the mouse Thy-1 promoter (19). These mice were termed VLW due to inclusion of the G272V, P301L and R406W mutations in the transgenic tau. Dystrophic neurites and hyperphosphorylated tau were detected in cortex and hippocampus. The lesions resembled pre-tangles in their lack of immunoreactivity with phospho-tau antibodies that recognise NFTs (phosphoserine 396/404). Electron microscopy revealed tau immunoreactive filamentous structures 2- to 8-nm in diameter that were negative for neurofilament. Presence of tau positive filaments was confirmed with ultrastructural analysis of sarkosyl insoluble tau; however, immunogold labeling with antibodies to tau phosphoepitopes was not reported in situ or in extracts. Increased lysosomal bodies were identified in the VLW animals, particularly in the neurons that were immunopositive for tau, as early as one month of age.

Tanemura and coworkers (30, 31) generated transgenic mice expressing V337M on 2N4R tau under the PDGFβ promoter. The construct contained myc and FLAG epitope tags at the amino- and carboxyl-terminal ends. Hippocampal neurons from 14-month transgenic mice displayed myc and phospho-tau immunoreactivity, which was lacking in non-transgenic littermates. The immunoreactive neurons were irregularly shaped and darkly stained with a variety of staining methods and ultrastructural studies showed organelles, lipofuscin pigment and cytoskeletal elements, but no definitive evidence of NFTs. Using a similar strategy, Tatebayashi and coworkers (32) generated transgenic mice expressing R406W mutation under the calcium calmodulin kinase-II promoter, again with myc and FLAG tags on amino and carboxyl terminal ends. Mutant tau was expressed from 7 to 18 fold over endogenous tau, and mutant tau was detected predominantly in forebrain neurons. In animals more than 18 months of age there was abnormal tau immunoreactivity in neurons, and some of the neurons had argyrophilia or weak Congo red birefringence. Ultrastructural studies showed cytoplasmic bundles of thin filaments that were different from thicker tubular fibrils that characterise human tauopathies. Transgenic animals also showed impairment in tests for contextual and cued fear conditioning.

Götz and coworkers generated transgenic mice with tetracycline-inducible expression of G272V tau under the mouse prion promotor (10). The expression was above endogenous levels and expressed in both neurons and glia. By 6 months of age thioflavin-S-positive oligodendroglial inclusions were detected in the spinal cord. The oligodendroglial inclusions were not argyrophilic with Gallyas stain, but at the electron microscopic level contained tubulofilamentous aggregates, with individual fibrils measuring 17 to 20 nm in width. Neurons formed tau-positive pretangles, but were not filamentous lesions and there was only a small amount of insoluble tau in formic acid extractable fractions.

Most recently, Allen and colleagues (2) utilised the mouse thy-1 promoter to drive expression of 0N4R human tau with the P301S mutation at approximately 2-fold the endogenous levels. Homozygous and hemizygous P301S mice developed paraparesis at approximately 6 and 12 months of age, respectively. Insoluble, hyperphosphorylated tau accumulated in the brains and spinal cords of the P301S animals that showed identical mobility to aggregated tau from human patients. Abnormally phosphorylated tau largely accumulated in nerve cells of the brainstem and spinal cords of the P301S animals with reduced immunoreactivity in the regions of the forebrain. Argyrophilic, thioflavin-S-positive neurons were also reported in the regions of concentrated tau pathology. Ultrastructurally, the lesions predominantly consisted of "half-twisted" ribbons that almost exclusively stained for human tau and lacked murine tau. Apoptosis did not appear to cause the neuronal loss (49%) that was reported in the ventral horn of the P301S mice. Interestingly, these mice shared many characteristics with the P301L 0N4R mice generated by Lewis and coworkers (18) including the development of frequent eye irritations.

Mice Expressing Transgenes that Alter Tau Kinase or Phosphatase Activity

The filamentous tau lesions observed in human neurodegenerative disease invariably contain tau that is hyperphosphorylated at specific residues (26). As a result there has been much speculation about the role of abnormal tau phosphorylation in the development of neurofibrillary pathology in AD and the tauopathies. To examine this question several groups have generated mice that overexpress transgenes designed to upregulate tau phosphorylation.

Transgenic mice were generated using a tetracycline-regulated system for conditional gene expression to express GSK-3β in adult animals thus avoiding possible deleterious effects of expression during development (21). Strong somatodendritic immuno-staining of hyperphosphorylated tau was detected in cortex and hippocampus, but no thioflavin-S fluorescence was detected. Western blotting with the phospho-tau antibodies (eg, PHF-1 and AD2) in cortex, striatum, hippocampus and cerebellum revealed increased levels of tau phosphorylation in the hippocampus. Increased TUNEL staining and astrogliosis further suggested that increased GSK-3β activity was initiating neurodegenerative changes in the mice; however, these changes occurred in the absence of neurofibrillary pathology (21). In a separate study, Ahlijanian and coworkers (1) overexpressed p25, a calpain cleavage product of p35, the endogenous regulator of another potential tau kinase, cdk5 (22). P25 lacks the regulatory region of p35 and thus causes constitutive activation of cdk5. P25 production has been suggested to underlie tau hyperphosphorylation in AD25. Mice expressing p25 developed hyperphosphorylated tau and silver-positive inclusions that also had neurofilament immunoreactivity, but again neurofibrillary pathology was not observed (1). Bian and colleagues (3) recently generated another transgenic mouse line, which overexpressed p25 in neurons. Despite the elevated cdk5 activity observed in these animals, axonal degeneration resulted in the absence of neurofibrillary tau pathology.

Kins and colleagues (15) addressed the role of tau hyperphosphorylation by generating mice that expressed a dominant negative mutant of the catalytic subunit of protein phosphatase 2A transgene in neurons. Abnormal tau phosphorylation (AT8 immunoreactivity) was observed in Purkinje cells of these transgenic mice. Ubiquitin immunoreactivity colocalised with the AT8 immunopositive aggregates; however, neurofibrillary lesions were not identified.

Transgenesis that resulted in altered tau kinase or phosphatase activity has produced some of the initial features of the tau pathology seen in human disease; however, the absence of neurofibrillary pathology or pronounced cell loss means that the relationship between tau hyperphosphorylation and tau-associated neurodegeneration remains uncertain. Pharmaceutical manipulation of tau kinases in both wild type and tau transgenic mice may provide additional clues on the role of hyperphosphorylation in the development neurofibrillary lesions and neurodegeneration.

Conclusion

Transgenic mice are now available that model both the tau pathological and biochemical changes that resemble different stages of human tauopathies. The availability of these models has allowed researchers to investigate potentially pathogenic interactions between tau and molecules such as Aβ, kinases, and phosphatases. With both proteomic and microarray technologies, it is now possible to examine variations in gene expression that accompany the progression of tau pathological and biochemical changes and to understand key events in the neurodegenerative process. These studies hold promise to identify potential therapeutic targets. Ablation of the endogenous mouse tau in these models (ie, humanising mice with respect to tau) may provide clues regarding interaction of tau isoforms. Comparisons of various tau transgenic mice should further our understanding of how strains or environmental factors may modify the progression of the tauopathy and allow us to determine which isoform and promoter combinations may lead to the next generation of models.

Inducible models of tauopathy should help determine what aspects of the disease process may be reversible and at which stage of the disease progression should therapeutic efforts be employed to give maximum benefits.

References

1. Ahlijanian MK, Barrezueta NX, Williams RD, Jakowski A, Kowsz KP, McCarthy S, Coskran T, Carlo A, Seymour PA, Burkhardt JE, Nelson RB, McNeish JD (2000) Hyperphosphorylated tau and neurofilament and cytoskeletal disruptions in mice overexpressing human p25, an activator of Cdk5. *Proc Natl Acad Sci U S A* 97: 2910-2915.

2. Allen B, Ingram E, Takao M, Smith MJ, Jakes R, Virdee K, Yoshida H, Holzer M, Craxton M, Emson PC, Atzori C, Migheli A, Crowther RA, Ghetti B, Spillantini MG, Goedert M (2002) Abundant tau filaments and nonapoptotic neurodegeneration in transgenic mice expressing human P301S tau protein. *J Neurosci* 22: 9340-9351.

3. Bian F, Nath R, Sobocinski G, Booher RN, Lipinski WJ, Callahan MJ, Pack A, Wang KK-W, Walker LC (2002) Axonopathy, tau abnormalities, and dyskinesia, but no neurofibrillary tangles in p25-transgenic mice. *J Comp Neurol* 446: 257-266.

4. Christi MA, Yang DS, Janus C, Phinney AL, Horne P, Pearson J, Strome R, Zuker N, Loukides J, French J, Turner S, Lozza G, Grilli M, Kunicki S, Morissette C, Paquette J, Gervais F, Bergeron C, Fraser PE, Carlson GA, George-Hyslop PS, Westaway D (2001). Early-onset amyloid deposition and cognitive deficits in transgenic mice expressing a double mutant form of amyloid precursor protein 695. *J Biol Chem* 276: 21562-21570.

5. D'Souza, I, Poorkaj P, Hong M, Nochlin D, Lee VM, Bird TD, Schellenberg GD (1999) Missense and silent tau gene mutations cause frontotemporal dementia with parkinsonism-chromosome 17 type, by affecting multiple alternative RNA splicing regulatory elements. *Proc Natl Acad Sci U S A* 96: 5598-5603.

6. Duff K, Knight H, Refolo LM, Sanders S, Yu X, Picciano M, Malester B, Hutton M, Adamson J, Goedert M, Bürki, K, Davis P (2000) Characterization of pathology in transgenic mice over-expressing human genomic and cDNA tau transgenes. *Neurobiol Dis* 7: 87-98.

7. Goedert M, Spillantini MG, Potier MC, Ulrich J, Crowther RA (1989) Cloning and sequencing of the cDNA encoding an isoform of microtubule-associated protein tau containing four tandem repeats: differential expression of tau protein mRNAs in human brain. *EMBO J* 8: 393-399.

8. Goedert M, Spillantini MG, Jakes R, Rutherford D, Crowther RA (1989) Multiple isoforms of human microtubule-associated protein tau: sequences and localization in neurofibrillary tangles of Alzheimer's disease. *Neuron* 3: 519-526.

9. Götz J, Chen F, Barmettler R, Nitsch RM (2001) Tau filament formation in transgenic mice expressing P301L tau. *J Biol Chem* 276: 529-534.

10. Götz J, Tolnay M, Barmettler R, Chen F, Probst A, Nitsch RM (2001) Oligodendroglial tau filament formation in transgenic mice expressing G272V tau. *Eur J Neurosci* 13: 2131-2140.

11. Higuchi M, Ishihara T, Zhang B, Hong M, Andreadis A, Trojanowski JQ, Lee V M-Y (2002) Transgenic mouse model of tauopathies with glial pathology and nervous system degeneration. *Neuron* 35: 433-446.

12. Hutton M, Lendon CL, Rizzu P, Baker M, Froelich S, Houlden H, Pickering-Brown S, Chakroverty S, Isaacs A, Grover A, Hackett J, Adamson J, Lincoln S, Dickson D, Davies P, Petersen RC, Stevens M, deGraaff E, Wauters E, van Baren J, Hillebrand M, Joosse M, Kwon JM, Nowotny P (1998) Association of missense and 5'-splice site mutations in tau with the inherited dementia FTDP-17. *Nature* 393: 702-705.

13. Ishihara T, Hong M, Zhang B, Nakagawa Y, Lee MK, Trojanowski JQ, Lee V M-Y (1999) Age-dependent emergence and progression of a tauopathy in transgenic mice overexpressing the shortest human tau isoform. *Neuron* 24: 751-762.

14. Ishihara T, Zhang B, Higuchi M, Yoshiyama Y, Trojanowski JQ, Lee VM (2001) Age-dependent induction of congophilic neurofibrillary tau inclusions in tau transgenic mice. *Am J Pathol* 158: 555-562.

15. Kins S, Crameri A, Evans DRH, Hemmings BA, Nitsch R, Gotz J (2001) Reduced PP2A activity induces tau hyperphosphorylation and altered compartmentalization of tau in transgenic mice. *J Biol Chem* 276: 38193-38200.

16. Kosik KS, Orecchio LD, Bakalis S, Neve RL (1989) Developmentally regulated expression of specific tau sequences. *Neuron* 2: 1389-1397.

17. Lee G, Neve RL, Kosik KS (1989) The microtubule binding domain of tau protein. *Neuron* 2: 1625-1624.

18. Lewis, J, McGowan E, Rockwood J, Melrose H, Nacharaju P, Van Slegtenhorst M, Gwinn-Hardy K, Murphy MP, Baker M, Yu X, Duff K, Hardy J, Corral A, Lin W-L, Yen S-H, Dickson DW, Davis P, Hutton M. (2000) Neurofibrillary tangles, amyotrophy and progressive motor disturbance in mice expressing mutant (P301L) tau protein. *Nat Genet* 25: 402-405.

19. Lim F, Hernandez F, Lucas JJ, Gomez-Ramos P, Moran MA, Avila J (2001) FTDP-17 Mutations in tau transgenic mice provoke lysosomal abnormalities and tau filaments in forebrain. *Mol Cell Neurosci* 18: 702-714.

20. Lin W-L, Lewis J, Yen S-H, Hutton M, Dickson DW (2003) Filamentous tau in oligodendrocytes and astrocytes of transgenic mice expressing the human tau isoform with the P301L mutation. *Am J Pathol* 162: 213-218.

21. Lucas JJ, Hernandez F, Gomez-Ramos P, Moran M, Hen R, Avila J (2001) Decreased nuclear β-catenin, tau hyperphosphorylation and neurodegeneration in GSK-3beta conditional transgenic mice. *EMBO J* 20: 27-39.

22. Patrick GN, Zukerberg L, Nikolic M, de la Monte S, Dikkes P, Tsai LH (1999) Conversion of p35 to p25 deregulates Cdk5 activity and promotes neurodegeneration. *Nature* 402: 615-622.

23. Poorkaj P, Bird TD, Wijsman E, Nemens E, Garruto RMm Anderson L, Andreadis A, Wiederholt WC, Raskind M, Schellenberg GD. (1998) Tau is a candidate gene for chromosome 17 frontotemporal dementia. *Ann Neurol* 43: 815-825.

24. Probst A, Götz J, Wiederhold KH, Tolnay M, Misti C, Jaton AL, HongM, Ishihara T, Lee VM-Y, Trojanowski JQ, Jakes R, Crowther RA, Spillantini MG, Bürki K, Goedert M (2000) Axonopathy and amyotrophy in mice transgenic for human four-repeat tau protein. *Acta. Neuropathol* 99: 469-481.

25. Spillantini MG, Bird TD, Ghetti B (1998) Frontotemporal dementia and parkinsonism linked to chromosome 17: a new group of tauopathies. *Brain Pathol* 8: 387-402.

26. Spillantini MG, Goedert M (1998) Tau protein pathology in neurodegenerative diseases. *Trends Neurosci* 21: 428-433.

27. Spillantini MG, Murrell JR, Goedert M, Farlow MR, Klug A, Ghetti (1998) Mutation in the tau gene in familial multiple system tauopathy with presenile dementia. *Proc Natl Acad Sci U S A* 95: 7737-7741.

28. Spittaels K, Van den Haute C, Van Dorpe J, Bruynseels K, Vandezande K, Laenen I, Geerts H, Mercken M, Sciot R, Van Lommel A, Loos R, van Leuven F (1999) Prominent axonopathy in the brain and spinal cord of transgenic mice overexpressing four-repeat human tau protein. *Am J Pathol* 155: 2153-2165.

29. Spittaels K, Van den Haute C, Van Dorpe J, Geerts H, Mercken M, Bruynseels K, Lasrado R, Vandezande K, Laenen I, Boon T, Van Lint J, Vandenheede J, Moechars D, Loos R, Van Leuven F (2000) Glycogen synthase kinase-3β phosphorylates protein tau and rescues the axonopathy in the central nervous system of human four-repeat tau transgenic mice. *J Biol Chem* 275: 41340-41349.

30. Tanemura K, Akagi T, Murayama M, Kikuchi N, Murayama O, Hashikama Y, Yoshiike Y, Park J-M, Matsuda K, Nakao S, Sun X, Sato S, Yamaguchi H, Takashima A (2001) Formation of filamentous tau aggregates in transgenic mice expressing V337M human tau. *Neurobiol Disease* 8: 1036-1045.

31. Tanemura K, Murayama M, Akagi T, Hashikawa T, Tominaga T, Ichikawa M, Yamaguchi H, Takashima A (2002) Neurodegeneration with tau accumulation in a transgenic mouse expressing V337M human tau. *J Neurosci* 22: 133-141.

32. Tatebayashi Y, Miyasaka T, Chui D-H, Akagi T, Mishima K-I, Iwasaki K, Fujiwara M, Tanemura K, Murayama M, Ishiguro K, Planel E, Sato S, Hashikawa T, Takashima A (2002) Tau filament formation and associative memory deficit in aged mice expressing mutant (R406W) human tau. *Proc Natl Acad Sci U S A* 99: 13896-13901.

CHAPTER 4

Synucleinopathies

Chapter Editor: Kurt Jellinger

4.1 Introduction to Synucleinopathies 156

4.2.1 Parkinson's Disease 159

4.2.2 Dementia with Lewy Bodies 188

4.2.3 Lewy Bodies in Conditions Other Than Disorders of α-Synuclein 200

4.3 Multiple System Atrophy 203

4.4 Experimental Models of Synucleinopathies 215

Introduction to Synucleinopathies

Maria Grazia Spillantini

BCSG1	breast cancer-specific gene1
GCI	glial cytoplasmic inclusion
LB	Lewy body
MSA	multiple system atrophy
NACP	non-amyloid β plaque component precursor

Parkinson's disease, one of the most common neurodegenerative diseases, was described by James Parkinson in 1817 (25). Its main neuropathological feature, the Lewy body (LB), was first described by Friederich Lewy in 1912 (19). Lewy bodies are eosinophilic inclusions that are particularly numerous in the substantia nigra (8). Although they were first described in Parkinson's disease, LB and Lewy neurites are also found in dementing disorders, such as dementia with Lewy bodies (23). Another disorder with eosinophilic inclusions is multiple system atrophy (MSA) where filamentous inclusions are found mainly in the cytoplasm and more rarely the nucleus of oligodendrocytes (24). These glial cytoplasmic inclusions (GCI) were first described by Papp and Lantos and have also been referred to as "Papp-Lantos inclusions."

The filamentous nature of the Lewy body was demonstrated in the 1960s (6). Although several proteins were found by immunohistochemistry in LBs, the biochemical nature of the characteristic filaments remained unknown. This situation changed in 1997, when 2 findings brought the little-studied protein α-synuclein to centre-stage. Firstly, a missense mutation in the α-synuclein gene was found to cause a rare, familial form of Parkinson's disease (26). Secondly, LBs and Lewy neurites present in cases of idiopathic Parkinson's disease and dementia with Lewy bodies were found to be strongly immunoreactive for α-synuclein (31). Subsequently, GCI were also shown to be immunoreactive for α-synuclein (22, 29). These findings were rapidly extended, with the identification of a second missense mutation in the α-synuclein gene in familial Parkinson's disease (17), and the finding that LB and GCI filaments were labelled by α-synuclein antibodies (2, 29, 30). It has since been shown that recombinant α-synuclein can form filaments in vitro that are structurally and antigenically similar to those extracted from the diseased human brain (28). Furthermore, α-synuclein staining is more widespread than ubiquitin staining making it the best marker for diseases with LBs (13, 27, 29, 30).

α-Synuclein belongs to a family of abundant brain proteins whose physiological functions are only incompletely known. The synuclein family consists of 3 members, named α-synuclein, β-synuclein and γ-synuclein, respectively (12). The first synuclein sequence was identified by Maroteoux et al in 1988 in *Torpedo californica* (20), and the name synuclein was used because the protein was found in both the nuclear envelope and synaptic terminals. In 1992, Tobe et al described a protein in rat and bovine brain, that they called phosphoneuroprotein 14 (32), and in 1993, Ueda et al reported the amino acid sequence of a human protein that they called "non-amyloid β plaque component precursor" (NACP), because they extracted a fragment of this protein, the NAC peptide, from Alzheimer's disease β-amyloid plaque preparations (34). However, later studies, failed to confirm the presence of NAC in amyloid plaques (5). In 1994, 2 homologous proteins from human brain were identified by virtue of the fact that they cross-reacted with an antibody raised against Alzheimer's disease paired helical filaments (14). One protein was identical to NACP, and the second protein was the human homologue of phosphoneuroprotein 14 (32, 34). Both proteins were homologous to synuclein from *Torpedo californica* and were consequently named α- and β-synuclein, respectively (14, 20). In 1997, Ji et al reported the sequence of a protein that they named breast cancer-specific gene1 (BCSG1), because of its abundance in human breast cancer tissue (15). Buchman et al identified the same protein and named it persyn (3). Because of its sequence similarities to α- and β-synucleins, BCSG1 (persyn) is now referred to as γ-synuclein.

The α-synuclein gene is located on chromosome 4, while the β- and γ-synuclein genes are on chromosomes 5 and 10, respectively (18). The synuclein proteins range from 127 to 140 amino acids in length, and their sequences are 55 to 62% identical. The α-synuclein gene is about 112 kb in length and consists of 7 exons, 5 of which make up the coding region of the protein (Figure 1). Alternatively spliced forms of α-synuclein lacking exon 3 or exon 5 exist, but their mRNAs are not abundant in brain, and their existence at the protein level has not been shown. Synucleins are characterised by the presence of imperfect 11 amino acid amino-terminal repeats that contain the KTKEGV consensus sequence and are separated by 5 to 8 amino acids (3, 14, 15, 20, 32, 34). The repeats constitute a lipid binding domain. The repeat region is followed by a hydrophobic stretch and a negatively charged carboxy-terminal region. In α-synuclein the hydrophobic stretch includes the NAC peptide, which has been demonstrated to be critical for fibril formation (11). Of the 3 synucleins, only α-synuclein is associated with the filamentous inclusions of the synucleinopathies. No genetic evidence linking β- and γ-synucleins to disease has been found, and these proteins have a reduced tendency to

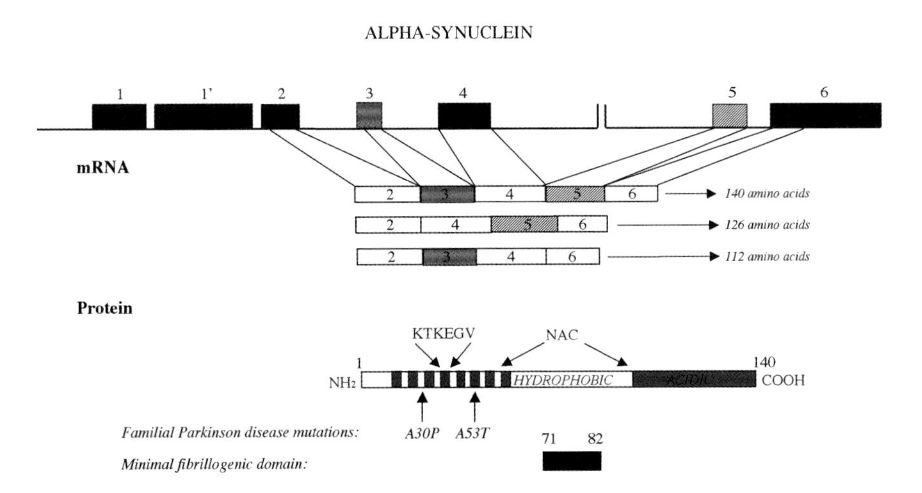

Figure 1. Diagrammatic representation of the SNCA gene, α-synuclein mRNAs and protein. The SNCA gene contains seven exons that through alternative splicing generate three mRNA transcripts. Only the existance of the protein derived from the longest mRNA trascript has been demonstrated.α-Synuclein protein contains 11 amino-acid repeats in the amino-terminal region that constitute the lipid binding domain. An intermediate hydrophobic area is present and the carboxy-terminus is acidic. The NAC region contains the 12 amino acids that are essential for α-synuclein aggregation. Genetic mutations found in α-synuclein in familial Parkinson's disease are shown.

aggregate (12). α-Synuclein is a potential phospho-protein, and phosphorylation could regulate its function. α-Synuclein deposits are phosphorylated at Ser129 in neurodegenerative diseases (9). Furthermore, in conditions of oxidative stress, α-synuclein can be nitrated in its amino-terminal part, and the presence of nitrated α-synuclein has been shown in LBs, Lewy neurites and GCI (10). The function of α-synuclein is not clear, it has been proposed that is involved in synaptic vesicle transport, that it is an inhibitor of phospholipase D2, and that it is an activity dependent negative regulator of dopamine release (1, 4). α-Synuclein is a natively unfolded protein that becomes structured upon binding to lipid membranes and in its unfolded form is degraded by the proteasome in a ubiquitin-independent manner (33). In diseases where it aggregates, α-synuclein changes conformation and aggregates to form fibrils with β-sheet structure similar to other amyloid proteins.

Although, it is now clear that α-synuclein is the major component of LBs and GCI, much more remains to be learned. In particular, the mechanisms by which dysfunction of α-synuclein leads to neuronal and glial cell degeneration remain to be identified. A crucial question is whether neurones and glial cells are damaged by conformationally altered, non-filamentous α-synuclein or by filamentous α-synuclein. Furthermore, it is important to determine what leads to α-synuclein assembly into filaments in sporadic idiopathic synucleiopathies. The answer to these questions will probably come from improved experimental animal models. The transgenic mice that are now available do not replicate many of the most important features of Lewy body diseases (16, 21, 35), and the production of transgenic mice as a model of MSA is still in progress. Only overexpression of α-synuclein in *Drosophila melanogaster* leads to neuronal death and Lewy body-like structure formation (7). The study of the 3 synucleins in animal models will also help in understanding their physiological functions. This knowledge will contribute to the design of drugs for the treatment of the synucleinopathies.

References

1. Abeliovich A, Schmitz Y, Farinas I, Choi-Lundberg D, Ho WH, Castillo PE, Shinsky N, Verdugo JM, Armanini M, Ryan A, Hynes M, Phillips H, Sulzer D, Rosenthal A (2000) Mice lacking α-synuclein display functional deficits in the nigrostriatal dopamine system. *Neuron* 25: 239-252.

2. Baba M, Nakajo S, Tu PH, Tomita T, Nakaya K, Lee VM, Trojanowski JQ, Iwatsubo T (1998) Aggregation of α-synuclein in Lewy bodies of sporadic Parkinson's disease and dementia with Lewy bodies. *Am J Pathol* 152: 879-884.

3. Buchman VL, Hunter HJ, Pinon LG, Thompson J, Privalova EM, Ninkina NN, Davies AM (1998) Persyn, a member of the synuclein family, has a distinct pattern of expression in the developing nervous system. *J Neurosci* 18: 9335-9341.

4. Clayton DF, George JM (1999) Synucleins in synaptic plasticity and neurodegenerative disorders. *J Neurosci Res* 58: 120-129.

5. Culvenor JG, McLean CA, Cutt S, Campbell BC, Maher F, Jakala P, Hartmann T, Beyreuther K, Masters CL, Li QX (1999) Non-Aβ component of Alzheimer's disease amyloid (NAC) revisited. NAC and alpha-synuclein are not associated with Abeta amyloid. *Am J Pathol* 155: 1173-1181.

6. Duffy PE, Tennyson VM (1965) Phase and electron microscopic observations of Lewy bodies and melanin granules in the substantia nigra and locus coeruleus in Parkinson's disease. *J Neuropathol Exp Neurol* 24: 398-414

7. Feany MB, Bender WW (2000) A Drosophila model of Parkinson's disease. *Nature* 404: 394-398.

8. Forno LS (1996) Neuropathology of Parkinson's disease. *J Neuropathol Exp Neurol* 55: 259-272

9. Fujiwara H, Hasegawa M, Dohmae N, Kawashima A, Masliah E, Goldberg MS, Shen J, Takio K, Iwatsubo T (2002) α-Synuclein is phosphorylated in synucleinopathy lesions. *Nat Cell Biol* 4: 160-164.

10. Giasson BI, Duda JE, Murray IV, Chen Q, Souza JM, Hurtig HI, Ischiropoulos H, Trojanowski JQ, Lee VM (2000) Oxidative damage linked to neurodegeneration by selective α-synuclein nitration in synucleinopathy lesions. *Science* 290: 985-989.

11. Giasson BI, Murray IV, Trojanowski JQ, Lee VM (2001) A hydrophobic stretch of 12 amino acid residues in the middle of α-synuclein is essential for filament assembly. *J Biol Chem* 276: 2380-2386.

12. Goedert M (2001) α-Synuclein and neurodegenerative diseases. *Nat Rev Neurosci* 2: 492-501.

13. Gomez-Tortosa E, Newell K, Irizarry MC, Sanders JL, Hyman BT (2000) α-Synuclein immunoreactivity in dementia with Lewy bodies: morphological staging and comparison with ubiquitin immunostaining. *Acta Neuropathol (Berl)* 99: 352-357.

14. Jakes R, Spillantini MG, Goedert M (1994) Identification of two distinct synucleins from human brain. *FEBS Lett* 345: 27-32.

15. Ji H, Liu YE, Jia T, Wang M, Liu J, Xiao G, Joseph BK, Rosen C, Shi YE (1997) Identification of a breast cancer-specific gene, BCSG1, by direct differential cDNA sequencing. *Cancer Res* 57: 759-764.

16. Kahle PJ, Neumann M, Ozmen L, Muller V, Jacobsen H, Schindzielorz A, Okochi M, Leimer U, van Der Putten H, Probst A, Kremmer E, Kretzschmar HA, Haass C (2000) Subcellular localization of wild-type and Parkinson's disease-associated mutant α-synuclein in human and transgenic mouse brain. *J Neurosci* 20: 6365-6373.

17. Kruger R, Kuhn W, Muller T, Woitalla D, Graeber M, Kosel S, Przuntek H, Epplen JT, Schols L, Riess O (1998) Ala30Pro mutation in the gene encoding α-synuclein in Parkinson's disease. *Nat Genet* 18: 106-108.

18. Lavedan C (1998) The synuclein family. *Genome Res* 8: 871-880.

19. Lewy FH (1912) In *Handbuch der Neurologie*, M Lewandowski, G Abelsdorff (eds). Springer Verlag: Berlin. pp. 920-933

20. Maroteaux L, Campanelli JT, Scheller RH (1988) Synuclein: a neuron-specific protein localized to the nucleus and presynaptic nerve terminal. *J Neurosci* 8: 2804-2815.

21. Masliah E, Rockenstein E, Veinbergs I, Mallory M, Hashimoto M, Takeda A, Sagara Y, Sisk A, Mucke L (2000) Dopaminergic loss and inclusion body formation in α-synuclein mice: implications for neurodegenerative disorders. *Science* 287: 1265-1269.

22. Mezey E, Dehejia AM, Harta G, Tresser N, Suchy SF, Nussbaum RL, Brownstein MJ, Polymeropoulos MH (1998) α-Synuclein in neurodegenerative disorders: murder or accomplice? *Nature Med* 4: 755-757.

23. McKeith IG, Ballard CG, Perry RH, Ince PG, O'Brien JT, Neill D, Lowery K, Jaros E, Barber R, Thompson P, Swann A, Fairbairn AF, Perry EK (2000) Prospective validation of consensus criteria for the diagnosis of dementia with Lewy bodies. *Neurology* 54: 1050-1058.

24. Papp MI, Kahn JE, Lantos PL (1989) Glial cytoplasmic inclusions in the CNS of patients with multiple system atrophy (striatonigral degeneration, olivopontocerebellar atrophy and Shy-Drager syndrome). *J Neurol Sci* 94: 79-100.

25. Parkinson J (1817) *An essay on the shaking palsy.* Whittingham and Rowland for Sherwood, Neely and Jones: London.

26. Polymeropoulos MH, Lavedan C, Leroy E, Ide SE, Dehejia A, Dutra A, Pike B, Root H, Rubenstein J, Boyer R et al (1997) Mutation in the α-synuclein gene identified in families with Parkinson's disease. *Science* 276: 2045-2047.

27. Schneider JA, Bienias JL, Gilley DW, Kvarnberg DE, Mufson EJ, Bennett DA (2002) Improved detection of substantia nigra pathology in Alzheimer's disease. *J Histochem Cytochem* 50: 99-106.

28. Serpell LC, Berriman J, Jakes R, Goedert M, Crowther RA (2000) Fiber diffraction of synthetic α-synuclein filaments shows amyloid- like cross-beta conformation. *Proc Natl Acad Sci U S A* 97: 4897-4902.

29. Spillantini MG, Crowther RA, Jakes R, Cairns NJ, Lantos PL, Goedert M (1998) Filamentous α-synuclein inclusions link multiple system atrophy with Parkinson's disease and dementia with Lewy bodies. *Neurosci Lett* 251: 205-208.

30. Spillantini MG, Crowther RA, Jakes R, Hasegawa M, Goedert M (1998) α-Synuclein in filamentous inclusions of Lewy bodies from Parkinson's disease and dementia with Lewy bodies. *Proc Natl Acad Sci U S A* 95: 6469-6473.

31. Spillantini MG, Schmidt ML, Lee VM, Trojanowski JQ, Jakes R, Goedert M (1997) α-Synuclein in Lewy bodies. *Nature* 388: 839-840.

32. Tobe T, Nakajo S, Tanaka A, Mitoya A, Omata K, Nakaya K, Tomita M, Nakamura Y (1992) Cloning and characterization of the cDNA encoding a novel brain-specific 14-kDa protein. *J Neurochem* 59: 1624-1629.

33. Tofaris GK, Layfield R, Spillantini MG (2001) α-Synuclein metabolism and aggregation is linked to ubiquitin- independent degradation by the proteasome. *FEBS Lett* 509: 22-26.

34. Ueda K, Fukushima H, Masliah E, Xia Y, Iwai A, Yoshimoto M, Otero DA, Kondo J, Ihara Y, Saitoh T (1993) Molecular cloning of cDNA encoding an unrecognized component of amyloid in Alzheimer disease. *Proc Natl Acad Sci U S A* 90: 11282-11286.

35. van der Putten H, Wiederhold KH, Probst A, Barbieri S, Mistl C, Danner S, Kauffmann S, Hofele K, Spooren WP, Ruegg MA, Lin S, Caroni P, Sommer B, Tolnay M, Bilbe G (2000) Neuropathology in mice expressing human α-synuclein. *J Neurosci* 20: 6021-6029.

Parkinson's Disease

Kurt A. Jellinger
Yoshikuni Mizuno

3-OMD	3-O-methyldopa	**MAP**	microtubule associated protein
5-HT	5-hydroxydopamine (serotonin)	**M-Enk**	metenkephalin
5-HIAA	5-hydroxyindolic acid	**MHPG**	3-methoxy-4-hydroxyphenylglycole
6-OHDA	6-hydroxydopamine	**MPP+**	1-methyl-4-phenyl-2, 3-dihydropyridinium
8-OHG	8-hydroxydeoxyguanosine	**MPTP**	1-methyl-4-phenyl-1, 2, 3, 6-tetrahydropyridine
AChE	acetylcholinesterase	**MSA**	multiple system atrophy
AD	Alzheimer's disease	**NBM**	nucleus basalis of Meynert
AGE	advanced glycation products	**NE**	norepinephrine
APP	amyloid precursor protein	**NFT**	neurofibrillary tangle
BDNF	brain derived neurotrophic factor	**NMDA**	N-methyl-D-aspartate
CAB	calbindin	**NO**	nitric oxide
CBD	corticobasal degeneration	**NOS**	nitric oxide synthase
ChAT	choline acetyltransferase	**NPpc**	nucleus pedunculopontinus pars compacta
COMT	catechol-o-methyl-transferase	**NTF**	tumor necrosis factor
D1R	D1 receptor	**OS**	oxidative stress
DAT	dopamine transporter	**PCD**	programmed cell death
DOPAC	3, 4-dihydroxyphenyl acetic acid	**PD**	Parkinson's disease
DRN	dorsal raphe nucleus	**PH-8**	phenylalanine hydroxylase
EO	early onset Parkinson's disease	**PSP**	progressive supranuclear palsy
ER	endoplasmic reticulum	**ROS**	reactive oxygen species
ERAD	endoplasmic reticulum-associated protein degradation	**SN**	substantia nigra
GABA	gamma amino butyric acid	**SNpc**	substantia nigra pars compacta
GAD	glutamin-decarboxylase	**SNpr**	substantia nigra pars reticulata
GDNF	glia-derived neurotrophic factor	**SOD**	superoxide dismutase
GP	globus pallidus	**SP**	substance P
GPe	external globus pallidus	**STN**	subthalamic nucleus
GPi	internal globus pallidus	**TH**	tyrosine hydroxylase
GSH	glutathion	**UCH-L1**	ubiquitin carboxy-terminus hydrolase L1
HVA	homovanillic acid	**UPS**	ubiquitin protease system
IR	immunoreactive	**VMAT2**	vesicular monoamine transporter
LB	Lewy body	**VTA**	ventral tegmental area
LC	locus coeruleus		
L-dopa	levodopa		
LN	Lewy neurite		
MAO	monoaminoxidase		

Definition

Parkinson's disease (PD) is a frequent neurodegenerative movement disorder characterised clinically by rigidity, akinesia, resting tremor, and postural instability due to progressive degeneration of the dopaminergic nigrostriatal system and other neuronal networks mainly caused by loss of pigmented neurones in the substantia nigra pars compacta (SNpc) and associated with widespread occurrence of intracytoplasmic Lewy bodies (LBs) and dystrophic Lewy neurites (LN). The resulting striatal dopamine deficiency and other biochemical deficits cause the clinical picture of this disorder.

There are many causes of parkinsonism (Table 1) and accepted clinical diagnostic criteria (71) provide a high sensitivity for identifying PD with a specificity of 75 to 90% (98, 98a, 111). For the diagnosis of definite PD histopathological confirmation is required. Genetic and environmental factors in the aetiology of PD are discussed. While mutations in α-synuclein and parkin genes have been identified in rare familial forms, for the majority of sporadic PD cases the aetiology is unknown,although a significant familial component in late onset PD suggests genetic factors without ruling out the possibility of a coexisting environmental component (200a).

Synonyms and Historical Annotation

In 1817 Parkinson (198) defined the disease which bears his name in his *Essay on the Shaking Palsy*, in 1913 Lewy (142) first described the concentric hyaline cytoplasmic inclusions, and in 1919 Trétiakoff (242) first observed the characteristic lesions of the SN. Description of *kampavata* presenting with tremor and akinesia probably representing PD was found in the ancient ayurvedic literature in India (4500-1000 BCE [134, 135]). Synonyms are *paralysis agitans*, *idiopathic parkinsonism*, *PD of the LB type* or *brainstem Lewy body disease* (162).

Epidemiology

PD occurs throughout the world and affects both sexes roughly equally or with a slight preponderance among males, but its prevalence has racial differences (134, 135). It is higher among whites, low among blacks, and intermediate in Asians. The prevalence of PD among whites is between 150 and 200 per 100000 population (53, 131), while a much higher prevalence (414 per 100000) was reported from Australia (160). In Japan, the prevalence is approximately 100 per 100000 (132). In Africa, one study reported a prevalence of 59 per 100000 in Nigeria (216). The prevalence among blacks in the United States was 105 per 100000, while 150 per 100000 among whites living in the same region. Blacks in the United States have a much higher prevalence compared to Nigerian people, as have people in Taiwan (130/100 000) as compared to those in China (18-57 per 100000) (31). The incidence of PD, according to a recent systemic review, is 16 to 19/100000 per year, only Italy showing a much lower incidence (8.6/100000 per year) (242a). These data may suggest the importance of environmental factors rather than racial and genetic factors in

1. Neurodegenerative disorders manifesting Parkinsonism
- Parkinson's disease (sporadic and familial)
- Progressive supranuclear palsy
- Multiple system atrophy (SND, OPCA, Shy-Drager syndrome)
- Dementia with Lewy bodies
- Corticobasal degeneration
- Pallidonigroluysian atrophy
- Frontotemporal dementia and parkinsonism
- Parkinsonism-Dementia complex of Guam and Kii Peninsula
- Hallervorden-Spatz disease
- Spinocerebellar ataxia 2
- Spinocerebellar ataxia 3
- Rigid type Huntington's disease
- Advanced Alzheimer's disease

2. Symptomatic Parkinsonism
- Vascular (pseudo)parkinsonism (lacunar state and/or leukoaraiosis)
- Drug-induced parkinsonism
  - Phenothiazines, Butyrophenones, Benzamide derivatives, Flunraridine, Reserpine
- Toxic parkinsonism
  - Manganese
  - Carbon monooxide
  - Carbon disulfide
  - MPTP
- Metabolic disorder
  - Wilson's disease
- Infectious and post-infectious disorders
  - Post-encephalitic parkinsonism (Von Economo encephalitis)
  - Other encephalitides (Japanese B encephalities and other viral encephalitis)
  - Creutzfeldt-Jakob disease
  - Neurosyphilis
- Other disorders
  - Normal pressure hydrocephalus
  - Frontal lobe tumor
  - Post-traumatic parkinsonism – Boxer's encephalopathy (dementia pugilistica)

Table 1. Differential diagnosis of Parkinson's disease.

the aetiology of PD. Its prevalence increases exponentially with age: between 65 and 90 years, about 0.3% of the general population and 3% of people over the age of 65 have PD (134, 135).

Genetics

The frequency of PD among relatives of index patients is 2 to 3 times higher than in the control population (52); however, results of twin studies are not convincing. A recent study revealed a high concordance rate in monozygotic twins with onset before 50 years of age (100%) and low in those with onset after 50 years of age (10.4%). In dizygotic twins, the concordance rate was 16.7% and 10.2%, respectively (236). With PET scanning for evaluation of the nigrostriatal involvement, the concordance rate in monozygotic twins was much higher (55.6%) than in dizygotic twins (18.8%) (200). Pathology of 2 monozygotic twins with a 20-year discordance interval revealed typical LB type of PD with very few cortical LBs and more severe lesions in the twin with longer duration of illness (44). The importance of genetic factors in early onset patients has been confirmed by recent discoveries of different forms of familial PD, where a single gene mutation can cause nigral degeneration with or without involvement of other structures. So far, 9 disease-causing loci and mutations in 3 genes, as well as several allelic associations have been linked to PD (Table 2). Mutant proteins are derived from causal mutations: *i)* α-synuclein which is linked to an autosomal dominant form of PD, *ii)* parkin, linked to an autosomal recessive form of early-onst PD, and *iii)* ubiquitin carboxy-terminus hydrolase L1 (UCH-L1) linked to an autosomal dominant form of typical PD. Association of single-nucleotide polymorphisms in a tau intron on chromosome 17q21 implicates tau as a susceptibility gene for late-onset PD (154) with increasing risk of PD for persons with the H1/H1 genotype (151). Genome screening suggests multiple genetic loci for the common adult-onset PD (217).

PARK1, linked to the long arm of chromosome 4, is parkinsonism caused by point mutations in the α-synuclein gene (128, 204). Clinical features are similar to those of sporadic PD, with good response to L-dopa, but the age of onset is younger and dementia is more frequent (231). Pathology includes SN and locus coeruleus (LC) degeneration and LBs with some cortical LBs. Two mutations have been reported: Ala53Thr (in families of Greek and Italian origin) and Ala30Pro (in families of German origin). Mutated forms of α-synuclein show increased tendency for self-aggregation and accumulation in the cytoplasm and neurites of nigral neurones and may interfere with axonal transport, but are also major components of LBs in sporadic PD (45). Recent examination of a brain of the Conturski kindred (Ala53 Thr mutation of the α-synuclein gene) disclosed concurrence of α-synuclein (neurites and few LBs) and neuritic and perikaryal tau inclusions, suggesting differences from the pathology of IPD (50a).

PARK 2 is autosomal recessive parkinsonism linked to the long arm of chromosome 6 (158). The clinical features are early onset (<40 years) L-dopa responsive parkinsonism with sleep benefit. Pathology shows severe neuronal loss in the SN and the locus coeruleus (LC) with absence of LBs (234). One patient with exon 4 deletion of the parkin gene showed accumulation of tau protein in the remaining SN neurones (172), but this is not a common pathological feature of PARK2. The causative gene was identified and named *parkin* (125). Various kinds of

Name	Chromosome	Gene Locus	Gene	Inheritance	Clinical phenotype	Neuropathology	References
PARK1	4	4q21-23	α-syn.	AD	EOP similar to SPD + dementia	Neuronal loss in SN and LC Subcortical and few cortical LBs	204 128
PARK2	6	6q25.2-27	parkin	AR	EOP similar to SPD		158 125 147
PARK3	2	2p13	unknown	AD	EOP similar to SPD + dementia	Neuronal loss in SN and LC (+ NFT and SP)	69
PARK4	4	4p16.3	unknown	AD	EOP L-dopa responsive PD + dementia	similar to LBD	176 56
PARK5	1	1p32-33	unknown	AR	EOP similar to SPD, no dementia	NA	244, 244a
PARK6	1	1p35-36					
PARK7	1	1p36	unknown	AR	EOP ?	NA	245
PARK8	12	12p11.2-p13.1	unknown	AD	E+AOP L-dopa responsive PD	extensive SN degeneration, no LBs	64a
PARK 9	1	1p32	unknown				91b
UCH-L1	4	4p14-15.1	UCH-L1	AD	similar to SPD	NA	140
FTDP-17	17	17q21-23	tau	AD	see Hutton & Miller (this book)		
Dys-Pa	19	19q13	unknown	AD	EOP	NA	
Lubag	X	Xq13.1	unknown	XR	EOP	Neurone loss + mosaic gliosis in caudate and lat. putamen	137
FTDP-17	17	17q21-22	Tau				

Dys-Pa: dystonia-parkinsonism, AD: autosomal dominant, AR: autosomal recessive, EOP: early onset parkinsonism, SP: sporadic PD, AOP: adult onset parkinsonism, NA: not available, XR: X chromosome related

Table 2. Familial forms of Parkinson's disease.

mutations—both exonic deletions and point mutations—have been observed (89). Duplications and a triplication of exons were reported in European families (146, 147). Recent studies in 2 American kindreds with early-onset parkinsonism (<41 years) revealed a novel 40 bp exon deletion on chromosome 6q.25.2.27 in one and an additional 7R275W substitition in the smaller kindred. Autopsy in a proband of the latter showed LB pathology. These data suggest that heterozygous parkin mutations and loss of parkin protein may lead to early-onset parkinsonism with LB pathology, while a hemizygous mutation may confer increased susceptibility to typical PD (55). Parkin contains 12 exons encompassing over 1.5 Mb and encodes a protein consisting of 465 amino acids. It is expressed in the Golgi, cytosol, and microsomal fractions, but not in the mitochondrial and nuclear fractions in human brain (223). It is associated with synaptic vesicle membranes and is transported to nerve terminals by the axoplasmic flow (130). Parkin is an ubiquitin E3 ligase involved in ATP-dependent endoplasmic reticulum-associated protein degradation (ERAD) (222). Candidate substrates are CDCrel-1, a synaptic vesicle protein (262); α-synuclein 22 (especially a 22 kDa glycosylated form of α-synuclein that is accumulated as a non-ubiquitinated form in AR-PD brains) (224): and Pael receptor, an endoplasmic reticulum (ER) protein (102). Cotransfection of parkin, α-synuclein, and synphylin results in the formation of ubiquitinated α-synuclein inclusions that is associated with cellular degeneration (32).

PARK3 is autosomal dominant parkinsonism linked to the short arm of chromosome 2 (69) which is phenotypically very similar to sporadic PD. Its penetrance is only 40%. Only 6 families have been reported to date, with dementia in two of them. Pathologically, SN and LC degeneration have been observed. In demented patients widespread neurofibrillary tangles and senile plaques were observed in the hippocampus, entorhinal cortex or neocortex.

PARK4 is autosomal dominant parkinsonism linked to the short arm of chromosome 4 (56). Clinical features are L-dopa responsive parkinsonism and dementia. The age of onset ranges from 25 to 48 years (176). Pathological changes are similar to that of dementia with LBs (DLB). Essential tremor phenotypes are seen in the pedigree with the same haplotypes.

PARK6 is autosomal recessive parkinsonism linked to the short arm of chromosome 1 very close to the PARK5 (244), with a wide range of ages at onset (244a) and a reduction of dopamine uptake in the dorsal putamen that is slower than in sporadic PD (119b). Linkage to the short arm was found among the families not linked to chromosome 6 (PARK6).

PARK7 is autosomal recessive parkinsonism that is also linked to the short arm of chromosome 1, very close, but not identical to the PARK6 locus (227, 245).

PARK8 is the most recently mapped autosomal dominant form of parkinsonism linked to chromosome 12q11.2-p.13.1 (64a). The age of onset ranges from 38 to 68 years. Clinical features are similar to those of sporadic PD with good response to L-dopa (185). Despite extensive SN degeneration, LBs are absent.

A new susceptibility gene for late onset PD in many Icelandic families was designated PARK10 (91b).

UCH-L1 (ubiquitin carboxyterminal hydrolase-L1) is a deubiquitinating enzyme. A point mutation (Lie93Met) was found in an autosomal dominant German family linked to the UCH-L1 locus located in the short arm of chromosome 4 was reported (140). It causes loss of the enzymatic activity of UCH-LI to about 50%. The clinical features are similar to those of spo-

1. Resting tremor (4-6 Hz)
2. Cogwheel rigidity
3. Bradykinesia (akinesia) and related symptoms
Difficulty in initiating movements
Slowness of movements
Difficulty in rolling over in bed
Micrographia
Loss of finger dexterity
Small voice
4. Loss of righting reflex
Stooped posture
Small step gait
Pulsion (retro-, ante-, and latero-)
Start hesitation and freezing
Festination
5. Loss of automatic movements
Loss of blinking (leptile atare)
Loss of automatic occular movement
Masked face
Loss of automatic swallowing (drooling of saliva)
Loss of arm swing
Difficulty of two motor acts
6. Autonomic dysfunction
Constipation
Seborrhoic face
Dysphagia
Impotence
Urinary frequency
Orthostatic hypotension
Increased sweating
7. Others
Myerson's sign
Westphal phenomenon

Table 3. Clinical features of Parkinson's disease.

radic PD. No autopsy report is available and the linkage to PD is not known.

Clinical features

Age of onset and the initial symptom. The age of onset of sporadic PD varies from 20 to 80 years, with a peak between 55 and 65 years. The most frequent initial symptom is resting tremor in one hand or leg first. It is the presenting symptom in about 50% of the patients and can occur in up to 80% during the course of illness. Asymmetric presentation is usual. Tremor first appears on one side, and then spreads to other limbs. Second most common are gait disturbances, usually starting in one leg. If they are symmetrical, other diseases such as progressive supranuclear palsy (PSP) should be considered. The third common presenting symptom is bradykinesia, which causes difficulties in performing fine finger movements and is often associated with micrographia.

Clinical manifestations. It is relatively easy for clinicians to diagnose patients with the full complement of clinical features of PD. Symptoms and signs, which may be seen in PD, are summarized in Table 3.

Tremor. In PD there is a resting tremor with a frequency of 4 to 6 Hz. It is usually more prominent in one hand. It may also be seen in the foot, jaw and tongue, but it almost never involves the head. If the head has a rotatory tremor, essential tremor is more likely.

Rigidity. This occurs in the form of a form of resistance to the passive stretch of skeletal muscles with a cogwheel-like resistance when passively extending and flexing the skeletal muscles in the limbs; its intensity is usually asymmetric.

Akinesia and bradykinesia. They are absence and slowness of movements. In PD, it takes more time before starting motor acts and these are conducted more slowly. Bradykinesia, one of the most important disabilities in PD, impairs the activities and quality of daily life, manifesting as micrographia, hypophonia, loss of finger dexterity, and difficulty in rolling over in bed, among others.

Loss of righting reflex. The righting reflex enables the patient to restore and maintain the posture when an external force is given suddenly to cause a perturbation of the balance. Loss of the reflex manifests initially as retropulsion and later as anteropulsion and lateropulsion.

Gait disturbances. The typical parkinsonian gait is a small stepped, slow, shuffling gait. The posture is stooped, and the arm swing is lost. In advanced stages of illness, start hesitation and freezing of gait may be seen. Its pathophysiologic mechanism is not known. It may be due to disturbance in the rhythm formation in the CNS, which is important in repetitive movements.

Loss of automatic movements. Some movements of the skeletal muscles are conducted automatically and unconsciously, eg, eye blinking, ocular or facial expressive movements, unconscious swallowing of saliva, and arm swing during walking. Loss of automatic movements gives rise to many of the typical features of PD such as masked face and reptile stare (loss of eye blinking and ocular movements).

Disturbance of two simultaneous motor acts. PD patients are often unable to perform two motor acts simultaneously, while one of the two motor acts is ignored.

Autonomic dysfunction. Among autonomic dysfunctions recognized in PD, constipation is one of the most common. Others include oily skin and seborrhoic face due to increase in apocrine secretion rich in lipids. Episodic perspiration may occur. Orthostatic hypotension is not common in untreated PD patients, although the blood pressure tends to be lower. Urinary frequency is not uncommon, but autonomous and atonic bladders are very uncommon. If these symptoms are seen early, disorders such as multiple system atrophy (MSA) should be considered.

Intellectual function. Overt dementia is not a usual feature in the early stage of PD, but patients may develop it during the course of the disease. Its reported frequency varies from 10 to 30%, increasing to about 50% with disease duration (1). The risk of dementia in PD is lower in those with a tremor-dominant form of PD (209). If dementia precedes parkinsonism or severe dementia follows within one year from the onset of parkinsonism, one should consider dementia with Lewy bodies (DLB).

Cognitive impairment. Cognitive deficits in the absence of overt dementia are common in PD. Diminished set-shifting ability is one of the characteristic cognitive disturbances of PD (49, 209). It can be examined by neuropsychological testing and is ascribed to the dysfunction of the basal ganglia-frontal lobe network.

Depression. Depression is a common feature in PD. Its frequency ranges from 30 to 50% (139, 232). A

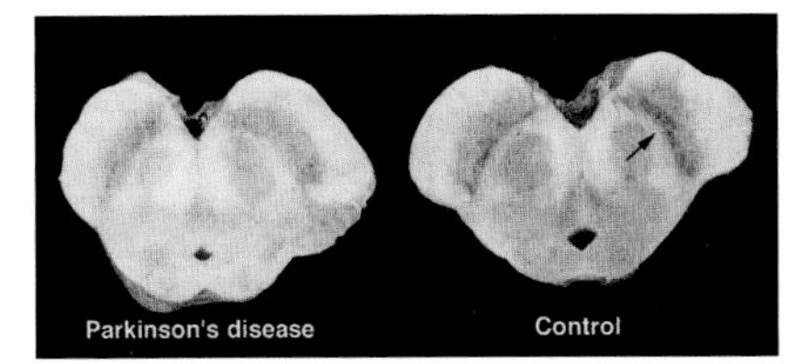

Figure 1. *Pallor of substantia nigra* (arrow) in Parkinson's disease compared to control.

recent global survey on the quality of life of PD patients revealed that the frequency of depression was 50%, and it represented an important factor after motor disability in determining the quality of life.

Neuroimaging. In uncomplicated PD, neuroimaging such as cranial CT and MRI is normal. These studies are useful to exclude other parkinsonian syndromes such as vascular forms of parkinsonism, MSA, PSP, etc. [^{123}I] MIBG (meta-iodobenzylguanidine) myocardial scintigraphy indicating cardiac sympathetic denervation from early stages of PD separates it from MSA and PSP (23, 48, 235). Progressive loss of cardiac sympathetic innervation in PD is also shown by decrease in radioactivity of the left ventricle and septum in serial [^{18}F] fluorodopamine PET scans (142a).[^{18}F] Fluorodopa uptake PET scanning (104), β-CIT SPECT (25, 235), and [^{18}F] CFT PET studies (186, 188) are useful in the early diagnosis of PD. Striatal uptake diminishes starting in the posterior putamen. Increased echo-genicity of the SN in patients with PD due to increased iron content has been demonstrated by transcranial ultrasound (14).

Laboratory findings. There are no specific abnormalities in the routine laboratory findings. CSF homovanillic acid (HVA), a dopamine metabolite, may be decreased. Synuclein has been detected in the CSF, but since both substances show an overlap between PD and normal controls, they cannot be used for diagnostic purposes (19). Electroencephalography (EEG) in most nondemented PD patients is either normal or shows nonspecific abnormalities and fails to differentiated PD from

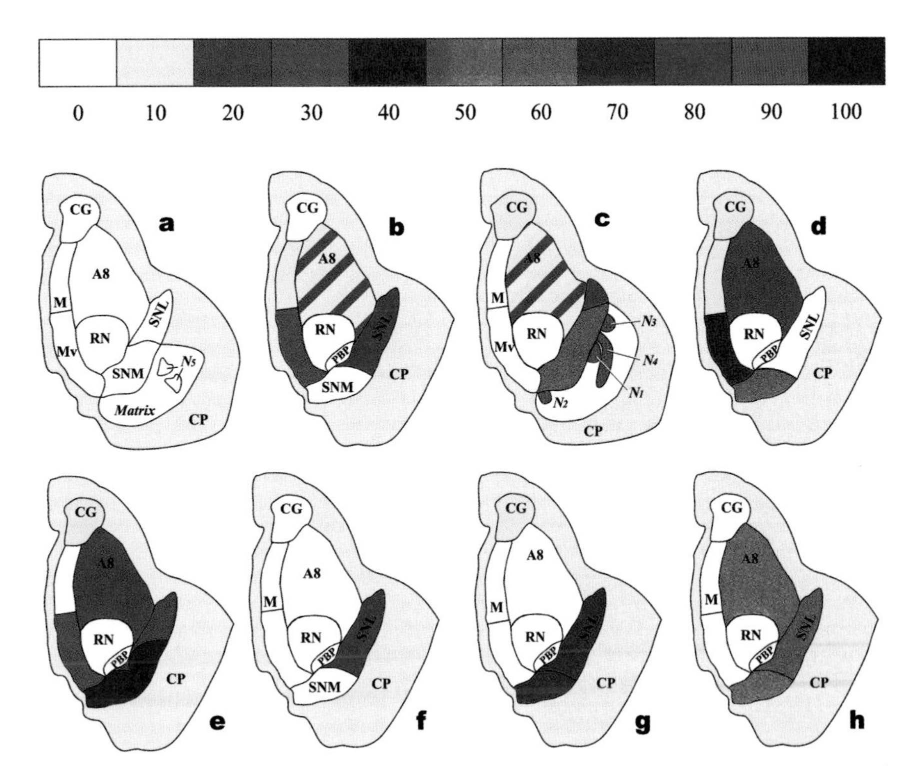

Figure 2. *Neuronal loss in catecholaminergic nuclei of midbrain (intermediate level) in Parkinson's disease.* **A.** Distribution of catecholaminergic nuclei; **B.** Distribution of melanized, TH-IR neurones (%) in normal controls; **C.** Average loss of TH-IR neurones in 5 PD cases (duration of illness 7-32 years); **D.** Percent average loss of TH-IR neurones in PD (no specific clinical type); **E.** Percent loss of TH-IR neurones in akinetic-rigid PD; **F.** percent loss of caspase-3 positive pigmented neurones in PD; **G.** Percent loss of TH-IR neurones in tremor-dominant subtype of PD; **H.** Percent loss of calbindin-IR neurones in Parkinson's disease.
A8: dopaminergic cell group A8; CG: central gray substance; CP: cerebral peduncle; M: medial group; Mv: medioventral group; N: nigrosome; RN: red nucleus, SNM: SN pars medialis; SNL: SN pars lateralis, PBP: parabrachial pigmented nucleus.

atypical parkinsonism (253), but increased alpha activity in REM sleep has been observed in de novo PD patients (254).

Macroscopy

Macroscopically, the brain is unremarkable or may show cortical atrophy and enlargement of the ventricles. On cut surface, pallor of the substantia nigra (SN) and locus ceruleus (LC) often is evident (Figure 1). An important negative finding is the normal appearance of the striatum and globus pallidus (GP).

Histopathology

General findings. Histopathology of PD is featured by the presence of numerous LBs and LNs in association with variable neurone loss in the midbrain and other subcortical nuclei, in particular the SN and LC (112, 134, 135). There is severe depletion of melanized neurones (45-66%) and of dopaminergic neurones immunoreactive (IR) for tyrosine hydroxylase (TH) (60-85%) in the A9 group of substantia nigra pars compacta (SNpc) (81, 149), particularly in the ventrolateral tier (area a, 91-97%) followed by the medioventral, dorsal and lateral areas (Figure 2). Susceptibility of dopaminergic neurones to degeneration has recently been shown to depend upon their distribiution within compartments of the substantia nigra defined by calbindin (CAB) immunostaining (39). A CAB-rich matix can be separated from 5 distinct CAB-poor zones or "nigrosomes." Neuronal loss is greater in nigrosomes than matrix in the caudal and mediolateral region. From there, it spreads to other nigrosomes and finally to the matrix along a caudo-rostral, latero-medial, and ventro-dorsal progression (39). This temporo-spatial order corresponds to a somatotopic pattern of dopaminergic terminal loss

	Neuronal system	Reduction vs. controls %
1.	Mesocortical dopaminergic systems	
	VTA: loss of melanized TH-IR neurons	40-86
	Ventral mesencephalon: dopamine/TH-IR loss	75
	Limbic areas and neocortex: dopamine loss	40-60
2.	Noradrenergic system	
	Locus coeruleus: pigmented cell loss	45-50
	Motor vagal nucleus: neuron loss (TH-IR, SP-IR)	5-77
	Supraoptic, paraventricular nucleus: cell loss	0
	Neocortex, limbic areas: norepinephrine loss	40-75
3.	Serotonergic system	
	Dorsal raphe nucleus: neuron loss	20-40
	Striatum, neocortex: serotonin loss	20-60
	Striatum, neocortex: 5-HT S-1, S-2 binding sites	reduced
4.	Cholinergic system	
	Nucleus basalis of Meynert: neuron loss	32-93
	Neocortex, hippocampus: ChAT, AChE loss	50-60
	Neocortex, hippocampus: nicotinic receptor loss	30-55
	Pedunculopontine tegmental nucleus: neuron loss	36-57
	Westphal-Edinger nucleus: neuronal loss	~50
5.	Peptidergic systems	
	Cholecystokinin-IR cell loss s. nigra	30-40
	Met-enkephalin loss: nigra, putamen, pallidum	50
	Substance P loss: nigra, globus pallidus	30-40
	SP-IR cell loss: nigra, pallidum	0
	brainstem, nuclei, cell loss	57-85
	Somatostatin: cortex, hippocampus (PD + AD)	30-60
	Neuropeptide Y-medulla; neuronal loss	70
	IR cell reduction: cortex, hippocampus	10-30

IR = immunoreactive; SP = substance P; ChAT = choline acetyltransferase; AchE = acetylcholine esterase

Table 4. Lesions of subcortical ascending systems in Parkinson's disease (108).

in the striatum that is more severe in the dorsal and caudal putamen than in the caudate nucleus (124).

There is a similar distribution of both reduced intensity of dopamine transporter (DAT) messenger (m) RNA in the remaining SNpc neurones (36) and decreased α-synuclein mRNA expression in the SN and cortex (181). Most telencephalic neurones in the A-9 and A-10 cell groups express high levels of DAT, while parts of the mesencephalic and all hypothalamic dopamine cell groups express little or no DAT (166). The degree of SNpc cell loss and loss of basal ganglia DAT immunoreactivity, show close correlation to the duration and severity of motor dysfunction (148). Decreases in the vesicular monoamine transporter (VMAT2), reflecting residual monoaminergic terminals, occur in early stages of PD in the striatum and amygdala, but not in the SN (34, 166).

The A-10 group of dopaminergic neurones, ventral tegmental area (VTA), nucleus parabrachialis and parabrachialis pigmentosus, projecting to cortical and limbic areas (mesocortico-limbic dopaminergic system), shows less involvement (40-50% cell loss), while the peri-retrorubral A-8 region, which contains only a few dopaminergic neurones but rather CAB-rich neurones, and the central periventricular grey either show little (20-32% cell loss in A-8) or no degeneration (164) (Figure 2). Cell depletion in these nuclei does not correlate with the duration of illness (150). Recent studies in cases with incidental LB pathology showed that PD lesions begin with the formation of α-synuclein IR neurites and LBs in the non-catechomalimnergic dorsal glossopharyngeus-vagus complex, in projection neurones of the intermediate reticular zone, and in neurones of the gain setting system (nucleus coeruleus-subcoeruleus, olfactory tract and nucleus) in the absence of nigral involvement. As in age-matched controls, in these initial cases, Lewy pathology does not occur in any of the later affected prosencephalitic sites (eg, hippocampus, amygdala, basal nucleus) (41a).

Lewy bodies and neurites. The characteristic, although not pathognomonic, finding in PD are LBs occurring in one of two general morphologic types: the classical or brainstem type and the cortical type (Figure 4A-C).

Classical LBs are intraneuronal, spherical cytoplamic inclusions ranging from 8 to 30 μm in diameter with a hyaline eosinophilic core and a narrow, pale-stained halo. The core region may develop a pattern of concentric lamellar bands (61, 145). A single neuron may contain several inclusions. Cortical LBs are eosino-philic, rounded, angular or reniform structures without an obvious halo. They are found in neurones of the cerebral cortex, particularly in layers V and VI of temporal, insular and cingulate regions. "Pale bodies" (synonyms: glassy degeneration, hyaline or colloid inclusion bodies), rounded areas of granular pale-staining eosinophilic material displacing neuromelanin in SN and LC neurones, have been proposed as precursors of LBs (38). Recent studies suggest an initial intraneuronal appearance of dust-like particles related to neuromelanin or lipofuscin, with homogeneous deposition of α-synuclein and ubiquitin in the central core of the LB (20, 68) Extraneuronal LBs are related to death and disappearance of the involved neurones (61).

Although LBs are not specific to PD and may occur in a variety of conditions as a secondary pathology (see below), a positive diagnosis of PD can usually be made by inspecting 2 unilateral sections from the mid-part of the SN and finding LBs. If no LBs are found, 2 further sections should be examined. If LBs are not seen in either SN or LC, then the diagnosis of PD of the LB type can be excluded. In case of cell loss from the SN and LC in the absence of LBs an alternative cause for parkinsonism should be pursued.

LBs are associated with coarse dystrophic neurites, *Lewy neurites*, with a similar immunohistochemical profile as LBs (45, 145). They are most frequent in the central and accessory cortical nuclei of the amygdala, in the CA 2-3 region of the hippocampus (Figure 4D) and the periamygdaloid cortex, but can also be detected in certain brainstem nuclei, the olfactory bulb, intermediolateral columns of the spinal cord, in sympathetic and parasympathetic ganglia, enteric, cardiac, and pelvic neurones (Table 5). They have also been described in the adrenal medulla. Absence of TH-IR in LNs suggests that the dystrophic neuritic processes are not necessarily derived from dopaminergic neurones.

Affected Region[a]	Major (putative) neuromediators[b]	Frequent	Rare
Cerebral cortex	Multiple		+
Anterior cingulate gyrus		++	
Temporal, insular		+	
Allocortex			+
Amygdala, central accessory cort. nucleus		++	
Basal nuclei			+
Nucleus basalis of Meynert	Acetylcholine	++	
Thalamus, midline nuclei		++	
Hypothalamus, lateral nucleus		++	
Lateral posterior nucleus	Norepinephrine		+
Paraventricular nucleus	Multiple		+
Tuberomamillar nucleus		++	
Subthalamic nucleus	Dopamine		+
Periaqueductal gray	Multiple		+
Substantia nigra zona compacta	Dopamine	++	
Nucleus parabrachialis pigmentosus	Dopamine	++	
Nucleus paranigralis	Dopamine	++	
Westphal-Edinger nucleus	Acetylcholine	+	
Darkschewitsch nucleus	Acetylcholine		+
Supratrochlear nucleus	Serotonin	+	
Nucleus tegmenti pedunculopontinus	Acetylcholine	+	
Central pontine gray	Multiple		+
Locus ceruleus	Norepinephrine	++	
Nucleus subceruleus	Norepinephrine	+	
Nucleus pontis centralis oralis	Serotonin	+	
Central superior nucleus of raphe	Serotonin		+
Processus griseum pontis supralemniscalis	?	+	
Dorsal motor nucleus of vagus	Norepinephrine	++	
Nucleus of Roller	?		+
Nucleus gigantocellularis	Serotonin		+
Nucleus paragigantocellularis lateralis	?		+
Nucleus medullae oblongatae centralis	Serotonin		+
C1 and C2 groups in medulla oblongata [31]	Epinephrine	++	
Olfactory bulb			
Spinal cord, intermediolateral column	Multiple		+
Spinal cord, intermediomedial column	Acetylcholine		+
Spinal cord, anterior horn			+
Autonomic (symp. and parasymp.) ganglia	Catecholamines	++	
Enteric nerve plexuses	Catecholamines		+
Adrenal medulla	Catecholamines		+

[a] Nomenclature of the brain stem nuclei (192).
[b] ref. 183
+ mild; ++ severe

Table 5. Distribution of Lewy bodies in Parkinson's disease (modified from ref. 112).

Neuronal vulnerability. Immunohistochemical methods have been used in an attempt to determine the nature of the selective vulnerability of neurons in PD. These studies show that PD neurones express calpain II, a calcium-dependent protease, which is not compensated for by its endogenous inhibitory protein calpastatin (175). In addition, fibroblastic growth factor-1 (FGF-1) and its binding activity are retained in SNpc neurones (251) and there is reduced expression of brain-derived neurotrophic factor (BDNF) (96). The number of trkB mRNA (a high-affinity BDNF-receptor) containing cells in SNpc and VTA is also decreased without a decrease in trkB mRNA in the remaining ones (13). While biochemistry revealed no difference of glial cell line-derived neurotrophic factor (GDNF) in the nigrostriatal regions in PD (168), immunohistochemistry showed 20% reduction of GDNF, and much less of BDNF in both neurones and neuropil (30), but increased numbers of BDNF and neurotrophin-3 (NT-3)-IR micro-glia around damaged neurones (125a). Reduced expression of the ND 1 subunit of mitochondrial complex I and of aldolase C in melanized SN neurones showed no relationship to disease duration or L-dopa treatment. However, recent PCR studies showed slective increase of mitochondrial DNA deletions/rearrangements in the SN but also in other regions of the PD brain compared with other movement disorders, AD and age-matched controls, indicating that mitochondrial dysfunction, a relative specific characteristic of PD, is not limited to the SN (77a). The reductions were specific to SN neurones, with no such changes in the pontine and LC neurones. The results suggest that dopaminergic SN neurones are more dependent on mitochondrial energy metabolism and oxidative phosphorylation than other brainstem populations (121).

Evidence suggests that selective vulnerability of SN melanized neurones, which have high expression of DAT mRNA (243), is unrelated to their intrinsic capacity of dopamine synthesis (123). On the other hand, they have low levels of calcium binding proteins, which have a neuroprotective role by buffering effects of Ca^{2+}-influx into cells. They also have weaker trophic support by neurotrophins and BDNF. Neurones that are not affected in PD, such as neurones in the subthalamic nucleus (STN) and GABAergic neurones in the SN pars reticulata (SNpr) are rich in calcium binding proteins (82).

In summary, the majority of midbrain dopaminergic neurones that are severely affected in PD are *i)* melainzed neurones located in the densely populated ventral tier of the SNpc, *ii)* rich in DAT and poor in gly-

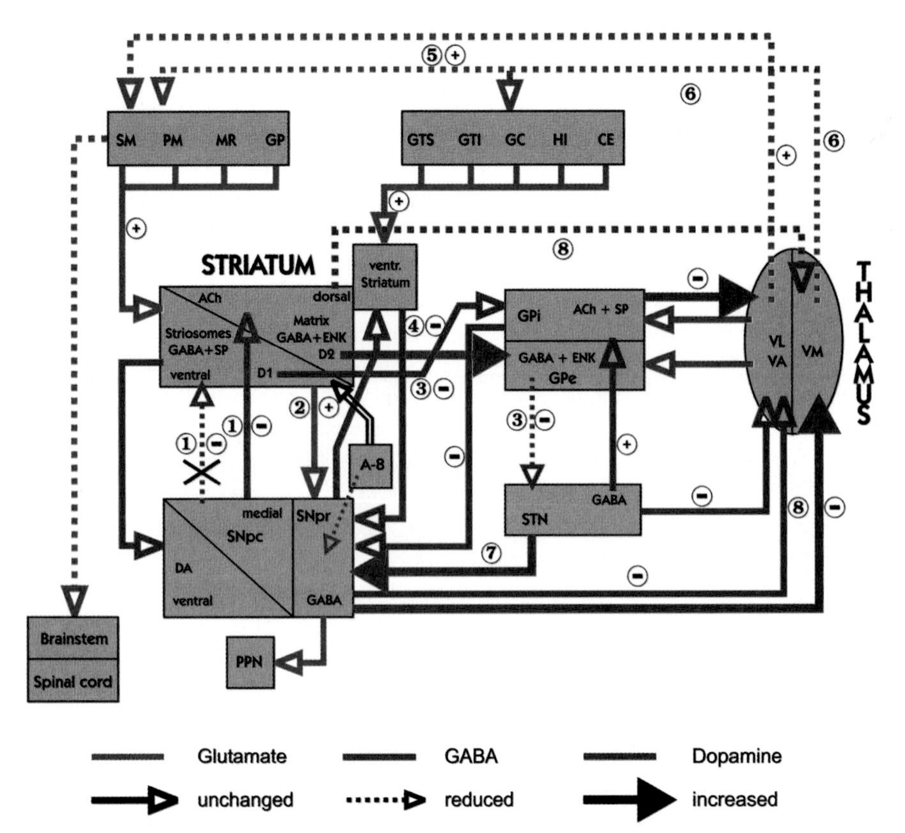

Figure 3. Schematic diagram of basal ganglia-thalamocortical circuitry under normal conditions and in Parkinson's disease. Cortex: SM supplementary motor field; PM premotor field; MR motor cortex, GP postcentral gyrus, GC gyrus cinguli; HI hippocampus; CE entorhinal cortex: Basal ganglia: SNpc SN zona compacta; SNpr SN reticulata, STN subthalamic nucleus, A-8 retrorubral field, GPi internal globus pallidus, GPe external globus pallidus, PAN peduriculopontine nucleus; VL, VLM ventro-lateral/medial thalamus; Vm medioventral thalamus; CS superior colliculus; MPT mesopontine tegmentum; ACh acetyl choline; SP substance P; ENK enkephalin; DA dopamine.
1 nigrostriatal dopaminergic pathway; 2 striato-nigral pathway; 3 "indirect" loop; 4 "direct" loop; 5 motor or complex loop; 6 thalamocortical pathway; 7 pallido-subthalamic pathway; + excitatory, – inhibitory. Adapted from Jellinger (1998).

colytic enzymes and calbindin, and *iii)* arborize densely in the striatum and sparsely in the extrastriatal structures. Conversely, most dopaminergic neurones that resist degeneration in PD are *i)* located in the scantily populated dorsal tier of the SNpc, *ii)* contain calbindin and glycolytic enzymes but are poor in DAT, and *iii)* arborize profusely in the extrastriatal components of the basal ganglia and sparsely in the striatum.

Glial and inflammatory reactions. Recent studies have shown widespread occurrence of argyrophilic, α-synuclein positive, tau-negative glial inclusions in both oligodendroglia and astrocytes in PD brain (Figure 4E). They differ from α-synuclein positive glial cytoplasmic inclusions (GCI) in MSA and from tau-positive glial fibrillary tangles in many tauopathies, eg, progressive supranuclear palsy (PSP) and corticobasal degeneration (CBD) (248, 249). Glial inclusions are found in regions with, eg, SNpc and LC neuronal loss and gliosis as well as regions without such pathology, eg, cerebral cortex, thalamus, white matter, cerebellum, spinal cord. They may appear early in the pathological process even at stages without apparent neuronal loss; their distribution pattern correlates with the appearance of LBs, eg, in the cerebral cortex and with TH-positive catecholaminergic neurones and fibres (92). They may be an early and important feature of PD, but their pathogenic impact needs further elucidation.

Neuronal loss in PD is accompanied by extracellular release of neuromelanin with uptake into macrophages (61), astroglial reaction and increase in major histocompatibility complex (MHC) class II positive microglia. The latter are capable of releasing proinflammatory cytokines, such as interleukin 1β (IL-1β), as well as interferon δ (IFδ), CD23, nitric oxide (NO), and other substances that mediate inflammatory or immune reactions. While the microglial reaction may be a reaction to neuronal death, it may also contribute to neuronal death (26, 161). Activated microglia can trigger neuronal apoptosis through the secretion of proteases such as cathepsin (120). In PD, the large number of activated microglia and perivascular iron-laden macrophages, free neuromelanin and extracellular LBs support a role of neuroinflammation in the pathogenesis of PD (107, 108).

Symptom-related lesion pattern in PD. The progressive degeneration of the nigrostriatal system is associated with dopaminergic denervation of the striatum. In early stages of PD, loss of dopamine uptake and of the presynaptic DAT is detected first in the posterior putamen (about 50%) with little involvement of the ventral putamen and the caudate nucleus. These changes are preceded by a preclinical phase, the duration and progression of which are still under discussion (104). From SPECT and PET studies, the estimated preclinical period ranges from 4.6 to 6.5 years, with an annual decline of striatal dopamine uptake of 8 to 10% (187) and of DAT between 5.7 to 6.4% or 10 to 13% (187, 203a, 205). Reduction in putamen 18F-dopa uptake after 2 years treatment (ropinirole or L-dopa) was 13% and 18%, respectively (204a). Hemi-parkinsonism shows a bilateral reduction, more severe contralateral to the clinical symptoms (239). As the disease progresses, dopamine loss is detected in the ventro-rostral putamen, but even in late stages it shows only about 30% reduction. The onset of motor symptoms of PD has been estimated to occur with loss of about 50% of SNpc neurones and a reduction of striatal dopamine uptake by 57 to 80% (15). In other studies motor symptoms of PD were noted with striatal dopamine uptake of 79% in the anterior and 70% in the posterior putamen without decrease in the caudate nucleus (207) or with 56% loss of DAT in the putamen (173). Thus, about 50% of dopaminergic striatal innervation appears sufficient for normal function (111, 113). IPD shows a marked heterogeneity in the clinical phenotype (60a).

The major clinical subtypes of PD are associated with specific lesion patterns with pathophysiological and therapeutic relevance (112, 113, 199):

Akinetic-rigid type. In this type the ventrolateral part of SNpc, which projects to the dorsal putamen, degenerates more severely than the medial part, which projects to the caudate and anterior putamen (Figure 3). Consequently, there is a correlation between SN neurone loss, severity of akinesia-rigidity, and dopamine loss in the posterior putamen (15). Abundant α-synuclein pathology in the striatum indicates involvement of the previously suggested "normal" striatum (50b). Dopaminergic denervation of the striatum affects the synaptic transmission of the output striatal GABAergic neurones with severe loss of dendrites on type I medium spiny neurones, the major targets of the dopaminergic input. In early stages of PD, the striatal efflux system via the GP, SNpr and thalamus to the cortex and the parallel nigro-pallido-cortical loop to the premotor cortex remain intact. The gradual loss of TH-IR and DAT-IR fibres and synpatic endings progresses from dorsal to ventral putamen. There is predominant involvement of metenkephalin (M-Enk)/substance P (SP) rich, acetylcholinesterase (AChE) poor striosomes that project to the ventrolateral SNpc. Preservation of the CAB-positive, somatostatin rich striatal matrix, which has increased somatostatin mRNA expression (54) and projects to GABAergic neurones of the SNpr and motor thalamus, suggests that the nerve endings that are richest in DAT are most sensitive to degeneration (166).

Striatal D1 receptors are predominantly located at striatonigral projection neurones ("direct pathway"), but are also present at endings of GABA neurones of SNpr that regulate dopamine release via dendrites of nigrostriatal neurones. The SP-IR endings are in contact with D2 receptor-IR dendrites and Enk-IR endings with D1 receptor-IR dendrites by which the axon collaterals forming the "direct loop" are in synaptic contact with neurones of the "indirect loop" and vice versa. Thus, both information loops of the neostriatum are in mutual synaptic contact (259).

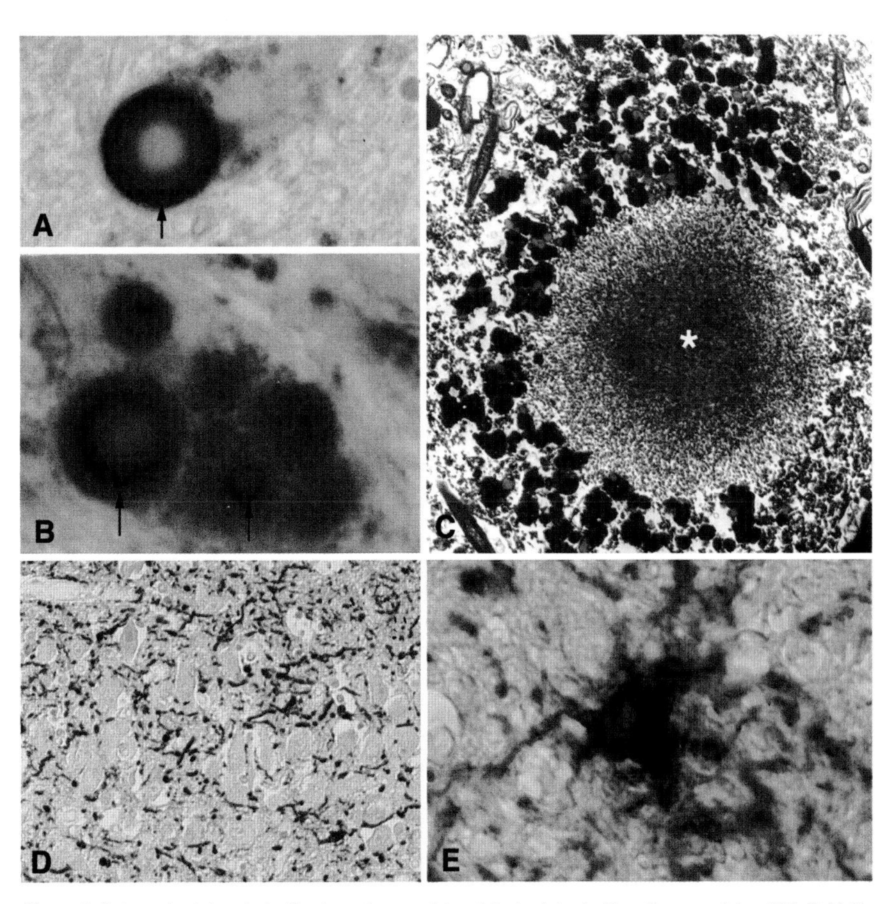

Figure 4. A. Lewy body in substantia nigra whose peripheral rim is stained with anti-α-synuclein ×300, **B.** Multiple Lewy bodies in nigral neuron ×1200, **C.** Electron microscopy of nigral LB showing a central electron dense filamentous core with a loosely fibrillary rim (x 2.500), **D.** Dystrophic Lewy neurites in the hippocampal C2/3 region, anti-α-synuclein ×150, **E.** Astrocytic inclusion in substantia nigra of PD brain labeled with anti-α-synuclein (blue) and GFAP (brown) ×900 (Courtesy Dr K. Wakabayashi).

Caudate nucleus biopsies in PD patients revealed reduced M-Enk staining in addition to reduced TH immunostaining that correlated with the severity of motor symptoms (40). Ultrastructural analyses in the caudate nucleus of L-dopa treated PD patients showed a 50% increase in the number of perforated synapses making contact with dendritic spines of D1 receptor (D1R) bearing neurones, but no changes in those on non-D1R spines. Slight increase in the surface area of the corticostriatal afferent fibres and of their mitochondria suggests a hyperactivity of these fibres in contact with D1R-bearing neurones of the direct pathway possibly involved in compensatory mechanisms (179). However, ultrastructural findings (133) and progressive loss of TH-and DAT-IR nigrostriatal fibres indicate transsynaptic degeneration as a possible substrate for the severity of motor deficits and decreased efficacy of dopamine treatment in late stages of PD (104).

Putamen D1 receptor binding shows negative correlation with the duration of disease and L-dopa treatment (233) while progressive loss of striatal D 2 receptors preserved for a long time may also contribute to doparesistence in late stages of PD.

Reference	DX	N	pm Time (h)	Method	% Neurons
47	PD	3	?	TU	0
167	juv PD	4	3-12.6	TU	0
	Late PD	7	1-5	TU	0-4.2 (m 1.2)
	Co	6	1-3	TU	0
6	PD	3	8.3±2.3	EM	3.7
240	PD	5	1.7-31	TU	6.9±2.2
	DLB	7	2.5-24.3	TU	11.46±1.3
	AD/PD	4	5.5-20	TU	7.8±2.45
	AD	5	11-16	TU	1.7±0.65
	Co	3	3-8	TU	0.93±0.47
126	PD	22	?	TU	"few" 1/22 brains
9	PD	3	7-30	TU	0
189	PD	3	?	TU+	1.5
	Co	3	?	YO	0.1
122	PD	16	5-3	TU	0-12.8 (m=2.0)
	MSA	4	8.5-35	TU	0-19.4 (m=9.0)
	DLB	1	16	TU	9.3
	PSP	1	25.5	TU	0
	Co	14	5.5-48	TU	0-10.5 (m=1.0)
257	PD	3	20-38	TU	0
	Co	4	4-42	TU	0
	PD	3	20-38	TU	2.0±1.2
	Co	4	4-42	(prol)	1.3±1.1
115	PD	5	4-12	TU	0/1080
	DLB	2	18-24	TU	0/1010
	PSP	3	12-24	TU	0/1080
	CBD	3	14-24	TU	0/1010
	Co	4	16-24	TU	0
237	PD	8	2,75-7	ISEL	9.0±5.0
	Co	4	8-11	YO	0.4±0.1

AD=Alzheimer's disease; iuv=iuvenile; Co=Controls; PD=Parkinson's disease; DLB=Dementia with Lewy bodies; MSA=multiple system atrophy; PSP=progressive supranuclear palsy; TU=TUNEL; CBD=corticobasal degeneration; YO=YOYO 1; pm=post mortem

Table 6. Incidence of DNA fragmentation in substantia nigra in variuos neurodegenerative disorders.

Reduced dopaminergic input to the putamen causes increased activity of the GABAergic inhibitory "indirect" striatal efferent loop via substantia nigra pars reticulata (SNpr) and globus pallidus interna (Gpi) (168) leading to increased GABA output to the ventrolateral thalamus projecting to the cortex-thalamo-cortical motor loop (Figure 3). The increased inhibition of thalamic premotor neurones as a result of excessive excitatory glutamatergic drive from the STN to the GPi/SNpr leads to an akinetic-rigid syndrome via reduced cortical activation. Disinhibition of the indirect pathway leads to a marked hypoactivity of the globus pallidus externa (Gpe) followed by a disinhibition of the STN (82, 134, 135, 195). Additional if not alternative mechanisms may underlie STN hyperactivity. Given the reciprocal innervation on the SNpc and the STN, the dopaminergic deficit may influence the STN activity directly, while the increased excitatory drive to the nigral neurones originating from the hyperactive STN might sustain the progression of the degenerative process (17).

The increased striatal GABAergic activity tends to disappear in the course of the disease and is reduced by L-dopa treatment. Alterations in signaling systems linking dopaminergic and glutamatergic receptors within the GABAergic efferent neurones may induce NMDA receptor changes resulting in long-term changes in glutamatergic synaptic efficacy which leads to alterations in the cortical input to the striatum and modifies striatal GABAergic output, favouring motor complications (29). Since the striatal matrix and its efferences remain intact, restitution of the dopaminergic transmission by L-DOPA substitution maintains the function of the "motor loop," but progressive degeneration with transgression to non-dopaminergic systems in later stages causes loss and reduced stimulation of postsynaptic D2 and muscarinic cholinergic receptors in the striatum by dopamine with unchanged antagonist binding. This uncoupling of receptor systems is considered a major cause of drug resistance of motor symptoms and adverse L-DOPA effects (dyskinesia, fluctuation) (16).

Tremor-dominant. This type of PD shows less severe total neuronal SN loss (mean 52.8% vs 69%) and less severe depletion in the lateral than in the medial SNpc (199). This may correlate with an inverse relation of domaine-uptake between the caudate nucleus and putamen to the severity of tremor, while such an index does not exist in relation to the degree of rigidity and bradykinesia (193). In addition, there is damage to the retrorubral A-8 field (Figure 3) that is usually preserved in akinetic-rigid PD (39). The A-8 area which, in contrast to A-9 and A-10, contains only few TH-IR and DAT-IR, but mainly calretinin-IR neurones (174), is independent of striatal influences but projects to the matrix of the dorsolateral striatum and ventromedial thalamus (197). Both the A-8 and A-10 areas directly influence the striatal efflux via SNpr and thalamus to the prefrontal cortex (64, 77) (Figure 3).

While necropsy cases of essential tremor, in general, show no pathological changes except for mild SN cell loss (137), PET studies suggest increased activity of ventral thalamic projections to cortical motor regions (8) and bilateral overactivity of cerebellar connections (43, 146a). MPTP (1-methyl-4-phenyl-1, 2, 3, 6-tetrahydropyridine)-lesioned monkeys with tremor show significant decrease of dopamine in the striatum suggesting that nigrostriatal degeneration contributes to tremor (51), while 4-6 Hertz tremor activity in GPi neurons point to its role role for rest tremor (100).

Figure 5. *Distribution pattern of lesions in Parkinson's disease.*
green: severe neuronal loss and Lewy bodies; red: Lewy bodies and mild neurone loss; yellow: Lewy bodies *ab* accessory basal nucleus of amygdala, *ac* accessory cortical nucleus of amygdala, *ad* anterodorsal nucleus of amygdala, *am* anteromedial nucleus of thalamus, *an* abducens motor nucleus, *ba* basal nucleus of amygdala, *bn* basal nucleus of Meynert, *ca1* first Ammon's horn sector, *ca2* second Ammon's horn sector, *ca* caudate nucleus, *cc* corpus callosum, *ce* central nuclei of amygdala, *cg* central grey of mesencephalon, *cl* claustrum, *co* cortical nuclei of amygdala, *cr* central nucleus of raphe, *db* nucleus of the diagonal band, *dm* dorsomedial hypothalamic nucleus, *dr* dorsal nucleus of raphe, *ds* decussation of superior cerebellar peduncles, *dv* dorsal nuclear complex of vagal nerve, *en* entorhinal region, *fn* facial motor nucleus, *fo* fornix, *gi* gigantocellular reticular nucleus, *gr* granular nucleus of amygdala, *hn* hypoglossal motor nucleus, *in* infundibular nucleus, *ir* intermediate reticular zone, *lc* locus coeruleus, *ld* laterodorsal nucleus of the thalamus, *lg* lateral geniculate body, *li* nucleus limitans thalami, *lt* lateral nuclei of the thalamus, *md* mediodorsal nuclei of thalamus, *me* medial nuclei of amygdala, *mf* medial longitudinal fasciculus, *mg* medial geniculate body, *ml* medial lemniscus, *mm* medial mamillary nucleus, *ms* medial septal nucleus, *mt* mamillothalamic tract, *mv* dorsal motor nucleus of vagal nerve, *oi* oliva inferior, *os* oliva superior, *ot* optic tract, *pe* external pallidum, *pf* parafascicular nucleus, *ph* posterior hypothalamic nucleus, *pi* internal pallidum, *po* pontine grey, *pr* praepositus nucleus, *pu* putamen, *pv* paraventricular nucleus, *re* reticular nucleus of the thalamus, *rm* nucleus raphes magnus, *ru* nucleus ruber, *sb* subiculum, *sc* superior cerebellar peduncle, *sf* solitary fascicle, *so* supraoptic nucleus, *sn* substantia nigra, *sp* subpeduncular nucleus, *st* nucleus of the stria terminalis, *sn* subthalamic nucleus, *te* transentorhinal region, *tl* lateral tuberal nucleus, *tm* tuberomamillary nucleus, *tp* tegmental pedunculopontine nucleus, *vl* ventro-lateral nuclei of thalamus, *vm* ventromedial hypothalamic nucleus, *vn* vestibular nuclei, *vt* dopaminergic nuclei of ventral tegmentum (paranigral nucleus and pigmented parabrachial nucleus), *zi* zona incerta.

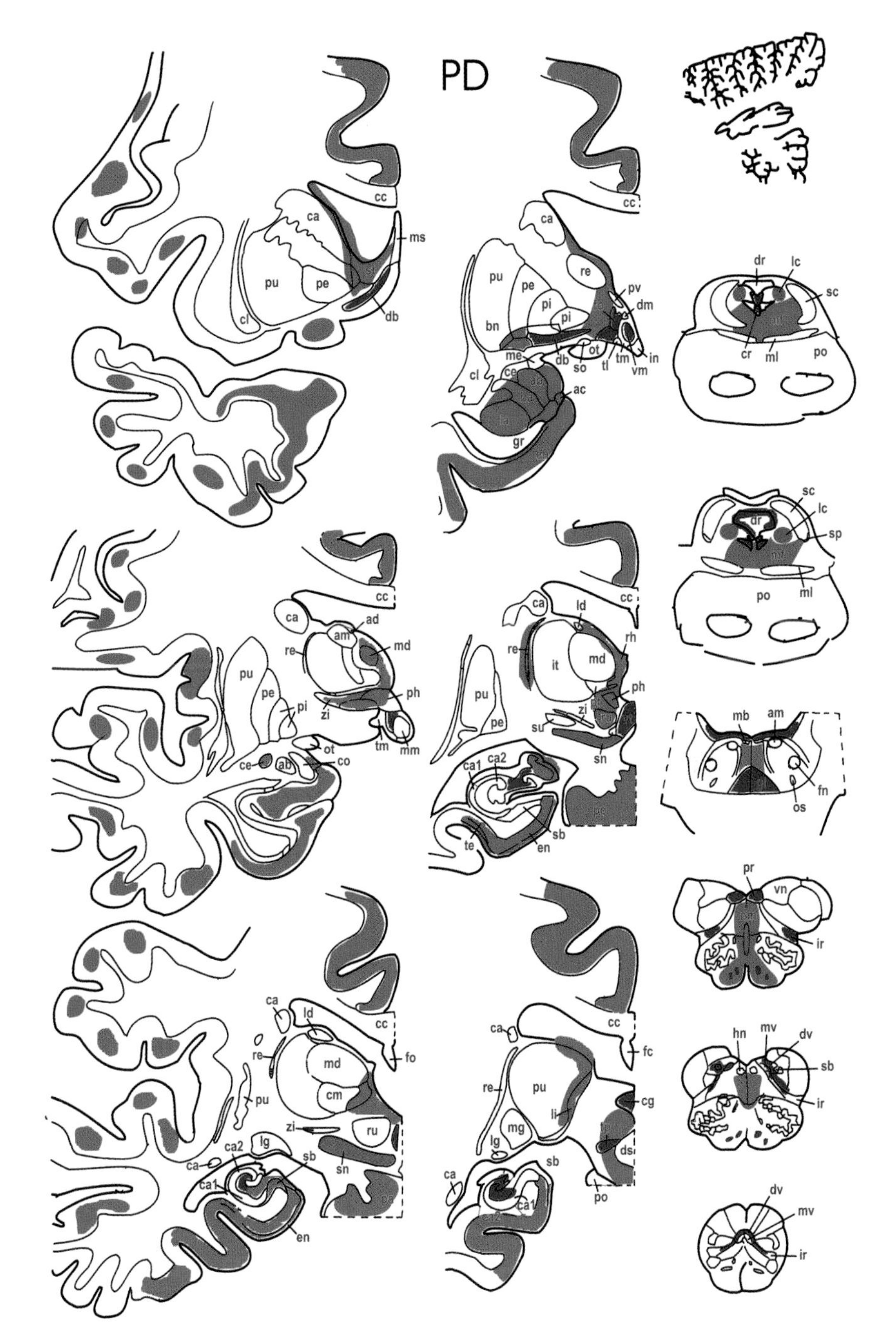

Distinction between PD and ageing brain. The distribution of SNpc lesions in PD differs from those seen in aging. In aging the dorsal tier is preferentially affected (39), while this region is involved only in late stages of PD (81). One study showed a 35 to 41% reduction in pigmented SN cells and severe loss of neuronal DAT-IR in the aged (148). The age-related neuronal loss was estimated to be a decrease of 9.8% per decade in total cell number, 7.4% in cell density, and 4.4% in neuronal volume (150). However, another recent study did not detect any significant loss of TH-IR neurones in the SN or other midbrain nuclei in very old subjects (129). While neuromelanin shows a continous accumulation in SNpc with ageing, in PD it is severely depleted compared to age-matched controls (260), which correlates with dropout of SNpc neurones (39).

Dementia in PD. Neuropathology findings in PD with dementia (PDD) include *i)* coexistent AD pathology, *ii)* involvement of various subcortico-cortical neuronal systems, or *iii)* cortical LB pathology. Concurrent AD pathology is seen in over 50% of PDD cases (111). While non-demented PD patients have AD pathology largely restricted to the limbic system, corresponding to a Braak stage of IV or less (21), PDD usually have more advanced AD pathology (Braak stage V and VI), with large amounts of tau-pathology in frontal, temporal and entorhinal cortices (41). Recent clinico-pathological studies showed a significant correlation between dementia and cortical AD-pathology that caused a signfiicantly shorter survival (average 4.5 versus 10 years) (114).

Parameter	Brain region	Reduction vs. controls %
Dopamine and metabolites		
Dopamine	SN	17
	Caudate nucleus	10
	Putamen	4
DOPAC	SN	2
	Putamen	10
HVA	SN	48
	Putamen	29
Dopamine metabolizing enzymes		
Tyrosine hydroxylase	SN	46
	Caudate nucleus	60
	Putamen	16
DOPA-Decarboxylase	Caudate nucleus	9
	Putamen	4
Catechol-O-Methyl-Transferase	SN	82
	Caudate nucleus	70
	Putamen	78
Monoamin-oxidase, type B	SN	125
Dopamine reuptake sites		
[^{3}H]Mazindol-binding	Caudate nucleus	32
	Putamen	16
[^{3}H]GBRI2935-binding	Caudate nucleus	13
	Putamen	33
[^{3}H]Win35,428-binding	Caudate nucleus	45
	Putamen	13
DAT-protein	Caudate nucleus	31
	Putamen	3
DAT-mRNA density in remaining neurons	SN	57
	SNC	86
Vesicular monoamin-transporter		
[^{3}H]Dihydroxytetrabenazin-binding	Caudate nucleus	30
	Putamen	15
	Caudate nucleus	49
	Putamen	23
mRNA-density in remaining neurons	SN	82

Table 7. Neurochemical findings in Parksinson's disease indicating damage to the dopaminergic nigro-striatal system (73).

Evidence that subcortical neuronal system pathology may account for dementia in PD includes studies showing that cognitive decline in PD is associated with reduced ChAT activity in the prefrontal cortex, dopaminergic hypofunction, and decreased numbers of dopaminergic D1 receptors in the caudate nucleus even in the absence of AD pathology (24, 157).

Widespread cortical LBs, demonstrated by α-synuclein immunohistochemistry, is increasingly considered to play a significant role in PDD. While some have reported correlations between cognitive impairment and the numbers of cortical LBs (99, 155) and of LNs in the amygdala and hippocampus (33), others have not found such an association (80). On the other hand, the density of both limbic LBs and of neuritic plaques correlated well with dementia severity, suggesting that both LB and neuritic pathology independently contribute to dementia (80, 110). Other recent studies in PD patients with late developing dementia and loss of the L-dopa response suggest that diffuse or transitional LBD is the major pathological substrate, while Alzheimer pathology often being modest is highly correlated with LB pathology, suggesting common origins or mutual triggering (8a).

Involvement of extranigral systems. PD is a multisystem disorder with involvement of many extranigral systems (Figure 5) (22, 107, 108). Lesions in PD are not random, but rather region-specific. Not all neurones of a given neurotransmitter type are vulnerable to LBs (Table 7), which may contribute to the complex patterns of functional, biochemial, and clinical deficits of this disorder.

Mesocortical dopaminergic system. Degeneration of dopaminergic fibres, originating from the SNpc (area A-9), the VTA (A-10), and the retrorubral area (A-8), innervating the striatum and the prefrontal, motor and premotor areas, and the thalamus, affects the functions of both the basal ganglia and cerebral cortex (64). The mesocorticolimbic system, which originates in the VTA and medial SNpc and projects to limbic and prefrontal areas and to the upper brainstem (196) is involved in PD. In demented subjects, the medial portion of SNpc shows greater neuronal loss than the lateral (199, 263). Cognitive and behavioural dysfunction in PD without concurrent AD have been related to cell depletion in VTA, reduction of TH-IRy in the prefrontal cortex, and neocortical monoamine terminal loss (152, 171).

Noradrenergic system. The *locus coeruleus* (LC area A-6), the main source of noradrenergic innervation of the rostral mesencephalon, hypothalamus, motor vagal nucleus, hippocampus, and neocortex (183), is involved in PD. Cell loss averages 40 to 50%, with predominant damage to the caudal, compact parts that project to the cerebellum and spinal cord. It is more severe in patients with depression or dementia or both, and can approach the loss seen in AD (263). PD cases without depression or dementia suffer a 39% decrease of large pigmented cells, while AD shows a decrease of both large (82%) and small neurons (39%). Cell loss in the rostral parts of the LC, which project to temporal cortex and hippocampus, correlates with the density of AD neuritic pathology, possibly consistent with a retrograde degeneration due to pathology in their cortical target areas. In contrast, LC cell loss in PD without a relationship to cortical pathology suggests a primary degeneration (94). LC damage causes deprivation of noradrenergic innervation of the forebrain and neocortex and has been related to dementia, depression, and autonomic dysfunction (73).

The pigmented neurones of the arcuate and periventricular hypothalamic nuclei are preserved (159), but

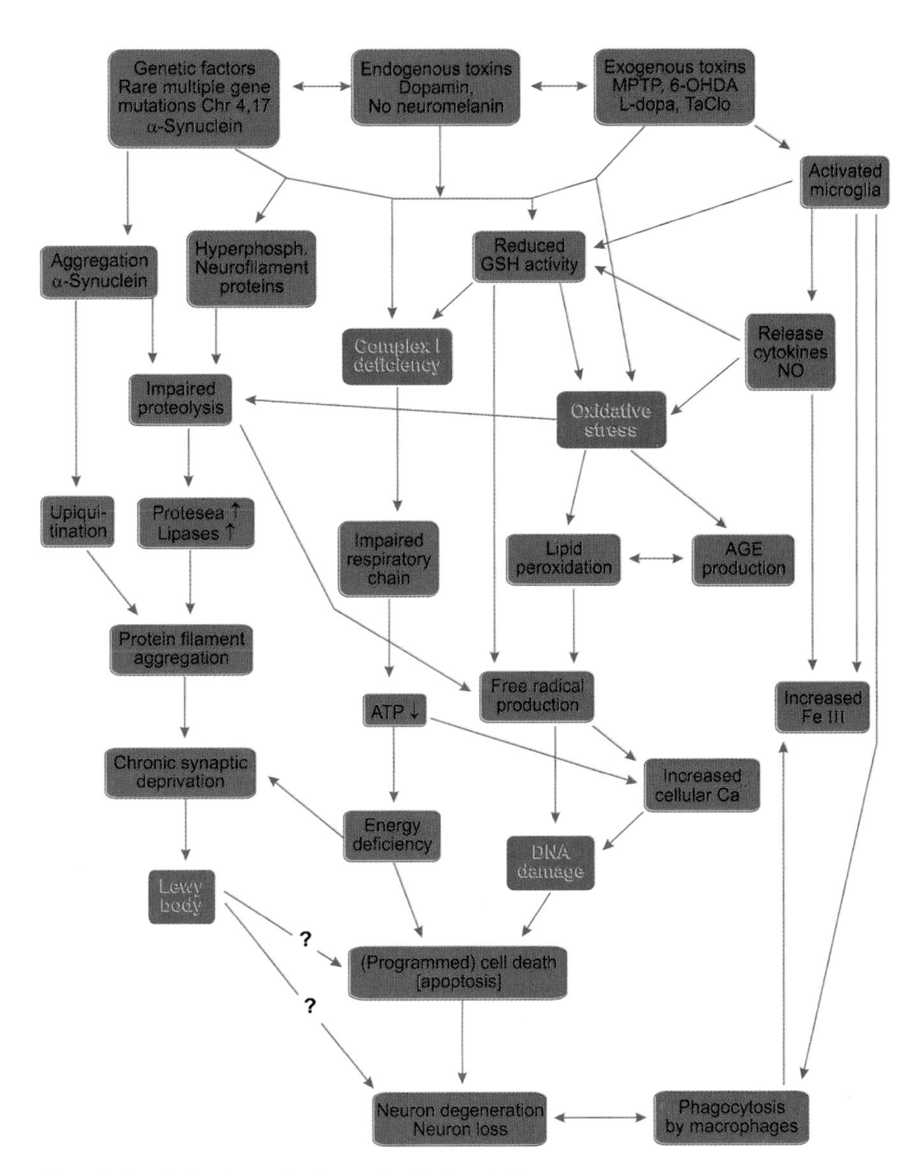

Figure 6. *Hypothetic scheme of pathogenesis of Parkinson's disease.*

decreased nucleolar volume and cytoplasmic RNA and a loss of TH-IR cells in the paraventricular and supraoptic nuclei indicate reduction in noradrenergic input.

The noradrenergic *dorsal vagal nucleus* shows no or only very little changes in aged controls and PD patients, with 5 to 17% cell loss, but frequent occurrence of LBs (78). They reported a 77% loss in SP-IR preganglionic cells of the dorsal motor vagal nucleus, whereas the noradrenergic TH-IR neurones, although often harbouring LBs, are not affected (<5% reduction).

The presence of many LBs in non-catecholaminergic neurones may indicate that their degeneration is caused by a primary process and is not secondary to damage to related pathways (78). Loss of substance P (SP)-IR vagal neurones, LBs of peripheral autonomic neurones in enteric plexuses, and reduced TH-IR in adrenal medulla with strong decrease of dopamine indicate damage to the sympathetic noradrenergic system that may contribute to vegetative symptoms in PD (73, 79). The adrenergic nuclei A-1 and A-2 in the medulla oblongata containing poorly pigmented neurones suffer no cell loss in PD, while a loss of NE synthesizing cells was observed on the Cl area of the medulla (66).

Serotonergic system. The *dorsal raphe nucleus* (DRN) or nucleus supratrochlearis and the central superior (raphe) nucleus, corresponding to cell groups B6-8, gives rise to ascending serotonergic pathways and is connected with many CNS centres (183). Neurons in the DRN are lost in PD, especially TH-IR neurones, while the phenylalanine hydroxylase (PH-8)-IR neurones are unaffected. By contrast, there is about 60% reduction of PH-8 serotonin-synthesizing cells in caudal midbrain and pons (79). Many of the remaining neurones contain LBs or LNs.

Cholinergic system. The cholinergic system shows cell loss and shrinkage in the magnocellular part of the Ch4 region of the *nucleus basalis of Meynert* (NBM) projecting to the neocortex and other cholinergic brainstem nuclei. NBM cell depletion, which averages 30 to 40%, does not correlate to age or duration of illness. NBM neuronal loss is higher in PDD, approaching values seen in AD (50-70%), and is more than in PD without dementia or aged controls (0-40%) (Table 3). On the other hand, about 50% neuronal loss was also detected in non-demented PD subjects, with no relation between cell counts and mental status (110, 199). LBs in NBM occur in 100% and NFTs in 30 to 65% of all PD brains.

The decrease of cholinergic innervation of the cortex and hippocampus may or may not correlate with the severity of NBM cell loss and with the mental status, although both deficits are usually higher in demented PD patients (203). In nondemented cases NBM cell loss ranging from 15 to 62% and is associated with no or little cortical Alzheimer pathology, while in demented PD subjects, NBM cell depletion between 64 and 90% is often accompanied by severe cortical AD lesions. These data suggest that degeneration of the ascending cholinergic system may precede the onset of mental changes and that there is a critical threshold of 75 to 80% neuronal loss and/or shrinkage within the NBM with equivalent cortical cholinergic denervation before dementia becomes apparent (109). The loss of cholinergic neurones in the NBM and in the brainstem may affect hippocampal and prefrontal structures and may thus contribute to cognitive impairment and behavioural changes (49).

The variability in NBM cell depletion and loss of cholinergic markers in the neocortex and hippocampus, irrespective of cortical lesions, suggest primary degeneration of the cholinergic forebrain system in PD, while secondary degeneration with defective retrograde transport of NGF is thought in AD (177).

The *nucleus tegmenti pedunculopontinus*, pars compacta (PPNc), an important cholinergic loop nucleus in the dorsolateral part of the caudal mesencephalic tegmentum, receives fibres and provides projections to the thalamus, SNpc, STN, striopallidum, pontine tegmentum, basal forebrain, and to widespread cortical areas (212). It is the centre of balance between cholinergic and dopaminergic basal ganglia functions (76). In PD, cell loss in the PPNc ranges from 36 to 57%, with loss of 57% of the SP-IR cells (106), and strong correlation to neurone loss in the SNpc, but not to the patients' age, duration of illness, and LB counts. Unaltered parameters of cholinergic transmission in the thalamus and STN in PD suggest that the lesion to the PPNc is a retrograde phenomenon rather than part of a systemic fibre degeneration.

Overactivity of the PPNc in MPTP parkinsonism could indicate dysfunctions in the tegmento-nigro-subthalamo-cortical pathways, but its clinical significance in PD remains unclear. Damage to the PPNc may contribute to disorders of locomotor activities, abnormalities of gait and posture, coordination of the sleeping-waking cycle, or cognitive disturbances (194).

The *Westphal-Edinger nucleus*, a visceral subdivision of the oculomotor complex, giving rise to cholinergic fibers to the ciliary ganglion regulating pupilloconstriction, suffers a 54% neuronal loss in PD, but only few cells are affected by LBs or neurofibrillary tangles (NFTs) (106). Damage to this and other brainstem nuclei including the periaqueductal grey, and nucleus interstitialis of Cajal may explain neuro-ophthalmic and REM sleep dysfunctions in PD (138).

Pathological lesions in the amygdala. This limbic structure, interconnected with the prefrontal cortex, hippocampus, basal forebrain, brainstem, and other areas regulating behavioural and autonomic functions (246) is affected in PD. LBs and LNs mainly involve the accessory cortical and lateral, less severe the basal and lateral nuclei (22). The central accessory nucleus integrates information from brainstem and hypothalamus to the basal forebrain and centres controlling endocrine or autonomic functions, but amygdala damage appears not to be a major cause of mental impairment in PD.

Other systems involved. Other areas involved in PD are the reticular brainstem nuclei controlling somatomotor and autonomic systems (12, 20, 22), posterolateral hypothalamus, the centre median-parafascicular thalamus (91), and the intermediolateral nuclei and Clarke's column in the spinal cord (250).

The *histaminergic system* is also affected in PD. The density of histaminic fibres in the middle portion of the SNpc and SNpr is increased, but the histaminic fibres are thinner than in controls and have enlarged vesicles, which could be a compensatory event due to deficiency of dopamine or a putative growth inhibitory factor (7). Histamine concentrations in postmortem PD brain but not in MSA are significantly increased in the putamen, SNPC, and globus pallidus, while the histamine metablite tele-methylhistamine concentrations are unchanged in PD (206b).

Peptidergic systems. While some neuropeptides are severely decreased, others are unchanged. There is considerable reduction of Met- and Leu-enkephalin with increase of somatostatin mRNA expression in the basal ganglia (54) of somatostatin in the striatum and SN in PD and, to a lesser degree, in "incidental LB disease." SP is diminished in the putamen. Some experimental models of PD show increased glutamatergic activity in the striatum (18) but brain glutamate and aspartate are unchanged in human PD, while GABA is mildly reduced in the medial thalamus and NMDA receptors are decreased in the caudate nucleus (73).

Immunohistochemistry and Ultrastructural Findings

Ultrastructural findings. In the SNpc of PD patients, electron microscopic studies reveal: *i)* normal cells with normal nuclei, *ii)* neurones with an aggregation of the normal indentation of the nucleoplasm or with other minor nuclear abnormalities, and *iii)* nerve cells with obvious nuclear abnormalities consisting either of an abnormal diffuse or focal electron density of the nucleus, contrasting with a relatively preserved cytoplasm or an electron dense remnant of a nucleus with still visible cytoplasm. Type 3 changes represent a dying cell, which may indicate either apoptosis or necrosis (62). Although some SN neurones in PD ultrastructurally reveal a loose and finely granular nuclear chromatin structure, only exceptional cells desplay a reduction in cell size and clumping of nuclear chromatin resembling apoptosis (75).

LBs ultrastructurally are composed of radially arranged 7 to 20 nm filaments associated with a granular electron-dense coating material and vesicular structures, while the core contains densely packed filaments and dense granular material (Figure 4C). Cortical LBs are formed from felt-like arranged filaments and granular material (61).

Immunohistochemistry. The precise biochemical composition of LBs and LNs is still unknown. Immunocytochemistry has shown the following major components: phosphorylated neurofilament proteins present in both core and periphery, synaptophysin and chromgranin A (vesicular structures may be degenerating nerve endings), the prosynaptic nerve terminal protein α-synuclein (Figure 4C) which can be extensively nitrated (230), synphilin, an α-synuclein interacting protein, located in the central and peripheral parts of LBs, gelsolin-related amyloid protein, amyloid β peptide (Aβ), amyloid preocursor protein (APP), actin-like protein, ubiquitin, and ubiqutin-pathway associated enzymes (UCH-L1, protease, ligase, and kinases), α-microglobulin, immunoglobulins, α-B crystallin (in about 10% of cortical LBs) probably mediating the aggregation of microfilaments, Cu/Zn superoxide dismutase, cytosolic and microtubule-associated proteins including tau protein, MAP-2, MAP-5, calbindin, tubulin, TH, G7 and G9 proteins (68, 145, 163). In addition, LBs contain lipids and redox-active iron (28). Colocalization of α-synuclein, synphilin and parkin, a known E3 ubiquitin ligase, and its E2-binding partner UbcH7 suggests that parkin proteins may play a role in the posttranslational procession and ubiqutination of α-synculein and may be required during LB formation (60, 215a, 224). This may explain why some forms of EOPD mutations lack LBs. They further contain 14-3-3- proteins that are involved in numerous signal transduction pathways and interact with α-synuclein (119a), and torsin, a novel protein in which a mutation causes dominant, early onset torsion dystonia, which may serve as a chaperone for misfolded proteins that require refilding or degradation (218). LBs have a distinc central ubiquitin-positive domain, while α-synuclein primarily occurs in the periphery, suggesting that these 2 proteins do not have the same compartment, with ubiquitination being the later event (67). However, not all LBs contain ubiquitin and 7 to 10% contain only α-synuclein, which is one of the best markers to differentiate LBs and LNs from negative neurofibrillary tangles (NFT) or Pick bodies (50). Staining for α-syunclein rather than ubiquitin is now the preferred method for detecting LBs and LNs. Several immunocytochemical studies have shown presence of α-synuclein (230), (Figure 4C), ubiquitin and phosphorylated neurofilament proteins. They have a distinct central ubiquitin-positive domain, while α-synuclein primarily occurs in the periphery suggesting that these two proteins do not have the same compartment (67).

α-Synuclein is one of the best markers to differentiate LBs and LNs from neurofibrillary tangles (NFTs) or Pick bodies (50). Staining for α-synuclein has replaced that for ubiquitin as the preferred method for detecting LBs and LNs. Altered α-synuclein is incorporated into LBs, their precursors ("pale bodies") and dystrophic LNs before ubiquitination. It is aggregated and fibrillated in vitro, resembling LB-like fibrils (88). Extracted filaments from SNpc in PD are labelled by antibodies against the carboxy-terminal region of α-synuclein in their entire length, while an antibody against its amino-terminal region labels only one filament end (37). α-Synuclein is more compact and in closer association with other molecules in LBs than in the neuropil, and its N-terminus shows a close intermolecular interaction to ubiquitin, suggesting that α-synuclein adopts an altered 3-dimensional structure and undergoes N-terminal ubiquitination (219). The mechanisms of its aggregation that may serve as a nidus for LB formation in vivo has not yet been elucidated, while in vitro it is modulated by various factors (229). The conformation of α-synuclein can be modulated by metals, with iron promoting aggregation and magnesium inhibiting aggregation (74a). Mutant and wild-type α-synuclein interact with the mitochondrial complex IV enzyme, cytochrome C oxidase (COX), and a COX inhibitor enhanced the sensitivity of SH-SY5Y neuroblastoma cells to dopamine induced cell death, suggesting that α-synuclein aggregation may contribute to enhance the mitochondrial dysfunction, which may be a key factor in the pathogenesis of PD (52a).Dopamine-dependent neurotoxicity is mediated by soluble protein complexes containing α-synuclein and 14-3-3 protein which are selectively elevated in the PD SN. Thus, these α-synuclein complexes can render endogenous dopamine toxic (257a).

Aggregation of α-synuclein may produce neuronal death due to promotion of mitochondrial energy deficit and oxidative stress (97, 210). Immunoreactivity for cytochrome c, located in the intramembrane of mitochondria and released upon apoptotic stimuli into the cytoplasm, is detected in LBs and defects in cytochrome oxidase c have been described in SNpc (105). In addition to decreases in cytochrome c oxidase, SNpc cell degeneration is also preceded by loss of neurofilament, DAT and TH proteins, as well as decreases in TH, DAT and neurofilament mRNA (105, 123). Further evidence that LBs show oxidative damage is the presence of advanced glycation endproducts (AGE) in LBs. AGE are thought to play a role in neurodegeneration since they are markers of transitional metal-induced oxidative stress and they induce protein crosslinking and free radical formation (178).

Despite the evidence that α-synuclein aggregates and LBs may be cytotoxic, it is not certain if they might also be harmless side-products or markers of cell damage. The UPS renders mutated or damaged proteins less toxic than their soluble forms, which suggests that the ubiquitinated proteins in LBs may be a manifestation of a cytoprotective response designed to eliminate damaged cellular components and to delay the onset of neuronal degeneration (32, 74). LBs may be indicators of neuronal dysfunction, a consequence of impaired degradation of abnormal cytoskeletal elements and a reaction to unknown degenerative processes (50).

Programmed cell death and neurodegeneration. Although the cause of neuronal death in PD is still enigmatic, several mechanisms are under discussion: apoptosis, (oncotic) necrosis, excitotoxic neurodegeneration, and autophagy (6, 109, 190, 238, 240). DNA fragmentation and an upregulation of pro-apoptotic and cell regulating proteins and enzymes (85, 153) suggest that *apoptosis*, a specific gene-directed form of programmed cell death (PCD), may represent a major pathway in the selective degeneration of specific neuronal populations. In

Increased	Decreased
Iron	Ferritin ?
Ferritin ?	GSH (GSSG unchanged); GSH/GSSG ratio)
Lactoferrin receptor expression	GSH-peroxidase activity
Ratio of oxidized to reduced glutathione (GSSG/GSH)	Catalase activity
Polyunsaturated fatty acids	Mitochondrial complex !
Mitochondrial monoaminoxidase B	Calcium binding protein (calbindin 28)
Lipofuscin	Transferrin receptor
Ubiquitin	Vitamins E and C
Cu/Zn-superoxide dismutase	Copper
Cytotoxic cytokines (TNF-_, IL-1, IL-6)	
Inflammatory transcription factor NFÍB	
Heme oxygenase-1	
Nitric oxide	
Thiobarbituric acid	
8-hydroxy-2-deoxy guanosine	

Table 8. Biochemical alterations in substantia nigra in Parkinson's disease indicating oxidative stress.

contrast to experimental and in vitro studies, however, conflicting results have been reported for human PD. DNA fragmentation, demonstrated by TUNEL and related techniques, and definite histological features of apoptosis are extremely rare in SNpc neurones, ranging from 0 to 12% (with a means of 1-2%) of the total dopaminergic SN cell population as compared to 0 to 1% in controls (122, 237, 240). On the other hand, some groups did not find any evidence of apoptosis in PD brains (9, 109, 126, 257). Occasionally, a combination of apoptosis and autophagic degeneration of SN neurones has been found (6).

Very few neurones show a mild to moderate expression of some pro-apoptotic proteins, eg, c-Jun, AP1, ASP, and Bax, and only occasionally express activated caspase-3 (85, 169, 237), suggesting a pro-apoptotic environment. In contrast, increased levels of anti-apoptotic factors such as Bcl-2 and Bcl-X in basal ganglia and SN have been reported (153). Others have found no differences in the immunoreactiviy of Bcl-2 and Bcl-X and in the expression of Bcl-2mRNA in SN neurones (111, 182). Some post mortem data suggest that Bax is expressed in SNpc neurones (247), although the intensity of Bax-IR was identical in LB and non-LB bearing neurones, suggesting that Bax does not contribute directly to LB formation (241). Bcl-xL mRNA, which labeled all dopaminergic neurones in human SNpc, was 1.8 times higher in PD than in controls. It was also detected in neurones with LBs, suggesting that surviving cells may be protected by this anti-apoptotic protein (85).

Reduced Fas and Fas-L in SN neurones with and without LBs, but increased Fax and Fas-L in reactive astroglia indicate that the Fas/Fas-L pathway does not play an essential role in regulating SN cell loss (59). A positive correlation between the degree of neuronal loss and the percentage of caspase-3 positive pigmented SN cells, with a 76% decrease in PD, suggests that this central effector enzyme of apoptosis may contribute to regional vulnerability of pigmented SN neurones (84, 86). Ultrastructurally activated caspase-3 staining was observed in dopaminergic cells displaying the morphological features of increased protein synthesis, but not in cells with the signs of apoptosis (85). Increased numbers of SN neurones expressing activated caspase-8, a proximal effector protein of the tumor necrosis factor (TNF) receptor family death pathway, suggest its activation in early stages of cell demise(87, 88). Elevated caspase activities and tumor necrosis factor recepter R 1 (p53) in SN and increased caspase-3 and Bax IRy accompany nuclear GAPDH (glyceraldehyde-3-phosphate dehydrogenase) translocation and neuronal apoptosis (237, 247). Activated forms of both caspase-8 and -9, upstream proteases known to cleave and activate caspase-3, have been demonstrated in SN neurones in PD (5). SN neurones also show translocation of DNA repair enzymes (PARP and DNA-PKCs) from the cytoplasm to the nucleus (144). On the other hand, no relationship between in situ labeling of nuclear DNA fragmentation or caspase-3 activation and MAPK has been observed (60), although recent studies have shown increased expression and redistribution of the anti-apoptotic molecule Bcl-x in PD (85a). The function of parkin protein that is important for the survival of the neurones that degenerate in PD, is cleaved during apoptosis by increased caspase activation, which was not significinatly affected by the disease-causing mutations K161N, G238E, T415N, and G430D and the polymorphism in R366W but is abrogated by mutation of Asp-126 alone. Cleavage is a membrane-associated event, and proteolysis has been shown to be sensitive to inhibitors of caspase. This suggests that parkin function is compromised in neuropathological states associated with an increased caspase activation, further adding to the cellular stress (117a). Furthermore, LBs in brainstem are consistently negative for apoptosis-related proteins, including activated caspase-3 (112), MAPK-P, p38Pn and SAPK/JNK, but they are stained with anti-ERK-2 antibodies (60). These data suggest that nuclear DNA damage, contribution of Bcl family proteins, and activation of the caspase cascade may be involved in the degeneration of dopaminergic neurones in PD, but they rarely indicate actual neuronal apoptosis.

Biochemistry

A large variety of neurochemical changes have been described in PD brains, including changes in neurotransmitters and other pathobiochemical pathways (Tables 7, 8).

Dopaminergic system. The striatonigral system, in addition to severe loss of dopamine in the putamen, less in the caudate and SN, shows considerable reduction of the dopamine metabolites 3, 4-dihydroxyphenyl acetic acid (DOPAC) and homovanillic acid (HVA) Table 7). The dopamine synthesizing enzyme tyrosine hydroxylase (TH) that catalyses the conversion of L-tyrosine to L-dopa and is the rate-limiting step in dopamine synthesis and DOPA decarboxylase are both decreased, whereas the activity of catechol-o-methyl-transferase (COMT) is only mildly reduced. Activity of monoamine oxidase B (MAO-B), which is found primarily in astroglia, is increased in PD. Decreases in dopamine in the striatum are disproportionate to decreases in DOPAC, HVA, and TH activity in mild to moderate PD, which indicates that surviving neurones are overactive (95). This compensatory phase is replaced in advanced stages of the disease by decreases in all these substances. Dopamine reuptake and DAT protein are reduced in the striatum, while DOPA decarboxylase mRNA, TH mRNA, DAT mRNA, and VMAT2 are reduced in the SN (243, 255). Less severe changes are seen in other dopaminergic systems, with 40 to 60% dopamine loss in the limbic and prefrontal cortex, hypothalamus, olfactory cortex and amygdala (72, 73). Reduction of dopamine in the retina (83) of both dopamine and TH activity in the adrenal medulla (73) and in other organs suggest that PD represents a generalized disorder of the dopaminergic system.

The postsynaptic dopaminergic D2 receptors are relatively unchanged in the striatum. A slight increase in their density and increases in the expression of mRNA in de novo PD patients could be due to reduced presynaptic dopaminergic activity "supersensitive dopamine receptors." By contrast, no modification of D1 receptor density in the striatum has been reported in de novo PD. In contrast, after L-DOPA treatment, D1 receptor density increases (179), suggesting that treatment changes the equilibrium between D1 and D2 receptors. Free endogenous dopamine may induce a "relative hyperstimulation" of the D1 receptors; subsequent internalization of dopamine receptors in response to excess stimulation may account for the development of motor fluctuations and dyskinesias after L-DOPA treatment (16, 29). The D2-3 receptor types outside the striatum are not involved in the early stages of PD, but only in advanced stages of the disease, particularly in the anterior cingulate and dorsolateral prefrontal cortex, and the thalamus (117). The role of the other dopaminergic receptors (D3-5) in the striatum of PD brain is still unclear.

Drugs	Recommended daily dosage	Main side effects
Dopamine precursors		
Levodopa + Carbidopa	300-1200 mg	anorexia, nausea, vomiting,
Levodopa + Benserazide	300-1200 mg	dyskinesia, hallucination, delusion,
Levodopa	1500-4500 mg	agitation, confusion
Dopamine agonists		
Bromocriptine	15-30 mg	anorexia, nausea, vomiting, constipation,
Pergolide	1.5-4.5 mg	diarrhea, dyspepsia, dry mouth, abdominal
Cabergoline	2-6 mg	pain, dyskinesia, dizziness, dystonia,
Talipexole	1.2-3.6 mg	hallucination, delusion, agitation,
Ropinilole	6-24 mg	confusion, drowsiness, skin rash,
Pramipexole	1.5-4.5 mg	edema, pleural effusion, postural hypotension
Piribedil	150-200 mg	
Monoamine Oxidase B inhibitor		
Deprenyl (Selegiline)	5-10 mg	nausea, dizziness, abdominal pain
COMT inhibitor		
Entacapone	200 mg/dose	dyskinesia, hallucination, confusion, liver dysfunction, rhabdomyolysis
Anti-cholingergics		
Trihexyphenidyl	4-6 mg	dry mouth, anorexia, constipation,
Biperidine	1 – 3 mg	confusion, delusion, agitation,
Piroheptine	2-6 mg	disturbed accomodation,
Benztropine	1-3 mg	increase in ocular pression, urinary retension, abdominal pain
Amantadine HCl	150-300 mg	hallucination, revedo reticularis
Norepinephrine precursor		
Droxydopa	300-900 mg	anorexia, nausea, hallucination

Table 9. Anti-Parkinson drugs.

Noradrenergic system. Degeneration of the noradrenergic neurones in the LC and other nuclei, with significant decrease of TH mRNA expression, causes a considerable decrease of norepinephrine (NE) in many brain regions, ranging from 22 to 88% of control, with variable changes in the major metabolite of norepinephrine, 3-methoxy-4-hydroxyphenylglycole (MHPG). The activity of dopamine-β-hydroxylase, the major synthesizing enzyme of NE, is decreased in PD. Noradrenergic dysfunction has been related to dementia, depression, and autonomic symptoms, eg, orthostatic hypotension in PD (72).

Serotonergic system. Serotonergic deficiency, related to degeneration of the DRN system, is reflected by reduced levels (40-50% of controls) of serotonin (5-HT) and its major metabolite 5-hydroxy-indolic acid (5-HIAA) in the striatum, medial frontal cortex and in other brain regions (73). Reduction of 5-HT and its receptors in the striatum and frontal cortex have been related to cognitive disorders and depression. Decreased serotonergic activity in the CSF related to accumulation of 3-O-methyldopa (3-OMD) in the brain may be associated with akinesia and with levodopa failure syndrome in advanced PD (143).

Cholinergic system. Damage to the cholinergic forebrain system is associated with reduced activities ChAT, the acetylcholine-synthesizing enzyme, in the cerebral cortex and hippocampus. In contrast, the binding densities of the muscarinic receptors are normal and there is increased binding for ^{3}H-hemicholinium, a marker of presynaptic high affinity choline-uptake (160% in the frontal cortex and caudate; 245% in the putamen), suggesting compensatory mechanisms (208).

GABAergic systems. The neuronal loss in SNpc affects the function of the output striatal GABAergic neurones, the major targets of dopamine-containing cells (228). Reduced activity of glutamate-decarboxylase (GAD), the GABA synthetic enzyme, is detected in basal ganglia and cerebral cortex. Levels of GABA are slighty increased in the striatum and mildly reduced in the medial thalamus in PD (95) . Although the GP is structurally preserved, the functional imbalance resulting from the disruption of the nigrostriatal pathways leads to 50% reduction of GAD mRNA in the GPe, which exerts an inhibitory influence on the STN via GABAergic fibers (184). Expression of GAD mRNA varies, but may increase after L-DOPA therapy. The GABA and flunitrazepam binding sites at GABA receptors and the density of 3H-flunitrazepam receptors in the SN and striatum are only slightly reduced (77), probably due to degeneration of dopaminergic neurones having GABA receptors and their downregulation due to increased activity of GABAergic striatal cells (72). The dopaminergic denervation of the striatum increases the GABAergic activity in early stages of PD, while it tends to spontaneously disappear in the course of illness and is reduced after L-DOPA therapy (141).

Excitatory amino acids. While some experimental models show increased glutamatergic activity in the striatum (17) in human PD brain the concentrations of aspartate and glutamate are unchanged (72). Binding experiments with selective NMDA antagonists revealed only mild reduction (about 40%) in the caudate nucleus and putamen (165). Autoradiography, however, showed severe reduction of ^{3}H-glutamate binding in the SN (252), since these receptors are localized at dopaminergic striatal neurones.

Peptidergic systems. The concentrations of most neuropeptides (eg, neuropeptide Y, thyrotropin-releasing hormone, vasopressin, neurotensin and vasoactive intestinal polypeptide) are unchanged (73). There is a considerable reduction of Met- and Leu-enkephalin in the VTA (70%), putamen, GP, and SN (30%) in PD. Decreases are less in "incidental" LB disease in VTA, with no changes in the caudate nucleus and nucleus accumbens. SP is reduced by 30 to 40% in the SN and GP in PD, but not in incidental LB disease. The reduction of peptides in the basal ganglia is considered an integral part of PD and not secondary to either loss of dopaminergic neurones or prolonged L-DOPA therapy (58). Somatostatin is decreased in the striatum and SN, and in the frontal cortex and hippocampus of demented PD patients. Neuropeptide receptors show a variable pattern of changes in the basal ganglia. Neurotensin binding density is reduced in the GPi and GPe; SP-binding is reduced in the GPi and putamen; D-Ala(2)-D-Leu(5)Enk binding is reduced in the posterior putamen; and Tyr-D-Ala-Gly-(Nme)-Phe-Glycol binding is reduced in both the putamen and caudate nucleus, while binding sites in SN were unchanged (58). Preproenkephalin mRNA levels are significantly increased in the lateral putamen of PD patients with L-dopa induced dyskinesias compared to nondyskinetic patients, while no change was observed in the medial putamen and caudate nucleus. These data suggest that increased synthesis of preproenkephalin in the medium spiny output neurones of the striopallidal pathway play a role in the development of L-dopa induced dyskinesias in PD (26a)

Free radicals and oxidative stress. There are many biochemical changes in the PD brain that indicate a compromised antioxidant system, which may underlie cellular vulnerability to progressive oxidative stress (OS) (Table 9). Selective increase in OS in the SN generates reactive oxygen species (ROS) or free radicals (eg, superoxide anions and hydroxyl radicals) that subsequently produce cellular damage that is non-selective and associated with oxidation of proteins, DNA, lipids, and fatty acids (73, 226, 258). Among the biochemical changes consistent with OS hypothesis are the following:

i) A significant increase of iron is observed in the SNpc of PD brains with a shift of Fe^{2+}:Fe^{3+} of about 2:1 as compared to 1:2 in controls. This metal appears in reactive microglia/macrophages, oligodendrocytes, astrocytes, and pigmented neurones where it is bound to neuromelanin (107, 108). Reactive and free tissue iron are capable of catalyzing oxidative reactions that initiate membrane lipid peroxidation due to interaction with available hydrogen peroxide via the Fenton reaction. It also acts as a catalyst to the Haber-Weiss reaction, leading to further production of hydroxyl radicals from hydrogen peroxide and exacerbation of OS and tissue damage. Iron is normally bound to ferritin, which exists in H and L form. Most brain ferritin is in the H form. There are conflicting data on ferritin levels in PD, but it has such a high iron-binding capacity that the increase of iron in PD may not require any increased buffering capacity from ferritin (226). In addition, neuromelanin, a product of dopamine auto-oxidation, is capable of forming a complex with iron, thereby potentiating the generation of free radicals and the aggregation of α-synuclein (14, 258).

ii) Glutathione in its reduced form (GSH) is an important antioxidant defense molecule and is involved in the repair of oxidized proteins. It is oxidized to its disulphid, GSSG, while GSSG reductase converts GSSG to GSH. Reduced levels of GSH, decreased ratio of reduced to oxidized glutathione (GSH/GSSG), and of glutathione peroxidase activity (destroys hydrogen peroxide, a precursor of the hydrogen oxide radicals) have been found in PD (225). Reduced GSH levels in SN of patients with PD and incidental LBD probably precedes loss of both complex I and dopamine and may be a marke for presymptomic PD (101, 238).

iii) Levels of superoxide dismutase (SOD), an enzyme important in dismuting superoxide ions, are indicative of superoxide generation. SOD exists in several isoenzymes, including copper-zinc (Cu-Zn)SOD which is cytosolic, and manganese (Mn)SOD, which is mitochondrial. Increased SOD activity leads to hydrogen peroxide formation. Both SOD isoenzymes are elevated in the SN of PD brain suggesting that SN neurones are exposed to increased superoxide generation.

iv) Levels of polyunsaturated fatty acids, malondialdehyde (MDA), a by-product of membrane lipid peroxidation, and hydroperoxide are increased in the SN of PD brain (101). These products of free radical damage to lipid membranes imply oxidative damage.

v) Intracellular 8-hydroxydeoxyguanosine, (8-OHG), produced by free-radical damage in DNA, is elevated in the nuclear and mDNA fractions in many PD brain regions (211). Increase in 8-OHG in SN neurones corresponding to their pattern of degeneration is consistent with increased oxidative damage to cytoplasmic DNA and RNA (261).

vi) The free-radical gas nitric oxide (NO), present in many tissues including the CNS, is generated by the conversion of L-arginine to L-citrulline by nitric oxide synthetase (NOS). NO, acting as an atypical molecular messenger at low conentrations, has cytotoxic properties at higher concentrations. As a free radical, NO may induce increased lipid peroxidation, release of Fe^{2+}, damage DNA or inhibit a number of enzymes, such as cytochrome c oxidase and SOD. It also affects mitochondrial function by inhibiting complexes II, III, and IV. While animal studies have shown increased NO in striatonigral neurones, attempts to demonstrate changes of NO in human PD brain have been inconclusive, with both decreased and increased levels of CSF nitrate, a marker for NOS activity (170). Overexpression of neuronal NOS was recently reported in the basal ganglia and in neutrophils of PD patients (70). Increased expression of NOS mRNA in Gpi and STN and reduced expression in the striatum may indicate compensatory mechanisms in increasing striatal dopamine release.

Metabolic ratios in the striatum. The results of proton magnetic resonance spectroscopy (MRS) of the striatum in PD as well as in MSA and PSP are controversy, but the majority of studies failed to show any differences in the A-acetylaspartate-choline (NAA/Cho) and /creatine (NAA/Cr) ratios, except for a recent study that found an increase in Cho with no changes in NAA in L-dopa treated PD patients (35).

Dysfunction of protein degradation. The occurrence of elevated levels of oxidatively damaged proteins, increased protein aggregation, and impaired proteolysis in the SNpc in sporadic PD may suggest that impaired protein degradation is a crucial factor in the pathogenesis of cell death (163).

Mitochondrial deficiency. A specific mitochondrial defect, characterized by a 35% deficiency of complex I but not other complexes in the respiratory chain, has been reported in the SN, but not other areas of the PD brain (215). Inhibition of the respiratory chain, particularly at complex I or III, results in generation of free radicals and reduced ATP synthesis. These in turn are prediucted to cause disturbance in cellular energy metabolism, DNA damage, and increased formation of mitochondrially generated ROS. They all contribute to neuronal cell death via decreased protein pumping and reduced voltage differential across the inner mitochondrial membrane. The latter would elicit opening of the mitochondrial permeability transition pore and initiation of cell death (190, 214, 237). Respiratory chain abnormalities have been also described in skeletal muscle mitochondria from PD patients (213), although MR spectroscopy studies have produced conflicting results (202).

Complex I deficiency has also been identified in platelet mitochondria, but this deficiency is modest (20-25%) and not viable as a biomarker of PD. No deletions or mutations have been detected in mitochnodiral DNA (mtDNA) in the SN or other parts of the PD brain (214); however, mtDNA transferred from PD patients induced a complex I deficit in recipient cybrid cells (126). These results indicate that mtDNA it causes complex I deficiency through yet to be detecxted inherited or somatic mutations in mtDNA.

The relationship between mitochondrial and free radical abnormalities is not fully understood, but both defects may form part of a self-amplifying cycle of events, since a defect of complex I can generate increased superoxide ions that enhance OS and cell damage in the presence of elevated concentrations of iron (115a).

Differential Diagnosis.

The clinical diagnosis of PD is usually based on the presence of parkinsonism, absence of specific abnormalities in MRI, and good response to L-dopa or to a dopamine agonist (71). Disorders which manifest parkinsonism are many (Table 1): *i) Progressive supranuclear palsy* pathologically shows severe degeneration of the SN, dentate nucleus, STN, and the GP with globose NFTs (3, 90); *ii) Multiple system atrophy* presents as parkinsonism similar to PD (136); *iii) Dementia with Lewy bodies* presents either with dementia or parkinsonism as the initial symptoms and differential diagnosis from PDD may be difficult (103); *iv) Corticobasal degeneration* consists of parkinsonism, dementia, and apraxia (46); *v) Vascular pseudo-parkinsonism* presents lower body parkinsonism with predominant gait disturbances, rare resting tremor and poor L-DOPA response. MRI shows multiple lacunar infarctions and/or leukoaraiosis. (42, 256); and *vi) Pure autonomic failure*, a progressive, adult-onset, degenerative disorder, clinically featured by orthostatic hypotension and bladder and sexual dysfunction without other accompanying neurological deficit, neuropathologically shows ubiquitin- and α-synuclein-positive LB-like intracytoplasmic inclusions in neurones of the SNpc, LC, spinal cord, sympathetic ganglia, and within autonomic nerves in the epicardial fat and bladder wall (119).

Pathogenesis

Although the aetiology of PD remains obscure, current pathogenetic hypotheses favor environmental and genetic factors (Figure 5) (220). There is increasing evidence that nigrostriatal cell death involves multiple processes that are a final pathway that may be common to many neurodegenerative diseases. They have been related to a cascade of multiple noxious factors including OS and free radical generation with increased NO formation and the generation of nitrotyrosine residues, neuromelanin-iron interaction with abnormal iron accumulation, alteration of iron-binding proteins, of cellular iron homoeostasis, and its interaction with α-synuclein. Free radical scavenger and neuroprotective systems such a glutathione are suboptimal, while SOD inducing an ever-increasing cycle of OS with increased activity of MDA, 8-OHG and production of AGEs, indicate increased oxidative damage to lipids, DNA and protein in SN neurones. The metabolism of endogenous dopamine may also produce a number of toxic byproducts that could contribute to increased OS (18, 116, 214). Other mechanisms include complex I deficiency and compromises of mitochondrial function, leading to decreased ATP production and bioenergetic defects, disorders of intracellular calcium homeo-stasis, and subsequent PCD which may be related to inadequate levels of neurotrophic factors, activation of the caspase cascade and several protein kinases, contribution of Bcl-family members, and aggregation of α-synuclein with formation of LBs. Additional immune factors and inflammatory changes promoted by microglia may contribute to or accelerate these processes. Each of these factors may form part of the pathogenesis of cell death, as well as being potential aetiological factors in themselves.

Research has attempted to determine whether these abnormalities are primary or secondary and whether they may be related to each other in a single sequence of events. Manipulation of these processes may lead to neuroprotective agents that could slow the rate of neuronal loss.

The presence of LBs in late-onset sporadic PD and their relative absence in young-onset familial PD patients leads to the speculation that LB formation may actually be a protective process that delays the onset of neuronal degeneration. The relative paucity or absence of LBs in patients with parkin mutations might deprive them from a natural defence mechanism that segregates abnormal proteins, and protects other cellular structures from their cytotoxic effects. This might account for the severe degeneration and early age of disease onset in these cases.

There is normally an age-related decline in mitochondrial function and activity of the UPS that might promote the accumulation of poorly degraded proteins (65). It is possible that these proteins might continue to accumulate within cells, and render them more sensitive to toxic insults. This could explain why the frequency of sporadic PD increases with age. The progressive accumulation of intracellualr proteins may further account for the presence of incidental LBs in the brains of around 10% of people over the age of 60 who are thought to be in a preclinical stage of PD (57). This is supported by reduced levels of GSH and complex I activity in these people (190). The sequestration and compartmentalization of poorly degraded and cytotoxic proteins as insoluble aggregates in LBs could serve as defence mechanism that reduces neurodegeneration and prevents the onset of clinical symptoms in patients with incidental LBs.

It is unclear why the SNpc preferentially degenerates in PD. The oxidative metabolism of dopamine, and its propensity to yield oxidative species, could cause local damage to intracellular proteins and components of the UPS over time. In the aged human brain, proteasomal function is lower in the SNpc compared with other brain regions, and dopamine cells are more vulnerable than GABA-releasing neurones to proteasome inhibition in culture (163). This could explain the unique vulnerability of the SNpc in PD, and its preferential degeneration in α-synuclein/parkin-linked familial PD, even though the expression of these proteins is altered throughout the brain in these disorders. Whereas genetic defects relating to the ubiquitin-proteasome system were reported in familial PD, in sporadic PD, proteasome peptidase activities are normal in brain areas without neuronal loss, but were mildly reduced in the striatum of MSA. These data suggest that a systemic, global disturbance in the catalytic activity and degradation ability of the proteasome itself is unlikely to be causally related wth PD (64b).

The key question that remains is what triggers the final common pathway in PD. Available data imply that multiple aetiologies are more likely than a single factor. This hypothesis may include the combination of genetic and environmental factors, where the contribution of each may vary between patients. Genetic susceptibility may be determined in part through impaired metabolism of free radicals or complex I activity, which in turn may be the product of nuclear or mitochondrial genomic deficits. Environmental interactions may include exogenous compounds with uptake and conversion similar to MPTP, such that they are targeted to the SN or endogenously generated neurotoxin(s) such as the tetrahydroisoquinoline or α-carbolines when a susceptbile background exists. The progressive neurodegeneration after a brief exposure to a neurotoxin earlier in life, combined with other evidence such as the occurrence of delayed onset progressive parkinsonism after encephalitis lethargica (91a), suggests that PD may arise as a consequence of either a single event or an ongoing process related to predetermined genetic susceptibility.

Evidence is emerging that genetic factors may be more important in PD than previously thought and that failure of the UPS system could cause or contribute to the development of both familial and sporadic PD. This might help to explain clinical and pathological differences and similarities in these disorders.

Future Directions and Therapy

Medical treatment. (Table 9) Drug therapy is the main treatment of PD, and L-DOPA administered with a peripheral DOPA decarboxylase inhibitor is still the gold standard. However, long-term use of levodopa produces various problems such as wearing off, on-off or no on/delayed on phenomena, dyskinesias, hallucinations and delusions, as well as autonomic dysfunction (135). Recent randomized controlled studies revealed that early use of a dopamine agonist and later L-dopa supplementation delayed the onset of motor complications such as wearing off and dyskinesias (206). Current recommendations are to start treatment with a dopamine agonist, when the patient does not have prominent cognitive impairment (166a, 191). Those with cognitive impairment tend to develop psychiatric side effects, eg, hallucinations, delusions, agitations, and confusion from dopamine agonists, and should be treated with L-DOPA. Other drugs are being used as adjunctive means when dopamine agonists or L-DOPA cannot alleviate parkinsonian symptoms adequately.

Surgical treatment. The first successful surgical treatment was thalamotomy for tremor and rigidity. The target for tremor was the ventralis intermedius nucleus and that for rigidity was the ventrolateralis (180). Grouping discharge with tremor frequency was recorded in the ventralis intermedius nucleus. Loss of the grouping discharge by electrocoagulation coincided with clinical disappearance of the tremor (11). Posterolateral pallidotomy was introduced as the treatment for motor complications such as wearing off and dyskinesia (10). "On" time disability did not change much after surgery, but "off" time disability improved significantly. Motor complications may recur after initial improvement in a considerable number of patients (4).

Deep brain stimulation of the STN was introduced more recently (118). In PD, the neuronal activity of the glutamatergic neurones in the STN is increased. High frequency electric stimulation to this nucleus results in a similar effect as blocking of this hyperactivity by destruction. Normally subthalamic glutamatergic neurones make excitatory synapses with GABAergic neurones of the Gpi which make inhibitory synapses with neurones in the ventralis anterior and the ventrolateral nuclei of the thalamus. Stimulation of the STN reduces the overactive pallidal inhibitory output to the thalamus and is suggested to have neuroprotective effects (27, 208). Deep brain stimulation to the GPi also produces similar effects as subthalamic stimulation (127). The recent trend is to perform subthalamic stimulation rather than pallidal stimulation, which is believed to be as good as STN stimulation in the treatment of dyskinesias.

Prognosis. The prognosis of patients with PD improved markedly since the introduction of L-DOPA treatment (93). Today the life expectancy of PD patients is nearly that of the general population (93, 156). L-DOPA treatment in PD does not enhance the degenerative process by the production of free radicals as previously suggested (2), although recent studies showed that chronic oral L-DOPA administration in normal monkeys can provoke dyskinesias and that this effect is dose-related (201).

Future directions. Future PD research will be devoted to the elucidation of the molecular mechanism of SN neuronal death. Molecular cloning of disease genes for familial forms of PD will be an important step to understanding pathogenesis. Today only two genes have been identified (α-synuclein and parkin), and there appears to be an interaction between these molecules (224). It is likely that proteins that are responsible for familial forms of PD are mutually related rather than unrelated and independent. Determination of the relationship between PD gene-derived proteins and other biochemical changes that are known in PD should provide a clearer understanding of neurodegeneration. These insights should lead to a more focused effort in the quest for therapeutic agents and strategies that can slow, halt or prevent the onset of neurodegeneration in PD.

Future treatment includes neuroprotective strategies, transplantation, and gene therapy. Neuroprotective treatment involves various drugs, which are expected to interrupt the cell death process. Antioxidants, anti-apoptotic agents, neurotrophic factors are under investigation (220). Up to now, no drug has yet been shown to delay the progression of PD. Transplantion has been tried in a limited number of institutes. Human fetal midbrain, porcine SN, and autologous adrenal medulla have been used, but the clinical efficacy has been unpredictable and long-lasting effects have been reported only in a limited number of patients (63, 171). Moreover, persistent dyskinesias in the absence of dopaminergic medication have been reported after dopamine cell implantation in PD which are caused by DOPA increase in the ventral putamen that preoperatively was relatively preserved (150a).

Gene therapy appears to be a promising approach. Introduction of genes regulating the synthesis of dopamine, eg, TH, DOPA decarboxylase, and GPT cyclohydrolase 1 was successful in improving parkinsonism in a monkey MPTP model (221). Combined gene therapy was more efficacious than single gene therapy. GTP cyclohydrolase 1 is the rate-limiting enzyme of the synthesis of biopterin, which is a co-factor of TH. If safety concerns can be resolved, gene therapy may be worthwhile in PD.

A more interesting approach may be gene therapy of familial forms of PD. α-Synuclein, which is mutated in PARK1, is believed to result in a gain of pathologic function and has increased tendency for self-aggregation and accumulation in the cytoplasm. If one can knock out the mutated gene without affecting the normal gene, one may be able to stop the disease process. Parkin-mutated PD, caused by a loss of function of parkin protein, which functions as an ubiquitin ligase, may be a better target for gene therapy. Introducing a parkin gene to restore parkin protein, with introduction of a gene into the striatum may be a goal.

References

1. Aarsland D, Andersen K, Larsen JP, Lolk A, Nielsen H, Kragh-Sorensen P (2001) Risk of dementia in Parkinson's disease: a community-based, prospective study. *Neurology* 56: 730-736.

2. Agid Y, Ahlskog E, Albanese A, Calne D, Chase T, De Yebenes J, Factor S, Fahn S, Gershanik O, Goetz C, Koller W, Kurth M, Lang A, Lees A, Lewitt P, Marsden D, Melamed E, Michel PP, Mizuno Y, Obeso J, Oertel W, Olanow W, Poewe W, Pollak P, Tolosa E, et al. (1999) Levodopa in the treatment of Parkinson's disease: a consensus meeting. *Mov Disord* 14: 911-913.

3. Albers DS, Augood SJ (2001) New insights into progressive supranuclear palsy. *Trends Neurosci* 24: 347-353.

4. Alkhani A, Lozano AM (2001) Pallidotomy for parkinson disease: a review of contemporary literature. *J Neurosurg* 94: 43-49.

5. Andersen JK (2001) Does neuronal loss in Parkinson's disease involve programmed cell death? *Bioessays* 23: 640-646.

6. Anglade P, Vyas S, Javoy-Agid F, Herrero MT, Michel PP, Marquez J, Mouatt-Prigent A, Ruberg M, Hirsch EC, Agid Y (1997) Apoptosis and autophagy in nigral neurons of patients with Parkinson's disease. *Histol Histopathol* 12: 25-31.

7. Anichtchik OV, Rinne JO, Kalimo H, Panula P (2000) An altered histaminergic innervation of the substantia nigra in Parkinson's disease. *Exp Neurol* 163: 20-30.

8. Antonini A, Moeller JR, Nakamura T, Spetsieris P, Dhawan V, Eidelberg D (1998) The metabolic anatomy of tremor in Parkinson's disease. *Neurology* 51: 803-810.

8a. Apaydin H, Ahlskog JE, Parisi JE, Boeve BF, Dickson DW (2002) Parkinson disease neuropathology: later-developing dementia and loss of the levodopa response. *Arch Neurol* 59: 102-112.

9. Banati RB, Daniel SE, Blunt SB (1998) Glial pathology but absence of apoptotic nigral neurons in long-standing Parkinson's disease. *Mov Disord* 13: 221-227.

10. Baron MS, Vitek JL, Bakay RA, Green J, Kaneoke Y, Hashimoto T, Turner RS, Woodard JL, Cole SA, McDonald WM, DeLong MR (1996) Treatment of advanced Parkinson's disease by posterior GPi pallidotomy: 1-year results of a pilot study. *Ann Neurol* 40: 355-366.

11. Benabid AL, Pollak P, Gao D, Hoffmann D, Limousin P, Gay E, Payen I, Benazzouz A (1996) Chronic electrical stimulation of the ventralis intermedius nucleus of the thalamus as a treatment of movement disorders. *J Neurosurg* 84: 203-214.

12. Benarroch EE, Schmeichel AM, Parisi JE (2000) Involvement of the ventrolateral medulla in parkinsonism with autonomic failure. *Neurology* 54: 963-968.

13. Benisty S, Boissiere F, Faucheux B, Agid Y, Hirsch EC (1998) trkB messenger RNA expression in normal human brain and in the substantia nigra of parkinsonian patients: an in situ hybridization study. *Neuroscience* 86: 813-826.

14. Berg D, Siefker C, Becker G (2001) Echogenicity of the substantia nigra in Parkinson's disease and its relation to clinical findings. *J Neurol* 248: 684-689.

15. Bernheimer H, Birkmayer W, Hornykiewicz O, Jellinger K, Seitelberger F (1973) Brain dopamine and the syndromes of Parkinson and Huntington. Clinical, morphological and neurochemical correlations. *J Neurol Sci* 20: 415-455.

15a. Betarbet R, Sherer TB, Di Monte DA, Greenamyre JT (2002) Mechanistic approaches to Parkinson's disease pathogenesis. *Brain Pathol* 12: 499-510.

16. Bezard E, Brotchie JM, Gross CE (2001) Pathophysiology of levodopa-induced dyskinesia: potential for new therapies. *Nat Rev Neurosci* 2: 577-588.

17. Blandini F, Nappi G, Tassorelli C, Martignoni E (2000) Functional changes of the basal ganglia circuitry in Parkinson's disease. *Prog Neurobiol* 62: 63-88.

18. Blum D, Torch S, Lambeng N, Nissou M, Benabid AL, Sadoul R, Verna JM (2001) Molecular pathways involved in the neurotoxicity of 6-OHDA, dopamine and MPTP: contribution to the apoptotic theory in Parkinson's disease. *Prog Neurobiol* 65: 135-172.

19. Borghi R, Marchese R, Negro A, Marinelli L, Forloni G, Zaccheo D, Abbruzzese G, Tabaton M (2000) Full length alpha-synuclein is present in cerebrospinal fluid from Parkinson's disease and normal subjects. *Neurosci Lett* 287: 65-67.

20. Braak E, Sandmann-Keil D, Rub U, Gai WP, de Vos RA, Steur EN, Arai K, Braak H (2001) alpha-synuclein immunopositive Parkinson's disease-related inclusion bodies in lower brain stem nuclei. *Acta Neuropathol (Berl)* 101: 195-201.

21. Braak H, Braak E (1991) Neuropathological stageing of Alzheimer-related changes. *Acta Neuropathol* 82: 239-259.

22. Braak H, Braak E, Yilmazer D, de Vos RA, Jansen EN, Bohl J (1996) Pattern of brain destruction in Parkinson's and Alzheimer's diseases. *J Neural Transm* 103: 455-490.

23. Braune S, Reinhardt M, Schnitzer R, Riedel A, Lucking CH (1999) Cardiac uptake of [123I]MIBG separates Parkinson's disease from multiple system atrophy. *Neurology* 53: 1020-1025.

24. Bruck A, Portin R, Lindell A, Laihinen A, Bergman J, Haaparanta M, Solin O, Rinne JO (2001) Positron emission tomography shows that impaired frontal lobe functioning in Parkinson's disease is related to dopaminergic hypofunction in the caudate nucleus. *Neurosci Lett* 311: 81-84.

25. Brucke T, Djamshidian S, Bencsits G, Pirker W, Asenbaum S, Podreka I (2000) SPECT and PET imaging of the dopaminergic system in Parkinson's disease. *J Neurol* 247 Suppl 4: IV/2-7.

26. Calingasan NY, Park LC, Calo LL, Trifiletti RR, Gandy SE, Gibson GE (1998) Induction of nitric oxide synthase and microglial responses precede selective cell death induced by chronic impairment of oxidative metabolism. *Am J Pathol* 153: 599-610.

26a. Calon F, Birdi S, Rajput AH, Hornykiewicz O, Bedard PJ, Di PT (2002) Increase of preproenkephalin mRNA levels in the putamen of Parkinson disease patients with levodopa-induced dyskinesias. *J Neuropathol Exp Neurol* 61: 186-196.

27. Carvalho GA, Nikkhah G (2001) Subthalamic nucleus lesions are neuroprotective against terminal 6-OHDA- induced striatal lesions and restore postural balancing reactions. *Exp Neurol* 171: 405-417.

28. Castellani RJ, Siedlak SL, Perry G, Smith MA (2000) Sequestration of iron by Lewy bodies in Parkinson's disease. *Acta Neuropathol (Berl)* 100: 111-114.

29. Chase TN, Oh JD (2000) Striatal mechanisms and pathogenesis of parkinsonian signs and motor complications. *Ann Neurol* 47: S122-129; discussion S129-130.

30. Chauhan NB, Siegel GJ, Lee JM (2001) Depletion of glial cell line-derived neurotrophic factor in substantia nigra neurons of Parkinson's disease brain. *J Chem Neuroanat* 21: 277-288.

31. Chen RC, Chang SF, Su CL, Chen TH, Yen MF, Wu HM, Chen ZY, Liou HH (2001) Prevalence, incidence, and mortality of PD: a door-to-door survey in Ilan county, Taiwan. *Neurology* 57: 1679-1686.

32. Chung KKK, Dawson VL, Dawson TM (2001) The role of the ubiquitin-proteasomal pathway in Parkinson's disease and other neurodegenerative disorders. *TINS* 24 (Suppl): S7-S14.

33. Churchyard A, Lees AJ (1997) The relationship between dementia and direct involvement of the hippocampus and amygdala in Parkinson's disease. *Neurology* 49: 1570-1576.

34. Ciliax BJ, Drash GW, Staley JK, Haber S, Mobley CJ, Miller GW, Mufson EJ, Mash DC, Levey AI (1999) Immunocytochemical localization of the dopamine transporter in human brain. *J Comp Neurol* 409: 38-56.

35. Clarke CE, Lowry M (2001) Systematic review of proton magnetic resonance spectroscopy of the stria-

tum in parkinsonian syndromes. *Eur J Neurol* 8: 573-577.

36. Counihan TJ, Penney JB, Jr. (1998) Regional dopamine transporter gene expression in the substantia nigra from control and Parkinson's disease brains. *J Neurol Neurosurg Psychiatry* 65: 164-169.

37. Crowther RA, Daniel SE, Goedert M (2000) Characterisation of isolated alpha-synuclein filaments from substantia nigra of Parkinson's disease brain. *Neurosci Lett* 292: 128-130.

38. Dale GE, Probst A, Luthert P, Martin J, Anderton BH, Leigh PN (1992) Relationships between Lewy bodies and pale bodies in Parkinson's disease. *Acta Neuropathol* 83: 525-529.

39. Damier P, Hirsch EC, Agid Y, Graybiel AM (1999) The substantia nigra of the human brain. II. Patterns of loss of dopamine-containing neurons in Parkinson's disease. *Brain* 122: 1437-1448.

40. De Ceballos ML, Lopez-Lozano JJ (1999) Subgroups of parkinsonian patients differentiated by peptidergic immunostaining of caudate nucleus biopsies. *Peptides* 20: 249-257.

41. Delacourte A, David JP, Sergeant N, Buee L, Wattez A, Vermersch P, Ghozali F, Fallet-Bianco C, Pasquier F, Lebert F, Petit H, Di Menza C (1999) The biochemical pathway of neurofibrillary degeneration in aging and Alzheimer's disease. *Neurology* 52: 1158-1165.

41a. Del Tredici K, Rub U, De Vos RA, Bohl JR, Braak H (2002) Where does parkinson disease pathology begin in the brain? *J Neuropathol Exp Neurol* 61: 413-426.

42. Demirkiran M, Bozdemir H, Sarica Y (2001) Vascular parkinsonism: a distinct, heterogeneous clinical entity. *Acta Neurol Scand* 104: 63-67.

43. Deuschl G, Wenzelburger R, Loffler K, Raethjen J, Stolze H (2000) Essential tremor and cerebellar dysfunction clinical and kinematic analysis of intention tremor. *Brain* 123: 1568-1580.

44. Dickson D, Farrer M, Lincoln S, Mason RP, Zimmerman TR, Jr., Golbe LI, Hardy J (2001) Pathology of PD in monozygotic twins with a 20-year discordance interval. *Neurology* 56: 981-982.

45. Dickson DW (2001) Alpha-synuclein and the Lewy body disorders. *Curr Opin Neurol* 14: 423-432.

46. Dickson DW, Litvan I (2002) Corticobasal degeneration. In *Neurodegeneration The molecular pathology of dementia and movement disorders*, DW Dickson (eds). ISN Neuropath Press: Basel.

47. Dragunow M, Faull RL, Lawlor P, Beilharz EJ, Singleton K, Walker EB, Mee E (1995) In situ evidence for DNA fragmentation in Huntington's disease striatum and Alzheimer's disease temporal lobes. *Neuroreport* 6: 1053-1057.

48. Druschky A, Hilz MJ, Platsch G, Radespiel-Troger M, Druschky K, Kuwert T, Neundorfer B (2000) Differentiation of Parkinson's disease and multiple system atrophy in early disease stages by means of I-123-MIBG-SPECT. *J Neurol Sci* 175: 3-12.

49. Dubois B, Malapani C, Verin M, Rogelet P, Deweer B, Pillon B (1994) [Cognitive functions and the basal ganglia: the model of Parkinson disease]. *Rev Neurol (Paris)* 150: 763-770.

50. Duda JE, Lee VM, Trojanowski JQ (2000) Neuropathology of synuclein aggregates. *J Neurosci Res* 61: 121-127.

50a. Duda JE, Giasson BI, Mabon ME, Miller DC, Golbe LI, Lee VM, Trojanowski JQ (2002) Concurrence of alpha-synuclein and tau brain pathology in the Contursi kindred. *Acta Neuropathol (Berl)* 104: 7-11.

50b. Duda JE, Giasson BI, Mabon ME, Lee VM, Trojanowski JQ (2002) Novel antibodies to synuclein show abundant striatal pathology in Lewy body diseases. *Ann Neurol* 52: 205-210.

51. Eberling JL, Pivirotto P, Bringas J, Bankiewicz KS (2000) Tremor is associated with PET measures of nigrostriatal dopamine function in MPTP-lesioned monkeys. *Exp Neurol* 165: 342-346.

52. Elbaz A, Grigoletto F, Baldereschi M, Breteler MM, Manubens-Bertran JM, Lopez-Pousa S, Dartigues JF, Alperovitch A, Tzourio C, Rocca WA (1999) Familial aggregation of Parkinson's disease: a population-based case- control study in Europe. EUROPARKINSON Study Group. *Neurology* 52: 1876-1882.

52a. Elkon H, Don J, Melamed E, Ziv I, Shirvan A, Offen D (2002) Mutant and wild-type alpha-synuclein interact with mitochondrial cytochrome C oxidase. *J Mol Neurosci* 18: 229-238.

53. Errea JM, Ara JR, Aibar C, de Pedro-Cuesta J (1999) Prevalence of Parkinson's disease in lower Aragon, Spain. *Mov Disord* 14: 596-604.

54. Eve DJ, Nisbet AP, Kingsbury AE, Temlett J, Marsden CD, Foster OJ (1997) Selective increase in somatostatin mRNA expression in human basal ganglia in Parkinson's disease. *Brain Res Mol Brain Res* 50: 59-70.

55. Farrer M, Chan P, Chen R, Tan L, Lincoln S, Hernandez D, Forno L, Gwinn-Hardy K, Petrucelli L, Hussey J, Singleton A, Tanner C, Hardy J, Langston JW (2001) Lewy bodies and parkinsonism in families with parkin mutations. *Ann Neurol* 50: 293-300.

56. Farrer M, Gwinn-Hardy K, Muenter M, DeVrieze FW, Crook R, Perez-Tur J, Lincoln S, Maraganore D, Adler C, Newman S, MacElwee K, McCarthy P, Miller C, Waters C, Hardy J (1999) A chromosome 4p haplotype segregating with Parkinson's disease and postural tremor. *Hum Mol Genet* 8: 81-85.

57. Fearnlley J, Lees AJ (1997) Parkinson's disease: Neuropathology. In *Movement Disorders*, RL Watts, WC Koller (eds). McGraw-Hill: New York. pp. 263-278.

58. Fernandez A, de Ceballos ML, Rose S, Jenner P, Marsden CD (1996) Alterations in peptide levels in Parkinson's disease and incidental Lewy body disease. *Brain* 119: 823-830.

59. Ferrer I, Blanco R, Cutillas B, Ambrosio S (2000) Fas and Fas-L expression in Huntington's disease and Parkinson's disease. *Neuropathol Appl Neurobiol* 26: 424-433.

60. Ferrer I, Blanco R, Marmona M, Puig B, Barrachina M, Gomec C, Ambrosio S (2001) Active, phosphorylation-dependent mitogen-activated protein kinase (MAPK/ERK), stress-activated protein kinase/c-jun, N-terminal kinase (SAPK/JNK) and p38 kinase expression in Parkinson's disease and dementia with Lewy bodies. *J Neural Transm* (in press).

60a. Foltynie T, Brayne C, Barker RA (2002) The heterogeneity of idiopathic Parkinson's disease. *J Neurol* 249: 138-145.

61. Forno LS (1996) Neuropathology of Parkinson's disease. *J Neuropathol Exp Neurol* 55: 259-272.

62. Forno LS, Norville RL, Langston JW (2001) EM study of nerve cell degeneration in substantia nigra in Parkinson's disease. *Park Dis Relat Disord* 7: S8.

63. Freed CR, Greene PE, Breeze RE, Tsai WY, DuMouchel W, Kao R, Dillon S, Winfield H, Culver S, Trojanowski JQ, Eidelberg D, Fahn S (2001) Transplantation of embryonic dopamine neurons for severe Parkinson's disease. *N Engl J Med* 344: 710-719.

64. Freeman A, Ciliax B, Bakay R, Daley J, Miller RD, Keating G, Levey A, Rye D (2001) Nigrostriatal collaterals to thalamus degenerate in parkinsonian animal models. *Ann Neurol* 50: 321-329.

64a. Funayama M, Hasegawa K, Kowa H, Saito M, Tsuji S, Obata F (2002) A new locus for Parkinson's disease (PARK8) maps to chromosome 12p11.2-q13.1. *Ann Neurol* 51: 296-301.

64b. Furukawa Y, Vigouroux S, Wong H, Guttman M, Rajput AH, Ang L, Briand M, Kish SJ, Briand Y (2002) Brain proteasomal function in sporadic Parkinson's disease and related disorders. *Ann Neurol* 51: 779-782.

65. Gaczynska M, Osmulski PA, Ward WF (2001) Caretaker or undertaker? The role of the proteasome in aging. *Mech Ageing Dev* 122: 235-254.

66. Gai WP, Vickers JC, Blumbergs PC, Blessing WW (1994) Loss of non-phosphorylated neurofilament immunoreactivity, with preservation of tyrosine hydroxylase, in surviving substantia nigra neurons in Parkinson's disease. *J Neurol Neurosurg Psychiatry* 57: 1039-1046.

67. Gai WP, Yuan HX, Li XQ, Power JT, Blumbergs PC, Jensen PH (2000) In situ and in vitro study of colocalization and segregation of alpha- synuclein, ubiquitin, and lipids in Lewy bodies. *Exp Neurol* 166: 324-333.

68. Galvin JE, Lee VM, Trojanowski JQ (2001) Synucleinopathies: clinical and pathological implications. *Arch Neurol* 58: 186-190.

69. Gasser T, Muller-Myhsok B, Wszolek ZK, Oehlmann R, Calne DB, Bonifati V, Bereznai B, Fabrizio E, Vieregge P, Horstmann RD (1998) A susceptibility locus for Parkinson's disease maps to chromosome 2p13. *Nat Genet* 18: 262-265.

70. Gatto EM, Riobo NA, Carreras MC, Chernavsky A, Rubio A, Satz ML, Poderoso JJ (2000) Overexpression of neutrophil neuronal nitric oxide synthase in Parkinson's disease. *Nitric Oxide* 4: 534-539.

71. Gelb DJ, Oliver E, Gilman S (1999) Diagnostic criteria for Parkinson disease. *Arch Neurol* 56: 33-39.

72. Gerlach M, Jellinger K, Riederer P (1994) The possible role of noradrenergic deficits in selected signs of Parkinson's disease. In *Noradrenergic mechanism in Parkinson's disease* (eds). CRC Press: Rota Raton, FL. pp. 59-71.

73. Gerlach M, Reichmann H, Riederer P (2001) Die Parkinson-Krankheit. In *Grundlagen, Klinik, Therapie* (eds). Springer-Verlag: Wien-New York.

74. Goldberg MS, Lansbury PT, Jr. (2000) Is there a cause-and-effect relationship between alpha-synuclein fibrillization and Parkinson's disease? *Nat Cell Biol* 2: E115-119.

74a. Golts N, Snyder H, Frasier M, Theisler C, Choi P, Wolozin B (2002) Magnesium inhibits spontaneous and iron-induced aggregation of α-synuclein. *J Biol Chem* 277: 16116-16123.

75. Graeber MB, Grasbon-Frodl E, Abell-Aleff P, al. e (1999) Nigral neurons are likely to die of a mechanism other than classical apoptosis in Parkinson´s disease. *Parkinsonism Rel Disord* 5: 187-192.

76. Greenamyre JT, MacKenzie G, Peng TI, Stephans SE (1999) Mitochondrial dysfunction in Parkinson's disease. *Biochem Soc Symp* 66: 85-97

77. Groenewegen HJ (1997) Cortical-subcortical relationships and the limbic foreBrain. In *Contemporary Behavioral Neurology*, MR Timble, JL Cummings (eds). Butterworth-Heinemann: Boston, MA. pp. 29-48

77a. Gu G, Reyes PF, Golden GT, Woltjer RL, Hulette C, Montine TJ, Zhang J (2002) Mitochondrial DANN deletions/rearrangements in Parkinson disease and related neurodegenerative disorders. J Neuropathol Exp Neurol 61: 634-639.

78. Halliday GM, Li YW, Blumbergs PC, Joh TH, Cotton RG, Howe PR, Blessing WW, Geffen LB (1990b) Neuropathology of immunohistochemically identified brainstem neurons in Parkinson's disease. *Ann Neurol* 27: 373-385.

79. Halliday GM, McRitchie DA, Cartwright HR, Pamphlett HS, Hely MA, Morris JGL (1996) Midbrain neuropathology in idiopathic Parkinson's disease and diffuse Lewy body disease. *J Clin Neurosci* 3: 52-60.

80. Harding AJ, Halliday GM (2001) Cortical Lewy body pathology in the diagnosis of dementia. *Acta Neuropathol (Berl)* 102: 355-363.

81. Hardman CD, Halliday GM (1999) The external globus pallidus in patients with Parkinson's disease and progressive supranuclear palsy. *Mov Disord* 14: 626-633.

82. Hardman CD, Halliday GM, McRitchie DA, Morris JG (1997) The subthalamic nucleus in Parkinson's disease and progressive supranuclear palsy. *J Neuropathol Exp Neurol* 56: 132-142.

83. Harnois C, Di Paolo T (1990) Decreased dopamine in the retinas of patients with Parkinson's disease. *Invest Ophthalmol Vis Sci* 31: 2473-2475.

84. Hartmann A, Hirsch EC (2001) Parkinson's disease. The apoptosis hypothesis revisited. *Adv Neurol* 86: 143-153.

85. Hartmann A, Hunot S, Michel PP, Muriel MP, Vyas S, Faucheux BA, Mouatt-Prigent A, Turmel H, Srinivasan A, Ruberg M, Evan GI, Agid Y, Hirsch EC (2000) Caspase-3: A vulnerability factor and final effector in apoptotic death of dopaminergic neurons in Parkinson's disease. *Proc Natl Acad Sci U S A* 97: 2875-2880.

85a. Hartmann A, Mouatt-Prigent A, Vita M, Abbas N, Perier C, Faucheus BA, Vyas S, Hirsch EC (2002) Increased expression and redistribution of the anti-apoptotic molecule Bcl-x in Parkinson's disease. *Neurobiol Dis* 10: 26-32.

86. Hartmann A, Troadec JD, Hunot S, Kikly K, Faucheux BA, Mouatt-Prigent A, Ruberg M, Agid Y, Hirsch EC (2001) Caspase-8 is an effector in apoptotic death of dopaminergic neurons in Parkinson's disease, but pathway inhibition results in neuronal necrosis. *J Neurosci* 21: 2247-2255.

87. Hashimoto M, Masliah E (1999) Alpha-synuclein in Lewy body disease and Alzheimer's disease. *Brain Pathol* 9: 707-720.

88. Hashimoto M, Takeda A, Hsu LJ, Takenouchi T, Masliah E (1999) Role of cytochrome c as a stimulator of alpha-synuclein aggregation in Lewy body disease. *J Biol Chem* 274: 28849-28852.

89. Hattori N, Kitada T, Matsumine H, Asakawa S, Yamamura Y, Yoshino H, Kobayashi T, Yokochi M, Wang M, Yoritaka A, Kondo T, Kuzuhara S, Nakamura S, Shimizu N, Mizuno Y (1998) Molecular genetic analysis of a novel Parkin gene in Japanese families with autosomal recessive juvenile parkinsonism: evidence for variable homozygous deletions in the Parkin gene in affected individuals. *Ann Neurol* 44: 935-941.

90. Hauw J-J, Agid Y (2002) Progressive supranuclear palsy. In *Neurodegeneration The molecular pathology of dementia and movement disorders*, DW Dennis (eds). ISN Neuropath Press: Basel.

91. Henderson JM, Carpenter K, Cartwright H, Halliday GM (2000) Degeneration of the centre median-parafascicular complex in Parkinson's disease. *Ann Neurol* 47: 345-352.

91a. Henry J, Jellinger K (2003) Post-encephalitic Parkinsonism. In *Neurodegeneration The molecular pathology of dementia and movement disorders*, D Dennis (eds). ISN Neuropath Press: Basel.

91b. Hicks AA, Petursson H, Jonsson T, Stefansson H, Johannsdottir HS, Sainz J, Frigge ML, Kong A, Gulcher JR, Stefansson K, Sveinbjornsdottir S (2002) A susceptibility gene for late-onset idiopathic Parkinson's disease. *Ann Neurol* 52: 549-555.

92. Hishikawa N, Hashizume Y, Yoshida M, Sobue G (2001) Widespread occurrence of argyrophilic glial inclusions in Parkinson's disease. *Neuropathol Appl Neurobiol* 27: 362-372.

93. Hoehn MM, Yahr MD (1967) Parkinsonism: onset, progression and mortality. *Neurology* 17: 427-442.

94. Hoogendijk WJ, Pool CW, Troost D, van Zwieten E, Swaab DF (1995) Image analyser-assisted morphometry of the locus coeruleus in Alzheimer's disease, Parkinson's disease and amyotrophic lateral sclerosis. *Brain* 118: 131-143.

95. Hornykiewicz O (2001) Chemical neuroanatomy of the basal ganglia--normal and in Parkinson's disease. *J Chem Neuroanat* 22: 3-12.

96. Howells DW, Porritt MJ, Wong JY, Batchelor PE, Kalnins R, Hughes AJ, Donnan GA (2000) Reduced BDNF mRNA expression in the Parkinson's disease substantia nigra. *Exp Neurol* 166: 127-135.

97. Hsu LJ, Sagara Y, Arroyo A, Rockenstein E, Sisk A, Mallory M, Wong J, Takenouchi T, Hashimoto M, Masliah E (2000) alpha-synuclein promotes mitochondrial deficit and oxidative stress. *Am J Pathol* 157: 401-410.

98. Hughes AJ, Daniel SE, Lees AJ (2001) Improved accuracy of clinical diagnosis of Lewy body Parkinson's disease. *Neurology* 57: 1497-1499.

98a. Hughes AJ, Daniel SE, Ben-Shlomo Y, Lees AJ (2002) The accuracy of diagnosis of parkinsonian syndromes in a specialist movement disorder service. *Brain* 125: 861-870.

99. Hurtig HI, Trojanowski JQ, Galvin J, Ewbank D, Schmidt ML, Lee VM, Clark CM, Glosser G, Stern MB, Gollomp SM, Arnold SE (2000) Alpha-synuclein cortical Lewy bodies correlate with dementia in Parkinson's disease. *Neurology* 54: 1916-1921.

100. Hutchison WD, Lozano AM, Tasker RR, Lang AE, Dostrovsky JO (1997) Identification and characterization of neurons with tremor-frequency activity in human globus pallidus. *Exp Brain Res* 113: 557-563.

101. Iha N, Jurma O, Lalli G, Y. L, H. PE, T. GJ, M. LR, J. FH, K. AJ (2000) Gluthathione depletion in PC12 results in selective inhibitation of mitochondrial complex I activity: implications for Parkinson's disease. *J Biol Chem* 275: 26096-26101

102. Imai Y, Soda M, Inoue H, Hattori N, Mizuno Y, Takahashi R (2001) An unfolded putative transmembrane polypeptide, which can lead to endoplasmic reticulum stress, is a substrate of Parkin. *Cell* 105: 891-902.

103. Ince P, McKeith I (2002) Dementia with Lewy bodies. In *Neurodegeneration The molecular pathology of dementia and movement disorders*, DW Dennis (eds). ISN Neuropath Press: Basel.

104. Ito K, Morrish PK, Rakshi JS, Uema T, Ashburner J, Bailey DL, Friston KJ, Brooks DJ (1999) Statistical parametric mapping with 18F-dopa PET shows bilaterally reduced striatal and nigral dopaminergic function in early Parkinson's disease. *J Neurol Neurosurg Psychiatry* 66: 754-758.

105. Itoh K, Weis S, Mehraein P, Muller-Hocker J (1997) Defects of cytochrome c oxidase in the substantia nigra of Parkinson's disease: and immunohistochemical and morphometric study. *Mov Disord* 12: 9-16.

106. Jellinger KA (1991) Pathology of Parkinson's disease. Changes other than the nigrostriatal pathway. *Mol Chem Neuropathol* 14: 153-197.

107. Jellinger KA (1999) Post mortem studies in Parkinson's disease--is it possible to detect brain areas for specific symptoms? *J Neural Transm* Suppl 56: 1-29.

108. Jellinger KA (1999) The role of iron in neurodegeneration: prospects for pharmacotherapy of Parkinson's disease. *Drugs Aging* 14: 115-140.

109. Jellinger KA (2000a) Cell death mechanisms in Parkinson's disease. *J Neural Transm* 107: 1-29.

110. Jellinger KA (2000b) Morphological substrates of mental dysfunction in Lewy body disease: an update. *J Neural Transm* Suppl 59: 185-212.

111. Jellinger KA (2001a) The pathology of Parkinson's disease. *Adv Neurol* 86: 55-72.

112. Jellinger KA (2001b) Cell death mechanisms in neurodegeneration. *J Cell Mol Med* 5: 1-17.

113. Jellinger KA (2002) Recent developments in the pathology of Parkinson's disease. *J Neural Transm* Suppl (62): 347-376.

114. Jellinger KA, Seppi K, Wenning GK, Poewe W (2002) Impact of coexisting Alzheimer pathology on the natural history of Parkinson's disease. *J Neural Transm* 109: in press.

115. Jellinger KA, Stadelmann CH (2000) The enigma of cell death in neurodegenerative disorders. *J Neural Transm* Suppl 60: 21-36.

116. Jenner P (1998) Oxidative mechanisms in nigral cell death in Parkinson's disease. *Mov Disord* 13: 24-34.

117. Kaasinen V, Nagren K, Hietala J, Oikonen V, Vilkman H, Farde L, Halldin C, Rinne JO (2000) Extrastriatal dopamine D2 and D3 receptors in early and advanced Parkinson's disease. *Neurology* 54: 1482-1487.

117a. Kahns S, Lykkebo S, Jakobsen LD, Nielsen MS, Jensen PH (2002) Caspase-mediated parkin cleavage in apoptotic cell death. *J Biol Chem* 277: 15303-15308.

118. Katayama Y, Kasai M, Oshima H, Fukaya C, Yamamoto T, Ogawa K, Mizutani T (2001) Subthalamic nucleus stimulation for Parkinson disease: benefits observed in levodopa-intolerant patients. *J Neurosurg* 95: 213-221.

119. Kaufmann H, Hague K, Perl D (2001) Accumulation of alpha-synuclein in autonomic nerves in pure autonomic failure. *Neurology* 56: 980-981.

119a. Kawamoto Y, Akiguchi I, Nakamura S, Honjyo Y, Shibasaki H, Budka H (2002) 14-3-3 proteins in Lewy bodies in Parkinson disease and diffuse Lewy body disease brains. *J Neuropathol Exp Neurol* 61: 245-253.

119b. Khan NL, Brooks DJ, Pavese N, Sweeney MG, Wood NW, Lees AJ, Piccini P (2002) Progression of nigrostriatal dysfunction in a parkin kindred: an [18F]dopa PET and clinical study. *Brain* 125: 2248-2256.

120. Kingham PJ, Pocock JM (2001) Microglial secreted cathepsin B induces neuronal apoptosis. *J Neurochem* 76: 1475-1484.

121. Kingsbury AE, Cooper M, Schapira AH, Foster OJ (2001) Metabolic enzyme expression in dopaminergic neurons in Parkinson's disease: an in situ hybridization study. *Ann Neurol* 50: 142-149.

122. Kingsbury AE, Mardsen CD, Foster OJ (1998) DNA fragmentation in human substantia nigra: apoptosis or perimortem effect? *Mov Disord* 13: 877-884.

123. Kingsbury AE, Marsden CD, Foster OJ (1999) The vulnerability of nigral neurons to Parkinson's disease is unrelated to their intrinsic capacity for dopamine synthesis: an in situ hybridization study. *Mov Disord* 14: 206-218.

124. Kish SJ, Shannak K, Hornykiewicz O (1988) Uneven pattern of dopamine loss in the striatum of patients with idiopathic Parkinson's disease. Pathophysiologic and clinical implications. *N Engl J Med* 318: 876-880.

125. Kitada T, Asakawa S, Hattori N, Matsumine H, Yamamura Y, Minoshima S, Yokochi M, Mizuno Y, Shimizu N (1998) Mutations in the parkin gene cause autosomal recessive juvenile parkinsonism. *Nature* 392: 605-608.

125a. Knott C, Stern G, Kingsbury A, Welcher AA, Wilkin GP (2002) Elevated glial brain-derived neurotrophic factor in Parkinson's diseased nigra. *Parkinsonism Relat Disord* 8: 329-341.

126. Kosel S, Hofhaus G, Maassen A, Vieregge P, Graeber MB (1999) Role of mitochondria in Parkinson disease. *Biol Chem* 380: 865-870.

127. Krack P, Pollak P, Limousin P, Hoffmann D, Benazzouz A, Le Bas JF, Koudsie A, Benabid AL (1998) Opposite motor effects of pallidal stimulation in Parkinson's disease. *Ann Neurol* 43: 180-192.

128. Kruger R, Kuhn W, Muller T, Woitalla D, Graeber M, Kosel S, Przuntek H, Epplen JT, Schols L, Riess O (1998) Ala30Pro mutation in the gene encoding alpha-synuclein in Parkinson's disease. *Nat Genet* 18: 106-108.

129. Kubis N, Faucheux BA, Ransmayr G, Damier P, Duyckaerts C, Henin D, Forette B, Le Charpentier Y, Hauw JJ, Agid Y, Hirsch EC (2000) Preservation of midbrain catecholaminergic neurons in very old human subjects. *Brain* 123: 366-373.

130. Kubo SI, Kitami T, Noda S, Shimura H, Uchiyama Y, Asakawa S, Minoshima S, Shimizu N, Mizuno Y, Hattori N (2001) Parkin is associated with cellular vesicles. *J Neurochem* 78: 42-54.

131. Kuopio AM, Marttila RJ, Helenius H, Rinne UK (1999) Changing epidemiology of Parkinson's disease in southwestern Finland. *Neurology* 52: 302-308.

132. Kusumi M, Nakashima K, Harada H, Takahashi K, Nakayama H (1994) Epidemiology of Parkinson's disease in Yonago city, Japan. *Mov Disord* 9 (Suppl 1): 95 (Abs)

133. Lach B, Grimes D, Benoit B, Minkiewicz-Janda A (1992) Caudate nucleus pathology in Parkinson's disease: ultrastructural and biochemical findings in biopsy material. *Acta Neuropathol* 83: 352-360.

134. Lang AE, Lozano AM (1998 a) Parkinson's disease. First of two parts. *N Engl J Med* 339: 1044-1053.

135. Lang AE, Lozano AM (1998 b) Parkinson's disease. Second of two parts. *N Engl J Med* 339: 1130-1143.

136. Lantos PL, Quinn NP (2002) Multiple system atrophy. In *Neurodegeneration The molecular pathology of dementia and movement disorders*, DW Dennis (eds). ISN Neuropath Press: Basel.

137. Lee MS, Kim YD, Im JH, Kim HJ, Rinne JO, Bhatia KP (1999) 123I-IPT brain SPECT study in essential tremor and Parkinson's disease. *Neurology* 52: 1422-1426.

138. Leigh J, Zee D (1991) *The Neurology of Eye Movement*. FA Davies: Philadelphia.

139. Leonard BE (1999) Prevalence and psychopathology of depression in Parkinson´s disease. In *Mental Dysfunction in Parkinson´s disease* II, EC Wolters, P Scheltens, HW Berendse (eds). Academic Pharmaceutical Productions: Utrecht. pp. 248-253

140. Leroy E, Boyer R, Auburger G, Leube B, Ulm G, Mezey E, Harta G, Brownstein MJ, Jonnalagada S, Chernova T, Dehejia A, Lavedan C, Gasser T, Steinbach PJ, Wilkinson KD, Polymeropoulos MH (1998) The ubiquitin pathway in Parkinson's disease. *Nature* 395: 451-452.

141. Levy R, Herrero MT, Ruberg M, Villares J, Faucheux B, Guridi J, Guillen J, Luquin MR, Javoy-Agid F, Obeso JA, et al. (1995) Effects of nigrostriatal denervation and L-dopa therapy on the GABAergic neurons in the striatum in MPTP-treated monkeys and Parkinson's disease: an in situ hybridization study of GAD67 mRNA. Eur *J Neurosci* 7: 1199-1209.

142. Lewy FH (1913) Zur pathologischen Anatomie der Paralysis agitans. *D Z Nervenheilk* 50: 50-55.

142a. Li S-T, Dendi R, Holmes C, Goldstein DS (2002) Progressive loss of cardiac sympathetic innervation in Parkinson disease (Brief Comm.). *Ann Neurol* in press.

143. Liu H, Iacono RP, Schoonenberg T, Kuniyoshi S, Buchholz J (1999) A comparative study on neurochemistry of cerebrospinal fluid in advanced Parkinson's disease. *Neurobiol Dis* 6: 35-42.

144. Love S (2001) Damage to nuclear DNA in Lewy body disease. *Neuroreport* 12: 2725-2729.

145. Lowe J, Leigh PN (2002) Disorders of movement and system degenerations. In *Greenfield's Neuropathology*, 7th Ed., D Graham, PL Lantos (eds). E. Arnold: London. pp. 389-391.

145a. Lozza C, Marie RM, Baron JC (2002) The metabolic substrates of bradykinesia and tremor in uncomplicated Parkinson's disease. *Neuroimage* 17: 688-699.

146. Lucking CB, Brice A (2000) Alpha-synuclein and Parkinson's disease. *Cell Mol Life Sci* 57: 1894-1908.

147. Lucking CB, Durr A, Bonifati V, Vaughan J, De Michele G, Gasser T, Harhangi BS, Meco G, Denefle P, Wood NW, Agid Y, Brice A (2000) Association between early-onset Parkinson's disease and mutations in the parkin gene. French Parkinson's Disease Genetics Study Group. *N Engl J Med* 342: 1560-1567.

148. Ma SY, Ciliax BJ, Stebbins G, Jaffar S, Joyce JN, Cochran EJ, Kordower JH, Mash DC, Levey AI, Mufson EJ (1999a) Dopamine transporter-immunoreactive neurons decrease with age in the human substantia nigra. *J Comp Neurol* 409: 25-37.

149. Ma SY, Rinne JO, Collan Y, Röyttä M, Rinne UK (1995) A quantitative morphometrical study of the neuron degeneration in the substantia nigra in patients with Parkinson's disease. *J Neurol Sci* 140: 40-45.

150. Ma SY, Roytt M, Collan Y, Rinne JO (1999b) Unbiased morphometrical measurements show loss of pigmented nigral neurones with ageing. *Neuropathol Appl Neurobiol* 25: 394-399.

150a. Ma Y, Feigin A, Dhawan V, Fukuda M, Shi Q, Greene P, Breeze R, Fahn S, Freed C, Eidelberg D (2002) Dyskinesia after fetal cell transplantation for parkinsonism: a PET study. *Ann Neurol* 52: 628-634.

151. Maraganore DM, Hernandez DG, Singleton AB, Farrer MJ, McDonnell SK, Hutton ML, Hardy JA, Rocca WA (2001) Case-Control study of the extended tau gene haplotype in Parkinson's disease. *Ann Neurol* 50: 658-661.

152. Marie RM, Barre L, Rioux P, Allain P, Lechevalier B, Baron JC (1995) PET imaging of neocortical monoaminergic terminals in Parkinson's disease. *J Neural Transm Park Dis Dement Sect* 9: 55-71.

153. Marshall KA, Daniel SE, Cairns N, Jenner P, Halliwell B (1997) Upregulation of the anti-apoptotic protein Bcl-2 may be an early event in neurodegeneration: studies on Parkinson's and incidental Lewy body disease. *Biochem Biophys Res Commun* 240: 84-87.

154. Martin ER, Scott WK, Nance MA, Watts RL, Hubble JP, Koller WC, Lyons K, Pahwa R, Stern MB, Colcher A, Hiner BC, Jankovic J, Ondo WG, Allen FH, Jr., Goetz CG, Small GW, Masterman D, Mastaglia F, Laing NG, Stajich JM, Ribble RC, Booze MW, Rogala A, Hauser MA, Zhang F, Gibson RA, Middleton LT, Roses AD, Haines JL, Scott BL, Pericak-Vance MA, Vance JM (2001) Association of single-nucleotide polymorphisms of the tau gene with late-onset Parkinson disease. *JAMA* 286: 2245-2250.

155. Marttila RJ, Rinne JO, Helenius H, Dickson DW, Roytta M (2000) Alpha-synuclein-immunoreactive cortical Lewy bodies are associated with cognitive impairment in Parkinson's disease. *Acta Neuropathol* 100: 285-290.

156. Marttila RJ, Rinne UK, Siirtola T, Sonninen V (1977) Mortality of patients with Parkinson's disease treated with levodopa. *J Neurol* 216: 147-153.

157. Marttila RJ, Röyttä M, Lonnberg P, M*rjama*ki P, Helenius H, O. RJ (2001) Choline acetyltransferase activity and striatal dopamine receptors in Parkinson's disease in relation to cognitive impairment. *Acta Neuropathol* 102: 160-166.

158. Matsumine H, Saito M, Shimoda-Matsubayashi S, Tanaka H, Ishikawa A, Nakagawa-Hattori Y, Yokochi M, Kobayashi T, Igarashi S, Takano H, Sanpei K, Koike R, Mori H, Kondo T, Mizutani Y, Schaffer AA, Yamamura Y, Nakamura S, Kuzuhara S, Tsuji S, Mizuno Y (1997) Localization of a gene for an autosomal recessive form of juvenile Parkinsonism to chromosome 6q25.2-27. *Am J Hum Genet* 60: 588-596.

159. Matzuk MM, Saper CB (1985) Preservation of hypothalamic dopaminergic neurons in Parkinson's disease. *Ann Neurol* 18: 552-555.

160. McCann SJ, LeCouteur DG, Green AC, Brayne C, Johnson AG, Chan D, McManus ME, Pond SM (1998) The epidemiology of Parkinson's disease in an Australian population. *Neuroepidemiology* 17: 310-317.

161. McGeer PL, Yasojima K, McGeer EG (2001) Inflammation in Parkinson's disease. *Adv Neurol* 86: 83-89.

162. McKeith IG, Galasko D, Kosaka K, Perry EK, Dickson DW, Hansen LA, Salmon DP, Lowe J, Mirra SS, Byrne EJ, Lennox G, Quinn NP, Edwardson JA, Ince PG, Bergeron C, Burns A, Miller BL, Lovestone S, Collerton D, Jansen EN, Ballard C, de Vos RA, Wilcock GK, Jellinger KA, Perry RH (1996) Consensus guidelines for the clinical and pathologic diagnosis of dementia with Lewy bodies (DLB): report of the consortium on DLB international workshop. *Neurology* 47: 1113-1124.

163. McNaught KS, Olanow CW, Halliwell B, Isacson O, Jenner P (2001) Failure of the ubiquitin-proteasome system in Parkinson's disease. *Nat Rev Neurosci* 2: 589-594.

164. McRitchie DA, Cartwright HR, Halliday GM (1997) Specific A10 dopaminergic nuclei in the midbrain degenerate in Parkinson's disease. *Exp Neurol* 144: 202-213.

165. Meoni P, Bunnemann BH, Kingsbury AE, Trist DG, Bowery NG (1999) NMDA NR1 subunit mRNA and glutamate NMDA-sensitive binding are differentially affected in the striatum and pre-frontal cortex of Parkinson's disease patients. *Neuropharmacology* 38: 625-633.

166. Miller GW, Staley JK, Heilman CJ, Perez JT, Mash DC, Rye DB, Levey AI (1997) Immunochemical analysis of dopamine transporter protein in Parkinson's disease. *Ann Neurol* 41: 530-539.

166a. Miyasaki JM, Martin W, Suchowersky O, Weiner WJ, Lang AE (2002) Practice parameter: initiation of treatment for Parkinson's disease: an evidence-based review: report of the Quality Standards Subcommittee of the American Academy of Neurology. *Neurology* 58: 11-17.

167. Mochizuki H, Mori H, Mizuno Y (1997) Apoptosis in neurodegenerative disorders. *J Neural Transm* Suppl 50: 125-140.

168. Mogi M, Togari A, Kondo T, Mizuno Y, Kogure O, Kuno S, Ichinose H, Nagatsu T (2001) Glial cell line-derived neurotrophic factor in the substantia nigra from control and parkinsonian brains. *Neurosci Lett* 300: 179-181.

169. Mogi M, Togari A, Kondo T, Mizuno Y, Komure O, Kuno S, Ichinose H, Nagatsu T (2000) Caspase activities and tumor necrosis factor receptor R1 (p55) level are elevated in the substantia nigra from parkinsonian brain. *J Neural Transm* 107: 335-341.

170. Molina JA, Jimenez-Jimenez FJ, Navarro JA, Vargas C, Gomez P, Benito-Leon J, Orti-Pareja M, Cisneros E, Arenas J (1996) Cerebrospinal fluid nitrate levels in patients with Parkinson's disease. *Acta Neurol Scand* 93: 123-126.

171. Monza D, Soliveri P, Radice D, Fetoni V, Testa D, Caffarra P, Caraceni T, Girotti F (1998) Cognitive dysfunction and impaired organization of complex motility in degenerative parkinsonian syndromes. *Arch Neurol* 55: 372-378.

172. Mori H, Kondo T, Yokochi M, Matsumine H, Nakagawa-Hattori Y, Miyake T, Suda K, Mizuno Y (1998) Pathologic and biochemical studies of juvenile parkinsonism linked to chromosome 6q. *Neurology* 51: 890-892.

173. Morrish PK, Rakshi JS, Bailey DL, Sawle GV, Brooks DJ (1998) Measuring the rate of progression and estimating the preclinical period of Parkinson's disease with [18F]dopa PET. *J Neurol Neurosurg Psychiatry* 64: 314-319.

174. Mouatt-Prigent A, Agid Y, Hirsch EC (1994) Does the calcium binding protein calretinin protect dopaminergic neurons against degeneration in Parkinson's disease? *Brain Res* 668: 62-70.

175. Mouatt-Prigent A, Karlsson JO, Yelnik J, Agid Y, Hirsch EC (2000) Calpastatin immunoreactivity in the monkey and human brain of control subjects and patients with Parkinson's disease. *J Comp Neurol* 419: 175-192.

176. Muenter MD, Forno LS, Hornykiewicz O, Kish SJ, Maraganore DM, Caselli RJ, Okazaki H, Howard FM, Jr., Snow BJ, Calne DB (1998) Hereditary form of parkinsonism--dementia. *Ann Neurol* 43: 768-781.

177. Mufson EJ, Conner JM, Kordower JH (1995) Nerve growth factor in Alzheimer's disease: defective retrograde transport to nucleus basalis. *Neuroreport* 6: 1063-1066.

178. Munch G, Luth HJ, Wong A, Arendt T, Hirsch E, Ravid R, Riederer P (2000) Crosslinking of alpha-synuclein by advanced glycation endproducts--an early pathophysiological step in Lewy body formation? *J Chem Neuroanat* 20: 253-257.

179. Muriel MP, Bernard V, Levey AI, Laribi O, Abrous DN, Agid Y, Bloch B, Hirsch EC (1999) Levodopa induces a cytoplasmic localization of D1 dopamine receptors in striatal neurons in Parkinson's disease. *Ann Neurol* 46: 103-111.

180. Narabayashi H, Ohye C (1980) Importance of microstereoencephalotomy for tremor alleviation. *Appl Neurophysiol* 43: 222-227.

181. Neystat M, Lynch T, Przedborski S, Kholodilov N, Rzhetskaya M, Burke RE (1999) Alpha-synuclein expression in substantia nigra and cortex in Parkinson's disease. *Mov Disord* 14: 417-422.

182. Nicotra A, Parvez SH (2000) Cell death induced by MPTP, a substrate for monoamine oxidase B. *Toxicology* 153: 157-166.

183. Nieuwenhuys R, Voogel J, Van Huizen C (1988) *The human central nervous system. A synopsis and atlas.* Springer: Berlin, Heidelberg, New York, Tokyo.

184. Nisbet AP, Eve DJ, Kingsbury AE, Daniel SE, Marsden CD, Lees AJ, Foster OJ (1996) Glutamate decarboxylase-67 messenger RNA expression in normal human basal ganglia and in Parkinson's disease. *Neuroscience* 75: 389-406.

185. Nukada H, Kowa H, Saitoh T, Tazaki Y, Miura S (1978) [A big family of paralysis agitans (author's transl)]. *Rinsho Shinkeigaku* 18: 627-634.

186. Nurmi E, Bergman J, Eskola O, Solin O, Hinkka SM, Sonninen P, Rinne JO (2000) Reproducibility and effect of levodopa on dopamine transporter function measurements: a [18F]CFT PET study. *J Cereb Blood Flow Metab* 20: 1604-1609.

187. Nurmi E, Ruottinen HM, Bergman J, Haaparanta M, Solin O, Sonninen P, Rinne JO (2001) Rate of progression in Parkinson's disease: a 6-[18F]fluoro-L-dopa PET study. *Mov Disord* 16: 608-615.

188. Nurmi E, Ruottinen HM, Kaasinen V, Bergman J, Haaparanta M, Solin O, Rinne JO (2000) Progression

in Parkinson's disease: a positron emission tomography study with a dopamine transporter ligand [18F]CFT. *Ann Neurol* 47: 804-808.

189. Olanow CW, Jenner P, Tatton N, Tatton WG (1998) Neurodegeneration. In *Parkinson's disease and movement disorders*, J Jankovic, E Tolosa (eds). Williams & Wilikins: Baltimore. pp. 67-103

190. Olanow CW, Tatton WG (1999) Etiology and pathogenesis of Parkinson's disease. *Annu Rev Neurosci* 22: 123-144.

191. Olanow CW, Watts RL, Koller WC (2001) An algorithm (decision tree) for the management of Parkinson's disease (2001): treatment guidelines. *Neurology* 56: S1-S88.

192. Olszewski J, Baxter D (1982) *Cytoarchitecture of the human brain stem.* S. Karger: Basel, München, Paris, London, New York, Sidney.

193. Otsuka M, Ichiya Y, Kuwabara Y, Hosokawa S, Sasaki M, Yoshida T, Fukumura T, Masuda K, Kato M (1996) Differences in the reduced 18F-Dopa uptakes of the caudate and the putamen in Parkinson's disease: correlations with the three main symptoms. *J Neurol Sci* 136: 169-173.

194. Pahapill PA, Lozano AM (2000) The pedunculopontine nucleus and Parkinson's disease. *Brain* 123: 1767-1783.

195. Parent A, Cossette M (2001) Extrastriatal dopamine and Parkinson's disease. *Adv Neurol* 86: 45-54.

196. Parent A, Hazrati LN (1995) Functional anatomy of the basal ganglia. I. The cortico-basal ganglia- thalamo-cortical loop. *Brain Res Brain Res* Rev 20: 91-127

197. Parent A, Parent M, Levesque M (1999) Basal ganglia and Parkinson´s disease: an anatomical perspective. *Neurosci News* 2: 19-26.

198. Parkinson J (1817) *An essay on the shaking palsy.* Whittingham and Rowland for Sherwood, Neely and Jones: London.

199. Paulus W, Jellinger K (1991) The neuropathologic basis of different clinical subgroups of Parkinson's disease. *J Neuropathol Exp Neurol* 50: 743-755.

200. Payami H, Larsen K, Bernard S, Nutt J (1994) Increased risk of Parkinson's disease in parents and siblings of patients. *Ann Neurol* 36: 659-661.

200a. Payami H, Zareparsi S, James D, Nutt J (2002) Familial aggregation of Parkinson disease: a comparative study of early-onset and late-onset disease. *Arch Neurol* 59: 848-850.

201. Pearce RK, Heikkila M, Linden IB, Jenner P (2001) L-Dopa induces dyskinesia in normal monkeys: behavioural and pharmacokinetic observations. *Psychopharmacology (Berl)* 156: 402-409.

202. Penn AM, Roberts T, Hodder J, Allen PS, Zhu G, Martin WR (1995) Generalized mitochondrial dysfunction in Parkinson's disease detected by magnetic resonance spectroscopy of muscle. *Neurology* 45: 2097-2099.

203. Perry EK, Irving D, Kerwin JM, McKeith IG, Thompson P, Collerton D, Fairbairn AF, Ince PG, Morris CM, Cheng AV, et al. (1993) Cholinergic transmitter and neurotrophic activities in Lewy body dementia: similarity to Parkinson's and distinction from Alzheimer disease. *Alzheimer Dis Assoc Disord* 7: 69-79.

203a. Pirker W, Djamshidian S, Asenbaum S, Gerschlager W, Tribl G, Hoffmann M, Brucke T (2002) Progression of dopaminergic degeneration in Parkinson's disease and atypical parkinsonism: a longitudinal beta-CIT SPECT study. *Mov Disord* 17: 45-53.

204. Polymeropoulos MH, Lavedan C, Leroy E, Ide SE, Dehejia A, Dutra A, Pike B, Root H, Rubenstein J, Boyer R, Stenroos ES, Chandrasekharappa S, Athanassiadou A, Papapetropoulos T, Johnson WG, Lazzarini AM, Duvoisin RC, Di Iorio G, Golbe LI, Nussbaum RL (1997) Mutation in the alpha-synuclein gene identified in families with Parkinson's disease. *Science* 276: 2045-2047.

204a. Rakshi JS, Pavese N, Uema T, Ito K, Morrish PK, Bailey DL, Brooks DJ (2002) A comparison of the progression of early Parkinson's disease in patients started on ropinirole or L-dopa: an (18)F-dopa PET study. *J Neural Transm* 109: 1433-1443.

205. Ransmayr G, Seppi K, Donnemiller E, Luginger E, Marksteiner J, Riccabona G, Poewe W, Wenning GK (2001) Striatal dopamine transporter function in dementia with Lewy bodies and Parkinson's disease. *Eur J Nucl Med* 28: 1523-1528.

206. Rascol O, Brooks DJ, Korczyn AD, De Deyn PP, Clarke CE, Lang AE (2000) A five-year study of the incidence of dyskinesia in patients with early Parkinson's disease who were treated with ropinirole or levodopa. 056 Study Group. *N Engl J Med* 342: 1484-1491.

206a. Righini A, Antonini A, Ferrarini M, de Notaris R, Canesi M, Triulzi F, Pezzoli G (2002) Thin section MR study of the basal ganglia in the differential diagnosis between striatonigral degeneration and Parkinson disease. *J Comput Assist Tomogr* 26: 266-271.

206b. Rinne JO, Anichtchik OV, Eriksson KS, Kaslin J, Tuomisto L, Kalimo H, Roytta M, Panula P (2002) Increased brain histamine levels in Parkinson's disease but not in multiple system atrophy. *J Neurochem* 81: 954-960.

207. Rinne JO, Nurmi E, Ruottinen HM, Bergman J, Eskola O, Solin O (2001) [F-18]FDOPA and [F-18]CFT are both sensitive PET markers to detect presynaptic dopaminergic hypofunction in early Parkinson's disease. *Synapse* 40: 193-200.

208. Rodriguez-Puertas R, Pazos A, Pascual J (1994) Cholinergic markers in degenerative parkinsonism: autoradiographic demonstration of high-affinity choline uptake carrier hyperactivity. *Brain Res* 636: 327-332.

209. Roos RA, Jongen JC, van der Velde EA (1996) Clinical course of patients with idiopathic Parkinson's disease. *Mov Disord* 11: 236-242.

210. Saha AR, Ninkina NN, Hanger DP, Anderton BH, Davies AM, Buchman VL (2000) Induction of neuronal death by alpha-synuclein. *Eur J Neurosci* 12: 3073-3077.

211. Sanchez-Ramos JR, Overvik E, Ames BN (1994) A marker of oxyradical-mediated DNA damage (8-hydroxy-2-deoxyguanosin) is increased in nigro-striatum of Parkinson's disease brain. *Neurodegeneration* 3: 197-204.

212. Scarnati E, Gasbarri A, Campana E, Pacitti C (1987) The organization of nucleus tegmenti pedunculopontinus neurons projecting to basal ganglia and thalamus: a retrograde fluorescent double labeling study in the rat. *Neurosci Lett* 79: 11-16.

213. Schapira AH (1994) Evidence for mitochondrial dysfunction in Parkinson's disease--a critical appraisal. *Mov Disord* 9: 125-138.

214. Schapira AH (2001) Causes of neuronal death in Parkinson's disease. *Adv Neurol* 86: 155-162.

215. Schapira AH, Cooper JM, Dexter D, Clark JB, Jenner P, Marsden CD (1990) Mitochondrial complex I deficiency in Parkinson's disease. *J Neurochem* 54: 823-827.

215a. Schlossmacher MG, Frosch MP, Gai WP, Medina M, Sharma N, Forno L, Ochiishi T, Shimura H, Sharon R, Hattori N, Langston JW, Mizuno Y, Hyman BT, Selkoe DJ, Kosik KS (2002) Parkin localizes to the Lewy bodies of Parkinson disease and dementia with Lewy bodies. *Am J Pathol* 160: 1655-1667.

216. Schoenberg BS, Osuntokun BO, Adeuja AO, Bademosi O, Nottidge V, Anderson DW, Haerer AF (1988) Comparison of the prevalence of Parkinson's disease in black populations in the rural United States and in rural Nigeria: door-to- door community studies. *Neurology* 38: 645-646.

217. Scott WK, Nance MA, Watts RL, Hubble JP, Koller WC, Lyons K, Pahwa R, Stern MB, Colcher A, Hiner BC, Jankovic J, Ondo WG, Allen FH, Jr., Goetz CG, Small GW, Masterman D, Mastaglia F, Laing NG, Stajich JM, Slotterbeck B, Booze MW, Ribble RC, Rampersaud E, West SG, Gibson RA, Middleton LT, Roses AD, Haines JL, Scott BL, Vance JM, Pericak-Vance MA (2001) Complete genomic screen in Parkinson disease: evidence for multiple genes. *JAMA* 286: 2239-2244.

218. Sharma N, Hewett J, Ozelius LJ, Ramesh V, McLean PJ, Breakefield XO, Hyman BT (2001a) A close association of torsinA and alpha-synuclein in Lewy bodies: a fluorescence resonance energy transfer study. *Am J Pathol* 159: 339-344.

219. Sharma N, McLean PJ, Kawamata H, Irizarry MC, Hyman BT (2001b) Alpha-synuclein has an altered conformation and shows a tight intermolecular interaction with ubiquitin in Lewy bodies. *Acta Neuropathol (Berl)* 102: 329-334.

220. Shastry BS (2001) Parkinson disease: etiology, pathogenesis and future of gene therapy. *Neurosci Res* 41: 5-12.

221. Shen Y, Muramatsu SI, Ikeguchi K, Fujimoto KI, Fan DS, Ogawa M, Mizukami H, Urabe M, Kume A, Nagatsu I, Urano F, Suzuki T, Ichinose H, Nagatsu T, Monahan J, Nakano I, Ozawa K (2000) Triple transduction with adeno-associated virus vectors expressing tyrosine hydroxylase, aromatic-L-amino-acid decarboxylase, and GTP cyclohydrolase I for gene therapy of Parkinson's disease. *Hum Gene Ther* 11: 1509-1519.

222. Shimura H, Hattori N, Kubo S, Mizuno Y, Asakawa S, Minoshima S, Shimizu N, Iwai K, Chiba T,

Tanaka K, Suzuki T (2000) Familial Parkinson disease gene product, parkin, is a ubiquitin-protein ligase. *Nat Genet* 25: 302-305.

223. Shimura H, Hattori N, Kubo S, Yoshikawa M, Kitada T, Matsumine H, Asakawa S, Minoshima S, Yamamura Y, Shimizu N, Mizuno Y (1999) Immunohistochemical and subcellular localization of Parkin protein: absence of protein in autosomal recessive juvenile parkinsonism patients. *Ann Neurol* 45: 668-672.

224. Shimura H, Schlossmacher MG, Hattori N, Frosch MP, Trockenbacher A, Schneider R, Mizuno Y, Kosik KS, Selkoe DJ (2001) Ubiquitination of a new form of alpha-synuclein by parkin from human brain: implications for Parkinson's disease. *Science* 293: 263-269.

225. Sian J, Gerlach M, Youdim MB, Riederer P (1999) Parkinson's disease: a major hypokinetic basal ganglia disorder. *J Neural Transm* 106: 443-476.

226. Silva MT, Schapira AHV (2001) Parkinson's disease. In *Pathogenesis of Neurodegenerative disorders*, MP Mattson (eds). Human Press: Totowa, NJ. pp. 53-79.

227. Slooter AJ, Cruts M, Van Broeckhoven C, Hofman A, van Duijin CM (2001) Apolipoprotein E and longevity: the Rotterdam Study. *J Am Geriatr Soc* 49: 1258-1259.

228. Smith AD, Bolam JP (1990) The neural network of the basal ganglia as revealed by the study of synaptic connections of identified neurones. *Trends Neurosci* 13: 259-265.

229. Spillantini M (2002) Introduction. In *Neurodegeneration The molecular pathology of dementia and movement disorders*, DW Dennis (eds). ISN Neuropath Press: Basel.

230. Spillantini MG, Schmidt ML, Lee VM, Trojanowski JQ, Jakes R, Goedert M (1997) Alpha-synuclein in Lewy bodies. *Nature* 388: 839-840.

231. Spira PJ, Sharpe DM, Halliday G, Cavanagh J, Nicholson GA (2001) Clinical and pathological features of a Parkinsonian syndrome in a family with an Ala53Thr alpha-synuclein mutation. *Ann Neurol* 49: 313-319.

232. Starkstein SE, Petracca G, Chemerinski E, Teson A, Sabe L, Merello M, Leiguarda R (1998) Depression in classic versus akinetic-rigid Parkinson's disease. *Mov Disord* 13: 29-33.

233. Stoessl AJ, Ruth TJ (1998) Neuroreceptor imaging: new developments in PET and SPECT imaging of neuroreceptor binding (including dopamine transporters, vesicle transporters and post synaptic receptor sites). *Curr Opin Neurol* 11: 327-333.

234. Takahashi H, Ohama E, Suzuki S, Horikawa Y, Ishikawa A, Morita T, Tsuji S, Ikuta F (1994) Familial juvenile parkinsonism: clinical and pathologic study in a family. *Neurology* 44: 437-441.

235. Takatsu H, Nishida H, Matsuo H, Watanabe S, Nagashima K, Wada H, Noda T, Nishigaki K, Fujiwara H (2000) Cardiac sympathetic denervation from the early stage of Parkinson's disease: clinical and experimental studies with radiolabeled MIBG. *J Nucl Med* 41: 71-77.

236. Tanner CM, Ottman R, Goldman SM, Ellenberg J, Chan P, Mayeux R, Langston JW (1999) Parkinson disease in twins: an etiologic study. *JAMA* 281: 341-346.

237. Tatton NA (2000) Increased caspase 3 and Bax immunoreactivity accompany nuclear GAPDH translocation and neuronal apoptosis in Parkinson's disease. *Exp Neurol* 166: 29-43.

238. Tatton WG, Olanow CW (1999) Apoptosis in neurodegenerative diseases: the role of mitochondria. *Biochim Biophys Acta* 1410: 195-213.

239. Tissingh G, Bergmans P, Booij J, Winogrodzka A, van Royen EA, Stoof JC, Wolters EC (1998) Drug-naive patients with Parkinson's disease in Hoehn and Yahr stages I and II show a bilateral decrease in striatal dopamine transporters as revealed by [123I]beta-CIT SPECT. *J Neurol* 245: 14-20.

240. Tompkins MM, Basgall EJ, Zamrini E, Hill WD (1997) Apoptotic-like changes in Lewy-body-associated disorders and normal aging in substantia nigral neurons. *Am J Pathol* 150: 119-131.

241. Tortosa A, Lopez E, Ferrer I (1997) Bcl-2 and Bax proteins in Lewy bodies from patients with Parkinson's disease and Diffuse Lewy body disease. *Neurosci Lett* 238: 78-80.

242. Trétiakoff MC (1919) Contribution à l'étude de l'anatomie pathologique du locus niger de Soemmering., (eds). Universit´t de Paris: Thése.

242a. Twelves D, Perkins KSM, Counsell C (2003) Systemic review of incidence studies of Parkinson's disease. *Mov Disord* 18: 19-21.

243. Uhl GR (1998) Hypothesis: the role of dopaminergic transporters in selective vulnerability of cells in Parkinson's disease. *Ann Neurol* 43: 555-560.

244. Valente EM, Bentivoglio AR, Dixon PH, Ferraris A, Ialongo T, Frontali M, Albanese A, Wood NW (2001) Localization of a novel locus for autosomal recessive early-onset parkinsonism, PARK6, on human chromosome 1p35-p36. *Am J Hum Genet* 68: 895-900.

244a. Valente EM, Brancati F, Ferraris A, Graham EA, Davis MB, Breteler MM, Gasser T, Bonifati V, Bentivoglio AR, De Michele G, Durr A, Cortelli P, Wassilowsky D, Harhangi BS, Rawal N, Caputo V, Filla A, Meco G, Oostra BA, Brice A, Albanese A, Dallapiccola B, Wood NW (2002) PARK6-linked parkinsonism occurs in several European families. *Ann Neurol* 51: 14-18.

245. van Duijn CM, Dekker MC, Bonifati V, Galjaard RJ, Houwing-Duistermaat JJ, Snijders PJ, Testers L, Breedveld GJ, Horstink M, Sandkuijl LA, van Swieten JC, Oostra BA, Heutink P (2001) Park7, a novel locus for autosomal recessive early-onset parkinsonism, on chromosome 1p36. *Am J Hum Genet* 69: 629-634.

246. Vereecken TH, Vogels OJ, Nieuwenhuys R (1994) Neuron loss and shrinkage in the amygdala in Alzheimer's disease. *Neurobiol Aging* 15: 45-54.

247. Vila M, Jackson-Lewis V, Vukosavic S, Djaldetti R, Liberatore G, Offen D, Korsmeyer SJ, Przedborski S (2001) Bax ablation prevents dopaminergic neurodegeneration in the 1-methyl- 4- phenyl-1,2,3,6-tetrahydropyridine mouse model of Parkinson's disease. *Proc Natl Acad Sci U S A* 98: 2837-2842.

248. Wakabayashi K, Engelender S, Yoshimoto M, Tsuji S, Ross CA, Takahashi H (2000) Synphilin-1 is present in Lewy bodies in Parkinson's disease. *Ann Neurol* 47: 521-523.

249. Wakabayashi K, Hayashi S, Yoshimoto M, Kudo H, Takahashi H (2000) NACP/alpha-synuclein-positive filamentous inclusions in astrocytes and oligodendrocytes of Parkinson's disease brains. *Acta Neuropathol (Berl)* 99: 14-20.

250. Wakabayashi K, Takahashi H (1997) The intermediolateral nucleus and Clarke's column in Parkinson's disease. *Acta Neuropathol (Berl)* 94: 287-289.

251. Walker DG, Terai K, Matsuo A, Beach TG, McGeer EG, McGeer PL (1998) Immunohistochemical analyses of fibroblast growth factor receptor-1 in the human substantia nigra. Comparison between normal and Parkinson's disease cases. *Brain Res* 794: 181-187.

252. Weihmuller FB, Ulas J, Nguyen L, Cotman CW, Marshall JF (1992) Elevated NMDA receptors in parkinsonian striatum. *Neuroreport* 3: 977-980.

253. Wenning GK, Litvan I, Verny M, Ray-Chaudhuri K, Granata R, Poewe W, Jellinger K ((1998)) Is EEG useful in the differential diagnosis of parkinsonism? *Parkinsonism Rel Disord* 4: 79-80.

254. Wetter TC, Brunner H, Hogl B, Yassouridis A, Trenkwalder C, Friess E (2001) Increased alpha activity in REM sleep in de novo patients with Parkinson's disease. *Mov Disord* 16: 928-933.

255. Wilson JM, Levey AI, Rajput A, Ang L, Guttman M, Shannak K, Niznik HB, Hornykiewicz O, Pifl C, Kish SJ (1996) Differential changes in neurochemical markers of striatal dopamine nerve terminals in idiopathic Parkinson's disease. *Neurology* 47: 718-726.

256. Winikates J, Jankovic J (1999) Clinical correlates of vascular parkinsonism. *Arch Neurol* 56: 98-102.

257. Wullner U, Kornhuber J, Weller M, Schulz JB, Loschmann PA, Riederer P, Klockgether T (1999) Cell death and apoptosis regulating proteins in Parkinson's disease--a cautionary note. *Acta Neuropathol (Berl)* 97: 408-412.

257a. Xu J, Kao SY, Lee FJ, Song W, Jin LW, Yankner BA (2002) Dopamine-dependent neurotoxicity of α-synuclein: a mechanism for selective neurodegeneration in Parkinson disease. *Nat Med* 8: 600-606.

258. Youdim MBH, Drigues N, Mande S (2001) Oxidative stress indices in Parkinson's disease. In *Parkinson's disease: methods and protocols*, MM Mouradian (eds). Humana Press: Totowa, NJ. pp. 137-153.

259. Yung KK, Smith AD, Levey AI, Bolam JP (1996) Synaptic connections between spiny neurons of the direct and indirect pathways in the neostriatum of the rat: evidence from dopamine receptor and neuropeptide immunostaining. Eur *J Neurosci* 8: 861-869.

260. Zecca L, Gallorini M, Schunemann V, Trautwein AX, Gerlach M, Riederer P, Vezzoni P, Tampellini D (2001) Iron, neuromelanin and ferritin content in the substantia nigra of normal subjects at different ages: consequences for iron storage and neurodegenerative processes. *J Neurochem* 76: 1766-1773.

261. Zhang J, Perry G, Smith MA, Robertson D, Olson SJ, Graham DG, Montine TJ (1999) Parkinson's disease is associated with oxidative damage to cytoplasmic DNA and RNA in substantia nigra neurons. *Am J Pathol* 154: 1423-1429.

262. Zhang Y, Gao J, Chung KK, Huang H, Dawson VL, Dawson TM (2000) Parkin functions as an E2-dependent ubiquitin- protein ligase and promotes the degradation of the synaptic vesicle-associated protein, CDCrel-1. *Proc Natl Acad Sci U S A* 97: 13354-13359.

263. Zweig RM, Cardillo JE, Cohen M, Giere S, Hedreen JC (1993) The locus ceruleus and dementia in Parkinson's disease. *Neurology* 43: 986-991.

Dementia with Lewy Bodies

Paul G. Ince
Ian G. McKeith

5HT	serotonin
AD	Alzheimer's disease
BA	Brodmann area
CA	cornu ammonis
ChAT	choline acetyltransferase
CSF	cerebrospinal fluid
DLB	demenita with Lewy bodies
DLBD	diffuse Lewy body disease
GABA	gamma aminobutyric acid
LBV	Lewy body variant of Alzheimer's disease
L-DOPA	levo-dioxyphenylalamine
MMSE	Mini-Mental State Exam
MRI	magnetic resonance imaging
PAF	pure autonomic failure
PD	Parkinson's diseaes
PDD	Parkinson's disease dementia
PET	positron emmision tomography
RBD	REM behaviour disorder
REM	rapid eye movement
SDLT	senile dementia of Lewy body type
SPECT	single photo emmission computerized tomography

Definition

Dementia with Lewy bodies (DLB) is a relatively new term (95) for a progressive dementia syndrome in the elderly, associated clinically with the core neuropsychiatric features of fluctuating cognition and visual hallucinations, in association with neurological evidence of Parkinsonism. The pathological features include a variable burden of α-synuclein immunoreactive neuronal pathology and Alzheimer-type pathology. At present there is no specific pathologic definition of DLB, it being largely a clinical diagnosis. In the only prospectively-diagnosed series with postmortem confirmation, the pathology was heterogeneous (93). It is often assumed that DLB is synonymous with diffuse Lewy body disease (40), but this remains to be determined.

Synonyms and Historical Annotation

Dementia with Lewy bodies emerged as a distinctive clinical syndrome around 1990 (23, 31, 32, 40, 72, 109) with the advent of sensitive immunohistochemical methods to detect Lewy bodies. Previously the occurrence of dementia in Parkinson's disease (PD), and parkinsonism in patients with dementia, were well-recognised clinical observations. The pathological literature prior to 1990 emphasised the frequent co-existence of Lewy bodies and Alzheimer-type pathology. It is impossible to determine how many of these cases would now be reclassified as DLB. The syndrome emerged initially in the Japanese literature (68, 71, 100) as an atypical variant of Alzheimer's disease (AD) with particular pathological and clinical features (58). Various groups used different nomenclature including: senile dementia of Lewy body type (SDLT), Lewy body variant of Alzheimer's disease (LBV), cortical Lewy body disease, diffuse Lewy body disease, Parkinson's disease dementia (PDD), and Lewy body dementia. The Consensus Workshop on DLB proposed that the present name be adopted, but acknowledged the validity of some of the previous nomenclature in denoting particular clinical settings (95).

Epidemiology

Incidence and prevalence. The true incidence and prevalence of DLB is unknown. It is considered to be the second most common neurodegenerative dementia syndrome in the elderly. There is a wide range of prevalence estimates in the published literature depending on study design and clinical background. The highest estimates come from specialist secondary dementia referral centres and range up to 26% (77) of demented patients. Studies with a community-based epidemiological design are fewer. A Japanese study has quoted a population prevalence of 0.1% in the over 65-year-olds (c.f. 3.8% "dementia," 2.1% AD, 1.0% vascular dementia) but did not include autopsy verification (138). A European study of elderly respondents coming to autopsy from a community-based sample showed significant Lewy body disease in 9% of the demented individuals (55). These individuals showed a range of pathology from "pure DLB" to AD with "incidental" Lewy bodies. There are no published studies from which the incidence of DLB can be derived. Survival was originally thought to be shorter on average than for AD (109), but a recent survival analysis showed no statistically significant differences (130). Meta-analysis suggests that patients with parkinsonism at onset may have longer survival compared to those with dementia, hallucinations and Alzheimer-type pathology (133).

Estimation of the prevalence of DLB in clinical practice is potentially confounded by co-incident cerebrovascular disease since this is a specific exclusion criterion in the Consensus Guidelines for the clinical diagnosis of DLB (95), which were primarily formulated to achieve a homogenous cohort for research purposes. More recent work has shown that vascular pathology is at least as common in DLB as it is in AD (93).

Sex and age distribution. DLB has been described as a syndrome in the elderly (>65 years). Onset prior to 65 years is not unknown and there is no established lower age limit. The disorder may have a slight male preponderance compared to AD.

Risk factors. There are no known risk factors for this disorder other than increasing age.

Genetics

No single gene determinant of DLB has been described. A few families with autosomal dominant inheritance of DLB are described (61), but there is no evidence that these are related to the α-synuclein gene as occurs in a handful of autosomal dominant PD pedigrees (111).

Numerous studies have examined the relationship of DLB to known and hypothetical genetic risk factors for AD. The best evidence available for a positive effect relates to the apolipoprotein E allele ϵ4 (18, 46, 64, 66, 73, 81, 101). Positive associations between DLB and the following genetic factors have also been described: iNOS 2A (137), CYP2D6 B (36, 126), dipeptidyl carboxipeptidase 1 (90) and butyryl cholinesterase K (118). A negative association with DLB has been described for the following genetic risk factors: iNOS 2A, eNOS 3 (120), presenilin 1 (121), CYP2D genes (7, 135), α-1 antichymotrypsin (73), α-2 macroglobulin (119). In keeping with the frequent presence of significant Alzheimer-type pathology in DLB, it should be noted that Lewy bodies in cortical and subcortical regions are commonly reported in patients with familial, early-onset AD due to point mutations in the APP or presenilin genes (62, 78), and in ageing Down's syndrome with Alzheimer-type pathology (80), indicating a link with the genetic basis of familial AD.

1. The central feature required for a diagnosis of DLB is progressive cognitive decline of sufficient magnitude to interfere with normal social or occupational function. Prominent or persistent memory impairment may not necessarily occur in the early stages, but is usually evident with progression. Deficits on tests of attention and of frontal-subcortical skills and visuospatial ability may be especially prominent.

2. **Two** of the following core features are **essential** for a diagnosis of *probable* DLB, **one** is **essential** for *possible* DLB:
   a) Fluctuating cognition with pronounced variations in attention and alertness
   b) Recurrent visual hallucinations, which are typically well formed and detailed
   c) Spontaneous motor features of parkinsonism

3. Features **supportive** of the diagnosis:
   a) Repeated falls
   b) Syncope
   c) Transient loss of consciousness
   d) Neuroleptic sensitivity
   e) Systematised delusions
   f) Hallucinations in other modalities

4. A diagnosis of DLB is **less likely** in the presence of
   a) Stroke disease evident as a focal neurological sign or on brain imaging.
   b) Evidence of a physical or brain disorder sufficient to account for the clinical picture.

Table 1. Consensus guidelines for the clinical diagnosis of Dementia with Lewy bodies (95). These criteria are proposed as being able to predict with high likelihood that dementia is associated with cortical Lewy bodies. They are potentially applicable to patients with idiopathic Parkinson's disease who subsequently develop dementia. These criteria do not exclude the presence of concomitant Alzheimer pathology and many patients may simultaneously meet guidelines for the clinical diagnosis of Alzheimer's disease.

Clinical Features

Signs and symptoms. DLB is primarily a progressive dementia syndrome and comes within the clinical differential diagnosis of dementia (40, 94, 95, 109). In contrast to AD, impairment of episodic memory is often minimal in the early stages (24) so that clinical diagnosis must include evaluation of additional cognitive modalities, particularly attention, visual perception and visuospatial performance. The Consensus Consortium on DLB characterised "probable" DLB as comprising a progressive dementia with the presence of 2 or more of the 3 core clinical features, and the variable presence of several supportive features (Table 1) (95). All of these clinical manifestations can be present in AD, vascular cognitive impairment and other neurodegenerative dementia syndromes. It has been shown that the discriminating value of the diagnostic constellation indicating probable DLB is greatest at an early stage and should be considered at any new dementia presentation (93). The Consensus Consortium guidelines for clinical diagnosis of DLB have been shown to have prospective diagnostic reliability that is at least as good as those used for AD (93).

Core diagnostic features. Consensus criteria for the clinical diagnosis of DLB have been proposed (95) to include the following symptoms:

Cognitive decline. Global clinical instruments for evaluating cognitive decline in established DLB (eg, MMSE, CAMCOG) show equal impairment compared to AD. The rate of cognitive decline in patients diagnosed with AD, DLB and vascular dementia are similar (11). DLB, however, is associated with a distinctive constellation of neuropsychological impairments, including both "cortical" (eg, memory, language, visuospatial ability) and "subcortical" modalities (eg, learning, attention, visuoconstructive ability, psychomotor speed) (24, 37, 40, 113-116). Memory deficits occur in DLB and contrast with AD. In AD there is an early and profound impairment of episodic memory. In contrast, working memory is more affected in DLB, with equivalent impairment of semantic memory, and early preservation of episodic memory (24, 73). Cognitive decline is more prevalent at disease onset, and parkinsonism less prevalent, in those patients with pathological confirmation of significant Alzheimer-type pathology (Lewy body variant of Alzheimer's disease [LBV]) (85).

Visual hallucinations. A prominent feature both early in the course of DLB and persisting during progression (9, 15). These hallucinations are well-formed, recurrent, and frequently comprise people or animals. They may occur in the presence of retained insight into their lack of reality (67, 96, 97).

Fluctuating cognition. Patients with DLB characteristically experience fluctuation in their cognitive state and level of consciousness over periods ranging from a few minutes to weeks or longer (95). Such episodes are independent of normal diurnal variation. Fluctuating cognition appears to derive from continuous variations in attentional capacity and is associated with greater impairment of Activities of Daily Living scores (14). Deficits in cognitive reaction time may distinguish DLB from AD (10). A potential neuroanatomical correlate of fluctuating cognition is involvement of the thalamic intralaminar nuclei (50).

Parkinsonism. Up to 75% of patients with DLB develop an extrapyramidal movement disorder, strongly reminiscent of PD (8), but characterised by milder signs (84). This may be found at presentation in about 25% of cases (especially in those with milder Alzheimer-type changes) (85) and develops in a further 50% during the course of the dementing illness. Parkinsonism is, however, not essential for the clinical diagnosis of DLB. Resting tremor is less common in DLB than PD and may reflect differences in the underlying neurochemical abnormality. Some patients will only show features of facial immobility or other subtle manifestations of extrapyramidal rigidity. Parkinsonism is much less frequent in early AD or vascular dementia (12) where it is uncommon if the MMSE score is above 10. If a patient presents with PD more than 1 year prior to the diagnosis of dementia then an arbitrary assignment to a diagnosis of "Parkinson's disease plus dementia" (PDD) has been recommended (95). It is worth noting that several recent neuropathologic studies have shown that PDD is often associated with diffuse and transitional types of Lewy body disease (3, 52, 91), which is the usual pathologic findings in DLB (93).

Supportive diagnostic features. *Neuroleptic sensitivity.* Patients with DLB are characteristically sensitive to both conventional neuroleptics, and newer atypical D2 dopamine receptor antagonists, used to control behavioural and psychotic symptoms in dementia. This "neuroleptic sensitivity"syndrome may be severe and life-threatening such that advice on prescribing practice is to use such drugs in DLB with extreme caution (92).

Falls, syncope, loss of consciousness. Repeated, unexplained falls are a clinical characteristic of DLB. They are present in at least 10% of patients and are unrelated to overt parkinsonism (16, 53). There is an association between either DLB or PD and orthostatic hypotension (13). This is presumed to arise from α-synucleinopathy affecting peripheral nerves, autonomic ganglia and the sympathetic innervation of the myocardium (4, 53, 65).

Delusions and auditory hallucinations. Neuropsychiatric manifestations within these modalities are relatively common in DLB but are not regarded as significant diagnostic discriminants since they are also prominent in AD and other related disorders (95).

Depression. A 50% prevalence of depressive symptoms in DL B is similar to that in PD and generally higher than that reported for AD. There is extensive loss of the serotonin (5-HT) transporter or reuptake site, in both the striatum and the cortex of PD and DLB cases, although paradoxically this is even lower in patients without depression, consistent with the concept that depression is associated with compensatory regenerative activity in 5-HT neurones (103).

REM sleep behaviour disorder. Sleep abnormalities are increasingly considered to be an important symptom in PD and DLB, and may predate the onset of other clinical features. In PD rapid eye movement (REM) behaviour disorder (RBD) is said to occur in 15% of all patients. Up to 40% of patients with RBD may eventually develop PD (19, 134). Interference with the maintenance of REM sleep atonia also occurs in DLB.

Imaging. *Structural imaging.* Several MRI studies have emphasised the relative preservation of medial temporal lobe volume in DLB compared to AD (17, 48) although there is no significant difference in the overall rate of brain atrophy in DLB compared with other dementia syndromes (99). Postmortem pathological assessment of temporal lobe volume provides a clear correlate of this in vivo imaging data (79). Such studies involve comparison of group means and it is likely that individual cases within the range of DLB and AD will overlap. Equivalent medial temporal lobe atrophy to that encountered in AD has also been reported, together with selective frontal lobe atrophy in DLB and PD (35).

Functional imaging. PET and SPECT studies show consistent evidence of occipital hypometabolism (reduced O_2 uptake and reduced glucose utilisation) compared with AD (51, 54, 82). The degeneration of the nigrostriatal dopaminergic projection in DLB is demonstrable by SPECT imaging of the pre-synaptic dopamine uptake site (131, 132). This investigation has been proposed as a diagnostic procedure to distinguish DLB from AD (131).

Laboratory findings. No clinically useful laboratory tests have been proposed based on plasma or CSF analysis for the diagnosis of DLB; however, several studies have been reported on the value of CSF tau and Aβ in differentiating AD from DLB (2, 102). In particular, CSF tau, especially phospho-tau, may be lower in DLB than in Alzhiemer's disease, although both show decreased levels of Aβ.

Macroscopy

There are no characteristic or specific macroscopic abnormalities for DLB. Some degree of diffuse cerebral atrophy is likely to be present, but may not be significantly outside the range encountered in non-demented elderly individuals. Cases with the "common form" of DLBD are more likely to have significant atrophy of the medial temporal lobe structures, especially parahippocampal gyrus and hippocampal formation, than cases of pure DLBD. A trend towards increased frontal and hippocampal atrophy related to the burden of Lewy body pathology has been reported (27). Circumscribed medial temporal lobe atrophy has been reported in some cases (89).

Deep grey nuclei of the cerebral hemispheres show mild and proportionate atrophy and the cerebral white matter is usually unremarkable. Lesions of cerebrovascular disease may be present and do not exclude co-existent Lewy body disease. In the diencephalon there is variable pallor of the substantia nigra, which may appear normal. Marked nigral pallor is likely to be correlated with a clinical history of overt parkinsonian signs and symptoms. In contrast, the locus ceruleus is usually depigmented.

Cortical region	BA	Anatomy	Score		
Entorhinal cortex	29	medial flank of collateral sulcus	0	1	2
Cingulate gyrus	24	whole gyral cortex	0	1	2
Mid-frontal cortex	8/9	lateral flank of superior frontal sulcus	0	1	2
Mid-temporal cortex	21	inferior surface of superior temporal sulcus	0	1	2
Inferior parietal lobule	40	lateral flank of parietal sulcus	0	1	2

Table 2. *Consensus pathological guidelines for reporting Lewy body distribution.* For each region Lewy bodies are counted from the depth of the sulcus to the lip. Counts are not made over the crest of the gyri except for the cingulate gyrus. Lewy bodies are predominantly located in deeper cortical layers (layers 5 and 6). In each region a count of up to 5 Lewy bodies in the cortical ribbon gives a score of 1 in the Table. Counts greater than 5 score as 2. The sum of the five areas is used to derive the category of cortical spread (maximum score 10). BA = Brodmann cortical area.
Cortical Lewy body score: 0-2 Brainstem-predominant, 3-6 Limbic or 'transitional', 7-10 Neocortical

Histopathology

Lewy bodies. There is no accepted "gold standard" for the pathological diagnosis of DLB, such as has been proposed for AD. The hallmark pathology of DLB is α-synucleinopathy, manifested as Lewy bodies of both classical and cortical types and neuritic degeneration. Cortical Lewy bodies appear to affect various subgroups of neurones including pyramidal cells and GABA-ergic interneurons (38, 122, 129). The severity and extent of these changes is variable and no thresholds have been widely accepted for diagnostic guidelines. In theory a patient with clinical features corresponding to the Consensus Guidelines for the Clinical Diagnosis of DLB (95) in whom any Lewy bodies can be demonstrated in the brain could be diagnosed as DLB.

The Consensus Pathological Guidelines (Table 2) were formulated to provide a method of scoring the severity and anatomical distribution of Lewy bodies in the cerebral cortex. They did not provide diagnostic criteria as it is sometimes mistakenly assumed. It was hoped that this method could be adapted to be included in the "CERAD" protocol (98) although this has not yet been achieved. This system of scoring cortical Lewy body pathology is based on 5 cortical areas: transentorhinal cortex Brodman area 29 (BA29), anterior cingulate gyrus (BA24), mid-frontal gyrus (BA8/9), superior aspect of middle temporal gyrus (BA21), and inferior parietal lobule (BA40). These areas were chosen on the basis of their frequent involvement by Lewy body pathology. The Consensus scoring system gives three categories within which cases can be assigned: "brainstem predominant," limbic (or transitional), and neocortical.

While there is an expectation that DLB cases will more likely fall into the limbic and neocortical categories there is no absolute requirement for this. Some cases diagnosed clinically as DLB according to the Consensus Guidelines fall into the "Brainstem-predominant" category (93). It has been proposed that the Consensus protocol be altered to exclude the frontal region because of the common finding of occasional Lewy bodies in this region in PD in the absence of dementia (45). This proposal assumes that it is desirable to have criteria that are able to distinguish demented cases with Lewy body disease on the basis of categorisation to at least the limbic category. However it is likely that PD and DLB represent a clinical and pathological spectrum so that individual cases will inevitably include overlapping anatomical spread of α-synuclein pathology. Recent studies has demonstrated that the number of Lewy bodies in the frontal gyri is the most statistically significant predictor of cognitive status in PD (91), and that cortical Lewy bodies are a better predictor of cognitive impairment in PD than Alzheimer-type pathology (3, 52).

The Consensus Pathological Guidelines were formulated prior to the discovery of the role of α-synuclein in Lewy body formation. The quantitative thresholds for allocating scores (ie, 0, 1-4, and 5+ Lewy bodies per region) are therefore based on ubiquitin immunocytochemistry or conventional staining (eg, H&E). While it is not clear that immunocytochemistry for α-synuclein is more sensitive than immunocytochemistry for ubiquitin in detecting Lewy bodies, it is definitely more specific (38). A single published study comparing ubiquitin and α-synuclein immunostaining reported that this is not the case, and that the increased burden of pathology demonstrated by α-synuclein immuno-staining comprised neuritic lesions not Lewy bodies (38).

The anatomical distribution of Lewy bodies in DLB, and all other neurodegenerative disorders in which they are found, does not follow a hierarchical pattern of spread analagous to the hypothesis of Braak in relation to neurofibrillary tangles (21). They are most frequently encountered in the pigmented midbrain and brainstem nuclei, the dorsal efferent nucleus of the vagus in the medulla, the basal forebrain cholinergic nuclei (eg, nucleus basalis of Meynert) and in limbic cortical regions especially the amygdala, entorhinal and anterior cingulate cortices (1, 20, 22, 28, 30, 41, 59, 69, 109). In contrast they are rarely encountered in the occipital cortex (109). Occasional cases in which limbic, especially amygdala Lewy bodies were present in the absence of demonstrable nigral involvement (39) are reported and highlight the difficulty in establishing the absence of lesions in any region in which they are present at very low frequency. The exclusion of Lewy body pathology is best-achieved using immunocytochemistry for α-synuclein.

Microvacuolation. Although cortical Lewy bodies are predominantly located in the deeper cortical layers there is frequently a significant degree of spongiosis affecting cortical layers 1, 2, and 3 (43). These changes may be sufficiently intense as to raise the possibility of a spongiform encephalopathy (86, 123). Immunoreactivity to prion protein should be normal in such cases, although the possibility of 2 co-existing disease processes might occur. There has been no detailed ultrastructural study of this finding and the cause remains undetermined. It has been demonstrated that up to 70% of pyramidal cells may be lost in DLB (129), together with other classes of neurons. The subsequent loss of apical dendritic permeation in the upper cortical layers is a plausible substrate for attenuation and spongiosis.

Alzheimer-type pathology. *Senile plaques.* The most difficult problem in defining DLB is its relationship with AD (see Differential Diagnosis). The disorder was first appreciated as a variant of AD (40, 109) and significant Alzheimer-type pathology is a consistent, but not universal, finding in DLB at autopsy.

Amyloid plaques, including neuritic plaques, are frequently present at a burden which is quantitatively equivalent to AD patients (109) and which would be associated with a diagnosis of Definite AD using the CERAD protocol (41, 44, 93, 98). However, many cases have predominantly diffuse amyloid palques with few neuritic elements (3). Despite this there is a subgroup of patients in whom the clinical picture is that of DLB, but who have minimal cerebral amyloid deposition (49, 70). Such patients emphasise the difficulty in ascribing the cognitive deficits and neuropsychological profile of DLB exclusively to senile plaque formation. Kosaka proposed that DLBD cases can be divided into two subgroups: A "common form of DLBD" is characterised by abundant neocortical senile plaques and with significant neurofibrillary tangles in medial temporal lobe cortex; while "pure DLBD" comprises the subgroup of patients in whom Alzheimer-type pathology is minimal (69). However the process of assigning cases to these groups is dependent on the criteria used to define AD, so that adopting different approaches in the same autopsy cohort generates differing proportions within each category (44).

Neurofibrillary tangles. Neurofibrillary tangles are present in the cortex of many patients with DLB and are usually restricted to limbic regions and especially the hippocampal pyramidal cell layers (40, 56, 109). In the hippocampal formation there is frequently a diffuse neuritic blush of hyper-phosphorylated tau immunoreactivity throughout the pyramidal sectors, especially CA1 and 2. Several biochemical studies have shown that extensive neocortical tau pathology, with the characteristics of AD, is absent in DLB (47, 125). If numerous neuritic plaques and neocortical neurofibrillary tangles are present in a case with Lewy bodies and a clinical picture of DLB then it may be equally valid to assign diagnoses of both DLB and AD. This pathological constellation represents the extreme end of the concept "Lewy body variant of Alzheimer's disease," which is a satisfactory diagnostic label for such cases.

Other lesions. Congophilic angiopathy may be present, especially in cases with significant senile plaque formation (136). Hippocampal pathology is usually less prominent that in AD, but includes Hirano bodies and granulovacuolar degeneration.

Immunocytochemistry and Ultrastructural Findings

The most important diagnostic tool in the pathological diagnosis of DLB is immunocytochemistry for α-synuclein (124). The advantage of using an antibody to ubiquitin compared to conventional stains to demonstrate Lewy bodies has also been established (76). These techniques are of particular value in demonstrating cortical Lewy bodies, which are inconspicuous in conventionally stained sections. Since the co-existence of Lewy bodies and neurofibrillary tangles is frequent in the ageing brain, the use of α-synuclein has the particular benefit of distinguishing between them. All other methods are less likely to achieve definite distinction between cortical Lewy bodies and small globular tangles.

The Lewy bodies of DLB show no immunochemical or morphological differences compared to PD. A wide range of epitopes has been demonstrated immunocytochemically within Lewy bodies and their ultrastructure has been described (chapter 4.2.1). Some neuronal inclusions may show immunoreactivity to both α-synuclein and tau, are morphologically intermediate between Lewy bodies and neurofibrillary tangles and show ultrastructural features of both paired helical filaments and a-synuclein fibrils (6).

Lewy neurites. The presence of diffuse neuritic lesions in DLB and PD was first demonstrated in the CA2/3 region of the hippocampus (33, 34). In practice these lesions are most prominent at the interface between pyramidal sectors CA1 and CA2. They are immunoreactive for α-synuclein, ubiquitin and variably for phosphorylated tau (AT8 and Tau2). They are not found in AD and were initially regarded as a means to discriminate DLBD from more restricted forms of Lewy body disease, but this remains to be proven (33). Immunohistochemistry with antibody to α-synuclein reveals extensive neuritic pathology throughout the brain. This technique will routinely demonstrate diffuse cytoplasmic reactivity, Lewy body–type lesions including so-called "neuritic Lewy bodies" and Lewy neurites. These are present in regions that were not previously associated with Lewy body pathology such as the caudate nucleus, putamen, claustrum, and thalamus. Detailed analysis of the relative fre-

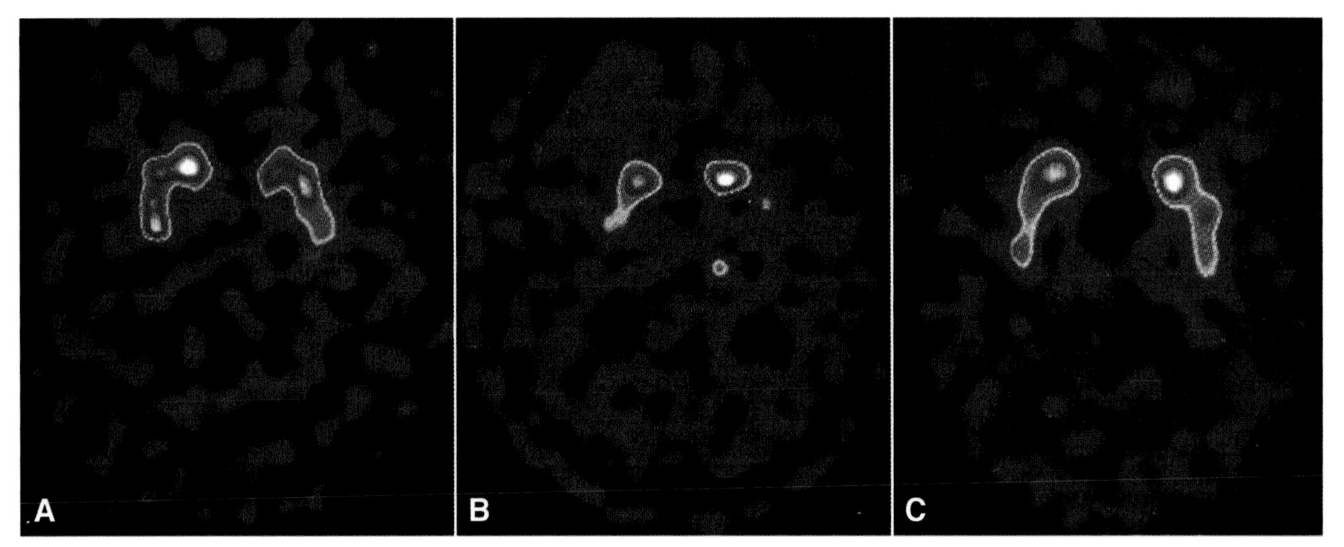

Figure 1. SPECT images of FP-CIT uptake in the corpus striatum. This ligand labels the dopamine re-uptake transporter and is a marker of pre-synaptic afferent nerve terminals. **A.** Normal elderly control showing similar uptake in the caudate and putamen. **B.** Dementia with Lewy bodies showing loss of uptake in the putamen. **C.** Alzheimer's disease patients show preservation of the putamen uptake signal.

quency of α-synuclein pathology in such sub-cortical regions, and the clinical correlation with such involvement, is not yet published, but preliminary studies suggest that density of Lewy neurites, particularly those in the amygdala, correaltes with cognitive impairment (26).

Synaptic loss and glial pathology. Synaptic loss is a consistent feature of DLB and is of equal severity to that demonstrable in AD. It is equally severe in the presence or absence of co-existent Alzheimer-type pathology (25, 42). The presence of synaptic loss may correlate with dementia, but has no value in diagnostic discrimination of the dementing disorders.

Glial lesions have been described in Lewy body disease and these have the morphology of thorn shaped astrocytes or coiled bodies and are immunoreactive for α-synuclein (127). Glial lesions are sparse in Lewy body disease and the concurrent presence of Lewy bodies should allow differentiation from multiple system atrophy in which synuclein-immunoreactive oligodendroglial cytoplasmic inclusions are a major histopathologic feature (75).

The role of microglia and inflammatory pathology in the evolution of DLB is unresolved and is diagnostically unhelpful (60, 112, 128).

Biochemistry

Cholinergic systems. Neocortical choline acetyltransferase (ChAT) in DLB is similar to that in demented PD and lower than in AD (32, 105). Cortical cholinergic activity is lower in hallucinating compared with non-hallucinating DLB cases, while 5-HT activity is relatively preserved (106). Loss of striatal ChAT in DLB (74), probably due to pathology of intrinsic local circuit neurons, may correlate with milder extrapyramidal clinical symptoms even in DLB cases that have equivalent loss of dopaminergic substantia nigra neurons compared with PD (107). In DLB and PD the muscarinic M1 subtype is elevated in the neocortex (108) due to up-regulation of postsynaptic receptors. DLB contrasts with AD in that muscarinic MI and M2 receptors are differentially affected (117) which may reflect differences in the underlying extent of pathology in the cholinergic projection from the basal forebrain (63). Normal receptor coupling via G proteins suggests that cholinoceptive neurons are intact in DLB and provides a rationale for cholinergic therapy. The α4β2 nicotinic receptor is reduced in the cortex in DLB, AD and PD, in contrast the α7 subunit is not affected in the cortex in DLB or Alzhiemer's disease (87).

Dopaminergic systems. DLB is associated with disruption of the dopaminergic input to the striatum, eg, reduced dopamine, and reduced homovanillic acid:dopamine ratio in autopsy tissue in DLB (74, 107). The dopamine transporter is low in DLB in comparison to AD and is demonstrable using FP-CIT SPECT imaging. Autopsy studies show no alteration in D1, D2, or D3 subtypes in DLB patients who have not been treated with L-DOPA (104, 110). The absence of D2 up-regulation, in contrast to PD may reflect differences in the nature or extent of basal ganglia pathology.

Differential Diagnosis

The concept of DLB is essentially syndromic. Difficulty in assimilating it into the clinicopathological diagnosis of dementing syndromes, and the neurodegenerative diseases, largely stems from a failure to appreciate that all the disorders which are traditionally regarded as diseases (including AD) are really syndromes within complex overlapping spectra of clinical presentations, and underlying pathological substrates. Within this field the concepts of "disease" which are most historically entrenched (eg, PD and AD) are the most difficult to realign to accommodate new findings.

The main differential diagnoses, on the basis of clinical overlap with DLB

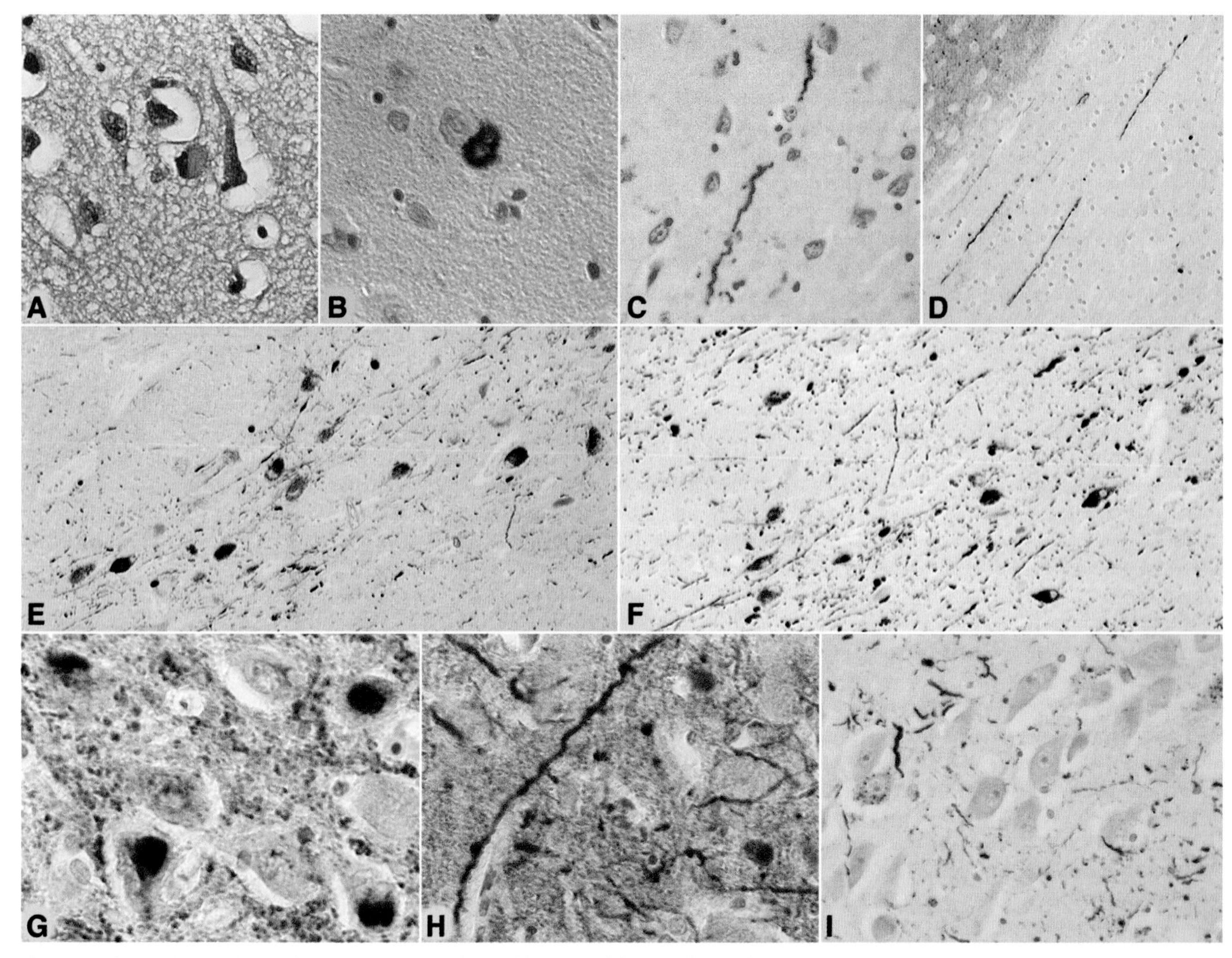

Figure 2. A. Cortical Lewy bodies are inconspicuous in conventional H&E stains but (**B**) are readily identified using immunocytochemistry to α-synuclein. **C.** α-synuclein antibodies also show abnormal neurites in the neocortex (**C**) and white matter (**D**, external capsule, note the diffuse staining of the insula cortex neuropil). In the substantia nigra of DLB patients (**E**) there is greater neuronal preservation and fewer Lewy neurites than in Parkinson's disease (**F**) although there are no absolute thresholds. In the hippocampus α-synuclein inclusions are found in pyramidal cells of all the CA sectors (**G**, CA2 neurons). Lewy neurites are usually abundant in the CA1/2 junction (**H**, α-synuclein) and may be co-immunoreactive for tau (**I**) in some cases.

have been AD, PD, vascular dementia, and Creutzfeldt-Jakob Disease. A recent prospective evaluation of the Consensus Guidelines for the clinical diagnosis of DLB (95) showed sensitivity and specificity of a clinical diagnosis of DLB of 0.83 and 0.95, respectively (93). Other studies have shown lower sensitivity, especially when there was concurrent AD (83).

Alzheimer's disease. Alzheimer-type pathology is a major component in most cases with the clinical diagnosis of DLB. There are no absolute criteria by which to judge the relative contributions of α-synucleinopathy, cerebral amyloidosis and tauopathy to the clinical phenotype in individual cases. Nor should the possibility of assigning two diagnoses in one patient be excluded. If the clinical picture is typical of DLB, then a small proportion of such cases will be false positives, in that they may not have Lewy bodies, but rather vacular or Alzheimer-type pathology (93). Conversely, the presence of Lewy bodies, including cortical Lewy bodies, may present with clinically probable AD and be more compatible with a diagnosis of LBV. As noted above many patients with genetically determined AD will have some degree of α-synucleinopathy (78, 80). It has also been noted that up to 57% of elderly sporadic AD patients have Lewy bodies (39) or synuclein filamentous aggregates in neurons with neurofibrillary tangles (5, 88), especially in the amygdala.

It has been proposed that patients with pathologic findings sufficient to warrant a diagnosis of AD as well as Lewy bodies be considered as two groups: those with the clinical features of DLB should be diagnosed as "LBV"; those with more prominent Alzheimer-type pathology and minimal Lewy bodies (eg, limited to the amygdala) and a clinical picture of typical AD should be diagnosed as "Alzheimer's disease with incidental Lewy bodies" (29).

Dementia in Parkinson's disease. Both PD and DLB are predominantly

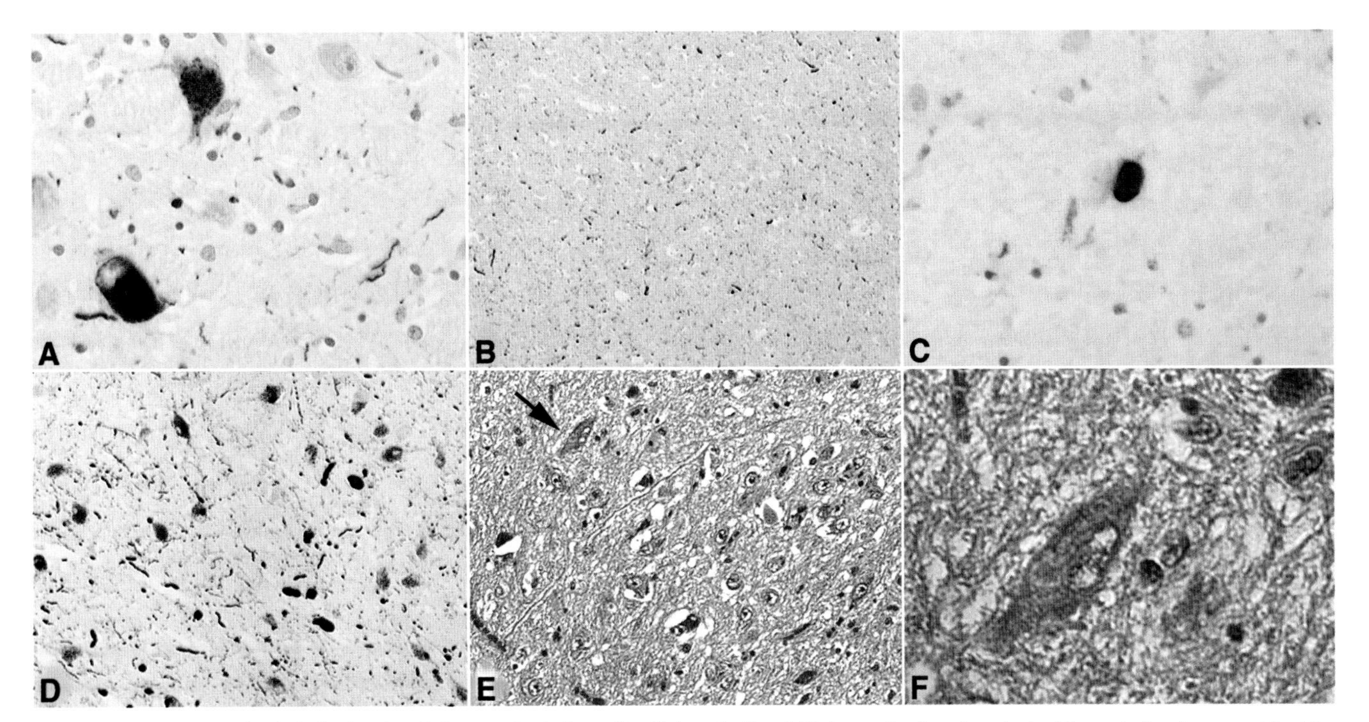

Figure 3. Lewy body related pathologies in subcortical grey matter in Dementia with Lewy bodies. **A.** Thalamus showing a Lewy body, diffuse cytoplasmic α-synuclein staining, and abundant Lewy neurites. **B.** The putamen shows few or absent perikaryal inclusions but widespread neuritic a-synuclein pathology; Lewy bodies and neuritic pathology in cholinergic nuclei—pedunculopontine tegmental nucleus (**C**) and nucleus basalis of Meynert (**D**). Occasional Lewy bodies are present in sympathetic and parasympathetic nuclei both centrally and in the periphery—Edinger Westphal nucleus (**E, F,** oculomotor complex). The neuron arrowed in **E** is shown enlarged in **F**.

characterised by α-synucleinopathy. The consensus workshop on DLB recommended an arbitrary distinction between DLB (predominantly a dementia syndrome) and dementia arising in a patient who initially presented with PD (predominantly a movement disorder syndrome) with initially preserved cognitive function (95). This is defined as a period in excess of 1 year between diagnosis of PD and the onset of cognitive impairment or behavioural dysfunction. Many patients with PD develop clinical features associated with DLB in the later stages of their illness. This does not invalidate the concept of DLB. It does illustrate the purpose of Table 3, which is to emphasise that α-synucleinopathy causes different clinical syndromes depending on anatomical extent and severity, and the presence of co-existent pathologies, within the central and peripheral nervous system. The concept of "PD" has no greater validity in defining a distinct disorder than does that of "DLB."

Syndrome	Neocortex	Limbic cortex & nbM	Substantia nigra	Dorsal motor n. of X	Lateral grey horn	Myenteric & sympathetic ganglia
DLB	++ to +++	+++	+ to ++	+ to +++	?	?
PD	+ to ++	++ to +++	+++	+ to +++	+ to ++	+ to ++
PAF	0	++	+	+++	++ to +++	+++
LB dysphagia	0	0	0 to +	0	?	+++

Table 3. Hypothetical spectrum of Lewy body disorders. Adapted from Ince et al 2000 (57). n = nucleus, LB = Lewy body, nbM = nucleus basalis of Meynert; PD = Parkinson's disease; PAF = pure autonomic failure, ? = no data available.

Vascular dementia. Early studies of DLB using retrospective case ascertainment show that vascular causes were frequently sited as the likely cause of cognitive decline (94). Vascular lesions are present in some cases of DLB and may warrant a diagnosis of a mixed dementia (DLB/vascular dementia). The frequency of less severe vascular lesions in DLB is likely to be no less common than for AD (93).

Creutzfeldt-Jakob disease. The 2 factors that raise this possibility in the differential diagnosis of DLB are clinical, rapid deterioration, and pathological, cortical spongiosis. Rapid progression is very likely to be due to injudicious use of neuroleptic therapy and the clinical history should be assessed for this possibility (92). Cortical microvacuolation is a consistent finding in DLB, but is unrelated to prion disease (86, 123), which can be excluded by anti-prion immunocytochemistry.

Pathogenesis

The pathogenesis of DLB concerns 3 major issues. The first is the molecular pathogenesis of α-synuclein aggregation and inclusion body formation. This topic is discussed in detail in chapter 4.2.1 on PD. The second concerns the molecular pathogenesis of Alzheimer-type pathology, albeit in a more limited distribution and reduced severity compared with AD. The basic mechanisms of cerebral amyloidosis and tau-inclusion body formation are discussed in chapter 2 on AD. The third relates to the different patterns of anatomical susceptibility in the nervous system that is found among the spectrum of the α-synucleinopathies (Table 3). This spectrum is based on the hypothesis that the disorders listed represent conditions in which there is a common underlying molecular pathogenesis giving rise to α-synucleinopathy, the clinical manifestation of which is dependent on the anatomical regions of the central and peripheral nervous system that are affected (57). No explanation for this spectrum has been proposed although it is presumed to arise from the particular genetic predisposition of individuals, in combination with the environmental insults sustained during life.

Future Directions and Therapy

Clinico-pathological studies will continue to refine understanding of the neuroanatomical factors and neurochemical pathology underlying the constellation of clinical features in DLB. Pathological verification of the diagnosis is an essential part of the validation of clinical diagnostic tests and advances in neuroimaging of brain pathology and abnormal function. The therapeutic implications of the cholinergic neurochemical pathology so far identified in DLB can be summarised as follows:

i) Cortical cholinergic deficits with functionally intact muscarinic M1 receptors suggest a potential value for cholinergic replacement therapy.

ii) Cortical cholinergic deficits in DLB relate more to psychiatric than cognitive symptoms and cholinergic replacement therapy may be effective in alleviating these.

iii) A randomised double blind clinical trial of cholinesterase inhibitors in patients with DLB showed marked improvements in attention, apathy, anxiety, hallucinations and delusions (93).

References

1. Alvord EC, Jr., Forno LS, Kusske JA, Kauffman RJ, Rhodes JS, Goetowski CR (1974) The pathology of Parkinsonism: a comparison of degenerations in cerebral cortex and brainstem. *Adv Neurol* 5: 175-193

2. Andreasen N, Minthon L, Davidsson P, Vanmechelen E, Vanderstichele H, Winblad B, Blennow K (2001) Evaluation of CSF-tau and CSF-Abeta42 as diagnostic markers for Alzheimer disease in clinical practice. *Arch Neurol* 58: 373-379.

3. Apaydin H, Ahlskog JE, Parisi JE, Boeve BF, Dickson DW (2002) Parkinson disease neuropathology: later-developing dementia and loss of the levo-dopa response. *Arch Neurol* 59: 102-112

4. Arai K, Kato N, Kashiwado K, Hattori T (2000) Pure autonomic failure in association with human alpha-synucleinopathy. *Neurosci Lett* 296: 171-173.

5. Arai Y, Yamazaki M, Mori O, Muramatsu H, Asano G, Katayama Y (2001) Alpha-synuclein-positive structures in cases with sporadic Alzheimer's disease: morphology and its relationship to tau aggregation. *Brain Res* 888: 287-296.

6. Arima K, Mizutani T, Alim MA, Tonozuka-Uehara H, Izumiyama Y, Hirai S, Ueda K (2000) NACP/alpha-synuclein and tau constitute two distinctive subsets of filaments in the same neuronal inclusions in brains from a family of parkinsonism and dementia with Lewy bodies: double-immunolabeling fluorescence and electron microscopic studies. *Acta Neuropathol* 100: 115-121.

7. Atkinson A, Singleton AB, Steward A, Ince PG, Perry RH, McKeith IG, Fairbairn AF, Edwardson JA, Daly AK, Morris CM (1999) CYP2D6 is associated with Parkinson's disease but not with dementia with Lewy Bodies or Alzheimer's disease. *Pharmacogenetics* 9: 31-35.

8. Ballard C, McKeith I, Burn D, Harrison R, O'Brien J, Lowery K, Campbell M, Perry R, Ince P (1997) The UPDRS scale as a means of identifying extrapyramidal signs in patients suffering from dementia with Lewy bodies. *Acta Neurol Scand* 96: 366-371.

9. Ballard C, McKeith I, Harrison R, O'Brien J, Thompson P, Lowery K, Perry R, Ince P (1997) A detailed phenomenological comparison of complex visual hallucinations in dementia with Lewy bodies and Alzheimer's disease. *Int Psychogeriatr* 9: 381-388.

10. Ballard C, O'Brien J, Gray A, Cormack F, Ayre G, Rowan E, Thompson P, Bucks R, McKeith I, Walker M, Tovee M (2001) Attention and fluctuating attention in patients with dementia with Lewy bodies and Alzheimer disease. *Arch Neurol* 58: 977-982.

11. Ballard C, O'Brien J, Morris CM, Barber R, Swann A, Neill D, McKeith I (2001) The progression of cognitive impairment in dementia with Lewy bodies, vascular dementia and Alzheimer's disease. *Int J Geriatr Psychiatry* 16: 499-503.

12. Ballard C, O'Brien J, Swann A, Neill D, Lantos P, Holmes C, Burn D, Ince P, Perry R, McKeith I (2000) One year follow-up of parkinsonism in dementia with Lewy bodies. *Dement Geriatr Cogn Disord* 11: 219-222.

13. Ballard C, Shaw F, McKeith I, Kenny R (1998) High prevalence of neurovascular instability in neurodegenerative dementias. *Neurology* 51: 1760-1762.

14. Ballard C, Walker M, O'Brien J, Rowan E, McKeith I (2001) The characterisation and impact of 'fluctuating' cognition in dementia with Lewy bodies and Alzheimer's disease. *Int J Geriatr Psychiatry* 16: 494-498.

15. Ballard CG, O'Brien JT, Swann AG, Thompson P, Neill D, McKeith IG (2001) The natural history of psychosis and depression in dementia with Lewy bodies and Alzheimer's disease: persistence and new cases over 1 year of follow-up. *J Clin Psychiatry* 62: 46-49.

16. Ballard CG, Shaw F, Lowery K, McKeith I, Kenny R (1999) The prevalence, assessment and associations of falls in dementia with Lewy bodies and Alzheimer's disease. *Dement Geriatr Cogn Disord* 10: 97-103.

17. Barber R, McKeith IG, Ballard C, Gholkar A, O'Brien JT (2001) A comparison of medial and lateral temporal lobe atrophy in dementia with Lewy bodies and Alzheimer's disease: magnetic resonance imaging volumetric study. *Dement Geriatr Cogn Disord* 12: 198-205.

18. Benjamin R, Leake A, Ince PG, Perry RH, McKeith IG, Edwardson JA, Morris CM (1995) Effects of apolipoprotein E genotype on cortical neuropathology in senile dementia of the Lewy body and Alzheimer's disease. *Neurodegeneration* 4: 443-448.

19. Boeve BF, Silber MH, Ferman TJ, Kokmen E, Smith GE, Ivnik RJ, Parisi JE, Olson EJ, Petersen RC (1998) REM sleep behavior disorder and degenerative dementia: an association likely reflecting Lewy body disease. *Neurology* 51: 363-370.

20. Braak E, Sandmann-Keil D, Rub U, Gai WP, de Vos RA, Steur EN, Arai K, Braak H (2001) alpha-synuclein immunopositive Parkinson's disease-related inclusion bodies in lower brain stem nuclei. *Acta Neuropathol* 101: 195-201.

21. Braak H, Braak E (1991) Neuropathological stageing of Alzheimer-related changes. *Acta Neuropathol* 82: 239-259

22. Braak H, Braak E, Yilmazer D, de Vos RA, Jansen EN, Bohl J, Jellinger K (1994) Amygdala pathology in Parkinson's disease. *Acta Neuropathol* 88: 493-500

23. Byrne EJ, Lennox G, Lowe J, Godwin-Austen RB (1989) Diffuse Lewy body disease: clinical features in 15 cases. *J Neurol Neurosurg Psychiatry* 52: 709-717.

24. Calderon J, Perry RJ, Erzinclioglu SW, Berrios GE, Dening TR, Hodges JR (2001) Perception, attention, and working memory are disproportionately impaired in dementia with Lewy bodies compared with Alzheimer's disease. *J Neurol Neurosurg Psychiatry* 70: 157-164.

25. Campbell BC, Li QX, Culvenor JG, Jakala P, Cappai R, Beyreuther K, Masters CL, McLean CA (2000) Accumulation of insoluble alpha-synuclein in dementia with Lewy bodies. *Neurobiol Dis* 7: 192-200.

26. Churchyard A, Lees AJ (1997) The relationship between dementia and direct involvement of the hippocampus and amygdala in Parkinson's disease. *Neurology* 49: 1570-1576.

27. Cordato NJ, Halliday GM, Harding AJ, Hely MA, Morris JG (2000) Regional brain atrophy in progressive supranuclear palsy and Lewy body disease. *Ann Neurol* 47: 718-728.

28. de Vos RA, Jansen EN, Stam FC, Ravid R, Swaab DF (1995) 'Lewy body disease': clinico-pathological correlations in 18 consecutive cases of Parkinson's disease with and without dementia. *Clin Neurol Neurosurg* 97: 13-22.

29. Del Ser T, Hachinski V, Merskey H, Munoz DG (2001) Clinical and pathologic features of two groups of patients with dementia with Lewy bodies: effect of coexisting Alzheimer-type lesion load. *Alzheimer Dis Assoc Disord* 15: 31-44.

30. Den Hartog Jager W, Bethlem J (1960) The distribution of Lewy bodies in the central and autonomic nervous system in idiopathic paralysis agitans. *J Neurol Neurosurg Psychiatry* 23: 283-290

31. Dickson DW, Crystal H, Mattiace LA, Kress Y, Schwagerl A, Ksiezak-Reding H, Davies P, Yen SH (1989) Diffuse Lewy body disease: light and electron microscopic immunocytochemistry of senile plaques. *Acta Neuropathol* 78: 572-584

32. Dickson DW, Davies P, Mayeux R, Crystal H, Horoupian DS, Thompson A, Goldman JE (1987) Diffuse Lewy body disease. Neuropathological and biochemical studies of six patients. *Acta Neuropathol* 75: 8-15

33. Dickson DW, Ruan D, Crystal H, Mark MH, Davies P, Kress Y, Yen SH (1991) Hippocampal degeneration differentiates diffuse Lewy body disease (DLBD) from Alzheimer's disease: light and electron microscopic immunocytochemistry of CA2-3 neurites specific to DLBD. *Neurology* 41: 1402-1409.

34. Dickson DW, Schmidt ML, Lee VM, Zhao ML, Yen SH, Trojanowski JQ (1994) Immunoreactivity profile of hippocampal CA2/3 neurites in diffuse Lewy body disease. *Acta Neuropathol* 87: 269-276

35. Double KL, Halliday GM, McRitchie DA, Reid WG, Hely MA, Morris JG (1996) Regional brain atrophy in idiopathic parkinson's disease and diffuse Lewy body disease. *Dementia* 7: 304-313.

36. Furuno T, Kawanishi C, Iseki E, Onishi H, Sugiyama N, Suzuki K, Kosaka K (2001) No evidence of an association between CYP2D6 polymorphisms among Japanese and dementia with Lewy bodies. *Psychiatry Clin Neurosci* 55: 89-92.

37. Galloway PH, Sahgal A, McKeith IG et al (1992) Visual pattern recognition memory and learning deficits in senile dementias of Alzheimer and Lewy body types. *Dementia* 3: 101-107

38. Gomez-Tortosa E, Newell K, Irizarry MC, Sanders JL, Hyman BT (2000) alpha-Synuclein immunoreactivity in dementia with Lewy bodies: morphological staging and comparison with ubiquitin immunostaining. *Acta Neuropathol* 99: 352-357.

39. Hamilton RL (2000) Lewy bodies in Alzheimer's disease: a neuropathological review of 145 cases using alpha-synuclein immunohistochemistry. *Brain Pathol* 10: 378-384.

40. Hansen L, Salmon D, Galasko D, Masliah E, Katzman R, DeTeresa R, Thal L, Pay MM, Hofstetter R, Klauber M et al (1990) The Lewy body variant of Alzheimer's disease: a clinical and pathologic entity. *Neurology* 40: 1-8.

41. Hansen LA (1997) The Lewy body variant of Alzheimer disease. *J Neural Transm* Suppl 51: 83-93

42. Hansen LA, Daniel SE, Wilcock GK, Love S (1998) Frontal cortical synaptophysin in Lewy body diseases: relation to Alzheimer's disease and dementia. *J Neurol Neurosurg Psychiatry* 64: 653-656.

43. Hansen LA, Masliah E, Terry RD, Mirra SS (1989) A neuropathological subset of Alzheimer's disease with concomitant Lewy body disease and spongiform change. *Acta Neuropathol* 78: 194-201

44. Hansen LA, Samuel W (1997) Criteria for Alzheimer's disease and the nosology of dementia with Lewy bodies. *Neurology* 48: 126-132.

45. Harding AJ, Halliday GM (1998) Simplified neuropathological diagnosis of dementia with Lewy bodies. *Neuropathol Appl Neurobiol* 24: 195-201.

46. Harrington CR, Louwagie J, Rossau R, Vanmechelen E, Perry RH, Perry EK, Xuereb JH, Roth M, Wischik CM (1994) Influence of apolipoprotein E genotype on senile dementia of the Alzheimer and Lewy body types. Significance for etiological theories of Alzheimer's disease. *Am J Pathol* 145: 1472-1484.

47. Harrington CR, Perry RH, Perry EK, Hurt J, McKeith IG, Roth M, Wischik CM (1994) Senile dementia of Lewy body type and Alzheimer type are biochemically distinct in terms of paired helical filaments and hyperphosphorylated tau protein. *Dementia* 5: 215-228.

48. Harvey GT, Hughes J, McKeith IG, Briel R, Ballard C, Gholkar A, Scheltens P, Perry RH, Ince P, O'Brien JT (1999) Magnetic resonance imaging differences between dementia with Lewy bodies and Alzheimer's disease: a pilot study. *Psychol Med* 29: 181-187.

49. Hely MA, Reid WG, Halliday GM, McRitchie DA, Leicester J, Joffe R, Brooks W, Broe GA, Morris JG (1996) Diffuse Lewy body disease: clinical features in nine cases without coexistent Alzheimer's disease. *J Neurol Neurosurg Psychiatry* 60: 531-538.

50. Henderson JM, Carpenter K, Cartwright H, Halliday GM (2000) Loss of thalamic intralaminar nuclei in progressive supranuclear palsy and Parkinson's disease: clinical and therapeutic implications. *Brain* 123: 1410-1421.

51. Higuchi M, Tashiro M, Arai H, Okamura N, Hara S, Higuchi S, Itoh M, Shin RW, Trojanowski JQ, Sasaki H (2000) Glucose hypometabolism and neuropathological correlates in brains of dementia with Lewy bodies. *Exp Neurol* 162: 247-256.

52. Hurtig HI, Trojanowski JQ, Galvin J, Ewbank D, Schmidt ML, Lee VM, Clark CM, Glosser G, Stern MB, Gollomp SM, Arnold SE (2000) Alpha-synuclein cortical Lewy bodies correlate with dementia in Parkinson's disease. *Neurology* 54: 1916-1921.

53. Imamura T, Hirono N, Hashimoto M, Kazui H, Tanimukai S, Hanihara T, Takahara A, Mori E (2000) Fall-related injuries in dementia with Lewy bodies (DLB) and Alzheimer's disease. *Eur J Neurol* 7: 77-79.

54. Imamura T, Ishii K, Hirono N, Hashimoto M, Tanimukai S, Kazui H, Hanihara T, Sasaki M, Mori E (2001) Occipital glucose metabolism in dementia with lewy bodies with and without Parkinsonism: a study using positron emission tomography. *Dement Geriatr Cogn Disord* 12: 194-197.

55. Ince P, Esiri M, Matthews F (2001) Pathological correlates of late-onset dementia in a multicentre, community-based population in England and Wales. *Lancet* 357: 169-175

56. Ince P, Irving D, MacArthur F, Perry RH (1991) Quantitative neuropathological study of Alzheimer-type pathology in the hippocampus: comparison of senile dementia of Alzheimer type, senile dementia of Lewy body type, Parkinson's disease and non-demented elderly control patients. *J Neurol Sci* 106: 142-152.

57. Ince P, Perry R, Perry E (2000) Pathology of Dementia with Lewy bodies. In *Dementia*, J O'Brien, A Byrne: 2nd Edition, Oxford University Press, Oxford, UK.

58. Ince PG, Perry EK, Morris CM (1998) Dementia with Lewy bodies. A distinct non-Alzheimer dementia syndrome? *Brain Pathol* 8: 299-324.

59. Iseki E, Kato M, Marui W, Ueda K, Kosaka K (2001) A neuropathological study of the disturbance of the nigro-amygdaloid connections in brains from patients with dementia with Lewy bodies. *J Neurol Sci* 185: 129-134.

60. Iseki E, Marui W, Akiyama H, Ueda K, Kosaka K (2000) Degeneration process of Lewy bodies in the brains of patients with dementia with Lewy bodies using alpha-synuclein-immunohistochemistry. *Neurosci Lett* 286: 69-73.

61. Ishikawa A, Takahashi H, Tanaka H, Hayashi T, Tsuji S (1997) Clinical features of familial diffuse Lewy body disease. *Eur Neurol* 38: 34-38.

62. Janssen JC, Lantos PL, Fox NC, Harvey RJ, Beck J, Dickinson A, Campbell TA, Collinge J, Hanger DP, Cipolotti L, Stevens JM, Rossor MN (2001) Autopsy-confirmed familial early-onset Alzheimer disease caused by the I153V presenilin 1 mutation. *Arch Neurol* 58: 953-958.

63. Jellinger K (1997) Morphological substrates of dementia in parkinsonism. A critical update. *J Neural Transm* 52, suppl: 57-82

64. Katzman R, Galasko D, Saitoh T, Thal LJ, Hansen L (1995) Genetic evidence that the Lewy body variant is indeed a phenotypic variant of Alzheimer's disease. *Brain Cogn* 28: 259-265.

65. Kaufmann H, Hague K, Perl D (2001) Accumulation of alpha-synuclein in autonomic nerves in pure autonomic failure. *Neurology* 56: 980-981.

66. Kawanishi C, Suzuki K, Odawara T, Iseki E, Onishi H, Miyakawa T, Yamada Y, Kosaka K, Kondo N, Yamamoto T (1996) Neuropathological evaluation and

apolipoprotein E gene polymorphism analysis in diffuse Lewy body disease. *J Neurol Sci* 136: 140-142.

67. Klatka LA, Louis ED, Schiffer RB (1996) Psychiatric features in diffuse Lewy body disease: a clinicopathologic study using Alzheimer's disease and Parkinson's disease comparison groups. *Neurology* 47: 1148-1152.

68. Kosaka K (1978) Lewy bodies in cerebral cortex, report of three cases. *Acta Neuropathol* 42: 127-134.

69. Kosaka K, Iseki E (1996) Diffuse Lewy body disease within the spectrum of Lewy body disease. In *Dementia with Lewy Bodies*, RH Perry, IG McKeith, EK Perry (eds). Cambridge Universtity Press: Cambridge. pp. 238-247

70. Kosaka K, Iseki E, Odawara T, al. e (1996) Cerebral type of Lewy body disease. *Neuropathol Appl Neurobiol* 16: 32-35

71. Kosaka K, Mehraein P (1979) Dementia-Parkinsonism syndrome with numerous Lewy bodies and senile plaques in cerebral cortex. *Arch Psychiatr Nervenkr* 226: 241-250.

72. Kosaka K, Tsuchiya K, Yoshimura M (1989) Lewy body disease with and without dementia: a clinicopathological study of 35 cases. *Clin Neuropathol* 7: 299-305

73. Lamb H, Christie J, Singleton AB, Leake A, Perry RH, Ince PG, McKeith IG, Melton LM, Edwardson JA, Morris CM (1998) Apolipoprotein E and alpha-1 antichymotrypsin polymorphism genotyping in Alzheimer's disease and in dementia with Lewy bodies. Distinctions between diseases. *Neurology* 50: 388-391.

74. Langlais PJ, Thal L, Hansen L, Galasko D, Alford M, Masliah E (1993) Neurotransmitters in basal ganglia and cortex of Alzheimer's disease with and without Lewy bodies. *Neurology* 43: 1927-1934.

75. Lantos PL (1998) The definition of multiple system atrophy: a review of recent developments. *J Neuropathol Exp Neurol* 57: 1099-1111.

76. Lennox G, Lowe J, Morrell K, Landon M, Mayer RJ (1989) Anti-ubiquitin immunocytochemistry is more sensitive than conventional techniques in the detection of diffuse Lewy body disease. *J Neurol Neurosurg Psychiatry* 52: 67-71.

77. Lennox G, Lowe JS, Godwin-Austen RB, Landon M, Mayer RJ (1989) Diffuse Lewy body disease: an important differential diagnosis in dementia with extrapyramidal features. *Prog Clin Biol Res* 317: 121-130

78. Lippa CF, Fujiwara H, Mann DM, Giasson B, Baba M, Schmidt ML, Nee LE, O'Connell B, Pollen DA, St George-Hyslop P, Ghetti B, Nochlin D, Bird TD, Cairns NJ, Lee VM, Iwatsubo T, Trojanowski JQ (1998) Lewy bodies contain altered alpha-synuclein in brains of many familial Alzheimer's disease patients with mutations in presenilin and amyloid precursor protein genes. *Am J Pathol* 153: 1365-1370.

79. Lippa CF, Johnson R, Smith TW (1998) The medial temporal lobe in dementia with Lewy bodies: a comparative study with Alzheimer's disease. *Ann Neurol* 43: 102-106.

80. Lippa CF, Schmidt ML, Lee VM, Trojanowski JQ (1999) Antibodies to alpha-synuclein detect Lewy bodies in many Down's syndrome brains with Alzheimer's disease. *Ann Neurol* 45: 353-357.

81. Lippa CF, Smith TW, Saunders AM, Crook R, Pulaski-Salo D, Davies P, Hardy J, Roses AD, Dickson D (1995) Apolipoprotein E genotype and Lewy body disease. *Neurology* 45: 97-103.

82. Lobotesis K, Fenwick JD, Phipps A, Ryman A, Swann A, Ballard C, McKeith IG, O'Brien JT (2001) Occipital hypoperfusion on SPECT in dementia with Lewy bodies but not AD. *Neurology* 56: 643-649.

83. Lopez OL, Becker JT, Kaufer DI, Hamilton RL, Sweet RA, Klunk W, DeKosky ST (2002) Research evaluation and prospective diagnosis of dementia with Lewy bodies. *Arch Neurol* 59: 43-46.

84. Louis ED, Klatka LA, Liu Y, Fahn S (1997) Comparison of extrapyramidal features in 31 pathologically confirmed cases of diffuse Lewy body disease and 34 pathologically confirmed cases of Parkinson's disease. *Neurology* 48: 376-380.

85. Luginger E, Seppi K, Litvan I (2000) Associated Alzheimer pathology modifies the natural history of dementia with Lewy bodies (DLB): a clinicopathological study. *Mov Disord* 15, suppl: 226

86. Mancardi GL, Mandybur TI, Liwnicz BH (1982) Spongiform-like changes in Alzheimer's disease. An ultrastructural study. *Acta Neuropathol* 56: 146-150

87. Martin-Ruiz C, Court J, Lee M, Piggott M, Johnson M, Ballard C, Kalaria R, Perry R, Perry E (2000) Nicotinic receptors in dementia of Alzheimer, Lewy body and vascular types. *Acta Neurol Scand Suppl* 176: 34-41

88. Marui W, Iseki E, Ueda K, Kosaka K (2000) Occurrence of human alpha-synuclein immunoreactive neurons with neurofibrillary tangle formation in the limbic areas of patients with Alzheimer's disease. *J Neurol Sci* 174: 81-84.

89. Masliah E, Galasko D, Wiley CA, Hansen LA (1990) Lobar atrophy with dense-core (brain stem type) Lewy bodies in a patient with dementia. *Acta Neuropathol* 80: 453-458

90. Mattila KM, Rinne JO, Roytta M, Laippala P, Pietila T, Kalimo H, Koivula T, Frey H, Lehtimaki T (2000) Dipeptidyl carboxypeptidase 1 (DCP1) and butyrylcholinesterase (BCHE) gene interactions with the apolipoprotein E epsilon4 allele as risk factors in Alzheimer's disease and in Parkinson's disease with coexisting Alzheimer pathology. *J Med Genet* 37: 766-770.

91. Mattila PM, Rinne JO, Helenius H, Dickson DW, Roytta M (2000) Alpha-synuclein-immunoreactive cortical Lewy bodies are associated with cognitive impairment in Parkinson's disease. *Acta Neuropathol* 100: 285-290.

92. McKeith I, Fairbairn A, Perry R, Thompson P, Perry E (1992) Neuroleptic sensitivity in patients with senile dementia of Lewy body type. *BMJ* 305: 673-678.

93. McKeith IG, Ballard CG, Perry RH, Ince PG, O'Brien JT, Neill D, Lowery K, Jaros E, Barber R, Thompson P, Swann A, Fairbairn AF, Perry EK (2000) Prospective validation of consensus criteria for the diagnosis of dementia with Lewy bodies. *Neurology* 54: 1050-1058.

94. McKeith IG, Fairbairn AF, Perry RH, Thompson P (1994) The clinical diagnosis and misdiagnosis of senile dementia of Lewy body type (SDLT). *Br J Psychiatry* 165: 324-332.

95. McKeith IG, Galasko D, Kosaka K, Perry EK, Dickson DW, Hansen LA, Salmon DP, Lowe J, Mirra SS, Byrne EJ, Lennox G, Quinn NP, Edwardson JA, Ince PG, Bergeron C, Burns A, Miller BL, Lovestone S, Collerton D, Jansen EN, Ballard C, de Vos RA, Wilcock GK, Jellinger KA, Perry RH (1996) Consensus guidelines for the clinical and pathologic diagnosis of dementia with Lewy bodies (DLB): report of the consortium on DLB international workshop. *Neurology* 47: 1113-1124.

96. McKeith IG, Perry RH, Fairbairn AF, Jabeen S, Perry EK (1992) Operational criteria for senile dementia of Lewy body type (SDLT). *Psychol Med* 22: 911-922.

97. McShane R, Gedling K, Reading M, McDonald B, Esiri MM, Hope T (1995) Prospective study of relations between cortical Lewy bodies, poor eyesight, and hallucinations in Alzheimer's disease. *J Neurol Neurosurg Psychiatry* 59: 185-188.

98. Mirra SS, Heyman A, McKeel D, Sumi SM, Crain BJ, Brownlee LM, Vogel FS, Hughes JP, van Belle G, Berg L (1991) The Consortium to Establish a Registry for Alzheimer's Disease (CERAD). Part II. Standardization of the neuropathologic assessment of Alzheimer's disease. *Neurology* 41: 479-486.

99. O'Brien JT, Paling S, Barber R, Williams ED, Ballard C, McKeith IG, Gholkar A, Crum WR, Rossor MN, Fox NC (2001) Progressive brain atrophy on serial MRI in dementia with Lewy bodies, AD, and vascular dementia. *Neurology* 56: 1386-1388.

100. Okazaki H, Lipkin LS, Aronson SM (1961) Diffuse intracytoplasmic ganglionic inclusions (Lewy type) associated with progressive dementia and quadriparesis in flexion. *J Neuropathol Exp Neurol* 20: 237-244

101. Olichney JM, Hansen LA, Galasko D, Saitoh T, Hofstetter CR, Katzman R, Thal LJ (1996) The apolipoprotein E epsilon 4 allele is associated with increased neuritic plaques and cerebral amyloid angiopathy in Alzheimer's disease and Lewy body variant. *Neurology* 47: 190-196.

102. Parnetti L, Lanari A, Amici S, Gallai V, Vanmechelen E, Hulstaert F (2001) CSF phosphorylated tau is a possible marker for discriminating Alzheimer's disease from dementia with Lewy bodies. Phospho-Tau International Study Group. *Neurol Sci* 22: 77-78.

103. Perry E, Piggott M, Johnson M, Ballard C, McKeith I, Burn D (2002) Neurotransmitter correlates of neuropsychiatric symptoms in dementia with Lewy bodies. In press.

104. Perry EK, Ballard C, Spurden D (1998) Cholinergic systems in the human brain: psychopharmacology and psychosis. *Alz Dis Rev* in press.

105. Perry EK, Haroutunian V, Davis KL, Levy R, Lantos P, Eagger S, Honavar M, Dean A, Griffiths M, McKeith IG, et al. (1994) Neocortical cholinergic activities differentiate Lewy body dementia from classical Alzheimer's disease. *Neuroreport* 5: 747-749.

106. Perry EK, Marshall E, Kerwin J, Smith CJ, Jabeen S, Cheng AV, Perry RH (1990) Evidence of a monoaminergic-cholinergic imbalance related to visual hallucinations in Lewy body dementia. *J Neurochem* 55: 1454-1456.

107. Perry EK, Marshall E, Perry RH, Irving D, Smith CJ, Blessed G, Fairbairn AF (1990) Cholinergic and dopaminergic activities in senile dementia of Lewy body type. *Alzheimer Dis Assoc Disord* 4: 87-95.

108. Perry EK, Smith CJ, Court JA, Perry RH (1990) Cholinergic nicotinic and muscarinic receptors in dementia of Alzheimer, Parkinson and Lewy body types. *J Neural Transm Park Dis Dement Sect* 2: 149-158.

109. Perry RH, Irving D, Blessed G, Fairbairn A, Perry EK (1990) Senile dementia of Lewy body type. A clinically and neuropathologically distinct form of Lewy body dementia in the elderly. *J Neurol Sci* 95: 119-139.

110. Piggott MA, Marshall EF, Thomas N, Lloyd S, Court JA, Jaros E, Burn D, Johnson M, Perry RH, McKeith IG, Ballard C, Perry EK (1999) Striatal dopaminergic markers in dementia with Lewy bodies, Alzheimer's and Parkinson's diseases: rostrocaudal distribution. *Brain* 122: 1449-1468.

111. Polymeropoulos MH, Lavedan C, Leroy E, Ide SE, Dehejia A, Dutra A, Pike B, Root H, Rubenstein J, Boyer R, Stenroos ES, Chandrasekharappa S, Athanassiadou A, Papapetropoulos T, Johnson WG, Lazzarini AM, Duvoisin RC, Di Iorio G, Golbe LI, Nussbaum RL (1997) Mutation in the alpha-synuclein gene identified in families with Parkinson's disease. *Science* 276: 2045-2047.

112. Rozemuller AJ, Eikelenboom P, Theeuwes JW, Jansen Steur EN, de Vos RA (2000) Activated microglial cells and complement factors are unrelated to cortical Lewy bodies. *Acta Neuropathol* 100: 701-708.

113. Sahgal A, Galloway PH, McKeith IG, Lloyd S, Cook JH, Ferrier IN, Edwardson JA (1992) Matching-to-sample deficits in patients with senile dementias of the Alzheimer and Lewy body types. *Arch Neurol* 49: 1043-1046.

114. Sahgal A, Gallowy PH, McKeith IG, Edwardson JA, Lloyd S (1992) A comparative study of attentional deficits in senile dementias of Alzheimer and Lewy body types. *Dementia* 3: 350-354

115. Sahgal A, McKeith IG, Galloway PH, Tasker N, Steckler T (1995) Do differences in visuospatial ability between senile dementias of the Alzheimer and Lewy body types reflect differences solely in mnemonic function? *J Clin Exp Neuropsychol* 17: 35-43.

116. Salmon DP, Galasko D, Hansen LA, Masliah E, Butters N, Thal LJ, Katzman R (1996) Neuropsychological deficits associated with diffuse Lewy body disease. *Brain Cogn* 31: 148-165.

117. Shiozaki K, Iseki E, Uchiyama H, Watanabe Y, Haga T, Kameyama K, Ikeda T, Yamamoto T, Kosaka K (1999) Alterations of muscarinic acetylcholine receptor subtypes in diffuse lewy body disease: relation to Alzheimer's disease. *J Neurol Neurosurg Psychiatry* 67: 209-213.

118. Singleton AB, Gibson AM, Edwardson JA, McKeith IG, Morris CM (1998) Butyrylcholinesterase K: an association with dementia with Lewy bodies. *Lancet* 351: 1818.

119. Singleton AB, Gibson AM, McKeith IG, Ballard CA, Perry RH, Ince PG, Edwardson JA, Morris CM (1999) Alpha2-macroglobulin polymorphisms in Alzheimer's disease and dementia with Lewy bodies. *Neuroreport* 10: 1507-1510.

120. Singleton AB, Gibson AM, McKeith IG, Ballard CG, Edwardson JA, Morris CM (2001) Nitric oxide synthase gene polymorphisms in Alzheimer's disease and dementia with Lewy bodies. *Neurosci Lett* 303: 33-36.

121. Singleton AB, Lamb H, Leake A, McKeith IG, Ince PG, Perry RH, Morris CM (1997) No association between a polymorphism in the presenilin 1 gene and dementia with Lewy bodies. *Neuroreport* 8: 3637-3639.

122. Smith MC, Mallory M, Hansen LA, Ge N, Masliah E (1995) Fragmentation of the neuronal cytoskeleton in the Lewy body variant of Alzheimer's disease. *Neuroreport* 6: 673-679.

123. Smith TW, Anwer U, DeGirolami U, Drachman DA (1987) Vacuolar change in Alzheimer's disease. *Arch Neurol* 44: 1225-1228.

124. Spillantini MG, Schmidt ML, Lee VM, Trojanowski JQ, Jakes R, Goedert M (1997) Alpha-synuclein in Lewy bodies. *Nature* 388: 839-840.

125. Strong C, Anderton BH, Perry RH, Perry EK, Ince PG, Lovestone S (1995) Abnormally phosphorylated tau protein in senile dementia of Lewy body type and Alzheimer disease: evidence that the disorders are distinct. *Alzheimer Dis Assoc Disord* 9: 218-222.

126. Tanaka S, Chen X, Xia Y, Kang DE, Matoh N, Sundsmo M, Thomas RG, Katzman R, Thal LJ, Trojanowski JQ, Saitoh T, Ueda K, Masliah E (1998) Association of CYP2D microsatellite polymorphism with Lewy body variant of Alzheimer's disease. *Neurology* 50: 1556-1562.

127. Terada S, Ishizu H, Haraguchi T, Takehisa Y, Tanabe Y, Kawai K, Kuroda S (2000) Tau-negative astrocytic star-like inclusions and coiled bodies in dementia with Lewy bodies. *Acta Neuropathol* 100: 464-468.

128. Togo T, Iseki E, Marui W, Akiyama H, Ueda K, Kosaka K (2001) Glial involvement in the degeneration process of Lewy body-bearing neurons and the degradation process of Lewy bodies in brains of dementia with Lewy bodies. *J Neurol Sci* 184: 71-75.

129. Wakabayashi K, Hansen LA, Masliah E (1995) Cortical Lewy body-containing neurons are pyramidal cells: laser confocal imaging of double-immunolabeled sections with anti-ubiquitin and SMI32. *Acta Neuropathol* 89: 404-408

130. Walker Z, Allen RL, Shergill S, Mullan E, Katona CL (2000) Three years survival in patients with a clinical diagnosis of dementia with Lewy bodies. *Int J Geriatr Psychiatry* 15: 267-273.

131. Walker Z, Costa DC, Ince P, McKeith IG, Katona CL (1999) In-vivo demonstration of dopaminergic degeneration in dementia with Lewy bodies. *Lancet* 354: 646-647.

132. Walker Z, Costa DC, Janssen AG, Walker RW, Livingstone G, Katona CL (1997) Dementia with lewy bodies: a study of post-synaptic dopaminergic receptors with iodine-123 iodobenzamide single-photon emission tomography. *Eur J Nucl Med* 24: 609-614.

133. Wenning G, Seppi K, Jellinger K (2000) Survival of patients with Dementia with Lewy bodies: a meta-analysis of 236 post-mortem confirmed cases. *Neurology* 54, suppl: A391-392

134. Wetter TC, Trenkwalder C, Gershanik O, Hogl B (2001) Polysomnographic measures in Parkinson's disease: a comparison between patients with and without REM sleep disturbances. *Wien Klin Wochenschr* 113: 249-253.

135. Woo SI, Hansen LA, Yu X, Mallory M, Masliah E (1999) Alternative splicing patterns of CYP2D genes in human brain and neurodegenerative disorders. *Neurology* 53: 1570-1572.

136. Wu E, Lipton RB, Dickson DW (1992) Amyloid angiopathy in diffuse Lewy body disease. *Neurology* 42: 2131-2135.

137. Xu W, Liu L, Emson P, Harrington CR, McKeith IG, Perry RH, Morris CM, Charles IG (2000) The CCTTT polymorphism in the NOS2A gene is associated with dementia with Lewy bodies. *Neuroreport* 11: 297-299.

138. Yamada T, Hattori H, Miura A, Tanabe M, Yamori Y (2001) Prevalence of Alzheimer's disease, vascular dementia and dementia with Lewy bodies in a Japanese population. *Psychiatry Clin Neurosci* 55: 21-25.

Lewy Bodies in Conditions Other Than Disorders of α-Synuclein

Carol F. Lippa

AD	Alzheimer disease
ALS	amyotrophic lateral sclerosis
ChAT	choline acetyl transform
CNS	central nervous system
DLB	dementia with Lewy bodies
LB	Lewy body
LBVAD	Lewy body variant of AD
MSA	multiple system atrophy
PD	Parkinson disease

There is increasing evidence that Lewy bodies (LBs) have clinical or biological significance in neurodegenerative diseases that are not primary synucleinopathies. Although traditionally considered the hallmark pathological feature of Parkinson's disease (PD) and unusual in other diseases, the increasing use of ubiquitin and α-synuclein immunohistochemistry has facilitated the realisation that LBs are common in a variety of CNS disorders (6, 7, 16, 28). In addition to disease states (Table 1), LBs occur in the substantia nigra in a small number of neurologically normal individuals with up to 10% of neurologically normal aged having brainstem LBs (17, 27). It is arguable that some individuals with brainstem LBs have an incipient synucleinopathy; however, the reasons for formation of LBs in otherwise normal aged subjects are unknown. In elderly patients with advanced degenerative diseases, small numbers of LBs may be a manifestation of end-stage disease with little clinical significance, or suggesting that PD is present concurrently in some cases (3, 4). Whether one considers LBs a pathologic feature related to the primary disease or an indicator of a second diagnosis, large numbers of LBs are hard to dismiss as being biologically irrelevant. Recent studies reported α-synuclein pathology (both cortical and subcortical) in up to 14% of subjects over 40 years of age, with an average of 11% in non-demented and of 23% in clinically demented subjects, suggesting that LB pathology is of importance for the pathogenesis of dementia (17, 27).

LBs have been described in numerous neurological diseases including Pick's disease and other forms of frontotemporal dementia, Creutzfeldt-Jakob disease, ataxia telangectasia, multiple system atrophy (MSA), corticobasal degeneration, pure autonomic failure, dystonia, progressive supranuclear palsy, neuroaxonal dystrophy, Hallervorden-Spatz disease, subacute sclerosing panencephalitis, amyotrophic lateral sclerosis (ALS), and in the ALS-dementia complex of Guam, Mege's syndrome and postpartum states (Table 1) (1, 5, 6, 8-16, 20, 23-26, 33).

The nonsynucleinopathy where LBs are most frequently described is Alzheimer's disease (AD). Cortical LBs are common in both familial and sporadic forms of AD and Down's syndrome (3, 4, 7, 10, 13, 14, 17, 18), estimates ranging from 7 to 60.7% of sporadic AD cases (7, 10) and even 71% of 45 AD cases with cortical LBs (Figure 1) (17, 27). It is argued that AD subjects with LBs comprise a distinct subset, which has been termed the Lewy body variant (LBVAD, [11]), as well as other names. These AD cases have more neuronal loss and pallor of pigmented brainstem nuclei, lower neocortical ChAT levels, and less intense neurofibrillary pathology com-

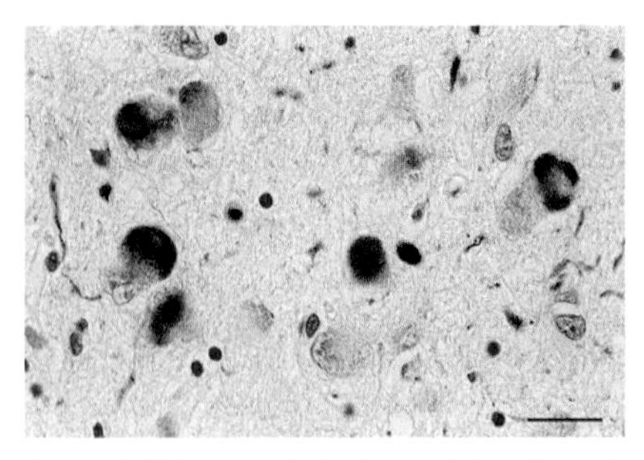

Figure 1. High power photomicrograph from the periamygdalar entorhinal cortex of a case with the LBVAD using double-label immunohistochemistry for tau (DAB, brown) and alpha-synuclein (new fuscin; red) demonstrating a LB in a neurone adjacent to a neurofibrillary tangle-bearing neurone.

Disorder	Relative frequency of LBs
Ageing and Alzheimer's disease	
Sporadic Alzheimer's disease	Often
Familial Alzheimer's disease	Often
Down's syndrome	Often
Tauopathies	
Pick's disease	Rarely
Progressive supranuclear palsy	Rarely
Corticobasal degeneration	Rarely
Parkinson-dementia complex of Guam	Rarely
Synucleinopathies	
Parkinson's disease	Always
Dementia with Lewy bodies	Always
Multiple system atrophy	Sometimes
Neurodegeneration with brain iron (Hallervorden-Spatz disease)	Sometimes
Pure autonomic failure	Sometimes
Meige's syndrome	Sometimes
Frontotemporal lobar degeneration	Rarely
Motor neurone disease (amyotrophic lateral sclerosis)	Rarely
Miscellaneous disorders	
Neuroaxonal dystrophy	Rarely
Subacute sclerosing panencephalitis	Rarely
Ataxia telangiectasia	Rarely

Table 1. Conditions associated with Lewy bodies.

pared with subjects with pure AD. Neuropsychological testing shows greater impairment in attention and visuospatial skills than AD subjects lacking LBs. However, some SPECT and gross pathological studies show similar changes in the brain compared with pure AD (13, 16, 30).

There is a large group of patients with numerous LBs in the amygdala, often in the absence of LBs elsewhere, even the substantia nigra (Figure 2) (7, 10, 13, 17). This occurs in over 60% of familial forms of AD including those with mutations of the amyloid precursor protein, presenilin-1 and presenilin-2 genes (13, 17) and in over 50% of aged Down's syndrome patients and sporadic AD subjects (7, 10, 14, 18). At this time, the nosology of this group is unknown. It is unclear if symptoms in subjects with LBs in the amygdala differ from those of patients with pure AD or AD patients with a wider distribution of neocortical LBs, as is classically described in the LBVAD. Although early studies indicate that features of DLB are not typically present in cases where LB are restricted to the amygdala, studies looking specifically for signs of amygdala dysfunction have not been done. When present, LBs in the amygdala are usually numerous, occurring either uniformly distributed in all amygdaloid nuclei in densities that may exceed 20 LBs per ×20 field (13, 14, 17, 18) or more prominent in the corticomedial nuclei. Since the amygdala is heavily involved with neuritic pathology in AD, these findings suggest that the process of LB formation may be triggered (at least in this susceptible region) by the AD process.

LBs are common in the amygdala in synucleinopathies including PD and DLB (2, 3, 19, 31), but also have been described in tauopathies including classical Pick's disease and the ALS-dementia complex of Guam (11, 20, 33), while LBs in the amygdala are not common in neurodegenerative diseases where the amygdala is spared such as ALS or normal aging (18, 29). It is speculated that these LBs form in diseases where the process of neuronal degeneration directly involves neurones in the amygdala. LBs in the amygdala are not common in MSA (18, 29), a condition where α-synuclein aggregates occur within glial cells, eg, in the white matter of the surrounding medial temporal lobe structures (4, 5, 6), while the gray matter of the amygdala is not heavily involved. This data indicates that LBs in the amygdala are not an obligatory feature in all synucleinopathies. One pilot series suggests that LBs in the amygdala may not occur in forms of frontotemporal dementia lacking specific histopathological features (18, 29), where the amygdala is often heavily involved, but cytoplasmic inclusions are not present. The absence of LBs is compatible with the notion that they form in an attempt to remove abnormal proteins (6, 7). If verified in a larger series, it would indicate that the process that promotes LB formation in the amygdala may be triggered by the presence of the cytoplasmic protein (aggregate) rather than other aspects of the degenerative cascade. In support of this, double label studies indicate that LBs in the amygdala in AD and Pick's disease often co-localise with neurofibrillary tangles and Pick bodies (13, 17, 18, 29).

Comparative analysis of the biochemical features of LBs in synucleinopathies and nonsynucleinopathies has focused on analysis of amygdala extracts due to the high density of LBs in this area. LBs in nonsynucleinopathies show the biological properties of LBs similar to those in other diseases. LBs from AD subjects demonstrate equal amounts of α-synuclein to those of control subjects in the soluble fraction (13, 17). This is also similar to the soluble α-synuclein fraction from synucleinopathy cases (1, 2). Using Western blot analysis of formic acid extracts, (insoluble) high molecular weight α-synuclein aggregates occur in familial AD cases with LBs (13, 17), which are not seen in control cases or in AD cases lacking LBs in the amygdala. These high molecular weight aggregates are also identical to the insoluble α-synuclein aggregates

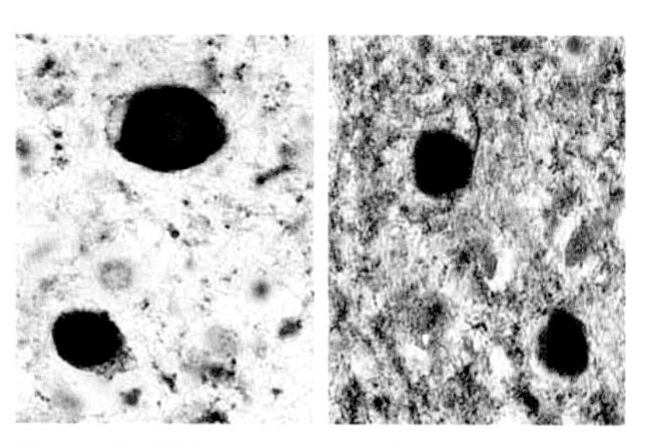

Figure 2. High-power photomicrograph from the amygdala of a familial AD case using double-label immunohistochemistry for tau (brown) and alpha-synuclein (red) demonstrating the co-occurrence of neurofibrillary tangles and Lewy bodies in one neurone.

that occur in synucleinopathies (1, 2). Thus, loss of α-synuclein solubility is important in the biological process by which LBs form in synucleinopathies and nonsynucleinopathies. However, other studies of brain homogenates from MSA, DLB, PD and normal aged controls, in PD and DLB detected substantial amounts of detergent-soluble and insoluble α-synuclein compared with controls, while MSA cases had significantly higher levels of α-synuclein in the detergent-soluble fraction of brain samples from pons and white matter with no detectable insoluble α-synuclein. The differences in solubility of α-syunclein between grey and white matter were suggested to result from different processing of α-synuclein in neurones compared with oligodendrocytes. Since highly insoluble α-synuclein is not involved in the pathogenesis of MSA, it is possible that buffered saline-soluble or detergent-soluble forms of α-synuclein may be involved in other synucleinopathies (4, 5). Characterising biochemical and metabolic changes that influence the solubility of α-synuclein is an area of intense investigation.

To further address the question of whether LB formation occurs by the same mechanism in all LBs, regardless of the underlying disease process, epitope mapping studies for α-synuclein have been performed. One study used a panel of α-synuclein antibodies that are well characterised and have been used extensively to characterise features of the aggregated protein in other synucleinopathies (4, 5). In MSA, α-synuclein aggregates show nonuniform mapping for the α-synuclein epitopes, whereas in disorders with neuronal α-synuclein aggregates (PD and DLB, Pick's disease and familial and sporadic AD) the epitope mapping pattern is uniform (5, 6, 11, 12, 20, 21). These data suggest that there may be conformational differences in the aggregated α-synuclein protein when the aggregate forms within glial cells. Overall, the pattern of epitope mapping is similar in LBs of all origins, but different from glial α-synuclein aggregates.

In summary, LBs occur commonly in a variety of neurodegenerative diseases. When present in high numbers, LBs are likely to be of biological or clinical significance. Evidence from biochemical and immunohistochemical studies indicates that the morphology of α-synuclein filaments in neuronal LBs show basic similarities, regardless of the underlying disease. Although investigators argue about whether LBs represent a concurrent disease state, all LBs studied thus far contain the full length α-synuclein protein and have uniform exposure of α-synuclein epitopes, regardless of whether the primary disease is an amyloidopathy, synucleinopathy or tauopathy. Therefore, one might envision LB formation in nonsynucleinopathies as a common reaction or process generated in response to differing biological triggers.

References

1. Agamanolis DP, Greenstein JI (1979) Ataxia-telangiectasia Report of a case with Lewy bodies and vascular abnormalities within cerebral tissue. *J Neuropathol Exp Neurol* 38: 475-489.

2. Baba M, Nakajo S, Tu PH, Tomita T, Nakaya K, Lee VM, Trojanowski JQ, Iwatsubo T (1998) Aggregation of α-synuclein in Lewy bodies of sporadic Parkinson's disease and dementia with Lewy bodies. Am J Pathol 152: 879-884.

3. Braak H, Braak E, Yilmazer D, Schultz C, de Vos RA, Jansen EN (1995) Nigral and extranigral pathology in Parkinson's disease. *J Neural Transm Suppl* 46: 15-31.

4. Brown DF, Dababo MA, Bigio EH, Risser RC, Eagan KP, Hladik CL,White CL (1998) Neuropathologic evidence that the Lewy body variant of Alzheimer disease represents coexistence of Alzheimer disease and idiopathic Parkinson disease. *J Neuropathol Exp Neurol* 57: 39-46.

5. Campbell BC, McLean CA, Culvenor JG, Gai WP, Blumbergs PC, Jakala P, Beyreuther K, Masters CL, Li QX (2001) The solubility of α-synuclein in multiple system atrophy differs from that of dementia with Lewy bodies and Parkinson's disease. *J Neurochem* 76: 87-96.

6. Duda JE, Giasson BI, Gur TL, Montine TJ, Robertson D, Biaggioni I, Hurtig HI, Stern MB, Gollomp SM, Grossman M, Lee VM, Trojanowski JQ (2000) Immunohistochemical and biochemical studies demonstrate a distinct profile of α-synuclein permutations in multiple system atrophy. *J Neuropathol Exp Neurol* 59: 830-841.

7. Galvin JE, Lee VM, Trojanowski JQ (2001) Synucleinopathies: clinical and pathological implications. *Arch Neurol* 58: 186-190.

8. Gibb WR, Lees AJ (1989) The significance of the Lewy body in the diagnosis of idiopathic Parkinson's disease. *Neuropathol Appl Neurobiol* 15:2 7-44.

9. Gibb WR Scaravilli F and Michund J (1990) Lewy bodies and subacute sclerosing panencephalitis. *J Neurol NeurosurgPsychiatry* 53: 710-711.

10. Hamilton RL (2000) Lewy bodies in Alzheimer's disease: a neuropathological review of 145 cases using α-synuclein immunohistochemistry. *Brain Pathol* 10: 378-384.

11. Hansen L, Salmon D, Galasko D, Masliah E, Katzman R, DeTeresa R, Thal L, Pay MM, Hofstetter R, Klauber, M et al (1990) The Lewy body variant of Alzheimer's disease: a clinical and pathologic entity. *Neurology* 40: 1147-50.

12. Hayashi S, Akasaki Y, Morimura Y, Takauchi S, Sato M, Miyoshi K (1992) An autopsy case of late infantile and juvenile neuroaxonal dystrophy with diffuse Lewy bodies and neurofibrillary tangles. *Clin Neuropathol* 11: 1-5.

13. Kaufmann H, Hague K, Perl D (2001) Accumulation of alpha-synuclein in autonomic nerves in pure autonomic failure. *Neurology* 56: 980-981.

14. Kazee AM, Han LY (1995) Cortical Lewy bodies in Alzheimer's disease *Arch Path Lab Med* 119: 448-453.

15. Leigh PN, Whitwell H, Garofalo O, Buller J, Swash M, Martin JE, Gallo JM, Weller RO, Anderton BH (1991) Ubiquitin-immunoreactive intraneuronal inclusions in amyotrophic lateral sclerosis. Morphology distribution and specificity. *Brain* 114: 775-788.

16. Lippa CF, Johnson R, Smith TW (1998) The medial temporal lobe in dementia with Lewy bodies: A comparative study with Alzheimer's disease. *Ann Neurol* 43: 102-106.

17. Lippa CF, Fujiwara H, Mann DM, Giasson B, Baba M, Schmidt ML, Nee LE, O'Connell B, Pollen DA, StGeorge-Hyslop P, Ghetti B, Nochlin D, Bird TD, Cairns NJ, Lee VM, Iwatsubo T, Trojanowski JQ (1998) Lewy bodies contain altered --synuclein in brains of many familial Alzheimer's disease patients with mutations in presenilin and amyloid precursor protein genes. *Am J Pathol* 153: 1365-1370.

18. Lippa CF, Schmidt ML, Lee VM, Trojanowski JQ (1999) Antibodies to α-synuclein detect Lewy bodies in many Down's syndrome brains with Alzheimer's disease. *Ann Neurol* 45: 353-357.

19. Lippa CF, Schmidt ML, Lee VM, Trojanowski JQ (2001a) α-Synuclein in familial Alzheimer's disease Epitope mapping parallels DLB and Parkinson's disease. *Arch Neurol* 58: 1817-20.

20. Lippa CF, Schmidt M, Lee VM, Trojanowski JQ (2001b) Lewy bodies in familial Alzheimer's disease: α-synuclein epitope mapping parallels dementia with Lewy bodies and Parkinson's disease but differs from multisystem atrophy. *Neurology* 56: 299-300.

21. Lippa CF, Schmidt ML, Lee VM, Trojanowski JQ (2001c): α-Synuclein-containing Lewy bodies in Pick's disease. Epitope mapping of Lewy body filaments is similar regardless of the underlying disease. *Ann Neurol* 50: S15.

22. Lowe J, Lennox G, Leigh PN (1997) Disorders of movement and system degenerations In Graham D Lantos PL (eds): *Greenfield's Neuropathology* 6th ed London E Amold pp 280-366.

23. Miura H, Tsuchiya K, Kubodera T, Shimamura H, Matsuoka T (2001) An autopsy case of pure autonomic failure with pathological features of Parkinson's disease. *Rinsho Shinkeigaku* 41: 40-44.

24. Monaco S, Nardelli E, Moretto G, Cavallaro T, Rizzuto N (1988) Cytoskeletal pathology in ataxia-telangiectasia. *Clin Neuropathol* 7: 44-46.

25. Mori H, Yoshimura M, Tomonaga M, Yamanouchi H (1986) Progressive supranuclear palsy with Lewy bodies. *Acta Neuropathol* 71: 344-346.

26. Murayama S, Ookawa Y, Mori H, Nakano I, Ihara Y, Kuzuhara S, Tomonaga M (1989) Immunocytochemical and ultrastructural study of Lewy body-like hyaline inclusions in familial amyotrophic lateral sclerosis. *Acta Neuropathol* 78: 143-152.

27. Perry RH, Irving D, Tomlinson BE (1990) Lewy body prevalence in the aging brain: relationship to neuropsychiatric disorders Alzheimer-type pathology and catecholaminergic nuclei. *J Neurol Sci* 100: 223-233.

28. Parkkinen L, Soininen H, Laakso M, Alafuzoff I (2001) α-Synuclein pathology is highly dependent on the case selection. *Neuropathol Appl Neurobiol* 27: 314-25.

29. Popescu A, Lippa CF (2001) Lewy bodies in the amygdala: α-Synuclein expression is increased in specific neurodegenerative diseases. *Neurology* 177-178.

30. Read SL, Miller BL, Mena I, Kim R, Itabashi H, Darby A (1995) SPECT in dementia: clinical and pathological correlation. *J Am Geriatr Soc* 43: 1243-1247.

31. Rezaie P, Cairns NJ, Chadwick A, Lantos PL (1996) Lewy bodies are located preferentially in limbic areas in diffuse Lewy body disease. *Neurosci Lett* 212: 111-114.

32. Schmidt ML, Martin JA, Lee VM, Trojanowski JQ (1996) Convergence of Lewy bodies and neurofibrillary tangles in amygdala neurones of Alzheimer's disease and Lewy body disorders. *Acta Neuropathol* 91: 475-481.

33. Yamazaki M, Arai Y, Baba M, Iwatsubo T, Mori O, Katayama Y, Oyanagi K (2000) --Synuclein inclusions in amygdala in the brains of patients with the parkinsonism-dementia complex of Guam. *J Neuropathol Exp Neurol* 59: 585-591.

Multiple System Atrophy

Peter L. Lantos
Niall Quinn

EMSA-SG	European MSA study group, http://*www.emsa-sg.org*
GCI	glial cytoplasmic inclusion
ICARS	International Comparative Ataxia Scale
ILOCA	idiopathic late-onset cerebellar ataxia
MED	male erectile dysfunction
MSA	multiple system atrophy
MSA-P	multiple system atrophy, predominant parkinsonian
MSA-C	multiple system atrophy, predominant cerebellar
NAMSA-SG	North American MSA study group
OPCA	olivopontocerebellar atrophy
PAF	progressive autonomic failure
PSP	progerssive supranuclear palsy
RBD	REM sleep behaviour disorder
SCA	spinocerebellar ataxia
SDA	Shy-Drager syndrome
SND	striatonigral degeneration
SSR	sympathetic skin response
QSART	quantitative sudomotor axonal response test

Definition, Diagnostic Criteria and Terminology

Until relatively recently, the definition and the diagnostic criteria of multiple system atrophy (MSA) have been fraught with difficulty, hindering epidemiological, clinical, and neuropathological studies. However, the disease can now be defined as a sporadic, adult onset degenerative disease of the nervous system of unknown cause, histologically characterised by α-synuclein positive glial cytoplasmic inclusions.

A Consensus Conference on MSA, held in April 1998 in Minneapolis, Minn, proposed new diagnostic criteria (27), based on 4 clinical domains of autonomic failure/urinary dysfunction, parkinsonism, cerebellar ataxia and corticospinal dysfunction, and distinguished, according to the level of diagnostic certainty possible, probable and definite MSA (see Clinical Features).

Recent studies revealed that application of either Quinn or Consensus criteria was superior to actual clinical diagnosis made early in disease, but there was little difference by the last clinical visit (53a). While application of the ICARS appears to be a useful tool to rate the severity of cerebellar signs in MSA, it is clearly contaminated by parkinsonian features (78a).

The diagnosis of definite MSA requires neuropathological confirmation by the presence of glial cytoplasmic inclusions. The Consensus Conference also recommended that the term MSA should be used only for this well-defined clinicopathological entity and the confusing term of multisystem degeneration is inappropriate for MSA. Moreover, patients should be designated as MSA-P or MSA-C, according to their predominant motor disorder—parkinsonian or cerebellar (27)

Synonyms and Historical Annotation

Originally, MSA was described as 3 apparently separate disorders. First, when cerebellar features predominated, as olivopontocerebellar atrophy (OPCA [18]); second, when parkinsonism predominated, as striatonigral degeneration (SND [1]); and third, when autonomic failure predominated, as the Shy-Drager syndrome (SDS [73]). Graham and Oppenheimer in 1969 (28), first introduced the term multiple system atrophy to encompass cases previously described as SDS, SND and OPCA. In subsequent years it became clear that the many cases of hereditary OPCA (now included under the classification of spinocerebellar ataxias) were distinct from MSA, a condition that, so far, has always been sporadic. In late-onset sporadic cerebellar ataxia—once recognised causes have been excluded—there remains a group of so-called idiopathic late-onset cerebellar ataxia (ILOCA); an estimated 25% of these cases turn out to have MSA (26, 43).

The final pathological justification for Graham and Oppenheimer's clinical classification (28) came with the description of glial cytoplasmic inclusions (GCIs) by Papp et al in 1989 (55, see below, under Histopathology). These specific inclusions, to be called Papp-Lantos inclusions, later found to be α-synuclein positive, were present in the brains of MSA cases, regardless of whether in life they have been labelled SDS, SND, or sporadic OPCA, but not in cases of hereditary OPCA, or other neurodegenerative disorders.

Epidemiology

Precise figures for incidence and prevalence of MSA are not known, although it is certain, from brain bank studies, that MSA is grossly underrecognised and misdiagnosed. A retrospective case note study in Olmsted County in Minnesota between 1976 and 1990 indicated an average incidence rate of 3.0 new cases per 100 000 per annum for the ages between 50 to 99 years (9). In a cross-sectional study in 15 general practices in London, United Kingdom, in which all suspect cases were examined, the age-adjusted prevalence per 100000 was 4.4 for MSA, compared to 6.4 for progressive supranuclear palsy (PSP) (68). In this population, there were 2.2 cases of MSA for every 100 with PD.

The disease appears to be more common in males. Thus, a review of 203 neuropathologically verified cases from the literature revealed a male to female ratio of 1.3:1.0 (90). MSA is an adult-onset disease—there has never been a proven case with onset before 30 years of age. Thereafter, incidence rises to a peak (and average) at around age 53, and appears to decline thereafter with advancing age, although this may be artefactual, as was the case in some early studies of PD.

Risk Factors

The cause of MSA is unknown. Abnormalities of mitochondrial chain function, oxidative stress, neurotoxicity and genetic susceptibility have all been considered. Analysis of mitochondrial function in the substantia nigra and in platelets of patients with MSA failed to identify any respiratory chain defect relative to controls (29). As potential evidence of oxidative stress and neurotoxicity, Dexter et al (19) found increased iron and ferritin content in the substantia nigra and striatum. The iron content of the putamen increased 5-fold: there were coarse electron-dense granules, fine granular and fibrillary material and lamellated structures (39). So far, 2 case-control studies of MSA have been reported (30, 83). The first, reviewing 100 patients who fulfilled the clinical diagnostic criteria of MSA in Houston, Tex, has revealed that 11 had been exposed to environmental toxins, including *N*-hexane, benzene, methyl isobutyl ketone and pesticides, thus raising the possible causative role of such agents (30). The second suggested an increased risk to MSA associated with occupational exposure to organic solvents, plastic monomers and additives, pesticides and metals, and a negative association with smoking (83).

Genetics

No instance of pathologically verified familial MSA has ever been recorded. Molecular genetic analysis again has not revealed any abnormality, although a novel cytochrome P-4502D6 mutant gene may be associated with MSA. In 10 patients the frequency of mutation in exon 6, causing an amino acid change from Arg296 to Cys296 was significantly higher than in controls (37). However, these results have not been confirmed in a larger series of 74 patients, including 15 autopsy-proven cases, and these conflicting results may reflect ethnic differences of the populations screened (5). In another study, 80 MSA patients were analysed for a range of genetic abnormalities, including spinocerebellar ataxia type 1 and 3 genes, the H5 pore region (the human homologue of the weaver mouse gene), insulin-like growth factor 1 (known to be reduced in lurcher mice), the ciliary neurotrophic factor and human leukocyte antigen HLA 32. However, consistent genetic associations have not been found (4). Moreover, nucleotide alterations were not found in the entire coding region of the α-synuclein gene, excluding a possible role of these genetic abnormalities in the pathogenesis of MSA (54). In addition, we have not found any effect of tau, apoliporotein E ϵ4, or synphylin gene variability on the development of MSA (52).

Clinical Features

Signs and symptoms. The core clinical features of MSA, which are used to diagnose the condition, are parkinsonism, cerebellar and pyramidal signs, and autonomic failure. In one clinical series of 100 patients with MSA (86), 80% had MSA-P (30% with, 50% without, cerebellar features), and 20% MSA-C (10% with, 10% without, parkinsonian features). Overall, about 90% of patients had some degree of parkinsonism, and about the same proportion some degree of autonomic failure, with cerebellar or pyramidal features in 50% each. MSA-P may have been over-represented in this series, from a centre with a special interest in movement disorders. Cerebellar clinics see a different picture. In addition, there are suggestions that the Western predominance of MSA-P over MSA-C may be reversed in Japan. Outside of the core features used in the official diagnostic criteria there are many other clinical pointers ("red flags") that may be useful in diagnosis.

A very early feature in many patients is REM sleep behaviour disorder (RBD), during which patients talk or shout, and strike out in their sleep, sometimes injuring their bed-partner or actually falling out of bed (59). If they awake or are woken, they report frightening nightmares. RBD occurs in at least 60% of MSA patients, usually as an early feature, and often disappears after one to 2 years. It also occurs in about one third of PD patients, usually later in the disease. Other common disorders of sleep or breathing in MSA include increased snoring, sleep apnoea, inspiratory sighs, gasps, or stridor (35).

The earliest symptom in many males with MSA is male erectile dysfunction (MED) often, like RBD, elicited retrospectively rather than being recognised at the time as a presenting complaint. Almost all patients of either sex develop urinary disturbance, comprising varying combinations of urinary frequency, urgency and nocturia (also relatively common in PD), but also incontinence, retention, or double micturition, secondary to incomplete bladder emptying, seen particularly in MSA (6). Inappropriate prostatectomy with MSA commonly leads to incontinence. Uro-neurologists maintain that these alterations are not, strictly speaking, autonomic, and deserve to be considered as a separate clinical domain. Constipation is frequent (as in PD), but primary faecal incontinence is rare in both PD and MSA.

Cardiovascular autonomic failure in MSA is variable. Although postural hypotension and postural faintness are relatively common, especially after introducing dopaminergic medication, they are only incapacitating in a minority of patients. In one series (86), only 15% of patients had experienced more than 3 syncopal episodes.

Parkinsonism in MSA is often just as asymmetric as in PD. Tremor is also common, being seen in two thirds of patients. However, it is usually an irregular postural or action tremor, and a classical-pill rolling rest tremor is distinctly uncommon in MSA (about 8% of cases). This irregular tremor may, on close inspection, turn out to be partly or even wholly, due to (often touch-or stretch-sensitive) myoclonic jerks of the hands and fingers, present in about one third of patients (64). The response to L-dopa in MSA is often poor or absent, and thus a helpful clue to distinguish it from PD. However, a moderate or even good, albeit waning, response to L-dopa occurs in up to 30% of patients (86). Peak-dose dyskinesias, if they occur, are usually dystonic, predominantly involving the neck and the face, as opposed to the typically choreo-dystonic, predominantly limb dyskinesias in PD.

Pyramidal dysfunction causes signs but few symptoms in MSA. Spasticity may be super-imposed in rigidity, but is rarely severe, and significant pyramidal weakness or scissors gait are not seen.

Cerebellar dysfunction in MSA may manifest as an eye movement disorder (jerky pursuit or nystagmus), ataxic dysarthria, limb ataxia, or gait ataxia. Depending on the degree of akinesia present, it can be difficult specifically to identify superimposed ataxia. Moreover, it can be difficult to decide whether to ascribe the postural instability that develops relatively early in MSA to cerebellar or basal ganglia dysfunction.

Rapid disease progression and early imbalance are characteristic of MSA, although falls within the first year are uncommon, and more suggestive of progressive supranuclear palsy (PSP). Speech in MSA is often characteristic. In addition to the characteristic monotony of parkinsonism, the voice is often more hypophonic, with an increase in pitch, and a super-imposed quivery, croaky, strained element. Dysphagia is also earlier and more prominent than in PD.

Other clinical "red flags" are cold, dusky violaceous extremities with poor circulatory return on blanching (41), Raynaud's phenomenon (50), disproportionate antecollis (62), leaning of the trunk to one side (the Pisa syndrome [16]), limb contractures, emotional incontinence, and the use of a rolator or wheelchair. There may be electrical evidence (usually sub-clinical) of a mild peripheral neuropathy or anterior horn cell involvement (60).

Although some frontal deficits can be found on detailed neuropsychological testing, dementia is not a feature of MSA (63). A combination of parkinsonism, dementia and autonomic failure is much more suggestive of Lewy body pathology.

Unfortunately, MSA is relentlessly progressive. Survival from first symptom is about 6 years in post-mortem cases reported in the literature (7), but 9 to 10 years in recent clinical case series, and similar between males and females, and between MSA-P and MSA-C. Death is usually secondary to bronchopneumonia, but sudden death, presumably from cardiovascular autonomic disturbance, can occur.

Imaging

Structural. CT scans may reveal cerebellar and sometime pontine atrophy, mainly in MSA-C cases, but are not very sensitive. MRI scans may demonstrate a variety of changes (Figure 1). Supratentorially (MSA-P>C) putaminal atrophy, slit-like hyperintensity at the lateral putaminal border, or posterior putaminal hypointensity (relative to globus pallidus on T2) are seen (Figure 1A), while infratentorally, (MSA-C>P), cerebellar atrophy, pontine atrophy, with a hot-cross-bun sign, and hyperintensity of the middle cerebellar peduncles are the lesions (Figure 1B) (44, 66, 69 71).

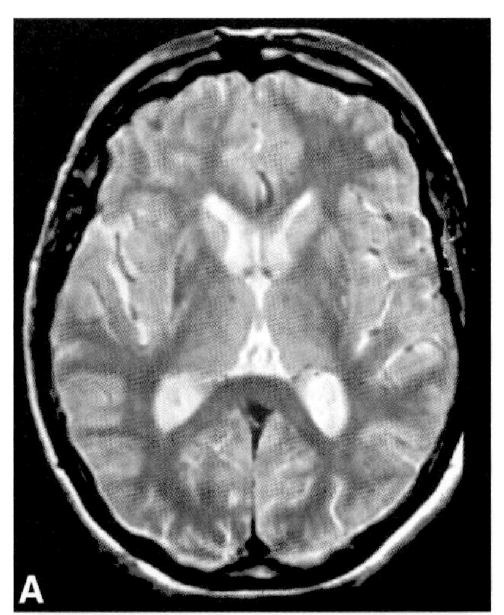

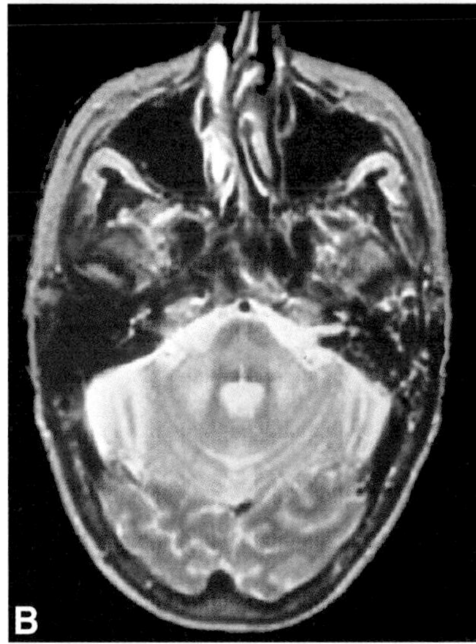

Figure 1. MRI of MSA **A**. Putaminal atrophy, hyperintense rim and putaminal hypointensity in comparison with the globus pallidus on T2-weighted images (1.5 T). **B**. Infratentorial atrophy and signal change in the pons ("hot-cross bun sign"), middle cerebellar peduncles and cerebellum on T2-weighted images (1.5 T).

Functional. Striatal glucose metabolism, as revealed by FDG PET, is often deficient in MSA relative to PD (22). Striatal D2 receptor binding, as revealed by raclopride PET or IBZM SPECT, is often decreased in untreated MSA versus PD patients (67, 70). However, L-dopa down-regulates these receptors, so reducing the difference in treated patients.

The terminals of nigrostriatal neurons, as revealed by F-DOPA PET and dopamine transporter SPECT scans, show decreased uptake and binding of tracer, but these techniques cannot at present discriminate between MSA and PD in individual patients (11, 58).

Laboratory findings. Cardiovascular autonomic function tests may reveal evidence of sympathetic or parasympathetic dysfunction, or both. However, similar results can be found in a minority of patients with PD, albeit usually only late in the disease course. I-123-MIBG cardiac scintigraphy can help to differentiate between pre- (as in MSA) and post- (as in PD) ganglionic cardiac denervation and may prove a useful diagnostic test (10).

The growth hormone response to a brief infusion of clonidine has been reported to be defective in MSA (40). Whether it is always normal, or often also abnormal, in PD remains controversial. The sympathetic skin response (SSR) and quantitative sudomotor axonal response test (QSART) are also

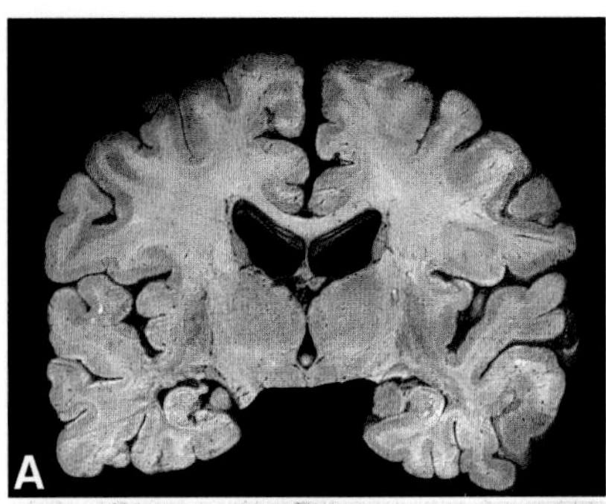

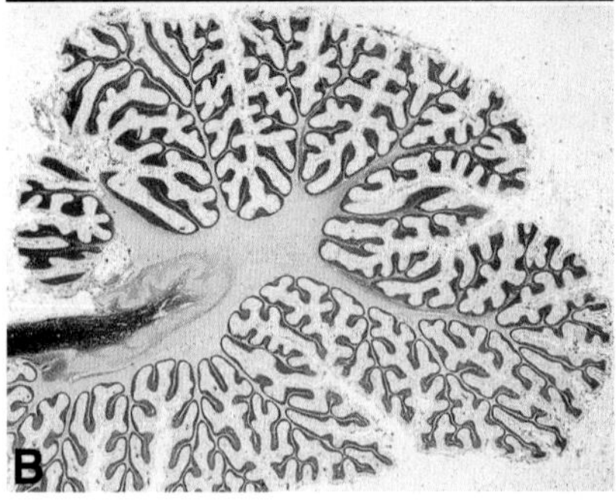

Figure 2. A. Coronal slice of a brain with MSA showing atrophy and greyish discoloration of both putamina. **B.** The cerebellum shows moderate atrophy and myelin pallor with preservation of the superior cerebellar peduncle (Luxol fast blue/cresyl violet).

claimed by some to distinguish reliably MSA from PD (65), but others find them less useful.

Urodynamic studies can reveal evidence of detrusor hyperreflexia (almost universal in MSA and present in 37% of PD [76]), but may also reveal evidence of bladder atony (more suggestive of MSA). Demonstration (by catheterisation or by ultrasound) of an abnormally high post-micturition residual volume, indicating incomplete bladder emptying, is more common in MSA. Urethral or anal sphincter EMG may reveal evidence of denervation and reinnervation (increased amplitude, duration, and polyphasia) secondary to loss of anterior horn cells from Onufrowicz's nucleus. This test is very frequently abnormal in MSA, and also frequently in PSP (82), but infrequently in PD or other neurodegenerative disorders, provided it is correctly interpreted (84). Thus, the satellite components of potentials must be included when measuring duration, and previous multiple or traumatic childbirth, abdominal surgery (which may cause a false positive result on either urethral or anal sphincter testing) or haemorrhoidectomy (which may affect anal but not urethral sphincter EMG), should be taken into consideration.

Moreover, there is also abnormal nerve conduction in 40% of cases, including mixed sensorimotor axonal neuropathy in 17.5% (60). In the muscles, the respiratory chain complex I (NADH:ubiquinone reductase) is reduced (8) and there is abnormal EMG suggesting partial denervation in 22.5% of the cases (60).

Macroscopy

Macroscopical appearance range from normal to focal atrophy of the affected structures, but generalised severe tissue loss is not a feature. Naked eye observation often confirms the neuroimaging and follows the clinical pattern. Thus in MSA-P (SND) the putamen may show atrophy and greyish discoloration (Figure 2A). In cases of MSA-C (OPCA), tissue loss usually occurs from the cerebellum (Figure 2B), the middle cerebellar peduncles and from the brainstem, particularly from the pons. However, the overall brain weight may not be substantially affected. The pigmented nuclei of the brainstem, the substantia nigra and the locus coeruleus, are often pale as a result of pigment loss. There may be cortical atrophy, particularly the motor and the premotor cortices, but these changes are difficult to assess. The preferential tissue loss of the content of the posterior fossa may result in a shift of the normal ratio of the total brain weight in relation to the weight of the brain stem and cerebellum of 8:1 in favour of the cerebral hemispheres. Nevertheless, an MRI study of 40 patients has shown progressive cerebral atrophy, occurring in all clinical sub-types and reflecting the duration of the disease rather than the age of patients (32). The spinal cord appears to be little affected even in cases of severe autonomic dysfunction.

Histopathology

The histological hallmark lesion of MSA is the GCI (Figure 3 A-D): this oligodendroglial inclusion will be discussed in detail below together with other cytoskeletal pathology. In addition, MSA is characterised by neuronal loss, astrocytosis, and loss of myelin from the affected areas together with activation of microglial cells (72). In a review of 203 pathologically verified cases, the most severe lesions were found in the substantia nigra, the locus coeruleus, the putamen, the inferior olives, the pontine nuclei, the Purkinje cells, and the intermediolateral columns of the spinal cord. In contrast, the cerebral cortex, the thalamus, the subthalamic nucleus, the caudate nucleus, the globus pallidus, the dentate nucleus, the nucleus ambiguous, the vestibular nuclei, the anterior horn cells, and the pyramidal tracts were relatively well preserved (90). Most of these observations in the past were based on subjective assessments, whereas some of the more recent analyses used sophisticated methods of morphometry.

Neuronal loss occurs in the striatonigral system, being most severe in the dorsal lateral zone of the caudal putamen and the lateral zone of the caudal nigra. This latter loss, amounting to some 80%, may cause demise of the calbindin-IR matrix cells in the caudal putamen, suggesting trans-synaptic degeneration of the striatonigral fibres (36). In addition, damage to the globus pallidus, the substantia nigra and the subthalamic nucleus may lead to dysfunction of these inhibitory nuclei projecting to the motor thalamus, a mechanism similar to that of progressive supranuclear palsy (31). In less severe cases the rostral parts are preserved (45). In the cerebellum the Purkinje cells are affected and their loss is more pronounced in the vermis than in the hemispheres. In the olivary nucleus the reduction is more severe in the accessory than in the inferior nucleus. The degree of neuronal loss appears to be related to the duration of illness and to the type of MSA (46, 80). Based on semi-quantitative assessments of neuronal loss, astrocytosis and GCIs in the substantia nigra and striato-pallidum in MSA-P, three degrees of severity can be distinguished reflecting disease pro-

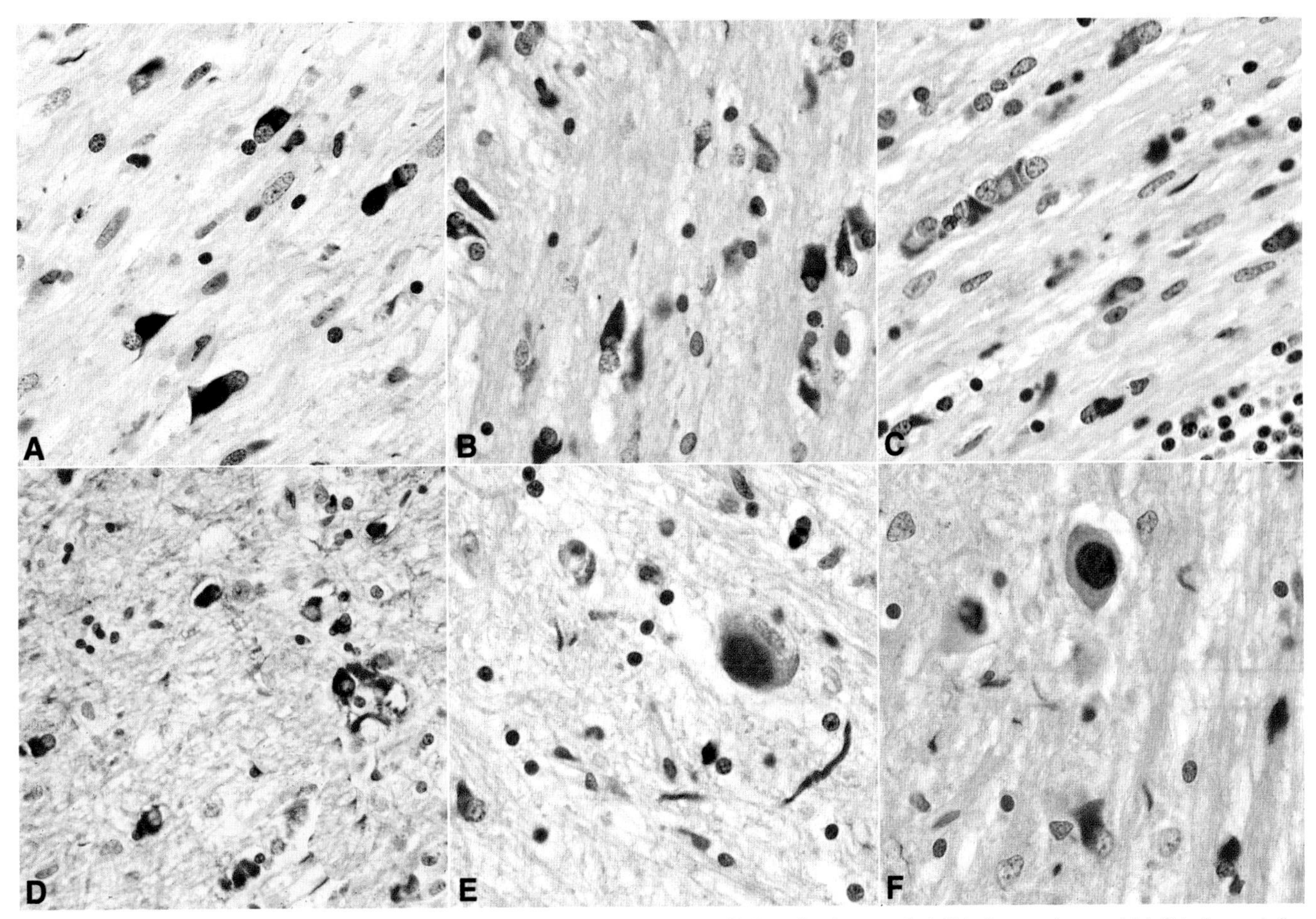

Figure 3. A-D. Glial cytoplasmic inclusions (Papp-Lantos inclusions) **A**. in the globus pallidus (Gallyas silver impregnation), **B**. in the pons (α-synuclein), **C**. in the cerebellar white matter (ubiquitin), **D**. in the white matter of the frontal lobe (unphosphorylated tau). **E**. Neuronal cytoplasmic inclusion and neurites in the pons (α-synuclein). **F**. Neuronal nuclear inclusions in the pons (α-synuclein) (All immunohistochemistry by ABC method, DAKO, using immunoperoxidase with haematoxylin).

gression (89). In addition, there is neuronal loss in the hypothalamus affecting the large histaminergic neurons in the tuberomammillary nucleus and the arginine-vasopressin immunopositive neurons in the suprachiasmatic nucleus, in the medulla oblongata involving the tyrosine hydrolase immunoreactive neurons and the arcuate nucleus, and in the spinal cord, affecting both the lateral horns and the intermediate zone of the anterior horns. These assessments of neuronal reduction in various areas of the central nervous system are particularly pertinent in clinicopathological correlations: the depletion of catechoaminergic neurons in the rostral ventrolateral portion of the medulla oblongata may explain some of the autonomic and endocrine manifestations of MSA (for review, see 48).

The neuropathology of MSA is more extensive than hitherto thought to involve certain areas of the cerebral cortex. An analysis of neuronal populations, using a robust stereological probe, the disector, shows that there is neuronal loss in the primary and supplementary motor cortex with accompanying increase of glial cells (74). The severe involvement of the motor cortex has been subsequently confirmed (77, 79).

The mechanism of neuronal cell death has been recently investigated. Apoptosis was observed in oligodendrocytes, but not in neurons (61). Since gene upregulation of p53 and CD95 precedes apoptosis, another study, investigating p53 and CD95 expression in various neurodegenerative diseases, found higher levels of CD95 in the temporal lobe in MSA compared to Parkinson's disease and aged-matched controls. Moreover increased p53 immunoreactivity was noted in neuronal and glial nuclei, neuronal perikarya, and in dystrophic and glial cell processes in the striatum and the midbrain. These findings indicate that p53- and CD95-associated apoptosis may be the mechanism of cell death in MSA, in common with other neurodegenerative disease (17). Diminished calcium binding capacity of Purkinje cells in MSA might lead to a change in the regulation of proteins of the bcl-2 family to favour the pathological initiation of apoptosis (91).

Glial cytoplasmic inclusions (Papp-Lantos inclusions). The histological hallmark lesion of MSA is the GCI, first reported and comprehensively characterised in 1989 (55). These oligodendroglial inclusions are argyrophilic (Figure 3A) and, although the Gallyas method yields superior results by its selective staining of abnormal inclusions, other silver impregnation techniques, including modified Bielschowsky, will demonstrate GCIs. Their shape varies from triangular, sickle, half-moon, oval or conical, to being occasionally flame-shaped to resemble superficially neurofibrillary tangles. They are of variable size, often completely occupying the cytoplasm to displace the nucleus eccentrically, and thus they are usually more voluminous than the "coiled bodies," observed also in oligodendrocytes in a various neurodegenerative diseases (15). To avoid confusion with other oligodendroglial inclusions of the coiled-body type to be found in various neurodegenerative diseases (20), glial cytoplasmic inclusions diagnostic of MSA should be referred to as Papp-Lantos inclusions. While they are easily visible in silver impregnations, they do not stain with any of the Holzer's, phosphotungstic acid haematoxylin, luxol fast blue and cresyl violet (Klüver-Barrera), Masson's trichrome, Mallory's azan, alcian blue, Nile blue, thioflavine S, oil red O, Sudan black, periodic acid Schiff and Congo red methods (48).

GCIs are not distributed haphazardly in the central nervous system, but are system-related (57). A semi-quantitative mapping has revealed that the structures rich in GCIs include the suprasegmental motor systems (primary motor and higher motor areas of the cerebral cortex, the "pyramidal," "extrapyramidal," and corticocerebellar systems), the supraspinal autonomic systems, and their targets. In contrast, the visual and auditory pathways, olfactory structures, somatosensory systems, association and limbic cortical areas, and subcortical limbic structures contain none or only a few GCIs. Structures with high GCI density (more than 300/mm^2) include the supplementary motor and primary motor cortical areas, with their subjacent white matter, the dorsolateral larger part of the putamen, the dorsolateral, smaller part of the caudate nucleus, the ponticuli substantiae griseae, the globus pallidus, the internal and the external capsules, the reticular formation, the basis pontis, the middle cerebellar peduncles and the cerebellar white matter. The distribution and density of GCIs have been correlated with the severity of MSA. GCI density in the corticopontine tracts correlates with the severity of MSA-C (OPCA), but not with that of MSA-P (SND). In the pyramidal tracts it correlates with both, while in the pencil fibres of the putamen it correlates with the severity of MSA-P, but not with that of MSA-C (34).

In addition to Papp-Lantos inclusions, neuronal inclusions have also been observed in MSA; indeed, inclusions were described in 5 cellular sites: in oligodendroglial cytoplasm and nucleus, in neuronal cytoplasm (Figure 3E) and nucleus (Figure 3F), and in axons (Figure 3E) (56). However, of these only GCIs occur consistently and in great density to be the hallmark lesion of MSA. Comparison of the severity of oligodendroglial degeneration (GCI density) with that of neuronal alterations (neuronal cytoplasmic and nuclear inclusions, degenerated neuronal processes, and loss of nerve cells) reveals a striking preponderance of oligodendroglial lesions. This finding indicates that degeneration of neither axons, nor neuronal cell bodies is a prerequisite for the formation of GCIs.

In MSA, not only the central nervous system is affected. Sural nerve biopsy shows a reduction of unmyelinated fibres 23%, whereas in Parkinson's disease and amyotrophic lateral sclerosis the density of these fibres remains unchanged (38).

Immunohistochemistry

Glial cytoplasmic and neuronal inclusions are positively immunostained with both α-synuclein (Figure 3B) and ubiquitin (Figure 3C), with the former giving superior results. In the first study of GCIs, they were found to be positive for ubiquitin, tau protein, and for α- and β-tubulin (55). The immunohistological staining with antibodies to tau appeared to be more controversial, until an immunohistochemical study using a panel of phosphorylation-independendent, dephosphorylation-dependent and phosphorylation-dependent tau antibodies has revealed that the tau in GCIs (Figure 3D) is different from the abnormally phosphorylated tau of Alzheimer's disease. It is also more like normal adult tau (12). Moreover, MSA-tau is different from the tau pattern of both progressive supranuclear palsy and corticobasal degeneration (13, 78).

The most important recent development in the characterisation of GCI has been the discovery of α-synuclein in MSA by several groups (3, 23, 51, 75, 51, 85). However, only one study (75) has described α-synuclein positivity in all 5 cellular sites as originally reported: oligodendroglial cytoplasm and nucleus, neuronal cytoplasm and nucleus, and axons corresponding to abnormal neurites. Double immunolabelling with antibodies to both α-synuclein and ubiquitin has convincingly demonstrated a more abundant and extensive staining pattern with the former antibody. Using different α-synuclein antibodies, the same study has also established that most or all the α-synuclein molecule is present in the neuronal and glial inclusions (75), although antibodies to the carboxy terminal of α-synuclein has revealed previously overlooked GCIs in the hippocampal formation (21). In contrast, β- and γ-synucleins are absent from these inclusions (21, 75).

Monoclonal antibodies against microtubule-associated protein-5 also gave positive reaction (2). Cyclin-dependent kinase 5 (cdk5), mitogen-activated protein kinase (MAPK) have been recently detected in GCIs (53) and 14-3-3 protein, which mediates several types of signal transduction pathways (39a).

However, the inclusions of MSA are negative with antibodies to neurofilaments, cytokeratin, vimentin, glial fibrillary acidic protein, actin, desmin, myelin basic protein and myosin. The cells containing GCIs give positive staining with oligodendroglial markers, including carbonic anhydrase isoenzyme II, Leu-7 and transferrin (for review, see 48).

Ultrastructure

In low-power electron micrographs, the main components of GCIs appear to be randomly distributed loose filaments, while higher magnification reveals tubular profiles, as indicated by their longitudinal view (Figure 4). In cross sections they are tubular structures composed of a round or ovoid wall with an outer diameter of 20 to 30 nm, enclosing a clear centre (55). Since the filaments are coated with dense granular material, accurate measurement of their diameter is fraught with problems (20). However, a recent study, using sarcosyl-extracted material, reported filaments with 2 distinct morphologies: twisted and straight. The width of the former alternated between 5 nm and 18 nm with a periodicity of 70 to 90 nm, whereas the second class of filaments had a uniform width of about 10 nm (Figure 5). Most importantly, both types of filaments were α-synuclein-positive by immuno-electron microscopy (75),

Although light microscopy, using silver impregnations and immunohistochemical techniques, has clearly indicated that the host cells are oligodendrocytes, electron microscopy has unequivocally confirmed this cellular localization. Moreover, these studies have also revealed that GCIs are present in all 3 types of oligodendrocytes: in the satellite cells adjacent to neurons in the grey matter, in the interfascicular variant in the white matter and in the perivascular oligodendrocytes of the affected areas (57).

Biochemistry

While the immunohistochemical profile of Papp-Lantos inclusions has been comprehensively characterized, very little is known about their precise biochemical composition. However, there is now increasing evidence to suggest that the physicochemical properties of α-synuclein in MSA are significantly changed, including both molecular weight and solubility (20, 81). Western blots have demonstrated detergent insoluble monomeric and high molecular weight α-synuclein in the cerebellar white matter rich in GCIs (21). The increase of α-synuclein in higher molecular weight species of 29 to 36 kDa and 45 to 55 kDa may represent aggregates (20). By contrast, another study found high levels of α-synuclein in the detergent-soluble fraction of brain samples from the pons and white matter of MSA cases (14). Density gradient enrichment and an anti-α-synuclein immunomagnetic technique, used to isolate pure and morphologically intact oligodendroglial inclusions from the white matter of MSA brains, have shown the inclusions to comprise multiple protein bands after separation by polyacrylamide gel electrophoresis. Further immunoblotting has demonstrated that these proteins include α-synuclein, αB-crystallin, tubulins, ubiquitin and prominent, possibly truncated α-synuclein species as high molecular weight aggregates (20).

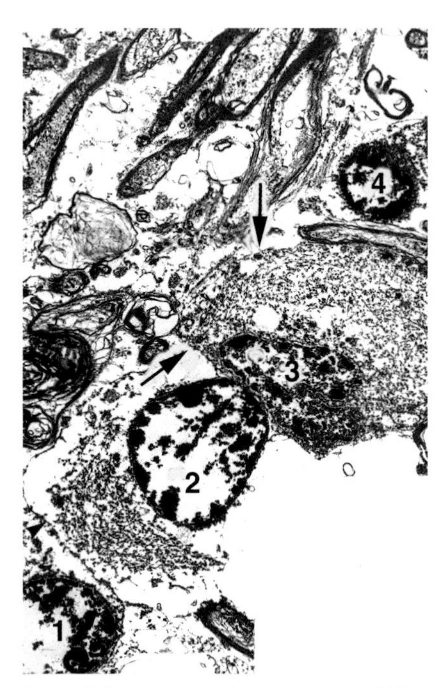

Figure 4. Low power electron micropgraph of interfascicular oligodendrocytes with nuclei (1, 2, 3, 4) in the external capsule. There is a GCI in the cytoplasm of cell 3 and another one in the vicinity of nucleus 2. Scale bar = 2.5 μm. (Reproduced by kind permission of Elsevier Science from J Neurol Sci 1988; 94:79-100)

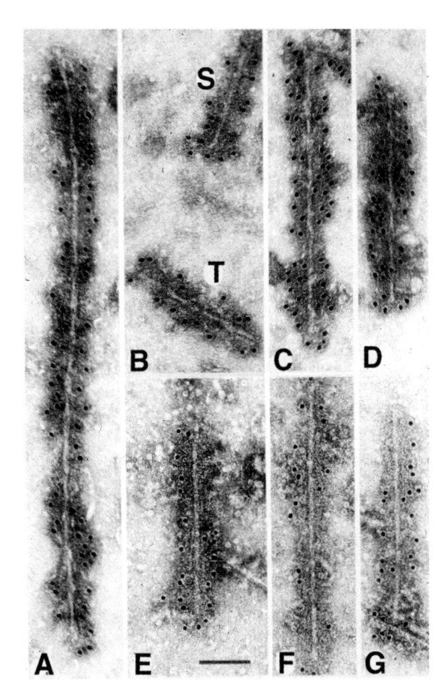

Figure 5. Immuno-electron microscopy of filaments from the frontal cortex and cerebellum, labelled of antibody to α-synuclein (PER4). The second antibody is conjugated to colloidal gold particles and appears as black dots. Panels **A**, **C** and **D** show "twisted" filaments, **E**, **F** and **G** "straight" filaments, while panel B shows both (T = twisted, S = straight). (Reproduced by kind permission from Spillantini et al. Neurosci Lett 1998; 251:205-208) Scale bar = 100nm.

Differential Diagnosis

Clinical. The main condition with which MSA-P is most often confused is PD. Many more cases of MSA are misdiagnosed as PD than vice-versa. Thus, PD may be associated with cardiovascular autonomic failure, MED or urinary frequency and urgency, although less often and usually later in the disease than in MSA-P (49), and with retention due to prostatic hypertrophy in males. PD may also be associated with pyramidal or cerebellar signs when there is additional cerebrovascular disease, or with pyramidal signs when there is additional cervical spondylotic myelopathy. The minority of L-dopa-responsive cases of MSA pose particular difficulties.

If the patient's parkinsonism is atypical and levodopa-unresponsive, a frequent problem is the distinction between MSA and PSP. Thus, the eye movement disorder of the latter may be subtle or late, and it is also a rapidly progressive disease associated with early falls, bladder symptoms, an abnormal sphincter EMG, and sometimes pyramidal signs, but not prominent cardiovascular autonomic dysfunction. However, PSP starts on average a decade later than MSA, very rarely before 45 years of age, and never before age 40. Cases of MSA with marked asymmetry and limb contractures can be confused with corticobasal degeneration (CBD), but limb apraxia is usually also present in this disorder.

MSA-C can be confused with hereditary spinocerebellar ataxias, but in these disorders a positive family history is usually present, onset is usually younger, and progression less rapid than MSA-C, and autonomic failure and parkinsonian features are uncommon (42). However, SCA2 and SCA3 may manifest as parkinsonism, sometimes L-dopa responsive, with mild or absent cerebellar signs, and patients with SCA-6 present later than other SCAs, sometimes without a positive family history, usually as a pure cerebellar syndrome, without autonomic failure, but sometimes with additional pyramidal signs.

It can be more difficult to determine which cases of ILOCA have, or will turn out to have, MSA. However, autonomic failure is uncommon in non-MSA cases of ILOCA, and the infratentorial atrophy on MRI usually spares the pons.

At an early stage, before other neurological signs develop, MSA can be mistaken for PAF. Although motor signs usually follow autonomic failure within 5 years in MSA, rarely the interval can be longer. Although most cases of "PAF" that die without developing motor signs have Lewy body pathology, MSA has been the cause in a couple of cases in the literature.

Pathological. The recent Consensus Statement on the diagnosis of MSA, while distinguishing possible, probable, and definite categories, is unequivocal that definite diagnosis can be made only after the neuropathological confirmation of the presence of a high density of GCIs in association with a combination of degenerative changes in the nigrostriatal and olivopontocerebellar pathways (27). However, since the Consensus Conference has defined diagnostic criteria from a clinical point of view, it did not make recommendations for a standardised neuropathological examination.

The European Brain Banking Network, considering the need for standardised neuropathological criteria for various neurodegenerative diseases, has proposed that the demonstration of GCIs by immunohistochemistry and/or silver impregnation in the frontal cortex, the lentiform nucleus, the pons, the cerebellum, the midbrain, the medulla oblongata and in the spinal cord provides a reliable and consistent neurohistological criterion for the diagnosis of MSA. Depending on clinical symptomatology, the examination of even fewer areas may secure the diagnosis (47). However, until the pathology, including phenotypic variation of MSA, is not fully characterized, a more comprehensive neurohistological examination, including both sampling and staining, is recommended both for clinicopathological correlations and research purposes. Thus, in addition to the frontal lobe, the temporal, parietal and occipital lobes should also be sampled, as well as other structures of the deep grey matter, including hippocampal formation, the amygdala, the caudate nucleus and the thalamus with the subthalamic region. Arguably, GCIs are one of the most reliable diagnostic hallmarks: they occur consistently and in high density only in MSA.

Following the original description of GCIs in MSA, oligodendroglial inclusions have been reported in Alzheimer's disease, Pick's disease, argyrophilic grain dementia, PSP and CBD and in other rare neurodegenerative diseases, including spinocerebellar ataxia type 1, familial progressive limbic lobe sclerosis and in cases of dementia linked to chromosome 17 (48). However, these oligodendroglial cytoplasmic inclusions, the so-called coiled bodies have a different morphology, distribution and antigenicity from GCIs. The 2 neurodegenerative diseases in which glial pathology usually is particularly prominent, PSP and CBD, the most severe glial pathology is clearly astroglial, in the form of astrocytic tangles and thorn-shaped astrocytes in PSP, and astrocytic plaques in CBD, while oligodendroglial changes develop in the less spectacular form of coiled bodies. Moreover, these inclusions are tau-positive (including phosphorylated tau), but more importantly they are α-synuclein negative.

Experimental Models

Although an experimental model unique to MSA does not exist, there are several rodent and primate models of Parkinson's disease and Huntington's disease mimicking nigral and striatal pathology, respectively with sufficient similarities to the striatonigral subtype of MSA to provide an animal model. These include sequential injections of 6-hydroxydopamine and quinolinic acid into the medial forebrain bundle and ipsilateral striatum, respectively. Intrastriatal injections of mitochondrial toxins, 3-nitropropionic acid and 1-methyl-4-phenylpyridinium in rodents cause striatal lesions and subtotal neuronal degeneration of the pars compacta of the ipsilateral substantia nigra, resulting in rat and primate models of striatonigral degeneration (24, 87).

Pathogenesis

The importance of GCIs in the pathogenesis of MSA remains to be established. However, the evidence that they play a central role in the disease mechanism, although circumstantial, is compelling. The pathogenetic mechanisms for different neurodegenerative diseases may considerably vary, but the formation of intraneuronal inclusions (eg, neurofibrillary tangles, Pick inclusions, Lewy bodies) and/or the deposition of abnormal extracellular proteins (βA4 amyloid, prion protein) herald the obvious neuropathological abnormalities. Based on our current knowledge, MSA is the only neurodegenerative disease in which oligodendroglial pathology is the predominant lesion. For this reason it is tempting to hypothesize that in MSA the formation of GCIs is the primary lesion which through the oligodendroglia-myelin-axon-neuron complex secondarily will affect nerve cells. This notion is supported by 2 "minimal-change" cases of MSA whose brains showed neuronal loss restricted to the substantia nigra and locus coeruleus, but with more widespread presence of GCIs (88). The close spatial and metabolic association between oligodendroglia and neuron is well-known and extends well beyond the age of myelin formation in the central nervous system. This presumptive pathogenetic mechanism in MSA is fundamentally different from that proposed for other neurodegenerative diseases in which neurons rather than oligodendroglial cells play the pivotal role.

The precise molecular mechanism by which GCIs are formed is unknown. Since cdk5 phoshorylating both tau and MAP2 and MAPK, phosphorylating MAP2 are predominantly neuronal enzymes. Their occurrence in GCIs suggests that their ectopic or aberrant expression may cause abnormal phosphorylation of microtubular proteins of the cytoskeleton, leading to GCI formation (53). An alternative biochemical model emphasises the importance of abnormal α-synuclein. Nitrated α-synuclein is present not only in Lewy bodies, but also in the inclusions of MSA and in the insoluble fractions of the affected brain regions of α-synucleinopathies, suggesting a link between the selective and specific nitration of α-synuclein and the development of degenerative changes (25).

Future Directions and Therapy

As mentioned earlier, many cases of MSA-P show at least some response to L-dopa, which should always be given an adequate therapeutic trial. However, many patients tolerate L-dopa poorly, because it makes them feel nauseated, ill or faint, or because it causes unacceptable facial and neck dystonia. Some of these patients can better tolerate dopamine agonists (often with domperidone cover), which also cause less dystonia. Amantadine should always be given a trial, and can provide useful, and sometimes striking, benefit in a minority (20-30%) of cases.

Thus far, functional stereotactic neurosurgery (pallidal or subthalamic), and also nigral cell grafting into striatum, have been largely ineffective. At present, there is no medical therapy for the cerebellar disorder of MSA. Spasticity and myoclonus are rarely severe enough to merit treatment with antispasticity or antimyoclonic drugs, but in some such cases may improve with baclofen, or with clonazepam or sodium valproate.

Postural hypotension can be ameliorated by support stockings, behavioural modifications, high-salt diet, or head-up tilt of the bed at night. If these do not suffice, fludrocortisone, ephedrine, midrodrine, DDAVP, or L-threo-DOPA can be helpful. MED may respond to sildenafil, but this may provoke or worsen orthostatic hypotension (33). Urinary frequency and urgency may be helped by peripherally acting anticholinergics such as oxbutynin, but these can provoke retention, especially when residual volume is 100 ml or more, when additional intermittent self-catheterisation is often indicated.

RBD may be helped by clonazepam at bedtime. Stridor and sleep apnoea may need intervention with continuous positive airway pressure (35) and sometimes vocal cord lateralisation procedures or tracheostomy. A number of MSA patients develop depression. This, and also emotional incontinence, responds to treatment with either a tricyclic or an SSRI.

Although some individual symptoms may be helped by the above medical interventions, the condition is inexorably progressive. It is therefore crucial to refer patients with MSA for non-medical interventions: physiotherapy, occupational therapy (with a home visit), speech therapy (with particular attention to swallowing and communication aids), dietetic advice, and expert evaluation in wheelchair clinic. The many PD nurse specialists are also familiar with, and available to, patients with MSA, and there are now a small number of nurses with a specific remit for patients with MSA. Information and support are also available either through national or local patient organizations, mainly for PD, but also through the SDS support organization in the USA and the Sarah Matheson Trust in the UK. The palliative care movement has recently widened its remit for neurological disorders, and now provides valuable domiciliary, respite and terminal care for patients with not only motor neuron disease, but also with MSA and PSP.

Recently a European MSA Study Group (EMSA-SG, *http://www.emsa-sg.org*) and also a sister North American group (NAMSA-SG) have been established, and are developing, in concert, improved diagnostic criteria (39a), rating scales and collection of natural history data, hopefully leading to clinical trials of potentially disease-modifying treatment.

References

1. Adams RD, van Bogaert L, van der Eecken H. (1961) Dégénérescences nigro-striées et cérébello-nigro-striées. *Psychiat Neurol* 142: 219-259.

2. Arai N, Nishimura M, Oda , Morimatsu Y, Ohe R, Nagatomo H (1992) Immunohistochemical expression of microtubule-associated protein 5 (MAP5) in glial cells in multiple system atrophy. *J Neurol Sci* 109: 102-106.

3. Arima K, Ueda K, Sunohara N, Arakawa K, Hirai S, Nakamura M, Tonozuka-Uehara H, Kawai M (1998) NACP/α-synuclein immunoreactivity in fibrillary components of neuronal and oligodendroglial cytoplasmic inclusion in the pontine nuclei in multiple system atrophy. *Acta Neuropathol* 96: 439-444.

4. Bandmann O, Sweeny MG, Daniel SE, Wenning GK, Quinn N, Marsden CD, Wood NW (1997) Multiple-system atrophy is genetically distinct from identified inherited causes of spinocerebellar degeneration. *Neurology* 49: 1598-1604.

5. Bandmann O, Wenning GK, Quinn NP, Harding AE (1995) Arg296 to Cys296 polymorphism in exon 6 of cytochrome P-450-2D6 (CYP2D6) is not associated with multiple system atrophy. *J Neurol Neurosurg Psychiatry* 59: 557.

6. Beck RO, Betts CD, Fowler CJ (1994) Genitourinary dysfunction in multiple system atrophy: clinical features and treatment in 62 cases. *Urology* 151: 1336-1341.

7. Ben Shlomo Y, Wenning GK, Tison F, Quinn NP (1997) Survival of patients with pathologically proven

multiple system atrophy: a meta-analysis. *Neurology* 48: 384-393.

8. Blin O, Desnuelle C, Rascol O, Borg M, Peyro Saint Paul H, Azulay JP, Bille F, Figuresarella D, Coulom F, Pellissier JF et al (1994) Mitochondrial respiratory failure in skeletal muscle from patients with Parkinson's disease and multiple system atrophy. *J Neurol Sci* 125: 95-101.

9. Bower JH, Maraganore DM, McDonnell SK, Rocca WA (1997) Incidence of progressive supranuclear palsy and multiple system atrophy in Olmsted County, Minnesota, 1976 to 1990. *Neurology* 495: 1284-1288.

10. Braune S, Reinhardt M, Schnitzer R, Riedel A, Lucking CH (1999) Cardiac uptake of [1231] MIBG separates Parkinson's disease from multiple system atrophy. *Neurology* 53: 1020-1025.

11. Burn DJ, Sawle GV, Books DJ (1994) Differential diagnosis of Parkinson's disease, multiple system atrophy and Steele-Richardson-Olszewski syndrome: discriminant analysis of striatal ^{18}F-dopa PET. *J Neurol Neurosurg Psychiatry* 57: 278-284.

12. Cairns NJ, Atkinson PF, Hanger DP, Anderton BH, Daniel SE, Lantos PL (1997) Tau protein in the glial cytoplasmic inclusions of multiple system atrophy can be distinguished from abnormal tau in Alzheimer's disease. *Neurosci Lett* 230: 49-52.

13. Cairns NJ, Mackay D, Daniel SE, Lantos PL (1998) Tau-pathology of oligodendroglial inclusions in multiple system atrophy, progressive supranuclear palsy and corticobasal degeneration. *Neuropathol Appl Neurobiol* 24: 131.

14. Campbell BC, McLean CA, Culvenor JG, Gai WP, Blumbergs PC, Jakala P, Beyreuther K, Masters CL, Li QX (2001) The solubility of alpha-synuclein in multiple system atrophy differs from that of dementia with Lewy bodies and Parkinson's diseases. *J Neurochem* 76: 87-96.

15. Chin S-M, Goldman JE (1996) Glial inclusions in CNS degenerative diseases. *J Neuropathol Exp Neurol* 55: 499-508.

16. Colosimo C, Albanese A, Hughes AJ, de Bruin VM, Lees AJ (1995) Some specific clinical features differentiate multiple system atrophy (striatonigral variety) from Parkinson's disease. *Arch Neurol* 52: 294-298.

17. de la Monte SM, Sohn YK, Ganju N, Wands JR (1998) p53- and CD95-associated apoptosis in neurodegenerative diseases. *Lab Invest* 78: 401-411.

18. Déjerine J, Thomas AA (1900) L'atrophie olivo-ponto-cérébelleuse. *Nouv Iconog Salpêtrière* 13: 330-370.

19. Dexter DT, Jenner P, Schapira AHV, Marsden CD (1992) Alterations in levels of iron, ferritin, and other trace metals in neurodegenerative diseases affecting the basal ganglia. *Ann Neurol* 32: S94-S100.

20. Dickson DW, Lin W, Liu W-K, Yen S-H (1999) Multiple system atrophy: a sporadic synucleinopathy. *Brain Pathol* 9: 721-732.

21. Duda JE, Giasson BI, Gur TL, Montine TJ, Robertson D, Biaggioni I, Hurtig HI, Stern MB, Gollomp SM, Grossman M, Lee VM, Trojanowski JQ (2000) Immunohistochemical and biochemical studies demonstrate a distinct profile of alpha-synuclein permutations in multiple system atrophy. *J Neuropathol Exp Neurol* 59: 830-841.

22. Eidelberg D, Takikawa S, Moeller JR, Dhawan V, Redington K, Chaly T, Robeson W, Dahl JR, Margouleff D, Fazzini E et al (1993) Striatal hypometabolism distinguishes striatonigral degeneration from Parkinson's disease. *Ann Neurol* 33: 518-527.

23. Gai WP, Power JHT, Blumbergs PC, Blessing WW (1998) Multiple-system atrophy: A new α-synuclein disease? *Lancet* 352: 547-548.

24. Ghorayeb I, Fernagut PO, Aubert I, Bezard E, Poewe W, Wenning GK, Tison F (2000) Toward a primate model of L-dopa-unresponsive parkinsonism mimicking striatonigral degeneration. *Mov Disord* 15: 531-536.

25. Giasson BI, Duda JE, Murray IV, Chen Q, Souza JM, Hurtig HI, Ischiropoulos H, Trojanowski JQ, Lee VM (2000) Oxidative damage linked to neurodegeneration by selective alpha-synuclein nitration in synucleinopathy lesions. *Science* 290: 985-989.

26. Gilman S, Little R, Johanns J, Heumann M, Kluin KJ, Junck L, Koeppe RA, An H (2000) Evolution of sporadic olivopontocerebellar atrophy into multiple system atrophy. *Neurology* 55: 527-532.

27. Gilman S, Low PA, Quinn N, Albanese A, Ben-Shlomo Y, Fowler CJ, Kaufmann H, Klockgether T, Lang AE, Lantos PL, Litvan I, Mathias CJ, Oliver E, Robertson D, Schatz I, Wenning GK (1999) Consenssus statement on the diagnosis of multiple system atrophy. *J Neurol Sci* 163: 94-98.

28. Graham JG, Oppenheimer DR (1969) Orthostatic hypotension and nicotine sensitivity in a case of multiple system atrophy. *J Neurol Neurosurg Psychiatry* 32: 28-34.

29. Gu M, Gash T, Cooper JM, Wenning GK, Daniel SE, Quinn NP, Marsden CD, Schapira AH (1997) Mitochondrial respiratory chain function in multiple system atrophy. *Mov Disord* 12: 418-422.

30. Hanna PA, Jankovic J, Kirkpatrick JB (1999) Multiple system atrophy: the putative causative role of environmental toxins. *Arch Neurol* 56: 90-94.

31. Hardman CD, Halliday GM, McRitchie DA, Morris JG (1997) The subthalamic nucleus in Parkinson's disease and progressive supranuclear palsy. *J Neuropathol Exp Neurol* 56: 132-142.

32. Horimoto Y, Aiba I, Yasuda T, Ohkawa Y, Katayama T, Yokokawa Y, Goto A, Ito Y (2000) Cerebral atrophy in multiple system atrophy by MRI. *J Neurol Sci* 173: 109-112.

33. Hussain IF, Brady CM, Swinn MJ, Mathias CJ, Fowler CJ (2001) Treatment of erectile dysfunction with sildenafil citrate (Viagra) in parkinsonism due to Parkinson's disease or multiple system atrophy with observations on orthostatic hypotension. *J Neurol Neurosurg Psychiatry* 71: 371-374.

34. Inoue M, Yagishita S, Ryo M, Hasegawa K, Amano M, Matsushita M (1997) The distribution and dynamic density of oligodendroglial cytoplasmic inclusions (GCIs) in multiple system atrophy: A correlation between the density of GCIs and the degree of involvement of striatonigral and olivopontocerebellar systems. *Acta Neuropathol* 93: 585-591.

35. Iranzo A, Santamaria J, Tolosa E (2000) Continuous positive air pressure eliminates nocturnal stridor in multiple system atrophy. Barcelona Multiple System Atrophy Study Group. *Lancet* 356: 1329-1330

36. Ito H, Kusaka H, Matsumoto S, Imai T (1996) Striatal efferent involvement and its correlation to levodopa efficacy in patients with multiple system atrophy. *Neurology* 47: 1291-1299.

37. Iwahashi K, Miyatake R, Tsuneoka Y, Matsuo Y, Ichikawa Y, Hosokawa K, Sato K, Hayabara T (1995) A novel cytochrome P-450IID6 (CYPIID6) mutant gene associated with multiple system atrophy. *J Neurol Neurosurg Psychiatry* 58: 263-264.

38. Kanda T, Tsukagoshi H, Oda M, Miyamoto K, Tanabe H (1996) Changes of unmyelinated nerve fibers in sural nerve in amyotrophic lateral sclerosis, Parkinson's disease and multiple system atrophy. *Acta Neuropathol* 91: 145-154.

39. Kato S, Meshitsuka S, Ohama E, Tanaka J, Llena JF, Hirano A (1992) Increased iron content in the putamen of patients with striatonigal degeneration. *Acta Neuropathol* 84: 328-330.

39a: Kawamoto Y, Akiguchi I, Nakamura S, Budka H (2002) Accumulation of 14-3-3 proteins in glial cytoplasmic inclusions in multiple system atrophy. *Ann Neurol* 52: 722-731.

40. Kimber JR, Watson L, Mathias CJ (1997) Distinction of idiopathic Parkinson's disease from multiple system atrophy by stimulation of growth hormone release with clonidine. *Lancet* 349: 1877-1881.

41. Klein C, Brown R, Wenning GK, Quinn NP (1997) The "cold hands" sign in multiple system atrophy. *Mov Disord* 12: 514-518.

42. Klockgether T, Ludtke R, Kramer B, Abele M, Burk K, Schols L, Riess O, Laccone F, Boesch S, Lopes-Cendes I, Brice A, Inzelberg R, Zilber N, Dichgans J (1998) The natural history of degenerative ataxia: a retrospective study in 466 patients. *Brain* 121: 589-600.

43. Klockgether T, Schroth G, Diener H-C, Dichgans J (1990) Idiopathic cerebellar ataxia of late onset: natural history and MRI morphology. *J Neurol Neurosurg Psychiatry* 53: 297-305.

44. Konagaya M, Konagaya Y, Iida M (1994) Clinical and magnetic resonance imaging study of extrapyramidal symptoms in multiple system atrophy. *J Neurol Neurosurg Psychiatry* 57: 1528-1531.

45. Kume A, Takahashi A, Hashizume Y (1993) Neuronal cell loss of the striatonigral system in multiple system atrophy. *J Neurol Sci* 117: 33-40.

46. Kume A, Takahashi A, Hashizume Y, Asai J (1991) A histometrical and comparative study on Purkinje cells loss and olivary nucleus cell loss in multiple system atrophy. *J Neurol Sci* 101: 178-186

47. Lantos PL (1995) Neuropathological diagnostic criteria of multiple system atrophy: A review. In: Cruz-Sanchez FF, Ravid R, Cuzner ML, eds. *Neuropathological diagnostic criteria for brain banking.* Amsterdam: IOS Press 116-121.

48. Lantos PL (1998) The definition of multiple system atrophy: a review of recent developments. *J Neuropath Exp Neurol* 57: 1099-1111.

49. Magalhaes M, Wenning GK, Daniel SE, Quinn NP (1995) Autonomic dysfunction in pathologically confirmed multiple system atrophy and idiopathic Parkinson's disease—a retrospective comparison. *Acta Neurol Scand* 91: 98-102.

50. Mathias CJ, Bannister R (1992) Investigation of autonomic disorders. In Bannister R & Mathias CJ (eds) *Autonomic Failure. A Textbook of Clinical Disorders of the Autonomic Nervous System.* Oxford University Press: Oxford 3edn: pp 255-290.

51. Mezey E, Dehejia A, Harta G, Papp MI, Polymeropoulos MH, Brownstein MJ (1998) Alpha synuclein in neurodegenerative disorders: Murderer of accomplice? *Nature Medicine* 4: 755-757.

52. Morris HR, Vaughan JR, Datta SR, Bandopadhyay R, Rohan De Silva HA, Schrag A, Cairns NJ, Burn D, Nath U, Lantos PL, Daniel S, Lees AJ, Quinn NP, Wood NW (2000) Multiple system atrophy/progressive supranuclear palsy: α-synuclein, synphilin, tau, and APOE. *Neurology* 55: 1918-1920.

53. Nakamura S, Kawamoto Y, Nakano S, Akiguchi I, Kimura J (1998) Cyclin-dependent kinase 5 and mitogen-activated protein kinase in glial cytoplasmic inclusions in multiple system atrophy. *J Neuropathol Exp Neurol* 57: 690-698.

53a. Osaki Y, Wenning GK, Daniel SE, Hughes A, Lees AJ, Mathias CJ, Quinn N (2002) Do published criteria improve clinical diagnostic accuracy in multiple system atrophy? *Neurology* 59: 1486-1491.

54. Ozawa T, Takano H, Onodera O, Kobayashi H, Ikeuchi T, Koide R, Okuizumi K, Shimohata T, Wakabayashi K, Takahashi H, Tsuji S (1999) No mutation in the entire coding region of the alpha-synuclein gene in pathologically confirmed cases of multiple system atrophy. *Neurosci Lett* 270: 110-112.

55. Papp MI, Kahn JE, Lantos PL (1989) Glial cytoplasmic inclusions in the CNS of patients with multiple system atrophy (striatonigral degeneration, olivopontocerebellar atrophy and Shy-Drager syndrome). *J Neurol Sci* 94: 79-100.

56. Papp MI, Lantos PL (1992) Accumulation of tubular structures in oligodendroglial and neuronal cells as the basic alteration in multiple system atrophy. *J Neurol Sci* 107: 172-182.

57. Papp MI, Lantos PL (1994) The distribution of oligodendroglial inclusions in multiple system atrophy and its relevance to clinical symptomatology *Brain* 117: 235-243.

58. Pirker W, Asenbaum S, Bencsits G, Prayer D, Gerschlager W, Deecke L, Brucke T (2000) [123I] beta-CIT SPECT in multiple system atrophy, progressive supranuclear palsy, and corticobasal degeneration. *Mov Disord* 15: 1158-1167.

59. Plazzi G, Corsini R, Provini F, Pierangeli G, Martinelli P, Montagna P, Lugaresi E, Cortelli P (1997) REM sleep behavior disorders in multiple system atrophy. *Neurol* 48: 1094-1097.

60. Pramstaller PP, Wenning GK, Smith SJM, Beck RO, Quinn NP, Fowler CJ (1995) Nerve conduction studies, skeletal muscle EMG, and sphincter EMG in multiple system atrophy. *J Neurol Neurosurg Psychiatry* 458: 618-621.

61. Probst-Cousin S, Rickert CH, Schmid KW, Gullotta F (1998) Cell death mechanisms in multiple system atrophy. *J Neuropathol Exp Neurol* 57: 814-821.

62. Quinn N (1989) Disproportionate antecollis in multiple system atrophy. *Lancet* 1 8642: 844.

63. Robbins TW, James M, Lange KW, Owen AM, Quinn NP, Marsden CD (1992) Cognitive performance in multiple system atrophy. *Brain* 115: 271-291.

64. Salazar G, Valls-Sole J, Marti MJ, Chang H, Tolosa ES (2000) Postural and action myoclonus in patients with parkinsonian type multiple system atrophy. *Mov Disord* 15: 77-83.

65. Sandroni P, Ahlskog JE, Fealy RD, Low PA (1991) Autonomic involvement in extrapyramidal and cerebellar disorders. *Clin Autonom Res* 1: 147-155.

66. Savoiardo M, Strada L, Girotti F, Zimmerman RA, Grisoli M, Testa D, Petrillo R (1990) Olivopontocerebellar atrophy: MR diagnosis and relationship to multiple system atrophy. *Radiology* 174: 693-696.

67. Sawle GV, Playford ED, Brooks DJ, Quinn N, Frackowiak RS (1993) Postsynaptic changes in the striatal dopamine projection in dopa naive parkinsonism. Diagnostic implications of the D2 receptor status. *Brain* 116: 853-867.

68. Schrag A, Ben-Shlomo Y, Quinn NP (1999) Prevalence of progressive supranuclear palsy and multiple system atrophy. *Lancet* 354: 1771-1775.

69. Schrag A, Kingsley D, Phatouros C, Mathias CJ, Lees AJ, Daniel SE, Quinn NP (1998) Clinical usefulness of magnetic resonance imaging in multiple system atrophy. *J Neurol Neurosurg Psychiatry* 65: 65-71.

70. Schulz JB, Klockgether T, Petersen D, Jauch M, Muller-Schauenburg W, Spieker S, Voigt K, Dichgans J (1994) Multiple system atrophy: natural history, MRI morphology and dopamine receptor imaging with 123IBZM-SPECT. *J Neurol Neurosurg Psychiatry* 57: 1047-1056.

71. Schulz JB, Skalej M, Wedekind D, Luft AR, Abele M, Voigt K, Dichgans J, Klockgether T (1999) Magnetic resonance imaging - based volumetry differentiates idiopathic Parkinson's syndrome from multiple system atrophy and progressive supranuclear palsy. *Ann Neurol* 45: 65-74.

72. Schwarz SC, Seufferlien T, Liptay S, Schmid RM, Kasischke K, Foster OJ, Daniel S, Schwarz J (1998) Microglial activation in multiple system atrophy: a potential role for NF-kappaB/rel proteins. *Neuroreport* 9: 3029-3032.

73. Shy GM, Drager GA (1960) A neurologic syndrome associated with orthostatic hypotension. *Arch Neurol* 2: 511-527.

74. Spargo E, Papp MI, Lantos PL (1996) Decrease in neuronal density in the cerebral cortex in multiple system atrophy. *Eur J Neurol* 3: 450-456.

75. Spillantini MG, Crowther RA, Jakes R, Cairns NJ, Lantos PL, Goedert M (1998) Filamentous a-synuclein inclusions link multiple system atrophy with Parkinson's disease and dementia with Lewy bodies. *Neurosci Lett* 251: 205-208.

76. Stocchi F, Carbone A, Inghilleri M, Monge A, Ruggieri S, Berardelli A, Manfredi M (1997) Urodynamic and neurophysiological evaluation in Parkinson's disease and multiple system atrophy. *J Neurol Neurosurg Psychiatry* 62: 507-511.

77. Su M, Yoshida Y, Hirata Y, Watahiki Y, Nagata K (2001) Primary involvement of the motor area in association with the nigrostriatal pathway in multiple system atrophy: neuropathological and morphometric evaluations. *Acta Neuropathol* 101: 57-64.

78. Takeda A, Arai N, Komori T, Iseki E, Kato S, Oda M (1997) Tau immunoreactivity in glial cytoplasmic inclusions in multiple system atrophy. *Neurosci Lett* 234: 63-66.

78a. Tison F, Yekhlef F, Balestre E, Chrysostome V, Quinn N, Wenning GK, Poewe W (2002) Application of the International Cooperative Ataxia Scale rating in multiple system atrophy. *Mov Disord* 17: 1248-1254.

79. Tsuchiya K, Ozawa E, Haga C, Watabiki S, Ikeda M, Sano M, Ooe K, Taki K, Ikeda K (2000) Constant involvement of the Betz cells and pyramidal tract in multiple system atrophy: a clinicopathological study of seven autopsy cases. *Acta Neuropathol* 99: 628-636.

80. Tsuchiya K, Watabiki S, Sano M, Iobe H, Shiotsu H, Taki K, Hashimoto K (1998) Distribution of cerebellar cortical lesions in multiple system atrophy: A topographic neuropathological study of three autopsy cases in Japan. *J Neurol Sci* 155: 80-85.

81. Tu PH, Galvin JE, Baba M, Giasson B, Tomita T, Leight S, Nakajo S, Iwatsubo T, Trojanowski JQ, Lee VM (1998) Glial cytoplasmic inclusions in white matter oligodendrocytes of multiple system atrophy: brains contain insoluble alpha-synuclein. *Ann Neurol* 44: 415-422.

82. Valldeoriola F, Valls-Sole J, Tolosa ES, Marti MJ (1995) Striatal and sphincter denervation in patients with progressive supranuclear palsy. *Mov Disord* 10: 550-555.

83. Vanacore N, Bonifati V, Fabbrini G, Colosimo C, De Michele G, Marconi R, Nicholl D, Locuratolo N, Talarico G, Romano S, Stocchi F, Bonuccelli U, De Mari M, Vieregge P, Meco G (2001) Epidemiology of multiple system atrophy. ESGAP Consortium. European Study Group on Atypical Parkinsonisms. *Neurol Sci* 22: 97-99.

84. Vodusek DB (2001) Sphincter EMG and differential diagnosis of multiple system atrophy. *Mov Disord* 16: 600-607.

85. Wakabayashi K, Yoshimoto M, Tsuji S, Takahashi H (1998) a-Synuclein immunoreactivity in glial cytoplasmic inclusions in multiple system atrophy. *Neurosci Lett* 249: 180-182

86. Wenning GK, Ben-Shlomo Y, Magalhaes M, Daniel SE, Quinn NP (1994a) Clinical features and natural history of multiple system atrophy. An analysis of 100 patients. *Brain* 117: 835-845.

87. Wenning GK, Granata R, Puschban Z, Scherfler C, Poewe W (1999) Neural transplantation in animal models of multiple system atrophy: a review. *J Neural Transm* Suppl 55: 103-113.

88. Wenning GK, Quinn N, Magalhaes M, Mathias C, Daniel SE (1994) 'Minimal change' multiple system atrophy. *Mov Disord* 9: 161-166.

89. Wenning GK, Seppi K, Tison F, Jellinger K (2001) A novel grading scale for striatonigral degenration. *J Neural Transm* 109: 307-320.

90. Wenning GK, Tison F, Ben Shlomo Y, Daniel SE, Quinn NP (1997) A review of 203 pathologically proven cases. *Mov Disord* 12: 133-147.

91. Wullner U, Weller M, Kornhuber, Bornemann A, Schulz JB, Riederer P, Klockgether T (2000) Altered expression of calcium- and apoptosis-regulating proteins in multiple system atrophy Purkinje cells. *Mov Disord* 15: 269-275.

Experimental Models of Synucleinopathies

Kurt A. Jellinger

5-HT	5-hydroxydopamine (serotonin)
5-HIAA	5-hydroxyindolic acid
6-OHDA	6-hydroxydopamine
AMPH	amphetamine
BDNF	brain derived neurotrophic factor
DAT	dopamine transporter
DOPAC	3,4-dihydroxyphenyl acetic acid
GDNF	glia-derived neurotrophic factor
GSH	glutathion
LB	Lewy body
L-dopa	Levodopa
MAO	monoaminoxidase
MDMA	3-4-methylendioxymethamphetamine
METH	methamphetamine
MPP⁺	1-methyl-4-phenyl-2,3-dihydropyridinium
MPTP	1-methyl-4-phenyl-1,2,3,6-tetrahydropyridine
mRNA	messenger ribonucleic acid
NMDA	N-methyl-D-aspartate
OS	oxidative stress
Par-4	prostate apoptosis response 4
PD	Parkinson's disease
ROS	reactive oxygen species
SN	substantia nigra
SOD	superoxide dismutase
TaClo	1-trichloromethyl-1,2,3,4-tetrahydro-b-carboline
TH	tyrosine hydroxylase
UCH-L1	ubiquitin carboxy-terminus hydrolase L1
VMAT2	vesicular monoamine transporter
VTA	ventral tegmental area

Parkinson's Disease

Spontaneous Lewy body parkinsonism does not occur in animals, but some of the principal mechanisms of PD have been demonstrated with pharmacologic agents and neurotoxins adminstered to a wide variety of animal species and by generating genetically engineered animal models (5, 8, 12, 74, 79). However, it is worth noting that the chronic infusion of the mitochondrial poison, rotenone, in rats seems to be the best toxin-induced animal model of PD that shows Lewy-like intraneuronal inclusions (6).

Reserpine and a-methyl-p-tyrosine models. Systemic administration of reserpine, a pharmacological compound causing depletion of catecholamines in the brain and inhibiting vesicular storage of dopamine, and of a-methyl-p-tyrosine, an inhibitor of TH, leads to an akinetic state in rodents. The motor deficits induced by these compounds are temporary and can be reversed by adminstering L-dopa, amphetamine, and dopamine receptor agonists, indicating that functional recovery depends on dopamine replacement (16, 30). Although these agents do not induce morphological changes, the similarity of the akinetic syndrome in these models to that in PD led to the major breakthrough hypothesis that PD results from dopamine deficiency.

Neuroleptic-induced akinesia. Systemic administration of classical neuroleptics, such as haloperidol, blocks postsynaptic dopamine receptors and induces akinetic or cataleptic syndromes that are due to disorders of dopaminergic neurotransmission in the nigro-striatal system. At least in part, the deficits can be treated by anticholinergic, dopamine-releasing substances, dopamine receptor agonistis, L-dopa and NMDA receptor antagonists (66).

The 6-OHDA model. 6-Hydroxydopamine (6-OHDA), a hydroxylated analogue of dopamine, was the first agent discovered to have specific neurotoxic properties to catecholaminergic neurons. The 6-OHDA model has been produced in many species, most frequently rats. Using the same transport systems as dopamine and NE, it leads to neuronal damage via OS and mitochondrial dysfunction (63). OS induced by 6-OHDA may arise from the combined effects on MAO, autooxidation of 6-OHDA and elevation in iron content. Although 6-OHDA has been shown to induce ROS-related collapse in mitochondrial membrane potential and to be a strong uncoupler of oxidative phosphorylation, inhibition of mitochondrial respiration appears not to be the main mechanism underlying its toxicity (8).

Since it does not cross the blood-brain barrier, CNS lesions can be produced by 6-OHDA only after direct intracerebral or intraventricular injection. Blocking neuronal 6-OHDA uptake by systemic des-methyl imipramine or stereotactic targeting of 6-OHDA in the SN, ventral tegmentum, forebrain bundle or striatum specifically damage the dopaminergic system (55). This leads to long-term destruction of dopaminergic neurones, first detected as early as 24 hours after administration. There is loss of 80 to 90% of TH-IR neurones and striatal dopamine depletion 2 to 3 days later that persists for 180 days due to progressive retrograde degeneration of nigro-striatal neurones. Intracerebral 6-OHDA causes both apoptotic and necrotic cell death of SN neurones (18, 20, 33) but in cell cultures it produces only apoptosis. Decreased α-synuclein mRNA in the presence of preserved DAT and VMAT2 mRNA in rats following 6-OHDA (36) and in the SN of PD suggests that α-synuclein decrease is an early event during neuronal damage and one that preceeds changes in TH and dopamine (50).

Behavioural changes (circling) occur when striatal dopamine loss exceeds 70%. Unilateral lesions cause an asymmetrical and quantifiable motor behaviour (turning of head and neck or circling toward the lesion side, often correlated with the degree of lesioning) that also offers the advantage of being able to use the intact side as a control for the lesioned side (67). Circling can be spontaneous or elicited by amphetamine, apomorphine, or dopamine agonists and is presumably induced by dopamine release or inhibition of its reuptake from nonfunctional pools, resulting in contralateral circling. Later, ipsilateral circling arises because dopamine pools in the lesioned side are depleted, and its release in the unlesioned side is increased. Dopamine agonists stimulate the receptors, which are upregulated and hypersensitive.

Bilateral injections produce a hypokinetic, aphagic state due to massive loss of dopaminergic neurones, which can be reversed by long term compensatory mechanisms of dopa-minergic neurones or sprouting of 5-HT neurones that varies with age of the animal (59). Endogenous neurotrophic factors, BDNF and GDNF, are differentially affected by aging; young animals have significantly more BDNF and GDNF compared to aged animals (85).

Although 6-OHDA does not produce pathology in many regions of the brain that are affected in PD and is not associated with Lewy body formation, there are several features of the model that are appealing, such as the slowly progressive nature of neurodegeneration. It will remain a useful model for selective nigral damage.

Loss of dopaminergic neurones in SN, VTA and the retrorubal area after unilateral injection of 6-OHDA in rats may reflect changes in early PD (33a), although bilateral lesion of the ventrolateral caudate-putamen complex is considered a more suitable model of PD that mimics the human disease with respect to behavioral and neurochemical parameters.

Methamphetamine. Psychostimulants such as D-amphetamine (AMPH) or methamphetamine (METH) and its derivatives (3-4-methylendioxymethamphetamine—MDMA—"ecstasy") exert pleotropic effects on dopaminergic neurones. They result in a selective degeneration of striatal dopamine neurones, long-term depletion of striatal dopamine and serotonin nerve terminals, and rapid redistribution of dopamine from vesicular stores to the cytoplam, where dopamine undergoes reverse transport to the extracellular space by DAT. High doses of METH induce glutamate release in the striatum, suggesting that it also has a synergistic effect on presynaptic dopaminergic terminals. Toxicity is increased by low doses of neuronal nitric oxide synthase inhibitors (1). Dopamine is concurrently oxidized to produce a 3-fold increase in free radicals.

Intracellular depletion using the dopamine synthesis inhibitor o-methyl-p-tyrosine or the VMAT blocker reserpine prevents drug-induced free radical formation (44). Although AMPH usually spares dopaminergic cell bodies, under some conditions these drugs can induce cell death. Extrastriatal CNS regions are not involved. AMPH also induces an early burst of free radicals in CNS-derived dopaminergic cell lines, but AMPH-mediated attenuation of ATP production and mitochondrial function was not observed, indicating that neither metabolic dysfunction nor loss of viability are a direct consequence of AMPH. However, exposure of neuronal cultures to AMPH in the presence of subtoxic doses of the mitochondrial complex I inhibitor rotenone dramatically increased cell death, mimicking the effects of MPP^+ (44). Excitatory amino acids also play a key role in AMPH toxicity, since blocking ionotropic glutamate receptors is neuroprotective (52). Despite some gaps in the understanding of METH action, this model provides an excellent tool to investigate the pathophysiology of PD at the level of the dopaminergic terminals (43).

The MPTP model. In the early 1980s, several users of synthetic heroin in northern California developed acute parkinsonsm caused by the contaminating compound 1-methyl-4-phenyl-1,2,3,6-tetrahydropyridine (MPTP) (40). Intravenous injection of MPTP results in an akinetic-rigid syndrome with or without resting tremor within 7 to 14 days. The parkinsonism responds well to levodopa initially, with subsequent development of fluctuations and dyskinesias. F-DOPA PET scans in affected patients and in individuals erxposed to MPTP but without parkinsonanian signs showed reduced striatal DOPA uptake and a progressive loss over time (14). Neuropathology in a few cases surviving 3 to 16 years after exposure to MPTP showed severe, ongoing loss of SN neurones, but no evidence of classical LBs (41).

MPTP crosses the blood-brain barrier, where it is converted to 1-methyl-4-phenyl-2,3-dihydropyridinium (MPP+) by the enzyme MAO-B localized in astroglia and serotonergic neurones, which explains the protective effect of MAO-B inhibitors (17). Selective uptake of MPP+ into dopaminergic neurones via the energy-dependent dopamine uptake sites and VMAT with subsequent accumulation of the neurotoxin in synaptic vesicles accounts, at least in part, for its specificity to dopaminergic neurones (71). Free cytosolic MPP^+ enters the mitochondria by an energy-dependent mechanism. In the mitochondria MPP^+ inhibits NADH coenzyme Q10 reductase (complex I), decreases ATP production, alters calcium homoeostasis, and generates free radicals. The ROS subsequently leads to activation of caspase-8 and apoptotic cell death (8, 65). MPTP also induces decreases in GSH and increases in free iron levels in the SNpc. Its toxicity is potentiated by deficiencies in SOD and glutathione peroxide genes (87).

Administration of MPTP results in nigrostrital cell death and depletion of striatal dopamine in a wide variety of species including mice, rats, cats, dogs, sheep and primates. The susceptibility to MPTP varies due to species differential susceptibility and parameters such as administration mode, dosage, and the age of the animal (26). In some nonhuman primates and in the C57BL/6 mice, MPTP induces SN lesions with a topology similar to that in human PD. Pathology is not limited to the SN, but also affects area A-8, VTA, LC and the hypothalamus (26, 76). The animals have 86% striatal dopamine loss and behavioural changes similar to those of human PD. In elderly monkeys, eosinophilic inclusions have been described, but their ultrastructural and histochemical features differ from LBs (24). Systemic administration leads to bilateral, often symmetrical parkinsonian features with corresponding partial loss of striatal dopamine. Although animals may tend to spontaneously recover and usually do not show progressive lesions, stable parkinsonism has been achieved in human primates (*Macaca*) by repeated administration of small doses of MPTP, and these animals have a progressive loss of dopamine reuptake in longitudinal PET studies (73).

Unilateral lesions induced by stereotactic injection of MPP+ into the nigrostriatal system may cause circling behaviour. The behavioural changes in the MPTP lesioned non-human primates (bradykinesia, rigidity, freezing, balance impairment, and postural or resting tremor); their reversal by L-dopa; and the development of dyskinesias after long-term administration of L-dopa resemble human PD (73). After acute MPTP treatment in mice no changes of dopamine D1 receptors are detected in the striatum and SN; D2 receptors are reduced in the SN, but not in the striatum. In contrast, DA uptake sites are markedly reduced in both regions; dopamine and DA and DOPAC content in the striatum and the number of TH positive SN neurones are also reduced (4). Acute treatment in cats causes significant decrease of DAT and TH protein in the striatum. Increased TH protein and mRNA and suppression of DAT protein and mRNA in the striatum and ventral mesencephalon are associated with functional recovery from MPTP-induced parkinsonism (62).

Recent studies indicate that MPP^+-induced ROS are not mitochondrial in origin, but derived from intracellular DA oxidation. Concurrent with ROS formation, MPP^+ leads to redistribution of vesicular dopamine to the cytoplasm and eventual extrusion from the cell by reverse transport via the DAT. That cytosolic DA oxidation plays a role in MPP+ toxicyt is suggested by the fact that cells depleted of newly synthesized or stored dopamine have significantly less superoxide production and less MPP^+-induced cell death, whereas increasing intracellular DA content exacerbates sensitivity to MPP+ (43). Heterozygote DAT knockout mice, which express about 50% of DAT, display neurotoxicity that is approximantely half that in wild-type mice, while VMAT2 heterozygote mice show enhanced vulnerability (48).

It is controversial whether MPTP/MPP^+ toxicity is mediated by apoptosis or necrosis (8). It has been suggested that MPTP/MPP+ causes apoptosis in a low dose chronic neurotoxic paradigm and necrosis in high dose acute paradigms (51). Acute adminstation of MPTP induces necrotic cell death, but does not produce increases in α-synuclein, but chronic MPTP administration, which induces apoptosis, increases α-synuclein expression in SN of mice and baboons. This redistribution of α-synuclein from its normal synaptic location to the cytoplasm may favor its aggregation in degenerating neurones and may play a role in MPTP toxicity (39, 78). Levels of the proapoptotic proteins BAX and Par-4 increase dramatically in dopaminergic neurones of monkeys and mice after MPTP exposure (20), while expression of the anti-apopotic factor Bcl-2 is decreased. These changes, however, are not specific to PD and also occur in other neurodegenerative disorders. BAX-deficient mice are resistent to MPTP toxicity; in spite of the almost complete survival of SN cells, BAX-deficient mice show a marked dopamine reduction. These results clearly indicate that effects of MPTP on dopaminergic neurones is mediated by more than just neuronal death (77, 79). Recent data suggest that MPTP neurotoxicity is a multi-component process, including mitochondrial dysfunction and ROS generated by vesicular dopamine displacement. These results indicate that in the presence of a complex I defect, misregulation of dopamine storage could contribute to nigral cell loss.

Studies in the MPTP mice model using cDNA microarray detected changes in expression of genes involved in oxidative stress, inflammatory processes, signal transduction, and glutamate toxicity that appear to be compensated by elevated expression in trophic factors and antioxidant defense. This early gene cascade after short MPTP exposure occurs prior to late nigrostriatal dopaminergic neuronal cell death (44a).

The MPTP models have provided insight into the mechanisms of striatonigral neurodegeneration and lead to development of therapeutic strategies, particularly with use of genetically engineered animal models (77, 79). Mutant mice deficient in MAO-B fail to transform MPTP into the active metabolite MPP^+ (31), and as previsouly mentioned, those deficient in DAT are resistent to MPTP toxicity (7). In mice engineered to express lower levels of VMAT-2, greater MPTP toxicity is due to increased MPP^+ sequestration into synaptic vesicles (72). On the other hand, mice deficient in SOD1, the key protective enzyme against superoxide, are more sensitive to MPTP (87). NO derived from upregulation of NOS in activated microglia may also be important in toxicity since mice deficient in NO synthase are partially protected against MPTP (42). Likewise, ablation of the pro-apoptotic protein Bax in mutant mice or, conversely, overexpression of the anti-apoptotic protein Bcl-2 in mice, attenuates dopaminergic neuronal death caused by MPTP (77, 79). Thus, the combined approach has shed light on molecular mechanisms that could be important in the pathogenesis of PD.

Rotenone and pesticides. Chronic systemic administration of low doses of the lipophilic pesticide rotenone, an inhibitor of mitochondrial complex I, recently have been shown to produce straital dopamine deleption and subsequent degeneration and loss of nigral dopaminergic neurones associated with hypokinesia and rigidity (6). Degenerating nigral neurons develop fibrillary cytoplasmic inclusions immunoreactive for ubiquitin and α-

Transgenic type	Loss of SNpc cells	Striatal dopamine	Motor deficits	Behaviour changes	Reference
Tyrosine hydroxylase -/- mice	no	unchanged	no	aggressive	(61)
Monoaminoxidase -/- mice	no	unchanged	no	aggressive	(68)
Catechol-0-methyl-transferase -/- mice	no	unchanged	no	aggressive	(29)
Vesicularmonoaminetransporter -/- mice	no	unchanged	no	no	(82)
VMAT-2 + reinfected neurons		increased dopamine release		–	(54)
Dopamine transporter -/- mice	no	increased	hyperactivity	no	(28)
Dopamine receptor -/- mice	no	reduced response	hypoactivity	yes	(69)
Cu-Zn-Superoxide dismutase -/- mice			enhanced toxicity of MPTP		(87, 88)
Glutathioneperoxidase -/- mice					
Manganese-superoxide dismutase -/- mice			age-related increase of apoptose		(37)
Monoamineoxidase B transgenic mice			catecholaminergic cell atrophy		(3)
GDNF -/- mice	no		early postnatal death, loss of noradrenergic neurons		(49)
BDNF -/- mice	yes		(developmental neuronal death)		(34)
TGF- -/- mice	yes		(without involvement of other dopaminergic neurons)		(9)
Adenosine nucleotide translocator -/- mice	no		oxidative damage		(22)
Complex 1 "cybrids"	yes	?	?	?	(58)

Table 1. Engineered models of Parkinson's disease (modified from Vila et al (77, 79)). BDNF = brain-derived neurotrophic factor; GDNF: = glial-derived neurotrophic factor; TGF = transforming growth factor.

synuclein similar to human LBs (6). Several pesticides, including rotenone, the organochloride dieldrin and paraquat induce a conformational change in α-synuclein and accelerate the rate of formation of α-synuclein fibrils in vitro, suggesting a possible molecular basis for PD (13, 74a, 74b).

Chronic exposure to sublethal doses of rotenone further cause delayed oxidative damage and apoptosis due to peroxide-induced cytochrome C release and caspase 3 activation indicating mitochondrial impairment (67a).

TaClo. TaClo (1-trichloromethyl-1,2,3,4-tetra-hydro-β-carboline), an inhibitor of mitochondrial complex I with a chemical structure similar to MPTP, stimulates hydroxyl radical production and has neurotoxic effects (11). This compound, which is transformed in vivo and in vitro from tryptamine and chloral hydrate, together with endogeneous biogenic amines was detected in both rats and humans treated with the sedative chloral hydrate or the industrial solvent trichlorethylene (10). After chronic exposition to trichlorethylene, acute parkinsonism was reported (32). Intracerebral injection of Taclo induces selective SN cell loss and dopamine depletion in the striatum (25).

The herbicide paraquat produces a dose- and age-dependent loss of SN neurones and glial response without significant striatal DA depletion but enhanced DA synthesis suggested by increased TH activity (48a).

Genetic models. *Spontaneous models.* Among the number of spontaneous genetic rodent models characterised by locomotor problems is the Weaver mouse, which has an autosomal recessive mutation in a potassium channel gene that leads to neuronal cell loss in the cerebellum and the nigrostriatal system. It has significant decrease in TH-IR neurones in the SNpc and reduction in striatal dopamine (53). Other models are the mutant circling (ci) rat with abnormal and drug-induced circling behaviour (84) and the AS/AGU rat, a mutant from the Albino-Swiss (AS) rat strain, which has a staggering gait, hind limb rigidity, and difficulty inittiating movement due to loss of dopamine in the extracellular fluid of the striatum, suggesting dopaminergic neurone dysfunction (15). Mutation in the rat protein kinase C gamma causes a movement disorder and age-progressive loss of SNpc neurones, and it may be a candidate gene for human neurodegenerative disorders (19).

Engineered models. Transgenic and homologous recombination ("knock-out") technologies have been used to generate mice overexpressing or deficient in specific steps of dopamine metabolism (Table 1). Ablation of the key enzymes responsible for dopamine metabolism (TH, MAO, COMT) and heterozygosity for VMAT-2 do not change the brain dopamine levels or produce motor problems, although aggressive behavour changes have been described (29, 61, 68). VAMT-2 overexpression in transfected dopamine neurones induces increased vesicle size and DOPA release (54), demonstrating that VAMT2 is a critical regulator of the rate of transmitter accumulation. DAT deficient mice show hyperactivity and a dramatic increase in striatal dopamine (28). Dopaminergic D2 receptor deficient mice show decreased capacity to respond to dopamine and a motor

Species	Form of α-synuclein	Promotor	Loss of SNpc cells	Striatal dopaminic deficit	Inclusions	Motor deficits	Reference
Mouse	α-synuclein -/-	–	no	yes	no	yes	(2)
Mouse	wild-type	PDGF	no	yes	nuclear and cytoplasmic, non-fibrillar α-syn aggregates, in neocortex, hippocampus (rarely in SN)	yes	(45)
Mouse	wild-type and mutant (A53T)	Thy-1	no	no	Lewy-like pathology, especially in motor neurones + axonal damage	yes	(75)
Mouse	mutant (A30P)	Thy-1 and TH	no	no	somal and neuritic accumulation of mutant α-synuclein	no	(58)
Mouse	wild-type and mutant (A53T, A30P)	TH	no	no	no	no	(47)
Mouse	wild-type and mutant (A30P)	Thy-1	no	no	Abnormal accumulation of α-syn in cell bodies and neurites	no	(35)
Mouse	α-syn + APP double transgenic		no	no	fibrillar α-syn + inclusions + accumulation of β-amyloid	yes	(23)
Mouse	mutant (A53T)		?	?	neuronal cytoplasmic, containing 10 to 16 nm fibrils	yes	(27a)
Mouse	mutant	Thy-1			α-syn accumulation throughout the brain (basal ganglia, brainstem)	?	(61a)
Mouse	mutant	PD6F			α-syn accumulation in neocortex, limbic system, olfactory regions; neuronal inclusions in deep neocortex	?	(61a)
Mouse	mutant (line M)	PD6F	?	?	α-syn expression in glial cells	?	(61a)
Mouse	mutant (h α-syn)		yes	yes	α-syn expression in neurones, axons, terminals in striatonigral system	yes	(60)
Mouse	mutant (hm² α-syn)		yes	yes	α-syn expression in striatonigral system	yes	(60)
Mouse	mutant (A30P+Thy-1)	Thy-1	?	?	α-syn protein K resistant, serine 129 hyperphosphorylated, cytoskeletal neuronal inclusions and detergent-insoluble oligodendroglial inclusions	yes	(49a)
Drosophila	wild-type and mutant (A53T, A30P)	GAL4	yes	yes	yes	yes	(46)

Table 2. Transgenic α-synuclein animals.

impairment similar to PD, but one that cannot be improved with dopamine agonists (69). These data demonstrate that, in line with human PD, no gross motor dysfunctions arise unless there are conspicuous changes in the dopaminergic pathway.

D_2 dopamine receptor knockout mice show motor and behavioural deficits similar to PD particularly in older age (24a).

Mice lacking various key enzymes for scavenging reactive oxidative species (ROS) do not show overt SN neurodegeneration, but over expression of a mutant form of the enzyme superoxide dismutase 1 (SOD 1) leads to neuronal loss in the SNpc and spinal cord (38). Transgenic mice overexpressing MAO-B show no neuronal death, but striking atrophy of SNpc neurones, probably due to increased ROS production during dopamine deamination (3).

Mutant mice deficient in glial-derived neurotrophic factor (GDNF) or brain-derived neurotrophic factor (BDNF) show early postnatal death. GDNF deficient mice have major abnormalities of noradrenergic neurones, with preservation of midbrain dopamine neurones (34), while BDNF deficient mice have developmental SNpc neuronal death (34). Mutant mice deficient in transforming growth factor alpha (TGFα) have significantly fewer SNpc neurones than wild-type littermates without involvement of other midbrain dopaminergic nuclei (9). Mice lacking the orphan nuclear receptor Nur-1 fail to generate midbrain dopaminergic neurones and are hypoactive (86) as do mice lacking engraded genes En-1 and En-2, suggesting that these genes control survival of midbrain dopaminergic neurones and may regulate expression of α-synuclein (70). Estrogen receptor knockout mice show degeneration of SNpc neurones with ageing (81) and mice deficient in the ATM gene (involved in DNA repair) also develop severe degeneration of SNpc neurones (21).

Mice lacking α-synuclein show deficits in the nigrostriatal system with mildly reduced striatal dopamine content and attenuation of dopamine-dependent locomotor response to amphetamine, suggesting that α-synuclein is an essential presynaptic, activity-dependent negative regulator of dopaminergic transmission (2).

Transgenic mice overexpressing either wild-type or mutant human α-synuclein have had inconsistent phenotypes (Table 2). Overexpression of wild-type α-synuclein driven by the platelet-derived growth factor promoter is associated with loss of dopaminergic neurones in different brain regions and inclusion bodies composed of granular, non-filamentous material that are immunoreative for α-synuclein and ubiquitin. Inclusions are detected in neocortex, hippocampus and, rarely, in the SN (45). Aged transgenic mice expressing either wild-type or A53T mutant of human α-synuclein produced under control of the Thy1 promoter have motor deficits and degeneration in brainstem and motor, but not SN neurones. They also have axonal damage and denervation at neuromuscular junctions, suggesting that mutant α-synuclein may not function properly in synapse maintenance. Over expression of wild-type human α-synuclein produced a similar phenotype (75). Three other lines of transgenics mice, expressing wild-type or mutant α-synuclein driven by either Thy 1 or TH promoter, showed no SN pathology and no increased sensitivity to MPTP (35, 47, 58).

Human α-synuclein-harboring familial PD-linked Ala-53→Thr mutation causes a neurodegenerative disease with α-synuclein aggregation in tg mice (41a).

Thy-1 human α-synuclein tg mice accumulate α-synuclein in synapses and neurones throughout the brain including basal ganglia and brainstem, while expression of α-synuclein from the platelet-derived growth factor (PDGP) promoter results in accumulation of α-synuclein in synapses of neocortex, limbic system, and olfactory regions and neuronal cytoplasmic inclusions in deep neocortical layers (61a).

Mutant tg mice expressing A53T human α-synuclein develop severe movement disorders associated with age-dependent intracytoplasmic neuronal α-synuclein inclusions consisting of 10- to 16-nm wide fibrils similart to human pathological inclusions (27a). Transgenic wild-type (hw α-syn) mice express α-syunclein in nigrostriatal system neurons, axons and terminals and result in corresponding behavioral and neurochemical changes. Double mutant (hm^2 α-syn) mice show reduced locomotor response to repeated doses of amphetamine, age-related decline in locomotor behaviour, striatal dopamine level and SNZC neurone numbers as well as increased sensitivity to effects of pesticide exposure (60).

Transgenic mice expressing human α-synuclein with the A30P mutation under the control of Thy-1 promoter show age-dependent formation of protein kinase K resistent and on serine 129 hyperphosphorylated, argyrophilic and ubiquitinated inclusions either in neurones or in oligodendroglia, the latter mimicking GCIs in MSA (49a).

Unlike mice, overexpression of human wild-type or mutant α-synuclein in drosophila has produced a number of features of human PD, including selective dopaminergic neurone loss, filamentous intraneuronal inclusions, and an age-dependent locomotor dysfunction (23). Since α-synuclein can be damaged by oxidative stress (OS), it is noteworthy that drosophila have greater oxidative metabolism than mice, which may explain the different vulnerabilites of these animals to experimental manipulations.

From these and other studies, reviewed by Vila et al (77, 79) it is clear that engineered animal models have contributed and will continue to contribute to elucidation of the pathogenesis of PD. With several PD-linked mutations still to be tested using these technologies, progress will hopefully also be made in understanding its aetiology.

Dementia with Lewy Bodies

For DLB, no specific animal model exists; however, transgenic mice with neuronal expression of both human mutant amyloid precursor protein and α-synuclein show severe learning and memory impairments and motor deficits. They develop age-related degeneration of cholinergic neurones and synaptic terminals associated with fibrillar α-synuclein positive, Lewy body-like inclusions (46). These results suggest that that α-amyloid may contribute to the development of LBs by promoting aggregation of α-synuclein and exacerbating α-synuclein-dependent pathologies (46).

Multiple System Atrophy

Although an experimental model for MSA does not exist, there are several rodent and primate models of PD and Huntington's disease with nigral or striatal pathology, respectively, with sufficient similarities to the striatonigral subtype of MSA to be considered an animal model for some of the features of MSA. These models include sequential injections of 6-OHDA into the medial forebrain bundle and quinolinic acid into the ipsilateral striatum. Intrastriatal injections of the mitochondrial toxins, 3-nitropropionic acid and 1-methyl-4-phenyl-pyridinium in rodents cause striatal lesions and subtotal neuronal degeneration in the ipsilateral SNpc, resulting in rat and primate models of striatonigral degeneration (27, 83). The double-lesion rat model of striatonigral degeneration has also been used to test the effects of embryonic ventral mesencephalic, striatal, or co-grafts (56, 57, 64, 80). None of these models leads to production of synuclein-immunoreactive glial cytoplasmic inclusions, that hallmark of MSA.

Another animal model of apoptotic neurodegeneration with a corresponding multiple system atrophy that mimicks some features of MSA is the transgenic mouse engineered to overexpress either wild-type or constitutively active alpha-1B adrenergic receptors. All transgenic lines showed granulovacuolar neurodegeneration beginning in alpha-1B adrenergicreceptor expressing domains of the brain and progressing with age. The mice have an age-related progressive Parkinson-like hindlimb disorder, dysfunction of 3,4-dihydroxyphenylalanine and considerable dopaminergic neuronal degeneration in the substantia nigra. They also have grand mal seizures and histologic evidence of cerebral cortical dysplasia and neurodegeneration, which are features of human MSA (89).

Tg mice expressing human α-synuclein with the A30P mutation under the control of Thy-1 promotor slow age-dependent formation of protein kinase resitent and an serine 129 hyperphosphorylated argyrophilic and ubiquitinated inclusions in neurones and oligodendroglia, the latter mimicking GCIs in MSA (49a).

References

1. Abekawa T, Ohmori T, Honda M, Ito K, Koyama T (2001) Effect of low doses of L-NAME on methamphetamine-induced dopaminergic depletion in the rat striatum. *J Neural Transm* 108: 219-1230.

2. Abeliovich A, Schmitz Y, Farinas I, Choi-Lundberg D, Ho WH, Castillo PE, Shinsky N, Verdugo JM, Armanini M, Ryan A, Hynes M, Phillips H, Sulzer D, Rosenthal A (2000) Mice lacking alpha-synuclein display functional deficits in the nigrostriatal dopamine system. *Neuron* 25: 239-252.

3. Andersen JK, Frim DM, Isacson O, Breakefield XO (1994) Catecholaminergic cell atrophy in transgenic mouse aberrantly overexpressing MAO-B in neurons. *Neurodegeneration* 3: 97-109.

4. Araki T, Mikami T, Tanji H, Matsubara M, Imai Y, Mizugaki M, Itoyama Y (2001) Biochemical and immunohistological changes in the brain of 1-methyl-4-phenyl-1,2,3,6-tetrahydropyridine (MPTP)-treated mouse. *Eur J Pharm Sci* 12: 231-238.

5. Beal MF (2001) Experimental models of Parkinson's disease. *Nat Rev Neurosci* 2: 325-334.

6. Betarbet R, Sherer TB, MacKenzie G, Garcia-Osuna M, Panov AV, Greenamyre JT (2000) Chronic systemic pesticide exposure reproduces features of Parkinson's disease. *Nat Neurosci* 3: 1301-1306.

7. Bezard E, Gross CE, Fournier MC, Dovero S, Bloch B, Jaber M (1999) Absence of MPTP-induced neuronal death in mice lacking the dopamine transporter. *Exp Neurol* 155: 268-273.

8. Blum D, Torch S, Lambeng N, Nissou M, Benabid AL, Sadoul R, Verna JM (2001) Molecular pathways involved in the neurotoxicity of 6-OHDA, dopamine and MPTP: contribution to the apoptotic theory in Parkinson's disease. *Prog Neurobiol* 65: 135-172.

9. Blum M (1998) A null mutation in TGF-α leads to a reduction in midbrain dopaminergic neurons in the substantia nigra. *Nat Neurosci* 1: 374-377.

10. Bringmann G, God R, Fahr S, Feineis D, Fornadi K, Fornadi F (1999) Identification of the dopaminergic neurotoxin 1-trichloromethyl-1,2, 3,4-tetrahydro-beta-carboline in human blood after intake of the hypnotic chloral hydrate. *Anal Biochem* 270: 167-175.

11. Bringmann G, God R, Feineis D, Janetzky B, Reichmann H (1995) TaClo as a neurotoxic lead: improved synthesis, stereochemical analysis, and inhibition of the mitochondrial respiratory chain. *J Neural Transm Suppl* 46: 245-254.

12. Cadet JL (2001) Molecular neurotoxicological models of Parkinsonism: focus on genetic manipulation of mice. *Parkinsonism Relat Disord* 8: 85-90.

13. Calabresi P, Saiardi A, Pisani A, Baik JH, Centonze D, Mercuri NB, Bernardi G, Borrelli E (1997) Abnormal synaptic plasticity in the striatum of mice lacking dopamine D2 receptors. *J Neurosci* 17: 4536-4544.

14. Calne DB, Langston JW, Martin WR, Stoessl AJ, Ruth TJ, Adam MJ, Pate BD, Schulzer M (1985) Positron emission tomography after MPTP: observations relating to the cause of Parkinson's disease. *Nature* 317: 246-248.

15. Campbell JM, Gilmore DP, Russell D, Growney CA, Favor G, Weir J, Stone TW, Payne AP (1998) Extracellular levels of dopamine and its metabolite 3,4-dihydroxy-phenylacetic acid measured by microdialysis in the corpus striatum of conscious AS/AGU mutant rats. *Neuroscience* 85: 323-325.

16. Carlsson A, Lundqvist M, Magnusson T (1957) 3,4-Dihydroxyphenylalanine and 5-hydroxy-tryptophan as reserpine antagonists. *Nature* 180: 1200.

17. Chiba K, Trevor A, Castagnoli N, Jr. (1984) Metabolism of the neurotoxic tertiary amine, MPTP, by brain monoamine oxidase. *Biochem Biophys Res Commun* 120: 574-578.

18. Choi WS, Yoon SY, Oh TH, Choi EJ, O'Malley KL, Oh YJ (1999) Two distinct mechanisms are involved in 6-hydroxydopamine- and MPP+- induced dopaminergic neuronal cell death: role of caspases, ROS, and JNK. *J Neurosci Res* 57: 86-94.

19. Craig NJ, Duran Alonso MB, Hawker KL, Shiels P, Glencorse TA, Campbell JM, Bennett NK, Canham M, Donald D, Gardiner M, Gilmore DP, MacDonald RJ, Maitland K, McCallion AS, Russell D, Payne AP, Sutcliffe RG, Davies RW (2001) A candidate gene for human neurodegenerative disorders: a rat PKCgamma mutation causes a Parkinsonian syndrome. *Nat Neurosci* 4: 1061-1062.

20. Duan W, Zhang Z, Gash DM, Mattson MP (1999) Participation of prostate apoptosis response-4 in degeneration of dopaminergic neurons in models of Parkinson's disease. *Ann Neurol* 46: 587-597.

21. Eilam R, Peter Y, Elson A, Rotman G, Shiloh Y, Groner Y, Segal M (1998) Selective loss of dopaminergic nigro-striatal neurons in brains of Atm-deficient mice. *Proc Natl Acad Sci U S A* 95: 12653-12656.

22. Esposito LA, Melov S, Panov A, Cottrell BA, Wallace DC (1999) Mitochondrial disease in mouse results in increased oxidative stress. *Proc Natl Acad Sci U S A* 96: 4820-4825.

23. Feany MB, Bender WW (2000) A Drosophila model of Parkinson's disease. *Nature* 404: 394-398.

24. Forno LS, Norville RL, Langston JW (2001) EM study of nerve cell degeneration in substantia nigra in Parkinson's disease. *Park Dis Relat Disord* 7: S8.

24a. Fowler SC, Zarcone TJ, Vorontsova E, Chen R (2002) Motor and associative deficits in D2 dopamine receptor knockout mice. *Int J Dev Neurosci* 20: 309-321.

25. Gerlach M, Reichmann H, Riederer P (2001) Die Parkinson-Krankheit. In *Grundlagen, Klinik, Therapie* (eds). Springer-Verlag: Wien-New York.

26. German DC, Nelson EL, Liang CL, Speciale SG, Sinton CM, Sonsalla PK (1996) The neurotoxin MPTP causes degeneration of specific nucleus A8, A9 and A10 dopaminergic neurons in the mouse. *Neurodegeneration* 5: 299-312.

27. Ghorayeb I, Fernagut PO, Aubert I, Bezard E, Poewe W, Wenning GK, Tison F (2000) Toward a primate model of L-dopa-unresponsive parkinsonism mimicking striatonigral degeneration. *Mov Disord* 15: 531-536.

27a. Giasson BI, Duda JE, Quinn SM, Zhang B, Trojanowski JQ, Lee VM (2002) Neuronal α-synucleinopathy with severe movement disorder in mice expressing A53T human α-synuclein. *Neuron* 34: 521-533.

28. Giros B, Jaber M, Jones SR, Wightman RM, Caron MG (1996) Hyperlocomotion and indifference to cocaine and amphetamine in mice lacking the dopamine transporter. *Nature* 379: 606-612.

29. Gogos JA, Morgan M, Luine V, Santha M, Ogawa S, Pfaff D, Karayiorgou M (1998) Catechol-O-methyltransferase-deficient mice exhibit sexually dimorphic changes in catecholamine levels and behavior. *Proc Natl Acad Sci U S A* 95: 9991-9996.

30. Gossel M, Schmidt WJ, Loscher W, Zajaczkowski W, Danysz W (1995) Effect of coadministration of glutamate receptor antagonists and dopaminergic agonists on locomotion in monoamine-depleted rats. *J Neural Transm Park Dis Dement Sect* 10: 27-39.

31. Grimsby J, Toth M, Chen K, Kumazawa T, Klaidman L, Adams JD, Karoum F, Gal J, J.C. S (1997) Increased stress response and beta-phenylethylamine in MAOB-deficient mice. *Nat Genet* 17: 206-210.

32. Guehl D, Bezard E, Dovero S, Boraud T, Bioulac B, Gross C (1999) Trichloroethylene and parkinsonism: a human and experimental observation. *Eur J Neurol* 6: 609-611.

33. He Y, Lee T, Leong SK (2000) 6-Hydroxydopamine induced apoptosis of dopaminergic cells in the rat substantia nigra. *Brain Res* 858: 163-166.

33a. Heim C, Sova L, Kurz T, Kolasiewicz W, Schwegler H, Sontag KH (2002) Partial loss of dopaminergic neurons in the substantia nigra, ventrotegmental area and the retrorubral area—model of the early beginning of Parkinson's symptomatology? *J Neural Transm* 109: 691-709.

34. Jackson-Lewis V, Vila M, Djaldetti R, Guegan C, Liberatore G, Liu J, O'Malley KL, Burke RE, Przedborski S (2000) Developmental cell death in dopaminergic neurons of the substantia nigra of mice. *J Comp Neurol* 424: 476-488.

35. Kahle PJ, Neumann M, Ozmen L, Muller V, Jacobsen H, Schindzielorz A, Okochi M, Leimer U, van Der Putten H, Probst A, Kremmer E, Kretzschmar HA, Haass C (2000) Subcellular localization of wild-type

and Parkinson's disease-associated mutant alpha-synuclein in human and transgenic mouse brain. *J Neurosci* 20: 6365-6373.

36. Kholodilov NG, Oo TF, Burke RE (1999) Synuclein expression is decreased in rat substantia nigra following induction of apoptosis by intrastriatal 6-hydroxydopamine. *Neurosci Lett* 275: 105-108.

37. Kokoszka JE, Coskun P, Esposito LA, Wallace DC (2001) Increased mitochondrial oxidative stress in the Sod2 (+/-) mouse results in the age-related decline of mitochondrial function culminating in increased apoptosis. *Proc Natl Acad Sci U S A* 98.

38. Kostic V, Gurney ME, Deng HX, Siddique T, Epstein CJ, Przedborski S (1997) Midbrain dopaminergic neuronal degeneration in a transgenic mouse model of familial amyotrophic lateral sclerosis. *Ann Neurol* 41: 497-504.

39. Kowall NW, Hantraye P, Brouillet E, Beal MF, McKee AC, Ferrante RJ (2000) MPTP induces alpha-synuclein aggregation in the substantia nigra of baboons. *Neuroreport* 11: 211-213.

40. Langston JW, Ballard P, Tetrud JW, Irwin I (1983) Chronic Parkinsonism in humans due to a product of meperidine-analog synthesis. *Science* 219: 979-980.

41. Langston JW, Forno LS, Tetrud J, Reeves AG, Kaplan JA, Karluk D (1999) Evidence of active nerve cell degeneration in the substantia nigra of humans years after 1-methyl-4-phenyl-1,2,3,6-tetrahydropyridine exposure. *Ann Neurol* 46: 598-605.

41a. Lee MK, Stirling W, Xu Y, Xu X, Qui D, Mandir AS, Dawson TM, Copeland NG, Jenkins NA, Price DL (2002) Human α-synuclein-harboring familial Parkinson's disease-linked Ala-53→Thr mutation causes neurodegenerative disease with α-synuclein aggregation in transgenic mice. *Proc Natl Acad Sci U S A* 99: 8968-8973.

42. Liberatore GT, Jackson-Lewis V, Vukosavic S, Mandir AS, Vila M, McAuliffe WG, Dawson VL, Dawson TM, Przedborski S (1999) Inducible nitric oxide synthase stimulates dopaminergic neurodegeneration in the MPTP model of Parkinson disease. *Nat Med* 5: 1403-1409.

43. Lotharius J, O'Malley KL (2000) The parkinsonism-inducing drug 1-methyl-4-phenylpyridinium triggers intracellular dopamine oxidation. A novel mechanism of toxicity. *J Biol Chem* 275: 38581-38588.

44. Lotharius J, O'Malley KL (2000) Role of mitochondrial dysfunction and dopamine-dependent oxidative stress in amphetamine-induced toxicity. *Ann Neurol* 49: 79-89.

44a. Mandel S, Grünblatt E, Maor G, Youdim MBR (2002) Early and late gene changes in MPTP mice model of Parkinson's disease empolying cDNA microarray. *Neurochem Res* 27:1231-1242.

45. Masliah E, Rockenstein E, Veinbergs I, Mallory M, Hashimoto M, Takeda A, Sagara Y, Sisk A, Mucke L (2000) Dopaminergic loss and inclusion body formation in alpha-synuclein mice: implications for neurodegenerative disorders. *Science* 287: 1265-1269.

46. Masliah E, Rockenstein E, Veinbergs I, Sagara Y, Mallory M, Hashimoto M, Mucke L (2001) β-amyloid peptides enhance α-synuclein accumulation and neuronal deficits in a transgenic mouse model linking Alzheimer's disease and Parkinson's disease. *Proc Natl Acad Sci U S A* 98: 12245-12250

47. Matsuoka Y, Vila M, Lincoln S, McCormack A, Picciano M, LaFrancois J, Yu X, Dickson D, Langston WJ, McGowan E, Farrer M, Hardy J, Duff K, Przedborski S, Di Monte DA (2001) Lack of nigral pathology in transgenic mice expressing human alpha-synuclein driven by the tyrosine hydroxylase promoter. *Neurobiol Dis* 8: 535-539.

48. Miller GW, Wang Y-M, Gainetdinov RR, Caron MG (2001) Dopamine transporter and vesicular monoamine transporter knockout mice. In *Parkinson's disease: methods and protocols*, MM Mouradian (eds). Humana Press: Totowa, NJ. pp. 179-190.

48a. McCormack AL, Thiruchelvam M, Manning-Bog AB, Thiffault C, Langston JW, Cory-Slechta DA, Di Monte DA (2002) Environmental risk factors and Parkinson's disease: selective degeneration of nigral dopaminergic neurons caused by the herbicide paraquat. *Neurobiol Dis* 10: 119-127.

49. Moore MW, Klein RD, Farinas I, Sauer H, Armanini M, Phillips H, Reichardt LF, Ryan AM, Carver-Moore K, Rosenthal A (1996) Renal and neuronal abnormalities in mice lacking GDNF. *Nature* 382: 76-79.

49a. Neumann M, Kahle PJ, Ozmen L, Iwatsubo T, Haass C, Kretzschmar HA (2002) Gae-dependent formation of proteinase K resistance and hyperphosphorylation of α-synuclein in transgenic mouse models of synucleinopathies. J Neuropathol Exp Neurol 61: 484.

50. Neystat M, Lynch T, Przedborski S, Kholodilov N, Rzhetskaya M, Burke RE (1999) Alpha-synuclein expression in substantia nigra and cortex in Parkinson's disease. *Mov Disord* 14: 417-422.

51. Nicotra A, Parvez SH (2000) Cell death induced by MPTP, a substrate for monoamine oxidase B. *Toxicology* 153: 157-166.

52. Ohmori T, Abekawa T, Koyama T (1996) The role of glutamate in behavioral and neurotoxic effects of methamphetamine. *Neurochem Int* 29: 301-307.

53. Patil N, Cox DR, Bhat D, Faham M, Myers RM, Peterson AS (1995) A potassium channel mutation in weaver mice implicates membrane excitability in granule cell differentiation. *Nat Genet* 11: 126-129.

54. Pothos EN, Larsen KE, Krantz DE, Liu Y, Haycock JW, Setlik W, Gershon MD, Edwards RH, Sulzer D (2000) Synaptic vesicle transporter expression regulates vesicle phenotype and quantal size. *J Neurosci* 20: 7297-7306.

55. Przedborski S, Levivier M, Jiang H, Ferreira M, Jackson-Lewis V, Donaldson D, Togasaki DM (1995) Dose-dependent lesions of the dopaminergic nigrostriatal pathway induced by intrastriatal injection of 6-hydroxydopamine. *Neuroscience* 67: 631-647.

56. Puschban Z, Scherfler C, Granata R, Laboyrie P, Quinn NP, Jenner P, Poewe W, Wenning GK (2000) Autoradiographic study of striatal dopamine re-uptake sites and dopamine D1 and D2 receptors in a 6-hydroxydopamine and quinolinic acid double-lesion rat model of striatonigral degeneration (multiple system atrophy) and effects of embryonic ventral mesencephalic, striatal or co-grafts. *Neuroscience* 95: 377-388.

57. Puschban Z, Waldner R, Seppi K, Stefanova N, Humpel C, Scherfler C, Levivier M, Poewe W, Wenning GK (2000) Failure of neuroprotection by embryonic striatal grafts in a double lesion rat model of striatonigral degeneration (multiple system atrophy). *Exp Neurol* 164: 166-175.

58. Rathke-Hartlieb S, Kahle PJ, Neumann M, Ozmen L, Haid S, Okochi M, Haass C, Schulz JB (2001) Sensitivity to MPTP is not increased in Parkinson's disease-associated mutant alpha-synuclein transgenic mice. *J Neurochem* 77: 1181-1184.

59. Reader TA, Dewar KM (1999) Effects of denervation and hyperinnervation on dopamine and serotonin systems in the rat neostriatum: implications for human Parkinson's disease. *Neurochem Int* 34: 1-21.

60. Richfield EK, Thiruchelvam M, Ferderoff H, Cory-Slechta D (2002) A transgenic mouse model of the Parkinson's disease phenotype. 7th Europ Congress of Neuropathology, Helsinki, July 13-16, 2002: P G-45.

61. Rios M, Habecker B, Sasaoka T, Eisenhofer G, Tian H, Landis S, Chikaraishi D, Roffler-Tarlov S (1999) Catecholamine synthesis is mediated by tyrosinase in the absence of tyrosine hydroxylase. *J Neurosci* 19: 3519-3526.

61a. Rockenstein E, Mallory M, Hashimoto M, Song D, Shults CW, Lang I, Masliah E (2002) Differential neuropathological alterations in transgenic mice expressing ·-synuclein from the platelet-derived growth factor and Thy-1 promoters. *J Neurosci Res* 68: 568-578.

62. Rothblat DS, Schroeder JA, Schneider JS (2001) Tyrosine hydroxylase and dopamine transporter expression in residual dopaminergic neurons: potential contributors to spontaneous recovery from experimental Parkinsonism. *J Neurosci Res* 65: 254-266.

63. Sachs C, Jonsson G (1975) Mechanisms of action of 6-hydroxydopamine. *Biochem Pharmacol* 24:1-8.

64. Scherfler C, Puschban Z, Ghorayeb I, Goebel GP, Tison F, Jellinger K, Poewe W, Wenning GK (2000) Complex motor disturbances in a sequential double lesion rat model of striatonigral degeneration (multiple system atrophy). *Neuroscience* 99: 43-54.

65. Schmidt N, Ferger B (2001) Neurochemical findings in the MPTP model of Parkinson's disease. *J Neural Transm* 108: 895-1009.

66. Schmidt WJ, Bubser M, Hauber W (1992) Behavioural pharmacology of glutamate in the basal ganglia. *J Neural Transm Suppl* 38: 65-89.

67. Schwarting RK, Huston JP (1996) The unilateral 6-hydroxydopamine lesion model in behavioral brain research. Analysis of functional deficits, recovery and treatments. *Prog Neurobiol* 50: 275-331.

67a. Sherer TB, Betarbet R, Stout AK, Lund S, Baptista M, Panov AV, Cookson MR, Greenamyre JT (2002) An in vitro model of Parkinson's disease: linking mitochondrial impairment to altered α-synuclein metabolism and oxidative damage. *J Neurosci* 22:7006-7015.

68. Shih JC, Chen K, Ridd MJ (1999) Monoamine oxidase: from genes to behavior. *Annu Rev Neurosci* 22: 197-217.

69. Sibley DR (1999) New insights into dopaminergic receptor function using antisense and genetically altered animals. *Annu Rev Pharmacol Toxicol* 39: 313-341.

70. Simon HH, Saueressig H, Wurst W, Goulding MD, O'Leary DD (2001) Fate of midbrain dopaminergic neurons controlled by the engrailed genes. *J Neurosci* 21: 3126-3134.

71. Staal RG, Sonsalla PK (2000) Inhibition of brain vesicular monoamine transporter (VMAT2) enhances 1-methyl-4-phenylpyridinium neurotoxicity in vivo in rat striata. *J Pharmacol Exp Ther* 293: 336-342.

71a. Swerdlow RH, Parks JK, Miller SW, Tuttle JB, Trimmer PA, Sheehan JP, Bennett JP, Davis RE, Parker WD (1996) Origin and functional consequences of the complex I defect in Parkinson's disease. *Ann Neurol* 40: 663-671.

72. Takahashi N, Miner LL, Sora I, Ujike H, Revay RS, Kostic V, Jackson-Lewis V, Przedborski S, Uhl GR (1997) VMAT2 knockout mice: heterozygotes display reduced amphetamine-conditioned reward, enhanced amphetamine locomotion, and enhanced MPTP toxicity. *Proc Natl Acad Sci U S A* 94: 9938-9943.

73. Taylor JR, Elsworth JD, Roth RH, Sladek JRJ, Redmond DEJ (1997) Severe long-term 1-methyl-4-phenyl-1, 2, 3, 6-tetrahydropyridine-induced parkinsonism in the vervet monkey (Cercopithecus aethiops sabaeus). *Neuroscience* 81: 745-755.

74. Tolwani RJ, Jakowec MW, Petzinger GM, Green S, Waggie K (1999) Experimental models of Parkinson's disease: insights from many models. *Lab Anim Sci* 49: 363-371.

74a. Uversky VN, Li J, Fink AL (2001) Pesticides directly accelerate the rate of alpha-synuclein fibril formation: a possible factor in Parkinson's disease. *FEBS Lett* 500:105-108.

74b. Sherere TH, Kim J-H, Betarbet R, Greenamyre JT (2002) Subcutaneous rotenone exposure causes highly selective dopaminergic degeneration and α-synuclein aggregation. *Exp Neurol* 2002 179:9-16.

75. van der Putten H, Wiederhold KH, Probst A, Barbieri S, Mistl C, Danner S, Kauffmann S, Hofele K, Spooren WP, Ruegg MA, Lin S, Caroni P, Sommer B, Tolnay M, Bilbe G (2000) Neuropathology in mice expressing human alpha-synuclein. *J Neurosci* 20: 6021-6029.

76. Varastet M, Riche D, Maziere M, Hantraye P (1994) Chronic MPTP treatment reproduces in baboons the differential vulnerability of mesencephalic dopaminergic neurons observed in Parkinson's disease. *Neuroscience* 63: 47-56.

77. Vila M, Jackson-Lewis V, Vukosavic S, Djaldetti R, Liberatore G, Offen D, Korsmeyer SJ, Przedborski S (2001) Bax ablation prevents dopaminergic neurodegeneration in the 1-methyl-4-phenyl-1,2,3,6-tetrahydropyridine mouse model of Parkinson's disease. *Proc Natl Acad Sci U S A* 98: 2837-2842.

78. Vila M, Vukosavic S, Jackson-Lewis V, Neystat M, Jakowec M, Przedborski S (2000) Alpha-synuclein upregulation in substantia nigra dopaminergic neurons following administration of the parkinsonian toxin MPTP. *J Neurochem* 74: 721-729.

79. Vila M, Wu DC, Prezeborski S (2001) Engineered modeling and the secrets of Parkinon's disease. *TINS* 24 (suppl): 49-55.

80. Waldner R, Puschban Z, Scherfler C, Seppi K, Jellinger K, Poewe W, Wenning GK (2001) No functional effects of embryonic neuronal grafts on motor deficits in a 3-nitropropionic acid rat model of advanced striatonigral degeneration (multiple system atrophy). *Neuroscience* 102: 581-592.

81. Wang L, Andersson S, Warne rM, Gustafsson JA (2001) Morphological abnormalities in the brains of estrogen receptor beta knockout mice. *Proc Natl Acad Sci U S A* 98: 2792-2796.

82. Wang YM, Gainetdinov RR, Fumagalli F, Xu F, Jones SR, Bock CB, Miller GW, Wightman RM, Caron MG (1997) Knockout of the vesicular monoamine transporter 2 gene results in neonatal death and supersensitivity to cocaine and amphetamine. *Neuron* 19: 1285-1296.

83. Wenning GK, R. G, Laboyrie PM, Quinn N, Jenner P, Marsden CD (1996) Reversal of behavioural abnormalities by fetal allografts in a novel rat model of striatonigral degeneration. *Mov Disord* 11: 522-532.

84. Witt TC, Triarhou LC (1995) Transplantation of mesencephalic cell suspensions from wild-type and heterozygous Weaver mice into the denervated striatum: assessing the role of graft-derived dopaminergic dendrites in the recovery of function. *Cell Transplant* 4: 323-333.

85. Yurek DM, Fletcher-Turner A (2001) Differential expression of GDNF, BDNF, and NT-3 in the aging nigrostriatal system following a neurotoxic lesion. *Brain Res* 891: 228-235.

86. Zetterstrom RH, Solomin L, Jansson L, Hoffer BJ, Olson L, Perlmann T (1997) Dopamine neuron agenesis in Nurr1-deficient mice. *Science* 276: 248-250.

87. Zhang J, Graham DG, Montine TJ, Ho YS (2000) Enhanced N-methyl-4-phenyl-1,2,3,6-tetrahydropyridine toxicity in mice deficient in CuZn-superoxide dismutase or glutathione peroxidase. *J Neuropathol Exp Neurol* 59: 53-61.

88. Zhang Y, Gao J, Chung KK, Huang H, Dawson VL, Dawson TM (2000) Parkin functions as an E2-dependent ubiquitin-protein ligase and promotes the degradation of the synaptic vesicle-associated protein, CDCrel-1. *Proc Natl Acad Sci U S A* 97: 13354-13359.

89. Zuscik MJ, Sands S, Ross SA, Waugh DJ, Gaivin RJ, Morilak D, Perez DM (2000) Overexpression of the alpha1B-adrenergic receptor causes apoptotic neurodegeneration: multiple system atrophy. *Nat Med* 6: 1388-1394.

CHAPTER 5

Trinucleotide Repeat Disorders

Chapter Editor: Hidehiro Mizuzawa

5.1 Introduction to Trinucleotide Repeat Disorders 226

5.2 Huntington's Disease 229

5.3 Spinocerebellar Ataxias 242

5.4 Friedreich's Ataxia 257

5.5 Dentatorubral-pallidoluysian Atrophy 269

5.6 Spinal and Bulbar Muscular Atrophy 275

Introduction to Trinucleotide Repeat Disorders

Christopher A. Ross

DRPLA	dentatorubralpallidoluisian atrophy
HD	Huntington's disease
SBMA	spinal and bulbar muscular atrophy
SCA	spinocerebellar ataxia

The class of neurodegenerative disorders caused by expanding triplet repeats is itself rapidly expanding. Several different repeating units of three nucleotides can expand to cause disease. Strikingly almost all of the triplet repeat diseases prominently affect the nervous system. Some of the diseases are developmental such as fragile X syndrome, caused by an expanding CGG repeat. Some have peripheral components, such as myotonic dystrophy, which is caused by an expanding CTG repeat. However most of the diseases are neurodegenerative diseases, and many are caused by expanding CAG repeats coding for polyglutamine.

The characteristic genetic feature of triplet repeat diseases is "anticipation," or earlier age of onset in successive generations within a family. Anticipation was originally postulated to be feature of hereditary psychiatric disease and mental retardation, but in the absence of clear definitions of phenotype and a plausible genetic mechanism, the idea lapsed after the turn of the nineteenth century. In fact, the prominent geneticist Lionel Penrose wrote an article in 1948 dismissing anticipation as an artifact of ascertainment and other biases. It was only with the discovery of the expanding triplet repeats causing SBMA, Fragile X syndrome, myotonic dystrophy, and then a plethora of diseases including Huntington's disease and many forms of spinocerebellar ataxia, that the concept of anticipation regained scientific credit (for review, see 8).

The understanding of the mechanism of expanding triplet repeats explained the feature of anticipation and brought clarity and unity to the genetics to these disorders. However, despite substantial recent progress, their pathogenesis has remained less well understood. Triplet repeat disorders can have a variety of different forms of inheritance, including recessive, autosomal dominant, and X-linked. Similarly, there is considerable variety in pathogenesis. Some disorders, such as Fragile X syndrome and Friedreich's ataxia, appear to be caused by a straightforward loss of function mechanism, in the case of Friedreich's ataxia, correlating well with recessive inheritance. Thus for Friedreich's ataxia an understanding of the pathogenesis of the disorder will hinge upon a full understanding of the normal functions of the gene product, termed frataxin. Interesting clues are emerging regarding its potential role in mitochondrial function and iron metabolism.

By contrast, the class of diseases caused by expanding CAG coding for polyglutamine appears to have a predominantly gain of function mechanism (7, 12, 20, 21). Huntington's disease (HD), for instance, has classic autosomal dominant inheritance. It shows almost complete dominance, with two copies of the mutant allele giving rise to a phenotype very similar to (though perhaps slightly more severe than) that of patients with one copy. Similarly, cell and mouse models are very consistent with a gain of function mechanism. A striking phenotype bearing considerable resemblance to human HD can be produced by insertion of sequences coding for mutant huntingtin the HD gene product into the mouse genome; for reviews see (9, 15). Invertebrate transgenic models have yielded results similar to those in mice. Similarly, neuronal cell death can be produced by transient or stable transfection of mutant huntingtin in cells in culture (2, 11, 16). Similar data have been obtained for a number of the spino-cerebellar ataxias (SCAs). Furthermore, the pathologic hallmark of the disease, consisting of intranuclear inclusions in vivo and protein aggregation in a variety of locations in the cell including the nucleus both in vivo and in vitro, can be produced in these transgenic and cell transfection experiments (2, 3, 4, 16).

However, recent data have also suggested the possibility of loss of function contributing to the phenotype. While huntingtin knockouts are embryonic lethals, a conditional knockout in which huntingtin is deleted from the adult brain strikingly has striatal degeneration, the pathologic hallmark of HD (5). Furthermore, huntingtin may have a neurotrophic function promoting the synthesis of growth factors such as BDNF (22).

SBMA—which is the only polyglutamine disease whose gene product (the androgen receptor) has a well-understood function—may provide a good model for exploring loss of function versus gain of function mechanisms (13). The androgen receptor is a transcription factor and binds to known sequences in promoters. Genes regulated by androgen are becoming increasingly well understood. Models of SBMA, both vertebrate and invertebrate, suggest that loss of function is less critical than gain of function for this disease, and quite possibly for polyglutamine disease in general.

Assuming that a major mechanism for polyglutamine diseases involves a gain of function, what might be that function? Progress is beginning to be made on molecular mechanisms. Recent studies have suggested that interference with gene transcription may be one important mechanism of polyglutamine disease. This interference may involve direct polyglutamine interactions with other transcription factors such as CBP or others (10). Alternatively, there might be interactions not mediated directly by the expanded polyglutamine tract possibly with CBP possibly with transcription factors such as TAF130 p53 Sp1 or others (6, 18, 19). A mechanism involving gene transcription would be consistent with the observation that, for many of the polyglutamine disease gene products, nuclear localization appears to enhance toxicity (11, 16). In addition, if the pathogenesis involves a direct polyglutamine interaction, this could be a common molecular mechanism for all the polyglutamine neurodegenerative diseases.

Another very interesting mechanism, which could also be common to all of these diseases, might be interference with the proteasome (1). The proteasome is a multi-subunit enzyme which cleaves misfolded proteins or proteins targeted for degradation. It has been suggested that proteins with expanded polyglutamines assume a conformation, which can enter the proteasome, but cannot be cleaved, and therefore results in a blockade of proteasome function.

A common feature of all polyglutamine diseases appears to be aggregation of the expanded polyglutamine containing protein. This was first observed in vitro for huntingtin, in the pioneering studies of Erich Wanker's laboratory (17). Strikingly, the threshold for aggregation in vitro--at least for HD, which has been most studied--appears to correspond quite closely to the threshold for disease in vivo. Nevertheless the role of aggregation is still controversial, in part because the intranuclear inclusions, the pathologic hallmarks of the disease, are not necessarily enriched in neurons most vulnerable to the disorders.

The patterns of neuropathology of the different polyglutamine diseases show striking similarities, but also differences (13). In each disorder there are a set of regions preferentially affected. These regions are quite divergent among the different diseases. However there is an overall set of regions which are affected in polyglutamine diseases, but which tend not to be affected in other diseases, such as Alzheimer's disease and Parkinson's disease. For instance, the polyglutamine diseases tend to involve basal ganglia, spinal and brainstem motor nuclei, and cerebellar Purkinje cells or deep cerebellar nuclei. By contrast, they do not preferentially involve hippocampus or basal forebrain, and substantia nigra is less involved than other regions.

Clinically, the features of the diseases follow logically from the areas affected. For instance, Huntington's disease (14) is characterized by chorea, dystonia, incoordination and dementia, reflecting the preferential involvement of basal ganglia and cerebral cortex. Most of the spino-cerebellar ataxias involve prominent cerebellar ataxia, due to cerebellar degeneration plus or minus other syndromes relating to brainstem or other structures. Finally, SBMA involves motor weakness due to bulbar and spinal motor neuron degeneration

These common features highlight 2 of the major questions regarding the pathogenesis of these diseases. Why do they all have delayed onset and selective neuronal degeneration? Investigation into the pathogenesis of these disorders is likely to yield basic mechanistic insight, and ultimately lead to rational treatments. Advances made in the polyglutamine and other triplet repeat diseases are also likely to be applicable to other neurodegenerative diseases.

References

1. Bence NF, Sampat RM, Kopito RR (2001) Impairment of the ubiquitin-proteasome system by protein aggregation. *Science* 292: 1552-1555.

2. Cooper JK, Schilling G, Peters MF, Herring WJ, Sharp AH, Kaminsky Z, Masone J, Khan FA, Delanoy M, Borchelt DR, Dawson VL, Dawson TM, Ross CA (1998) Truncated N-terminal fragments of huntingtin with expanded glutamine repeats form nuclear and cytoplasmic aggregates in cell culture. *Hum Mol Gen* 7: 783-790.

3. Davies SW, Turmaine M, Cozens BA, DiFiglia M, Sharp AH, Ross CA, Scherzinger E, Wanker EE, Mangiarini L, Bates G P (1997) Formation of neuronal intranuclear inclusions (NII) underlies the neurological dysfunction in mice transgenic for the HD mutation. *Cell* 90: 537-548.

4. DiFiglia M, Sapp E, Chase KO, Davies SW, Bates GP, Vonsattel JP, Aronin N (1997) Aggregation of huntingtin in neuronal intranuclear inclusions and dystrophic neurites in brain. *Science* 27: 1990-1993.

5. Dragatsis I, Levine MS, Zeitlin S (2000) Inactivation of Hdh in the brain and testis results in progressive neurodegeneration and sterility in mice. *Nat Genet* 26: 300-306.

6. Dunah AW, Jeong H, Griffin A, Kim YM, Standaert DG, Hersch SM, Mouradian MM, Young AB, Tanese N, Krainc D (2002) Sp1 and TAFII130 transcriptional activity disrupted in early Huntington's disease. *Science* 296: 2238-2243.

7. MacDonald ME, Gusella, JF (1996) Huntington disease: Translating a CAG repeat into pathogenic mechanism. *Curr Opin Neurobiol* 6: 638-643.

8. Margolis RL, McInnis MG, Rosenblatt A, Ross C A (1999) Trinucleotide repeat expansion and neuropsychiatric disease. *Arch Gen Psychiatry* 56: 1019-1031.

9. Menalled LB, Chesselet MF (2002) Mouse models of Huntington's disease. *Trends Pharmacol Sci* 23: 32-39.

10. Nucifora FCJr, Sasaki M, Peters MF, Huang H, Cooper JK, Yamada M, Takahashi H, Tsuji S, Troncoso J, Dawson VL, Dawson TM, Ross CA (2001) Interference by huntingtin and atrophin-1 with cbp-mediated transcription leading to cellular toxicity 1. *Science* 291: 2423-2428.

11. Peters MF, Nucifora FCJr, Kushi J, Seaman HC, Cooper JK, Herring WJ, Dawson VL, Dawson TM, Ross CA (1999) Nuclear targeting of mutant Huntingtin increases toxicity 3. *Mol Cell Neurosci* 14: 121-128.

12. Ross CA (2002) Polyglutamine pathogenesis. Emergence of unifying mechanisms for Huntington's disease and related disorders. *Neuron* 35: 819.

13. Ross CA (1995) When more is less: Pathogenesis of glutamine repeat neurodegenerative diseases. *Neuron* 15: 493-496.

14. Ross CA, Margolis RL, Rosenblatt A, Ranen NG, Becher MW, Aylward E (1997) Reviews in molecular medicine: Huntington disease and the related disorder, dentatorubral-pallidoluysian atrophy (DRPLA). *Medicine* 76: 305-338.

15. Rubinsztein DC (2002) Lessons from animal models of Huntington's disease. *Trends Genet* 18:202-209.

16. Saudou F, Finkbeiner S, Devys D, Greenberg ME (1998) Huntingtin acts in the nucleus to induce apoptosis but death does not correlate with the formation of intranuclear inclusions. *Cell* 95: 55-66.

17. Scherzinger E, Lurz R, Turmaine M, Mangiarini L, Hollenbach B, Hasenbank R, Bates GP, Davies SW, Lerach H, Wanker EE (1997) Huntingtin-encoded polyglutamine expansions form amyloid-like protein aggregates in vitro and in vivo. *Cell* 90: 549-558.

18. Shimohata T, Nakajima T, Yamada M, Uchida C, Onodera O, Naruse S, Kimura T, Koide R, Nozaki K, Sano Y, Ishiguro H, Sakoe K, Ooshima T, Sato A, Ikeuchi T, Oyake M, Sato T, Aoyagi Y, Hozumi I, Nagat-

su T, Takiyama Y, Nishizawa M, Goto J, Kanazawa I, Davidson I, Tanese N, Takahashi H, Tsuji S (2000) Expanded polyglutamine stretches interact with TAFII130, interfering with CREB-dependent transcription. *Nat Genet* 26: 29-36.

19. Steffan JS, Kazantsev A, Spasic-Boskovic O, Greenwald M, Zhu YZ, Gohler H, Wanker EE, Bates GP, Housman DE, Thompson LM (2000) The Huntington's disease protein interacts with p53 and CREB-binding protein and represses transcription. *Proc Natl Acad Sci U S A* 97: 6763-6768.

20. Taylor JP, Hardy J, Fischbeck KH (2002) Toxic proteins in neurodegenerative disease. *Science* 296: 1991-1995.

21. Zoghbi HY, Orr HT (2000) Glutamine repeats and neurodegeneration. *Annu Rev Neurosci* 23: 217-247.

22. Zuccato C, Ciammola A, Rigamonti D, Leavitt BR, Goffredo D, Conti L, MacDonald M E, Friedlander RM, Silani V, Hayden MR, Timmusk T, Sipione S, Cattaneo E (2001) Loss of huntingtin-mediated BDNF gene transcription in Huntington's disease 3. *Science* 293: 493-498.

Huntington's Disease

John C. Hedreen
Raymund A. C. Roos

AMPA	alpha-amino-3-hydroxy-5methylisoxalate-4-proprionic acid
CAP	caudate, accumbens, putamen
CSF	cerebrospinal fluid
CT	computer tomography
DRPLA	dentatorubralpallidoluysian atrophy
GABA	gamma aminobutyric acid
GFAP	glial fibrillary acidic protein
GP	globus pallidus
HD	Huntington's disease
Htt	huntingtin
JHD	juvenile Huntington's disease
MRI	magnetic resonance imaging
NMDA	N-methyl-D-aspartate

Definition

Huntington's disease (HD) is an autosomal dominant neurodegenerative disorder clinically characterised by involuntary movements, cachexia, psychiatric symptoms and dementia. The mean age of onset is 40 years (range: 2-85 years), and the duration of illness is 17 years (range: 2-45 years). The gene for HD (known as IT15), on the short arm of chromosome 4, was discovered in 1993, and the HD mutation was found to be an expanded CAG repeat (79). The discovery of the gene initiated new research on the pathophysiology and provided for predictive presymptomatic testing for HD (66).

Synonyms and Historical Annotations

George Huntington first described HD in 1872 in an essay on chorea. He described a family with chorea in East Hampton, Long Island. He noted the hereditary nature of the disorder, onset in adult life and the tendency to "insanity." Chorea had been described earlier in the century, but Huntington's description linked the clinical syndrome to a hereditary disorder. Given the prominence of chorea as the characteristic motor symptom, it was initially referred to as Huntington's chorea. More recently, however, as the importance of other clinical features was recognised, the name was changed to Huntington's disease.

Epidemiology

HD has a prevalence of 5 to 10 per 100000 in the Western countries. In Japan and Africa the incidence and prevalence is lower compared to other areas of the world. In other parts of the world very little is known about incidence and prevalence of HD. Epidemiologic studies performed before 1993 were based upon the clinical picture, family history and post-mortem pathology and are less accurate, while those after 1993 have greater reliability due to genetic testing (138). Clinical awareness of HD and social and economic factors that promote longevity also influence the epidemiological figures. Based upon data on age at onset and duration of illness, the total number of individuals with the mutated gene is several-fold the number of symptomatic cases (67).

Genetics

HD is an autosomal dominant disorder, and men and women are equally affected. HD is caused by an expanded CAG-repeat in the HD gene on the short arm of chromosome 4 (4p16.3). Normal individuals have stable repeat lengths up to 26, and unstable repeat lengths from 27 to 35. HD is associated with repeat lengths of 36 and above, with lengths 36 to 39 demonstrating incomplete penetrance. Individuals without HD with repeat lengths from 27 to 39 may have children with repeat lengths in the symptomatic range (68). These are so-called "de novo" clinical cases, constituting up to 10% of incident cases (7, 45, 93).

Paternal inheritance is associated with increased likelihood of repeat-length expansion, which leads to an earlier age of onset in the next generation. This phenomenon is referred to as "anticipation" (106). While children from an affected person have a 50% risk at birth, the clinical presentation varies depending the repeat-length. In particular, those patients who develop symptoms before the age of 20 (6% of all cases), the so-called juvenile HD (JHD), more often inherited their gene (75%) from their father.

While an inverse relationship between the repeat-length and age of onset is found (very long repeats are found in JHD), it is not possible to accurately predict the age of onset from the repeat-length. Moreover, there is no clear relationship between the length of the CAG-repeat and other clinical features of HD.

The HD gene is 185 kb and contains 67 exons. Two mRNA transcripts (10.5 and 13.5 kb) encode for the protein huntingtin, a 348 kDa protein. The CAG repeat is in the coding region of the gene and the expansion leads to production of an abnormal huntingtin that contains an expanded polyglutamine stretch near the amino terminus. (CAG encodes for the amino acid glutamine). Huntingtin has a transport function, plays a role in the transcription and is important for neurogenesis. The mutated huntingtin interacts with other proteins (huntingtin associated proteins) probably playing a role in neuronal cell death. The abnormal huntingtin, together with ubiquitin, forms neuronal nuclear inclusions. The exact role of the inclusions is not known (37).

Clinical Features

Signs and symptoms. The patients develop unwanted, unnecessary movements of voluntary muscles termed chorea. Initially this leads to subtle changes in motor behaviour, often explained as nervousness or restlessness. There is an increase of blinking, as well as difficulties with speech and swallowing. Walking becomes unsta-

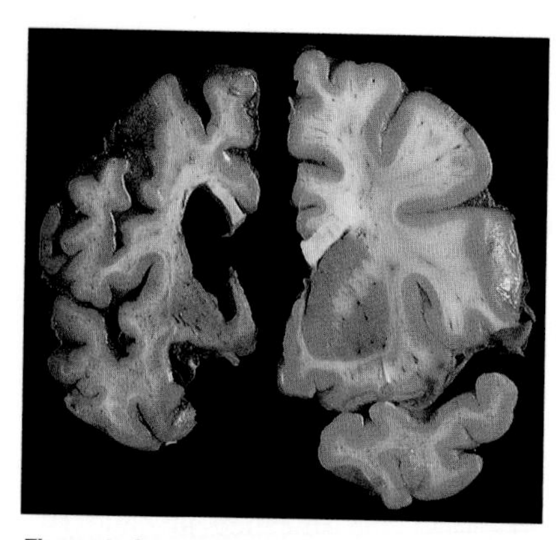

Figure 1. Coronal slices of fixed half-brains at the level of the nucleus accumbens. HD grade 4 is on the left and a normal brain from an individual of similar age is on the right. Note in the HD brain atrophy of cerebral cortex and white matter, severe atrophy of the neostriatum, and marked enlargement of the lateral ventricle.

ble, superficially resembling drunkenness; later leading to near falls and falling. Often the movements are enclosed in socially accepted movements.

In addition to hyperkinetic features, hypokinesia, akinesia, and bradykinesia develop in all stages and at all ages, and often dominate the clinical picture in juvenile HD. The balance between hypokinesia and hyperkinesia is individually determined. All patients in the end develop an akinetic-rigid disorder, making them immobile. Yet even in end stage disease, subtle choreatic movements in the face or extremities can be found. The progression of motor problems leads to clumsiness in daily activities. Activities of daily living are performed slower and eventually the patient becomes totally dependent. Dystonia, tics and myoclonus are also often observed.

On neurological examination, eye movement abnormalities (including disturbed and delayed saccades), motor impersistence of tongue and facial muscles, dysdiadochokinesia, difficulty in walking (especially line-walking), and speech and swallowing difficulties are the main features. All patients lose weight during the course of the disease due to wasting of energy by the movement disorder, difficulty in eating and swallowing, loss of interest in food and changes in hypothalamic function.

Particularly disturbing to patient and family are behavioural and cognitive disorders. In the very early stages of HD, the explanation for these behavioural symptoms may be difficult, because they are nonspecific. The psychiatric manifestations include anxiousness, depression, paranoia, schizophrenia, and phobia. The exact prevalence of the psychiatric symptoms is not known. Mood disorders, especially depression, are most frequent. Suicide is more common in HD than the general population. Patients also develop personality changes, including behaviour disorders thta may be characterised by verbal and physical aggression. Increased irritability can occur very early in the disease, often antedating choreatic movements by years. The personality changes may be characterised by increased assertiveness or apathy. Difficulties in performing job-related functions become manifest due to motor, behavioural and cognitive factors. Many patients retain insight into their mental dysfunction. Changes in language usage and impaired memory retrieval also frequently develop.

Imaging and Laboratory Findings

The diagnosis of HD is based on the clinical features, family history and DNA analysis. For clinical diagnosis, imaging and laboratory tests are not necessary. Atrophy of the basal ganglia and cortex on CT or MRI scans are not specific and not always proportional to the clinical severity. Research methods using SPECT and PET are not yet available for clinical usage.

Macroscopy

Gross findings (Figure 1) upon examination of the fixed postmortem brain depend on the stage of disease. Very early cases may show little or no gross changes. Very advanced cases display severe atrophy of the entire brain. Brain weight is often 900 to 1000 g, and may be as low as 800 g. Such advanced cases display extreme atrophy of the neostriatum, the brain region most affected in HD, whereas other regions of the brain manifest mild to moderate atrophy. As the neostriatum has a volume of no more than 60 cc, the loss of 300 g or more of brain weight clearly demonstrates major involvement of extra-striatal regions in HD. In late stages, atrophy of the cerebral cortex and white matter is evident, greater in frontal, parietal and occipital regions than in the temporal lobe (Figure 1). The globus pallidus, diencephalon, brainstem and cerebellum also display readily apparent atrophy in advanced disease, and the ventricular system is markedly dilated.

Little other gross pathology is noted in most cases. The substantia nigra is usually well pigmented, although the locus coeruleus may show a decrease in pigment in advanced cases. Atherosclerotic pathology of cerebral arteries and cerebral infarcts may be encountered. A few HD patients have received therapeutic intra-striatal transplants and at autopsy islands of transplanted tissue are observed in the striatum (21, 49).

Vonsattel grading. A system for grading pathological severity in postmortem HD brains was introduced in 1985 by Vonsattel et al (153), based partly on macroscopic atrophy of the neostriatum (Figure 2) and partly on microscopic changes in the neostriatum. Assignment of Vonsattel grade is essential for later research use of postmortem tissue. The gross coronal slices are inspected at three levels, and blocks are taken for paraffin embedding at these levels: Level of caudate, accumbens, and putamen (CAP); level of globus pallidus (GP); tail of caudate nucleus (with hippocampus) at the level of the lateral geniculate body. Vonsattel et al (153) described five grades of severity:

Grade 0. No gross changes from normal are noted. The diagnosis of HD is here based on clinical history, family history, and DNA test results. With a positive DNA test in an at-risk individual, the category of grade 0 may be extended to include those with the mutation who had not displayed clinical signs up to the time of death (122). It should be noted that quantitative measures of striatal volume in MRI studies have shown atrophy in preclinical stages (11-13). Absence of atrophy should therefore not be regarded as an absolute requisite criterion for grade 0 or grade 1.

Grade 1. Atrophy at the CAP level is still not obvious on gross inspection of brain slices, and assignment to grade 1 depends on microscopic changes. The tail and body of the caudate nucleus may show grossly appreciable atrophy at this stage.

Grade 2. Atrophy of the neostriatum at the CAP level is now clear-cut on gross inspection, although the head of the caudate retains a mildly bulging, convex border with the lateral ventricle.

Grade 3. Atrophy is marked, especially in dorsal (superior) regions of neostriatum, and there is now an approximately straight border between the head of the caudate nucleus and the lateral ventricle.

Grade 4. Further atrophy of the caudate nucleus and the putamen produces a concave, wrinkled, caudate-ventricular border. There is a greater degree of atrophy in dorsal than in ventral regions, reflecting relative preservation of the nucleus accumbens even at advanced stages.

The Vonsattel grade of disease severity in postmortem brains has a significant correlation with measures of clinical progression determined at the last clinical examination before death (113, 153). The introduction of the Vonsattel grading system proved to be a powerful aid to research for investigators using postmortem tissue, allowing more sophisticated experimental designs than simply comparing data from control and disease brains.

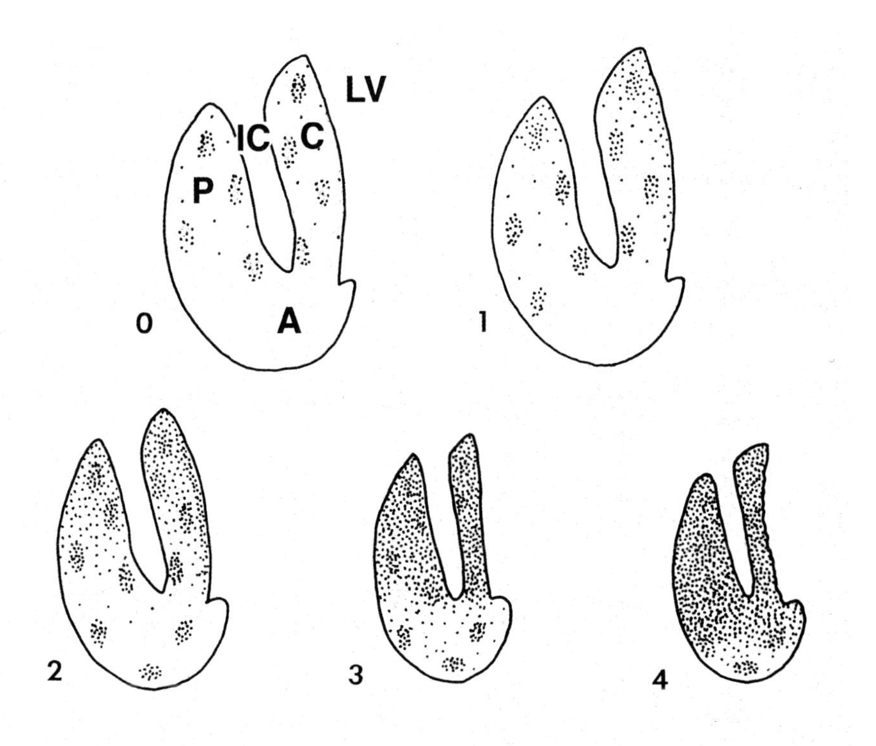

Figure 2. Diagram of neostriatum at the nucleus accumbens level showing Vonsattel grades 0 to 4. The lateral ventricle (LV) is on the right and the internal capsule (IC) separates the caudate nucleus (C) and the putamen (P). The nucleus accumbens (A) is below the internal capsule. Note progressive atrophy and change of the curve at the interface between head of caudate and lateral ventricle. Dots indicate loss of neostriatal medium spiny neurons with associated fibrillary astrocytosis. Striosome involvement (small groups of dots) and light matrix involvement is indicated from grade 0 forward. Severe involvement of the matrix begins at the top of the caudate nucleus and putamen in grade 1 and progresses ventrally through grade 4.

Histopathology

Histopathological findings also depend markedly on the stage of disease.

Neostriatum. The most severe histological changes in the brain occur in the neostriatum. Initially, medium spiny neurones are affected and other neurone types are relatively preserved until later stages (91, 150). Among medium spiny neurones, those in the striosomal compartment and those containing the peptide enkephalin are most susceptible. Neuronal loss is accompanied by reactive astrocytosis and microgliosis (71, 131, 153). The most thorough description of neostriatal histopathology is that of Vonsattel et al (153). These investigators examined 159 brains of individuals with HD and classified them by severity into 5 grades as described above (see also [150]). Histological changes that characterize the different grades are as follows:

Grade 0. Qualitative microscopic examination of H&E-stained sections at the 3 standard levels does not reveal any readily identifiable changes. As described below, immunocytochemical studies reveal neuronal and synaptic terminal loss limited to the striosomal compartment of the neostriatum (69, 71). Vonsattel et al (153), by cell counting, found that neuronal loss in the neostriatum was present in grade 0 cases before such cell loss was discernible on qualitative microscopic inspection. An increase in the density of oligodendroglia in the neostriatum is present at this stage, and immunohistochemistry will reveal intranuclear inclusions in neurons (55).

Grade 1. Neuronal loss and an accompanying fibrillary astrocytosis are present in the dorsomedial region of the head of the caudate nucleus, in the tail and body of the caudate nucleus, and in the dorsalmost putamen. Attempted diagnosis based on microscopic identification of apparently typical very early changes can be mistaken (55), perhaps because the dorsalmost parts of the normal head of the caudate and putamen contain many entering corticostriatal fibers and have a lower density of neurons, and because occasional reactive astrocytes may be present in non-HD postmortem neostriatum. Early grade 1 changes are better revealed by immunohistochemi-

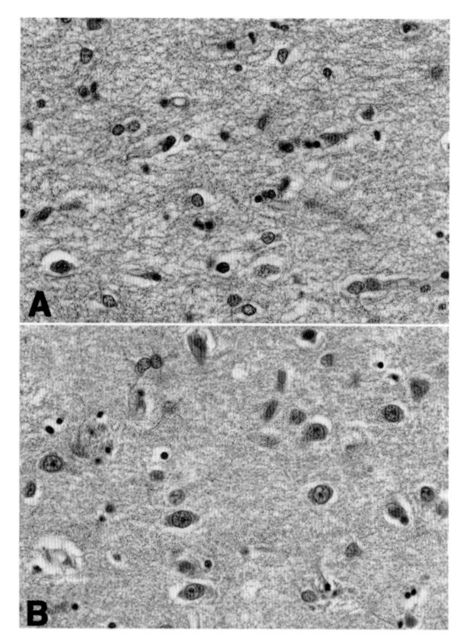

Figure 3. Photomicrographs of neostriatal matrix in upper (**A**) and lower (**B**) head of caudate nucleus in grade 2 HD. Note severe loss of neurons and prominent fibrillary astrocytosis in **A**, whereas **B** shows little change from normal neostriatum. Hematoxylin and eosin (H&E), ×400.

cal reaction for glial fibrillary acidic protein, huntingtin, or ubiquitin (55, 70, 71).

Grade 2. Changes seen in grade 1 extend ventrolaterally in the caudate nucleus and ventrally in the putamen, but the ventralmost putamen at the CAP level and the nucleus accumbens remain relatively free of these changes (Figure 3). Pencil bundles of Wilson are white matter bundles in the neostriatum that contain myelinated axons of medium spiny neurones. In the dorsal striatal regions depleted of most medium spiny neurones, the pencil bundles show marked myelin depletion and increased density of oligodendrocytes.

Grade 3. Severe neurone loss and astrocytosis now involves most of the caudate nucleus and putamen. The nucleus accumbens is still relatively intact, although some pathological changes may be evident, especially with immunohistochemical methods. Some regions of the ventral putamen at the CAP level remain relatively spared.

Grade 4. Severe atrophy, neuronal loss, and astrocytosis affect all of the caudate nucleus and putamen, and these changes extend to a variable

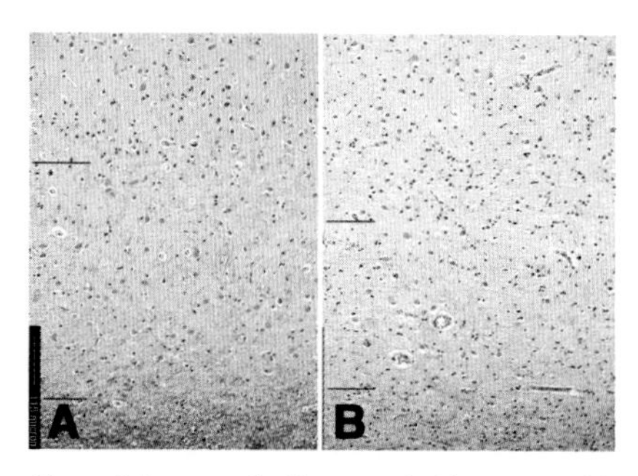

Figure 4. Lower cortical layers and white matter, middle frontal gyrus, in normal (**A**) and grade 4 HD (**B**) brains. The horizontal lines indicate the layer IV-V and Layer VI-white matter boundaries. Note significant atrophy of layers V-VI and loss of neurons in these layers in advanced HD. H&E, ×100, vertical bar in A is 115 μm.

extent down into the nucleus accumbens.

The distribution by grade of a series of postmortem brains is obviously arbitrary, the fraction in earlier grades depending on the incidence of accidents and other causes of death. Grades 0 and 1 represent early stages of the disease, whereas grades 3 and 4 represent terminal stages. Some grade 2 brains are from patients who would have progressed to grade 3 or 4 if their lives had not been cut short, but many are from older individuals with late onset disease whose clinical course was 15 years or more.

Severe neostriatal neuronal loss progresses from the tail of the caudate nucleus to the body to the head, and also in a dorsomedial to ventrolateral direction. The corresponding severe neurone loss in the putamen progresses from caudal to rostral and from dorsal to ventral (128, 151). The nucleus accumbens is relatively spared even at advanced stages. The caudal to rostral and dorsal to ventral progression of neostriatal pathology is a pathognomonic diagnostic feature of HD. There is as yet no pathophysiological explanation for this differential vulnerability. The severe neurone loss is accompanied by a prominent fibrillary astrocytosis. In early stages, neurone loss occur more prominently in the neostriatal striosomes (see section on immunohistochemistry) with fairly vigorous astrocytosis, and more subtly in the matrix, accompanied by scattered reactive astrocytes. The early neurone loss in the striosomes is difficult to discern in routinely stained preparations, but can readily be demonstrated in hematoxylin-counterstained sections immunostained for calbindin, a marker of the striosomal-matrix compartments (71) (Figure 5C).

Cerebral neocortex. Microscopic inspection of the cerebral neocortex in advanced cases will often show thinning of the cortical strip and readily discernible loss of neurons in deep layers (Figure 4). This finding is also observed in the entorhinal cortex. Morphometric studies show thinning of the cerebral cortex, thinning of cortical layers III, V, and especially VI, and neuron loss in the same layers, maximal in layer VI (38, 72, 75, 140). There is no readily apparent astrocytic response, but morphometry reveals an increase in glial size (125).

Hippocampal formation, including entorhinal cortex. Although this region of the brain was long thought to be highly resistant in HD, 2 studies have provided evidence of neuronal loss in advanced cases. Braak and Braak (23) described a severe depletion of neurones in the most basal layer of the entorhinal cortex, and Spargo et al (141) reported a significantly reduced neuronal density in the hippocampal CA1 field in HD compared to control brains.

Amygdala. The amygdala may undergo moderate atrophy in advanced HD with mild apparent neurone loss but no quantitative studies of neuronal number have been reported.

Basal forebrain. Neurones of the nucleus basalis of Meynert appear to be present in normal numbers in HD (32, 102, 144).

Globus pallidus. The globus pallidus is atrophic in advanced cases and is the site of considerable Wallerian degeneration of striatal axons consequent to death of medium spiny striatal neurones. A mild astrocytic reaction may be seen, presumably secondary to Wallerian degeneration, but possibly also associated with mild to moderate pallidal neuronal loss (94, 95). In advanced cases, in sections stained with H&E and Luxol fast blue a moderate to severe decrease in myelin staining is observed. This change is more prominent in the external than in the internal pallidal segment.

Thalamus and subthalamus. The small internuncial neurones of the ventrolateral nucleus of the thalamus are reported to undergo a marked decrease in number relative to the number of large thalamocortical neurones (41). Neurone loss in the mediodorsal nucleus and centromedian-parafascicular complex has also been described (73, 74). The subthalamic nucleus undergoes a modest decline in neuronal number, but this is not easily detected as it is accompanied by atrophy of similar degree (94).

Hypothalamus. The lateral tuberal nucleus shows a severe loss of neurones (92).

Substantia nigra and midbrain. The substantia nigra, like the globus pallidus, receives a heavy axonal input from neostriatal neurones that degenerate in HD and is the site of atrophy, Wallerian degeneration with associated myelin pallor, and astrocytosis. Both pigmented and nonpigmented nigral neurones are reported to be significantly lower in number in HD than in controls (119). Other midbrain regions show no obvious histological change, despite substantial atrophy in advanced disease.

Pons, medulla and spinal cord. The nucleus pontis centralis caudalis in HD brains has fewer large neurones than controls (90). Neurones of the locus coeruleus and dorsal raphe were reported to be normal in number (102), whereas another study (169) demonstrated loss of rostral locus coeruleus neurones but not dorsal raphe neurones in severely demented Huntington's disease patients, whereas mildly demented patients showed no neuronal loss. No histopathological changes in spinal cord have been described.

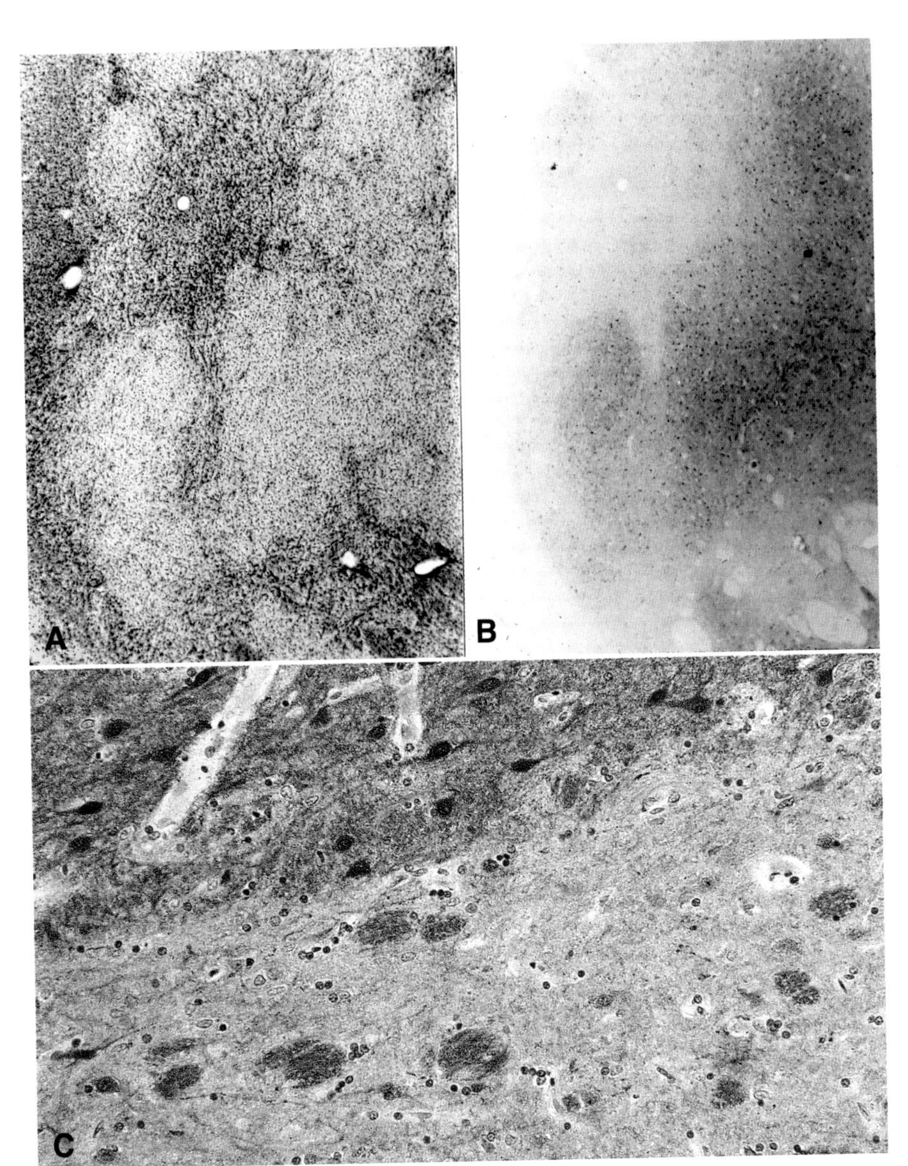

Figure 5. A, B. Adjacent sections from lower putamen at nucleus accumbens level in grade 2 HD. **A.** Glial fibrillary acidic protein (GFAP) immunocytochemistry, ×20. **B.** Calbindin immunocytochemistry, ×20. In both **A** and **B** the external capsule is on the left, and is well stained for GFAP. Striosomes in the putamen, indicated by lack of calbindin staining in **B**, are highly gliotic in **A**. **C.** Ventral putamen in grade 2 HD, immunostained for calbindin with hematoxylin counterstain. The matrix (above) is well stained, with many strongly immunoreactive medium spiny neurons. A striosome (below) contains glia, and some calbindin-immunoreactive bundles of white matter, but few neurons. ×200.

Cerebellum. The cerebellum is often atrophied and Purkinje cell density may be moderately decreased in advanced HD (83, 151).

Other pathological findings. Mild and occasionally advanced changes of Alzheimer's disease are present in a proportion of HD brains, just as in non-HD control brains in the same age range. Infarcts may be present, and may interfere with diagnostic evaluation when they occur in the neostriatum.

Immunohistochemistry and Ultrastructural Findings

The specific type of neostriatal neurone vulnerable in HD is the medium-spiny GABAergic projection neurone (59). This is the type-I neuron of Braak and Braak (22). These cells constitute ~95% of neostriatal neurones and contain either enkephalin or substance P; enkephalin-containing neurones send their axons principally to the external pallidum and substance P-containing neurones to the internal pallidum and substantia nigra pars reticulata and

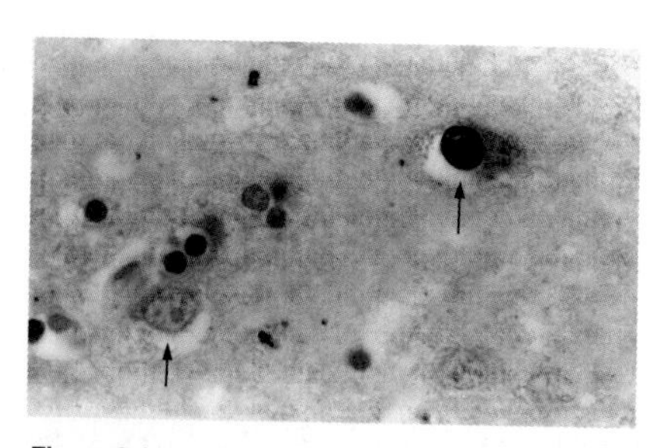

Figure 6. Intranuclear inclusion in neostriatal medium spiny neuron (upper right). Another medium spiny neuron (lower left) appears normal. Ubiquitin immunocytochemistry, with hematoxylin counterstain. ×400.

pars compacta (53). As judged by the relative decrease in immunostaining of terminals in target regions, the medium spiny neurones containing enkephalin suffer first (126).

Glial fibrillary acidic protein immunocytochemistry readily demonstrates the dorsal to ventral wave of progressive pathological change described by Vonsattel et al (71). In addition, small islands of neuronal loss and astrocytosis are seen throughout the caudate nucleus and putamen at the grade 0 stage and in later grades in the regions ventral to, and not yet affected by, the wave of severe, generalised neuronal loss. These islands were noted to be of the same size and distribution as the striosomes described by Graybiel and Ragsdale (60). The striosomal compartment contains neurones that receive input predominantly from limbic regions of cerebral cortex, and the striosomal medium spiny neurones project heavily to the pars compacta of the substantia nigra.

Immunocytochemical studies using antibodies to enkephalin and to calbindin, markers that differentiate striosomal and matrix compartments of neostriatum, demonstrated the identity of the islands with striosomes (Figure 5C). Thus the striosomal compartment loses a large fraction of its medium spiny neurones in advance of the matrix compartment (69). As the latter has a much larger number of neurones, it cannot be ruled out that early matrix loss may exceed in absolute numbers that in the striosomes. Goto et al (56, 57) described loss of the medium spiny neurone marker calcineurin and of the synaptic terminal marker synaptophysin in striosome-like neostriatal patches in early to middle stages of disease. Early loss of NADPH diaphorase neuropil in the striosomes was reported by Morton et al (112), and Augood et al (10) described a patchy loss of neostriatal enkephalin messenger RNA in very early HD that also likely reflects a striosome-specific pathology. Medium spiny neurones with DNA fragmentation can be demonstrated in the neostriatum in HD brain (124). They are maximal in superior parts of putamen and caudate nucleus in grade 3 cases, and therefore do not correlate with early changes.

Islands of relatively preserved neostriatum may be observed in the putamen in grade 3 cases (152). These islands occur in the matrix (71), and may represent "matrisomes" of Graybiel (46, 47).

The cerebral cortex in HD shows a decrease in immunoreactivity for synaptophysin (166), and a decrease in neurones immunopositive for non-phosphorylated neurofilament protein (36, 100).

Immunohistochemical studies with antibodies to the huntingtin protein have shown only minor differences in protein distribution between normal and HD brains (58, 133). The distribution of huntingtin mRNA and protein does not match that of the vulnerable neurones in HD. Studies with antibodies to N-terminal regions of huntingtin and to ubiquitin have revealed small intranuclear inclusions in some neurones of the neostriatum (Figure 6), cerebral cortex, and hippocampal formation (19, 40, 65, 70, 99, 137). A few nuclear inclusions were found also in neurones of the amygdala, red nucleus and dentate nucleus. They were absent in neurones of the thalamus, pallidum, substantia nigra, cerebellar cortex, and inferior olive, despite strong immunostaining for huntingtin in many of these neurones in normal and HD brains (58, 133).

Ultrastructural studies in HD have also revealed the neuronal intranuclear inclusions (40, 127). Neuronal intranuclear inclusions analogous to those of HD characterise other CAG triplet repeat expansion diseases and have been the subject of intensive recent investigation in animal and cell culture models (15, 104, 117, 130). The density of the intranuclear inclusions in the neocortex correlates with the CAG repeat length (19, 137). The intranuclear inclusions are present even in presymptomatic cases (55), and are diagnostically important in such cases.

Dystrophic neurites containing huntingtin and ubiquitin are found in the same regions of brain as the intranuclear inclusions, namely cerebral cortex, allocortex, and neostriatum (19, 27, 40, 58, 80, 99, 133). Both intranuclear inclusions and dystrophic neurites occur in regions affected by neurone loss in HD. The intranuclear inclusions are consequently suspected of being markers for an intracellular toxic process, and the dystrophic neurites markers for axonal dysfunction and degeneration.

Biochemistry

The dysfunction and eventual degeneration and disappearance of neurones lead directly to changes in levels of the receptors and neurotransmitters of these neurones, and indirectly to reactive changes in functional activity and levels of receptors and other biochemical moieties in other neurones of the same neural circuit. Thus, in HD a loss of enkephalin-containing striatopallidal GABAergic inhibitory neurones in the neostriatum leads directly to a decrease in enkephalin and GABA levels in the neostriatum and in the external pallidum (164). External pallidal neurones display increased levels of GABA receptors in reaction to loss of GABAergic input (54). Loss of neostriatal substance P-containing GABAergic neurons projecting to the substantia nigra pars reticulata results directly in lower levels of substance P and GABA in the striatum and pars reticulata, and indirectly to an increase in postsynaptic GABA receptors on pars reticulata neurones. Loss of striosomal neurones that project to the substantia nigra pars compacta would likely result directly in loss of GABA and substance P in the neostriatal striosomes and in the pars compacta. Being freed of inhibitory input, the postsynaptic neurones in globus pallidus and substantia nigra are presumed to become more active.

In the neocortex, the cause of neuronal loss in HD, as in the neostriatum, is uncertain, and its elucidation in relation to the abnormal huntingtin protein remains for the future. Participation of excitotoxicity via glutamatergic receptors in neuronal loss in HD has been a major theme in theories of pathogenesis. Wagster et al (155) found a depletion of kainate and AMPA but not NMDA glutamatergic receptors in deep layers of cerebral cortex, suggesting the special vulnerability of cortical neurones bearing the kainate and AMPA receptors. A similar vulnerability may exist in the neostriatum, although evidence has also been presented for selective vulnerability of NMDA receptor bearing neurones (151).

Differential Diagnosis

Because the pathological changes in HD are highly specific, and DNA studies of CAG repeat length during life are becoming more common, postmortem differential diagnosis does not often pose difficulties. The obvious exception is the very early case (grade 0 or early grade 1) without a definite clinical/DNA diagnosis. In addition to possible neurone loss and fibrillary astrocytosis in the tail of the caudate nucleus and dorsalmost head of caudate and putamen, such cases will likely display neuronal intranuclear inclusions in the neostriatum and cerebral cortex (55).

As a rule, other diseases that pathologically affect the neostriatum, including frontotemporal dementia and Pick's disease, do not display the characteristic preferential involvement of dorsal and caudal regions found in HD (150). In addition to very early cases, the neuropathologist will encounter differential diagnostic issues in 3 situations:

Clinical diagnosis of HD, another pathological diagnosis. Non-HD choreatic diseases such as benign familial chorea, senile chorea (50), mitochondrial chorea and dementia, Sydenham's chorea, neuroacanthocytosis, antiphospholipid antibody syndrome, and dentatorubral-pallidoluysian atrophy (DRPLA) may occasionally receive the clinical diagnosis of HD. These diseases have a distinct pattern of neuropathology and do not show the characteristic dorsal-predominant neostriatal pathology of HD.

Non-Huntington clinical diagnosis, pathological diagnosis of HD. The neuropathologist must also be alert for the occasional autopsy case of HD that has a non-HD premortem diagnosis, such as Alzheimer's disease, in individuals in whom the movement disorder is not prominent. Another category of cases that may yield an unexpected pathological diagnosis of early grade HD is that of the clinically unaffected at-risk HD family member (55, 122). Repeat length analysis is an invaluable additional test in both situations, even when the pathological changes appear to be pathognomonic, as the postmortem diagnosis will be an unwelcome surprise to both family and clinician. A diagnostic repeat length test must be arranged between family and clinician, and is not ordered independently by the pathologist (6, 121, 147).

Clinical and pathological HD phenotype, but normal repeat lengths. When the repeat length test became available, large-scale analyses of HD clinic populations revealed small numbers with a clinical diagnosis of HD but with normal CAG repeat lengths in the huntingtin gene. Some of these individuals were soon diagnosed by DNA studies with other diseases such as DRPLA, but others remain undiagnosed (7, 8, 85, 103, 122, 129, 154, 161, 162). Some have atypical or vague clinical histories, but three of these who came to autopsy had relatively typical HD-like postmortem pathology, including the requisite dorsoventral gradation, although cerebellar pathology was also noted in two (122). Some with HD-like histories who have come to autopsy have non-HD pathology, but one individual with HD-like symptoms but normal repeat lengths showed changes characteristic of grade 1 HD (162) and others showed neostriatal pathology at least somewhat similar to that of HD (103, 161). Repeat length test arranged between family and clinician is highly desirable in cases that have atypical clinical or pathological features, especially cerebellar signs or pathology (154).

Experimental Models

Prior to the discovery of the huntingtin gene, experimental animal models of HD replicated striatal medium spiny neurone death by injection of excitotoxins (25, 33). Recent work has concentrated on use of mitochondrial toxins that also preferentially affect medium spiny neurones (25).

After the discovery of the huntingtin gene, a considerable research effort began to elucidate the function of huntingtin protein and to determine the pathophysiological mechanisms by which the expanded glutamine stretch in about half of the protein produced is able to cause, over decades, a slowly progressive toxic effect on neostriatal and other neurones (148). Mouse models expressing huntingtin with the expanded glutamine stretch have been developed, initially by Bates et al (101). Non-mammalian in vivo models in Drosophila and Caenorhabditis elegans have recently been introduced. In vitro cell preparations have also been used extensively. The use of these models has been recently reviewed (17, 84, 96, 108, 117, 135, 139, 148, 167).

Pathogenesis

Clinicopathological correlation. Classic diagnostic features of the clinical syndrome of HD, including chorea, subtle non-choreatic movement difficulties, minor cognitive deterioration, and psychiatric or behavioral problems, are already present early in the disease course. Brains of patients with classic symptomatology who have died early in the course of their disease demonstrate only grade 0 or early grade 1 pathology. In contrast, the classically described postmortem pathology, grades 3 and 4, corresponds to late clinical stages. A characteristic feature of late pathology, the dorsal to ventral progression of severe neostriatal neurone loss, does not have a clinical counterpart. There is an inverted somatotopic motor representation in the putamen (4, 34, 35), but chorea does not affect legs first, then arms, and finally face. Furthermore, although advanced HD is characterized by massive loss of neostriatal neurons, it has been known for decades (39, 160) that a destructive lesion of the neostriatum in experimental animals does not cause chorea. These observations suggest that earlier, more subtle pathological and pathophysiological changes may give rise to the classical symptomatology, and that severe loss of neostriatal neurons, ie, classic late stage pathology, corresponds instead to the terminal, bedridden, rigid clinical state.

An explanation for early symptomatology in the face of minimal histopathology was provided by Young, Penney, Reiner, Albin, and colleagues (1, 3, 126). In immunocytochemical preparations, they found a decline compared to controls in enkephalin-labeled axons terminating in the external pallidum in grade 2 and even in grade 0 HD, whereas substance P-labeled axons in the internal pallidum were relatively intact. They concluded that there was initially a selective dysfunction and loss of enkephalin-containing striatal neurones followed later in the disease course by dysfunction and loss of substance P neurones. This finding suggested a functional mechanism whereby disinhibition of external pallidal neurones might lead to hyperexcitability of pallidoreceptive thalamocortical neurones, causing chorea. An influential model of pathologic basal ganglia circuit function in HD based on this finding was proposed by Albin et al (2). The possibility that early loss or dysfunction of enkephalin-containing neurones occurs primarily in the striosomal compartment was suggested by the findings of Augood et al (10), who reported striosome-like zones of decreased enkephalin mRNA in the neostriatum of early HD brains.

As the striosomal system undergoes degeneration in the early clinical stages of HD (71), this degeneration might be thought to be responsible for at least some of the early symptomatology. In contrast, the dorsal-to-ventral wave of severe degeneration described by Vonsattel et al (153) must involve predominantly matrix neurones and does not affect a significant portion of the neostriatum until grade 2. A modified model of altered function in the basal ganglia circuit in early stages based on the finding of early striosomal involvement was proposed by Hedreen and Folstein (71). This model postulates increased striatal dopamine release secondary to disinhibition of the nigral pars compacta caused by loss of GABAergic afferents from striosomal neurones. Some support for the presence of a hyperdopaminergic state in early HD has been provided by studies of dopamine metabolites in the cerebrospinal fluid (51), and dopamine receptor blockers are a commonly used therapy. Levels of striatal dopamine receptors are decreased in early stages (9, 24, 158), consistent with an effect of excessive striatal dopamine levels. In experimental studies, dopamine has been suggested to be part of the mechanism of cell death in HD (81, 123).

Regional vulnerability. It remains a mystery why neostriatal medium spiny neurones, especially those containing enkephalin, are more vulnerable than other neurones (110, 136), and both the differential striosome-matrix vulnerability and the dorsal-to-ventral progression of pathology are unexplained. As the huntingtin protein itself is widely distributed, it has been postulated that other proteins, that interact with huntingtin but do not share its wide distribution, may determine the regional vulnerability. In addition, different afferent synaptic connections of the more and less vulnerable neurone populations may play a part. One recent paper perhaps relevant to this issue reports that proteolysis of huntingtin produces different peptide products in striatum than in cerebral cortex (109). Another describes a failure by ailing corticostriatal neurones to deliver growth factors to medium spiny neurones in the neostriatum (168).

Excitotoxicity and mitochondrial damage. In support of the excitotoxic model, it has been shown that the relative susceptibility of the different types of neostriatal neurones to some excitotoxins is similar to that observed in HD (25). Striosomes have been shown to contain higher levels of kainate receptors (43, 44), suggesting the possible involvement of an excitotoxic mechanism in their early vulnerability. The putative excitotoxic effect may occur in the context of decreased ATP levels secondary to mitochondrial functional decline (61, 115). Interactions between mutant huntingtin, glutamatergic receptors, glutamate uptake, and excitotoxicity have been discovered (97, 143, 165). The timing of the appearance of mitochondrial abnormalities in human disease and in a mouse model has been studied (62). Candidate pathogenetic mechanisms involving energy depletion, oxidative stress, and excitotoxicity have recently been reviewed (25, 26, 61, 149)

Molecular pathogenesis. A variety of themes have been pursued in the various experimental models that express abnormal huntingtin protein and in studies using postmortem tissue (84, 117, 148). Subjects of investigation have included aggregation of proteins with long polyglutamine tracts (156, 157), caspases that cut a toxic fragment containing the expanded glutamine sequence from the mutated huntingtin protein (84, 89, 159), the interaction of normal and mutated huntingtin with other proteins (63, 120), their relation to cytoplasmic perikaryal, axonal, and synaptic functions (87, 98), their relationship to nuclear functions and the formation of nuclear aggregates (84, 88, 104, 117, 130, 148), altered glutamatergic receptor function in the neostriatum (28, 30), and dopamine as a potential neurotoxin (81, 123).

Attention has recently been focussed on 2 potential pathogenetic mechanisms, both of which are consistent with the long, slow course of neurotoxicity that takes place in human brain. One is the likely deterioration in normal cell functions consequent to binding of transcription factors and related proteins by huntingtin with an expanded glutamine tract (29, 52, 104, 105, 116). The second is the functional impairment of the proteasome-ubiquitin system by mutated huntingtin (20, 82, 84, 104). These 2 proposed mechanisms may overlap, as many transcription factors are regulated by ubiquitination (146).

Future Directions and Therapy

Current therapy of HD is directed at improving quality of life by symptomatic treatment with medication on the one hand and improving living circumstances on the other. Involuntary movements are treated with dopamine receptor blocking agents. The psychiatric symptoms are treated, depending on the kind of symptom and the severity with anxiolytics, antidepressants, and neuroleptic drugs. Besides medication, advice and support for patient and family are essential (48, 66, 114, 134).

New experimental developments include surgical implantation of foetal cells, and potentially of stem cells (14, 21, 42, 49). Current research on pathogenetic mechanisms using animal and cell culture models will continue, as elucidation of toxic mechanisms is the key to devising future therapeutic strategies (5, 18, 31, 76, 78, 86, 107, 108, 118, 142, 145, 163). Therapies are most beneficially aimed at the earliest pathogenic steps, and least at the endpoints of the pathogenetic process (64). Thus, potential therapies that prevent transcription and translation of the mutant allele would provide the most desirable approach. In contrast, therapies that merely attempt to replace neurotransmitters of dead and dying neurones or to adjust for transmitter imbalances would be less optimal, although they may still have very important symptomatic benefits.

In conclusion, the clinical aims in current research studies will be: *i)* preventing onset of clinical symptoms, *ii)* slowing or stopping progression of the disease, and *iii)* restoring function. Although the first trial interventions in patient groups are not yet successful, experimental studies in animal models give hope for the development of new compounds for use in patients with HD.

References

1. Albin RL, Reiner A, Anderson KD, Dure LS IV, Handelin B, Balfour R, Whetsell WO, Jr., Penney JB, Young AB (1992) Preferential loss of striato-external pallidal projection neurons in presymptomatic Huntington's disease. *Ann Neurol* 31: 425-430.

2. Albin RL, Young AB, Penney JB (1989) The functional anatomy of basal ganglia disorders. *Trends Neurosci* 12: 366-375.

3. Albin RL, Young AB, Penney JB, Handelin B, Balfour R, Anderson KD, Markel DS, Tourtellotte WW, Reiner A (1990) Abnormalities of striatal projection neurons and N-methyl-D-aspartate receptors in presymptomatic Huntington's disease. *N Engl J Med* 322: 1293-1298.

4. Alexander GE, DeLong MR (1985) Microstimulation of the primate neostriatum. II. Somatotopic organization of striatal microexcitable zones and their relation to neuronal response properties. *J Neurophysiol* 53: 1417-1430.

5. Alexi T, Borlongan CV, Faull RL, Williams CE, Clark RG, Gluckman PD, Hughes PE (2000) Neuroprotective strategies for basal ganglia degeneration: Parkinson's and Huntington's diseases. *Prog Neurobiol* 60: 409-470.

6. Almqvist EW, Bloch M, Brinkman R, Craufurd D, Hayden MR (1999) A worldwide assessment of the frequency of suicide, suicide attempts, or psychiatric hospitalization after predictive testing for Huntington disease. *Am J Hum Genet* 64: 1293-1304.

7. Almqvist EW, Elterman DS, MacLeod PM, Hayden MR (2001) High incidence rate and absent family histories in one quarter of patients newly diagnosed with Huntington disease in British Columbia. *Clin Genet* 60: 198-205.

8. Andrew SE, Goldberg YP, Kremer B, Squitieri F, Theilmann J, Zeisler J, Telenius H, Adam S, Almquist E, Anvret M, et al. (1994) Huntington disease without CAG expansion: phenocopies or errors in assignment? *Am J Hum Genet* 54: 852-863.

9. Andrews TC, Weeks RA, Turjanski N, Gunn RN, Watkins LH, Sahakian B, Hodges JR, Rosser AE, Wood NW, Brooks DJ (1999) Huntington's disease progression. PET and clinical observations. *Brain* 122: 2353-2363.

10. Augood SJ, Faull RL, Love DR, Emson PC (1996) Reduction in enkephalin and substance P messenger RNA in the striatum of early grade Huntington's disease: a detailed cellular in situ hybridization study. *Neuroscience* 72: 1023-1036.

11. Aylward EH, Brandt J, Codori AM, Mangus RS, Barta PE, Harris GJ (1994) Reduced basal ganglia volume associated with the gene for Huntington's disease in asymptomatic at-risk persons. *Neurology* 44: 823-828.

12. Aylward EH, Codori AM, Barta PE, Pearlson GD, Harris GJ, Brandt J (1996) Basal ganglia volume and proximity to onset in presymptomatic Huntington disease. *Arch Neurol* 53: 1293-1296.

13. Aylward EH, Codori AM, Rosenblatt A, Sherr M, Brandt J, Stine OC, Barta PE, Pearlson GD, Ross CA (2000) Rate of caudate atrophy in presymptomatic and symptomatic stages of Huntington's disease. *Mov Disord* 15: 552-560.

14. Bachoud-Lévi AC, Remy P, Nguyen JP, Brugieres P, Lefaucheur JP, Bourdet C, Baudic S, Gaura V, Maison P, Haddad B, Boisse MF, Grandmougin T, Jeny R, Bartolomeo P, Dalla Barba G, Degos JD, Lisovoski F, Ergis AM, Pailhous E, Cesaro P, Hantraye P, Peschanski M (2000) Motor and cognitive improvements in patients with Huntington's disease after neural transplantation. *Lancet* 356: 1975-1979.

15. Bates GP, Benn C (2002) Other polyglutamine diseases. In *Huntington's disease*, 3rd ed., G Bates, PS Harper, L Jones (eds). Oxford University Press: Oxford. pp. 429-472.

16. Bates G, Harper PS, Jones L, Eds. (2002) *Huntington's disease*, 3rd ed. Oxford University Press: Oxford .

17. Bates GP, Murphy KPSJ (2002) Mouse models of Huntington's disease. In *Huntington's disease*, 3rd ed., G Bates, PS Harper, L Jones (eds). Oxford University Press: Oxford. pp. 387-426.

18. Beal MF, Hantraye P (2001) Novel therapies in the search for a cure for Huntington's disease. *Proc Natl Acad Sci U S A* 98: 3-4.

19. Becher MW, Kotzuk JA, Sharp AH, Davies SW, Bates GP, Price DL, Ross CA (1998) Intranuclear neuronal inclusions in Huntington's disease and dentatorubral and pallidoluysian atrophy: correlation between the density of inclusions and IT15 CAG triplet repeat length. *Neurobiol Dis* 4: 387-397.

20. Bence NF, Sampat RM, Kopito RR (2001) Impairment of the ubiquitin-proteasome system by protein aggregation. *Science* 292: 1552-1555.

21. Björklund A, Lindvall O (2000) Cell replacement therapies for central nervous system disorders. *Nat Neurosci* 3: 537-544.

22. Braak H, Braak E (1982) Neuronal types in the striatum of man. *Cell Tissue Res* 227: 319-342.

23. Braak H, Braak E (1992) Allocortical involvement in Huntington's disease. *Neuropathol Appl Neurobiol* 18: 539-547.

24. Brooks DJ, Andrews T (2002) Imaging Huntington's disease. In *Huntington's disease*, 3rd ed., G Bates, PS Harper, L Jones (eds). Oxford University Press: Oxford. pp. 95-110.

25. Brouillet E, Conde F, Beal MF, Hantraye P (1999) Replicating Huntington's disease phenotype in experimental animals. *Prog Neurobiol* 59: 427-468.

26. Browne SE, Ferrante RJ, Beal MF (1999) Oxidative stress in Huntington's disease. *Brain Pathol* 9: 147-163.

27. Cammarata S, Caponnetto C, Tabaton M (1993) Ubiquitin-reactive neurites in cerebral cortex of subjects with Huntington's chorea: a pathological correlate of dementia? *Neurosci Lett* 156: 96-98.

28. Cepeda C, Ariano MA, Calvert CR, Flores-Hernandez J, Chandler SH, Leavitt BR, Hayden MR, Levine MS (2001) NMDA receptor function in mouse models of Huntington disease. *J Neurosci Res* 66: 525-539.

29. Cha JH (2000) Transcriptional dysregulation in Huntington's disease. *Trends Neurosci* 23: 387-392.

30. Cha JH, Kosinski CM, Kerner JA, Alsdorf SA, Mangiarini L, Davies SW, Penney JB, Bates GP, Young AB (1998) Altered brain neurotransmitter receptors in transgenic mice expressing a portion of an abnormal human Huntington disease gene. *Proc Natl Acad U S A* 95: 6480-6485.

31. Chen M, Ona VO, Li M, Ferrante RJ, Fink KB, Zhu S, Bian j, Guo L, Farrell LA, Hersch SM, Hobbs W, Vonsattel J-P, Cha J-H, Friedlander RM (2000) Minocycline inhibits caspase-1 and caspase-3 expression and delays mortality in a transgenic mouse model of Huntington disease. *Nature Med* 6: 797-801.

32. Clark AW, Parhad IM, Folstein SE, Whitehouse PJ, Hedreen JC, Price DL, Chase GA (1983) The nucleus basalis in Huntington's disease. *Neurology* 33: 1262-1267.

33. Coyle JT, Puttfarcken P (1993) Oxidative stress, glutamate, and neurodegenerative disorders. *Science* 262: 689-695.

34. Crutcher MD, DeLong MR (1984a) Single cell studies of the primate putamen. I. Functional organization. *Exp Brain Res* 53: 233-243.

35. Crutcher MD, DeLong MR (1984b) Single cell studies of the primate putamen. II. Relations to direction of movement and pattern of muscular activity. *Exp Brain Res* 53: 244-258.

36. Cudkowicz M, Kowall NW (1990) Degeneration of pyramidal projection neurons in Huntington's disease cortex. *Ann Neurol* 27: 200-204.

37. Davies SW, Beardsall K, Turmaine M, DiFiglia M, Aronin N, Bates GP (1998) Are neuronal intranuclear inclusions the common neuropathology of triplet-repeat disorders with polyglutamine-repeat expansions? *Lancet* 351: 131-133.

38. De la Monte SM, Vonsattel J-P, Richardson EP (1988) Morphometric demonstration of atrophic changes in the cerebral cortex, white matter, and neostriatum in Huntington's disease. *J Neuropathol Exp Neurol* 47: 516-525.

39. DeLong MR, Georgopoulos AP (1981) Motor functions of the basal ganglia. In *Handbook of Physiology The Nervous System Motor Control* JM Brookhart, VB Mountcastle, VB Brooks, SR Geiger (eds). American Physiological Society: Bethesda. pp. 1017-1061.

40. DiFiglia M, Sapp E, Chase KO, Davies SW, Bates GP, Vonsattel JP, Aronin N (1997) Aggregation of huntingtin in neuronal intranuclear inclusions and dystrophic neurites in brain. *Science* 277: 1990-1993.

41. Dom R, Malfroid M, Baro F (1976) Neuropathology of Huntington's chorea. Studies of the ventrobasal complex of the thalamus. *Neurology* 26: 64-68.

42. Dunnett SB, Rosser AE (2002) Cell and tissue transplantation. In *Huntington's disease*, 3rd ed., G Bates, PS Harper, L Jones (eds). Oxford University Press: Oxford. pp. 512-546.

43. Dure LS IV, Young AB, Penney JB (1991) Excitatory amino acid binding sites in the caudate nucleus and frontal cortex of Huntington's disease. *Ann Neurol* 30: 785-793.

44. Dure LS IV, Young AB, Penney JB, Jr. (1992) Compartmentalization of excitatory amino acid receptors in human striatum. *Proc Natl Acad Sci U S A* 89: 7688-7692.

45. Falush D, Almqvist EW, Brinkmann RR, Iwasa Y, Hayden MR (2000) Measurement of mutational flow implies both a high new-mutation rate for Huntington disease and substantial underascertainment of late-onset cases. *Am J Hum Genet* 68:373-385.

46. Flaherty AW, Graybiel AM (1993) Output architecture of the primate putamen. *J Neurosci* 13:3222-3237.

47. Flaherty AW, Graybiel AM (1994) Input-output organization of the sensorimotor striatum in the squirrel monkey. *J Neurosci* 14:599-610.

48. Folstein SE (1989) *Huntington's Disease. A Disorder of Families.* The Johns Hopkins Press: Baltimore.

49. Freeman TB, Hauser RA, Sanberg PR, Saporta S (2000) Neural transplantation for the treatment of Huntington's disease. *Prog Brain Res* 127: 405-411.

50. García Ruiz PJ, Gómez-Tortosa E, del Barrio A, Benítez J, Morales B, Vela L, Castro A, Requena I (1997) Senile chorea: a multicenter prospective study. *Acta Neurol Scand* 95: 180-183.

51. Garrett MC, Soares-da-Silva P (1992) Increased cerebrospinal fluid dopamine and 3,4-dihydroxyphenylacetic acid levels in Huntington's disease: evidence for an overactive dopaminergic brain transmission. *J Neurochem* 58: 101-106.

52. Gerber HP, Seipel K, Georgiev O, Hofferer M, Hug M, Rusconi S, Schaffner W (1994) Transcriptional activation modulated by homopolymeric glutamine and proline stretches. *Science* 263: 808-811.

53. Gerfen CR, Young WS, 3rd (1988) Distribution of striatonigral and striatopallidal peptidergic neurons in both patch and matrix compartments: an in situ hybridization histochemistry and fluorescent retrograde tracing study. *Brain Res* 460: 161-167.

54. Glass M, Dragunow M, Faull RL (2000) The pattern of neurodegeneration in Huntington's disease: a comparative study of cannabinoid, dopamine, adenosine and GABA(A) receptor alterations in the human basal ganglia in Huntington's disease. *Neuroscience* 97: 505-519.

55. Gomez-Tortosa E, MacDonald ME, Friend JC, Taylor SA, Weiler LJ, Cupples LA, Srinidhi J, Gusella JF, Bird ED, Vonsattel JP, Myers RH (2001) Quantitative neuropathological changes in presymptomatic Huntington's disease. *Ann Neurol* 49: 29-34.

56. Goto S, Hirano A (1990) Synaptophysin expression in the striatum in Huntington's disease. *Acta Neuropathol* 80: 88-91.

57. Goto S, Hirano A, Rojas-Corona RR (1989) An immunohistochemical investigation of the human neostriatum in Huntington's disease. *Ann Neurol* 25: 298-304.

58. Gourfinkel-An I, Cancel G, Trottier Y, Devys D, Tora L, Lutz Y, Imbert G, Saudou F, Stevanin G, Agid Y, Brice A, Mandel JL, Hirsch EC (1997) Differential distribution of the normal and mutated forms of huntingtin in the human brain. *Ann Neurol* 42: 712-719.

59. Graveland GA, Williams RS, DiFiglia M (1985) Evidence for degenerative and regenerative changes in neostriatal spiny neurons in Huntington's disease. *Science* 227: 770-773.

60. Graybiel AM, Ragsdale CW, Jr. (1978) Histochemically distinct compartments in the striatum of human, monkeys, and cat demonstrated by acetylthiocholinesterase staining. *Proc Natl Acad Sci U S A* 75: 5723-5726.

61. Grunewald T, Beal MF (1999) Bioenergetics in Huntington's disease. *Ann N Y Acad Sci* 893: 203-213.

62. Guidetti P, Charles V, Chen EY, Reddy PH, Kordower JH, Whetsell WO Jr, Schwarcz R, Tagle DA (2001) Early degenerative changes in transgenic mice expressing mutant huntingtin involve dendritic abnormalities but no impairment of mitochondrial energy production. *Exp Neurol* 169: 340-350.

63. Gusella JF, MacDonald ME (1998) Huntingtin: a single bait hooks many species. *Curr Opin Neurobiol* 8: 425-430.

64. Gusella JF, MacDonald ME (2000) Molecular genetics: unmasking polyglutamine triggers in neurodegenerative disease. *Nat Rev Neurosci* 1: 109-115.

65. Gutekunst C-A, Li S-H, Yi H, Mulroy JS, Kuemmerle S, Jones R, Rye D, Ferrante RJ, Hersch SM, Li X-J (1999) Nuclear and neuropil aggregates in Huntington's disease: relationship to neuropathology. *J Neurosci* 19: 2522-2534.

66. Harper PS (1996) *Huntington's Disease.* W.B. Saunders: London.

67. Harper PS (2002) the epidemiology of Huntington's disease. In *Huntington's disease*, 3rd ed., G Bates, PS Harper, L Jones (eds). Oxford University Press: Oxford. pp. 159-197.

68. Harper PS, Jones L (2002) Huntington's disease: genetic and molecular studies. In *Huntington's disease*, 3rd ed., G Bates, PS Harper, L Jones (eds). Oxford University Press: Oxford. pp. 113-158.

69. Hedreen JC (2002) Striosome and matrix pathology in Huntington disease. In *The Basal Ganglia VII*, LFB Nicholson, RLM Faull (eds). Plenum Press: New York. pp. 475-479.

70. Hedreen JC (2003) Neuronal intranuclear inclusions in neostriatal striosomes and matrix in Huntington's disease. In T*he Basal Ganglia VI*, AM Graybiel, MR DeLong, ST Kitai (eds). Plenum Press: New York. pp. 83-86.

71. Hedreen JC, Folstein SE (1995) Early loss of neostriatal striosome neurons in Huntington's disease. *J Neuropathol Exp Neurol* 54: 105-120.

72. Hedreen JC, Peyser CE, Folstein SE, Ross CA (1991) Neuronal loss in layers V and VI of cerebral cortex in Huntington's disease. *Neurosci Lett* 133: 257-261.

73. Heinsen H, Rub U, Bauer M, Ulmar G, Bethke B, Schuler M, Bocker F, Eisenmenger W, Gotz M, Korr H, Schmitz C (1999) Nerve cell loss in the thalamic mediodorsal nucleus in Huntington's disease. *Acta Neuropathol* (Berl) 97: 613-622.

74. Heinsen H, Rub U, Gangnus D, Jungkunz G, Bauer M, Ulmar G, Bethke B, Schuler M, Bocker F, Eisenmenger W, Gotz M, Strik M (1996) Nerve cell loss in the thalamic centromedian-parafascicular complex in patients with Huntington's disease. *Acta Neuropathol* 91: 161-168.

75. Heinsen H, Strik M, Bauer M, Luther K, Ulmar G, Gangnus D, Jungkunz G, Eisenmenger W, Götz M (1994) Cortical and striatal neurone number in Huntington's disease. *Acta Neuropathol* 88: 320-333.

76. Heiser V, Scherzinger E, Boeddrich A, Nordhoff E, Lurz R, Schugardt N, Lehrach H, Wanker EE (2000) Inhibition of huntingtin fibrillogenesis by specific antibodies and small molecules: implications for Huntington's disease therapy. *Proc Natl Acad Sci U S A* 97: 6739-6744.

77. Holmes SE, O'Hearn E, Rosenblatt A, Callahan C, Hwang HS, Ingersoll-Ashworth RG, Fleisher A, Stevanin G, Brice A, Potter NT, Ross CA, Margolis RL (2001) A repeat expansion in the gene encoding junctophilin-3 is associated with Huntington disease-like 2. *Nature Genet* 29: 377-378.

78. Hughes RE, Olson JM (2001) Therapeutic opportunities in polyglutamine disease. *Nat Med* 7: 419-423.

79. The Huntington's Disease Collaborative Research Group (1993) A novel gene containing a trinucleotide repeat that is expanded and unstable on Huntington's disease chromosomes. *Cell* 72: 971-983.

80. Jackson M, Gentleman S, Lennox G, Ward L, Gray T, Randall K, Morrell K, Lowe J (1995) The cortical neuritic pathology of Huntington's disease. *Neuropathol Appl Neurobiol* 21: 18-26.

81. Jakel RJ, Maragos WF (2000) Neuronal cell death in Huntington's disease: a potential role for dopamine. *Trends Neurosci* 23: 239-245.

82. Jana NR, Zemskov EA, Wang G, Nukina N (2001) Altered proteasomal function due to the expression of polyglutamine- expanded truncated N-terminal huntingtin induces apoptosis by caspase activation through mitochondrial cytochrome c release. *Hum Mol Genet* 10: 1049-1059.

83. Jeste DV, Barban L, Parisi J (1984) Reduced Purkinje cell density in Huntington's disease. *Exp Neurol* 85: 78-86.

84. Jones L (2002) The cell biology of Huntington's disease. In *Huntington's disease*, 3rd ed., G Bates, PS Harper, L Jones (eds). Oxford University Press: Oxford. pp. 348-386.

85. Kambouris M, Bohlega S, Al-Tahan A, Meyer BF (2000) Localization of the gene for a novel autosomal recessive neurodegenerative Huntington-like disorder to 4p15.3. *Am J Hum Genet* 66: 445-452.

86. Karpuj MV, Becher MW, Springer JE, Chabas D, Youssef S, Pedotti R, Mitchell D, Steinman L (2002) Prolonged survival and decreased abnormal movements in transgenic model of Huntington disease, with administration of the transglutaminase inhibitor cystamine. *Nature Med* 8: 143-149.

87. Kegel KB, Kim M, Sapp E, McIntyre C, Castaño, Aronin N, DiFiglia M (2000) Huntingtin expression stimulates endosomal-lysosomal activity, endosome tubulation, and autophagy. *J Neurosci* 20: 7268-7278.

88. Kegel KB, Meloni AR, Yi Y, Kim YJ, Doyle E, Cuiffo BG, Sapp E, Wang Y, Qin ZH, Chen JD, Nevins JR, Aronin N, DiFiglia M (2002) Huntingtin is present in the nucleus, interacts with the transcriptional corepressor C-terminal binding protein, and represses transcription. *J Biol Chem* 277: 7466-7476 .

89. Kim YJ, Yi Y, Sapp E, Wang Y, Cuiffo B, Kegel KB, Qin ZH, Aronin N, DiFiglia M (2001) Caspase 3-cleaved N-terminal fragments of wild-type and mutant huntingtin are present in normal and Huntington's disease brains, associate with membranes, and undergo calpain-dependent proteolysis. *Proc Natl Acad Sci U S A* 98: 12784-12789.

90. Koeppen AH (1989) The nucleus pontis centralis caudalis in Huntington's disease. *J Neurol Sci* 91: 129-141.

91. Kowall NW, Ferrante RJ, Martin JB (1987) Patterns of cell loss in Huntington's disease. *Trends Neurosci* 10: 24-29.

92. Kremer HP, Roos RA, Dingjan G, Marani E, Bots GT (1990) Atrophy of the hypothalamic lateral tuberal nucleus in Huntington's disease. *J Neuropathol Exp Neurol* 49: 371-382.

93. Laccone F, Engel U, Holinski-Feder E, Weigell-Weber M, Marczinek K, Nolte D, Morris-Rosendahl DJ, Zühlke C, Fuchs K, Weirich-Schwaiger H, Schlüter G, von Beust G, Vieira-Saecker A, Webere B, Riess O (1999) DNA analysis of Huntington's disease: Five years of experience in Germany, Austria and Switzerland. *Neurology* 53: 801-806.

94. Lange H, Thorner G, Hopf A, Schroder KF (1976) Morphometric studies of the neuropathological changes in choreatic diseases. *J Neurol Sci* 28: 401-425.

95. Lange HW (1981) Quantitative changes of telencephalon, diencephalon, and mesencephalon in Huntington's chorea, postencephalitic, and idiopathic parkinsonism. *Vehr Anat Ges* 75: 923-925.

96. Leavitt BR, Wellington CL, Hayden MR (1999) Recent insights into the molecular pathogenesis of Huntington disease. *Semin Neurol* 19: 385-395.

97. Li H, Li S-H, Johnston H, Shelbourne PF, Li X-J (2000) Amino-terminal fragments of mutant huntingtin show selective accumulation in striatal neurons and synaptic toxicity. *Nat Genet* 25: 385-389.

98. Li H, Li S-H, Yu Z-X, Shelbourne P, Li X-J (2001) Huntingtin aggregate-associated axonal degeneration is an early pathological event in Huntington's disease mice. *J Neurosci* 21: 8473-8481.

99. Maat-Schieman ML, Dorsman JC, Smoor MA, Siesling S, Van Duinen SG, Verschuuren JJ, den Dunnen JT, Van Ommen GJ, Roos RA (1999) Distribution of inclusions in neuronal nuclei and dystrophic neurites in Huntington disease brain. *J Neuropathol Exp Neurol* 58: 129-137.

100. Macdonald V, Halliday GM, Trent RJ, McCusker EA (1997) Significant loss of pyramidal neurons in the angular gyrus of patients with Huntington's disease. *Neuropathol Appl Neurobiol* 23: 492-495.

101. Mangiarini L, Sathasivam K, Seller M, Cozens B, Harper A, Hetherington C, Lawton M, Trottier Y, Lehrach H, Davies SW, Bates GP (1996) Exon 1 of the HD gene with an expanded CAG repeat is sufficient to cause a progressive neurological phenotype in transgenic mice. *Cell* 87: 493-506.

102. Mann DM (1989) Subcortical afferent projection systems in Huntington's chorea. *Acta Neuropathol* 78: 551-554.

103. Margolis RL, O'Hearn E, Rosenblatt A, Willour V, Holmes SE, Franz ML, Callahan C, Hwang HS, Troncoso JC, Ross CA (2001) A disorder similar to Huntington's disease is associated with a novel CAG repeat expansion. *Ann Neurol* 50: 373-380.

104. Margolis RL, Ross CA (2001) Expansion explosion: new clues to the pathogenesis of repeat expansion neurodegenerative diseases. *Trends Mol Med* 7: 479-482.

105. McCampbell A, Fischbeck KH (2001) Polyglutamine and CBP: fatal attraction? *Nat Med* 7: 528-530.

106. McKusick V Mendelian inheritance in man 143100. *http://www.ncbi.nlm.nih.gov/omim/*

107. McMurray CT (2001) Huntington's disease: new hope for therapeutics. *Trends Neurosci* 24 Suppl: S32-S38.

108. Menalled LB, Chesselet M-F (2002) Mouse models of Huntington's disease. *Trends Pharmacol Sci* 23: 32-39.

109. Mende-Mueller LM, Toneff T, Hwang SR, Chesselet MF, Hook VY (2001) Tissue-specific proteolysis of Huntingtin (htt) in human brain: evidence of enhanced levels of N- and C-terminal htt fragments in Huntington's disease striatum. *J Neurosci* 21: 1830-1837.

110. Mitchell IJ, Cooper AJ, Griffiths (1999) The selective vulnerability of striatopallidal neurons. *Progr Neurobiol* 59: 691-719.

111. Moore RC, Xiang F, Monaghan J, Han D, Zhang Z, Edstrom L, Anvret M, Prusiner SB (2001) Huntington disease phenocopy is a familial prion disease. *Am J Hum Genet* 69: 1385-1388.

112. Morton AJ, Nicholson LF, Faull RL (1993) Compartmental loss of NADPH diaphorase in the neuropil of the human striatum in Huntington's disease. *Neuroscience* 53: 159-168.

113. Myers RH, Vonsattel JP, Stevens TJ, Cupples LA, Richardson EP, Martin JB, Bird ED (1988) Clinical and

neuropathologic assessment of severity in Huntington's disease. *Neurology* 38: 341-347.

114. Nance MA, Westphal B (2002) Comprehensive care in Huntington's disease. In *Huntington's disease*, 3rd ed., G Bates, PS Harper, L Jones (eds). Oxford University Press: Oxford. pp. 475-500.

115. Novelli A, Reilly JA, Lysko PG, Henneberry RC (1988) Glutamate becomes neurotoxic via the N-methyl-D-aspartate receptor when intracellular energy levels are reduced. *Brain Res* 451: 205-212.

116. Nucifora FC, Jr., Sasaki M, Peters MF, Huang H, Cooper JK, Yamada M, Takahashi H, Tsuji S, Troncoso J, Dawson VL, Dawson TM, Ross CA (2001) Interference by huntingtin and atrophin-1 with cbp-mediated transcription leading to cellular toxicity. *Science* 291: 2423-2428.

117. Orr HT (2001) Beyond the Qs in the polyglutamine diseases. *Genes Dev* 15: 925-932.

118. Orr HT, Zoghbi HY (2000) Reversing neurodegeneration: a promise unfolds. *Cell* 101: 1-4.

119. Oyanagi K, Takeda S, Takahashi H, Ohama E, Ikuta F (1989) A quantitative investigation of the substantia nigra in Huntington's disease. *Ann Neurol* 26: 13-19.

120. Passani LA, Bedford MT, Faber PW, McGinnis KM, Sharp AH, Gusella JF, Vonsattel JP, MacDonald ME (2000) Huntingtin's WW domain partners in Huntington's disease post-mortem brain fulfill genetic criteria for direct involvement in Huntington's disease pathogenesis. *Hum Mol Genet* 9: 2175-2182.

121. Paulson GW, Prior TW (1997) Issues related to DNA testing for Huntington's disease in symptomatic patients. *Semin Neurol* 17: 235-238.

122. Persichetti F, Srinidhi J, Kanaley L, Ge P, Myers RH, D'Arrigo K, Barnes GT, MacDonald ME, Vonsattel JP, Gusella JF, et al. (1994) Huntington's disease CAG trinucleotide repeats in pathologically confirmed post-mortem brains. *Neurobiol Dis* 1: 159-166.

123. Petersen A, Larsen KE, Behr GG, Romero N, Przedborski S, Brundin P, Sulzer D (2001) Expanded CAG repeats in exon 1 of the Huntington's disease gene stimulate dopamine-mediated striatal neuron autophagy and degeneration. *Hum Mol Genet* 10: 1243-1254.

124. Portera-Cailliau C, Hedreen JC, Price DL, Koliatsos VE (1995) Evidence for apoptotic cell death in Huntington disease and excitotoxic animal models. *J Neurosci* 15: 3775-3787.

125. Rajkowska G, Selemon LD, Goldman-Rakic PS (1998) Neuronal and glial somal size in the prefrontal cortex: a postmortem morphometric study of schizophrenia and Huntington disease. *Arch Gen Psychiat* 55: 215-224.

126. Reiner A, Albin RL, Anderson KD, D'Amato CJ, Penney JB, Young AB (1988) Differential loss of striatal projection neurons in Huntington disease. *Proc Natl Acad Sci U S A* 85: 5733-5737.

127. Roizin L, Stellar S, Liu JC (1979) Neuronal nuclear-cytoplasmic changes in Huntington's chorea: electron microscopic investigations. *Adv Neurol* 23: 95-122.

128. Roos RAC, Pruyt JFM, de Vries J, Bots, GTAM (1985) Neuronal distribution in the putamen in Huntington's disease. *J Neurol Neurosurg Psychiat* 48:422-425.

129. Rosenblatt A, Ranen NG, Rubinsztein DC, Stine OC, Margolis RL, Wagster MV, Becher MW, Rosser AE, Leggo J, Hodges JR, ffrench-Constant CK, Sherr M, Franz ML, Abbott MH, Ross CA (1998) Patients with features similar to Huntington's disease, without CAG expansion in huntingtin. *Neurology* 51: 215-220.

130. Ross CA, Wood JD, Schilling G, Peters MF, Nucifora FC, Jr., Cooper JK, Sharp AH, Margolis RL, Borchelt DR (1999) Polyglutamine pathogenesis. *Philos Trans R Soc Lond B Biol Sci* 354: 1005-1011.

131. Sapp E, Kegel KB, Aronin N, Hashikawa T, Uchiyama Y, Tohyama K, Bhide PG, Vonsattel JP, DiFiglia M (2001) Early and progressive accumulation of reactive microglia in the Huntington disease brain. *J Neuropathol Exp Neurol* 60:161-172.

132. Sapp E, Penney J, Young A, Aronin N, Vonsattel J-P, DiFiglia M (1999) Axonal transport of N-terminal huntingtin suggests early pathology of corticostriatal projections in Huntington disease. *J Neuropathol Exp Neurol* 58:165-173.

133. Sapp E, Schwarz C, Chase K, Bhide PG, Young AB, Penney J, Vonsattel JP, Aronin N, DiFiglia M (1997) Huntingtin localization in brains of normal and Huntington's disease patients. *Ann Neurol* 42: 604-612.

134. Schrag A, Quinn N (1999) Disorders of the basal ganglia and their modern management. *J R Coll Physicians Lond* 33: 323-327.

135. Shelbourne PF (2000) Of mice and men: solving the molecular mysteries of Huntington's disease. *J Anat* 196: 617-628.

136. Sieradzan KA, Mann DM (2001) The selective vulnerability of nerve cells in Huntington's disease. *Neuropathol Appl Neurobiol* 27: 1-21.

137. Sieradzan KA, Mechan AO, Jones L, Wanker EE, Nukina N, Mann DM (1999) Huntington's disease intranuclear inclusions contain truncated, ubiquitinated huntingtin protein. *Exp Neurol* 156: 92-99.

138. Siesling S, de Vlis MV, Losekoot M, Belfroid RDM, Maat-Keivit JA, Kremer HPH, Roos RAC. Family history and DNA analysis in patients with suspected Huntington's disease (2000) *J Neurol Neurosurg Psychiat* 69: 54-59.

139. Sipione S, Cattaneo E (2001) Modeling huntington's disease in cells, flies, and mice. *Mol Neurobiol* 23: 21-51.

140. Sotrel A, Paskevich PA, Kiely DK, Bird ED, Williams RS, Myers RH (1991) Morphometric analysis of the prefrontal cortex in Huntington's disease. *Neurology* 41: 1117-1123.

141. Spargo E, Everall IP, Lantos PL (1993) Neuronal loss in the hippocampus in Huntington's disease: a comparison with HIV infection. *J Neurol Neurosurg Psychiatry* 56: 487-491.

142. Steffan JS, Bodai L, Pallos J, Poelman M, McCampbell A, Apostol BL, Kazantsev A, Schmidt E, Zhu YZ, Greenwald M, Kurokawa R, Housman DE, Jackson GR, Marsh JL, Thompson LM (2001) Histone deacetylase inhibitors arrest polyglutamine-dependent neurodegeneration in Drosophila. *Nature* 413: 739-743.

143. Sun Y, Savanenin A, Reddy PH, Liu YF (2001) Polyglutamine-expanded huntingtin promotes sensitization of N-methyl-D- aspartate receptors via post-synaptic density 95. *J Biol Chem* 276: 24713-24718.

144. Tagliavini F, Pilleri G (1983) Basal nucleus of Meynert. A neuropathological study in Alzheimer's disease, simple senile dementia, Pick's disease and Huntington's chorea. *J Neurol Sci* 62: 243-260.

145. Tarnopolsky MA, Beal MF (2001) Potential for creatine and other therapies targeting cellular energy dysfunction in neurological disorders. *Ann Neurol* 49: 561-574.

146. Thomas D, Tyers M (2000) Transcriptional regulation: Kamikaze activators. *Curr Biol* 10: R341-343.

147. Tibben A (2002) Genetic counseling and presymptomatic testing. In *Huntington's disease*, 3rd ed., G Bates, PS Harper, L Jones (eds). Oxford University Press: Oxford. pp. 198-248.

148. Tobin AJ, Signer ER (2000) Huntington's disease: the challenge for cell biologists. *Trends Cell Biol* 10: 531-536.

149. Turner C, Schapira AHV (2002) Energy metabolism and Huntington's disease. In *Huntington's disease*, 3rd ed., G Bates, PS Harper, L Jones (eds). Oxford University Press: Oxford. pp. 309-323.

150. Vonsattel J-PG, Ge P, Kelley L (1997) Huntington's disease. In *The Neuropathology of Dementia*, M M, Esiri, H J, Morris (eds). Cambridge University Press: Cambridge. pp. 214-240.

151. Vonsattel JP, DiFiglia M (1998) Huntington disease. *J Neuropathol Exp Neurol* 57: 369-384.

152. Vonsattel JP, Myers RH, Bird ED, Ge P, Richardson EP, Jr. (1992) [Huntington disease: 7 cases with relatively preserved neostriatal islets]. *Rev Neurol* 148: 107-116.

153. Vonsattel JP, Myers RH, Stevens TJ, Ferrante RJ, Bird ED, Richardson EP, Jr. (1985) Neuropathological classification of Huntington's disease. *J Neuropathol Exp Neurol* 44: 559-577.

154. Vuillaume I, Meynieu P, Schraen-Maschke S, Destee A, Sablonniere B (2000) Absence of unidentified CAG repeat expansion in patients with Huntington's disease-like phenotype. *J Neurol Neurosurg Psychiatry* 68: 672-675.

155. Wagster MV, Hedreen JC, Peyser CE, Folstein SE, Ross CA (1994) Selective loss of [3H]kainic acid and [3H]AMPA binding in layer VI of frontal cortex in Huntington's disease. *Exp Neurol* 127: 70-75.

156. Wanker EE (2000) Protein aggregation and pathogenesis of Huntington's disease: mechanisms and correlations. *Biol Chem* 381: 937-942.

157. Wanker EE, Dröge (2002) Structural biology of Huntington's disease. In *Huntington's disease*, 3rd ed., G Bates, PS Harper, L Jones (eds). Oxford University Press: Oxford. pp. 327-347.

158. Weeks RA, Piccini P, Harding AE, Brooks DJ (1996) Striatal D1 and D2 dopamine receptor loss in

asymptomatic mutation carriers of Huntington's disease. *Ann Neurol* 40: 49-54.

159. Wellington CL, Hayden MR (2000) Caspases and neurodegeneration: on the cutting edge of new therapeutic approaches. *Clin Genet* 57: 1-10.

160. Wilson SAK (1914) An experimental research into the anatomy and physiology of the corpus striatum. *Brain* 36: 427-492.

161. Xiang F, Almqvist EW, Huq M, Lundin A, Hayden MR, Edstrom L, Anvret M, Zhang Z (1998) A Huntington disease-like neurodegenerative disorder maps to chromosome 20p. *Am J Hum Genet* 63: 1431-1438.

162. Xuereb JH, MacMillan JC, Snell R, Davies P, Harper PS (1996) Neuropathological diagnosis and CAG repeat expansion in Huntington's disease. *J Neurol Neurosurg Psychiatry* 60: 78-81.

163. Yamamoto A, Lucas JJ, Hen R (2000) Reversal of neuropathology and motor dysfunction in a conditional model of Huntington's disease. *Cell* 101: 57-66.

164. Yohrling GJ, Cha J-HJ (2002) Neurochemistry of Huntington's disease. In *Huntington's disease*, 3rd ed., G Bates, PS Harper, L Jones (eds). Oxford University Press: Oxford. pp. 276-308.

165. Zeron MM, Chen N, Moshaver A, Lee AT, Wellington CL, Hayden MR, Raymond LA (2001) Mutant huntingtin enhances excitotoxic cell death. *Mol Cell Neurosci* 17: 41-53.

166. Zhan SS, Beyreuther K, Schmitt HP (1993) Quantitative assessment of the synaptophysin immuno-reactivity of the cortical neuropil in various neurodegenerative disorders with dementia. *Dementia* 4: 66-74.

167. Zoghbi HY, Orr HT (2000) Glutamine repeats and neurodegeneration. *Annu Rev Neurosci* 23: 217-247.

168. Zuccato C, Ciammola A, Rigamonti D, Leavitt BR, Goffredo D, Conti L, MacDonald ME, Friedlander RM, Silani V, Hayden MR, Timmusk T, Sipione S, Cattaneo E (2001) Loss of huntingtin-mediated BDNF gene transcription in Huntington's disease. *Science* 293: 493-498.

169. Zweig RM, Ross CA, Hedreen JC, Peyser C, Cardillo JE, Folstein SE, Price DL (1992) Locus coeruleus involvement in Huntington's disease. *Arch Neurol* 49: 152-156.

Spinocerebellar Ataxias

Hidehiro Mizusawa
H. Brent Clark
Arnulf H. Koeppen

ADCA	autosomal dominant cerebellar ataxia
AVED	ataxia with isolated vitamine E deficiency
CCA	cerebellar cortical atrophy
CSF	cerebrospinal fluid
DRPLA	dentatorubralpallidoluisian atrophy
EOAH	early onset ataxia with oculomotor apraxia and hypoalbuminaemia
FRDA	Friedreich's ataxia
LCCA	late cortical cerebellar atrophy
MSA-C	multiple system atrophy, cerebellar variant
MSA-P	multiple system atrophy, parkinsonian variant
MJD	Machado-Joseph disease
OPCA	olivopontocerebellar atrophy
SCA	spinocerebellar ataxia
SCD	spinocerebellar degeneration
SND	striatonigral degeneration

Definition

Spinocerebellar ataxia (SCA) is defined as a group of neurodegenerative diseases presenting with motor ataxia of the extremities and trunk, ataxic speech, nystagmus and ataxic gait as well as other symptoms, including motor weakness, sensory impairments, Parkinsonism, dysautonomia, and cognitive impairment. The pathological process involves mainly the cerebellum, brainstem and spinal cord. The cerebrum, including the basal ganglia, as well as the peripheral and autonomic nervous systems are also affected in some disorders.

Synonyms and historical annotations

Many students of hereditary ataxia credit Marie (66) with the first effort to distinguish several types of familial spinocerebellar degeneration. Prior to 1893, all cases were considered Friedreich's ataxia (FRDA). In numerous subsequent publications, the pattern of inheritance (dominant or recessive), age of onset, and clinical features formed the basis of classification (2). The name "spinocerebellar ataxia" (SCA) now implies dominant transmission but the great heterogeneity and unexplained "anticipation" (earlier onset and more severe clinical course in affected members of successive generations) raised doubts about the reliability of clinical criteria. Almost invariably, case reports included detailed descriptions and illustrations of the neuropathology, and it seemed that only morphological findings (38) or a combination of clinical features and pathology (33) would permit a firm classification. Menzel (72) observed a peculiar combined atrophy of basis pontis and cerebellum in hereditary ataxia, and "olivopontocerebellar atrophy" (OPCA) was thought to be equivalent to autosomal dominant ataxia. Actually, the name was first selected for two non-familial cases of ataxia (16), and the most common cause of OPCA is now known to be multiple system atrophy (MSA). Only 3 types of SCA (SCA1, SCA2, and SCA7) show OPCA while SCA6 and SCA17 belong to a group that was previously called "pure cerebellar" or "cerebello-olivary" atrophy.

Following a pioneering linkage study of Yakura and coworkers in 1974, in which a hereditary SCA was demonstrated to be linked with an HLA locus on chromosome 6 (120), Zoghbi and Ranum and their co-workers identified 6p22-23 as a genetic locus for autosomal dominant "OPCA" in 1991 (88, 129). This form of SCA was designated SCA type 1 (SCA1). Orr and coworkers identified the SCA1 gene (ataxin 1) in 1993 using molecular genetic methods (83). Subsequently, other genes and gene loci have been identified and designated sequentially as SCA2, SCA3 and so on. At present, SCA is first divided into sporadic and hereditary categories, and the latter is further classified by genes and genetic loci (Table 1).

Sporadic degenerative ataxic disorders diseases include cortical cerebellar atrophy (CCA) and MSA, the latter showing cerebellar (MSA-C) and parkinsonian (MSA-P) variants (27). CCA should be used for a SCA exhibiting pure cerebellar signs and symptoms without any evidence suggesting a hereditary disorder. There are many acquired or secondary cerebellar degenerations, such as alcoholic and paraneoplastic cerebellar degenerations, which should be ruled out before CCA is diagnosed. There are a few synonyms for SCA, including spinocerebellar degeneration (SCD), cerebellar ataxia and cerebellar degeneration. If the diseases are hereditary, hereditary ataxia has also been used.

Epidemiology

Incidence and prevalence. The prevalence of SCAs is reported to be around 5 per 100000 persons (86). According to a Japanese nationwide survey, approximately 60% of SCA patients are sporadic and 40% are hereditary (36). There are many forms of hereditary SCA (19). Among hereditary ataxias, FRDA is the most common in whites, but has not been found in Japan, where SCA1, SCA2 and Huntington's disease are also uncommon (110). In contrast, dentatorubropallidoluysial atrophy (DRPLA) and SCA6 are more common in Japan. In other words incidence and prevalence of SCAs differ among ethnic groups and geographic areas (20, 89, 96).

Sex and age distribution. Usually both sporadic and hereditary forms affect men and women equally. Ages of onset are usually after 40 to 50 years, although pediatric onset is seen in some forms. Many autosomal dominant ataxias have abnormally expanded CAG repeats in the causative genes, and the age of onset is inversely correlated with the repeat length (127) (Figure 1). The mean age of onset is oldest for SCA6.

Risk factors. No definite risk factors have been identified for SCAs.

Genetics

There are more autosomal dominant than autosomal recessive SCAs. Interestingly, most autosomal dominant forms of SCA have a common genetic mechanism—abnormal expansion of a CAG triplet repeat in the causative genes (19, 128). The normal ranges of repeats are from around 10 to around 30 and disease ranges are usually over 40 to 90, realizing that each disorder has its own normal and abnormal ranges (Figure 1). Clinical manifestations, including age of onset, are related to repeat length. Signs and symptoms are more marked with more severe atrophy of the brain associated with longer repeat lengths (81). Children often exhibit an earlier age of onset than the affected parent (genetic anticipation) and have more marked disease due to unstable expansion of the CAG repeat.

In most disorders the CAG repeat is located in the coding region of the gene and consequently is translated into polyglutamine tract within the protein. Therefore, these diseases are called either CAG-repeat or polyglutamine (polyQ) diseases. The precise pathologic mechanism of polyglutamine disease has not been elucidated, but mutant proteins containing abnormally expanded polyglutamine, which tend to form abnormal intranuclear and cytoplasmic aggregates, are believed to exert some toxic action (gain of toxic function) producing neuronal dysfunction or death (Figure 2).

In SCA 6 both normal and abnormal repeat lengths are so small that the largest expanded repeat is still within the normal range of the other CAG repeat diseases (Table 1). The smallness is probably related to the fact that the repeat is very stable; consequently, anticipation is not significant in SCA6. SCA 8 is reportedly caused by CTG expansion in the ataxin 8 gene, but this observation needs further confirmation because the mutation is also detected in normal controls. A pentanucleotide expansion causes SCA10 and a CAG repeat expansion in the 5′ untranslated region of the gene encoding a brain-specific regulatory subunit of protein phosphatase 2A is the etiology of SCA12.

Clinical Features

Signs and symptoms. Except for FRDA and ataxia associated with vitamin E deficiency (AVED), which present with ataxia due to spinal cord posterior column involvement, most spinocerebellar ataxias show ataxia of extremities and trunk of a cerebellar type. AVED is an autosomal recessive ataxia caused by mutations in the gene for the alpha-tocopherol transfer protein. Its recognition is important because it is a heritable ataxia that is also treatable (6, 84, 122, 123). Among various signs and symptoms of cerebellar ataxia, ataxic gait is often the initial symptom and most common. Other signs include gaze nystagmus, cerebellar dysarthria and ataxic speech. SCA6 is the most common autosomal dominat cerebellar ataxia with pure cerebellar signs and symptoms (128), but SCA5, SCA14 and SCA16 may also be included in this category. Other SCAs, particularly SCA1, SCA2, and SCA3 present with not only cerebellar, but also extracerebellar signs and symptoms due to involvement of multiple systems,

Sporadic SCAs

- cerebellar cortical atrophy (CCA)
- multiple system atrophy (MSA)
  - olivopontocerebellar atrophy (OPCA)
  - striatonigral degeneration (SND)
  - Shy-Drager syndrome (SDS)

Hereditary SCAs

Autosomal dominant

- spinocerebellar ataxia type 1 (SCA1) 6p22-23, ataxin 1
- spinocerebellar ataxia type 2 (SCA2) 12q23-24.1, ataxin 2
- spinocerebellar ataxia type 3 (MJD/SCA3) 14q24.3-32, ataxin 3
- spinocerebellar ataxia type 4 (SCA4) 16q24-ter
- spinocerebellar ataxia type 5 (SCA5) 11ctr
- spinocerebellar ataxia type 6 (SCA6) 19p13, CACNA1A
- spinocerebellar ataxia type 7 (SCA7) 3p14.1-21.3, ataxin 7
- spinocerebellar ataxia type 8 (SCA8) 13q21 ataxin 8
- spinocerebellar ataxia type 10 (SCA10) 22q13, ataxin 10
- spinocerebellar ataxia type 11 (SCA11) 15q14-21.3
- spinocerebellar ataxia type 12 (SCA12) 5q31-33, ataxin 12
- spinocerebellar ataxia type 13 (SCA13) 19q13.3-13.4
- spinocerebellar ataxia type 14 (SCA14) 19q13.4-ter
- spinocerebellar ataxia type 16 (SCA16) 8q22.1-24.1
- spinocerebellar ataxia type 17 (SCA17) 6q27, TBP
- dentatoruburopallidoluisian atrophy (DRPLA) 12q12-ter, atrophin
- episodic ataxia type 1 (EA1) 12p, KCNA1
- episodic ataxia type 2 (EA2) 19p13, CACNA1A

Autosomal recessive

- Friedreich's ataxia (FRDA) 9q13-21.1, frataxin
- ataxia with isolated vitamin E deficiency (AVED) 8q13.1-13.3, α-TTP
- early onset ataxia with oculomotor apraxia and hypoalbuminaemia (EOAH) 9q13, aprataxin

Table 1. *Classification of main spinocerebellar ataxias (SCAs).* Many mitochondrial encephaloneuromyopathies which are not included in the table could show ataxia due to the involvement of the cerebellum, spinal cord and peripheral nervous system. Spastic paraplegias and some paediatric ataxias including ataxia telangiextasia are not included in this table. TBP elsewhere in the chapter given as TATA-binding protein.

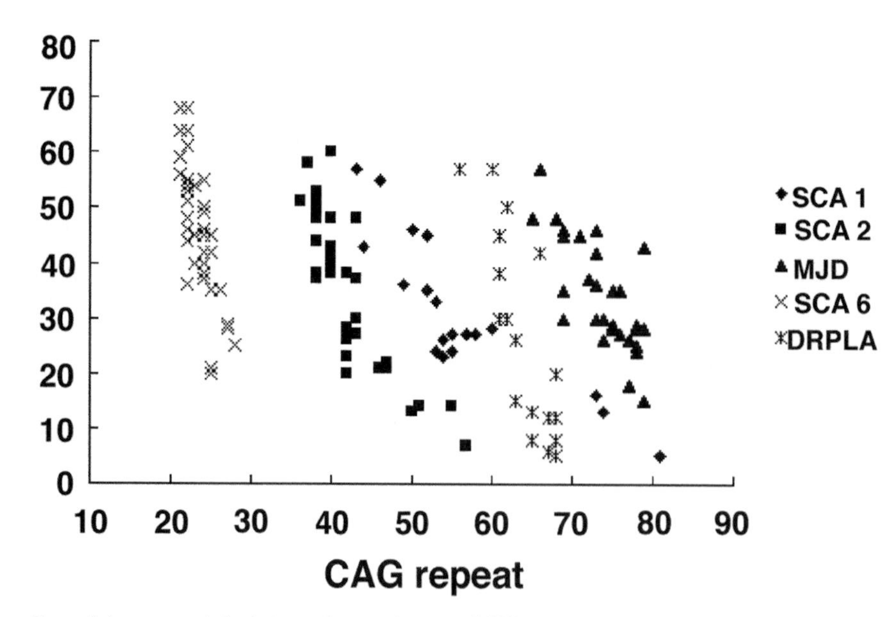

Figure 1. Inverse correlation between the age of onset and CAG repeat numbers. Data of SCA6 were added to the figures by Zoghbi et al, 1998.

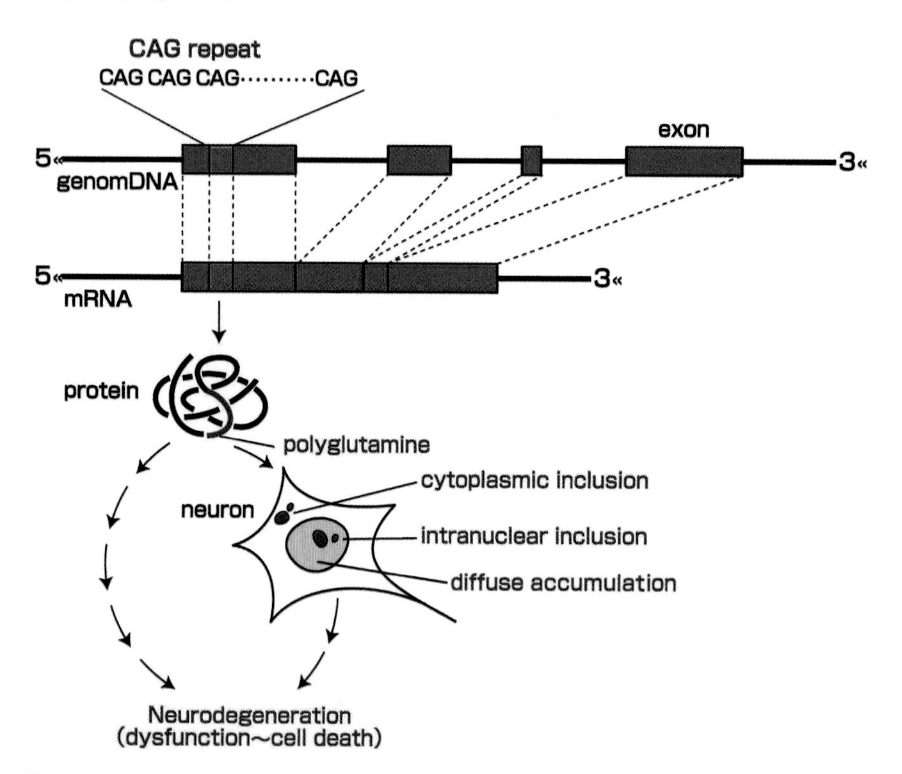

Figure 2. Hypothetical pathomechanisms of CAG-repeat diseases. Mutant proteins of their fragments containing abnormally expanded polyglutamine tracts play important roles in neurodegeneration.

including basal ganglia, brainstem and spinal cord in addition to the cerebellum.

SCA3 or Machado-Joseph disease (MJD) was originally described in families of Portuguese descent, but it has become apparent that MJD/SCA3 is found worldwide and may be the most common autosomal dominant ataxia (18, 68, 92, 113). SCA3/MJD shows a very wide spectrum of clinical manifestation and is classified into 3 clinical types, which are correlated to CAG repeat length. In type I (spastic-dystonic type), clinical manifestations start in the first 2 decades and include weakness and spasticity of the extremities, particularly the legs, dystonic posture of face, neck, trunk, and extremities. Tendon reflexes are active with clonus and pathological reflexes. Gait is mainly spastic and slightly ataxic. Gaze nystagmus, especially horizontal one, is prominent with saccadic eye movement and upward gaze limitation. Fasciculation and myokymia of face and tongue with very prominent, bulging eyes are very characteristic of MJD. In type II (ataxic type), cerebellar manifestation including nystagmus, dysarthria and ataxic gait appear in the second to fourth decades, associated with spasticity, rigidity and dystonia. Facial and lingual fasciculation and ophthalmoparesis are also common. In type III (ataxic-amyotrophic type), prominent cerebellar ataxia is accompanied by distal sensory loss of all modalities and amyotrophy. Tendon reflexes are diminished or absent. Although many cases have these typical features, some unusual phenotypes, such as pure cerebellar ataxia and spastic paraplegia, have also been reported. Dementia is usually not observed in SCA3/MJD.

SCA1 is characterised not only by cerebellar deficits, but also by Parkinsonism, pyramidal tract signs, external ophthalmoplegia, dysphagia and amyotrophy of the extremities (17, 54). Tendon reflexes are often hyperactive with extensor planter responses.

The gene for SCA2 was cloned 3 years after the gene locus had been determined in large Cuban families (28, 44, 87, 95). In SCA 2, slow eye movement is the most characteristic clinical features, along with cerebellar ataxia, extraocular paresis, hyporeflexia, diminished vibration sense and involuntary movements, including postural tremor, action myoclonus and chorea (1, 25, 97). A positive Babinski's sign with diminished tendon reflexes is also characteristic of SCA2.

SCA3/MJD, SCA1 and SCA2 share many signs and symptoms, although each has its characteristic features. The complete clinical assessment should include examination of other affected family members in order to ascertain whether substantial phenotypic differences reflect genetic anticipation.

Finally, the clinical diagnosis should be confirmed by gene analysis.

SCA7 was established by the assignment of the gene locus in 1995 (3, 32), later followed by identification of the gene in 1997 (13). SCA7 is characterised by disturbed visual acuity due to macular and retinal degeneration in addition to cerebellar ataxia, oculomotor and extrapyramidal signs (4, 13, 30, 80). Oculomotor involvement includes slow saccades and less frequently supranuclear ophthalmoplegia. Hyperreflexia with extensor plantar response, sensory disturbance and dementia are also described. The onset ranges very widely from the infantile period to the sixth decade depending on the repeat length. Retinal and cerebellar degeneration develop in transgenic mice expressing the mutant gene (125).

SCA6 is intriguing because the gene function is well known as voltage-dependent P/Q type alpha 1A-Ca channel (126). In SCA6, pure cerebellar ataxia is the cardinal feature (50), while diminished vibration sense, hyporeflexia, hyperreflexia and involuntary movement have been inconsistently detected in some individuals (26, 43, 69, 106). Occasionally, patients complain of episodic ataxia, vertigo or headache indicating a relationship to the allelic diseases, episodic ataxia type 2 and familial hemiplegic migraine (52, 53, 82). Vertical nystagmus with oscillopsia is not uncommon (31, 112). In SCA6, cerebellar Purkinje cells are predominantly affected with cytoplasmic, ubiquitin-negative inclusions (47, 49, 51), which distinct from the intranuclear, ubiquitin-positive inclusions in CAG repeat disorders. Moreover, SCA6 is associated with a channelopathy since cultured cells transfected with the SCA6 gene mutation have Ca-channel dysfunction (71, 91, 114).

SCA5 (90, 107) and SCA16 (73) are very rare.

SCA4 (21) is characterised by profound neuropathy and occasional pyramidal tract signs in addition to cerebellar symptoms, but the identical locus causes a pure cerebellar ataxia or ADCA-III in some families in Japan (77, 111).

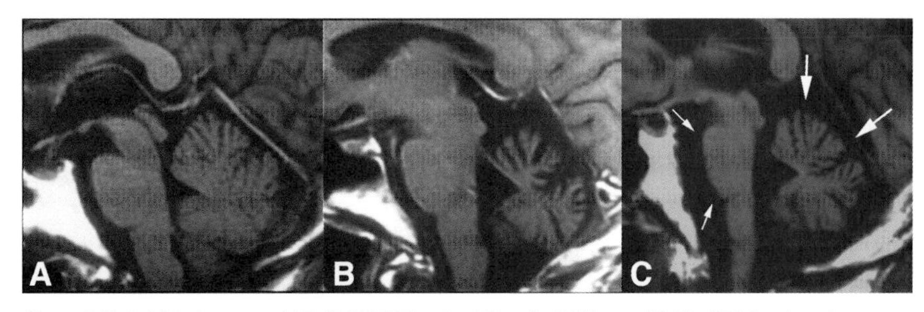

Figure 3. Brain MRIs from control (**A**), MJD/SCA3 patient (**C**) and a SCA6 case (**B**). The SCA6 patient shows atrophy restricted to the cerebellum whereas the MJD/SCA3 patient reveals atrophy of both the pons and cerebellum.

SCA8, which is reported to be due to an abnormal CTG repeat expansion, shows cerebellar ataxia and spasticity (14, 61); however, further clinicopathologic studies are necessary since the purported mutation has been detected in normal individuals as well as patients with other diseases (102, 105, 118, 119).

SCA10 is characterised by not only cerebellar ataxia, but also seizures (70). In SCA12, characteristic features include action tremor, hyperreflexia, and subtle Parkinsonism without disabling cerebellar dysfunction (40, 79). SCA13 is a childhood-onset cerebellar gait ataxia associated with moderate mental retardation and mild developmental delay in motor acquisition (35). In SCA14, there are episodic myoclonus-like involuntary movements as well as cerebellar ataxia (121). SCA17 is caused by abnormal expansion of the CAG repeat in a TATA binding protein and is clinically characterised by dementia, Parkinsonism, involuntary movements, hyperreflexia and cerebellar signs (78).

Imaging. In CCA and SCA6 only cerebellar atrophy, particularly cerebellar cortical atrophy is seen (76, 98), although rare pontine atrophy was reported (109). Other forms of SCAs that have involvement of extracerebellar systems may show atrophy or signal intensity changes or both in extracerebellar systems, including the pons, basal ganglia and cerebrum (29, 46) (Figure 3).

Laboratory findings. Usual examinations of the blood, urine, feces, and CSF are all within normal limits. In AVED (6, 84, 122, 123) and early onset ataxia with oculomotor apraxia and hypoalbuminemia (EOAH) (12, 75), there are laboratory signs of vitamin E deficiency and hypoalbuminemia, respectively. Neuro-otological examination reveals oculomotor, vestibular and cerebellar abnormalities such as nystagmus, ocular dysmetria, abnormal caloric test and so on in many SCAs.

Macroscopy

The neuropathology of hereditary ataxia represents a phenotype in the tissues, and the current task is the correct interpretation of the pathogenesis, taking into consideration the responsible mutations. The spectrum of morphological abnormalities in SCA is very wide. It includes the central and peripheral nervous systems (CNS, PNS), and in the CNS ranges from lesions of the retina to atrophy at all levels of the spinal cord. Neuropathological observations have been made on SCA1, SCA2, SCA3, SCA6, SCA7, and SCA17. The description that follows compares three common types (SCA2, SCA3/MJD and SCA6) and emphasises the lesions that cause the most prominent clinical feature, ataxia.

Brain weights in SCA2 are often below 1000 g whereas they are normal or modestly reduced in SCA3 and SCA6. Cerebral, cerebellar, and pontine atrophy in SCA2 is often dramatic (Figure 4A). All brain stem structures are smaller than normal, and there is often pigment loss in the substantia nigra. The atrophic pontine base stands in contrast to the preserved tegmentum. The normal contour of the inferi-

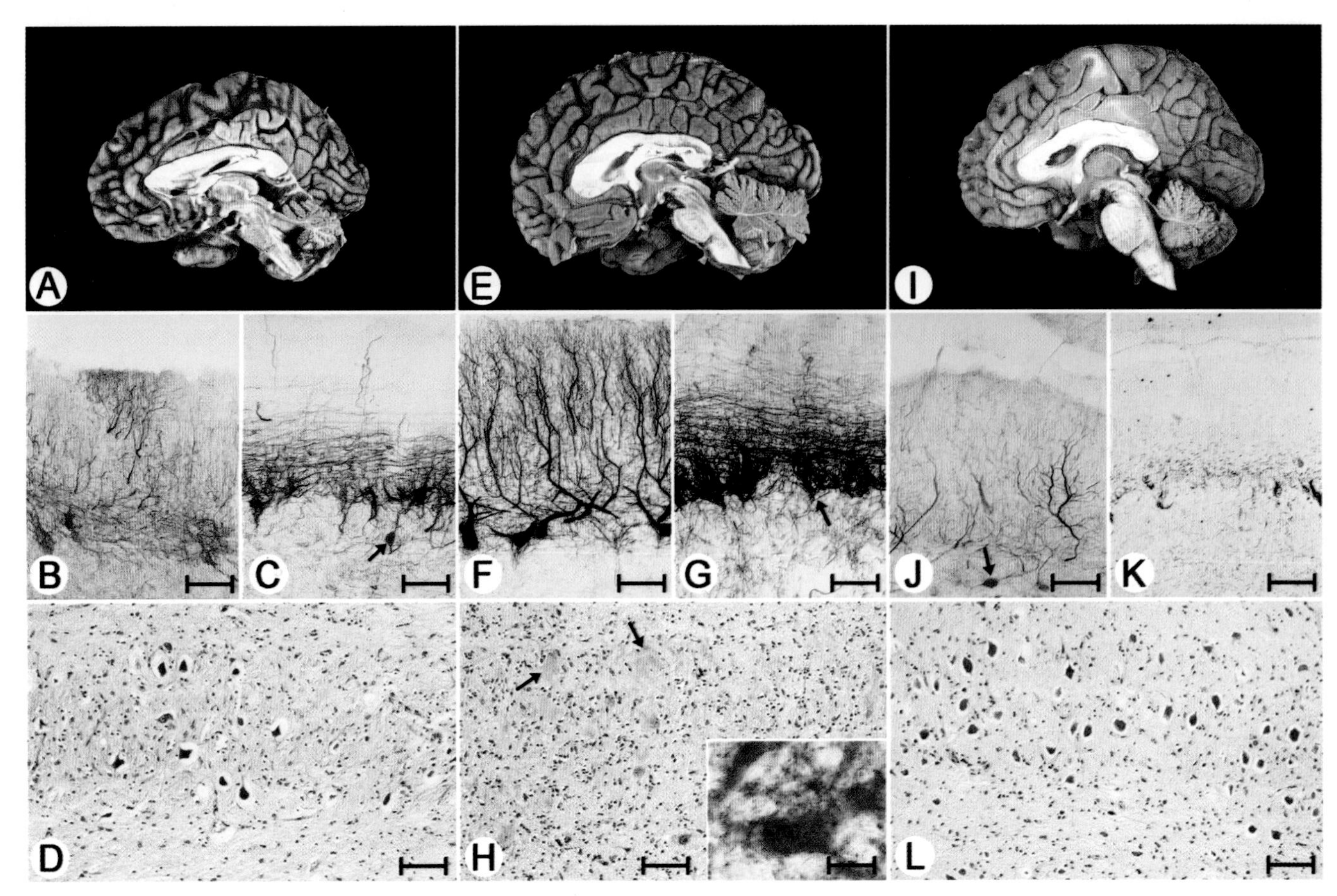

Figure 4. *Gross and microscopic pathology of SCA2, SCA3/MJD, and SCA6.* **A-D**: SCA2; **E-H**: SCA3/MJD; **I-L**: SCA6; **B, C, F, G, J, K**: Cerebellar cortex (immunostain for non-phosphorylated neurofilament protein in **B**, **F**, and **J**; immunostain for phosphorylated neurofilament protein in **C**, **G**, and **K**); **D**, **H**, **L**: dentate nucleus (cresyl violet; inset in **C**, immunostain for SNAP-25). The brain of the patient with SCA2 (**A**) shows striking atrophy of the basis pontis and the vermis, and the fourth ventricle is dilated. There is also cortical atrophy of the cerebrum. The gross specimen of SCA3/MJD (**E**) is normal. The cerebellum of the patient with SCA6 (**I**) is small. The immunostains for non-phosphorylated neurofilament protein of SCA2 (**B**) and SCA6 (**J**) show severe loss of Purkinje cell bodies and their dendrites while the dendritic arbor of these cells is intact in SCA3/MJD (**F**). Normal axonal filaments yield little if any reaction product with this antibody, and the axonal expansion in (arrow in **J**) is a pathological finding. Immunostaining for phosphorylated neurofilament protein in SCA2 (**C**) reveals preservation of many parallel fibers, empty baskets, and a torpedo (arrow in **C**). In SCA6, severe loss of Purkinje cells (**J**) is accompanied by atrophy of parallel fibers and lack of baskets (**K**). In contrast to SCA2 and SCA6, the cerebellar cortex in SCA3/MJD shows the expected density of parallel fibers and an abundance of baskets about normal Purkinje cells (**B**). Also, the "pinceaux" of the proximal Purkinje cell axons are visualised (arrow in **G**). The dentate nucleus in SCA2 (**D**) shows focal loss of nerve cells while it is normal in SCA6 (**L**). In SCA3/MJD, the lesion of the dentate consists of neuronal loss and grumose degeneration (arrows and insert in **H**). Magnification bars: 100 μm in B-L; 25 μm in the insert in H.

or olivary nucleus disappears, and on slices, the meandering chief olivary nuclei are indistinct. The fourth ventricle is dilated. There is no convincing gross cerebellar or pontine atrophy in SCA3/MJD (Figure 4E) but the specimen of a SCA6 patient shows a small cerebellum (Figure 4I).

Histopathology

The microphotographs of the cerebellar cortex of the three cases shown in Figure 4 are the results of immunocytochemical stains on 40 μm-thick vibratome sections. A monoclonal antibody to non-phosphorylated neurofilament protein was used to visualise Purkinje cell bodies and their dendritic expansions. Thinning of the molecular layer due to Purkinje cell atrophy is apparent in SCA2 (Figure 4B) and SCA6 (Figure 4J). In SCA3/MJD, the thickness of the molecular layer is normal (approximately 500 μm) (Figure 4F). Purkinje cells are abundant and display their elaborate dendritic expansions. In SCA6 (Figure 4J), this antibody produces abnormal staining of axons and axonal expansions in the granular layer (arrow in Figure 4J). Monoclonal antibodies to phosphorylated neurofilament protein are suitable to reveal normal and pathological axons (Figure 4C, G, K). The empty baskets shown in SCA2 (Figure 4C) are characteristic of many forms of familial and sporadic cerebellar cortical atrophy, and the partial preservation of many parallel fibers is also a common observation (Figure 4C). However, parallel fibers may be quite depleted as shown in the case of SCA6 (Figure 4K). In SCA3/MJD, parallel fibers, baskets, and pinceaux (arrow in Figure 4G) are normal.

The dentate nuclei in SCA2, SCA3/MJD, and SCA6 are shown in Figure 4D, H, and L, respectively. In SCA2, neuronal loss is patchy (Figure 4D). In contrast, neuronal size and density appear normal in SCA6 (Figure 4L). The dentate lesion in SCA3/MJD is remarkable for severe neuronal loss and "grumose" degeneration (Figure 4H). Immunocytochemical staining for the synaptosome-associated protein 25 (SNAP25) reveals

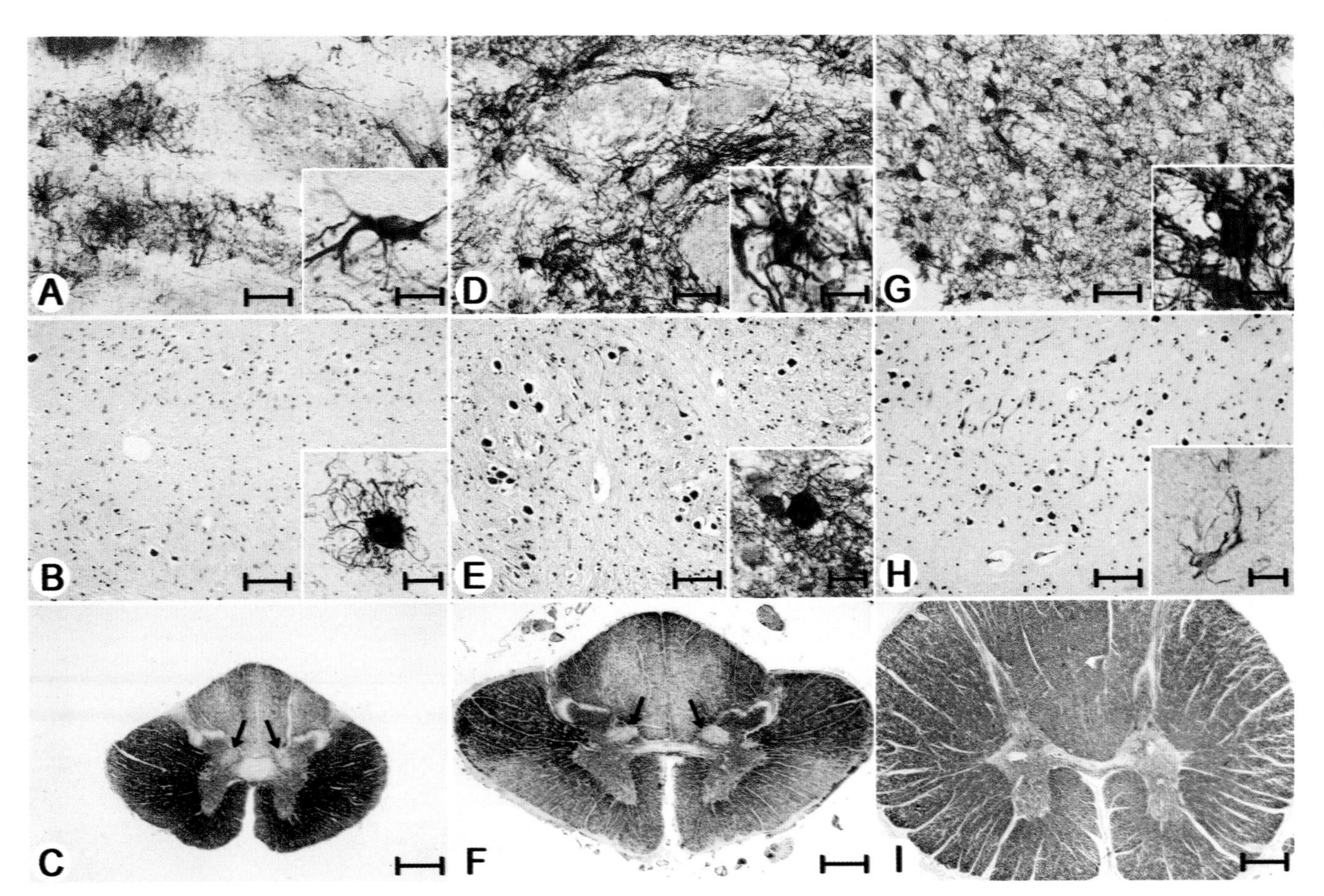

Figure 5. *Microscopic pathology of SCA2, SCA3/MJD, and SCA6.* **A-C**: SCA2; **D-F**: SCA3/MJD; **G-I**: SCA6; **A,D,G**: basis pontis (immunostain for non-phosphorylated neurofilament protein); **B,E,H**: inferior olivary nucleus (cresyl violet; insets, immunostain for non-phosphorylated neurofilament protein); **C,F,I**: thoracic spinal cord (immunostain for myelin basic protein). The neuropil of the basis pontis in SCA2 is greatly reduced (**A**), and many neurons have lost their stellate appearance (inset in **A**). The pontine neuropil in SCA3/MJD (**D** and inset) and SCA6 (**G** and inset) is normal. The inferior olivary nucleus in SCA2 (**B**) shows subtotal neuronal loss though the remaining nerve cells have a normal globular dendritic expanse (inset in **B**). The inferior olivary nucleus is normal in SCA3/MJD (**E** and inset). Olivary neurons are abundant in SCA6 (**H**) though their dendrites are greatly simplified (inset in **H**). The microphotographs of the spinal cord in **C**, **F**, and **I** were prepared at the same magnification and enlargement. The thoracic spinal cord in SCA2 (**C**) is very small (cross-sectional area = 16.7 mm^2) and shows fiber loss in the dorsal columns and the dorsal nuclei of Clarke (arrows). In SCA3/MJD, the cross-sectional area of the spinal cord is lower than normal for the illustrated upper lumbar level (31.6 mm^2) (**F**). There is fiber loss in the dorsal and anterolateral fasciculi, and in the dorsal nuclei (arrows in **F**). The spinal cord in SCA6 (**I**) is entirely normal. The cross-sectional area exceeds 50 mm^2. Magnification markers are 100 μm in **A, B, D, E, G**, and **H**; 25 μm in all insets; and 1 mm in **C**, **F**, and **I**.

that grumose degeneration is due to an overabundance of synaptic terminals (inset in Figure 4H).

Figure 5 illustrates findings in the pons, the inferior olivary nuclei, and the spinal cord. Severe neuronal loss in the basis pontis is characteristic of SCA2 (Figure 5A). The remaining neurons lack the normal stellate appearance and are often bipolar (inset in Figure 5A). In contrast, SCA3/MJD (Figure 5D) and SCA6 (Figure 5G) show abundant nerve cells with normal dendrites (insets in Figure 5D and G). The main inferior olivary nucleus in SCA2 is often totally devoid of nerve cells (Figure 5B). However, the few remaining nerve cells show the normal elaborate spherical dendritic arbor (inset in Figure 5B). In SCA3/MJD, the inferior olivary nucleus is preserved (Figure 5E and inset). In the illustrated case of SCA6, the cresyl violet stain shows numerous nerve cells in the inferior olivary nucleus (Figure 5H). However, immunostaining for cell bodies and dendrites reveals a greatly impoverished dendritic tree (inset in Figure 5H).

The size of the spinal cord in SCA2 is greatly reduced, and there is fiber loss in the dorsal columns (Figure 5C). The cross-sectional area in the illustrated section (Figure 5C) is only 16.7 mm^2 (Normal: 32-43 mm^2). There is some loss of myelinated fibers in the substance of the nucleus dorsalis of Clarke (arrows in Figure 5C). The spinal cord lesions in SCA3/MJD bear a superficial resemblance to the abnormalities in FRDA, ie, combined atrophy of the dorsal and lateral columns, and severe reduction of the number of nerve cells in Clarke's nucleus (arrows in Figure 5F). The cross-sectional area of the illustrated section is 31.6 mm^2, which is less than normal for the upper lumbar level. Spinal cord lesions in SCA6 are absent (Figure 4). The estimated area of the illustrated section exceeds 50 mm^2. For purposes of comparison, it should be pointed out that magnification and photographic enlargement in Figure 5C, F, and I are the same.

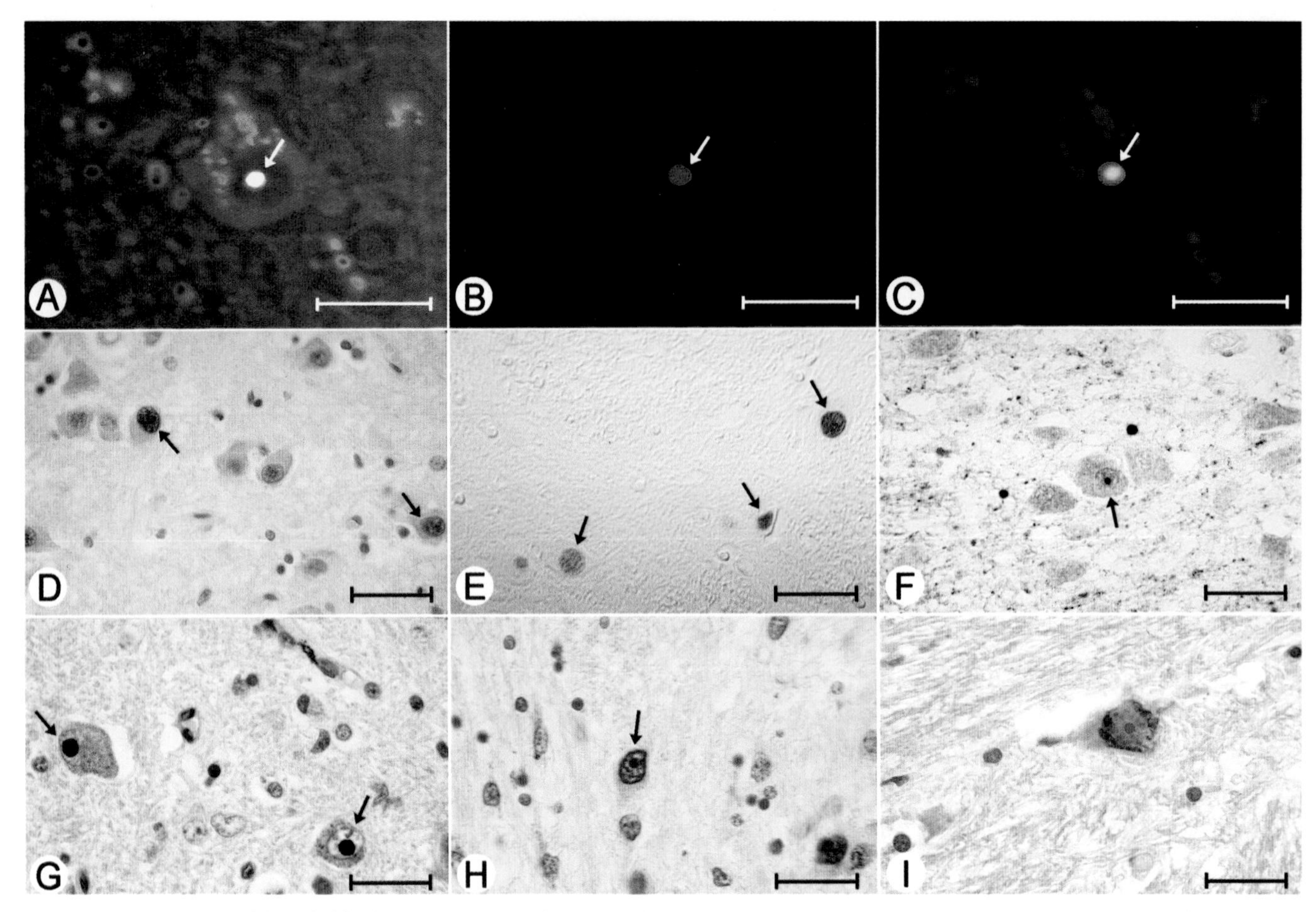

Figure 6. *Inclusion bodies in SCA.* **A-C**, SCA3/MJD. Double-label confocal immunofluorescence micro-scopy with anti-ataxin-3 (fluorescein isothiocyanate, **A**) and anti-ubiquitin (Quantum Red, **B**) shows co-localization (overlay in **C**) of the reaction products in an intranuclear inclusion (basis pontis) (arrows in **A-C**). Images in **B** and **C** were processed to suppress lipofuscin fluorescence. **D-F**, SCA17. Positive contrast immunocytochemistry shows pan-nuclear reaction product in nerve cells of the basis pontis with monoclonal anti-TATA-binding protein (arrows in **D**) and monoclonal anti-polyQ (1C2) (arrows in **E**) but a nucleoliform inclusion with anti-ubiquitin (arrow in **F**). Sections in **D** and **F** were counterstained with hematoxylin. The section in **E** was not counterstained but photographed with Nomarski interference optics. **G** (SCA1); **H** (SCA2); **I** (SCA6). Immunocytochemistry with monoclonal antibody 1C2 shows dense intranuclear inclusions of pontine neurons in SCA1 (arrows in **G**), mixed pan-nuclear and nucleoliform inclusions in SCA2 (arrow in **H**), and cytoplasmic reaction product in SCA6. Magnification markers in all microphotographs, 25 μm.

Immunocytochemistry

Figure 6 illustrates inclusion bodies in several forms of SCA that are known to be due to CAG expansions in the coding regions of their respective genes. The result of immunostaining often depends on the epitopes that the antibody recognises (99). In addition to the abnormal gene product, intranuclear inclusion bodies often contain ubiquitin and other proteins that may be termed "chaperones" (9, 11, 67, 103, 104). Figure 6A, B, and C show the confocal images of an intranuclear inclusion body in the basis pontis of a patient with SCA3/MJD. There is perfect co-localisation of the reaction products obtained with antisera to ataxin3 (Figure 6A) and ubiquitin, respectively (Figure 6B; overlay in Figure 6C).

A monoclonal antibody originally raised against the TATA-binding protein (65) recognises polyglutamine stretches in several proteins (45, 115, 116). The antibody, termed 1C2 (65), is now commercially available and can be used to advantage in known or suspected SCA with expanded CAG trinucleotides. The TATA-binding protein itself may be mutated due to CAG expansion, and the resulting autosomal dominant ataxia is now known as SCA17 (23, 59, 78). Figures 6D-F illustrate the immunocytochemical results in a patient with SCA17. The antibodies were a monoclonal anti-TATA-binding protein without defined epitope (Figure 6D), 1C2 (anti-polyglutamine) (Figure 6E), and monoclonal anti-ubiquitin (Figure 6F). The first two antibodies yielded a pan-nuclear reaction product (Figure 6D, E) whereas anti-ubiquitin visualised a nucleoliform intranuclear inclusion. The 1C2 antibody yielded large and rather dense intranuclear inclusions in SCA1 (Figure 6G), a mixture of pan-nuclear and nucleoliform reaction product in SCA2 (Figure 6H), and strictly cytoplasmic inclusions in SCA6 (Figure 6I).

Correlation of Genotype and Phenotype

New morphological methods provide improved neuroanatomical detail of the lesions but overlap generally precludes the identification of a specific form of SCA by gross inspection and the study of stained slides. A notable exception is SCA3/MJD. Its neuropathological phenotype is unique because of the combination of neuronal loss in the dentate nucleus, grumose degeneration, atrophy of the nucleus dorsalis of Clarke, and fiber loss in the dorsal and anterolateral columns of the spinal cord. In SCA7, the combination of pigmentary retinopathy and OPCA is also specific enough to allow a conclusion based on morphological observations.

The length of the CAG trinucleotide repeat affects the *clinical* phenotype, especially the age of onset and the severity of the illness. Borderline expansions may be clinically silent or cause late onset. Progressive expansion of unstable repeats in successive generations accounts for anticipation. Very long expansions, such as in SCA7, cause onset in infancy (4) or even intrauterine death (74). Only anecdotal evidence is available that larger CAG trinucleotide repeat expansions affect the *neuropathological* phenotype. The reason is the current lack of parameters that can be measured in specimens and correlated with the length of the expansion. In a review of hereditary ataxia, Koeppen illustrated the effect of a large expansion in SCA2 (56). In this family, the father's abnormal allele contained 41 CAG trinucleotide repeats. In the son, the CAG stretch had expanded to 58 repeats. Survivals were 22 and 9 years, respectively, and the affected son had much more severe atrophy of the basis pontis and cerebellum than the father. These observations suggest that only relatively simple measurements on the gross specimens, such as weight, diameters, or cross-sectional areas, may be needed to establish morphological "severity" of ataxia as a function of CAG trinucleotide repeat expansion. Autopsy specimens may be used in a manner similar to neuroradiological measurements. Onodera et al (81) measured magnetic resonance images of 21 patients with SCA3/MJD. They made multiple-regression analyses in which age and lengths of CAG trinucleotide repeats were the independent variables. Both age and lengths of the repeats correlated significantly with progressive atrophy of brain stem and cerebellum. In FRDA, the cross-sectional area of the thoracic spinal cord can be used to assess the effect of abnormal guanine-adenine-adenine (GAA) expansions. In homozygous patients with short GAA stretches, the area is less seriously reduced than in cases with longer GAA repeats (56). Spinocerebellar ataxia type 7 probably offers the best chance for successful morphometry on gross specimens. The disease has a very broad clinical and neuropathological spectrum, and pathological CAG trinucleotide repeat expansions range from 41 to 306 (4).

The Contribution of Immunocytochemistry to the Neuropathology of the Spinocerebellar Ataxias

Immunocytochemistry has replaced the traditional Golgi impregnation, which is fickle, time-consuming, and expensive. Successful staining depends on prompt autopsies and fixation at cold-room temperatures. Initial perfusion is preferred over immersion of large specimens in fixatives. Fixation times should be relatively short (less than one week), and tissue blocks can be stored for some time in buffer containing 15% sucrose and 15 mM sodium azide (for vibratome sections). Vibratome sections often show better retention of antigenic determinants though their processing is laborious. The thickness of vibratome sections (40-100 μm) permits 3-dimensional reconstruction of dendritic arbors in the confocal microscope but thinner, slide-mounted sections of paraffin- or polyethylene glycol-embedded tissues are more readily processed in batches and by automation. Antigen retrieval, monoclonal and polyclonal antibodies, single- or multiple-label confocal immunofluorescence microscopy provide much greater microscopic detail than was possible in the past.

In neuropathological studies of SCA1, SCA2, SCA6, SCA7, and SCA17, Purkinje cell atrophy has attracted most attention, and the clinical phenomenon of "ataxia" is often considered the direct result of this specific neuronal loss. However, the neuropil of the cerebellar cortex is complex, and the study of stellate, basket, and granule cells, and Golgi neurons is also needed. Antibodies to non-phosphorylated neurofilament protein show some selectivity for normal and atrophic Purkinje cells (Figure 1), and the reaction product rivals that of a successful Golgi impregnation (60). Similarly, anti-calbindin-D 28k visualises Purkinje cell dendrites in great detail (48, 117). A combination of antibodies to three calcium-binding proteins can be used to reveal Purkinje cells (calbindin-D 28k; parvalbumin), stellate and basket cells (parvalbumin), and parallel fibers (calretinin) (100). The immunocytochemical result after staining with antibodies to these proteins may provide some insight into calcium dysmetabolism in Purkinje cells, and immunoreactivity of calbindin-D 28k and parvalbumin in SCA may be lost before these neurons undergo atrophy (48, 117). Antibodies to the microtubule-associated protein 2 (MAP2) are useful to assess the state of stellate, basket, and Golgi neurons because Purkinje cells do not stain well with anti-MAP2. Koeppen et al (60) reported that in SCA2 the small neurons of the molecular layer survive despite subtotal loss of Purkinje cells.

Antibodies to non-phosphorylated neurofilament protein and MAP1 show the remarkable dendritic arrangement in the dentate nucleus. Multiple dendrites arise directly and asymmetrically from one side of the neuronal cell body. They stream toward the dendrites of neighboring cells and thus form a dense interlacing network of processes. This distribution presumably offers a wide receptive field for incoming terminals that resembles the dendritic expansion of Purkinje cells (60).

In the inferior olivary nucleus, antibodies to non-phosphorylated neurofilament, MAP1, and MAP2 show the full spherical dendritic expanse of the normal nerve cell (Figure 5E) and are useful to assess dendritic atrophy (inset in Figure 5H) and neuronal loss. The same antibodies can also be used for the visualization of normal and atrophic neurons in the basis pontis (Figure 5A, D, G).

Antibodies to phosphorylated neurofilament protein are useful in immunocytochemical methods for axons, Purkinje cells baskets (Figure 4C, G), and torpedoes (Figure 4C). They also reveal grumose degeneration in SCA3/MJD (not illustrated).

Synapses are of obvious importance in the study of all neurodegenerative diseases, and Koeppen et al (58) reported a comprehensive study in various SCA. Antibodies to SNAP-25, a protein of the presynaptic membrane, are especially useful for archival tissues. The antigenic determinants of the protein survive even prolonged storage in fixatives or paraffin. They are readily restored by antigen retrieval methods, such as microwave irradiation in citrate buffer (58). Vibratome sections of promptly fixed tissue may retain glutamic acid decarboxylase (GAD) antigenicity (60). The enzyme catalyzes the rate-limiting step in the biosynthesis of γ-amino-butyric acid (GABA), and GAD-reactivity in Purkinje cell bodies, their afferent synapses, parallel fibers arising from stellate and basket neurons, and Purkinje cell-derived afferents in the dentate nucleus allows insight into disturbed GABA-ergic microcircuitry in SCA (58). Stains for synapses also readily show the grumose degeneration of the dentate nucleus in SCA3/MJD (Figure 4H).

Clinico-anatomic Correlation

Ataxia, dysmetria, and dysarthria ultimately represent incorrectly processed signals from the motor cortex. Despite emphasis on Purkinje cell dysfunction in many SCA, the dentate nucleus is a critical way station that provides most cerebellar efferents. It also "diverts" some of its output to the inferior olivary nucleus on the opposite side. Olivocerebellar fibers cross the midline and issue collaterals to the dentate nucleus. Lapresle and Hamida (64) named this feedback loop the "triangle of Guillain and Mollaret." Discrete lesions of the dentate nucleus or the contralateral central tegmental tract in the pons cause olivary hypertrophy due to transsynaptic degeneration (22). A typical clinical manifestation of this lesion is palatal myoclonus. In addition, vascular lesions, tumors, or plaques of multiple sclerosis in the hilum of dentate nucleus also cause lasting ipsilateral dysmetria. It may be quite violent and has been likened to myoclonus ("action myoclonus"). In theory, the severe dentate lesion in SCA3/MJD in the presence of an intact cerebellar cortex should also cause olivary hypertrophy. However, a systematic comparison of progressive supranuclear palsy, DRPLA, and SCA3/MJD revealed that only the 2 first conditions generated olivary hypertrophy. It was absent in SCA3/MJD (34). All three conditions show grumose degeneration, and this phenomenon seems unrelated to the presence or the absence of olivary hypertrophy. The lack of transsynaptic olivary changes in SCA3/MJD is unexplained.

Purkinje cell dysfunction and atrophy cannot be interpreted without attention to the inferior olivary nuclei. De Zeeuw et al (15) reviewed the complex intraolivary circuitry and the three working hypotheses of olivocerebellar physiology. They are respectively named "timing hypothesis," "comparator hypothesis," and "learning hypothesis." The last is most attractive because it provides a relatively simple mechanism by which olivocerebellar fibers send error messages to Purkinje cells. Accordingly, ataxia may be the result of inadequate olivocerebellar input to "error-prone" Purkinje cells. Though it is widely accepted that destructive lesions of the cerebellar cortex cause retrograde contralateral atrophy of the inferior olivary nuclei, this process does not occur in a commensurate manner in all acquired or hereditary forms of Purkinje cell atrophy (eg, Figure 5H).

Gray and white matter lesions of the spinal cord in SCA2 and SCA3/MJD (Figure 5) add to the clinical phenotype of ataxia. In SCA3/MJD, neuronal loss in Clarke's nucleus (Figure 5F) and the long fiber tracts of the dorsal and anterolateral funiculi likely aggravate the dysfunction of the dentate nucleus.

Atrophy of the nuclei of the basis pontis causes ataxia in its own right and must be considered in SCA1, SCA2, and SCA7. It is not surprising that SCA2 shows the most severe clinical manifestations. This disease combines cerebellar cortical atrophy, loss of nerve cells in the dentate nucleus, pons, and inferior olivary nuclei with degeneration of the spinal cord.

Pathogenesis

The discovery of intranuclear inclusion bodies in several polyQ diseases raised the hope that a "primary" lesion of specific nerve cells could be detected by immunocytochemical methods. Such inclusions have now been reported in SCA1, SCA2, SCA3, SCA7, and SCA17. They can be detected by antibodies to the unmutated proteins (ataxin1, ataxin2, ataxin3, ataxin7, and TATA-binding protein [in SCA17]). The antibodies "recognise" mutated proteins even more readily than the normal cytoplasmic or nuclear analogues, and the presence of nucleoliform inclusions is generally interpreted as aggregation. In SCA6, the mutation expands the polyQ stretch of the α_{1A}-calcium channel protein, and 1C2-reaction product accumulates mostly in the cytoplasm rather than the nucleus (Figure 6I and (49)). While a "gain-of-function" impairment may be true for long polyQ expansions, the problem in SCA6 is more likely interference with normal calcium channel properties. Results in SCA2 have varied with the antibodies that were used to detect ataxin2. Inclusion bodies were reported as absent (41), present (62) or abundant (85).

Several observations temper enthusiasm over a possible common pathogenic mechanism in polyQ diseases. The apparent main disease target in SCA1, SCA2, SCA6, and SCA7 is the Purkinje cell but these neurons either show no intranuclear inclusions or only minute aggregates (SCA6; [49]). In SCA3/MJD, inclusions are present in greatest abundance in the neurons of the basis pontis (Figure 6A-C) though there is no pontine atrophy (Figure 5D). Nuclear reaction product is often pan-nuclear rather than nucleoliform (Figure 6D, E). Diffuse and nucleoliform reaction product may occur in the same cell (Figure 6H). Pan-nuclear 1C2-reactive antigens are not necessarily associated with ubiquitin (Figure 6F). Pang et al (85) found a numerical discrepancy between 1C2- and ubiquitin-reactive inclusions, and Holmberg et al (37) made similar observations in SCA7. The distribution of inclusion bodies in the CNS of various SCA is not the same, with SCA17 perhaps showing the most extensive involvement of cerebral cortex, diencephalon, brain stem, and cerebellum (59). In this type of SCA, inclusions are absent from Purkinje cells, the neurons of the dentate nucleus, the remaining neurons of the inferior olivary nuclei, the lentiform nucleus, and the spinal cord. Interestingly, they are present in the stellate and basket cells of the cerebellar molecular layer (59).

Inclusion bodies cannot be viewed as proof of "primary" atrophy of a specific neuronal cell type. Alternate explanations must be found, and it is appropriate to review the complex combination of lesions at various levels of the CNS and PNS in terms of traditional retrograde and transsynaptic degeneration. Invariably, SNAP25 reaction product in the molecular layer of the cerebellar cortex remains despite subtotal Purkinje cell loss (58). This observation implies that orphaned terminals survive despite loss of their main target. Also, the disappearance of Purkinje cells does not necessarily cause retrograde atrophy in stellate and basket neurons (60). In SCA with cortical cerebellar atrophy, the granular layer is often well preserved, accounting for the persistence of parallel fibers (Figure 4C). This exemption is not always true, and atrophy of the granular layer with disappearance of parallel fibers may occur in advanced cases, such as illustrated for SCA6 in Figure 4K.

The topistic relationship between cerebellar cortex and the inferior olivary nucleus has been known since 1908 (39), and the neurons of the inferior olive have often been considered dependent on the trophic effect of Purkinje cells. Retrograde atrophy of olivary neurons is not invariable after Purkinje cell loss. The olivocerebellar pathway shows impressive plasticity in experimental animals (108). The partial destruction of olivary nerve cells in rats by 3-acetylpyridine causes loss of climbing fiber input to Purkinje cells but surviving fibers gradually re-innervate the orphaned neurons by sprouting over substantial distances (93, 94). The regenerative potential of climbing fibers is not restricted to the developing nervous system (5). Axotomy in the adult rat affects the neurons of the contralateral principal olive much more severely than the medial and dorsal accessory nuclei (5). The preservation of the medial accessory olivary nucleus in several types of SCA may be the human equivalent to the experimental results in the rat. Buffo et al (5) offered the interpretation that olivary neurons belong to two or more subsets with differential vulnerability to axonal interruption.

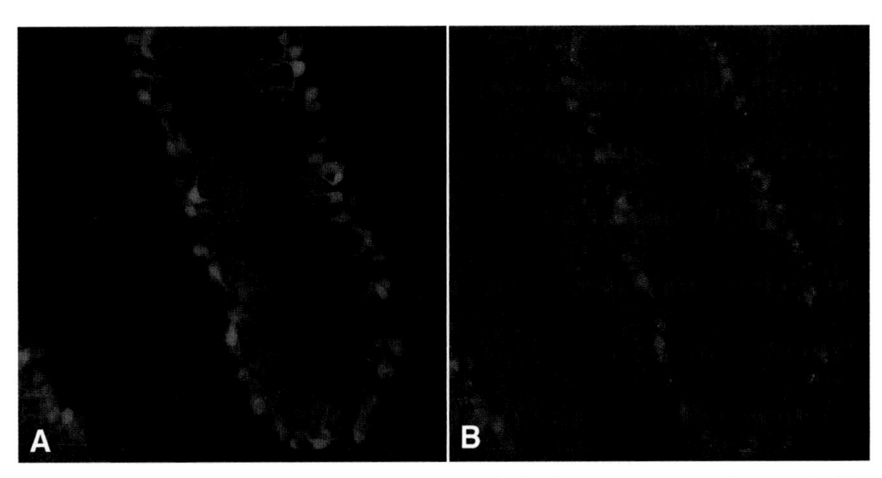

Figure 7. The cerebellum of an 18-week-old homozygous ataxin-1[82Q] transgenic mouse co-immunostained for calbindin (**A**) and for ataxin-1 (**B**). Note the dendritic atrophy of Purkinje cells and the presence of heterotopic Purkinje cells in the molecular layer. The ataxin-1 antibody labels intranuclear inclusions within these same Purkinje cells.

There are no spontaneously occurring human diseases with selective loss of nerve cells in the inferior olivary nuclei in which climbing fiber plasticity can be examined. Nevertheless, it may be suggested that in SCA with cerebellar cortical atrophy, functional failure of olivary neurons is a primary event. Two common observations in sporadic and hereditary atrophy of the cerebellar cortex have not been explained. They are the preservation of the uvula, the nodulus, and the adjacent tonsils in the cerebellum, and the medial accessory nuclei of the inferior olives. Holmes and Stewart (39) were aware of this phenomenon when they reported their case 7, a patient with "primary degeneration of the cerebellar cortex." The authors offered no explanation for the retention of some olivary nerve cells while others had undergone subtotal atrophy. It may be argued that integrity of olivary nerve cells accounts for the preservation of the cerebellar cortex, such as in SCA3/MJD (Figure 4F, G). However, the evidence in experimental animals favors the interpretation that at least during development Purkinje cells provide trophic factors, and climbing fibers have the matching receptors. A possible exception is the brain-derived neurotrophic factor that is transported in an anterograde fashion through climbing fibers (101). Under the concept of the triangle of Guillain and Mollaret, climbing fibers give off collaterals to the cerebellar nuclei. If dentate neurons remain intact, such as shown for SCA6 in Figure 4L, they may provide sufficient retrograde trophic influence to the neurons of the inferior olivary nucleus and thus compensate for the loss of Purkinje cells.

Purkinje cell atrophy removes most afferents to the dentate nucleus with consequent loss of GABA-ergic input (as shown for SCA2 by GAD immunocytochemistry; [60]). Staining for synapses with anti-SNAP-25 allows a quantitative assessment of synaptic loss in the dentate nucleus (58). Deafferentation of the dentate nucleus in the course of Purkinje cell atrophy does not necessarily cause loss of nerve cells. In SCA3/MJD, Purkinje cells and olivary neurons are intact, and neuronal loss in the dentate nucleus cannot be attributed to lack of afferent input. Accordingly, the dentate lesion should be considered "primary." The synaptic loss in this condition (58) must be interpreted as a secondary event.

The loss of neurons in the basis pontis may also be primary. It can be expected to cause depletion of mossy fiber terminals in the granular layer but it is unlikely that transneuronal atrophy affects Purkinje cell across one or two synapses (pons→granule cells→Purkinje cells; pons→granule cells→stellate/basket cells→Purkinje cells).

Many uncertainties remain. More by exclusion than by direct evidence, the following neuronal groups are likely to undergo primary atrophy: the dentate nucleus in SCA3/MJD and the basis pontis in SCA1, SCA2, and SCA7. Evidence is still insufficient to claim primary atrophy of Purkinje cells or the inferior olivary nucleus in SCA1, SCA2, SCA6, SCA7, and SCA17. At the level of the spinal cord, the nucleus dorsalis probably also undergoes primary atrophy in SCA3/MJD. In contrast to FRDA, the neurons in the ganglia of the dorsal root are generally preserved, and transsynaptic atrophy is unlikely. Both FRDA and SCA3/MJD show significant synaptic depletion in Clarke's nucleus but the mechanisms of this loss are different. It is anterograde in FRDA and retrograde in SCA3/MJD (58).

Experimental Models

The first animal model of spinocerebellar ataxia was developed by Orr and colleagues for SCA1. A transgenic murine model of SCA1 was made using a Purkinje cell-specific promoter to express full-length human ataxin1 (7). Lines expressing high levels of an expanded allele, ataxin1[82Q] developed severe ataxia and progressive Purkinje cell pathology within several months, while mice expressing a non-expanded allele, ataxin1[30Q], did not. Pathologically, Purkinje cells in the SCA1 transgenic mice develop two features seen in SCA1 patients; dendritic atrophy (10), and intranuclear ubiquitinated aggregates of mutant ataxin1 (104) (Figure 7); suggesting that the transgenic mice undergo a disease process very similar to that seen in the human condition. Loss of Purkinje cells in the transgenic mice was minimal at the time when ataxia was first apparent, indicating that the neurological deficits arise initially from neuronal dysfunction and atrophy, and only later from neuronal loss.

Other transgenic mice were generated that express expanded ataxin1[82Q] with a mutated nuclear localization sequence, ataxin1^{K772T} (55). Although these mice had levels of ataxin1 in Purkinje cells similar to those in the original ataxin1[82Q] transgenic mice, they never developed disease. Ataxin1 was present only in the cytoplasm and formed no aggregates, even at one year of age. These results indicate that it is the ataxin1 protein with an expanded polyglutamine tract that is pathogenic and not *SCA1* mRNA with an expanded number of CAG-repeats. Nuclear localization of the protein also appears to be critical for pathogenesis and formation of ataxin1 aggregates.

Additional lines of transgenic mice were made using an expanded ataxin1[77Q] gene with a deletion in a region essential for self-association of ataxin1 (55). These mice developed disease similar to the original ataxin1[82Q] transgenic mice, but they did not form intranuclear aggregates of ataxin1. When ataxin1[82Q] transgenic mice were crossed with mice lacking expression of *Ube3a*, a gene important for ubiquitin function (11), it was found that nuclear aggregates of ataxin1[82Q] were reduced in frequency and size, and the Purkinje cell pathology was more severe than that seen in the ataxin1[82Q] mice. These studies suggest that ataxin1-ubiquitination is important for the formation of the nuclear aggregates but also indicate that pathogenesis in these models of SCA1 is not dependent on the presence of those aggregates.

More recently, there have been reports of transgenic models of SCA2 (42) SCA7 (24, 63, 124, 125) and SCA3/MJD (8), all of which exhibit one or more of the neuropathological deficits found in the human counterpart of each disease, and are likely to serve as useful models of pathogenesis.

References

1. Babovic-Vuksanovic D, Snow K, Patterson MC, Michels VV (1998) Spinocerebellar ataxia type 2 (SCA 2) in an infant with extreme CAG repeat expansion. *Am J Med Genet* 79: 383-387.

2. Bell J, Carmichael EA (1939) On hereditary ataxia and spastic paraplegia. In *The treasury of human inheritance*, RA Fisher (eds). Cambridge University Press: Cambridge. pp. 141-281.

3. Benomar A, Krols L, Stevanin G, Cancel G, LeGuern E, David G, Ouhabi H, Martin JJ, Durr A, Zaim A (1995) The gene for autosomal dominant cerebellar ataxia with pigmentary macular dystrophy maps to chromosome 3p12-p21.1. *Nat Genet* 10: 84-88.

4. Benton CS, de Silva R, Rutledge SL, Bohlega S, Ashizawa T, Zoghbi HY (1998) Molecular and clinical studies in SCA7 define a broad clinical spectrum and the infantile phenotype. *Neurology* 51: 1081-1086.

5. Buffo A, Fronte M, Oestreicher AB, Rossi F (1998) Degenerative phenomena and reactive modification of the adult rat inferior olivary neurons following axotomy and disconnection from their targets. *Neuroscience* 85: 587-604.

6. Burck U, Goebel HH, Kuhlendahl HD, Meier C, Goebel KM (1981) Neuromyopathy and vitamin E deficiency in man. *Neuropediatrics* 12: 267-278.

7. Burright EN, Clark HB, Servadio A, Matilla T, Feddersen RM, Yunis WS, Duvick LA, Zoghbi HY, Orr HT (1995) SCA1 transgenic mice: a model for neurodegeneration caused by an expanded CAG trinucleotide repeat. *Cell* 82: 937-948.

8. Cemal CK, Carroll CJ, Lawrence L, Lowrie MB, Ruddle P, Al-Mahdawi S, King RH, Pook MA, Huxley C, Chamberlain S (2002) YAC transgenic mice carrying pathological alleles of the MJD1 locus exhibit a mild and slowly progressive cerebellar deficit. *Hum Mol Gen* 11: 1075-1094.

9. Chai Y, Koppenhafer SL, Shoesmith SJ, Perez MK, Paulson HL (1999) Evidence for proteasome involve-

ment in polyglutamine disease: localization to nuclear inclusions in SCA3/MJD and suppression of polyglutamine aggregation in vitro. *Hum Mol Genet* 8: 673-682.

10. Clark HB, Burright EN, Yunis WS, Larson S, Wilcox C, Hartman B, Matilla A, Zoghbi HY, Orr HT (1997) Purkinje cell expression of a mutant allele of SCA1 in transgenic mice leads to disparate effects on motor behaviors, followed by a progressive cerebellar dysfunction and histological alterations. *J Neuroscience* 17: 7385-7395.

11. Cummings CJ, Mancini MA, Antalffy B, DeFranco DB, Orr HT, Zoghbi HY (1998) Chaperone suppression of aggregation and altered subcellular proteasome localization imply protein misfolding in SCA1. *Nat Genet* 19: 148-154.

12. Date H, Onodera O, Tanaka H, Iwabuchi K, Uekawa K, Igarashi S, Koike R, Hiroi T, Yuasa T, Awaya Y et al (2001) Early-onset ataxia with ocular motor apraxia and hypoalbuminemia is caused by mutations in a new HIT superfamily gene. *Nat Genet* 29: 184-188.

13. David G, Abbas N, Stevanin G, Durr A, Yvert G, Cancel G, Weber C, Imbert G, Saudou F, Antoniou E, Drabkin H et al (1997) Cloning of the SCA7 gene reveals a highly unstable CAG repeat expansion. *Nat Genet* 17: 65-70.

14. Day JW, Schut LJ, Moseley ML, Durand AC, Ranum LP (2000) Spinocerebellar ataxia type 8: clinical features in a large family. *Neurology* 55: 649-657.

15. De Zeeuw CI, Simpson JI, Hoogenraad CC, Galjart N, Koekkoek SKE, Ruigrok TJH (1998) Microcircuitry and function of the inferior olive. *Trend Neurosci* 21: 391-400.

16. Dejerine J, Thomas A (1900) L'atrophie olivo-ponto-cérébelleuse. *Nouv Icon Salpêtrierè* 13: 330-370.

17. Dubourg O, Durr A, Cancel G, Stevanin G, Chneiweiss H, Penet C, Agid Y, Brice A (1995) Analysis of the SCA1 CAG repeat in a large number of families with dominant ataxia: clinical and molecular correlations. *Ann Neurol* 37: 176-180.

18. Dürr A, Stevanin G, Cancel G, Duyckaerts C, Abbas N, Didierjean O, Chneiweiss H, Benomar A, Lyon-Caen O, Julien J et al(1996) Spinocerebellar ataxia 3 and Machado-Joseph disease: clinical, molecular, and neuropathological features. *Ann Neurol* 39: 490-499.

19. Evidente VG, Gwinn-Hardy KA, Caviness JN, Gilman S (2000) Hereditary ataxias. *Mayo Clin Proc* 75: 475-490.

20. Filla A, Mariotti C, Caruso G, Coppola G, Cocozza S, Castaldo I, Calabrese O, Salvatore E, De Michele G, Riggio MC, Pareyson D et al (2000) Relative frequencies of CAG expansions in spinocerebellar ataxia and dentatorubropallidoluysian atrophy in 116 Italian families. *Eur Neurol* 44: 31-36.

21. Flanigan K, Gardner K, Alderson K, Galster B, Otterud B, Leppert MF, Kaplan C, Ptacek LJ (1996) Autosomal dominant spinocerebellar ataxia with sensory axonal neuropathy (SCA4): clinical description and genetic localization to chromosome 16q22.1. *Am J Hum Genet* 59: 392-399.

22. Foix C, Chavany J-A, Hillemand P (1926) Le syndrome myoclonique de la calotte: Étude anatomo-clinique du nystagmus du voile et des myoclonies rythmiques associées, oculaires, faciales, etc. *Rev Neurol* 45: 942-956.

23. Fujigasaki H, Martin J-J, De Deyn PP, Camuzat A, Deffond D, Stevanin G, Dermaut B, Von Broeckhoven C, Dürr A, Brice A (2001) CAG repeat expansion in the TATA box-binding protein gene causes autosomal dominant cerebellar ataxia. *Brain* 124: 1939-1947.

24. Garden GA, Libby RT, Fu YH, Kinoshita Y, Huang J, Possin DE, Smith AC, Martinez RA, Fine GC, Grote SK, Ware CB et al (2002) Polyglutamine-expanded ataxin-7 promotes non-cell-autonomous Purkinje cell degeneration and displays proteolytic cleavage in ataxic transgenic mice. *J Neurosci* 22: 4897-4905.

25. Geschwind DH, Perlman S, Figueroa CP, Treiman LJ, Pulst SM (1997) The prevalence and wide clinical spectrum of the spinocerebellar ataxia type 2 trinucleotide repeat in patients with autosomal dominant cerebellar ataxia. *Am J Hum Genet* 60: 842-850.

26. Geschwind DH, Perlman S, Figueroa KP, Karrim J, Baloh RW, Pulst SM (1997) Spinocerebellar ataxia type 6. Frequency of the mutation and genotype-phenotype correlations. *Neurology* 49: 1247-1251.

27. Gilman S, Low PA, Quinn N, Albanese A, Ben-Shlomo Y, Fowler CJ, Kaufmann H, Klockgether T, Lang AE, Lantos PL, Litvan I et al (1999) Consensus statement on the diagnosis of multiple system atrophy. *J Neurol Sci* 163: 94-98.

28. Gispert S, Twells R, Orozco G, Brice A, Weber J, Heredero L, Scheufler K, Riley B, Allotey R, Nothers C et al (1993) Chromosomal assignment of the second locus for autosomal dominant cerebellar ataxia (SCA2) to chromosome 12q23-24.1. *Nat Genet* 4: 295-299.

29. Giuffrida S, Saponara R, Restivo DA, Trovato Salinaro A, Tomarchio L, Pugliares P, Fabbri G, Maccagnano C (1999) Supratentorial atrophy in spinocerebellar ataxia type 2: MRI study of 20 patients. *J Neurol* 246: 383-388.

30. Giunti P, Stevanin G, Worth PF, David G, Brice A, Wood NW (1999) Molecular and clinical study of 18 families with ADCA type II: evidence for genetic heterogeneity and de novo mutation. *Am J Hum Genet* 64: 1594-1603.

31. Gomez CM, Thompson RM, Gammack JT, Perlman SL, Dobyns WB, Truwit CL, Zee DS, Clark HB, Anderson JH (1997) Spinocerebellar ataxia type 6: gaze-evoked and vertical nystagmus, Purkinje cell degeneration, and variable age of onset. *Ann Neurol* 42: 933-950.

32. Gouw LG, Kaplan CD, Haines JH, Digre KB, Rutledge SL, Matilla A, Leppert M, Zoghbi HY, Ptacek LJ (1995) Retinal degeneration characterizes a spinocerebellar ataxia mapping to chromosome 3p. *Nat Genet* 10: 89-93.

33. Greenfield JG (1954) *The spino-cerebellar degenerations.* Blackwell Sci Publ: Oxford.

34. Hanihara T, Amano N, Takahashi T, Itoh Y, S. Y (1998) Hypertrophy of the inferior olivary nucleus with progressive supranuclear palsy. *Eur Neurol* 39: 97-102.

35. Herman-Bert A, Stevanin G, Netter JC, Rascol O, Brassat D, Calvas P, Camuzat A, Yuan Q, Schalling M, Durr A, Brice A (2000) Mapping of spinocerebellar ataxia 13 to chromosome 19q13.3-q13.4 in a family with autosomal dominant cerebellar ataxia and mental retardation. *Am J Hum Genet* 67: 229-235.

36. Hirayama K, Takayanagi T, Nakamura R, Yanagisawa N, Hattori T, Kita K, Yanagimoto S, Fujita M, Nagaoka M, Satomura Y et al (1994) Spinocerebellar degenerations in Japan: a nationwide epidemiological and clinical study. *Acta Neurol Scand Suppl* 153: 1-22.

37. Holmberg M, Duyckerts C, Dürr A, Cancel G, Gourfinkel-An I, Damier P, Faucheux B, Trottier Y, Hirsch EC, Agid Y, Brice A (1998) Spinocerebellar ataxia type 7 (SCA7). A neurodegenerative disorder with neuronal intranuclear inclusions. *Hum Mol Genet* 7: 913-918.

38. Holmes G (1907) A form of familial degeneration of the cerebellum. *Brain* 30: 466-489.

39. Holmes G, Stewart TG (1908) On the connection of the inferior olives with the cerebellum in man. *Brain* 31: 125-137.

40. Holmes SE, O'Hearn EE, McInnis MG, Gorelick-Feldman DA, Kleiderlein JJ, Callahan C, Kwak NG, Ingersoll-Ashworth RG, Sherr M, Sumner AJ, Sharp AH et al (1999) Expansion of a novel CAG trinucleotide repeat in the 5' region of PPP2R2B is associated with SCA12. *Nat Genet* 23: 391-392.

41. Huynh DP, Del Bigio MR, Ho DH, Pulst S-M (1999) Expression of ataxin-2 in brains from normal individuals and patients with Alzheimer's disease and spinocerebellar ataxia 2. *Ann Neurol* 45: 232-241.

42. Huynh DP, Figueroa K, Hoang N, Pulst SM (2000) Nuclear localization or inclusion body formation of ataxin-2 are not necessary for SCA2 pathogenesis in mouse or human. *Nat Genet* 26: 44-50.

43. Ikeuchi T, Takano H, Koide R, Horikawa Y, Honma Y, Onishi Y, Igarashi S, Tanaka H, Nakao N, Sahashi K, Tsukagoshi H et al (1997) Spinocerebellar ataxia type 6: CAG repeat expansion in alpha1A voltage-dependent calcium channel gene and clinical variations in Japanese population. *Ann Neurol* 42: 879-884.

44. Imbert G, Saudou F, Yvert G, Devys D, Trottier Y, Garnier JM, Weber C, Mandel JL, Cancel G, Abbas N, Durr A et al (1996) Cloning of the gene for spinocerebellar ataxia 2 reveals a locus with high sensitivity to expanded CAG/glutamine repeats. *Nat Genet* 14: 285-291.

45. Imbert G, Trottier Y, Beckmann J, Mandel JL (1994) The gene for the TATA binding protein (TBP) that contains a highly polymorphic protein coding CAG repeat maps to 6q27. *Genomics* 21: 667-668.

46. Imon Y, Katayama S, Kawakami H, Murata Y, Oka M, Nakamura S (1998) A necropsied case of Machado-Joseph disease with a hyperintense signal of transverse pontine fibres on long TR sequences of magnetic resonance images. *J Neurol Neurosurg Psychiatry* 64: 140-141.

47. Ishikawa K, Fujigasaki H, Saegusa H, Ohwada K, Fujita T, Iwamoto H, Komatsuzaki Y, Toru S, Toriyama H, Watanabe M, Ohkoshi N, Shoji S, Kanazawa I, Tanabe T, Mizusawa H (1999) Abundant expression and cytoplasmic aggregations of [alpha]1A voltage-

dependent calcium channel protein associated with neurodegeneration in spinocerebellar ataxia type 6. *Hum Mol Genet* 8: 1185-1193.

48. Ishikawa K, Mizusawa H, Fujita T, Ohkoshi N, Doi M, Komatsuzaki Y, Iwamoto H, Ogata T, Shoji S (1995) Calbindin-D 28K immunoreactivity in the cerebellum of spinocerebellar degeneration. *J Neurol Sci* 129.

49. Ishikawa K, Owada K, Ishida K, Fujigasaki H, Shun Li M, Tsunemi T, Ohkoshi N, Toru S, Mizutani T, Hayashi M, Arai N et al (2001) Cytoplasmic and nuclear polyglutamine aggregates in SCA6 Purkinje cells. *Neurology* 56: 1753-1756.

50. Ishikawa K, Tanaka H, Saito M, Ohkoshi N, Fujita T, Yoshizawa K, Ikeuchi T, Watanabe M, Hayashi A, Takiyama Y et al (1997) Japanese families with autosomal dominant pure cerebellar ataxia map to chromosome 19p13.1-p13.2 and are strongly associated with mild CAG expansions in the spinocerebellar ataxia type 6 gene in chromosome 19p13.1. *Am J Hum Genet* 61: 336-346.

51. Ishikawa K, Watanabe M, Yoshizawa K, Fujita T, Iwamoto H, Yoshizawa T, Harada K, Nakamagoe K, Komatsuzaki Y, Satoh A, Doi M et al (1999) Clinical, neuropathological, and molecular study in two families with spinocerebellar ataxia type 6 (SCA6). *J Neurol Neurosurg Psychiatry* 67: 86-89.

52. Jen JC, Yue Q, Karrim J, Nelson SF, Baloh RW (1998) Spinocerebellar ataxia type 6 with positional vertigo and acetazolamide responsive episodic ataxia. *J Neurol Neurosurg Psychiatry* 65: 565-568.

53. Jodice C, Mantuano E, Veneziano L, Trettel F, Sabbadini G, Calandriello L, Francia A, Spadaro M, Pierelli F, Salvi F, Ophoff RA, Frants RR, Frontali M (1997) Episodic ataxia type 2 (EA2) and spinocerebellar ataxia type 6 (SCA6) due to CAG repeat expansion in the CACNA1A gene on chromosome 19p. *Hum Mol Genet* 6: 1973-1978.

54. Kameya T, Abe K, Aoki M, Sahara M, Tobita M, Konno H, Itoyama Y (1995) Analysis of spinocerebellar ataxia type 1 (SCA1)-related CAG trinucleotide expansion in Japan. *Neurology* 45: 1587-1594.

55. Klement IA, Skinner PJ, Kaytor MD, Yi H, Hersch SM, Clark HB, Zoghbi HY, Orr H (1998) Ataxin-1 nuclear localization and aggregation: role in polyglutamine-induced disease in SCA1 transgenic mice. *Cell* 95: 41-53.

56. Koeppen AH (1998) The hereditary ataxias. *J Neuropathol Exp Neurol* 57: 531-543.

57. Koeppen AH (2002) Neuropathology of the inherited ataxias. In *The cerebellum and its disorders*, U-B Manto, M Pandolfo (eds). Cambridge University Press: Cambridge. pp. 387-405.

58. Koeppen AH, Dickson AC, Lamarche JB, Robitaille Y (1999) Synapses in the hereditary ataxias. *J Neuropathol Exp Neurol* 58: 748-764.

59. Koeppen AH, Dickson AC, Riess O (2002) The neuropathology of spinocerebellar ataxia type 17 (SCA17). *Can J Neurol Sci* 29: 399.

60. Koeppen AH, Mitzen EJ, Hans MB, Barron KD (1986) Olivopontocerebellar atrophy: Immunocytochemical and Golgi observations. *Neurology* 36: 1478-1488.

61. Koob MD, Moseley ML, Schut LJ, Benzow KA, Bird TD, Day JW, Ranum LP (1999) An untranslated CTG expansion causes a novel form of spinocerebellar ataxia (SCA8). *Nat Genet* 21: 379-384.

62. Koyano S, Uchihara T, Fujigasaki H, Nakamura A, Yagishita S, Iwabuchi K (1999) Neuronal intranuclear inclusions in spinocerebellar ataxia type 2: triple-labeling immunofluorescent study. *Neurosci Lett* 273: 117-120.

63. La Spada AR, Fu YH, Sopher BL, Libby RT, Wang X, Li LY, Einum DD, Huang J, Possin DE, Smith AC, Martinez RA et al (2001) Polyglutamine-expanded ataxin-7 antagonizes CRX function and induces cone-rod dystrophy in a mouse model of SCA7. *Neuron* 31: 913-927.

64. Lapresle J, Hamida MB (1970) The dentato-olivary pathway. Somatotopic relationship between the dentate nucleus and the contralateral inferior olive. *Arch Neurol* 22: 135-143.

65. Lescure A, Lutz Y, Eberhard D, Jacq X, Krol A, Grummt I, Davidson I, Chambon P, Tora L (1994) The N-terminal domain of the human TATA-binding protein plays a role in transcription from TATA-containing RNA polymerase II and III promoters. *EMBO J* 13: 1166-1175.

66. Marie P (1893) Sur l'hérédo-ataxie cérébelleuse. *Sem Med* 13: 444-447.

67. Matilla A, Koshy BT, Cummings CJ, Isobe T, Orr HT, Zoghbi HY (1997) The cerebellar leucine-rich acidic nuclear protein interacts with ataxin-1. *Nature* 389.

68. Matilla T, McCall A, Subramony SH, Zoghbi HY (1995) Molecular and clinical correlations in spinocerebellar ataxia type 3 and Machado-Joseph disease. *Ann Neurol* 38: 68-72.

69. Matsumura R, Futamura N, Fujimoto Y, Yanagimoto S, Horikawa H, Suzumura A, Takayanagi T (1997) Spinocerebellar ataxia type 6. Molecular and clinical features of 35 Japanese patients including one homozygous for the CAG repeat expansion. *Neurology* 49: 1238-1243.

70. Matsuura T, Yamagata T, Burgess DL, Rasmussen A, Grewal RP, Watase K, Khajavi M, McCall AE, Davis CF, Zu L, Achari M, Pulst SM, Alonso E, Noebels JL, Nelson DL, Zoghbi HY, Ashizawa T (2000) Large expansion of the ATTCT pentanucleotide repeat in spinocerebellar ataxia type 10. *Nat Genet* 26: 191-194.

71. Matsuyama Z, Wakamori M, Mori Y, Kawakami H, Nakamura S, Imoto K (1999) Direct alteration of the P/Q-type Ca2+ channel property by polyglutamine expansion in spinocerebellar ataxia 6. *J Neurosci* 19: RC14.

72. Menzel P (1891) Beitrag zur Kenntnis der hereditaren Ataxie und Kleinhirnatrophie. *Arch Psychiat Nervenkrankh* 22: 160-190.

73. Miyoshi Y, Yamada T, Tanimura M, Taniwaki T, Arakawa K, Ohyagi Y, Furuya H, Yamamoto K, Sakai K, Sasazuki T, Kira J (2001) A novel autosomal dominant spinocerebellar ataxia (SCA16) linked to chromosome 8q22.1-24.1. *Neurology* 57: 96-100.

74. Monckton DG, Cayuela ML, Gould FK, Brock GJ, Silva R, Ashizawa T (1999) Very large (CAG)(n) DNA repeat expansions in the sperm of two spinocerebellar ataxia type 7 males. *Hum Mol Genet* 8: 2473-2478.

75. Moreira MC, Barbot C, Tachi N, Kozuka N, Uchida E, Gibson T, Mendonca P, Costa M, Barros J, Yanagisawa T et al (2001) The gene mutated in ataxia-ocular apraxia 1 encodes the new HIT/Zn-finger protein aprataxin. *Nat Genet* 29: 189-193.

76. Murata Y, Kawakami H, Yamaguchi S, Nishimura M, Kohriyama T, Ishizaki F, Matsuyama Z, Mimori Y, Nakamura S (1998) Characteristic magnetic resonance imaging findings in spinocerebellar ataxia 6. *Arch Neurol* 55: 1348-1352.

77. Nagaoka U, Takashima M, Ishikawa K, Yoshizawa K, Yoshizawa T, Ishikawa M, Yamawaki T, Shoji S, Mizusawa H (2000) A gene on SCA4 locus causes dominantly inherited pure cerebellar ataxia. *Neurology* 54: 1971-1975.

78. Nakamura K, Jeong SY, Uchihara T, Anno M, Nagashima K, Nagashima T, Ikeda S, Tsuji S, Kanazawa I (2001) SCA17, a novel autosomal dominant cerebellar ataxia caused by an expanded polyglutamine in TATA-binding protein. *Hum Mol Genet* 10: 1441-1448.

79. O'Hearn E, Holmes SE, Calvert PC, Ross CA, Margolis RL (2001) SCA12: Tremor with cerebellar and cortical atrophy is associated with a CAG repeat expansion. *Neurology* 56: 299-303.

80. Oh AK, Jacobson KM, Jen JC, Baloh RW (2001) Slowing of voluntary and involuntary saccades: an early sign in spinocerebellar ataxia type 7. *Ann Neurol* 49: 801-804.

81. Onodera O, Idezuka J, Igarashi S, Takiyama Y, Endo K, Takano H, Oyake M, Tanaka H, Inuzuka T, Hayashi T, Yuasa T, Ito J, Miyatake T, Tsuji S (1998) Progressive atrophy of cerebellum and brainstem as a function of age and the size of the expanded CAG repeats in the MJD1 gene in Machado-Joseph disease. *Ann Neurol* 43: 288-296.

82. Ophoff RA, Terwindt GM, Vergouwe MN, van Eijk R, Oefner PJ, Hoffman SM, Lamerdin JE, Mohrenweiser HW, Bulman DE, Ferrari M et al (1996) Familial hemiplegic migraine and episodic ataxia type-2 are caused by mutations in the Ca^{2+} channel gene CACNL1A4. *Cell* 87: 543-552.

83. Orr HT, Chung MY, Banfi S, Kwiatkowski TJJ, Servadio A, Beaudet AL, McCall AE, Duvick LA, Ranum LP, Zoghbi HY (1993) Expansion of an unstable trinucleotide CAG repeat in spinocerebellar ataxia type 1. *Nat Genet* 4: 221-226.

84. Ouahchi K, Arita M, Kayden H, Hentati F, Ben Hamida M, Sokol R, Arai H, Inoue K, Mandel JL, Koenig M (1995) Ataxia with isolated vitamin E deficiency is caused by mutations in the alpha-tocopherol transfer protein. *Nat Genet* 9: 141-145.

85. Pang JT, Giunti P, Chamberlain S, An SF, Vitaliani R, Scaravilli T, Martinian L, Wood NW, Scaravilli F, Ansorge O (2002) Neuronal intranuclear inclusions in SCA2: a genetic, morphological and immunohistochemical study of two cases. *Brain* 125: 656-663.

86. Plaitakis A (1992) Classification and epidemiology of cerebellar degenerations. In *Cerebellar degenerations: Clinical Neurobiology*, A Plaitakis (eds). Klüwer Acad Press: Boston. pp. 185-204.

87. Pulst SM, Nechiporuk A, Nechiporuk T, Gispert S, Chen XN, Lopes-Cendes I, Pearlman S, Starkman S, Orozco-Diaz G, Lunkes A et al (1996) Moderate expansion of a normally biallelic trinucleotide repeat in spinocerebellar ataxia type 2. *Nat Genet* 14: 269-276.

88. Ranum LP, Duvick LA, Rich SS, Schut LJ, Litt M, Orr HT (1991) Localization of the autosomal dominant HLA-linked spinocerebellar ataxia (SCA1) locus, in two kindreds, within an 8-cM subregion of chromosome 6p. *Am J Hum Genet* 49: 31-41.

89. Ranum LP, Lundgren JK, Schut LJ, Ahrens MJ, Perlman S, Aita J, Bird TD, Gomez C, Orr HT (1995) Spinocerebellar ataxia type 1 and Machado-Joseph disease: incidence of CAG expansions among adult-onset ataxia patients from 311 families with dominant, recessive, or sporadic ataxia. *Am J Hum Genet* 57: 603-608.

90. Ranum LP, Schut LJ, Lundgren JK, Orr HT, Livingston DM (1994) Spinocerebellar ataxia type 5 in a family descended from the grandparents of President Lincoln maps to chromosome 11. *Nat Genet* 8: 280-284.

91. Restituito S, Thompson RM, Eliet J, Raike RS, Riedl M, Charnet P, Gomez CM (2000) The polyglutamine expansion in spinocerebellar ataxia type 6 causes a beta subunit-specific enhanced activation of P/Q-type calcium channels in Xenopus oocytes. *J Neurosci* 20: 6394-6403.

92. Rosenberg RN (1992) Machado-Joseph disease: an autosomal dominant motor system degeneration. *Mov Disord* 7: 193-203.

93. Rossi F, Wiklund L, van der Want JJ, Strata P (1991) Reinnervation of cerebellar Purkinje cells by climbing fibers surviving a subtotal lesion of the inferior olive in the adult rat. I. Development of new collateral branches and terminal plexuses. *J Comp Neurol* 308: 513-535.

94. Rossi F, van der Want JJ, Wiklund L, Strata P (1991) Reinnervation of cerebellar Purkinje cells by climbing fibers surviving a subtotal lesion of the inferior olive in the adult rat. II. Synaptic organization on reinnervated Purkinje cells. *J Comp Neurol* 308: 536-554.

95. Sanpei K, Takano H, Igarashi S, Sato T, Oyake M, Sasaki H, Wakisaka A, Tashiro K, Ishida Y, Ikeuchi T, Koide R et al (1996) Identification of the spinocerebellar ataxia type 2 gene using a direct identification of repeat expansion and cloning technique, DIRECT. *Nat Genet* 14: 277-284.

96. Sasaki H, Fukazawa T, Yanagihara T, Hamada T, Shima K, Matsumoto A, Hashimoto K, Ito N, Wakisaka A, Tashiro K (1996) Clinical features and natural history of spinocerebellar ataxia type 1. *Acta Neurol Scand* 93: 64-71.

97. Sasaki H, Wakisaka A, Sanpei K, Takano H, Igarashi S, Ikeuchi T, Iwabuchi K, Fukazawa T, Hamada T, Yuasa T, Tsuji S, Tashiro K (1998) Phenotype variation correlates with CAG repeat length in SCA2--a study of 28 Japanese patients. *J Neurol Sci* 159: 202-208.

98. Satoh JI, Tokumoto H, Yukitake M, Matsui M, Matsuyama Z, Kawakami H, Nakamura S, Kuroda Y (1998) Spinocerebellar ataxia type 6: MRI of three Japanese patients. *Neuroradiology* 40: 222-227.

99. Schmidt T, Landwehrmeyer B, Schmitt I, Trottier Y, Auburger G, Laccone F, Klockgether T, Völpel M, Epplen JT, Schöls L, Riess O (1998) An isoform of ataxin-3 accumulates in the nucleus of neuronal cells in affected brain regions of SCA3 patients. *Brain Pathol* 8: 669-679.

100. Schwaller B, Meyer M, Schiffmann S (2002) 'New' functions for 'old' proteins: The role of the calcium-binding proteins calbindin D-28k, calretinin and parvalbumin, in cerebellar physiology. Studies with knockout mice. *Cerebellum* 1: 241-258.

101. Sherrard RM, Bower AJ (2002) Climbing fiber development: do neurotrophins have a part to play? *Cerebellum* 1: 225-276.

102. Silveira I, Alonso I, Guimaraes L, Mendonca P, Santos C, Maciel P, Fidalgo De Matos JM, Costa M, Barbot C, Tuna A et al (2000) High germinal instability of the (CTG)n at the SCA8 locus of both expanded and normal alleles. *Am J Hum Genet* 66: 830-840.

103. Sisodia SS (1998) Nuclear inclusions in glutamine repeat disorders: Are they pernicious, coincidental, or beneficial? *Cell* 95: 1-4.

104. Skinner PJ, Koshy B, Cummings CJ, Klement IA, Helin K, Servadio A, Zoghbi HY, Orr HT (1997) Ataxin-1 with expanded glutamine tracts alters nuclear matrix-associated structures. *Nature* 389: 971-977.

105. Sobrido MJ, Cholfin JA, Perlman S, Pulst SM, Geschwind DH (2001) SCA8 repeat expansions in ataxia: a controversial association. *Neurology* 57: 1310-1312.

106. Stevanin G, Durr A, David G, Didierjean O, Cancel G, Rivaud S, Tourbah A, Warter JM, Agid Y, Brice A (1997) Clinical and molecular features of spinocerebellar ataxia type 6. *Neurology* 49: 1243-1246.

107. Stevanin G, Herman A, Brice A, Durr A (1999) Clinical and MRI findings in spinocerebellar ataxia type 5. *Neurology* 53: 1355-1357.

108. Strata P, Rossi F (1998) Plasticity of the olivocerebellar pathway. *Trends Neurosci* 21: 407-413.

109. Sugawara M, Toyoshima I, Wada C, Kato K, Ishikawa K, Hirota K, Ishiguro H, Kagaya H, Hirata Y, Imota T, Ogasawara M, Masamune O (2000) Pontine atrophy in spinocerebellar ataxia type 6. *Eur Neurol* 43: 17-22.

110. Takano H, Cancel G, Ikeuchi T, Lorenzetti D, Mawad R, Stevanin G, Didierjean O, Durr A, Oyake M, Shimohata T, Sasaki R et al (1998) Close associations between prevalences of dominantly inherited spinocerebellar ataxias with CAG-repeat expansions and frequencies of large normal CAG alleles in Japanese and Caucasian populations. *Am J Hum Genet* 63: 1060-1066.

111. Takashima M, Ishikawa K, Nagaoka U, Shoji S, Mizusawa H (2001) A linkage disequilibrium at the candidate gene locus for 16q-linked autosomal dominant cerebellar ataxia type III in Japan. *J Hum Genet* 46: 167-171.

112. Takeichi N, Fukushima K, Sasaki H, Yabe I, Tashiro K, Inuyama Y (2000) Dissociation of smooth pursuit and vestibulo-ocular reflex cancellation in SCA6. *Neurology* 54: 860-866.

113. Takiyama Y, Nishizawa M, Tanaka H, Kawashima S, Sakamoto H, Karube Y, Shimazaki H, Soutome M, Endo K, Ohta S, et al. (1993) The gene for Machado-Joseph disease maps to human chromosome 14q. *Nat Genet* 4: 300-304.

114. Toru S, Murakoshi T, Ishikawa K, Saegusa H, Fujigasaki H, Uchihara T, Nagayama S, Osanai M, Mizusawa H, Tanabe T (2000) Spinocerebellar ataxia type 6 mutation alters P-type calcium channel function. *J Biol Chem* 275: 10893-10898.

115. Trottier L, Lutz Y, Stevanin G, Imbert G, Devys D, Cancel G, Saudou F, Weber C, David G, Tora L, Agid Y, Brice A, Mandel J-L (1995) Polyglutamine expansion as a pathological epitope in Huntington's disease and four dominant cerebellar ataxias. *Nature* 378: 403-406.

116. Trottier Y, Zeder-Lutz G, Mandel J-L (1998) Selective recognition of proteins with pathological polyglutamine tracts by a monoclonal antibody. In *Genetic instabilities and hereditary neurological diseases*, RD Wells, ST Warren (eds). Academic Press: San Diego. pp. 447-453.

117. Vig PJS, Fratkin JD, Desaiah D, Currier RD, Subramony SH (1996) Decreased parvalbumin immunoreactivity in surviving Purkinje cells of patients with spinocerebellar ataxia-1. *Neurology* 47: 249-253.

118. Vincent JB, Neves-Pereira ML, Paterson AD, Yamamoto E, Parikh SV, Macciardi F, Gurling HM, Potkin SG, Pato CN, Macedo A et al (2000) An unstable trinucleotide-repeat region on chromosome 13 implicated in spinocerebellar ataxia: a common expansion locus. *Am J Hum Genet* 66: 819-829.

119. Worth PF, Houlden H, Giunti P, Davis MB, Wood NW (2000) Large, expanded repeats in SCA8 are not confined to patients with cerebellar ataxia. *Nat Genet* 24: 214-215.

120. Yakura H, Wakisaka A, Fujimoto S, Itakura K (1974) Letter: Hereditary ataxia and HL-A. *N Engl J Med* 291: 154-155.

121. Yamashita I, Sasaki H, Yabe I, Fukazawa T, Nogoshi S, Komeichi K, Takada A, Shiraishi K, Takiyama Y et al (2000) A novel locus for dominant cerebellar ataxia (SCA14) maps to a 10.2-cM interval flanked by D19S206 and D19S605 on chromosome 19q13.4-qter. *Ann Neurol* 48: 156-163.

122. Yokota T, Shiojiri T, Gotoda T, Arita M, Arai H, Ohga T, Kanda T, Suzuki J, Imai T, Matsumoto H, Harino S et al (1997) Friedreich-like ataxia with retinitis pigmentosa caused by the His101Gln mutation of the alpha-tocopherol transfer protein gene. *Ann Neurol* 41: 826-832.

123. Yokota T, Wada Y, Furukawa T, Tsukagoshi H, Uchihara T, Watabiki S (1987) Adult-onset spinocerebellar syndrome with idiopathic vitamin E deficiency. *Ann Neurol* 22: 84-87.

124. Yvert G, Lindenber KS, Devys D, Helmlinger D, Landwehrmeyer GB, Mandel JL (2001) SCA7 mouse models show selective stabilization of mutant ataxin-7 and similar cellular responses in different neuronal cell types. *Hum Mol Gen* 10: 1679-1692.

125. Yvert G, Lindenberg KS, Picaud S, Landwehrmeyer GB, Sahel JA, Mandel JL (2000) Expanded polyglutamines induce neurodegeneration and trans-neuronal alterations in cerebellum and reti-

na of SCA7 transgenic mice. *Hum Mol Genet* 9: 2491-2506.

126. Zhuchenko O, Bailey J, Bonnen P, Ashizawa T, Stockton DW, Amos C, Dobyns WB, Subramony SH, Zoghbi HY, Lee CC (1997) Autosomal dominant cerebellar ataxia (SCA6) associated with small polyglutamine expansions in the alpha 1A-voltage-dependent calcium channel. *Nat Genet* 15: 62-69.

127. Zoghbi HY (1996) The expanding world of ataxins. *Nat Genet* 14: 237-238.

128. Zoghbi HY (2000) Spinocerebellar ataxias. *Neurobiol Dis* 7: 523-527.

129. Zoghbi HY, Jodice C, Sandkuijl LA, Kwiatkowski TJJ, McCall AE, Huntoon SA, Lulli P, Spadaro M, Litt M, Cann HM et al (1991) The gene for autosomal dominant spinocerebellar ataxia (SCA1) maps telomeric to the HLA complex and is closely linked to the D6S89 locus in three large kindreds. *Am J Hum Genet* 49: 23-30.

Friedreich's Ataxia

Yves Robitaille
Thomas Klockgether
Jacques B. Lamarche

FRDA1	Friedreich's ataxia

Definition

Friedreich's ataxia (FRDA1) is the most common autosomal recessive ataxia (6, 38). It is due to mutations of a gene encoding a mitochondrial protein named frataxin, localised on chromosome 9q13-21.1 (23). In most cases, the causative mutation is an homozygous, intronic GAA repeat expansion resulting in markedly reduced expression of frataxin (23). The clinical hallmarks of FRDA are pre-adolescent onset, ataxia, areflexia, proprioceptive sensory abnormalities, and cardiomyopathy. The classic FRDA phenotype is now referred to as FRDA1, which was linked to chromosome 9q13 mutations. A new locus on chromosome 9p23-11, is referred to in the literature as FRDA2 (28). The clinical phenotypes of both diseases have remained indistinguishable to this time.

FRDA is a progressive disease leading to disability and premature death. Median latency to the wheelchair-bound phase is 11 years. Life expectancy after disease onset averages 35 to 40 years (68). Age of onset and progression rate are partly determined by the GAA repeat length of the shorter allele: in patients with longer expansions, disease onset is earlier and progression to loss of ambulation faster (40).

Synonyms and Historical Annotations

In 1863, Nikolaus Friedreich was the first to report cases of an early-onset, hereditary ataxia, which was later named after him (45, 46). He described the salient clinical features of FRDA in 9 siblings of 3 families. To distinguish this disorder from tabes dorsalis, which used to be a common cause of familial and sporadic ataxia, was Friedreich's most remarkable achievement. In 1876, he described the degenerative spinal features classically associated with FRDA (4, 47). Generally acknowledged clinical diagnostic criteria were established by Geoffroy et al (49), and the British neurologist Harding (58). After unsuccessful attempts to identify the biochemical defect underlying FRDA, the molecular elucidation of FRDA started with the chromosomal localisation of the gene on chromosome 9q by Chamberlain in 1988 (26), which was more specifically targeted on chromosome 9q13 by Montermini et al in 1995 (96). In 1996, an European consortium identified an intronic GAA repeat expansion as the causative mutation (24).

Epidemiology

Incidence and prevalence. FRDA1 has the highest incidence/prevalence rate amongst recessive ataxias. It has been documented worldwide, with highest incidence/prevalence rates reported in Canada (7), United States (7, 9), France (31), Spain (106), Italy (84). There are a limited number of population-based studies which provided strong epidemiological data on prevalence rates. Leone et al. reported a prevalence rate of 1.7:100 000 in the Aosta valley, Italy (84). A similar survey in Cantabria, Spain yielded a prevalence rate of 4.7:100 000 (106). A multi-national European epidemiologic study evaluated the FRDA prevalence at 1:29 000, with a carrier rate of 1:85 (130). The carrier rate, based on molecular diagnostic techniques, was recorded at 1:60 to 1:90 in Germany (43). In general, the regional distribution of FRDA is uneven. Molecular studies showed that the GAA expansion causing FRDA is found only in individuals of European, North African, Middle Eastern, or Indian origin. In contrast, the GAA expansion was not found among sub-Saharan Africans, Amerindians, and people from China, Japan, and Southeast Asia (77). Despite an exhaustive epidemiologic study of a large Japanese cohort of ataxic subjects, which established the incidence of FRDA at 2.4 % in 1988-1989 (61), expanded GAA repeats have yet to be documented in Japan (125). Due to founder effects, the highest prevalence rates were recorded in few restricted regions, such as the Rimouski area in Quebec, Canada (7), to the point that pseudo-dominant inheritance may occur (59).

Sex and age distribution. FRDA1 equally affects both sexes. Mean age at onset is 15 years, ranging from 2 to 51 years (39). Approximately 85% of all FRDA1 patients have disease onset before 20 years of age. Mean age of onset of symptoms was 10.52 ± 7.4 years in Harding's cohort of 115 patients (57). Loss of ambulation occurs on average 10.8 ± 6.0 years after disease onset (39).

Risk factors. FRDA is an inherited disorder with no known environmental risk factors. Age of onset and disease progression are influenced by repeat length (40). In addition, female sex appears to accelerate disease progression (69).

Genetics

In more than 95% of patients, the causative mutation is an homozygous GAA repeat expansion in the first intron of the frataxin gene (22, 24). The gene spans 80 kb of genomic DNA, is composed of 7 exons and is highly conserved across the phylogenetic scale (Figure 1). Wild type frataxin is an 18 kd soluble mitochondrial protein with 210 amino acids. Crystallographic studies recently documented a protein fold (39, 99, 104).

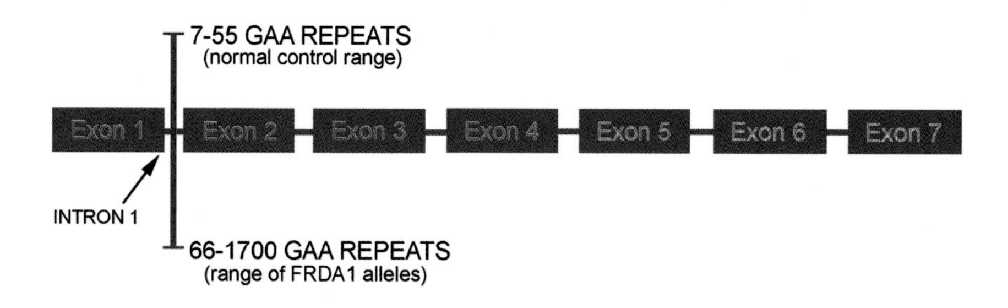

Figure 1. Drawing of the FRDA1 gene on chromosome 9q13.- 21.1. Exons are marked as boxes, introns as lines. Numbers of GAA repeats in Intron 1 are noted in normal and FRDA1 subjects.

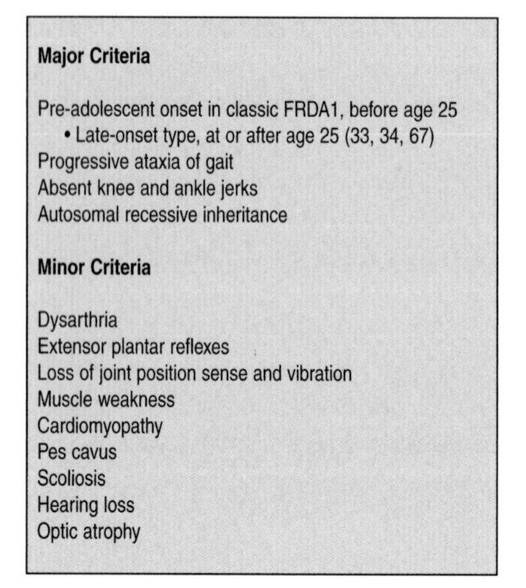

Major Criteria

Pre-adolescent onset in classic FRDA1, before age 25
- Late-onset type, at or after age 25 (33, 34, 67)

Progressive ataxia of gait
Absent knee and ankle jerks
Autosomal recessive inheritance

Minor Criteria

Dysarthria
Extensor plantar reflexes
Loss of joint position sense and vibration
Muscle weakness
Cardiomyopathy
Pes cavus
Scoliosis
Hearing loss
Optic atrophy

Table 1. Diagnostic clinical criteria for Friedreich's ataxia. Updated according to Geoffroy et al (48) and Harding (57).

Less than 4% of FRDA patients are compound heterozygotes with one allele carrying the GAA repeat expansion and the second a point mutation (24, 29). A summary of FRDA point mutations in compound heterozygous patients was recently updated (104).

In 2 different studies of normal controls, repeat lengths varied between 7 to 29 (43), and 9 to 55 repeat sequences (30). Disease-associated repeats contain 66 to more than 1700 trinucleotides, most commonly between 600 to 1000 (31, 44, 104) (Figure 1). More than 80% of all Europeans have short normal alleles in the range of 5 to 10 trinucleotides (31). It has also recently been proposed that these alleles expanded through 2 duplication steps to form very large normal alleles with a length of more than 30 trinucleotides (77). These very large normal alleles are unstable and serve as a reservoir for pathogenic expansions beyond the critical threshold of 66 repeats (31, 43). Haplotype studies which showed that all frataxin alleles containing more than 12 repeats have a common origin suggest that the 2 duplication steps have been extremely rare events (77).

Expanded alleles are unstable with a strong tendency to contraction with paternal transmission and both contraction and expansion with maternal transmission. The length of the shorter allele is inversely correlated with the age of onset, and with the amount of residual frataxin in patient's lymphocytes (90). Patients with earlier age of onset usually have a more severe phenotype and faster disease progression (40, 44).

The point mutations include truncating and missense mutations (104). Mutations of the carboxy-terminus part of frataxin are associated with a phenotype similar to that of patients homozygous for the GAA expansion. In contrast, 2 missense mutations in the amino-terminal part of frataxin (D122Y, G130V) caused a milder clinical presentation suggesting that frataxin function is less severely affected by these mutations (29). Recently, a second FRDA locus was mapped to chromosome 9p (FRDA2). The affected gene and causative mutations have yet to be identified (28, 75). The clinical phenotypes of FRDA2 are identical to the classic type of FRDA1.

Clinical Features

Signs and symptoms. Classic FRDA (FRDA1) has its onset in preadolescence, and is heralded by an ataxic gait (6, 22, 49, 104). Ocular nystagmus with saccades, and pyramidal tract involvement also appear early, usually with pes cavus. Upgoing plantar reflexes with abolished achillean reflex are the hallmark of FRDA1 in later years. Patients become wheelchair bound during adulthood. FRDA1 is compatible with a long life, but results into an earlier age range at death than the normal population (69). Cognitive skills are usually spared even into advanced age, although mental retardation was associated with the FRDA phenotype in few subjects, and is likely unrelated to the specific mutational effects of FRDA1 (69).

The prominent sign of FRDA is progressive ataxia, initially affecting gait and stance, and later also arm movements. Muscle reflexes of the legs are absent in about 90% of the patients. Approximately 80% of the patients have extensor plantar responses.

Diagnostic grids were expanded by Geoffroy in 1976 (49) and Harding in 1981 (58) before late onset FRDA phenotypes were ascertained (Table 1). They both provided major and minor criteria with an emphasis on early preadolescent onset, progressive ataxia, loss of proprioceptive sensory modalities, absent deep tendon reflexes, especially knee and ankle jerks, muscle weakness and autosomal recessive inheritance as major criteria. Extensor plantar reflexes, dysarthria, pes cavus, scoliosis and cardiomyopathy were considered as minor criteria. Currently validated criteria have basically undergone little change since the early accurate phenotypic descriptions by Friedreich (45, 46). In one study, however, up to 25% of FRDA1 subjects who were homozygous for a GAA expansion lacked one or more of the cardinal clinical signs often associated with the FRDA1 clinical phenotype: absent lower limb reflexes and/or presence of pyramidal tract signs (40).

All FRDA patients develop an ataxic speech disorder, usually within the first 5 years of their disease. Disorders of ocular motility are part of the clinical spectrum. Oculomotor disorders include square wave jerks during fixation and reduced gain of vestibulo-ocular reflex. Oculomotor disturbances pointing to cerebellar dysfunction such as gaze-evoked nystagmus or saccadic hypermetria are usually absent (132). Physical examination reveals pale discs in many FRDA patients. However, a loss of visual acuity is encountered in only 10 to 20% of the patients. Similarly, 10 to 20% develop sensorineural hearing problems.

Results of electrophysiologic tests will classically confirm the absence of sensory nerve action potentials and evoked spinal somatosensory potentials in true FRDA1, while motor or mixed nerve conduction velocities display less decrease than in sensory nerves (25, 93). FRDA1 subjects will progressively evolve into a severe sensory neuropathy which tends to predominate in lower limbs (119). Severe optic atrophy and hearing loss may also contribute to impair the neurologic status.

Lower motor neuron involvement has been reported, but its occurrence is rare and was not frequently reported as an associated sign in classic FRDA (21, 135). When present, amyotrophy is directly correlated with high GAA repeat expansions and disease duration as well (40). There are also well documented phenotypes with onset in late adulthood and retained lower tendon reflexes (69, 104).

With disease progression, distal wasting of both lower and upper extremities develops. Due to pyramidal involvement and muscle wasting, FRDA patients may have considerable weakness. In conjunction with ataxia, this often leads to considerable slowness of movements. Approximately half of the patients have skeletal deformities (scoliosis, pes cavus) which are due to muscle wasting starting early in life. Almost all patients will display some form of sensory disturbance with reduced vibration and/or positional sense (40, 49, 58).

In approximately 60% of FRDA1 patients, echocardiography reveals an hypertrophic cardiomyopathy. ECG abnormalities with disturbances of repolarisation are even more common, and may provide further systemic morbidity in the form of cardiac dysrythmias, especially atrial fibrillation. The FRDA1 cardiomyopathy and its releated complications are frequent causes of premature lethality. In one study, direct correlations were found between the thickness of the interventricular septum, left ventricular mass and GAA repeat expansions, but not with the type or severity of its cardiologic and/or neurologic complications (41). It differs significantly from the familial types of primary hypertrophic cardiomyopathies, which usually show larger volumetric increases of left ventricular size, and are prone to ventricular fibrillation (64).

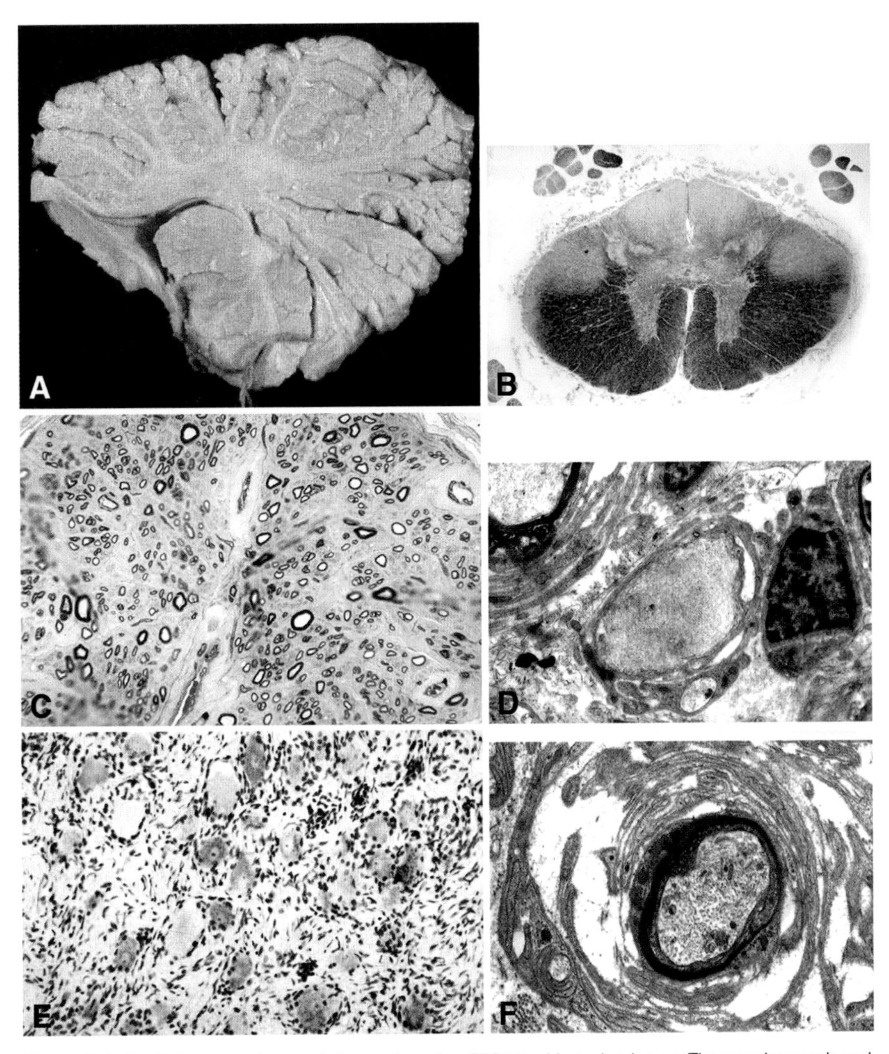

Figure 2. A. Sagittal paravermian cerebellar section of an FRDA1 subject, classic type. The superior vermis and posterior lobes display mild atrophy. ×20.**B.** Photomicrograph of a transverse cut of thoracic spinal cord, FRDA1 subject, classic type. Posterior roots are pale, indicating loss of myelinated fibers. There is severe wallerian degeneration of posterior and lateral columns with loss of myelinated fibers, which mostly extends into the dorsal spinocerebellar tract. ×25, Luxol Fast Blue stain. **C.** Semi-thin section of posterior root stained with Toluidine Blue, FRDA1 subject. There is marked loss of large myelinated fibers. ×212. **D.** Electron microphotograph of axonal swelling laden with neurofilaments in dorsal root ganglion, FRDA1. ×4384. **E.** HE stain of dorsal root ganglion. Numerous Nageotte nodules emphasise loss of ganglion cells. Some ganglion cells display chromatolysis. x 212. **F.** Electron microphotograph of dorsal root ganglion, which shows concentric hypertrophy of Schwann cell processes. ×4384.

FRDA1 is frequently complicated by adult onset diabetes mellitus (DM), which may be severe to the point of insulin dependence. Systemic lesions associated with DM type II, like premature arteriosclerosis, post-diabetic microangiopathy, peripheral neuropathy add up as additional risk factors to prolonged survival. Diabetes mellitus was ascertained in 10 to 32% of selected FRDA cohorts, in association with high GAA expansions (40, 44).

Major Criteria

Cerebellum
- Dentate nucleus atrophy, usually severe
- Wallerian degeneration of cerebellar central and hilar dentate white matter
- Wallerian degeneration of dentato-rubro-thalamic pathways, including superior cerebellar peduncles

Sub-Cortical
- Neuronal loss in gracile and cuneate sensory relay nuclei
- "Dying back" degeneration of pyramidal tracts distal to cerebral peduncles at pontine and bulbar levels

Spinal Cord
- Wallerian degeneration of dorsal and ventral spino-cerebellar tracts
- Degeneration of Clarke's columns, usually severe, with neuronal loss
- Wallerian degeneration of posterior columns, moderate to severe
- "Dying back" degeneration of crossed pyramidal tracts (lateral columns), severe, usually modest in anterior columns for uncrossed pyramidal tracts

Roots and Dorsal Root Ganglia
- Loss of large myelinated fibers
- Ganglion cell loss, moderate to severe, with Nageotte nodules

Peripheral Nerves
- Selective involvement of sensory nerves
- Distal axonopathy with loss of axonal densities
- Loss of large myelinated fibers with few myelin debris, likely secondary to axonopathy

Minor Criteria

Cerebral Hemispeheres
- Wallerian degeneration of optic nerves, chiasm and tracts
- Neuronal loss in ventral-posterior thalamic nuclei
- Loss of large pyramidal neurons with gliosis in motor strip

Subcortical
- Occasional hypertrophy of principal olivary nuclei, usually mild, most often absent
- Wallerian degeneration of inferior cerebellar peduncle
- Wallerian degeneration of median lemniscus, usually moderate

Cerebellum
- Cortical cerebellar atrophy, mild to moderate, secondary to loss of Purkinje cells
- Proximal axonal swellings (« torpedoes ») in Purkinje cell and molecular layers
- Hypertrophy of Bergmann's glia

Spinal
- Motor neuron disease with loss of anterior horn cells and gliosis, rarely documented

Roots and Dorsal Root Ganglia
- Loss of affinity for myelin stains and axonal densities of posterior roots
- Axonal swellings laden with neurofilaments in posterior roots
- "Onion-bulb"-like hypertrophy of Schwann cell processes
- Segmental demyelination with loss of myelinated fibers

Peripheral Nerves
- Segmental demyelination

Systemic
- Hypertrophic cardiomyopathy

Table 2. Diagnostic neuropathological criteria for Friedreich's ataxia.

Imaging. Magnetic resonance imaging typically shows atrophy of the cervical spinal cord. On average, reduction of the cross-sectional area of the cervical spinal cord approaches 50% of normal (68). The cerebellar cortex is often reported normal on MRI, but may display mild atrophy. A positron emission tomography study using fluoro-deoxyglucose showed widespread increase of glucose metabolism in the brains of ambulatory FRDA patients (51).

Laboratory findings. No diagnostic serology and/or biochemical assay is yet available for the diagnosis of FRDA. ^{31}P Magnetic Resonance spectroscopy has however disclosed lower mitochondrial ATP production rates in skeletal muscles compared to normal controls, which may provide further diagnostic clues (86). The specific diagnostic test for FRDA1 currently relies on molecular genetic methods aimed at the detection and measure of GAA triplet expansions and point mutations. FRDA genetic tests may be useful to establish prognosis and for genetic counselling. However, inter- and intrafamilial somatic mosaicism is well-documented and may contribute to making GAA expansion-based prognosis inaccurate (60, 95).

Macroscopy

Fresh brain weights are usually within normal limits compared with age-matched controls. At the base, the pontine curvature is normal as well as the olivary complexes. The vermis and cerebellar hemispheres on sagittal sections usually show no or little evidence of gross cortical cerebellar atrophy (72, 81). In the early onset phenotype with retained reflexes (FARR), cortical cerebellar atrophy may be more obvious in the absence of optic atrophy and cardiomyopathy (40). Occasionally however, vermian atrophy may be striking (81). Lateral and posterior columns may appear greyish on cross-sections, depending on the evolutionary stage of FRDA1 lesions. The dentate nucleus generally appears grayish and shrivelled (73) (Figure 2A). The spinal cord may display varying degrees of diffuse atrophy with normal spinal arteries and veins. Posterior columns may appear grayish on cross sections, depending on the stage of FRDA lesions. Posterior roots are thin and grey compared to anterior roots, which are spared in most cases. Although some evidence of motor neuron degeneration may be observed, it definitely remains a rare occurrence (81).

Histopathology

The lesions associated with the classic FRDA1 phenotype are mostly sub-cortical and spinal (72). They are classified as major and minor criteria in Table 2. There is usually little evidence of active myelin breakdown in any of the degenerated tracts. Pyramidal tracts undergo a predominantly "dying back" type of degeneration

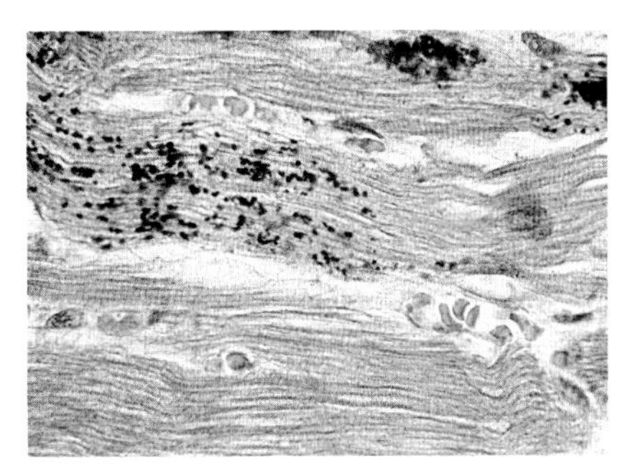

Figure 3. Prussian Blue stain. Myocardium of FRDA1 subject with cardiomyopathy. Myocardial cells are laden with aggregates of iron. ×450.

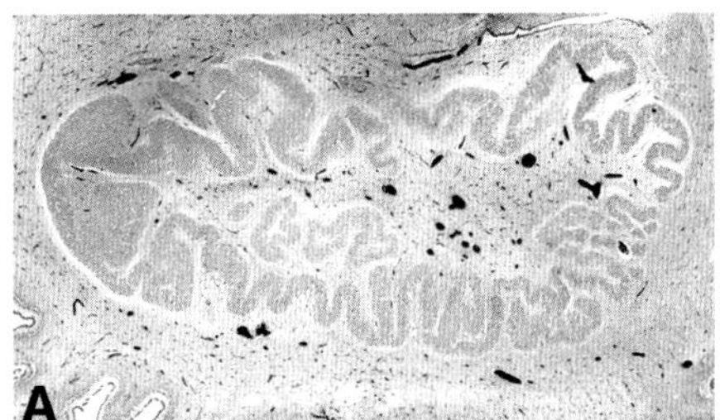

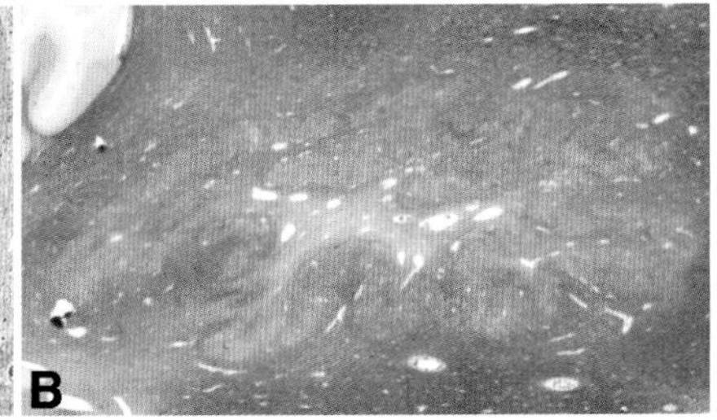

Figure 4. Dentate Nucleus in FRDA1 and control. **A.** ×25, HPS stain, 31-week-old fetus. The normal wavy pattern of Dentate Nucleus neurons is well developped. **B.** ×25, Klüver-Barrera stain, FRDA1 subject. The Dentate Nucleus is shrivelled, lacks the normal undulated pattern. Myelinated fibers within the hilum are pale.

which may have its origin within the motor strip (98, 102). Associative cortical areas largely remain unscathed by the primary FRDA lesions (81, 102).

In thalamic nuclei, especially ventro-lateral complexes, slight to marked focal loss of neurons, possibly due to the disease process or to anoxia is frequently observed. No consistent significant changes are seen in the pallidum. There may be a subtle loss of neurons with reactive gliosis, in the external pallidum, and sub-thalamic nuclei, which may rarely be severe in the latter (81, 102). Optic nerves and tracts may exhibit loss of myelinated fibers to a varying extent.

Cortico-spinal tract degeneration can usually be traced at pontine and bulbar levels, only very seldom at peduncular levels. The substantia nigra may display a moderate degree of pigment incontinence with mild loss of pigmented neurons. Such nigral lesions are however rare, as all brain stem pigmented nuclei, were always reported as normal in typical FRDA1. Nuclei pontis are spared. Although main olivary nuclei may undergo secondary hypertrophy, due to chronic denervation brought about by dentate nucleus degeneration, neuronal loss has seldom been documented. Despite the severity of the dentate nucleus atrophy (72), the incidence of olivary hypertrophy in FRDA is quite low. Accessory olivary nuclei may however be severely degenerated (102).

There is a consistent loss of myelinated fibers in superior cerebellar peduncles, while the restiform body is better preserved. Median lemnisci and solitary tracts may display moderate degres of myelinated fiber loss (81, 102, 134). Gracile, cuneate and accessory cuneate sensory nuclei are bound to show significant neuronal loss and gliosis, from deafferentation and trans-synaptic degeneration, which tend to be more severe within gracile nuclei (72, 81, 102, 134). Vestibular nuclei may also be affected by similar lesions. Red and cochlear nuclei as well as sensory trigeminal nuclei and midbrain colliculi are rarely involved.

The cerebellar cortex often reveals a mild to moderate degree of Purkinje cell loss with secondary hypertrophy of Bergmann's glia, and proximal axonal swellings ("torpedoes"), which may be patchy (81). Several axonal swellings may be observed within the molecular layer itself. The thickness of the cerebellar molecular layer may be significantly diminished in nearly half of autopsied FRDA1 subjects (73). Those subjects burdened by the highest GAA expansions may harbor a more diffusely distributed Purkinje cell attrition. Rarely, the vermis may exhibit substantial atrophy. The cerebellar white matter tends to display moderate degrees of wallerian degeneration, spreading within the hilum and periphery of the dentate nucleus (81). Dentate nuclei will classically show severe atrophy, which is usually directly correlated with the severity and extent of myelinated fiber loss in the hilum (72).

The brunt of FRDA lesions falls on the spinal cord, posterior roots and dorsal ganglia. Dorsal and ventral spino-cerebellar tracts also undergo severe attrition, usually in the form of wallerian degeneration, which is easily detectable on myelin stains and neurofilament immunopreparations (2). Dorsal spino-cerebellar tracts are classically more severely degenerated than the anterior (Figure 2B). There is moderate to severe loss of neurons in Clarke's columns, which also become severely atrophied (72, 102). Posterior columns undergo severe wallerian degeneration predominantly targeted on gracilis tracts, with lesser involvement of cuneate fasciculi (Figure 2B). Crossed cortico-spinal tracts also undergo severe wallerian degeneration starting at pontine and bulbar levels, which tends to be milder in anterior columns, in keeping with a "dying back" type of distal degeneration (74, 98). Moreover, there may be slight degeneration and loss of motor neurons with reactive gliosis in few FRDA subjects (71, 79).

Posterior roots will always show severe axonal and myelin loss (52) (Figure 2B, C). Axonal swellings filled with filamentous aggregates strongly immunoreactive for neurofilament markers will also be found within posterior roots and dorsal root ganglia (Figure 2D). The latter display somewhat pleomorphic ganglion cells, some of which often degenerate, leaving behind telltale footprints in the form of Nageotte nodules, made of residual satellite perineuronal cells (79) (Figure 2E).

Peripheral nerves lesions are characterised by a loss of large and moderate size myelinated fibers associated with a chronic axonopathy, which appears to have an early onset with relatively little progression after repeat sural nerve biopsies (103, 119). Segmental demyelination was observed, albeit inconstantly. Few or even no myelin

I. Non progressive recessively inherited ataxias

A. Hyper-reflexic

- **1.** congenital ataxic diplegia (Gustavson) (53)
- **2.** congenital dysequilibrium syndrome (Sanner) (122)
- **3.** non-progressive autosomal recessive ataxia, with mental retardation, optic atrophy and skin abnormalities (CAMOS), Lebanese type (36, 94)

B. Hypo-reflexic

- **1.** congenital, non-progressive, cerebellar ataxia (Batten-Lamy, or "recessive infantile spastic diplegia") (14)
- **2.** Recessive ataxia with ocular apraxia and hypoalbuminemia, Portuguese type (10, 97)
- **3.** Recessive ataxia with oculomotor apraxia and hypoalbuminemia, Japanese type (97)

II. Intermittent ataxias

A. Hereditary hyperammonaemias associated with ataxia

- **1.** congenital hyperammonaemia type II
- **2.** citrullinemia
- **3.** argeninosuccinic aciduria
- **4.** hyperornithinaemia

B. Hyperalaninaemic and hyperpyruvate states

- **1.** intermittent cerebellar ataxia
- **2.** necrotising encephalopathy (Leigh's disease)

C. Hartnup disease (11)

D. Branched-chain ketonuria (Maple syrup urine disease)

III. Progressive recessively inherited ataxias

A. Hyper or normo-reflexic

1. Early onset (Type I)

Type 1a
- **a.** Ataxia-telentegiectasia (Louis-Bar syndrome) (88)
- **b.** Amyotrophic familial spastic paraplegia (112)
- **c.** Troyer syndrome (33)
- **d.** Charlevoix-Saguenay syndrome (20)
- **e.** Lesh-Nyhan syndrome (85)

Type 1b :
- **a.** Behr's disease (62)
- **b.** Sjögren-Larsson syndrome (129)
- **c.** Congenital ataxia and aniridia (Gillespie Syndrome) (50)
- **d.** Marinesco-Sjögren syndrome (91)
- **e.** Progressive ophtalmoplegia, ataxia and neuropathy (32)
- **f.** Ataxia, deafness and mental retardation (ADR syndrome) (16)

2. Childhood and adolescence onset (Type II)

Type IIa:
- **a.** Hereditary recessive spastic ataxia (R-SCD, or recessive spino-cerebellar degeneration
- **b.** FARR, early onset with retained reflexes (92)

Type IIb:
- **a.** R-SCD with blindness and deafness (Hallgren's syndrome) (55)
- **b.** R-SCD and slow eye movements
- **c.** The Beauce R-SCD syndrome
- **d.** Ataxia, deafness, and oligophrenia syndrome (Jeune) (65)
- **e.** Familial ataxia with peroneal muscular atrophy and optic atrophy (17)
- **f.** Familial spino-cerebellar degeneration with cerebellar atrophy, neuropathy, increased serum creatine, gamma globulins and α-fetoproteins (137)
- **g.** Nephrophtisis with progressive ataxia and retinal pigmentation

3. Adult and late onset (Type III)

Type IIIa
- **a.** Fickler-Wickler, recessive cerebellar atrophy of late onset (71)

Type IIIb
- **a.** Spastic paraplegia, oligophrenia, amyotrophy and retinal degeneration (Kjellin syndrome) (67)
- **b.** Cerebellar ataxia and hypogonadism(Richards and Rundle syndrome) (113)
- **c.** Familial cerebellar ataxia with hypergonadotropic hypogonadism and sensorineural deafness (3)

B. Hypo-reflexic

1. Early onset (Type IV)

Type IVa
- **a.** Hereditary sensory neuropathy with ataxia

Type IVb
- **a.** HSN-Type E, with dysautonomia (Riley-Day syndrome) (115)

Type IVc
- **a.** Cerebellar ataxia, motor neuron disease, learning difficulties, and Dystonia (134)

Type IVd
- **a.** Infantile onset spino-cerebellar degeneration with sensory neuropathy (IOSCA) (87)

2. Childhood and adolescent onset (Type V)

Type Va
- **a.** FRDA1 classic type linked to Ch. 9q13 (49)
- **b.** FRDA1 with rapid progression (Rimouski sub-type) (7)
- **c.** FRDA1 with very slow progression (Acadian sub-type) (9)
- **d.** FRDA1 with neurogenic muscle atrophy (135)
- **e.** FRDA1, early onset with retained reflexes (57, 92)
- **f.** FRRR1, Friedreich's ataxia with retained reflexes (104)
- **g.** FRDA1 presenting as pure sensory ataxia (15)
- **h.** FRDA1 presenting as spastic paraparesis (48)
- **i.** FRDA1 with generalised chorea (56)
- **j.** FRDA1-like phenotype with vitamin E deficiency linked to Ch. 8q mutation (83)
- **k.** FRDA2 linked to 9p23-p11 (28, 75)
- **l.** Recessive HMSN (so-called "recessive Roussy-Levy Syndrome") (116)
- **m.** Childhood ataxia with musculo-skeletal coenzyme Q10 deficiency (100)

Type Vb
- **a.** Bassen-Kornzweig disease (13)
- **b.** Refsum's heredopathia atactica polyneuritiformis (107)
- **c.** Polyneuropathy, oligophrenia, premature menopause, and acromicra (Lundberg's Syndrome) (87)
- **d.** Unverrich-Lundborg disease, with myoclonic epilepsy and late onset ataxia

3. Adult and late onset (Type VI)

Type VIa
- **a.** Gamma-glutamylcysteine synthetase deficiency (113)
- **b.** LOFA, late onset Friedreich's ataxia (34, 35, 68)

debris are found within Schwann cell cytoplasm (63, 66, 103). Loss of myelinated fibers may reflect the severity of axonal damage. Degenerated axons show no specific ultrastructural features. GAA expansion had a significant inverse correlation with lost myelinated fibers as well as decreased amplitude of sensory action potentials in one study (123).

The cardiomyopathic lesions are classically associated with strikingly pleomorphic nuclei. Lamarche et al aptly demonstrated with iron stains (Prussian Blue, Perl's), the granular iron deposits scattered throughout the myocardium (80, 81, 121), often in chain-like distribution, now elucidated as the footprint lesions linked to frataxin mutations and abnormal metabolic turnover of mitochondrial iron (5, 107, 109) (Figure 3). It is frequently accompanied by a usually slight chronic non specific inflammatory response, which may include some siderophages (80, 82). Searches for similar iron-laden cell deposits throughout the CNS were generally unsuccessful, except by MRI spectroscopy in dentate nuclei (136). Recent studies by Bradley et al of iron staining in few autopsied FRDA1 subjects revealed similar iron deposits within hepatocytes, although inconstant, which were also observed within outer walls of hepatic sinusoids (22). They were also detected within the splenic red pulp's macrophages. None were however found in the cerebellum, dorsal root ganglia, spinal cord, skeletal muscles, peripheral nerves and pancreas (22).

Immunohistochemistry and Ultrastructural Findings

Ultrastructural observations of dorsal root ganglia yielded numerous lesions in the form of decreased axonal densities, and axonal swellings laden with 10-nm wide structures consistent with neurofilaments (79). These are associated with "onion-bulb"-like hypertrophy of Schwann cell processes (Figure 2F). Ganglion cells mostly display excess densities of lipofuscin and glycogen granules (79).

Heterogeneous ultrastructural abnormalities of Schmidt-Lantermann clefts were described in FRDA1 peripheral nerves as well as in several diseases unrelated to FRDA1, such as HSAN-1, HMSN 1-III, HMSN IV, tomaculous neuropathies, metachromatic leukodystrophies, ceroid lipofuscinosis, dysproteinemic neuropathies, and would therefore appear to be non specific (127).

Axonal degeneration and markedly decreased densities of large myelinated fibers are the main lesions observed in FRDA1 sural nerves (65, 124). Decreased axonal diameters and myelin thickness are frequent findings (18, 93). On teased nerve fiber preparations, some evidence of segmental demyelination may be observed, which tends to be subtle and could therefore suggest that hypomyelination may occur in the earliest cases (66, 119). Loss of large myelinated fibers would likely be secondary to a "dying back" type of axonal atrophy. Schwann cell hypertrophy with "onion-bulb"-like rings were occasionally described (12, 119). Lack of correlation of the severity of peripheral nerve lesions with disease duration was often reported, with a single exception (66, 124). In few studies, severity of the peripheral neuropathy was significantly inversely correlated with GAA repeat length (123). The pathophysiology appeared to be linked either to a progressive dying back process or maturational abnormality of axons (18, 103).

The sensory neuropathy of FRDA1 subjects is one in which little evidence of regenerative Bungner's bands (142), by comparison with selective vitamin E deficiency associated with the FRDA phenotype in whose sural nerves regeneration is likely to be more abundant. The FRDA phenotype associated with severe vitamin E deficiency is mapped to a chromosome 8q mutation in the alpha-tocopherol transfer protein gene (83), unlike FRDA1.

Biochemistry

A genetic test for the detection of the GAA repeat expansion is widely available and can be used to confirm a putative clinical diagnosis of FRDA1. Genetic testing is particularly useful in atypical cases with preserved muscle reflexes and late disease onset. Routine laboratory tests are usually normal in FRDA except elevated blood glucose in diabetic FRDA patients. 8-hydroxy-2′-deoxyguanosine, a marker of oxidative DNA damage, is increased in urine of FRDA patients (128). Mitochondrial malic enzyme deficiency has also been documented, but is now of little diagnostic value (133). However, increased serum levels of malondialdehyde, a marker of lipid peroxydation, were reported in FRDA pediatric subjects (42), suggesting that free radical products may constitute significant pathophysiological factors.

Differential Diagnosis

The differential diagnosis of recessive ataxias includes numerous entities, which were exhaustively reviewed by Barbeau et al (8) and recently updated (Table 3). Documentation of early and late onset FRDA sub-types (34, 35, 57, 68, 92, 110), as well as with retained reflexes (104), the well documented heterogeneity of disease progression with slower and more rapid sub-types all contribute to an increasingly challenging clinical diagnosis of FRDA, now made considerably easier by the widespread availability of highly specific molecular genetic tests (68). The molecular basis of FRDA phenotypic heterogeneity lies in the basic concept that GAA expansion sizes will ultimately drive phenotypic severity in an inversely proportional ratio to tissue decreases of frataxin levels (44, 104).

A newer item in the differential diagnosis involves detection of the autosomal recessive Charlevoix-Saguenay spastic ataxia (ARSACS), which has a higher incidence/prevalence rate than FRDA1 in Canada (20). ARSACS is the product of a 2 main

Table 3. (Opposing page) Classification of recessively inherited ataxias (8). Updated list of syndromes/diseases.

gene mutations in the *sacsin* locus on Chromosome 13q11. The specific function of *sacsin* is still unknown. ARSACS mutations have now been detected in French, Tunisian, and Turkish subjects (53).

The Roussy-Levy syndrome, a subtype of Charcot-Marie-Tooth disease, is an autosomal dominant degenerative disease which associates peripheral neuropathy with ataxia and tremor, whose features may be misleading because of tendon jerks may be abolished (116). Various forms of hereditary spastic paraparesis have also been confused with FRDA (33, 112). Several sub-types of autosomal dominant spino-cerebellar ataxias may be confused with FRDA during later stages of evolution due to overlapping phenotypic features, especially in SCA1, 2, and 3 variants (72).

Besides ataxia-telengiectasia, linked to mutations on locus Ch. 11q22-23 (88), several ataxic syndromes were recently genotyped: Unverricht-Lundborg disease, with myoclonic epilepsy and late onset ataxia on Ch. 21q (Cystatin B) (78), infantile onset spino-cerebellar degeneration with sensory neuropathy (IOSCA) on Ch. 10q24 (101), ataxia with oculo-motor apraxia and hypoalbunemia on Ch.9p13 (Aprataxin) (97), ataxia with neuropathy and high serum α-fetoprotein levels, on 9q33-34 (19), ataxia, deafness and optic atrophy, on Ch. 6p21-23 (19). A non-progressive form of congenital ataxia associated with mental retardation, optic atrophy and skin abnormalities was mapped to Ch. 15q24-q26 (36). A sub-type of childhood ataxia is associated with deficiency of co-enzyme Q10 (100).

Experimental Models

Few animal models could reproduce the full spectrum of the cell and molecular lesions observed in FRDA1. Seldom could they reproduce its natural progression to the point of claiming an exact phenocopy of the human disease (131). The yeast knockout model of frataxin, charaterised by a marked mitochondrial accumulation of iron, has yielded critical new insights on the role of frataxin on mitochondrial iron turnover by demonstrating a return to normal in vitro functional levels after frataxin gene replacement (5). In knockout transgenic mice by inactivation of the ataxia mouse gene through an exon 4 deletion, lethality occurred shortly after birth for homozygous animals, albeit without iron accumulation. Very numerous apoptotic and necrotic cells were observed (30).

Attempts to create transgenic mouse models of FRDA have recently become much more successful. Since complete absence of frataxin in mice leads to early murine lethality in the embryonic stage (30), a conditional gene targeting approach has been used to create a mouse line with frataxin deficiency restricted to striated muscle and another line with frataxin deficiency in neurons and cardiac muscle (108). The neuron-specific mutants have a progressive neurological phenotype and markedly reduced lifespan. Cardiac hypertrophy is a feature of both mouse lines (108). Biochemical studies in these models showed that the mitochondrial iron accumulation follows rather than precedes decline of the activity of mitochondrial enzyme complexes containing iron-sulphur clusters (108). These observations lend further support to the view that mitochondrial dysfunction in FRDA1 is a direct sequel of frataxin deficiency rather than caused by iron-induced oxidative stress.

FRDA1 fibroblasts were found to be more sensitive to oxydative stress compared to normal cell cultures, which displayed high levels of apoptosis when caspase 3 was activated by staurosporine. The fibroblasts could be rescued by in vitro anti-apoptotic inhibitors (141).

Pathogenesis

GAA repeats form DNA segments which are composed only of purines on one strand and pyrimidines on the complementary strand. These sequences are known to form triple helical structures which can combine as bimolecular complexes, which have been named sticky DNA. It has recently been shown that sticky DNA formation inhibits transcription of the frataxin gene (120). Indeed, frataxin tissue levels of FRDA patients are reduced to less than 10% of normals (23, 116). Frataxin has an expression pattern that correlates in part with the sites of pathology of the disease (23). The cellular specificity of the neurodegeneration in FRDA is thus at least partly explained by the distribution of frataxin. However, frataxin is also prominently expressed in a number of non-neuronal tissues such as liver, muscle, thymus and brown fat that are not affected in FRDA. The resistance of some of these tissues to the loss of frataxin may lie in their dividing nature and/or reduced sensitivity towards mitochondrial dysfunction.

At the cellular level, frataxin localises to mitochondria at the matrix side of the inner mitochondrial membrane (23, 76, 107). Yeasts with a targeted disruption of the frataxin homologue YFH1p abnormally accumulates iron within the mitochondria (5). This abnormal iron accumulation is reversed by reintroduction of the human frataxin gene (5). The mitochondrial iron overload is associated with increased oxidative stress and free radical synthesis as well as reduced activity of mitochondrial enzyme complexes containing iron-sulphur clusters (117, 128). Upon severe frataxin depletion, iron overload is also promoted by the mitochondrial intermediate peptidase (MIP), whose normal function involves maturation of specific proteins endowed with iron receptors within inner mitochondrial membranes (28). The process of oxydative phosphorylation is thus secondarily compromised. Impaired mitochondrial enzyme activity has been confirmed in myocardial biopsies of FRDA patients (114, 136).

The precise relationship between mitochondrial iron metabolism and mitochondrial dysfunction is not entirely clear. While initial studies suggested that frataxin is involved in mitochondrial iron efflux and that mitochondrial dysfunction is secondary to iron-induced oxidative stress (5, 109), more recent studies showed that frataxin binds iron in a high molecular weight form and keeps it in a reduced form (1). Consequently, it has been hypothesised that the decline of mitochondrial activity in FRDA1 is not only due to oxidative stress but also to impaired utilisation of iron for synthesis of iron-sulphur clusters (108).

While initial studies of frataxin function were performed in cellular and animal models, a number of patient studies lend further support to the hypothesis that FRDA1 is a mitochondrial disorder associated with abnormal deposition of iron. Waldvogel et al applied a newly developed multigradient echo magnetic resonance sequence, which allows to measure tissue iron levels in the brain (136). In the dentate nuclei of FRDA1 patients, iron content was significantly increased compared to controls while iron content was unchanged in the globus pallidus (136). Two studies indicated increased iron content in fibroblasts obtained from FRDA patients (37, 144). Lodi et al used postexercise phosphocreatine recovery as measured by phosphorus magnetic resonance spectroscopy of skeletal muscle to assess mitochondrial ATP production in vivo (86). Skeletal muscle mitochondrial ATP production was significantly reduced in FRDA1 patients compared to controls, in a manner directly dependent on GAA repeat length (86).

Future Directions and Therapy

Iron and calcium chelation would appear indicated in view of the pivotal role played by frataxin in mitochondrial iron turnover, which allows intramitochondrial accumulation of iron through the mutated frataxin isoforms. However, ascorbate and desferrioxamine trials have been complicated by significant in vitro iron-induced side effects (118). Moreover, the specificity of iron chelation in the context of normal serum iron and ferritin levels documented in FRDA1 subjects would likely be poorly effective (139). Desferrioxamine therapy may further be complicated by a marked decrease of the mitochondrial enzyme aconitase in presence of sharply reduced iron levels, which would sustain an even higher deficit in FRDA1 subjects, already well known to display low baseline values of serum aconitase (117).

Newer classes of iron chelators have been proven effective in vitro for high output mobilisation of mitochondrial iron from reticulocyte cultures. Isomers of the 2-pyridylcarboxaledehyde isonicotionoyl hydrazone class (PCIH) are potentially useful molecules for future clinical trials (114).

Anti-oxidant therapy trials with *idobenone* are on-going for some FDRA cohorts. They were the object of a preliminary report which provided evidence that the cardiac complications linked to the cardiomyopathy may be stabilised (118). Preliminary data on therapeutic trials with the free radical scavenger *idebenone* revealed a statistically significant volumetric reduction of heart size on echocardiography and simultaneous stabilisation and even reduction in the severity of ataxic symptoms in 8 of 11 FRDA pediatric subjects whose age ranged from 10- to 18-years-old (A. Fournier, M. Vanasse, personnal communication). In 3 FRDA subjects, patients treated with *idebenone* during 4 to 9 months eventually showed a reduction in the left ventricular mass index on echocardiography. In another recent *idebenone* trial protocol, no significant improvement of clinical scores was observed, either on the cardiomyopathy or neurologic signs (126).

Ascorbic acid and co-enzyme Q_{10} were used in recent therapy trials of small FRDA1 cohorts (86). Co-enzyme Q_{10} resulted in significantly improved skeletal muscle levels of mitochondrial ATP production simultaneously to an increased cardiac phosphocreatine/ATP ratio on spectroscopic MRI, albeit without improvement in the neurological and cardiac status (86). Such treatment protocols constitute a novel therapeutic approach of potential benefit to FRDA subjects.

Gene therapy remains a theoretical indication as human trials are not yet underway. These could aim at either the neurologic signs and/or the cardiomyopathy, the latter likely more accessible to efficient gene therapy protocols. However, until even more phenotypically reliable animal models of human FRDA can be obtained, development of gene therapy protocols will remain impeded.

Altogether, the encouraging results obtained in early trials of anti-oxidant drugs constitute a first step towards further validation with larger cohorts. Yet better transgenic models of FRDA would be helpful in the in vitro testing of more effective pharmacotherapeutic strategies.

References

1. Adamec J, Rusnak F, Owen WG, Naylor S, Benson LM, Gacy AM, Isaya G (2000) Iron-dependent self-assembly of recombinant yeast frataxin: implications for Friedreich ataxia. *Am J Hum Genet* 67: 549-562.

2. Agid Y, Blin J (1987) Nerve cell death in degenerative diseases of the central nervous system: clinical aspects. *Ciba Found Symp* 126: 3-29.

3. Amor DJ, Delatycki MB, Gardner RJ, Storey E (2001) New variant of familial cerebellar ataxia with hypergonadotropic hypogonadism and sensorineural deafness. *Am J Med Genet* 99: 29-33.

4. Andermann F (1976) Nicolaus Friedreich and degenerative atrophy of the posterior columns of the spinal cord. *Can J Neurol Sci* 3: 275-277.

5. Babcock M, de Silva D, Oaks R, Davis-Kaplan S, Jiralerspong S, Montermini L, Pandolfo M, Kaplan J (1997) Regulation of mitochondrial iron accumulation by Yfh1p, a putative homolog of frataxin. *Science* 276: 1709-1712.

6. Barbeau A (1978) Friedreich's Ataxia 1978--an overview. *Can J Neurol Sci* 5: 161-165.

7. Barbeau A (1980) Distribution of ataxia in Quebec. In *Spinocerebellar degenerations*, I Sobue (eds). University of Tokyo Press: Tokyo. pp. 121-141.

8. Barbeau A (1982) A tentative classification of recessively inherited ataxias. *Canad J Neurol Sci* 9: 96-98.

9. Barbeau A, Roy M, Sadibelouiz M, Wilensky MA (1984) Recessive ataxia in Acadians and "Cajuns". *Can J Neurol Sci* 11: 526-533.

10. Barbot C, Coutinho P, Chorao R, Ferreira C, Barros J, Fineza I, Dias K, Monteiro J, Guimaraes A, Mendonca P et al (2001) Recessive ataxia with ocular apraxia: review of 22 Portuguese patients. *Arch Neurol* 58: 201-205.

11. Baron DN, Dent CE, Harris H, Hart EW, Jepson JB (1956) Hereditary pellagra-like skin rash with temporary cerebellar ataxia, constant amino aciduria, and other bizarre biochemical features. *Lancet* 2: 421-428.

12. Barreira AA, Marques Junior W, Sweeney MG, Davis MB, Chimelli L, Paco-Larson ML, Wood NW (1999) A family with Friedreich ataxia and onion-bulb

formations at sural nerve biopsy. *Ann N Y Acad Sci* 883: 466-468.

13. Bassen FA, Kornzweig AL (1950) Malformation of the erythrocytes ina case of atypical retinitis pigmentosa. *Blood* 5: 381-386.

14. Batten FE (1905) Ataxia in childhood. *Brain* 28: 484-505.

15. Berciano J, Combarros O, De Castro M, Palau F (1997) Intronic GAA triplet repeat expansions in Friedreich's ataxia presenting with pure sensory ataxia. *J Neurol* 244: 390-391.

16. Berman W, Haslam RH, Koningsmark BW, Capute AJ, Migeon CJ (1973) A new familial syndrome with ataxia, hearing loss, and mental retardation. Report of three brothers. *Arch Neurol* 29: 258-261.

17. Bernabo'Brea G, Rathschuler R, Rasore-Quartino A (1966) Familial ataxia with peroneal muscular atrophy and optic atrophy. *Riv Oto-Neuro-Oftalmol* 41: 273-290.

18. Bilbao J, Midroni G, Cohen S (1995) "Genetically determined neuropathies". In *Biopsy diagnosis of peripheral neuropathy* (eds). Butterworth-Heinemann: Boston, New York, Toronto. pp. 353-409.

19. Bomont P, Watanabe M, Gershoni-Barush R, Shizuka M, Tanaka M, Sugano J, Guiraud-Chaumeil C, Koenig M (2000) Homozygosity mapping of spinocerebellar ataxia with cerebellar atrophy and peripheral neuropathy to 9q33-34, and with hearing impairment and optic atrophy to 6p21-23. *Eur J Hum Genet* 8: 986-990.

20. Bouchard JP, Barbeau A, Bouchard R, Bouchard RW (1978) Autosomal recessive spastic ataxia of Charlevoix-Saguenay. *Can J Neurol Sci* 5: 61-69.

21. Boudouresques J, Toga M, Khalil R, Gosset A, Vigouroux RA, Pellissier JF (1971) Amyotrophic form of a spinocerebellar degeneration. Anatomoclinical study and nosological discussion. *Rev Neurol (Paris)* 125: 25-38.

22. Bradley JL, Blake JC, Chamberlain S, Thomas PK, Cooper JM, Schapira AHV (2000) Clinical, biochemical and molecular genetics in Friedreich's ataxia. *Hum Mol Genet* 9: 275-282.

23. Campuzano V, Montermini L, Lutz Y, Cova L, Hindelang C, Jiralerspong S, Trottier Y, Kish SJ, Faucheux B, Trouillas P et al (1997) Frataxin is reduced in Friedreich ataxia patients and is associated with mitochondrial membranes. *Hum Mol Genet* 6: 1771-1780.

24. Campuzano V, Montermini L, Molto MD, Pianese L, Cossee M, Cavalcanti F, Monros E, Rodius F, Duclos F, Monticelli A et al (1996) Friedreich's ataxia: autosomal recessive disease caused by an intronic GAA triplet repeat expansion. *Science* 271: 1423-1427.

25. Caruso G, Santoro L, Perretti A, Massini R, Pelosi L, Crisci C, Ragno M, Campanella G, Filla A (1987) Friedreich's ataxia: electrophysiologic and histologic findings in patients and relatives. *Muscle Nerve* 10: 503-515.

26. Chamberlain S, Shaw J, Rowland A, Wallis J, South S, Nakamura Y, von Gabain A, Farrall M, Williamson R (1988) Mapping of mutation causing Friedreich's ataxia to human chromosome 9. *Nature* 334: 248-250.

27. Chew A, Sirugo G, Alsobrook JP, Isaya G (2000) Cloning, expression and chromosomal assignment of the human mitochondrial intermediate peptidase gene (MIPEP). *Genomics* 65: 104-112.

28. Christodoulou K, Deymeer F, Serdaroglu P, Ozdemir C, Poda M, Georgiou DM, Ioannou P, Tsingis M, Zamba E, Middleton LT (2001) Mapping of the second Friedreich's ataxia (FRDA2) locus to chromosome 9p23-p11: evidence for further locus heterogeneity. *Neurogenetics* 3: 127-132.

29. Cossée M, Durr A, Schmitt M, Dahl N, Trouillas P, Allinson P, Kostrzewa M, Nivelon-Chevallier A, Gustavson KH, Kohlschutter A et al (1999) Friedreich's ataxia: point mutations and clinical presentation of compound heterozygotes. *Ann Neurol* 45: 200-206.

30. Cossée M, Puccio H, Gansmuller A, Koutnikova H, Dierich A, LeMeur M, Fischbeck K, Dolle P, Koenig M (2000) Inactivation of the Friedreich ataxia mouse gene leads to early embryonic lethality without iron accumulation. *Hum Mol Genet* 9: 1219-1226.

31. Cossée M, Schmitt M, Campuzano V, Reutenauer L, Moutou C, Mandel JL, Koenig M (1997) Evolution of the Friedreich's ataxia trinucleotide repeat expansion: founder effect and premutations. *Proc Natl Acad Sci U S A* 94: 7452-7457.

32. Croft PB, Cutting JC, Jewesbury EC, Blackwood W, Mair WG (1977) Ocular myopathy (progressive external ophthalmoplegia) with neuropathic complications. *Acta Neurol Scand* 55: 169-197.

33. Cross HE, McKusick VA (1967) The Troyer syndrome. A recessive form of spastic paraplegia with distal muscle wasting. *Arch Neurol* 16: 473-485.

34. De Michele G, Filla A, Barbieri F, Perretti A, Santoro L, Trombetta L, Santorelli F, Campanella G (1989) Late onset recessive ataxia with Friedreich's disease phenotype. *J Neurol Neurosurg Psychiatry* 52: 1398-1401.

35. De Michele G, Filla A, Cavalcanti F, Di Maio L, Pianese L, Castaldo I, Calabrese O, Monticelli A, Varrone S, Campanella G et al (1994) Late onset Friedreich's disease: clinical features and mapping of mutation to the FRDA locus. *J Neurol Neurosurg Psychiatry* 57: 977-979.

36. Delague V, Bareil C, Bouvagnet P, Salem N, Chouery E, Loiselet J, Megarbane A, Claustres M (2001) Nonprogressive autosomal recessive ataxia maps to chromosome 9q34-9qter in a large consanguineous Lebanese family. *Ann Neurol* 50: 250-253.

37. Delatycki MB, Camakaris J, Brooks H, Evans-Whipp T, Thorburn DR, Williamson R, Forrest SM (1999) Direct evidence that mitochondrial iron accumulation occurs in Friedreich ataxia. *Ann Neurol* 45: 673-675.

38. Delatycki MB, Williamson R, Forrest SM (2000) Friedreich ataxia: an overview. *J Med Genet* 37: 1-8.

39. Dhe-Paganon S, Shigeta R, Chi Y-L, Ristow M, Bork P (2000) Crystal structure of human frataxin. *J Biol Chem* 275: 30753-30756.

40. Dürr A, Cossée M, Agid Y, Campuzano V, Mignard C, Penet C, Mandel JL, Brice A, Koenig M (1996) Clinical and genetic abnormalities in patients with Friedreich's ataxia. *N Engl J Med* 335: 1169-1175.

41. Dutka DP, Donnelly JE, Nihoyannopoulos P, Oakley CM, Nunez DJ (1998) Marked variation in the cardiomyopathy associated with Friedreich's ataxia. *Heart* 81: 141-147.

42. Émond M, Lepage G, Vanasse M, Pandolfo M (2000) Increased levels of plasma malondialdehyde in Friedreich ataxia. *Neurology* 55: 1752-1753.

43. Epplen C, Epplen JT, Frank G, Miterski B, Santos EJ, Schols L (1997) Differential stability of the (GAA)n tract in the Friedreich ataxia (STM7) gene. *Hum Genet* 99: 834-836.

44. Filla A, De Michele G, Cavalcanti F, Pianese L, Monticelli A, Campanella G, Cocozza S (1996) The relationship between trinucleotide (GAA) repeat length and clinical features in Friedreich ataxia. *Am J Hum Genet* 59: 554-560.

45. Friedreich N (1863) Über degenerative Atrophie der spinalen Hinterstränge. *Virchows Arch Pathol Anat Physiol Klin Med* 26: 391-419.

46. Friedreich N (1863) Über degenerative Atrophie der spinalen Hinterstränge. *Virchows Arch Pathol Anat Physiol Klin Med* 26: 433-459.

47. Friedreich N (1876) Über Ataxie mit besonderer Berücksichtigung der hereditären Formen. *Virchows Arch pathol Anat Physiol Klin Med* 68: 145-245.

48. Gates P, Paris D, Forrest S, Williamson R, Gardner R (1998) Friedreich's ataxia presenting as adult spastic ataxia. *Neurogenetics* 1: 297-299.

49. Geoffroy G, Barbeau A, Breton G, Lemieux B, Aube M, Leger C, Bouchard JP (1976) Clinical description and roentgenologic evaluation of patients with Friedreich's ataxia. *Can J Neurol Sci* 3: 279-286.

50. Gillespie FD (1965) Aniridia, cerebellar ataxia and oligophrenia in siblings. *Arch Ophtal* 73: 338-341.

51. Gilman S, Junck L, Markel DS, Koeppe RA, Kluin KJ (1990) Cerebral glucose hypermetabolism in Friedreich's ataxia detected with positron emission tomography. *Ann Neurol* 28: 750-757.

52. Goto S, Hirano A (1990) Immunohistochemical evidence for the selective involvement of dorsal root fibres in Friedreich's ataxia. *Neuropathol Appl Neurobiol* 16: 365-370.

53. Gucuyener K, Ozgul K, Paternotte C, Erdem H, Prud'homme JF, Ozguc M, Topaloglu H (2001) Autosomal recessive spastic ataxia of Charlevoix-Saguenay in two unrelated Turkish families. *Neuropediatrics* 32: 142-146.

54. Gustavson KH, Hagberg B, Sanner G (1969) Identical syndromes of cerebral palsy in the same family. *Acta Paediatr Scand* 58: 330-340.

55. Hallgren B (1959) Retinitis pigmentosa combined with congenital deafness, vestibulo-cerebellar ataxia and mental abnormality in a proportion of cases. *Acta Psychiat Scand Suppl* 34: 138.

56. Hanna MG, Davis MB, Sweeney MG, Noursadeghi M, Ellis CJ, Elliot P, Wood NW, D. MC (1998) Generalized chorea in two patients harboring the Friedreich's ataxia gene trinucleotide repeat expansion. *Mov Disord* 13: 339-340.

57. Harding AE (1981) Early onset cerebellar ataxia with retained tendon reflexes: a clinical and genetic study of a disorder distinct from Friedreich's ataxia. *J Neurol Neurosurg Psychiatry* 44: 503-508.

58. Harding AE (1981) Friedreich's ataxia: a clinical and genetic study of 90 families with an analysis of early diagnostic criteria and intrafamilial clustering of clinical features. *Brain* 104: 589-620.

59. Harding AE, Zilkha KJ (1981) 'Pseudo-dominant' inheritance in Friedreich's ataxia. *J Med Genet* 18: 285-287.

60. Hellenbroich Y, Schwinger E, Zuhlke C (2001) Limited somatic mosaicism for Friedreich's ataxia GAA triplet repeat expansions identified by small pool PCR in blood leukocytes. *Acta Neurol Scand* 103: 188-192.

61. Hirayama K, Takayanagi T, Nakamura R, Yanagisawa N, Hattori T, Kita K, Yanagimoto S, Fujita M, Nagaoka M, Satomura Y et al (1994) Spinocerebellar degenerations in Japan: a nationwide epidemiological and clinical study. *Acta Neurol Scand Suppl* 153: 1-22.

62. Horoupian DS, Zucker DK, Moshe S, Peterson HD (1979) Behr syndrome: a clinicopathologic report. *Neurology* 29: 323-327.

63. Hughes J, Brownell B, Hewer RL (1968) The peripheral sensory pathway in Friedreich's ataxia. *Brain* 91: 803-818.

64. James TN, Cobbs BW, Coghlan HC, McCoy WC, Fisch C (1987) Coronary disease, cardioneuropathy, and conduction system abnormalities in the cardiomyopathy of Friedreich's ataxia. *Br Heart J* 57: 446-457.

65. Jeune M, Tommasi M, Freycon F, Nivelon J (1963) Syndrôme familial associant ataxie, surdité et oligophrénie. Sclérose myocardique d'évolution fatale chez l'un des enfants. *Pédiatrie* 18: 984-987.

66. Jitpimolmard S, Small J, King RH, Geddes J, Misra P, McLaughlin J, Muddle JR, Cole M, Harding AE, Thomas PK (1993) The sensory neuropathy of Friedreich's ataxia: an autopsy study of a case with prolonged survival. *Acta Neuropathol* 86: 29-35.

67. Kjellin KG (1959) Familial spastic paraplegia with amyotrophy, oligophrenia and central retinal degeneration. *Arch Neurol* 1: 133-140.

68. Klockgether T, Chamberlain S, Wullner U, Fetter M, Dittmann H, Petersen D, Dichgans J (1993) Late-onset Friedreich's ataxia. Molecular genetics, clinical neurophysiology, and magnetic resonance imaging. *Arch Neurol* 50: 803-806.

69. Klockgether T, Lüdtke R, Kramer B, Abele M, Bürk K, Schöls L, Riess O, Laccone F, Boesch S, Lopes Cendes I et al (1998) The natural history of degenerative ataxia: a retrospective study in 466 patients. *Brain* 121: 589-600.

70. Klopstock T, Chahrokh-Zadeh S, Holinski-Feder E, Meindl A, Gasser T, Pongratz D, Muller-Felber W (1999) Markedly different course of Friedreich's ataxia in sib pairs with similar GAA repeat expansions in the frataxin gene. *Acta Neuropathol (Berl)* 97: 139-142.

71. Koenigsmark BW, Weiner LP (1970) The olivopontocerebellar atrophies: a review. *Medicine (Baltimore)* 49: 227-241.

72. Koeppen AH (1998) The hereditary ataxias. *J Neuropathol Exp Neurol* 57: 531-543.

73. Koeppen AH, Dickson AC, Lamarche JB, Robitaille Y (1999) Synapses in the hereditary ataxias. *J Neuropath Exp Neurol* 58: 748-764.

74. Kornyey S (1986) Some problems of the systemic degeneration and atrophies. *Acta Neuropathol* 72: 98-102.

75. Kostrzema M, Klockgether T, Damian MS, Muller U (1997) Locus heterogeneity in Friedreich ataxia. *Neurogenetics* 1: 43-47.

76. Koutnikova H, Campuzano V, Foury F, Dolle P, Cazzalini O, Koenig M (1997) Studies of human, mouse and yeast homologues indicate a mitochondrial function for frataxin. *Nat Genet* 16: 345-351.

77. Labuda M, Labuda D, Miranda C, Poirier J, Soong BW, Barucha NE, Pandolfo M (2000) Unique origin and specific ethnic distribution of the Friedreich ataxia GAA expansion. *Neurology* 54: 2322-2324.

78. Lafrenièere RG, Rochefort DL, Chrétien N, Rommens JM, Cochius JI, Kalviainen R, Nousiainen U, Patry G, Farrell K et al(1997) Unstable insertion of the 5-prime flanking region of the cystatin B gene is the most common mutation in progressive myoclonus epilepsy type 1, EPM1. *Nature Gen* 15: 298-302.

79. Lamarche J, Luneau C, Lemieux B (1982) Ultrastructural observations on spinal ganglion biopsy in Friedreich's ataxia: a preliminary report. *Can J Neurol Sci* 9: 137-139.

80. Lamarche JB, Côté M, Lemieux B (1980) The cardiomyopathy of Friedreich's ataxia. Morphological observations in three cases. *Can J Neurol Sci* 7: 389-396.

81. Lamarche JB, Lemieux B, Lieu HB (1984) The neuropathology of "typical" Friedreich's ataxia in Quebec. *Can J Neurol Sci* 11: 592-600.

82. Lamarche JB, Shapcott D, Côté M, Lemieux B (1993) Cardiac iron deposits in Friedreich's ataxia. In *Handbook of cerebellar disease*, R Lechtenberg: pp. 453-457.

83. Larnaout A, Belal S, Zouari M, Fki M, Ben Hamida C, Goebel HH, Ben Hamida M, Hentati F (1997) Friedreich's ataxia with isolated vitamin E deficiency: a neuropathological study of a Tunisian patient. *Acta Neuropathol (Berl)* 93: 633-637.

84. Leone M, Bottacchi E, D'Alessandro G, Kustermann S (1995) Hereditary ataxias and paraplegias in Valle d'Aosta, Italy: a study of prevalence and disability. *Acta Neurol Scand* 91: 183-187.

85. Lesch M, Nyhan WL (1964) A familial disorder of uric acid metabolism and central nervous system function. *Am J Med Genet* 36: 561-570.

86. Lodi R, Cooper JM, Bradley JL, Manners D, Styles P, Taylor DJ, Schapira AH (1999) Deficit of in vivo mitochondrial ATP production in patients with Friedreich ataxia. *Proc Natl Acad Sci U S A* 96: 11492-11495.

87. Lönnqvist T, Paetau A, Nikali K, von Boguslawski K, Pihko H (1998) Infantile onset spinocerebellar ataxia with sensory neuropathy (IOSCA): neuropathological features. *J Neurol Sci* 161: 57-65.

88. Louis-Bar D (1941) Sur un syndrôme progressif comprenant des télengiectasies capillaires cutanées et conjonctivales symétriques, à disposition naevoïde et de troubles cérébelleux. *Confin Neurol (Basel)* 4: 32-42.

89. Lundberg PO (1971) Hereditary polyneuropathy, oligophrenia, premature menopause and acromicria. A new syndrome. *Eur Neurol* 5: 84-98.

90. Machkhas H, Bidichandani SI, Patel PI, Harati Y (1998) A mild case of Friedreich ataxia: lymphocyte and sural nerve analysis for GAA repeat length reveals somatic mosaicism. *Muscle Nerve* 21: 390-393.

91. Marinesco G, Dragonesco S, Yasilin D (1931) Nouvelle maladie familiale caractérisée par une cataracte congénitale et un arrêt du développement somato-neuro-psychique. *Encéphale* 2: 97-109.

92. Marzouki N, Belal S, Benhamida C, Benlemlih M, Hentati F (2001) Genetic analysis of early onset cerebellar ataxia with retained tendon reflexes in four Tunisian families. *Clin Genet* 59: 257-262.

93. McLeod JG, Morgan JA (1976) Electrophysiological and pathological studies in spinocerebellar degenerations. *Proc Aust Assoc Neurol* 13: 113-117.

94. Megarbane A, Delague V, Ruchoux MM, Rizkallah E, Maurage CA, Viollet L, Rouaix-Emery N, Urtizberea A (2001) New autosomal recessive cerebellar ataxia disorder in a large inbred Lebanese family. *Am J Med Genet* 101: 135-141.

95. Montermini L, Kish SJ, Jiralerspong S, Lamarche JB, Pandolfo M (1997) Somatic mosaicism for Friedreich's ataxia GAA triplet repeat expansions in the central nervous system. *Neurology* 49: 606-610.

96. Montermini L, Rodius F, Pianese L, Molto MD, Cossee M, Campuzano V, Cavalcanti F, Monticelli A, Palau F, Gyapay G et al (1995) The Friedreich ataxia critical region spans a 150-kb interval on chromosome 9q13. *Am J Hum Genet* 57: 1061-1067.

97. Moreira MC, Barbot C, Tachi N, Kozuka N, Uchida E, Gibson J, Mendoca P, Costa M, Barros J, Yanagisawa T, Watanabe M, Ikeda Y, Aoki M, Nagata T, Coutinho P, Sequeiros J, Koenig M (2001) The gene mutated in ataxia-oculomotor apraxia 1 encodes the new HIT/Zn-finger protein aprataxin. Nature Gen 29: 189-193.

98. Murayama S, Bouldin TW, Suzuki K (1992) Pathological study of corticospinal-tract degeneration in Friedreich's ataxia. *Neuropathol Appl Neurobiol* 18: 81-86.

99. Musco G, Stier G, Kolmerere B, Adinolfi S, Martin S, Frenkiel T, Gibson T, Pastore A (2000) Towards a structural understanding of Friedreich's ataxia: the solution structure of frataxin. *Structure* 8: 695-707.

100. Musumeci O, Naini A, Slonim AE (2001) Familial cerebellar ataxia with coenzyme Q10 deficiency. *Neurology* 56: 849-855.

101. Nikali K, Isosomppi J, Lonnqvist T, Mao Ji, Suomalainen A, Peltonen L (1997) Toward cloning of a novel ataxia gene: refined assignment and physical map of the IOSCA locus on 10q24. *Genomics* 39:185-191.

102. Oppenheimer DR (1979) Brain lesions in Friedreich's ataxia. *Can J Neurol Sci* 6: 173-176.

103. Ouvrier RA, McLeod JG, Conchin TE (1982) Friedreich's ataxia. Early detection and progression of peripheral nerve abnormalities. *J Neurol Sci* 55: 137-145.

104. Palau F (2001) Friedreich's ataxia and frataxin: molecular genetics, evolution and pathogenesis (Review). *Int J Mol Med* 7: 581-589.

105. Patel PI, Isaya G (2001) Friedreich ataxia: from GAA triplet-repeat expansion to frataxin deficiency. *Am J Hum Genet* 69: 15-24.

106. Polo JM, Calleja J, Combarros O, Berciano J (1991) Hereditary ataxias and paraplegias in Cantabria, Spain. An epidemiological and clinical study. *Brain* 114: 855-866.

107. Priller J, Scherzer CR, Faber PW, MacDonald ME, Young AB (1997) Frataxin gene of Friedreich's ataxia is targeted to mitochondria. *Ann Neurol* 42: 265-269.

108. Puccio H, Simon D, Cossee M, Criqui-Filipe P, Tiziano F, Melki J, Hindelang C, Matyas R, Rustin P, Koenig M (2001) Mouse models for Friedreich ataxia exhibit cardiomyopathy, sensory nerve defect and Fe-S enzyme deficiency followed by intramitochondrial iron deposits. *Nat Genet* 27: 181-186.

109. Radisky DC, Babcock MC, Kaplan J (1999) The yeast frataxin homologue mediates mitochondrial iron efflux. Evidence for a mitochondrial iron cycle. *J Biol Chem* 274: 4497-4499.

110. Ragno M, De Michele G, Cavalcanti F, Pianese L, Monticelli A, Curatola L, Bolettini F, Cocozza A, Caruso G, Santoro I et al (1997) Broaded Friedreich's ataxia phenotype after gene cloning. Minimal GAA expansion causes late-onset spastic ataxia. *Neurology* 49: 1617-1620.

111. Refsum S (1946) Heredopathia atactica polyneuritiformis: a familial syndrome not hitherto described. A contribution to the clinical study of the hereditary diseases of the nervous system. *Acta Psychiat Scand Suppl* 38: 1-303.

112. Refsum S, Skillicorn SA (1954) Amyotrophic familial spastic paraplegia. *Neurology* 4: 40-47.

113. Richards F, Cooper MR, Pearce LA (1974) Familial spinocerebellar degeneration, hemolytic anemia and glutathione deficiency. *Arch Int Med* 134: 534.

114. Richardson DR, Mouralian C, Ponka P, Becker E (2001) Development of potential iron chelators for the treatment of Friedreich's ataxia: ligands that mobilize mitochondrial iron. *Biochim Biophys Acta* 1536: 133-140.

115. Riley CM, Day RL, Greelen DM, Langford WS (1949) Central autonomic dysfunction with defective lacrimation. I. Report of five cases. *Pediatrics* 3: 468.

116. Rombold CR, Riley HA (1926) The abortive type of Friedreich's disease. *Arch Neurol Psychiatry* 16: 301-312.

117. Rötig A, de Lonlay P, Chretien D, Foury F, Koenig M, Sidi D, Munnich A, Rustin P (1997) Aconitase and mitochondrial iron-sulphur protein deficiency in Friedreich ataxia. *Nat Genet* 17: 215-217.

118. Rustin P, von Kleist-Retzow JC, Chantrel-Groussard K, Sidi D, Munnich A, Rotig A (1999) Effect of idebenone on cardiomyopathy in Friedreich's ataxia: a preliminary study. *Lancet* 354: 477-479.

119. Said G, Marion MH, Selva J, Jamet C (1986) Hypotrophic and dying-back nerve fibers in Friedreich's ataxia. *Neurology* 36: 1292-1299.

120. Sakamoto N, Ohshima K, Montermini L, Pandolfo M, Wells RD (2001) Sticky DNA, a self-associated complex formed at long GAA*TTC repeats in intron 1 of the frataxin gene, inhibits transcription. *J Biol Chem* 276: 27171-27177.

121. Sanchez-Casis G, Cote M, Barbeau A (1976) Pathology of the heart in Friedreich's ataxia: review of the literature and report of one case. *Can J Neurol Sci* 3: 349-354.

122. Sanner G (1973) The dysequilibrium syndrome: A genetic study. *Neuropédiatrie* 4: 403-413.

123. Santoro L, De Michele G, Perretti A, Crisci C, Cocozza S, Cavalcanti F, Ragno M, Monticelli A, Filla A, Caruso G (1999) Relation between trinucleotide GAA repeat length and sensory neuropathy in Friedreich's ataxia. *J Neurol Neurosurg Psychiatry* 66: 93-96.

124. Santoro L, Perretti A, Crisci C, Ragno M, Massini R, Filla A, De Michele G, Caruso G (1990) Electrophysiological and histological follow-up study in 15 Friedreich's ataxia patients. *Muscle Nerve* 13: 536-540.

125. Sasaki H, Tashiro K (1999) Frequencies of triplet repeat disorders in dominantly inherited spinocerebellar ataxia (SCA) in Japan. *Nippon Rinsho* 57: 787-791.

126. Schols L, Vorgerd M, Schillings M, Skipka G, Zange J (2001) Idebenone in patients with Friedreich ataxia. *Neurosci Lett* 306: 169-172.

127. Schröder JM, Himmelmann F (1992) Fine structural evaluation of altered Schmidt-Lanterman incisures in human sural nerve biopsies. *Acta Neuropathol* 83: 120-133.

128. Schulz JB, Dehmer T, Schols L, Mende H, Hardt C, Vorgerd M, Burk K, Matson W, Dichgans J, Beal MF et al (2000) Oxidative stress in patients with Friedreich ataxia. *Neurology* 55: 1719-1721.

129. Sjögren T, Larsson T (1967) Oligophrenia in combination with congenital ichthyiosis and spastic disorders. *Acta Psychiatry Neurol Scand Suppl* 32 113: 1-112.

130. Skre H (1980) *Epidemiology of Spinocerebellar degeneration in Western Norway: Hereditary diseases.* University of Tokyo Press, Tokyo: 103.

131. Sotelo C, Guenet JL (1988) Pathologic changes in the CNS of dystonia musculorum mutant mouse: an animal model for human spinocerebellar degeneration. *Neurosci Lett* 27: 403-424.

132. Spieker S, Schulz JB, Petersen D, Fetter M, Klockgether T, Dichgans J (1995) Fixation instability and oculomotor abnormalities in Friedreich's ataxia. *J Neurol* 242: 517-521.

133. Stumpf DA, Parks JK, Eguren LA, Haas R (1982) Friedreich ataxia: III. Mitochondrial malic enzyme deficiency. *Neurology* 32: 221-227.

134. Urich H, Norman RM, Lloyd OC (1957) Suprasegmental lesions in Friedreich's ataxia. *Confin Neurol (Basel)* 17: 360-371.

135. van Boegert L, Moreau H (1939) Combinaison de l'amyotrophie de Charcot-Marie-Tooth et de la maladie de Friedreich chez plusiurs membres d'une même famille. *Encéphale* 34: 312-320.

136. Waldvogel D, van Gelderen P, Hallett M (1999) Increased iron in the dentate nucleus of patients with Friedrich's ataxia. *Ann Neurol* 46: 123-125.

137. Watanabe M, Sugai Y, Concannon P, Koenig M, Schmitt M, Sato M, Shizuka M, Mizushima K, Ikeda Y, Tomidokoro Y et al (1998) Familial spinocerebellar ataxia with cerebellar atrophy, peripheral neuropathy, and elevated level of serum creatine kinase, gamma-globulin, and alpha-fetoprotein. *Ann Neurol* 44: 265-269.

138. Wilmshurst JM, Surtees R, Cox T, Robinson RO (2000) Cerebellar ataxia, anterior horn cell disease, learning difficulties, and dystonia: a new syndrome. *Dev Med Child Neurol* 42: 775-779.

139. Wilson RB, Lynch DR, Fischbeck KH (1998) Normal serum iron and ferritin concentrations in patients with Friedreich's ataxia. *Ann Neurol* 44: 132-134.

140. Wilson RB, Roof DM (1997) Respiratory deficiency due to loss of mitochondrial DNA in yeast lacking the frataxin homologue. *Nat Genet* 16: 352-357.

141. Wong A, Yang J, Cavadini P, Gellera C, Lonnerdal B, Taroni F, Cortopassi G (1999) The Friedreich's ataxia mutation confers cellular sensitivity to oxidant stress which is rescued by chelators of iron and calcium and inhibitors of apoptosis. *Hum Mol Genet* 8: 425-430.

142. Zouari M, Feki M, Ben Hamida C, Larnaout A, Turki I, Belal S, Mebazaa A, Ben Hamida M, Hentati F (1998) Electrophysiology and nerve biopsy: comparative study in Friedreich's ataxia and Friedreich's ataxia phenotype with vitamin E deficiency. *Neuromuscul Disord* 8: 416-425.

Dentatorubral-pallidoluysian Atrophy

Hitoshi Takahashi
Mitsunori Yamada
Shoji Tsuji

CNS	central nervous system
DRPLA	dentatorubral-pallidoluisian atrophy
HD	Huntington's disease
MERRF	myoclonus epilepsy associated with ragged-red fibres
MJD	Machado–Joseph disease
MRI	magnetic resonance imaging
OMIM	Online Mendelian Inheritance in Man (*http:www.ncbi.nlm.nih.gov/omim*)
NII	neuronal intranuclear inclusion
NMI	nuclear membrane indentation
TBP	TATA-binding protein

Definition

Dentatorubral-pallidoluysian atrophy (DRPLA) is a rare autosomal dominant neurodegenerative disorder caused by an expansion of the CAG repeat in the DRPLA gene located on the short arm of chromosome 12 (12p13.31) (10, 14). The CAG repeats in patients with DRPLA were expanded to 54 to 79 repeat units, as compared to 6 to 35 repeat units in normal individuals (6).

Synonyms and Historical Annotations

The term DRPLA was originally used by Smith et al to describe a neuropathological condition associated with severe neuronal loss, particularly in the dentatorubral and pallidoluysian systems of the central nervous system, in a sporadic case without a family history (22). The hereditary form was first described in 1972 by Naito and colleagues (15).

Epidemiology

Incidence and prevalence. DRPLA has been reported to occur predominantly in Japanese individuals. However, it is now known that the disease may be found rarely in families in other ethnic backgrounds (1, 27). The prevalence rate of DRPLA in the Japanese population has been estimated to be 0.2 to 0.7 per 100 000, which is comparable with that of Huntington's disease (HD) in the Japanese population (8).

Sex and age distribution. Male and female patients are equally affected. The age at onset varies considerably from early childhood to late adulthood depending on the size of expanded CAG repeats.

Risk factor. Since DRPLA is a monogenic disease caused by expansion of CAG repeats of DRPLA gene, there have been no established risk factors that affect the clinical presentations of DRPLA.

Genetics

From the clinical genetic point of view, DRPLA is characterised by prominent anticipation (6, 10, 14). Paternal transmission results in more prominent anticipation (26-29 years/generation) than does maternal transmission (14-15 years/generation), indicating that the presence of the mechanisms underlie the intergenerational instability of the expanded CAG repeats during male gametogenesis.

The gene for DRPLA was mapped to 12p13.31 by in situ hybridisation (25). The human DRPLA gene spans approximately 20 kbp and consists of 10 exons, with the CAG repeats located in exon 5 (13). Putative nuclear localising signals have been identified near the amino-terminus of DRPLA protein (12), which is compatible with recent observations that DRPLA protein is translocated into nucleus preferentially in neuronal cells (18). The physiological functions of DRPLA protein, however, remain to be elucidated.

The previous studies indicate that CAG repeat expansion does not alter the transcription or translation efficiency of the mutant DRPLA gene (17, 35). Therefore, it seems likely that mutant DRPLA proteins with expanded polyglutamine stretches are toxic to neuronal cells ("gain of toxic functions").

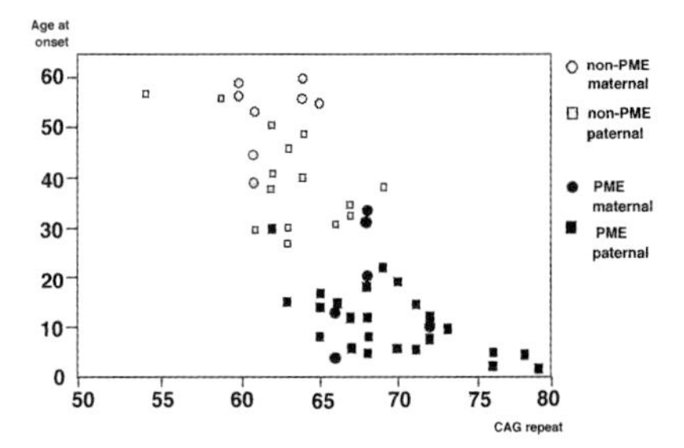

Figure 1. Correlation between the age of onset of DRPLA and the size of expanded CAG repeats. PME - progressive myoclonus epilepsy. Reproduced with permission from references 5 to 7.

Clinical Features

Signs and symptoms. The most striking clinical features of DRPLA are the considerable heterogeneity in the clinical presentation depending on the age at onset, and the prominent genetic anticipation (MIM#125370) (5-7, 15). Naito and Oyanagi reported that juvenile-onset patients (onset before the age of 20) frequently exhibit a phenotype of progressive myoclonus epilepsy (PME), characterised by ataxia, seizures, myoclonus, and progressive intellectual deterioration. Epileptic seizures are a feature in all patients with onset before the age of 20 and the frequency of seizures decreases with age after 20. Occurrence of seizures in patients with onset after the age of 40 is rare. Various forms of generalised seizures including tonic, clonic or tonic-clonic seizures are observed in DRPLA. Myoclonic epilepsy and absence or atonic seizures are occasionally observed in patients with onset before the age of 20.

In contrast, patients with onset after the age of 20 tend to develop cerebellar ataxia, choreoathetosis and dementia, thereby making this disease occasionally difficult to differentiate from HD and other spinocerebellar ataxias

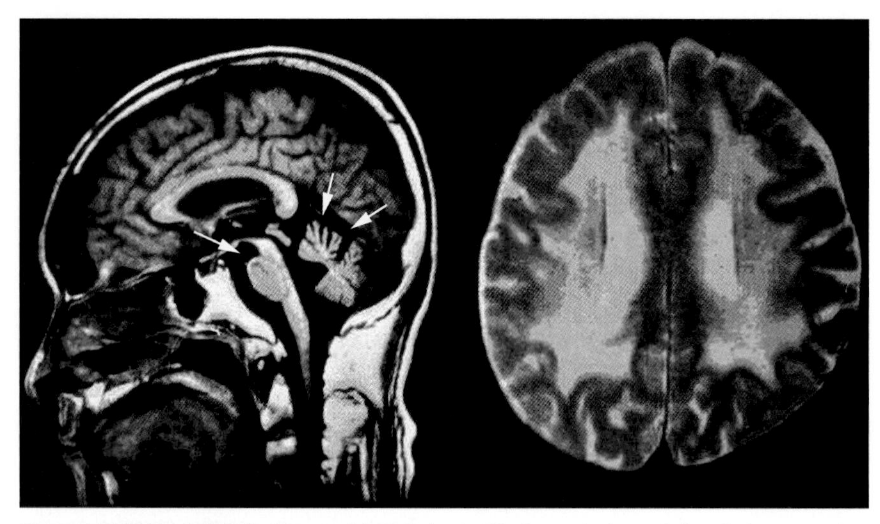

Figure 2. DRPLA is characterised neuroradiologically by atrophic changes in the cerebellum, brain stem particularly the pons and cerebrum.

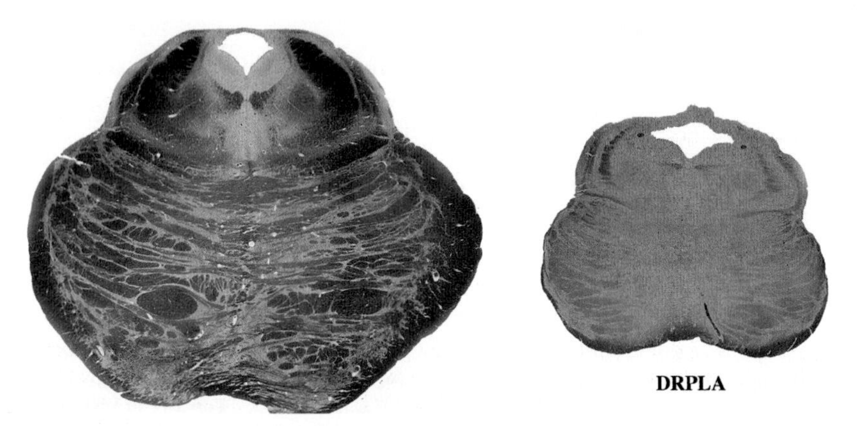

Figure 3. Comparison between one control and one DRPLA patient (right). The brain stem is markedly atrophic in the diseased patient. Same magnification, Klüver-Barerra stain.

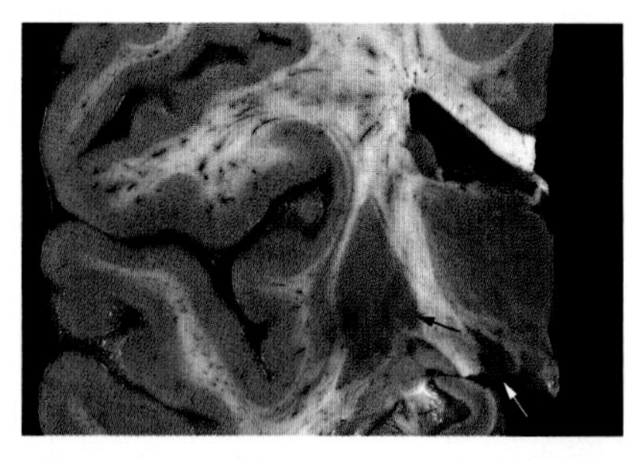

Figure 4. Brain section from a case with DRPLA. The globus pallidus (dark arrow), especially the lateral part and the subthalamic nucleus (light arrow) are atrophic with a brownish discoloration.

(15). Some patients were occasionally diagnosed as having HD, since the main clinical presentations were involuntary movements and dementia that masked the presence of ataxia. The evaluation of preceding ataxia and atrophy of the cerebellum and brainstem, in particular the pontine tegmentum, as detected by sagittal MRI scan is crucial for the differential diagnosis.

The discovery of the gene for DRPLA has made it possible to analyse the diverse clinical presentations based on the size of expanded CAG repeats (6).

Imaging. MRI findings of DRPLA are characterised by atrophic changes in cerebellum, pons, brain stem and cerebrum. High-signal lesions in the cerebral white matter, globus pallidus, thalamus, midbrain, and pons on T2-weighted MRI have been often found in adult patients with long disease duration (11).

Laboratory findings. Molecular diagnosis of DRPLA is made by analysis of the size of the CAG repeat in the DRPLA gene. Since PCR amplification may fail for largely expanded CAG repeats, careful interpretation of the analysis is required when only one allele is detected. There are no laboratory findings specific to DRPLA.

Macroscopy

The conventional neuropathology of DRPLA has been described repeatedly (15, 24, 26). At autopsy, the thickening of the skull is a significant feature of DRPLA: the patients had 2 to 3 times the thickness of normal skull bone. Macroscopically, the brain is small generally. At first glance, the cerebrum, brain stem and cerebellum are relatively well proportioned in external appearance. There is no correlation between brain weight and clinical factors such as age at onset, age at death and disease duration, and between brain weight and CAG repeat size. The spinal cord is proportionately small in size.

On cut surface, the brain reveals atrophy and brownish-tan discoloration of the globus pallidus, the subthalamic nucleus, and the dentate nucleus and its hilus. The atrophy of the brain stem tegmentum, being more marked in the pontine tegmentum, is also noted. The cerebral cortical atrophy is slight or negligible. However, almost every case shows mild to moderate dilatation of the lateral ventricle.

Histopathology

Combined degeneration of the dentatorubral and pallidoluysian systems is the major pathological feature of DRPLA. The globus pallidus, especially the lateral segment, and the dentate nucleus are consistently involved, showing loss of neurones, and astrocytosis. The subthalamic nucleus also shows loss of neurones. The loss of neurones is always milder than that of the lateral segment of the globus pallidus. The gliosis, which is more apparent than the neuronal loss, is considered to be mainly due to degeneration and loss of the pallidosubthalamic fibres originated from the lateral segment of the globus pallidus. In the dentate nucleus, the remaining neurones are often swollen or shrunken with so-called "grumose degeneration": numerous eosinophilic and argyrophilic granular materials, which represent the secondary change of the axon terminals of the Purkinje cells, accumulate around the somata and dendrites. Myelin pallor and astrocytosis are evident in the hilus. In the red nucleus, definite astrocytosis is seen, but loss of neurones is usually not evident. In general, pallidoluysian degeneration is more marked than dentatorubral degeneration in the juvenile-onset disease, and the reverse is seen in the adult-onset disease.

The population of the cerebral cortical neurones appears to be mildly or slightly decreased. Although usually mild in degree, the presence of reactive astrocytes is often found in the cerebral white matter. In some cases, especially in the adult-onset cases, diffuse myelin pallor is also evident in the white matter. In DRPLA, various other brain regions are also affected mildly or moderately, but it is also important to note that the substantia nigra, the locus coeruleus, the pontine nuclei, and the cranial nerve nuclei, with the exception of vestibular nuclei, are well preserved.

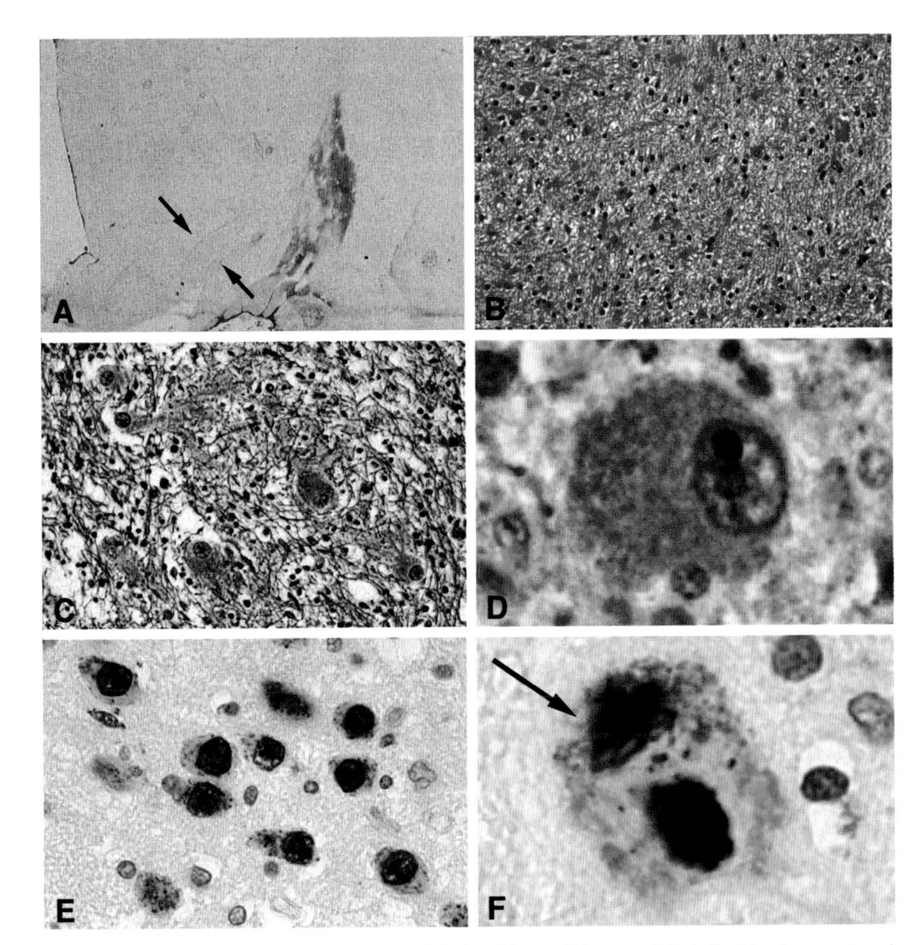

Figure 5. A. Staining showing fibrillary astrocytosis in the globus pallidus, especially in the lateral segment, and the subthalamic nucleus (arrows), being more severe in the former (Holzer). **B.** Neuronal loss and reactive astrocytosis in the lateral segment of the globus pallidus. **C.** Bodian staining showing the remaining dentate nucleus neurons with so-called grumose degeneration. **D.** A round ubiquitinated intranuclear inclusion in a dentate nucleus neuron. **E, F.** 1C2 immunostaining. Diffuse nuclear labeling with occasional intranuclear inclusions in neurons of the pontine nuclei (**E**). Immunoreactive intracytoplamic filamentous structures (arrow) in a dentate nucleus neuron (**F**).

Immunohistochemistry and Ultrastructural Findings

Neuronal intranuclear inclusions. Neuronal intranuclear inclusions (NIIs) have become the neuropathological signature common in all the CAG repeat diseases. In DRPLA, NIIs are eosinophilic round structures, which had long been overlooked in the previous histopathological studies. These NIIs are easily detectable by ubiquitin immunohistochemistry (3, 4), and also immunoreactive for expanded polyglutamine stretches as well as for atrophin-1, the DRPLA gene product (4, 32). They are mostly a single structure, but 2 or more inclusions are occasionally encountered in a cell nucleus (30). It is noteworthy that similar ubiquitinated intranuclear inclusions can also be detected in the glial cells (3).

Ultrastructurally, NIIs are often found in neuronal nuclei that exhibit nuclear membrane indentations (NMIs) (3, 4, 23). These inclusions are non-membrane bound, heterogeneous in composition, and contain a mixture of granular and filamentous structures. The filamentous composition is straight or slightly curved, approximately 10 to 20 nm in diameter, and is organised in random but sometimes parallel arrays. NIIs are occasionally surrounded by a single capsular structure, which is basically composed of granular materials and possesses immunoreactivity for PML (promyelocytic leukemia protein) (30). Intranuclear aggregate bodies experimentally formed in culture cells by transfection of DRPLA cDNA are dominantly composed of radially oriented filaments approximately 10 to 12 nm in diameter (4).

Diffuse intranuclear accumulation of expanded polyglutamine stretches. Immunohistochemistry with 1C2 monoclonal antibody reveals that, in addition to NIIs, expanded polyglutamine stretches accumulate diffusely in the neuronal nuclei (32). In contrast to the paucity of NII formation (3), the nuclear abnormality involves many neurones in a wide range of CNS regions far beyond the systems previously reported to be affected by conventional neuropathology (32). The novel lesion distribution may be responsible for a variety of clinical features such as dementia and epilepsy in DRPLA. The expansion of lesion distribution by the diffuse nuclear

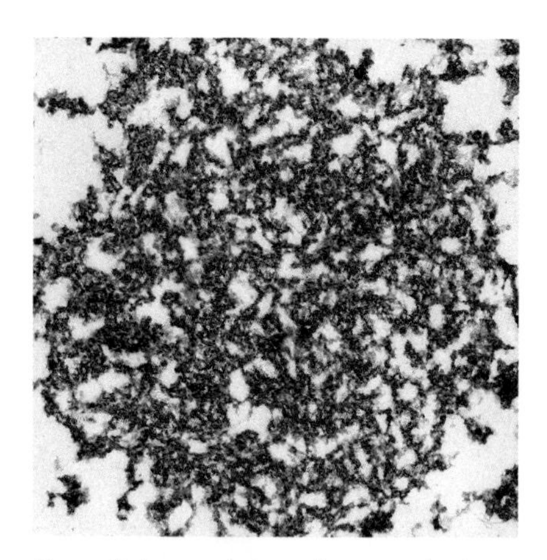

Figure 6. Immunoelectron microscopy showing a ubiquitinated intranuclear inclusion in a dentate nucleus neuron. The filamentous profile is evident. From ref. 14, with permission.

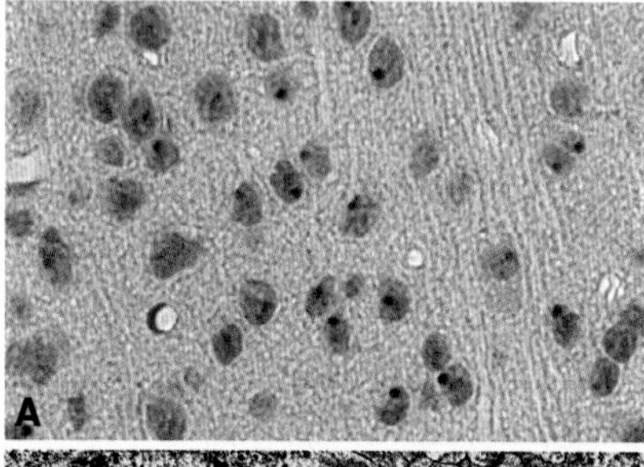

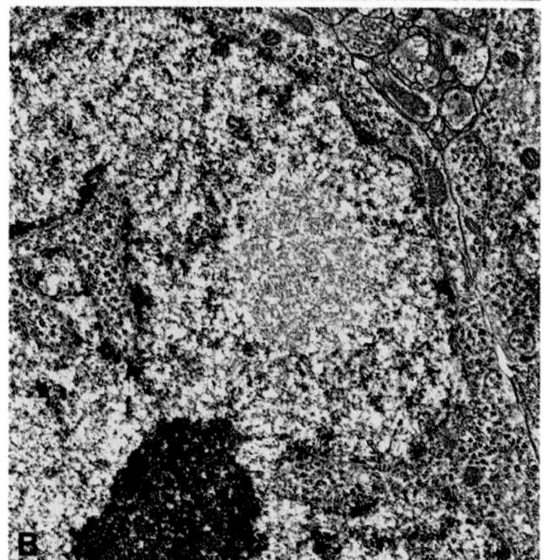

Figure 7. Transgenic mouse model of DRPLA. **A.** Ubiquitinated intranuclear inclusions in the cerebral cortical neurons. **B.** Electron microscopy showing a fine filamentous inclusion within a nucleus that exhibits strong nuclear membrane indentations.

labelling is also demonstrated in other CAG-repeat diseases, such as Huntington's disease (31) and Machado-Joseph disease (28).

Filamentous inclusions. In addition to the NII formation, ubiquitinated filamentous inclusions occur in the neuronal cytoplasm. These cytoplasmic inclusions are morphologically indistinguishable from the skein-like inclusions observed in the spinal anterior horn cells in amyotrophic lateral sclerosis. In DRPLA, however, these structures are formed exclusively in the dentate nucleus neurones (2). It is shown that they are also immunoreactive for expanded polyglutamine stretches (29). Moreover, they can be immunostained with an antibody against the C terminus of atrophin-1 (34), and with the antibody APG840 that recognises the region upstream to the polyglutamine stretch in atrophin-1 (32). Since the NIIs in DRPLA lack the antigenicity of the C terminus of atrophin-1 (34), the cytoplasmic filamentous inclusions seem to be unique structures in the molecular profile.

Nuclear enlargement. Recently, the nuclei of the cerebellar granule cells from patients with DRPLA were studied ultrastructurally and morphometrically (23). Even nuclei without NIIs or NMIs were significantly larger in the patients than in the controls, indicating that nuclear enlargement is a more prevalent abnormality than formation of NIIs or NMIs. Moreover, in the DRPLA patients there was a significant inverse correlation between the cross-sectional nuclear area and the disease duration: the degree of nuclear enlargement tended to decrease with time after the onset of the illness.

Biochemistry

As mentioned above, widespread ubiquitinated inclusions and diffuse accumulation of mutant atrophin-1 occur in the neuronal nuclei in various brain regions in DRPLA. Why are the dentatorubral and pallidoluysian systems most severely affected? It is possible that this is related to the physiological functions of atrophin-1 as a protein. The role of atrophin-1 in normal conditions has yet to be clarified.

Differential Diagnosis

Neuropathologically, Machado-Joseph disease (MJD/SCA3) and myoclonus epilepsy associated with ragged-red fibres (MERRF) are the main diagnostic contender (26). MJD/SCA3, which is also a CAG-repeat disease, involves multiple sites of the nervous system. Importantly, degeneration of the globus pallidus is marked in the medial segment of the globus pallidus. The subthalamic nucleus shows loss of neurones with astrocytosis, which is more severe than the medial side of the globus pallidus (subthlamo-pallidal degeneration). In MERRF, which is caused by point mutations in mitochondrial DNA, the pallidoluysian and dentatorubral systems are affected as seen in DRPLA. However, the substantia nigra, cerebellar cortex and spinocerbellar tract system also show marked degeneration. At present, all these disorders can be diagnosed genetically before the patients' deaths in practice.

Atrophy and degeneration of the globus pallidus, subthalamic nucleus, and dentate nucleus occur in several diseases in addition to DRPLA. In progressive supranuclear palsy and corticobasal degeneration, there exists tau-related pathology in the cerebral cortex, substantia nigra and various other brain regions (see chapter 3).

Experimental Models

To elucidate the molecular mechanisms of neuronal degeneration in DRPLA, transgenic mice harbouring a single copy of a full-length human mutant DRPLA gene with 76 or 129 CAG repeats have been generated (19, 20). These mice show intergenerational instability of CAG repeats similar to those observed in DRPLA pedigrees. The Q76 mice show no obvious phenotypes over 2 years, however, like the human brains affected by DRPLA, intranuclear diffuse accumulation of mutant protein can be observed in the mice brains. Interestingly, the accumulation first occurs in the restricted CNS regions such as the globus pallidus, subthalamic nucleus and cerebellar dentate nucleus beginning at around 4 weeks of age, and thereafter rapidly extends to multiple brain regions including the cerebral cortex. No NIIs are formed in this type of mouse. In contrast, the Q129 mice show clinical phenotypes similar to the DRPLA patients. Myoclonic movement appears at 3 weeks of age, followed by a rapid progress of ataxia and epilepsy by 12 weeks, and all the mice die by 16 weeks. The formation of NIIs is detectable after 9 weeks of age in the restricted CNS regions similar to those in the human DRPLA brain. The Q129 mice have revealed that the diffuse accumulation of mutant protein in neuronal nuclei is a phenomenon prior to the NII formation, and may be responsible for the onset of myoclonic movement.

Pathogenesis

Recent studies indicated the co-localisation of several transcription factors on NIIs, such as TATA-binding protein (TBP), TBP-associated factor ($TAF_{II}130$), Sp1, cAMP-responsive element-binding protein (CREB) and CREB-binding protein (CBP) (16, 21, 30, 32). These factors contain the glutamine-rich domains, and interaction of this domain with expanded polyglutamine stretches was demonstrated in an in vitro study (9). The findings strongly suggest that recruitment of several transcription factors into NIIs plays an important role in producing neuronal dysfunction, which may result in slowly progressive neuronal degeneration, and eventual neuronal cell death, probably apoptotic. It is also reported that NIIs interact with intranuclear domains such as PML nuclear bodies and coiled bodies (30), suggesting that intranuclear structural alteration is also induced by NII formation.

Further Directions and Therapy

It has recently been suggest that intranuclear accumulation of mutant proteins and transcriptional dysregulation are the primary pathogenic mechanisms of polyglutamine diseases. Given the reversibility of disease process in polyglutamine disease (33), there seems to be a wide time window for therapeutic approaches, and therapeutic strategies aimed against transcriptional dysregulation will be a challenging approach.

References

1. Burke JR, Wingfield MS, Lewis KE, Roses AD, Lee JE, Hulette C, Pericak-Vance MA, Vance JM (1994) The Haw River syndrome: dentatorubropallidpluysian atrophy (DRPLA) in an African-American family. *Nat Genet* 7: 521-524

2. Hayashi Y, Kakita A, Yamada M, Egawa S, Oyanagi S, Naito H, Tsuji S, Takahashi H (1998) Hereditary dentatorubral-pallidoluysian atrophy: Ubiquitinated filamentous inclusions in the cerebellar dentate nucleus neurones. *Acta Neuropathol* 95: 479-482

3. Hayashi Y, Kakita A, Yamada M, Koide R, Igarashi S, Takano H, Ikeuchi T, Wakabayashi K, Egawa S, Tsuji S, Takahashi H (1998) Hereditary dentatorubral-pallidoluysian atrophy: detection of widespread ubiquitinated neuronal and glial intranuclear inclusions in the brain. *Acta Neuropathol* 96: 547-552

4. Igarashi S, Koide R, Shimohata T, Yamada M, Hayashi Y, Takano H, Date H, Oyake M, Sato T, Egawa S, Ikeuchi T, Tanaka H, Nakano R, Tanaka K, Hozumi I, Inuzuka T, Takahashi H, Tsuji S (1998) Suppression of aggregate formation and apoptosis by transglutaminase inhibitions in cells expressing truncated DRPLA protein with an expanded polyglutamine stretch. *Nat Genet* 18: 111-117

5. Ikeuchi T, Koide R, Onodera O, Tanaka H, Oyake M, Takano H, Tsuji S (1995) Dentatorubral-pallidoluysian atrophy. Molecular basis for wide clinical features of DRPLA. *Clin Neurosci* 3:23-27

6. Ikeuchi T, Koide R, Tanaka H, Onodera O, Igarashi S, Takahashi H, Kondo R, Ishikawa A, Tomoda A, Miike T, Sato K, Ihara Y, Hayabara T, Isa F, Tanaka H, Tokiguchi S, Hayashi M, Shimizu N, Ikuta F, Naito H, Tsuji S (1995) Dentatorubral-pallidoluysian atrophy (DRPLA): Clinical features are closely related to unstable expansions of trinucleotide (CAG) repeat. *Ann Neurol* 37:769-775

7. Ikeuchi T, Onodera O, Oyake M, Koide R, Tanaka H, Tsuji S (1995) Dentatorubral-pallidoluysian atrophy (DRPLA): close correlation of CAG repeat expansions with the wide spectrum of clinical presentations and prominent anticipation. *Semin Cell Biol* 6:37-44.

8. Inazuki G, Kumagai K, Naito H (1990) Dentatorubral-pallidoluysian atrophy (DRPLA): Its distribution in Japan and prevalence rate in Niigata. *Seishin Igaku* 32:1135-1138

9. Kazantsev A, Preisinger E, Dranovsky A, Goldgaber D, Housman D (1999) Insoluble detergent-resistant aggregates form between pathological and nonpathological lengths of polyglutamine in mammalian cells. *Proc Natl Acad Sci U S A* 96: 11404-11409

10. Koide R, Ikeuchi T, Onodera O, Tanaka H, Igarashi S, Endo K, Takahashi H, Kondo R, Ishikawa A, Hayashi T, Saito M, Tomoda A, Miike T, Naito H, Ikuta F, Tsuji S (1994) Unstable expansion of CAG repeat in hereditary dentatorubral-pallidoluysian atrophy (DRPLA). *Nat Genet* 6:9-13

11. Koide R, Onodera O, Ikeuchi T, Kondo R, Tanaka H, Tokiguchi S, Tomoda A, Miike T, Isa F, Beppu H, Shimizu N, Watanabe Y, Horikawa Y, Shimohata T, Hirata K, Ishikawa A, Tsuji S (1997) Atrophy of the cerebellum and brainstem in dentatorubral pallidoluysian atrophy. Influence of CAG repeat size on MRI findings. *Neurology* 49:1605-1612

12. Miyashita T, Nagao K, Ohmi K, Yanagisawa H, Okamura-Oho Y, Yamada M (1998) Intracellular aggregate formation of dentatorubral-pallidoluysian atrophy (DRPLA) protein with the extended polyglutamine. *Biochem Biophys Res Commun* 249:96-102

13. Nagafuchi S, Yanagisawa H, Ohsaki E, Shirayama T, Tadokoro K, Inoue T, Yamada M (1994) Structure and expression of the gene responsible for the triplet repeat disorder, dentatorubral and pallidoluysian atrophy (DRPLA). *Nat Genet* 8:177-182

14. Nagafuchi S, Yanagisawa H, Sato K, Shirayama T, Ohsaki E, Bundo M, Takeda T, Tadokoro K, Kondo I, Maruyama N, Tanaka Y, Kikushima H, Umino D, Kurosawa H, Furukawa T, Nihei K, Inoue T, Sano A, Komure O, Takahashi M, Yoshizawa K, Kanazawa I, Yamada I (1994) Expansion of an unstable CAG trinucleotide on chromosome 12p in dentatorubral and pallidoluysian atrophy. *Nat Genet* 6:14-18

15. Naito H, Oyanagi S (1982) Familial myoclonus epilepsy and choreoathetosis: hereditary dentatorubral-pallidoluysian atrophy. *Neurology* 32:798-807

16. Nucifora FC Jr, Sasaki M, Peters MF, Huang H, Cooper JK, Yamada M, Takahashi H, Tsuji S, Troncoso J, Dawson VL, Dawson TM, Ross CA (2001) Interference by huntingtin and atrophin-1 with CBP-mediated transcription leading to cellular toxicity. *Science* 291: 2423-2428

17. Onodera O, Oyake M, Takano H, Ikeuchi T, Igarashi S, Tsuji S (1995) Molecular cloning of a full-length cDNA for dentatorubral-pallidoluysian atrophy and regional expressions of the expanded alleles in the CNS. *Am J Hum Genet* 57:1050-1060

18. Sato A, Shimohata T, Koide R, Takano,H, Sato T, Oyake M, Igarashi S, Tanaka K, Inuzuka T, Nawa H, Tsuji S (1999) Adenovirus-mediated expression of mutant DRPLA proteins with expanded polyglutamine stretches in neuronally differentiated PC12 cells. Preferential intranuclear aggregate formation and apoptosis. *Hum Mol Genet* 8:997-1006

19. Sato T, Oyake M, Nakamura K, Nakao K, Fukusima Y, Onodera O, Igarashi S, Takano H, Kikugawa K, Ishida Y, Shimohata T. Koide R, Ikeuchi T, Tanaka H, Futamura N, Matsumura R, Takayanagi T, Tanaka F, Sobue G, Komure O, Takahashi M, Sano A, Ichikawa Y, Goto J, Kanazawa I, Katsuki M, Tsuji S (1999) Transgenic mice harboring a full-length human mutant DRPLA gene exhibit age-dependent intergenerational and somatic instabilities of CAG repeats comparable with those in DRPLA patients. *Hum Mol Genet* 8: 99-106

20. Sato T, Yamada M, Oyake M, Nakao K, Nakamura K, Katsuki M, Takahashi H, Tsuji S (1999) Transgenic mice harboring a full-length human DRPLA gene with highly expanded CAG repeats exhibit severe disease phenotype. *Am J Hum Genet* 65 (suppl): A30

21. Shimohata T, Nakajima T, Yamada M, Uchida C, Onodera O, Naruse S, Kimura T, Koide R, Nizaki K, Sano Y, Ishiguro H, Sakoe K, Ooshima T, Sato A, Ikeuchi T, Oyake M, Sato T, Aoyagi Y, Hozumi I, Nagatsu T, Takiyama Y, Nishizawa M, Goto J, Kanazawa I, Davidson I, Tanese N, Takahashi H, Tsuji S (2000) Expanded polyglutamine stretches associated with CAG repeat diseases interact with TAFII130, interfering with CREB-dependent transcription. *Nat Genet* 26: 29-36

22. Smith JK, Gonda VE, Malamud N (1958) Unusual form of cerebellar ataxia: Combined dentato-rubral and pallido-Luysian degeneration. *Neurology* 8:205-209

23. Takahashi H, Egawa S, Piao-Y-S, Hayashi S, Yamada M, Shimohata T, Oyanagi K, Tsuji S (2001) Neuronal nuclear alterations in dentatorubral-pallidoluysian atrophy: ultrastructural and morphometric studies of the cerebellar granule cells. *Brain Res* 919:12-19

24. Takahashi H, Ohama E, Naito H, Takeda S, Nakashima S, Makifuchi T, Ikuta F (1982) Hereditary dentatorubral-pallidoluysian atrophy: clinical and pathologic variants in a family. *Neurology* 38:1065-1070

25. Takano T, Yamanouchi Y, Nagafuchi S, Yamada M (1996) Assignment of the dentatorubral and pallidoluysian atrophy (DRPLA) gene to 12p 13.31 by fluorescence in situ hybridization. *Genomics* 32:171-2.

26. Takeda S, Takahashi H (1996) Neuropathology of dentatorubopallidoluysian atrophy. *Neuropathology* 16:48-55

27. Warner TT, Williams L, Harding AE (1994) DRPLA in Europe. *Nat Genet* 6:225

28. Yamada M, Hayashi S, Tsuji S, Takahashi H (2001) Involvement of the cerebral cortex and autonomic ganglia in Machado-Joseph disease. *Acta Neuropathol* 101: 140-144

29. Yamada M, Piao Y-S, Toyoshima Y, Tsuji S, Takahashi H (2000) Ubiquitinated filamentous inclusions in the DRPLA cerebellar dentate nucleus neurones contain expanded polyglutamine stretches. *Acta Neuropathol* 99: 615-618

30. Yamada M, Sato T, Shimohata T, Hayashi S, Igarashi S, Tsuji S, Takahashi H (2001) Interaction between neuronal intranuclear inclusions and PML nuclear and coiled bodies in CAG repeat diseases. *Am J Pathol* 159:1785-1795

31. Yamada M, Wood JD, Shimohata T, Hayashi S, Tsuji S, Ross CA, Takahashi H (2001) Widespread occurrence of intranuclear atrophin-1 accumulation in the central nervous system neurones of patients with dentatorubral-pallidoluysian atrophy. *Ann Neurol* 49: 14-23

32. Yamada M, Tsuji S, Takahashi H (2000) Pathology of CAG repeat diseases. *Neuropathology* 20: 319-325

33. Yamamoto A, Lucas JJ, Hen R (2000) Reversal of neuropathology and motor dysfunction in a conditional model of Huntington's disease. *Cell* 101:57-66.

34. Yazawa I, Nakase H, Kurisaki H (1999) Abnormal dentatorubral-pallidoluysian atrophy (DRPLA) protein complex is pathologically ubiquitinated in DRPLA brains. *Biochem Biophys Res Commun* 260: 133-138

35. Yazawa I, Nukina N, Hashida H, Goto J, Yamada M, Kanazawa I (1995) Abnormal gene product identified in hereditary dentatorubral-pallidoluysian atrophy (DRPLA) brain. *Nat Genet* 10:99-103.

Spinal and Bulbar Muscular Atrophy

Gen Sobue
Hiroaki Adachi
Masahisa Katsuno

AR	androgen receptor
CBP	CREB-binding protein
DRPLA	dentatorubral-pallidoluisian atrophy
HD	Huntington's disease
MJD	Machado-Joseph disease
NI	nuclear inclusion
SBMA	spinal and bulbar muscular atrophy

Definition and Historical Annotations

Spinal and bulbar muscular atrophy (SBMA) was first described in a paper entitled "progressive bulbar palsy" in 1897 by Kawahara in Japan (14, 38). He reported the clinical characteristics of 2 brothers and their uncle on the maternal side with progressive atrophy of the tongue, dysarthria, dysphagia and gait disturbance. In 1953, Takikawa reported the clinical characteristics of one family with 6 patients, and classified SBMA as an inherited disease with a sex-linked recessive trait (39). The report by Kennedy et al on 2 families in 1968 has often been quoted as the first description of SBMA in Western countries (15). Since SBMA patients are frequently associated with gynecomastia, testicular failure and other feminized signs, this disease had been thought to be caused by an abnormality of androgen receptor (AR). The candidate gene was mapped to the proximal long arm of the X-chromosome in 1986 (10), and was determined to be the abnormal expansion of a CAG repeat in AR gene in 1991 (18).

Age at Onset

Many SBMA patients notice postural tremulous movements of the hands up to 20 years before muscle weakness appears. The tremor is usually not progressive; however, it does become worse with some patients. They also present occasional painful muscle cramps mainly in the lower legs and trunk when they are aware of muscle weakness or several years before that. The cramps can last for several years or even decades and decrease with the progress of the muscle weakness. It has been impossible for some patients to whistle since childhood. Limb muscle weakness, atrophy and fasciculation, and difficulty in swallowing and speech usually begin in the third to sixth decade of life, and only infrequently develop during adolescence.

Clinical Features

Neurological signs and symptoms. Consciousness and intelligence are not disturbed. Bilateral facial and masseter muscle weakness, poor uvula and soft palatal movements, and atrophy of the tongue with fasciculation are observed. Facial fasciculation is also characteristic. Repeated aspiration pneumonia due to dysphagia and the involvement of respiratory muscles may lead to premature death in some cases. The voice has a characteristic nasal quality. The muscle weakness and atrophy in the limbs are generalised or prominent in proximal muscles, and usually symmetrical. Although fasciculation in the extremities is rarely present at rest, it is easily induced as contraction fasciculation when patients hold their arms horizontally or bend their legs while lying on their backs. This contraction fasciculation is present in the early stage of the disease and is important for the diagnosis. Muscle tone is hypotonic. The motor involvement is slowly progressive and confines some patients to the wheel chair. SBMA patients may also have mild sensory impairment that usually remains subclinical. In most cases, the vibration sense is slightly diminished in the distal lower extremities, but occasionally all the sensory modalities are slightly disturbed. Deep tendon reflexes are hypoactive or absent. Pathological reflexes are not detected. Cerebellar and autonomic functions are normal.

Endocrinological abnormalities. Affected males show signs of androgen insensitivity, including gynecomastia, which frequently develops during adolescence, as well as testicular atrophy, impaired spermatogenesis, reduced fertility, impotence, and feminised skin changes. Serum testosterone levels are usually normal or increased.

Female heterozygous carriers. Female heterozygous carriers (36) are usually phenotypically normal, although mildly affected females have been reported. In addition, subclinical signs such as high-amplitude unit discharge and an elevated serum creatine kinase level are occasionally observed. It has been considered that female carriers may be protected by a favourable X-inactivation pattern or by low levels of circulating androgens.

Neurophysiological findings. Needle electromyography shows giant and polyphasic motor unit potentials of long duration in a diffuse distribution including limbs, trunk and tongue. Fibrillation potentials and positive sharp waves are occasionally observed. These abnormalities are frequently found in clinically unaffected muscles. The motor and sensory conduction velocities in the limbs are rarely prolonged. Terminal motor latencies are occasionally delayed. The sensory action potentials are reduced or absent in some cases.

Laboratory findings. Laboratory studies reveal an elevated serum creatine kinase level, impaired glucose tolerance or diabetes mellitus, slight hepatic dysfunction, and hyperlipi-

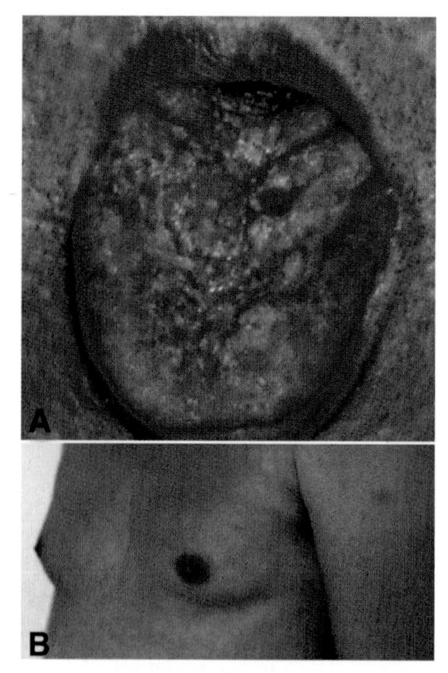

Figure 1. SBMA case showing **A.** atrophy of the tongue and **B.** gynecomastia.

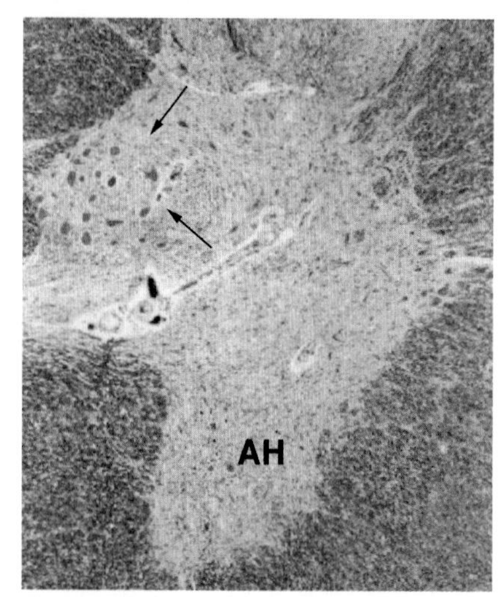

Figure 2. Reduction in the neuronal population of persisting nerve cells in the lumbar anterior horn (AH) and preservation of the posterior horn nerve cells (arrows). Klüver-Barrera, ×20.

demia. Usually, creatine kinase rises two to ten times the normal level and is thus a useful diagnostic indicator. Cerebrospinal fluid is normal. The test of genomic DNA is the most important one for the diagnosis.

Genetics

The molecular basis of SBMA is the expansion of a trinucleotide CAG repeat in the first coding exon of the AR gene, which encodes polyglutamine (polyQ) tract (18). A normally polymorphic CAG repeat ranges from

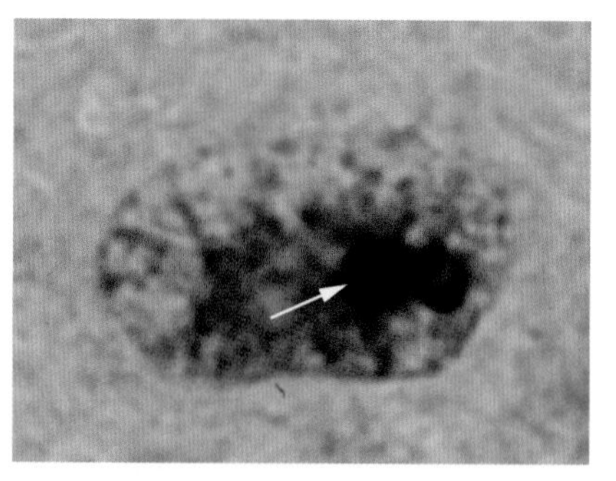

Figure 3. Nuclear inclusion (arrow) and diffuse nuclear staining of the mutant AR in the lumbar anterior horn cell of a SBMA patient stained with a monoclonal antibody (1C2) against abnormally expanded polyglutamine (polyQ). ×600.

14 to 32 CAGs, whereas a repeat in SBMA patients ranges from 40 to 62 CAGs (40). An inverse correlation has been reported between the CAG repeat size and the age at onset, or the degree of muscular weakness adjusted by the age at examination (8, 13, 19). Intergenerational CAG repeat expansion is observed, predominantly via paternal rather than maternal transmission, suggesting that the particular instability of the CAG repeat occurs in spermatogenesis (19, 33). The severity of the disease is different in each member of the same family.

Histopathology

The histopathology has been described repeatedly (11, 15, 21, 35). In SBMA, lower motor neurones are markedly depleted through all spinal segments and in brainstem motor nuclei except for the third, fourth and sixth cranial nerves. Many of the remaining anterior horn cells are remarkably atrophic and are accompanied by mild gliosis. The number of nerve fibres in the ventral spinal nerve roots is variably reduced. Neurones in the Onufrowicz nuclei, in the intermediolateral columns and in Clarke's columns of the spinal cord are generally well preserved.

Primary sensory neurones are also involved, but less severely affected. A quantitative study of primary sensory neurones at several levels in the peripheral nervous system shows a marked reduction in myelinated fibres and a preserved cellular population in the dorsal root ganglia. Evidence of regeneration is inconspicuous. Unmyelinated fibres are well preserved throughout all the nerves examined. These observations indicate that a primary sensory neuronopathy with a distally accentuated axonopathy is the salient sensory pathological process in SBMA. Muscle histopathology shows both neurogenic and myogenic findings. There are groups of atrophic fibres with a number of small angular fibres, fibre type grouping and clumps of pyknotic nuclei as well as variability in fibre size, scattered basophilic regenerating fibres and central nuclei. The neurogenic histopathology is consistent with chronic denervation.

Immunohistochemistry and Ultrastructural Findings

Nuclear inclusions (NIs) formed by the disease protein, are a pathologic hallmark of polyQ diseases, in which they have been shown to occur selectively in neurones of the affected brain regions. In the residual motor neurones of the SBMA spinal anterior horn, trigeminal nuclei and hypoglossal nuclei, there are AR-immunoreactive ubiquitinated NIs detected by antibodies that recognise a small portion of the N terminus of the AR protein. These NIs with expanded polyQ are also detected by antibodies to the abnormally expanded polyQ, many components of ubiquitine-proteasome and molecular chaperone pathways, but not by other immunoreactive AR epitopes. NIs are not observed in other nonaffected neural tissues. Similar NIs occurred not only in the motor neurones, but also in nonneural tissues including scrotal skin, dermis, kidney, heart, and testis.

Electron microscopic immunohistochemistry shows dense aggregates of AR-positive granular material without limiting membrane, both in the neural and nonneural inclusions. In other polyQ diseases such as HD and MJD, NIs show filamentous structures. This difference may suggest that the pathways of NIs formation are different among the different protein products.

Experimental Models

There are several AR transgenic mouse models with a truncated or full-version of AR gene driven by neurone-specific promoters including the AR, the prion protein (PrP) and the neurofilament light chain (NF-L) promoters (1, 3), a highly expanded 239 polyglutamine (polyQ) repeat under the control of human AR promoter (2) and AR-YAC transgenic mice (20). Neuronal phenotypes and NIs were documented in those with potent promoters of PrP or NF-L-driven truncated AR containing a highly expanded CAG repeat (1) and with a 239 polyQ repeat (2), which showed progressive neurological phenotypes of muscular weakness and ataxia, small body size and short life-span without neurone loss or astrogliosis. In these mouse models polyQ NIs were widespread but found in select regions of the central nervous system (CNS) such as the spinal cord, cerebrum and cerebellum as well as in certain peripheral visceral organs.

Efforts to create mouse models with a full-version of AR gene have failed to reproduce the disease phenotype because of low levels of protein expression (3). Expression levels of the mutant protein may contribute to the neuronal selectivity seen in these mouse models (41). Some other transgenic mouse models of polyQ diseases showed neuronal dysfunction without acute neurodegeneration resulting in neurone loss and astrogliosis (26, 32). Furthermore, even in the transgenic mouse models with neurone loss, a marked functional impairment of neurones such as an altered expression of transcriptional factors preceding the neurone loss has been documented (24). These findings suggested that polyQ can induce the functional impairment of neurones which precedes gross neuronal degeneration. The expanded polyQ may play a central role in such functional impairment. The neuronal dysfunction, which may precede neuronal cell death, is important from the therapeutic point of view.

Similarly, cell culture systems showed that the mutant AR formed NIs as a common link among the polyQ diseases (17, 28, 34, 37). Currently, it is considered that the polyQ NIs are not linked to neuronal cell death (16, 31). The evidence from cellular and transgenic mouse models indicated that nuclear localisation of the mutant protein is important in toxicity. These cellular models are useful for investigating the pathogenesis in SBMA.

Pathogenesis

To date, several polyQ diseases have been identified, including SBMA, Huntington's disease (HD), dentatorubralpallidoluysian atrophy (DRPLA), Machado-Joseph disease (MJD), and other spinocerebellar degenerations. The polyQ diseases have different disease-causing gene, but similar clinicopathological features, suggesting that these disorders share common pathological mechanisms leading to selective neuronal loss as the gain of a neurotoxic function. Transgenic mouse models that express cDNAs with an expanded CAG repeat for polyQ diseases reproduce many aspects of the associated neurodegenerative disease, confirming the gain of a neurotoxic function. Since the patients with complete androgen insensitivity syndrome never show neurologic deficits (25, 43), it has been considered that a novel neurotoxic function of the mutant AR causes neuronal dysfunction and degeneration in SBMA patients. On the other hand, SBMA patients show signs of partial androgen insensitivity, indicating that the mutant AR protein has either not completely normal ligand binding ability or low transcriptional activity (29). In addition, a partial loss of AR function may contribute to the neurodegenerative phenotype as well, given the evidence for a trophic effect of AR in neurones.

Although mutant AR proteins are expressed ubiquitously throughout the nervous system and often in other tissues as well (9), only a limited number of specific neuronal populations are prone to dysfunction and degeneration. NIs occurred not only in the motor neurones, but also in nonneural tissues in SBMA. An important question remains as to why the neurones are selectively affected despite the presence of NIs in both the affected neurones and nonaffected nonneural tissues. The cells of the nonneural tissues are mitotic cells in contrast to motor neurones. Hence, those cells with toxic effects associated with the mutant AR may be replaced by turnover. The difference in cell turnover rates could contribute to selective neuronal degeneration.

A common neuropathological feature of polyQ diseases is the presence of NIs containing the expanded polyQ in affected nervous regions. Although NIs may represent the final physical state of a misfolded protein, their role in disease pathogenesis remains unclear. The salient feature of NIs in SBMA is the finding that N-terminal epitopes are selectively detected. This absence of other immunoreactive AR epitopes within the NIs may be due to an altered AR configuration or the masking of AR epitopes by other proteins, or proteolytic cleavage of the AR. The fact that these NIs are ubiquitinated raises the possibility that alterations occur in the major intracellular system for degrading proteins. Processing of the polyQ containing protein by proteases may liberate the truncated polyQ tract. Indeed, a truncated, expanded-repeat AR is more toxic to cultured cells than a full-length form with the same repeat length (28).

Experimental studies using cell culture models or transgenic mice indicated the necessity of nuclear localisation of the mutant protein (16,31), suggesting that a critical nuclear factor or process is disrupted by the polyQ expansion. In SBMA, AR is confined to a multi-heteromeric inactive complex in the cell cytoplasm, and translocates into the nucleus in a ligand-dependent manner (42), which must be enhanced in male patients. The CREB-binding protein (CBP) is sequestered in the AR aggregates in tissues of SBMA patients and in neuronal cell lines expressing AR with expanded polyQ, leading to altered transcriptional activity (27). These alterations, particularly in trancriptional activity, may contribute to the impaired neuronal function and neuronal cell death. Soluble levels of CBP are reduced in cells expressing expanded polyQ despite increased levels of CBP mRNA. Overexpression of CBP rescues cells from polyglutamine-mediated toxicity in neuronal cell culture. The ability of over-expressed CBP to block polyQ-induced toxicity suggests that this sequestration may be an important step in the disease pathogenesis.

Future Directions and Therapy

Chaperone and PolyQ diseases. Recently, overexpression of chaperones has been reported to decrease aggregate formation in cellular polyQ disease models (37). Immunohistochemical studies revealed that polyQ-formed NIs colocalized with several chaperones and proteasome (5, 7). A combination of Hsp70 and Hsp40 or Hsp70 alone in the cell model of SBMA (17) has a favourable effect on cellular protection as well as on the suppression of aggregate formation; and the combination of Hsp70 and Hsp40 has the strongest effect among them. Chaperones have also been confirmed to suppress aggregate formation and cellular toxicity in other polyQ disease models (4, 6, 7). The overexpression of both Hsp70 and Hsp40 chaperones reduces cytotoxicity and aggregate formation with disease gene product in PolyQ disease. Molecular chaperones could be involved in the actual formation of expanded PolyQ by stabilising the unfolded protein in an intermediate conformation, which has the propensity to interact with itself or other proteins. In addition, chaperones may maintain proteins in an appropriate conformation (12). These evidences suggest that increasing the expression level or enhancing the function of chaperones may provide an avenue for the treatment of PolyQ diseases.

CBP. CBP is sequestered in AR-positive NIs, resulting in a decrease in soluble CBP and CBP-dependent transcription. This sequestration is toxic to the cells, and the toxicity is blocked by the over-expression of CBP (27, 30).

References

1. Abel A (2001) Expression of expanded repeat androgen receptor produces neurologic disease intransgenic mice. *Hum Mol Genet* 15: 107-116.

2. Adachi H (2001) Transgenic mice with an expanded CAG repeat controlled by the human AR promoter show polyglutamine nuclear inclusions and neuronal dysfunction without neuronal cell death. *Hum Mol Genet* 10: 1039-1048.

3. Bingham PM (1995) Stability of an expanded trinucleotide repeat in the androgen receptor gene in transgenic mice. *Nature Genet* 9: 191-196.

4. Carmichael J (2000) Bacterial and yeast chaperones reduce both aggregate formation and cell death in mammalian cell models of Huntington's disease. *Proc Natl Acad Sci U S A* 97: 9701-9705.

5. Chai Y (1999) Analysis of the role of heat shock protein (Hsp) molecular chaperones in polyglutamine disease. *J Neurosci* 19: 10338-10347.

6. Chan HY (2000) Mechanisms of chaperone suppression of polyglutamine disease: selectivity, synergy and modulation of protein solubility in Drosophila. *Hum Mol Genet* 9: 2811-2820.

7. Cummings CJ (1998) Chaperone suppression of aggregation and altered subcellular proteasome localization imply protein misfolding in SCA1. *Nat Genet* 19: 148-154.

8. Doyu M (1992) Severity of X-linked recessive bulbospinal neuronopathy correlates with size of the tandem CAG repeat in androgen receptor gene. Ann Neurol 32:707-710.

9. Doyu M (1994) Androgen receptor mRNA with increased size of tandem CAG repeat is widely expressed in the neural and nonneural tissues of X-linked recessive bulbospinal neuronopathy. *J Neurol Sci* 127: 43-47.

10. Fischbeck KH (1986) Localization of the gene for X-linked spinal muscular atrophy. *Neurology* 36: 1595-1598.

11. Harding AE (1982) X-linked recessive bulbospinal neuronopathy: a report of ten cases. *J Neurol Neurosurg Psychiatry* 45: 1012-1019.

12. Hendricks JP (1993) Molecular chaperone functions of heat-shock proteins. *Annu Rev Biochem* 62: 349-384.

13. Igarashi S (1992) Strong correlation between the number of CAG repeats in androgen receptor genes and the clinical onset of features of spinal and bulbar muscular atrophy. *Neurology* 42:2300-2302.

14. Kawahara H (1897) A family of progressive bulbar palsy. *Aichi Med J* 16: 3-4 (in Japanese).

15. Kennedy WR (1968) Progressive proximal spinal and bulbar muscular atrophy of late onset: a sex-linked recessive trait. *Neurology* 18:671-680.

16. Klement IA (1998) Ataxin-1 nuclear localization and aggregation: role in polyglutamine-induced disease in SCA1 transgenic mice. *Cell* 95: 41-53.

17. Kobayashi Y (2000) Chaperones Hsp70 and Hsp40 suppress aggregate formation and apoptosis in cultured neuronal cells expressing truncated androgen receptor protein with expanded polyglutamine tract. *J Biol Chem* 275: 8772-8778.

18. La Spada AR (1991) Androgen receptor gene mutations in X-linked spinal and bulbar muscular atrophy. *Nature* 352: 77-79.

19. La Spada AR (1992) Meiotic stability and genotype-phenotype correlation of the trinucleotide repeat in X-linked spinal and bulbar muscular atrophy. *Nat Genet* 2: 301-304.

20. La Spada AR (1998) Androgen receptor YAC transgenic mice carrying CAG 45 alleles show trinucleotide repeat instability. *Hum Mol Genet* 7: 959-967.

21. Li M (1995) Primary sensory neurones in X-linked recessive bulbospinal neuronopathy: histopathology and androgen receptor gene expression. *Muscle Nerve* 18: 301-308.

22. Li M (1998) Nuclear inclusions of the androgen receptor protein in spinal and bulbar muscular atrophy. *Ann Neurol* 44: 249-254.

23. Li M (1998) Nonneural nuclear inclusions of androgen receptor protein in spinal and bulbar muscular atrophy. *Am J Pathol* 153: 695-701.

24. Lin X (2000) Polyglutamine expansion down-regulates specific neuronal genes before pathologic changes in SCA1. *Nature Neurosci* 3: 157-163.

25. MacLean HE (1995) Defects of androgen receptor function: from sex reversal to motor neurone disease. *Mol Cell Endocrinol* 112: 133-141.

26. Mangiarini L (1996) Exon 1 of the HD gene with an expanded CAG repeat is sufficient to cause a progressive neurological phenotype in transgenic mice. *Cell* 87: 493-506.

27. McCampbell A (2000) CREB-binding protein sequestration by expanded polyglutamine. *Hum Mol Genet* 9: 2197-2202.

28. Merry D E (1998) Cleavage, aggregation and toxicity of the expanded androgen receptor in spinal and bulbar muscular atrophy. *Hum Mol Genet* 7: 693-701.

29. Mhatre AN (1993) Reduced transcriptional regulatory competence of the androgen receptor in X-linked spinal and bulbar muscular atrophy. *Nat Genet* 5: 184-188 .

30. Nucifora FC Jr (2001) Interference by huntingtin and atrophin-1 with cbp-mediated transcription leading to cellular toxicity. *Science* 291: 2423-2428.

31. Saudou F (1998) Huntingtin acts in the nucleus to induce apoptosis but death does not correlate with the formation of intranuclear inclusions. *Cell* 95: 55-66.

32. Shelbourne PF (1999) A Huntington's disease CAG expansion at the murine Hdh locus in unstable and associated with behavioural abnormalities in mice. *Hum Mol Genet* 8: 763-774.

33. Shimada N (1995) X-linked recessive bulbospinal neuronopathy: clinical phenotypes and CAG repeat size in androgen receptor gene. *Muscle Nerve* 18:1378-1384.

34. Simeoni S (2000) Motoneuronal cell death is not correlated with aggregate formation of androgen

receptors containing an elongated polyglutamine tract. *Hum Mol Genet* 9: 133-144.

35. Sobue G (1989) X-linked recessive bulbospinal neuronopathy, a clinicopathological study. *Brain* 112: 209-232.

36. Sobue G (1993) Subclinical phenotypic expressions in heterozygous females of X-linked recessive bulbospinal neuronopathy. *J Neurol Sci* 117: 74-78.

37. Stenoien DL (1999) Polyglutamine-expanded androgen receptors form aggregates that sequester heat shock proteins, peroteasome components and SRC-1, and are suppressed by the HDJ-2 chaperone. *Hum Mol Genet* 8: 731-741.

38. Takahashi A (2001) Hiroshi Kawahara (1858-1918). *J Neurol* 248: 241-242.

39. Takikawa K (1953) A pedigree with progressive bulbar paralysis appearing in sex-linked recessive inheritance. *Jpn J Genet* 28: 116-125 (in Japanese).

40. Tanaka F (1996) Founder effect in spinal and bulbar muscular atrophy (SBMA). *Hum Mol Genet* 5: 1253-1257.

41. Tanaka F (1999) Tissue-specific somatic mosaicism in spinal and bulbar muscular atrophy is dependent on CAG-repeat length and androgen receptor gene expression level. *Am J Hum Genet* 65: 966-973.

42. Zhou ZX (1994) The androgen receptor: an overview. *Recent Prog Horm Res* 49: 249-274.

43. Zoppi S (1993) Complete testicular feminization caused by an amino-terminal truncation of the androgen receptor with downstream initiation. *J Clin Invest* 91: 1105-1112.

CHAPTER 6

Prion Disorders

Chapter Editor: Catherine Bergeron

6.1 Introduction to Prion Diseases 282

6.2.1 Sporadic Creutzfeldt-Jakob Disease 287

6.2.2 Familial Creutzfeldt-Jakob Disease 298

6.2.3 Iatrogenic Prion Disorders 307

6.2.4 Variant Creutzfeldt-Jakob Disease 310

6.3 Gerstmann-Sträussler-Scheinker Disease 318

6.4 Fatal Insomnia: Familial and Sporadic 326

6.5 Kuru 333

6.6 In Vivo and In Vitro Models of Prion Disease 335

Introduction to Prion Diseases

Adriano Aguzzi

BSE	bovine spongiform encephalopathy
CWD	chronic wasting disease
fCJD	familial Creutzfeldt-Jakob disease
FDC	follicular dendritic cells
FFI	fatal familial insomnia
FSE	feline spongiform encephalopathy
GSS	Gerstmann-Sträussler-Scheinker syndrome
iCJD	iatrogenic Creutzfeldt-Jakob disease
PrP	prion protein
sCJD	spontaneaus Creutzfeldt-Jakob disease
TME	transmissible mink encephalopathy
TNF	tumour necrosis factor
TSE	transmissible spongiform encephalopathy
vCJD	new variant Creutzfeldt-Jakob disease

Prion diseases (3) are fatal neurodegenerative conditions affecting humans and a wide variety of animals (Table 1). Prion diseases are also called transmissible spongiform encephalopathies (TSEs), a term that underlines their infectious character. The most widely accepted hypothesis (4) on the nature of the infectious agent causing TSEs (the prion) predicates that it consists essentially of PrP^{res}, an abnormally folded, protease-resistant, beta-sheet rich isoform of a normal cellular protein termed PrP^{C} (Figure 1).

Molecular Biology of Prions

The prion may be defined as the agent that causes transmissible spongiform encephalopathies. This definition has proved useful operationally, but it says nothing about the true physical nature of the agent (4). A different definition centers on the structural biology of prions. According to this second definition, prions are proteins that can exist in at least two different conformations, one of which can induce the conversion of further prion molecules from one conformation into the other. Therefore, prions can act as true genetic elements—even though they do not contain informational nucleic acids—in that they are self-perpetuating and heritable (51). Two decades after Stanley Prusiner formulated the prion hypothesis, there is still uncertainty as to whether these 2 definitions coincide in the case of mammalian prions, since it has not yet been established which fraction of the protease-resistant PrP represents the infectious agent. Although all amyloid proteins and their precursors would fit the second definition, these proteins do not seem to be transmissible or infectious in vivo or in cell culture.

The normal mammalian prion protein is known as PrP^{C}. In vitro conversion of this protein can yield a moiety that has many of the physico-chemical properties characteristic of PrP^{res}. These include aggregation into higher-order complexes that are birefringent when stained with amyloid dyes such as Congo red, formation of fibrils identifiable by electron microscopy, and partial resistance to proteolytic enzymes, as identified by digestion with proteinase K (7, 34, 47).

An element common to the 2 definitions mentioned above, and absolutely required for the classification of a protein as a prion, is transmissibility. None of the experimental procedures reported so far has unambiguously accomplished transformation of the cellular prion protein PrP^{C} into a transmissible agent. Speculations abound as to why this has not been possible. The requirement for additional cellular factors distinct from PrP^{C}, for example, has been invoked on the basis of genetic evidence (55), but has never been proved. Universal consensus about the nature of the agent will predictably be reached only when a synthetic reconstitution has been done from non-infectious material.

Anatomy and Pathophysiology of Prion Neuroinvasion

In most cases of prion infection in both humans and animals, the point of entry is outside the nervous system, but how prions administered to the periphery of the body reach the CNS is

Disease	Host	Pathogenetic mechanism
iCJD	Human	Infection with prion-tainted growth hormone, gonadotropins, dura mater, etc.
vCJD	Human	Infection with BSE prions
fCJD	Human	Germ line mutation in the *PRNP* gene
sCJD	Human	Unknown
Kuru	Fore population	Infection through ritual cannibalism
GSS	Human	Germ line mutation in the *PRNP* gene
FFI	Human	Germ line mutation in the *PRNP* gene
FSI	Human	Unknown
Scrapie	Sheep	Infection of sheep with specific *Prnp* genotypes
BSE	Cow	Infection with tainted meat-and-bone meal
TME	Mink	Unknown
CWD	Mule, deer, elk	Unknown
FSE	cat	Infection with tainted meat-and-bone meal
Encephalopathy of exotic captive ungulated	Kudu, Nyala, Oryx	Infection with tainted meat-and-bone meal

Table 1. Prion diseases of humans and animals. iCJD: iatrogenic CJD; vCJD: new-variant CJD; fCJD: familial CJD; sCJD: sporadic CJD; GSS: Gerstmann-Sträussler-Scheinker syndrome; FFI: Fatal familial Insomnia; FSI: fatal sporadic insomnia; BSE: Bovine spongiform encephalopathy; TME: transmissible mink encephalopathy; CWD: chronic wasting disease; FSE: Feline spongiform encephalopathy.

unknown (Figure 2). Available evidence indicates that prions colonise the immune system; lymphocytes (13) and follicular dendritic cells (30) in germinal centers (specialised areas of lymphoid organs important for affinity maturation of B-lymphocytes) express considerable amounts of PrP^C. Extracerebral prion protein is required for neuroinvasion (10). Prion knockout (*Prnp*$^{0/0}$) mice harbouring a PrP^C-expressing graft in their brains consistently develop spongiform encephalopathy (restricted to the graft) upon intracerebral inoculation with the infectious agent (9). The mice do not, however, develop such encephalopathies upon intraocular, intraperitoneal or even intravenous administration of the agent (8, 10). Therefore, the absence of PrP^C prevents the spread of the infectious agent within the body (1).

Reconstitution of the hematopoietic and lymphopoietic system with stem cells derived from wild-type or transgenic mice overexpressing PrP^C does not restore neuroinvasion (19), implying that the crucial compartment is sessile, and that it cannot be transferred by adoptive bone-marrow reconstitution (8). There are at least 2 likely candidates for this compartment—peripheral nerves (45) and follicular dendritic cells (30).

What are the molecular mechanisms by which FDCs could capture prions? Capture of conventional antigens by FDCs occurs via Fcγ receptors and complement receptors: the same systems are operational in prion capture when limiting amounts of infectivity are introduced (33, 36), but additional molecules are likely to play a role in this process.
On the other hand, neuroinvasion—the development of brain disease after peripheral challenge—is unaffected in TNF-R1 (31) and lymphotoxin β (38) knockout mice, and cannot even be fully repressed by treatment with an antibody against the lymphotoxin β receptor (37, 39). Therefore, although the lack of signalling from lymphotoxin β to FDCs probably accounts for some of the protection from peripheral prion inoculation observed in B-cell deficient mice, lymphocytes probably have an additional role in prion neuroinvasion. This function is independent of PrP expression (32) and probably distinct from lymphotoxin β/TNF signalling. Peripheral autonomic nerves play a major role (6, 23) in transport from germinal centers to the central nervous system, and lymphocytes may be involved in the migration of prions from FDCs to peripheral nerves.

"Refolding" model

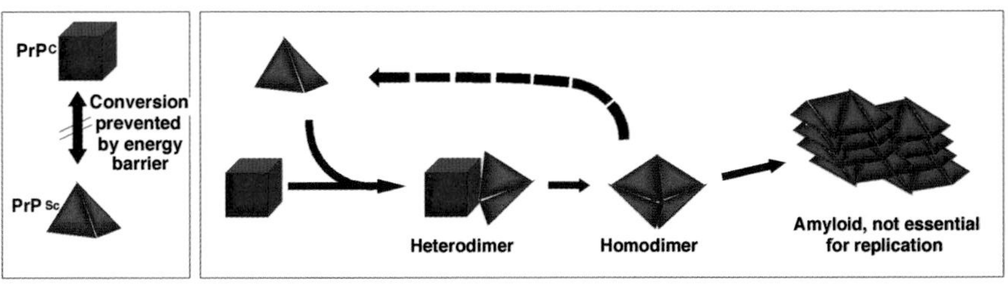

"Seeding" model

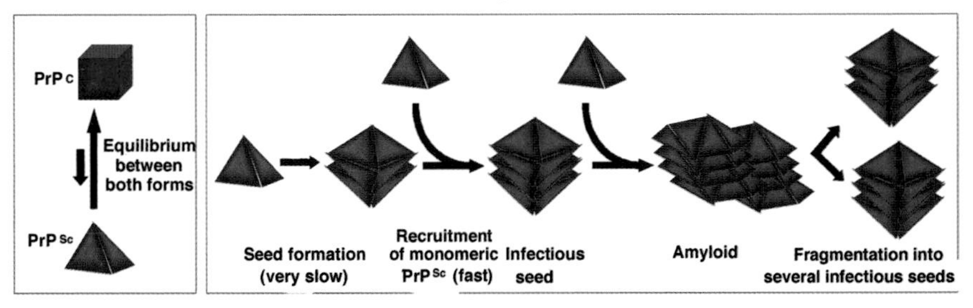

Figure 1. The 2 currently most popular hypotheses on the replication of prions. **A.** Presents the refolding model, which was proposed by Dr. Stanley Prusiner. According to this model, the disease-associated prion protein PrP^{Sc} binds the physiological, normal prion protein (PrP^C). Binding may be assisted by one or more chaperons provisionally designated as "protein x." The conversion process occurs during this binding and leads to transformation of PrP^C into a copy ofPrP^{Sc}. The newly formed PrP^{Sc} feeds back into the vicious circle, and will lead to further replication of itself—as long as the substrate, PrP^C, is available. As a final step, PrP^{Sc} aggregates and forms amyloid-fibrils; however, these are not essential for prion replication.

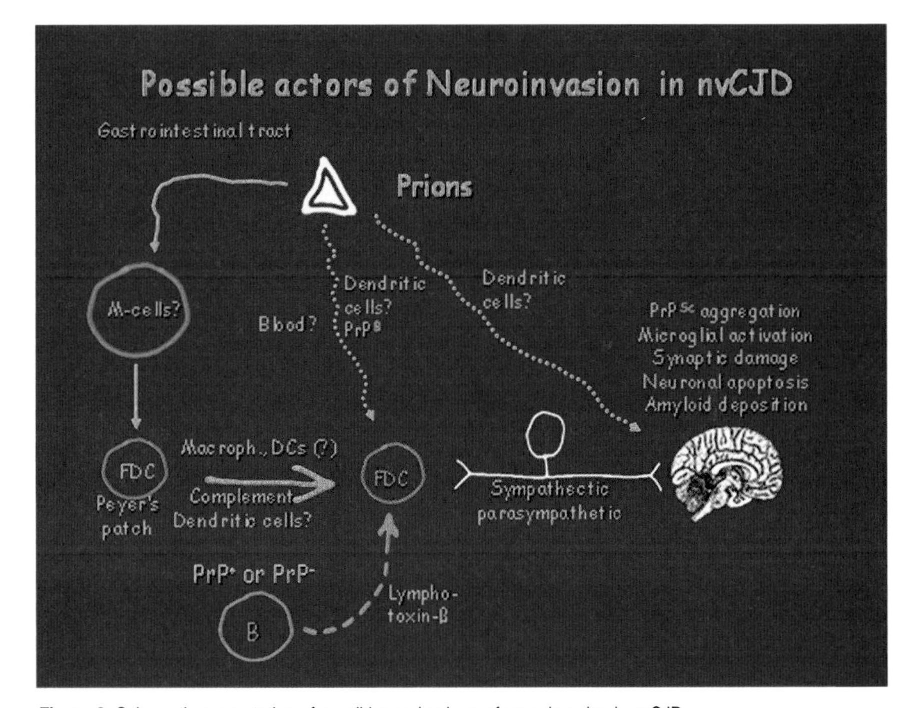

Figure 2. Schematic presentation of possible mechanisms of neuroinvasion in nvCJD.

Prion: Agent of transmissible spongiform encephalopathy. According to the terminology adopted here, the term "prion" does not have structural implications other than that a protein is an essential component.

"Protein only" hypothesis: States that the prion is devoid of informational nucleic acid and consists of protein (or glycoprotein) as essential pathogenic component. Genetic evidence strongly suggests that the protein is an abnormal form of PrP (perhaps congruent with PrP^{Sc}). The association with other "non-informational" molecules (for example lipids or glycosamino glycans) is not excluded.

PrP^{c} or PrP-sen: The naturally occurring form of the mature *Prnp* gene product. It is glycosylated, anchored to the plasma membrane by a GPI residue and poor in β-sheet structure. Its presence in a given cell type is necessary, but not sufficient, for the replication of the prion.

PrP^{Sc} or PrP-res: An "abnormal" form of the mature *Prnp* gene product found in tissue of TSE sufferers, operationally defined as being partly resistant to proteinase K digestion under defined reaction conditions. It is believed to differ from PrP^{c} only (or mainly) conformationally and is rich in β sheet structure. Within the framework of the "protein only" hypothesis it is often considered to be the transmissible agent or prion.

Prion strains: Prion strains have different phenotypes—for example, incubation times, distribution of lesions in the brain, relative abundance of mono-, di- and unglycosylated PrPSc, and electrophoretic mobility of the protease-resistant part of PrP^{Sc}. But they can all be propagated in the same inbred mouse strain, indicating that, within the framework of the protein-only hypothesis, the same polypeptide chain can mediate different strain phenotypes.

From Bench to Clinic

Since prions can be detected in lymphoreticular tissues (eg, spleen, lymph nodes, tonsils, and appendix) of patients with vCJD, is there a risk of iatrogenic transmission though blood or tissues from people with preclinical vCJD, or from contaminated surgical instruments? Epidemiological surveys over the past 2 decades have not implicated transfusions, or administration of plasma fractions, as risk factors for prion diseases; however, a small increase in relative risk for sporadically occurring disease (sCJD) is associated with surgery of all kinds (16), and it may indeed indicate unrecognised iatrogenic transmission. With vCJD the situation may not be as simple. We do not know as much about the epidemiology and iatrogenic transmissibility of this new disease as we do about sCJD.

Another question relates to the possibility of chronic sub-clinical disease or a permanent "carrier" status in cows as well as in humans. There is evidence that such a carrier status may be produced by the passage of the infectious agent across species (5, 44) between hamsters and mice. Immune deficiency can also lead to a similar situation, even when there is no species barrier (20). Therefore, the problem of animal transmissible spongiform encephalopathies could be more widespread than is assumed. Moreover, people carrying the infectious agent may transmit it horizontally (2) and the risks associated with this possibility can be met only if we know more about how the agent is transmitted and how prions reach the brain from peripheral sites.

Preventive Measures

What can be done to prevent spread of the disease? vCJD seems to be much more "lympho-invasive" than sCJD. In particular, vCJD prions can be easily detected in lymphatic organs such as tonsils and the appendix (26-28). This is also the case for scrapie of sheep (49, 50, 56), but not for sCJD prions.

Although prion infectivity of circulating lymphocytes seems to be at least two logs lower than that detected in splenic lymphocytes (46), the possibility that circulating lymphocytes may be in equilibrium with their splenic siblings call for cautionary measures when dealing with blood products. But what should these be? Leukodepletion—a filtering process that aims at reducing the number of leukocytes in transfused blood units—has been advocated, but there is still no certainty about its efficacy. In addition, even if blood prion infectivity is initially contained in lymphocytes in vivo, lysis of cells may possibly lead to contamination of blood units with infectious "microparticles" (22) which may be difficult to remove by any method (short of ultracentrifugation). Many of the virus-removal steps involved in the manufacture of stable blood products have some positive effects on prion removal, so the possibility of such contamination can be regarded as a worst-case scenario.

A final consideration applies to secondary prophylaxis. Given the large amount of infectious BSE material that has entered the human food chain, it is possible that many people harbor pre-clinical vCJD. Unfortunately, the distribution of pre-clinical disease is unknown, and most available prion assays are very insensitive. Once sub-clinical carriers are identified, it will be imperative to develop strategies that will help to control spread of the agent and prevent the outbreak of symptoms in these people.

Interventional approaches to prion diseases. There are no reports of cure in patients suffering from clinically manifest TSE. It would be unrealistic to expect that the enormous amount of damage that is already visible in the early clinical phase of the disease could be easily reversed by pharmacological treatment. A more realistic goal may be deceleration of disease. Many attempts at prion therapy have gone towards inhibition of accumulation of PrP^{res}. Many compounds are effective in clearing PrP^{res} and prion infectivity in vitro, such as chlorpromazine, quinacrine (17, 35, 48), Congo red (14), amphotericin B (41), anthracycline derivatives (54), sulfated polyanions (15), pentosan polysulphate (18), soluble lymphotoxin-β receptors (39), porphyrins (42), branched polyamines (53), and beta-sheet breaker peptides (52). Sadly, none of these substances have, so far, proved particularly effective for actual therapy of overtly sick animals—let alone human patients.

The sympathetic nervous system appears to play a role in transmission of infectivity from the lymphoreticular to the central nervous compartment. Injection of 6-hydroxydopamine, or of anti-nerve-growth factor antibodies, causes efficient and protracted sympathectomy, and significantly delays development of scrapie upon intraperitoneal inoculation (24). While sympathectomy is far too invasive to represent a viable option for post-exposure prophylaxis, the sympathetic nervous system may be worth being explored as a target for halting neuroinvasion.

Pre-exposure prophylaxis and immunization strategies. For many conventional viral agents, vaccination is the most effective method of infection control. In vitro pre-incubation with anti-PrP antisera was reported to reduce the prion titer of infectious hamster brain homogenates by up to 2 log units (21) and an anti-PrP antibody was found to inhibit formation of PrP^{Sc} in a cell-free system (29). Further, antibodies (33) and F(ab) fragments raised against certain domains of PrP (40) can suppress prion replication in cultured cells; however, it is difficult to induce humoral in vivo immune responses against PrP^{C}. This is most likely due to tolerance of the mammalian immune system to PrP^{C}, which is an endogenous protein expressed rather ubiquitously. Ablation of the *Prnp* gene (12), which encodes PrP^{C}, renders mice highly susceptible to immunization with prions (10), and many of the best available monoclonal antibodies to the prion protein have been generated in $Prnp^{0/0}$ mice (43). $Prnp^{0/0}$ mice are not suitable for testing vaccination regimens since they do not support prion pathogenesis (11). Instead, transgenic introduction of an anti-PrP heavy chain into the germ line of mice produced high anti-PrP^{C} titers. This sufficed to confer protection from scrapie upon intraperitoneal prion inoculation (25).

A Perspective for the Near Future

Many promising approaches are being developed towards post-exposure and pre-exposure prophylaxis. They involve small therapeutic molecules and cytokine antagonists (post-exposure) as well as specific anti-PrP^{C} immunity (pre-exposure), but prophylaxis only makes sense if one can define the population at risk. This is why progress in this field must go hand-in-hand with progress in prion diagnostics. The latter is proceeding at a speedy pace. Therapy, however, is unlikely to be profitable for any time to come, since the number of CJD patients is exceedingly small and will hopefully not increase too much.

References

1. Aguzzi A (1997) Neuro-immune connection in spread of prions in the body? *Lancet* 349: 742-743.

2. Aguzzi A (2000) Prion diseases, blood and the immune system: concerns and reality. *Haematologica* 85: 3-10.

3. Aguzzi A, Montrasio F, Kaeser PS (2001) Prions: health scare and biological challenge. *Nat Rev Mol Cell Biol* 2: 118-126.

4. Aguzzi A, Weissmann C (1997) Prion research: the next frontiers. *Nature* 389: 795-798.

5. Aguzzi A, Weissmann C (1998) Spongiform encephalopathies. The prion's perplexing persistence. *Nature* 392: 763-764.

6. Baldauf E, Beekes M, Diringer H (1997) Evidence for an alternative direct route of access for the scrapie agent to the brain bypassing the spinal cord. *J Gen Virol* 78 (Pt 5): 1187-1197.

7. Bessen RA, Kocisko DA, Raymond GJ, Nandan S, Lansbury PT, Caughey B (1995) Non-genetic propagation of strain-specific properties of scrapie prion protein. *Nature* 375: 375-700.

8. Blattler T, Brandner S, Raeber AJ, Klein MA, Voigtlander T, Weissmann C, Aguzzi A (1997) PrP-expressing tissue required for transfer of scrapie infectivity from spleen to brain. *Nature* 389: 69-73.

9. Brandner S, Isenmann S, Kuhne G, Aguzzi A (1998) Identification of the end stage of scrapie using infected neural grafts. *Brain Pathol* 8: 19-27.

10. Brandner S, Isenmann S, Raeber A, Fischer M, Sailer A, Kobayashi Y, Marino S, Weissmann C, Aguzzi A (1996) Normal host prion protein necessary for scrapie-induced neurotoxicity. *Nature* 379: 339-343.

11. Bueler H, Aguzzi A, Sailer A, Greiner RA, Autenried P, Aguet M, Weissmann C (1993) Mice devoid of PrP are resistant to scrapie. *Cell* 73: 1339-1347.

12. Bueler H, Fischer M, Lang Y, Bluethmann H, Lipp HP, DeArmond SJ, Prusiner SB, Aguet M, Weissmann C (1992) Normal development and behaviour of mice lacking the neuronal cell-surface PrP protein. *Nature* 356: 577-582.

13. Cashman NR, Loertscher R, Nalbantoglu J, Shaw I, Kascsak RJ, Bolton DC, Bendheim PE (1990) Cellular isoform of the scrapie agent protein participates in lymphocyte activation. *Cell* 61: 185-192.

14. Caughey B, Race RE (1992) Potent inhibition of scrapie-associated PrP accumulation by congo red. *J Neurochem* 59: 768-771.

15. Caughey B, Raymond GJ (1993) Sulfated polyanion inhibition of scrapie-associated PrP accumulation in cultured cells. *J Virol* 67: 643-650.

16. Collins S, Law MG, Fletcher A, Boyd A, Kaldor J, Masters CL (1999) Surgical treatment and risk of sporadic Creutzfeldt-Jakob disease: a case-control study. *Lancet* 353: 693-697.

17. Doh-Ura K, Iwaki T, Caughey B (2000) Lysosomotropic agents and cysteine protease inhibitors inhibit scrapie-associated prion protein accumulation. *J Virol* 74: 4894-4897.

18. Farquhar C, Dickinson A, Bruce M (1999) Prophylactic potential of pentosan polysulphate in transmissible spongiform encephalopathies. *Lancet* 353: 117.

19. Fischer M, Rulicke T, Raeber A, Sailer A, Moser M, Oesch B, Brandner S, Aguzzi A, Weissmann C (1996) Prion protein (PrP) with amino-proximal deletions restoring susceptibility of PrP knockout mice to scrapie. *Embo J* 15: 1255-1264.

20. Frigg R, Klein MA, Hegyi I, Zinkernagel RM, Aguzzi A (1999) Scrapie pathogenesis in subclinically infected B-cell-deficient mice. *J Virol* 73: 9584-9588.

21. Gabizon R, McKinley MP, Groth D, Prusiner SB (1988) Immunoaffinity purification and neutralization of scrapie prion infectivity. *Proc Natl Acad Sci U S A* 85: 6617-6621.

22. Gidon-Jeangirard C, Hugel B, Holl V, Toti F, Laplanche JL, Meyer D, Freyssinet JM (1999) Annexin V delays apoptosis while exerting an external constraint preventing the release of CD4+ and PrPc+ membrane particles in a human T lymphocyte model. *J Immunol* 162: 5712-5718.

23. Glatzel M, Aguzzi A (2000) PrP(C) expression in the peripheral nervous system is a determinant of prion neuroinvasion. *J Gen Virol* 81 Pt 11: 2813-2821.

24. Glatzel M, Heppner FL, Albers KM, Aguzzi A (2001) Sympathetic innervation of lymphoreticular organs is rate limiting for prion neuroinvasion. *Neuron* 31: 25-34.

25. Heppner FL, Musahl C, Arrighi I, Klein MA, Rulicke T, Oesch B, Zinkernagel RM, Kalinke U, Aguzzi A (2001) Prevention of scrapie pathogenesis by transgenic expression of anti-prion protein antibodies. *Science* 294: 178-182.

26. Hill AF, Butterworth RJ, Joiner S, Jackson G, Rossor MN, Thomas DJ, Frosh A, Tolley N, Bell JE, Spencer M, King A, Al-Sarraj S, Ironside JW, Lantos PL, Collinge J (1999) Investigation of variant Creutzfeldt-Jakob disease and other human prion diseases with tonsil biopsy samples. *Lancet* 353: 183-189.

27. Hill AF, Zeidler M, Ironside J, Collinge J (1997) Diagnosis of new variant Creutzfeldt-jakob disease by tonsil biopsy. *Lancet* 349: 99-100.

28. Hilton DA, Fathers E, Edwards P, Ironside JW, Zajicek J (1998) Prion immunoreactivity in appendix before clinical onset of variant Creutzfeldt-Jakob disease. *Lancet* 352: 703-704.

29. Horiuchi M, Caughey B (1999) Specific binding of normal prion protein to the scrapie form via a localized domain initiates its conversion to the protease-resistant state. *Embo J* 18: 3193-203.

30. Kitamoto T, Muramoto T, Mohri S, Doh-Ura K, Tateishi J (1991) Abnormal isoform of prion protein accumulates in follicular dendritic cells in mice with Creutzfeldt-Jakob disease. *J Virol* 65: 6292-6295.

31. Klein MA, Frigg R, Flechsig E, Raeber AJ, Kalinke U, Bluethmann H, Bootz F, Suter M, Zinkernagel RM, Aguzzi A (1997) A crucial role for B cells in neuroinvasive scrapie. *Nature* 390: 687-690.

32. Klein MA, Frigg R, Raeber AJ, Flechsig E, Hegyi I, Zinkernagel RM, Weissmann C, Aguzzi A (1998) PrP expression in B lymphocytes is not required for prion neuroinvasion. *Nat Med* 4: 1429-1433.

33. Klein MA, Kaeser PS, Schwarz P, Weyd H, Xenarios I, Zinkernagel RM, Carroll MC, Verbeek JS, Botto M, Walport MJ, Molina H, Kalinke U, Acha-Orbea H, Aguzzi A (2001) Complement facilitates early prion pathogenesis. *Nat Med* 7: 488-492.

34. Kocisko DA, Come JH, Priola SA, Chesebro B, Raymond GJ, Lansbury PT, Caughey B (1994) Cell-free formation of protease-resistant prion protein. *Nature* 370: 471-474.

35. Korth C, May BC, Cohen FE, Prusiner SB (2001) Acridine and phenothiazine derivatives as pharmacotherapeutics for prion disease. *Proc Natl Acad Sci U S A* 98: 9836-9841.

36. Mabbott NA, Bruce ME, Botto M, Walport MJ, Pepys MB (2001) Temporary depletion of complement component C3 or genetic deficiency of C1q significantly delays onset of scrapie. *Nat Med* 7: 485-487.

37. Mabbott NA, Mackay F, Minns F, Bruce ME (2000) Temporary inactivation of follicular dendritic cells delays neuroinvasion of scrapie. *Nat Med* 6: 719-720.

38. Manuelidis L, Zaitsev I, Koni P, Lu ZY, Flavell RA, Fritch W (2000) Follicular dendritic cells and dissemination of Creutzfeldt-Jakob disease. *J Virol* 74: 8614-8622.

39. Montrasio F, Frigg R, Glatzel M, Klein MA, Mackay F, Aguzzi A, Weissmann C (2000) Impaired prion replication in spleens of mice lacking functional follicular dendritic cells. *Science* 288: 1257-1259.

40. Peretz D, Williamson RA, Kaneko K, Vergara J, Leclerc E, Schmitt-Ulms G, Mehlhorn IR, Legname G, Wormald MR, Rudd PM, Dwek RA, Burton DR, Prusiner SB (2001) Antibodies inhibit prion propagation and clear cell cultures of prion infectivity. *Nature* 412: 739-743.

41. Pocchiari M, Schmittinger S, Masullo C (1987) Amphotericin B delays the incubation period of scrapie in intracerebrally inoculated hamsters. *J Gen Virol* 68 (Pt 1): 219-223.

42. Priola SA, Raines A, Caughey WS (2000) Porphyrin and phthalocyanine antiscrapie compounds. *Science* 287: 1503-1506.

43. Prusiner SB, Groth D, Serban A, Koehler R, Foster D, Torchia M, Burton D, Yang SL, DeArmond SJ (1993) Ablation of the prion protein (PrP) gene in mice prevents scrapie and facilitates production of anti-PrP antibodies. *Proc Natl Acad Sci U S A* 90: 10608-10612.

44. Race R, Chesebro B (1998) Scrapie infectivity found in resistant species. *Nature* 392: 770.

45. Race R, Oldstone M, Chesebro B (2000) Entry versus blockade of brain infection following oral or intraperitoneal scrapie administration: role of prion protein expression in peripheral nerves and spleen. *J Virol* 74: 828-833.

46. Raeber AJ, Klein MA, Frigg R, Flechsig E, Aguzzi A, Weissmann C (1999) PrP-dependent association of prions with splenic but not circulating lymphocytes of scrapie-infected mice. *Embo J* 18: 2702-2706.

47. Raymond GJ, Hope J, Kocisko DA, Priola SA, Raymond LD, Bossers A, Ironside J, Will RG, Chen SG, Petersen RB, Gambetti P, Rubenstein R, Smits MA, Lansbury PT, Jr., Caughey B (1997) Molecular assessment of the potential transmissibilities of BSE and scrapie to humans. *Nature* 388: 285-288.

48. Roikhel VM, Fokina GI, Pogodina VV (1984) Influence of aminasine on experimental scrapie in mice. *Acta Virol* 28: 321-324.

49. Schreuder BE, van Keulen LJ, Smits MA, Langeveld JP, Stegeman JA (1997) Control of scrapie eventually possible? *Vet Q* 19: 105-113.

50. Schreuder BE, van Keulen LJ, Vromans ME, Langeveld JP, Smits MA (1998) Tonsillar biopsy and PrPSc detection in the preclinical diagnosis of scrapie. *Vet Rec* 142: 564-568.

51. Serio TR, Cashikar AG, Kowal AS, Sawicki GJ, Moslehi JJ, Serpell L, Arnsdorf MF, Lindquist SL (2000) Nucleated conformational conversion and the replication of conformational information by a prion determinant. *Science* 289: 1317-1321.

52. Soto C, Kascsak RJ, Saborio GP, Aucouturier P, Wisniewski T, Prelli F, Kascsak R, Mendez E, Harris DA, Ironside J, Tagliavini F, Carp RI, Frangione B (2000) Reversion of prion protein conformational changes by synthetic beta-sheet breaker peptides. *Lancet* 355: 192-197.

53. Supattapone S, Wille H, Uyechi L, Safar J, Tremblay P, Szoka FC, Cohen FE, Prusiner SB, Scott MR (2001) Branched polyamines cure prion-infected neuroblastoma cells. *J Virol* 75: 3453-3461.

54. Tagliavini F, McArthur RA, Canciani B, Giaccone G, Porro M, Bugiani M, Lievens PM, Bugiani O, Peri E, Dall'Ara P et al (1997) Effectiveness of anthracycline against experimental prion disease in Syrian hamsters. *Science* 276: 1119-1122.

55. Telling GC, Scott M, Mastrianni J, Gabizon R, Torchia M, Cohen FE, DeArmond SJ, Prusiner SB (1995) Prion propagation in mice expressing human and chimeric PrP transgenes implicates the interaction of cellular PrP with another protein. *Cell* 83: 79-90.

56. van Keulen LJ, Schreuder BE, Meloen RH, Mooij-Harkes G, Vromans ME, Langeveld JP (1996) Immunohistochemical detection of prion protein in lymphoid tissues of sheep with natural scrapie. *J Clin Microbiol* 34: 1228-1231.

Sporadic Creutzfeldt-Jakob Disease

Herbert Budka
Mark W. Head
James W. Ironside
Pierluigi Gambetti
Piero Parchi
Martin Zeidler
Fabrizio Tagliavini

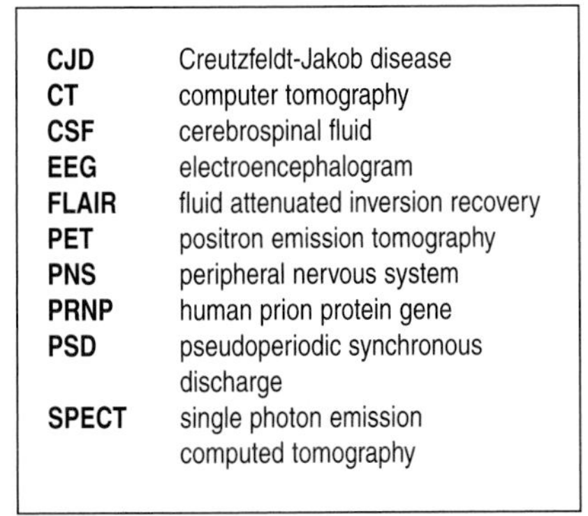

CJD	Creutzfeldt-Jakob disease
CT	computer tomography
CSF	cerebrospinal fluid
EEG	electroencephalogram
FLAIR	fluid attenuated inversion recovery
PET	positron emission tomography
PNS	peripheral nervous system
PRNP	human prion protein gene
PSD	pseudoperiodic synchronous discharge
SPECT	single photon emission computed tomography

Definition

Most cases (85%) of Creutzfeldt-Jakob disease (CJD) are sporadic, arising for no obvious reason. The typical clinical picture of sporadic CJD is a rapidly progressive dementia with ataxia and myoclonus, associated with pseudoperiodic synchronous discharges (PSD) on the electroencephalogram (EEG) and a positive CSF 14-3-3 test. The disease is neuropathologically characterised by spongi-form degeneration, neuronal loss, gliosis, and the presence of altered forms of the prion protein, termed PrP^{res}, which are protease resistant. In recent years, advances in diagnostic procedures have allowed for the identification of previously unrecognised, atypical cases, which account for approximately 10% of the sporadic CJD population.

Synonyms and Historical Annotations

In 1920, Hans Gerhard Creutzfeldt reported the case of a 22-year-old woman who died following a history of progressive cerebral dysfunction (13). A year later, another German neuroscientist, Alfons Maria Jakob, described 5 further cases (29), and in 1922 the term Creutzfeldt-Jakob disease was coined. Nomenclature was problematic over the ensuing decades, with more than 50 synonyms used to describe the disease now known as CJD. To confuse matters further, CJD was sometimes employed as a convenient diagnosis for any unexplained rapidly progressive dementia, and many cases (including Creutzfeldt's original patient) would not have met modern criteria for CJD. Eponymous terms are still occasionally used today: Heidenhain syndrome for patients in which visual symptoms predominate in the early stages, and Brownell-Oppenheimer variant for cases with a mainly cerebellar presentation.

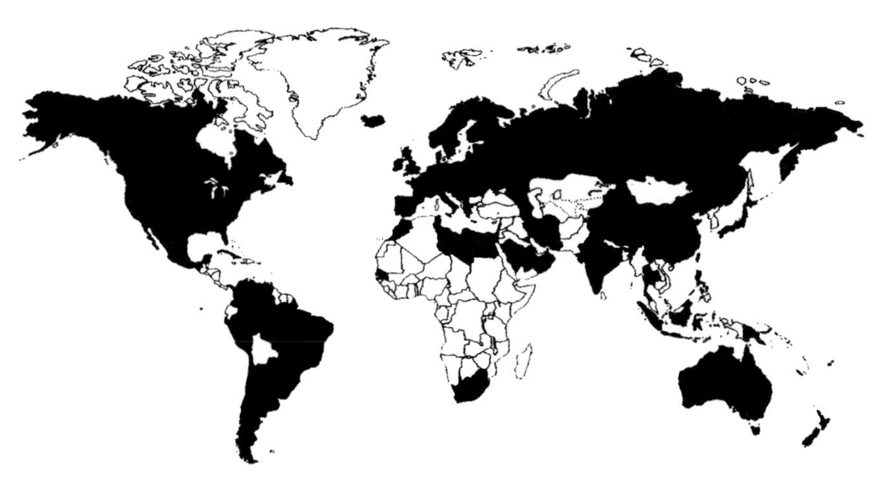

Figure 1. Countries reporting CJD (black).

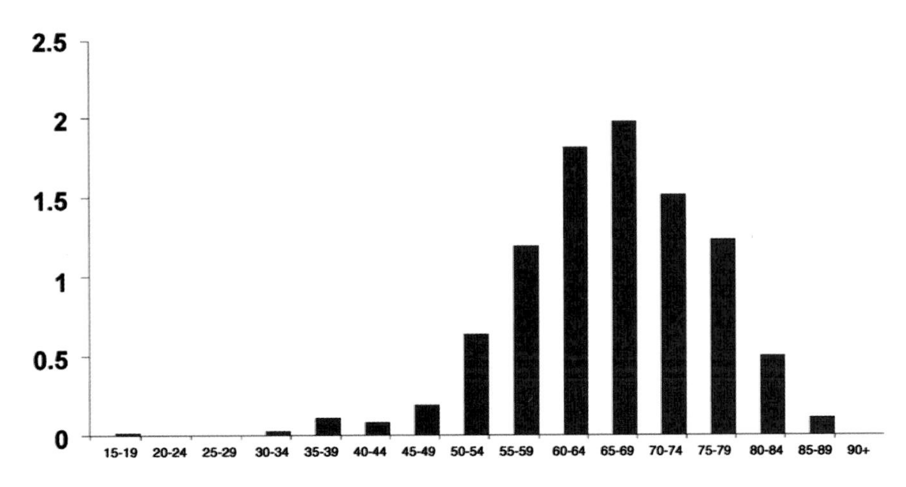

Figure 2. Age-specific incidence (cases per million per year) of sporadic CJD.

Epidemiology

Incidence and prevalence. The incidence is approximately 1 case per million population per year. The disease occurs worldwide at a roughly similar rate in countries where surveillance has occurred (Figure 1).

Sex and age distribution. The sex incidence is equal and mean age of onset is about 65 years (range 14-92) as shown in Figure 2.

Risk factors. One previously popular hypothesis for the cause of sporadic CJD was that the disease resulted from acquisition of the scrapie agent, for example through eating sheep eyeballs or brain. Perhaps the strongest argument against this theory is that there is a relatively consistent incidence of

A. Definite
Diagnosed by standard neuropathological techniques; and/or
Immunocytochemically and/or Western blot confirmed PrPres and/or
Presence of scrapie-associated fibrils.

B. Probable
Progressive dementia; and
At least two out of the following four clinical features:
- Myoclonus
- Visual or cerebellar disturbance
- Pyramidal/extrapyramidal dysfunction
- Akinetic mutism;

and
A typical EEG during an illness of any duration and/or
A positive 14-3-3 CSF assay and a clinical duration to death <2 years;
Routine investigations should not suggest an alternative diagnosis.

C. Possible
Progressive dementia; and
At least two out of the following four clinical features:
- Myoclonus
- Visual or cerebellar disturbance
- Pyramidal/extrapyramidal dysfunction
- Akinetic mutism;

and
No EEG or atypical EEG; and
Duration <2 years.

Table 1. Diagnostic criteria for CJD surveillance.

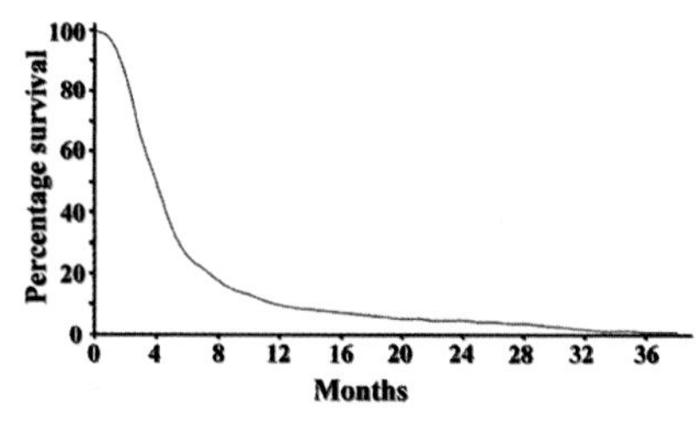

Figure 3. Survival curve of sporadic CJD.

CJD around the world, including in countries with a low or no incidence of scrapie. Uncontrolled studies and case reports have suggested a number of other potential risk factors, including contact with ferrets, eating squirrel brains, craniotomy, medical/paramedical profession and a family history of dementia. Clearly these findings have to be interpreted cautiously due to the small number of cases involved and the lack of a control group. Case-control studies conducted in Japan, the United States, Australia, the United Kingdom, and the European Union have each identified a number of apparent risks for the development of sporadic CJD, although no factor has been consistently implicated. A meta-

Clinical feature	Onset (%)	Course (%)
Cognitive impairment	69	100
Memory loss	48	100
Behavioural abnormalities	29	57
Cerebellar	33	71
Visual	19	42
Pyramidal	2	62
Extrapyramidal	0.5	56
Akinetic mutism	0	75
Seizures	0	19
Myoclonus	1	78

Table 2. Clinical features of CJD present at either onset or during the course of the illness.

analysis of 3 of these studies failed to identify any statistically significant dietary, occupational, or past medical risk factors (66).

Genetics

Codon 129 of the human prion protein gene (*PRNP*) contains a common polymorphism (ATG/GTG), which encodes for methionine or valine. In the normal white population, the allele frequencies are 62% methionine (M) and 38% valine (V), and the genotype frequencies are 37% MM, 51% MV and 12% VV (12). This polymorphism is not pathogenic in itself; however, homozygosity for methionine increases the susceptibility to sporadic CJD (45); furthermore, the genotype at codon 129 has a striking influence on the clinical and pathological phenotype.

Clinical Features

Signs and symptoms. Patients usually present (in order of decreasing frequency) with cognitive decline, ataxia or visual disturbance, either alone or in combination (6, 49). The diagnostic criteria for sporadic CJD produced by WHO for clinical surveillance purposes (68) are listed in Table 1. Dementia is invariably present during the course of the illness and myoclonus, although a rare presenting feature, is observed at some stage in most cases. The frequency of various clinical features are listed in Table 2. As the disease progresses multi-focal CNS failure occurs with increasing global cognitive dysfunction, ataxia, dependency and urinary incontinence, culminating in the patient becoming bed bound, mute and unresponsive. Terminally, the patients are usually rigid, frequently cortically blind, dysphagic (predisposing to aspiration and pneumonia, the commonest cause of death) and may develop Cheyne-Stokes respiration. Physical signs correspond with the global CNS involvement and may include a combination of cerebellar, pyramidal, and extrapyramidal signs. Primitive reflexes and paratonic (*gegenhalten*) rigidity are also common, whereas lower motor neuron signs are rarely observed. The median and mean duration of illness are approximately 4.5 and 8 months respectively (Figure 3). About 10% of patients survive more than a year and 5% longer than 2 years. Exceptionally, cases with illness duration greater than 5 years have been described. The shortest illness course is around 2 weeks.

Approximately 50% of cases suspected to have CJD have a final alternative diagnosis. A wide spectrum of diseases may produce, although uncommonly, a subacute encephalopathy with cognitive deterioration, ataxia and myoclonus (52). The most common condition that clinically imitates CJD (in series of pathologically verified cases) is Alzheimer's disease, followed by vascular dementia and Lewy body disease. Disorders that mimic CJD most closely are some metabolic conditions, such as Hashimoto's encephalopathy. A minority of CJD suspects recover without a diagnosis being established.

Imaging. The main role of neuroimaging in patients with suspected CJD has traditionally been to exclude other conditions. Computerised tomography (CT) is reported to be normal in 57 to 80% of cases. The most frequent CT abnormality in CJD is cerebral atrophy, which occurs particularly in those with a protracted illness. The potential for cerebral MRI to be a useful tool in the diagnosis of CJD is becoming increasingly recognised. A number of case reports since 1985 have described bilateral striatal high signal on T2 or proton density weighted imaging (Figure 4). A recent study of 162 sporadic CJD cases and 58 controls found that this appearance had a sensitivity of 67% and specificity of 93% (60). Other less common MRI features of sporadic CJD include cortical, thalamic, or globus pallidus hyperintensity. T1-weighted imaging does not usually show any signal change and there is typically no gadolinium enhancement. Fluid attenuated inversion recovery (FLAIR) and diffusion-weighted imaging are reported to be more sensitive at detecting grey matter abnormalities compared to conventional MRI sequences. The usefulness of positron emission tomography (PET) and single photon emission computed tomography (SPECT) in establishing a diagnosis of CJD is debatable. Claims that there is a characteristic appearance in CJD that may be diagnostically useful should be interpreted with caution as no study has attempted to evaluate SPECT or PET as a diagnostic tool for CJD using a suitable control group.

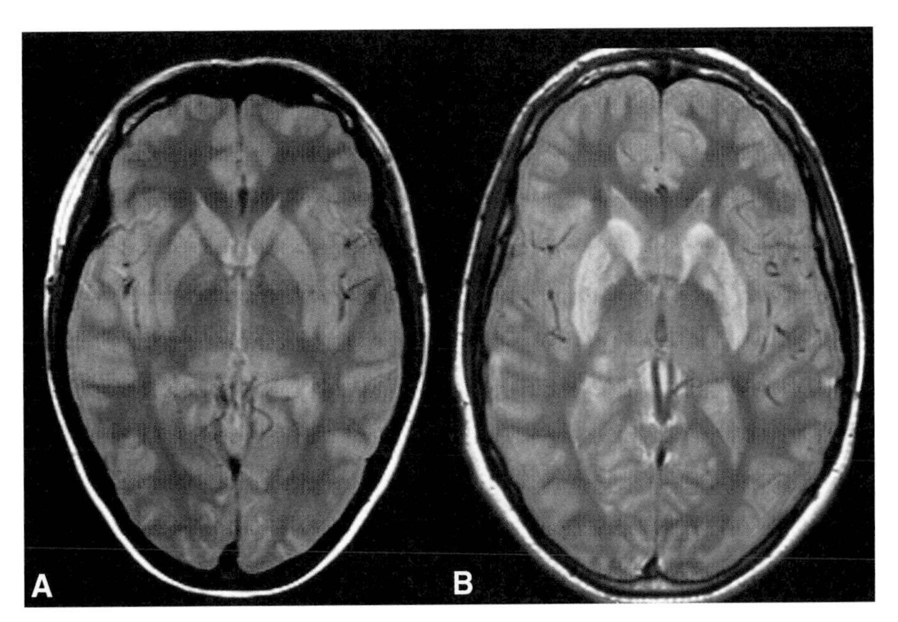

Figure 4. Axial proton density-weighted MRI. A. Normal appearance and B. sporadic CJD showing homogeneous hyperintensity in the putamen and caudate head.

Laboratory findings. Routine haematological and biochemical investigations, including inflammatory markers, are usually normal in sporadic CJD, although elevation of serum liver enzymes or bilirubin or both has been reported in 40 to 52% of cases. The cause of this observation is uncertain, but perhaps most likely this is an epiphenomenon, resulting from debility, drug effects or secondary infection.

Routine CSF analysis in CJD is also usually normal. About one-third of cases have a protein ≥0.5 g/L, and rarely values between 1.5 to 2.0 g/L have been documented. Oligoclonal IgG bands confined to the CSF are not usually found in CJD, although this has been documented in a small number of case reports. A number of studies (including a study of 300 cases) have reported that CSF pleocytosis was never seen. One report described a patient with a white cell count as high as 16×10^6, but this was after a seizure and the count was normal a few days later. Jacobi noted a mild pleocytosis (5-11 cells) in 6 (5.4%) of 110 definite CJD cases (28). The clinical features of these 6 patients were not stated and no mention was made of the results of any previous or later spinal taps.

14-3-3 is a neuronal phosphoserine-binding protein named for its mobility on 2-dimensional gel electrophoresis, and found in a high concentration in the CNS. This protein is released into the CSF as a consequence of extensive destruction of brain tissue. In a study of 222 definite CJD cases and 307 controls the sensitivity and specificity of the detection of the 14-3-3 for the diagnosis of CJD were both 93% (71). As a result of the high accuracy of the test it has been incorporated into criteria for a probable case of CJD (68). A recent study has suggested that an elevated CSF tau may have a comparable accuracy to 14-3-3 (44).

EEG abnormalities characterised by generalised, pseudoperiodic synchronous discharges of sharp waves, or di-/triphasic slow waves recurring at 0.5 to 1.5 Hz (Figure 5) have traditionally been considered the most important paraclinical finding and some studies reported that >90% of patients develop these changes. A recent large prospective case-control analysis found that only 144 (66%) of 219 pathologically confirmed CJD cases had a typical EEG, as did 11 (26%) of 43 non-CJD cases initially classified as possible or probable CJD (71). Another study compared the sensitivity and specificity of the EEG, MRI and CSF 14-3-3 and found that the latter was the best discriminator between CJD and other rapidly progressive dementias (52).

Macroscopy

Gross inspection of the brain may not reveal obvious abnormalities. More commonly, however, there is some degree of cerebral atrophy, which can be diffuse or have focal accentuations. Based on preferential involvement of specific regions, occipital (23), striatal, thalamic and cerebellar (7) variants have been described (56). The hippocampal formation is usually well preserved even in cases of severe brain atrophy, at variance with other degenerative dementias including Alzheimer's disease.

Histopathology

The *triad* of spongiform change, neuronal loss, and gliosis involving both astrocytes and microglia is the neuropathological hallmark of CJD. Extensive sampling from various brain areas (including frontal, temporal, and occipital lobes, basal ganglia, and cerebellum) is mandatory in every suspected case; however, one block of tissue with typical histological changes

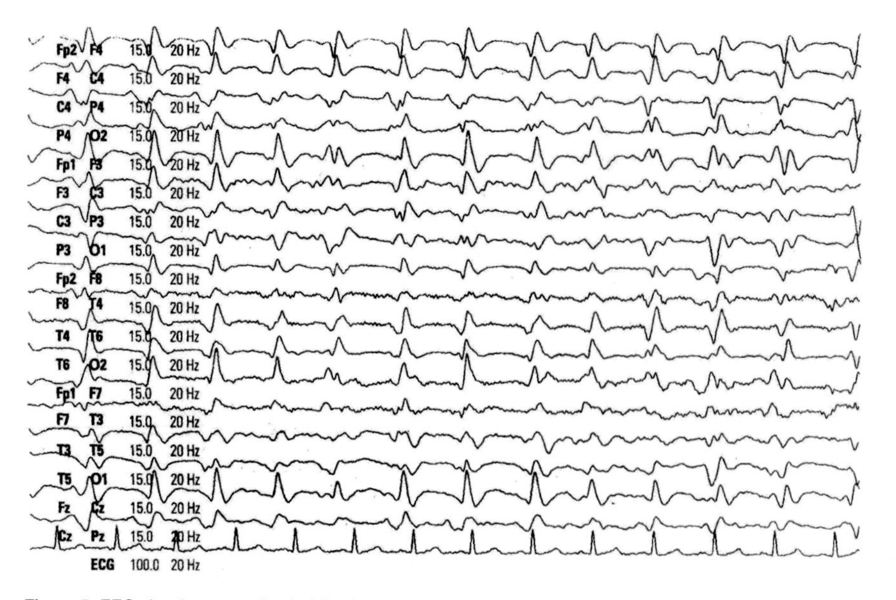

Figure 5. EEG showing generalized triphasic pseudoperiodic complexes in a case of sporadic CJD.

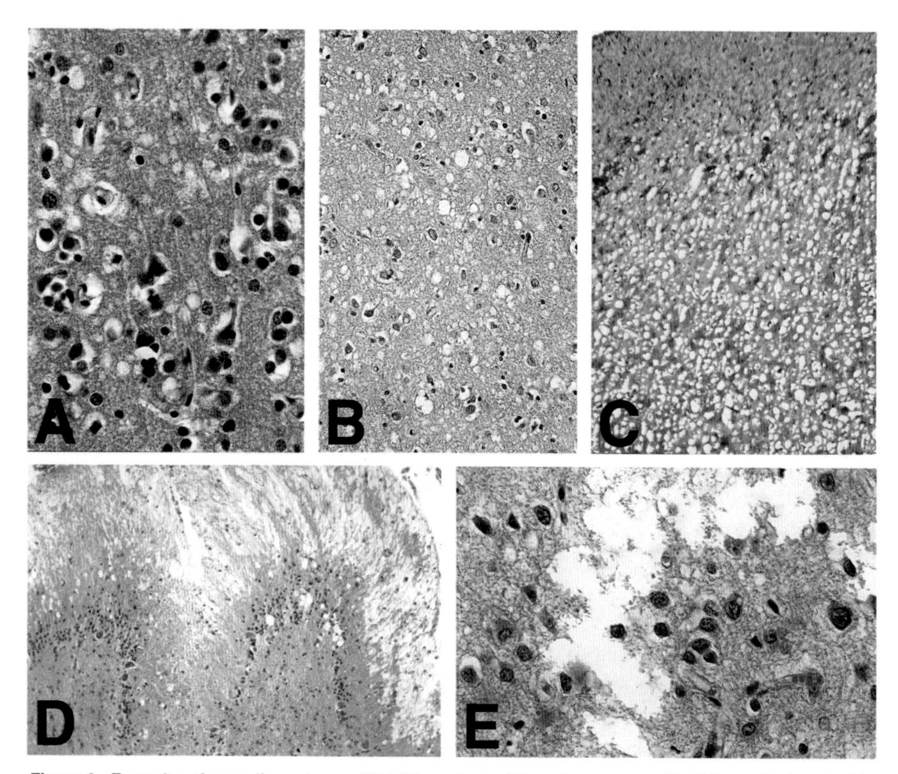

Figure 6. Examples of spongiform change. Mild (**A**), moderate (**B**), and very severe (**C, D**) in cerebral cortex (**A-C**) and cerebellum (**D**), to be differentiated from nonspecific "status spongiosus" (**E**).

and/or unambiguous PrP immunoreactivity is sufficient for a definite diagnosis. Brain biopsy has been found to be diagnostic in 95% of CJD cases in which the disease has been confirmed at autopsy or by experimental transmission (6). This procedure, however, should be restricted to rare instances where a treatable alternative diagnosis is suggested by clinical or laboratory findings.

While neuronal loss and gliosis are common to many other CNS disorders, *spongiform change* is relatively specific to CJD, but may differ in severity (Figure 6) between cases and from region to region in the brain. This alteration is characterised by diffuse or focally clustered, small, round or oval vacuoles in the neuropil of the cerebral cortex (whole thickness or deep layers), the subcortical grey matter and the cerebellar molecular layer. An almost constant location is the head of the caudate nucleus (55). By contrast, spongiform changes are rarely present in the brainstem and spinal cord, although PrP accumulation can be demonstrated at these sites. Extent, morphology and distribution of spongiform changes vary greatly between patients and disease subtypes as specified below. However, CJD brains with equivocal, little or no spongiosis are very rare. In these cases, PrP immunohistochemistry and Western blot analysis have a decisive diagnostic role (19). In contrast with transmissible spongiform encephalopathies of animals, the presence of vacuoles in nerve cell bodies is uncommon. Ballooning of neurons observed in some instances is related to accumulation of neurofilament proteins. Spongiform changes and astocytosis may also involve the white matter (10, 41, 51). Extensive white matter degeneration distinguishes the "pan-encephalopathic" form of CJD, which is particularly frequent in Japan (43).

Neuronal loss in the affected cortical and subcortical regions appears to follow an apoptotic pathway which seems to correlate with microglial activation and axonal damage rather than local deposition of PrP^{res} (16). Specific vulnerability of a peculiar, parvalbumin-expressing subset of inhibitory GABAergic neurons has been observed (3, 18). The granular layer of the cerebellum is frequently depleted. The involvement of the basal nucleus of Meynert, either primarily or secondarily to cortical neuronal loss, is variable (2, 11). The existence of an "amyotrophic" form of CJD combining motor neuron loss with dementia has been doubted and remains to be proven, since experimental transmission of such cases has been unsuccessful (58). On the other hand, amyotrophy may occasionally be a prominent feature of proven CJD (69). It is noteworthy that a significant portion of histopathologically typical CJD patients—including 43% of familial cases—did not transmit disease to laboratory animals, and that absence of spongiform change was an almost 100% predictive indicator of non-transmissibility (6).

A minority of CJD brains have classical compact "kuru type" plaques with fringed outline. They also stain with periodic acid-Schiff, alcian blue, Congo red (staining disappears after formic acid treatment) and thioflavine S. Kuru plaques of CJD are most frequent in the cerebellar cortex where they are usually confined to the granular layer. CJD brains may also show age-related Alzheimer-type amyloid deposits immunoreactive for the β-peptide, with or without PrP co-localisation (21). Neuroaxonal dystrophy may be widespread in some CJD brains (36). Furthermore, "antler"-type dendritic hypertrophy and axonal torpedoes may occur in the cerebellar cortex.

Immunohistochemistry and Ultrastructure

Use and significance. In recent years, immunohistochemistry for disease-associated PrP has emerged as an indispensable adjunct to classical methods, particularly in cases with equivocal histopathology (9, 34). Since cross-linking fixatives such as formaldehyde affect PrP antigenicity, effective pre-treatment and staining protocols have been developed for formalin-fixed, paraffin-embedded tissue. Another possibility to visualize PrP and map its distribution is the "histoblot" (cryostat sections blotted onto nitrocellulose membranes, treated with proteinase K and immuno-stained). This procedure provides impressive preparations of rodent brain (64) but is difficult to apply to the much larger human brain sections. More recently developed techniques such as the paraffin-embedded tissue (PET) blot (61) or the use of Carnoy's fixative (ie, ethanol:chloroform:acetic acid, 6:3:1) instead of formalin (14) offer powerful alternatives for detection of disease-associated PrP.

PrP immunohistochemistry has been also used as surrogate marker for infectivity in peripheral tissues, such as lymphoid organs (25) and peripheral nervous system (20), that are important for considerations of infectivity risks. Moreover, PrP is a central marker for development, spread and distribution of pathology, although the extent of PrP deposits does not always correlate with type and severity of local tissue damage (19). Local deposition of PrP requires the presence of neuronal but not glial elements. PrP immunoreactivity is absent in preexisting brain lesions such as infarctions in which neuronal elements had been focally destroyed and replaced by a gliotic scar (8).

Technique and pitfalls. Since the anti-PrP antibodies that are currently available for immunohistochemistry—including the widely used 3F4 (30)—do not distinguish between normal and disease-specific PrP, it is crucial to abolish the immunoreactivity of PrP^C and enhance that of PrP^{res}. Various protocols have been developed for formalin-fixed, paraffin-embedded sections, including hydrolytic or hydrated autoclaving, microwaving, and formic acid and/or guanidine thiocyanate treatment. Among these protocols, a procedure combining hydrated autoclaving, formic acid and guanidine thiocyanate (4) and a minor modification thereof (65) has been found to be the most effective for all types of PrP deposits, including the "synaptic" type which is the most difficult to reveal. On the other hand, the histoblot, the PET blot and the immunohistochemistry on Carnoy-fixed, paraffin-embedded tissue provide the highest sensitivity and specificity, since the sections are subjected to proteinase K digestion with complete degradation of the normal PrP and the effect of formic acid and/or guanidine thiocyanate treatment on PrP^{res} is more pronounced (14, 61).

A recent study on the effectiveness of various anti-PrP antibodies and pretreatment protocols showed that none of the antibodies labelled given CJD subtypes exclusively, but the intensity of immunoreactivity varied among morphologically distinct types of deposit (33). In particular, fine granular or synaptic deposits stained weakly or not at all with antibodies against the N-terminus of PrP, while coarser and plaque-type deposits were labelled by all antibodies. It must be noted that the possibility of pitfalls requires extensive experience in technique and interpretation. Labelling of neuronal somata in all cases, irrespective of type of disease, and staining at the periphery (dystrophic neurites) and/or throughout the senile plaques of Alzheimer patients were observed with most antibodies, except 6H4 and 12F10 which recognize epitopes comprising residues 144 to 152 and 142 to 160, respectively; accordingly, 6H4 and 12F10 are less likely to recognise the normal PrP in immunohistochemistry (33). Thus interpretation of positive labelling has to be made by experienced observers and must consider the morphology of obtained signals.

Patterns and distribution of PrP deposition in the CNS. PrP^{res} accumulates in the CNS of CJD patients following different patterns—ie, synaptic, patchy/perivacuolar, perineuronal and plaque-like (Figure 7)—which may overlap in the individual brain (8, 9, 19). The occurrence and/or the prevalence of these patterns are related—at least in part—to PrP^{res} type, polymorphism at *PRNP* codon 129 and brain region, as specified below. The diffuse synaptic pattern (31) comprises usually abundant, tiny immunolabelled dots, occasionally accompanied by coarser and bigger deposits, throughout the neuropil. In some patients, PrP immunoreactivity in the cerebral cortex is limited to only few small dots and is hardly detectable; however, in these cases, the cerebellum is usually clearly involved. In the cerebellar cortex, the granular layer is most frequently affected with coarse granules, with additional but variable fine stippling of the molecular layer.

Many cases with very prominent spongiform change exhibit a striking patchy PrP immunoreactivity around

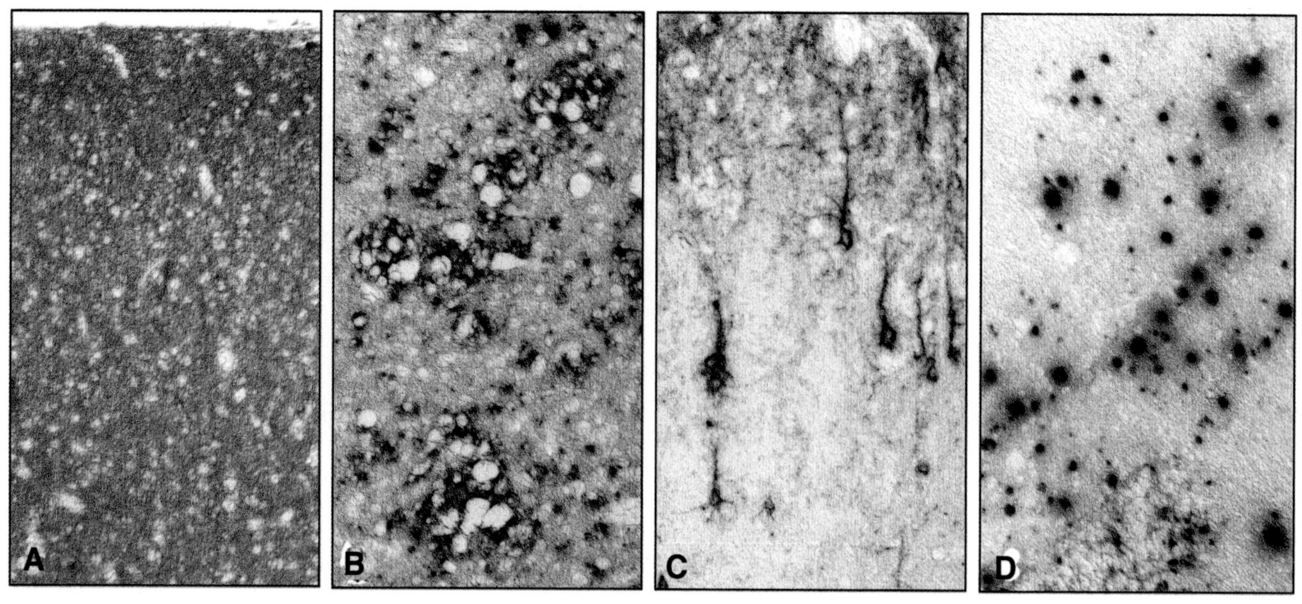

Figure 7. Patterns of PrP immunoreactivity: synaptic (**A**), perivacuolar (**B**), perineuronal (**C**) and plaque-like (**D**).

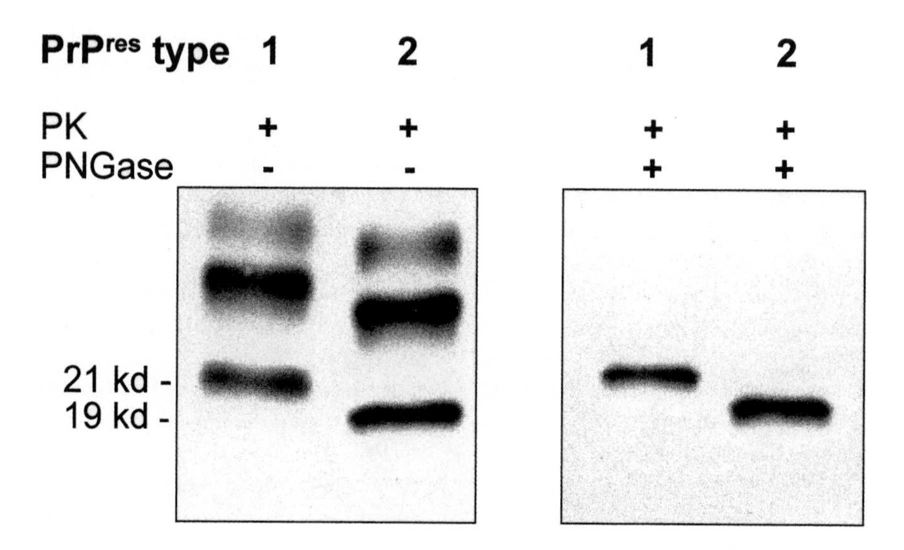

Figure 8. Western blot analysis of brain homogenates from patients with sporadic CJD showing type 1 and type 2 PrP^{res} (48) after proteinase K (PK) digestion (left panel) and PK digestion followed by deglycosylation (right panel)with glycopeptide N-glycosidase F (PNGase) Antibody 3F4 (1:50 000).

the vacuoles. The submicroscopic structures involved in this type of PrP deposition (which is non-fibrillar) remain to be elucidated. Interestingly, ubiquitin is deposited in a similar pattern, suggesting accumulation of both proteins within lysosomes (27). Plaque-like deposits are the only type of PrP deposit extending to the subcortical white matter (19) and are more frequent than true congophilic kuru plaques which are well visible already without immunohistochemistry. The PrP plaques are often surrounded by ubiquitin-positive profiles (27, 63). Some patients exhibit both "plaque" and "non plaque" (synaptic, perivacuolar) staining patterns. "Florid" or "daisy-like" plaques—a prominent feature of variant CJD (67)—are absent in sporadic CJD. It is noteworthy that, as for the spongiform change, PrP deposition may be focal, and in rare instances the detection of PrP immunoreactivity may require staining of several blocks.

PrP deposition in the PNS. Most recently, new patterns of granular ganglionic and tiny adaxonal PrP deposits were described in spinal and autonomic ganglia, spinal roots and peripheral nerves in rare CJD cases (20) and experimental scrapie (17). It remains to be established by sequential studies whether this PNS involvement reflects centripetal or centrifugal spread of PrP^{res} and follows the spreading pathways of the infectious agent.

Electron microscopy. Ultrastructurally, the spongiform changes correspond to enlarged cell processes (mainly neurites) containing curled membrane fragments and amorphous material (38). Further, peculiar tubulovesicular structures have been described as a specific ultrastructural marker of CJD (37).

Biochemistry

The molecular signature of CJD is the presence of altered forms of PrP, which are partially resistant to proteinase K digestion under conditions where the normal PrP is completely degraded. In CJD, the protease-resistant fragment of PrP^{res} shows 2 distinct patterns of electrophoretic mobility, named type 1 and 2 (Figure 8), which result from cleavage of PrP^{res} at different sites by proteinase K (47, 48). Type 1 has a relative molecular mass of 21 kDa and the primary cleavage site at residue 82, while type 2 has a relative molecular mass of 19 kDa and the primary cleavage site at residue 97 (48, 50). Further heterogeneity of PrP^{res} may be related to differences in the glycans carried by the abnormal protein isoforms (46). Description of additional PrP^{res} types resulted in another nomenclature (11a) than that (48) described above.

Subtypes of sporadic CJD: clinicopathological profile and molecular basis of heterogeneity. Six phenotypic subtypes—5 of sporadic CJD and one of the sporadic form of fatal familial insomnia—have been recently characterised based on a comprehensive clinical, pathological and molecular analysis of a large series of cases (Table 3) (49). The 6 subtypes largely correlate at the molecular level with the genotype at codon 129 (MM, MV, VV) and the physicochemical properties of PrP^{res} (type 1 or type 2 PrP^{res}). This molecular classification has been based on a considerable number of cases for the more common subtypes, but on relatively few cases for the rarer subtypes.

Codon 129 genotype PrP type	Previous terminology	Frequency (%)	Onset (yrs)/ Duration (mo)	Distinctive features
		sCJD		
M/M 1 M/V 1	Myoclonic or Heidenhain	72	63.2/3.9	Typical CJD, clinically and pathologically. Typical EEG (83%). "Synaptic" pattern of PrP immunostain.
V/V 1	Unavailable	1	39.0/15.3	Early onset. No typical EEG. Cerebellum spared. Weak "synaptic" PrP immunostain.
M/M 2 Cortical	Long duration	2	65.3/17.0	No typical EEG. Coarse spongiosis and PrP immunostain. Cerebellum spared.
M/V2	Cerebellar or ataxic CJD Kuru plaque variant	8	59.0/18.0	Ataxia at onset. Rarely typical EEG. Kuru plaques.
V/V 2	Cerebellar or ataxic CJD	15	60.3/6.6	As M/V 2, but no kuru plaques or cerebellar atrophy. Plaque-like PrP immunostain.
		SFI		
M/M 2 Thalamic	Thalamic CJD or Fatal Insomnia	2	60.3 / 14.0	Clinically and pathologically indistinguishable from FFI.

Table 3. Classification of sporadic CJD and FI (49).

The most common subtype, which accounts for over 70% of all sporadic CJD cases affects subjects who are either homozygous for methionine or heterozygous at codon 129 and have PrP^{res} type 1 (MM1 and MV1) (48, 49). The mean age at onset of symptoms is about 65 years and the average clinical duration is about 4 months. Signs at onset may vary and often involve multiple systems. They include cognitive decline in about two-thirds of the cases, gait or limb ataxia in approximately one-third, mental disturbances, visual signs of central origin, myoclonus or other involuntary movements, each occurring in about one-fourth of patients. Neurological signs are unilateral at onset in about 25% of cases. PSD are recorded at EEG in about 80% of cases, usually within the first 3 months of symptoms (49). The histopathology is characterised by a variable degree of spongiform change, gliosis, and neuronal loss affecting mainly the cerebral cortex, striatum, medial thalamus and cerebellum, whereas the hippocampus, hypothalamus and brain stem are relatively spared. In the cerebral cortex, the vacuolisation is seen in all layers and is often more prominent in the occipital lobe. Immunohistochemistry demonstrates a synaptic pattern of PrP staining, involving most grey structures of the cerebrum with relative sparing of the hippocampal formation (Figure 9).

The second most common phenotype comprises about 15% of the sporadic CJD population and includes subjects who are homozygous for valine at codon 129 and have PrP^{res} type 2 (VV2) (48, 49). The mean age at onset and clinical duration are 60 years and about 7 months, respectively. Clinically, the VV2 patients show prominent gait ataxia at onset, while dementia often occurs later in the course of the illness. Prominent myoclonus is absent in about one third of the cases, and most patients also lack PSD on EEG. Pathologically, the VV2 subjects show a moderate to severe spongiform change and gliosis with variable neuronal loss in the limbic structures, striatum, thalamus, hypothalamus, cerebellum, and brain stem nuclei. In contrast, the participation of the neocortex is a function of the disease duration, particularly in the occipital lobe, and it is often spared in cases with a relatively rapid course. Moreover, the spongiform change is often laminar and mainly involves the deep cortical layers. Immunostaining is characterised by the presence of plaque-like, focal PrP deposits which are not visible with routine staining procedures and do not contain PrP amyloid, since they are Congo red and thioflavine S negative. Another distinctive immunostaining features is the strong reaction around some neuronal perikaria, while the neuropil shows the punctuate pattern. Moreover, cases with a less than one-year duration are characterized by a laminar distribution of the immunostaining in the deep cortical layers corresponding to the spongiform degeneration (Figure 9). The distribution of the PrP^{res}, like the distribution of the spongiform degeneration, is affected by the duration of the disease (48). In cases of less than 5-month duration, PrP^{res} is present in relatively large and similar amounts

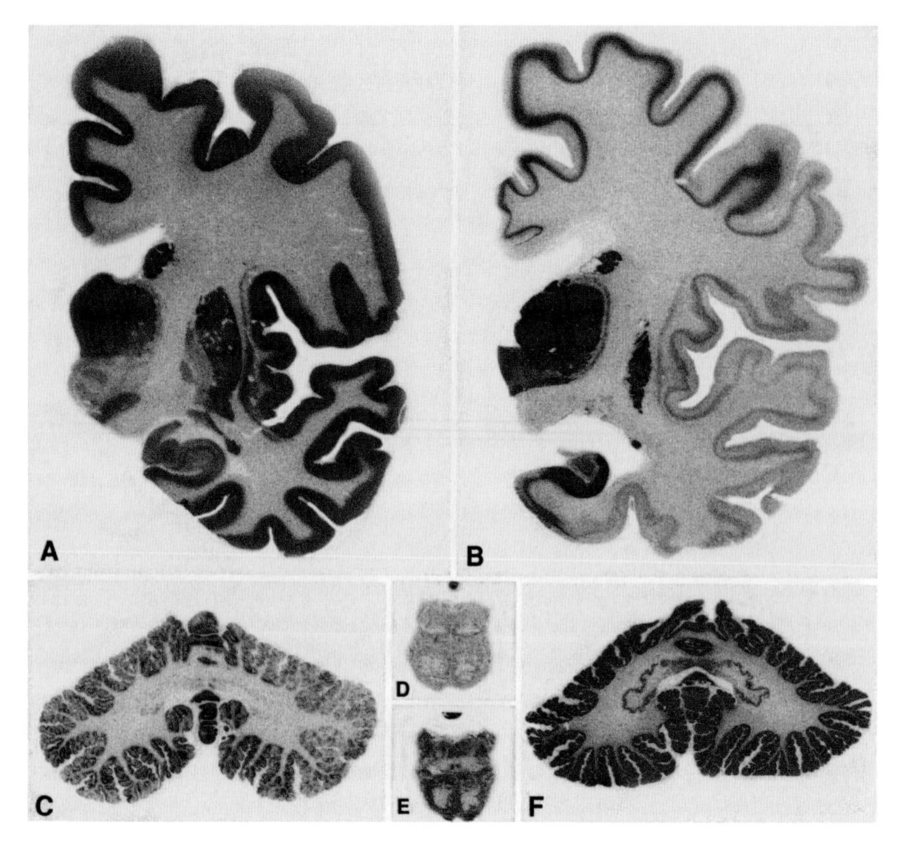

Figure 9. PrPres immunohistochemistry in MM1 (**A, C, D**) and VV2 (**B, E, F**) CJD brains. Note the striking difference in brain regional distribution of the abnormal protein. The immunostaining was carried out with the antibody 3F4 (1:5000) on Carnoy-fixed, paraplast-embedded sections.

throughout the brain except for the neocortex where it is barely detectable. This distribution is quite different from that of the MM1 and MV1 subjects in which the PrP^{res} is most abundant in the neocortex. In cases over 1 year duration PrP^{res} also markedly increases in the neocortex so that it becomes homogeneously distributed in all grey matter regions.

The third most common phenotype affects about 8% of cases, and comprises the kuru plaque variant, which is linked to MV at codon 129 and PrP^{res} type 2 (MV2) (48, 49). The mean age at onset and clinical duration are 59 years and 18 months, respectively. This subtype shows striking similarities with the VV2 phenotype, including the frequent absence of typical EEG changes, the widespread subcortical spongiform change, and the presence of numerous focal plaque-like PrP deposits. It is characterised by a longer mean duration, a higher frequency of cognitive impairment at onset, and a more significant involvement of the cerebral cortex. Furthermore, a unique feature of the MV2 subjects is the presence of amyloid plaques of the kuru type. These plaques are always seen in the cerebellum, typically in the upper region of the granular layer, but they can also be detected in other regions such as the cerebral cortex, striatum, and thalamus, in the cases with the longest duration.

Two distinct phenotypes affect subjects who are homozygous for methionine at codon 129 and show PrP^{res} type 2 (48, 49) The first (MM2-cortical) comprises about 2% of the sporadic CJD population. The mean age at onset in these subjects is 65 years, and the average disease duration 17 months. Clinically, these subjects present with cognitive impairment, while sustained myoclonus, visual signs, and the typical EEG changes are usually absent. Cerebellar signs are mild or absent, even late in the course of the disease. The lesion profile of the MM2-cortical subjects is similar to that of the MM1 or MV1 group, with the exception of the cerebellum, which lacks significant spongiform change despite the long duration of symptoms. Moreover, the spongiform change typically consists of large and coarse vacuoles. PrP immunohistochemistry shows a coarse pattern of staining, which is often called perivacuolar (9), because of its prevalent localization at the rim of the large vacuoles. Occasionally, a spotted pattern with PrP positive rounded structures is seen. The second phenotype that is linked to PrP^{res} type 2 and methionine homozygosity also affects about 2% of the sporadic human prion disease population (49). This variant (MM2-thalamic) is virtually indistinguishable from fatal familial insomnia (FFI), and there is now convincing evidence that both the sporadic MM2-thalamic variant and FFI are caused by the same prion strain. Thus, this phenotype, for which the term sporadic fatal insomnia or sFI has been proposed, is described in detail in the chapter on fatal insomnia.

The finding that the MM2-cortical subtype of sporadic CJD and sFI are phenotypically quite distinct but share the same genotype at codon 129 and the same PrP^{res} type raises questions concerning the molecular basis of phenotypic diversity. However, recent studies (46) have shown that the PrP^{res} present in these 2 conditions differ in the glycans they carry, providing a possible mechanism for the different phenotypes.

Finally, a rare phenotype that affects about 1% of the sporadic CJD population is linked to PrP^{res} type 1 and homozygosity for valine at codon 129 (49). The VV1 subjects show a mean age at onset of 39 years, which is by far the youngest among the sporadic CJD variants, and a mean duration of 15 months. Although the VV1 subjects identified to date are limited in number, they appear to show a quite homogeneous and consistent phenotype, both clinically and pathologically. Symptoms at onset include progressive dementia, mainly of the frontotemporal type, which may evolve for some months without significant motor signs, such as ataxia or myoclonus. In addition, typical changes are absent on EEG examination. The pathology in these subjects predominantly affects the corticostriatal regions, while other subcortical structures, including the cerebellum, are relatively spared. Additional pathological features are the relative sparing of the occipital lobe in comparison to the frontal and temporal lobes, and the presence of numerous ballooned neurons in the cerebral cortex. Routine PrP immunohistochemistry is characteristically unrevealing in these subjects, and is limited to a faint punctate staining in the cerebral cortex, despite the severe spongiform degeneration.

sCJD with mixed type 1 and type 2 features. Up to 20 to 25% of sporadic CJD cases may have both types of PrP^{res} in their brain (49, 54) (Figure 10). Usually, type 1 appears to dominate over type 2 in homozygotes for methionine at codon 129, while the opposite occurs in homozygotes for valine. In support of the molecular/phenotype association outlined above, the clinical-pathological profile in individual cases depends on the predominant type of PrP^{res}, which accumulates in the central nervous system (49, 54). Accordingly, the phenotype of most MM1+2 CJD patients largely overlaps with that of the MM1, whereas the clinical and pathological features of VV1+2 cases resemble those of VV2 patients. PrP immunohistochemistry shows a mixed synaptic and perivacuolar reactivity in the MM1+2, and is useful to distinguish these cases. In contrast, the histopathological recognition of the VV1+2 subjects is more difficult, since type 1 in the VV cases is not associated with a specific staining pattern.

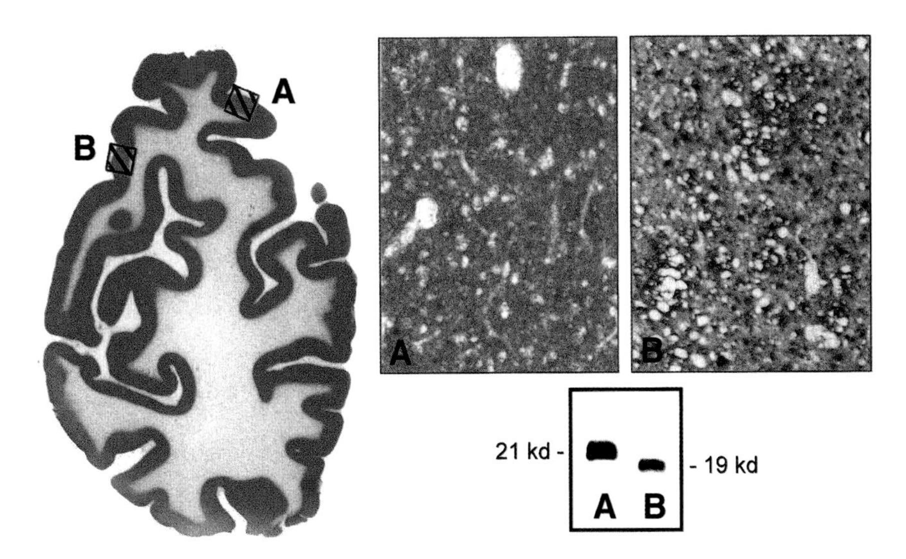

Figure 10. Immunohistochemistry and Western blot analysis with the antibody 3F4 showing the co-occurrence of type 1 (**B**) and type 2 (**A**) PrP^{res} in the same CJD patient. The distinct PrP^{res} types are associated with different patterns of PrP deposition and severity of spongiform changes. The immunoblot analysis was carried out after deglycosylation.

Differential Diagnosis

Spongiform change should not be confused with non-specific spongiosis or status spongiosus (Figure 6E) observed in brain oedema, metabolic encephalopathies and in gliotic neuropil following extensive neuronal loss. Focal changes qualitatively similar to the spongiform change of CJD may occur in some cases of Alzheimer's disease, diffuse Lewy body disease, Pick's disease, and dementia lacking specific histological features (9, 35). Perineuronal or perivascular vacuolation is seen in brain tissue following recent hypoxic/ischaemic damage. Superficial cortical, perineuronal, perivascular, and perinuclear-oligodendroglial vacuolation is most commonly an artefact related to inappropriate tissue processing, in particular fixation or embedding procedures.

Pathogenesis

Most investigators accept a central role for the prion protein in TSE pathophysiology. The prion hypothesis suggests that PrP^{res} once present in the brain initiates a wave of self-propagating conformational conversion of endogenous PrP^{C} (53). In principle the ensuing neurodegeneration might result from the loss of an essential function performed by PrP^{C} or a toxic gain of function by PrP^{res}. A growing body of work implicates PrP^{C} in stress (particularly oxidative stress) resistance and a role in copper metabolism. This potentially links CJD to the oxidative stress hypothesis invoked as an explanation for a variety of other neurodegenerative conditions. Alternatively there is strong evidence to suggest that a particular region of PrP, which spontaneously adopts a β-sheet conformation ($PrP^{106-126}$), is toxic to neurones and recapitulates many of the cellular effects seen in the central nervous system (63a). These data and the β-sheet-rich amyloid-like properties of PrP^{res} link CJD to other brain disorders resulting from protein aggregation, such as Alzheimer's disease. The oxidative stress and amyloid models of pathogenesis are generic to all TSE and have been reviewed recently (15, 22, 26).

Future Directions and Therapy

No safe effective therapies currently exist for any form of CJD or indeed for any of the related animal TSE. While the pharmacological, clinical and logistical problems might seem insurmountable, there nevertheless exists several reasons for a degree of optimism regarding the possibility of developing therapies, especially for variant CJD. Blood and urine tests for PrP^{Sc} or surrogate markers of disease have been reported for animal TSEs that appear to work during the clinical phase at least (42, 59, 62). A recently described method for amplifying PrP^{Sc} is likely to increase the sensitivity of such detection methods markedly (57).

A wide variety of structurally unrelated compounds have been shown to inhibit PrP^{Sc} accumulation in cell free and in vitro model systems. Some of these have also been shown to prolong the incubation period in animal models of TSE disease although their beneficial effects are often restricted to administration closely following peripheral exposure (1, 5, 22). The possibilities of targeting agent replication in the lymphoreticular system or harnessing the immune system to clear PrP^{Sc} are also therapeutic avenues currently under investigation for TSE (24, 39, 40).

In practice the immediate aim must be to find pharmacological agents or treatments that give some benefit to those diagnosed with all forms of CJD and suffering neurological symptoms and irreversible decline. The screening of existing licensed pharmacological agents that are known to cross the blood-brain barrier, for effects in model systems and their subsequent introduction in controlled clinical trials must be a high priority (32). In this context, the objective assessment of the effects of quinacrine and chlorpromazine treatment of CJD patients is awaited with great interest.

References

1. Aguzzi A, Glatzel M, Montrasio F, Prinz M, Heppner FL (2001) Interventional strategies against prion diseases. *Nat Rev Neurosci* 2: 745-749.

2. Arendt T, Bigl V, Arendt A (1984) Neurone loss in the nucleus basalis of Meynert in Creutzfeldt-Jakob disease. *Acta Neuropathol (Berl)* 65: 85-88.

3. Belichenko PV, Miklossy J, Belser B, Budka H, Celio MR (1999) Early destruction of the extracellular matrix around parvalbumin-immunoreactive interneurons in Creutzfeldt-Jakob disease. *Neurobiol Dis* 6: 269-279.

4. Bell JE, Gentleman SM, Ironside JW, McCardle L, Lantos PL, Doey L, Lowe J, Fergusson J, Luthert P, McQuaid S, Allen IV (1997) Prion protein immunocytochemistry—UK five centre consensus report. *Neuropathol Appl Neurobiol* 23: 26-35.

5. Brown P (2001) The pathogenesis of transmissible spongiform encephalopathy: routes to the brain and the erection of therapeutic barricades. *Cell Mol Life Sci* 58: 259-265.

6. Brown P, Gibbs C, Rodgers-Johnson P, Asher DM, Sulima MP, Bacote A, Goldfarb LG, Gajdusek DC (1994) Human spongiform encephalopathy: the National Institute of Health series of 300 cases of experimentally transmitted disease. *Ann Neurol* 35: 513-529.

7. Brownell B, Oppenheimer D (1965) An ataxic form of presenile polioencephalopathy (Creutzfeldt-Jakob disease). *J Neurol Neurosurg Psychiat* 28: 350-361.

8. Budka H (2000) Histopathology and immunohistochemistry of human transmissible spongiform encephalopathies (TSEs). *Arch Virol* Suppl 135-142.

9. Budka H, Aguzzi A, Brown P, Brucher JM, Bugiani O, Gullotta F, Haltia M, Hauw JJ, Ironside JW, Jellinger K, et al. (1995) Neuropathological diagnostic criteria for Creutzfeldt-Jakob disease (CJD) and other human spongiform encephalopathies (prion diseases). *Brain Pathol* 5: 459-466.

10. Bugiani O, Tagliavini F, Giaccone G, Boeri R (1989) Creutzfeldt-Jakob disease: astrocytosis and spongiform changes of the white matter, in *Unconventional virus diseases of the central nervous system*, Court L, Dormont D, Brown P, Kingsbury D (eds). Lefrancq: Candè, France. pp. 172-183.

11. Cartier L, Verdugo R, Vergara C, Galvez S (1989) The nucleus basalis of Meynert in 20 definite cases of Creutzfeldt-Jakob disease. *J Neurol Neurosurg Psychiatry* 52: 304-309.

11a. Collinge J, Sidle KCL, Meads J, Ironside J, Hill AF (1996) Molecular analysis of prion strain variation and the aetiology of "new variant" CJD. *Nature* 383: 685-690.

12. Collinge J, Palmer MS, Dryden AJ (1991) Genetic predisposition to iatrogenic Creutzfeldt-Jakob disease. *Lancet* 337: 1441-1442.

13. Creutzfeldt H (1920) Über eine eigenartige herdförmige Erkrankung des Zentralnervensystems. *Z ges Neurol Psychiat* 57: 1-18.

14. Giaccone G, Canciani B, Puoti G, Rossi G, Goffredo D, Iussich S, Fociani P, Tagliavini F, Bugiani O (2000) Creutzfeldt-Jakob disease: Carnoy's fixative improves the immunohistochemistry of the proteinase K-resistant prion protein. *Brain Pathol* 10: 31-37.

15. Giese A, Kretzschmar HA (2001) Prion-induced neuronal damage—the mechanisms of neuronal destruction in the subacute spongiform encephalopathies. *Curr Top Microbiol Immunol* 253: 203-217.

16. Gray F, Chretien F, Adle-Biassette H, Dorandeu A, Ereau T, Delisle MB, Kopp N, Ironside JW, Vital C (1999) Neuronal apoptosis in Creutzfeldt-Jakob disease. *J Neuropathol Exp Neurol* 58: 321-328.

17. Groschup MH, Beekes M, McBride PA, Hardt M, Hainfellner JA, Budka H (1999) Deposition of disease-associated prion protein involves the peripheral nervous system in experimental scrapie. *Acta Neuropathol (Berl)* 98: 453-457.

18. Guentchev M, Hainfellner JA, Trabattoni GR, Budka H (1997) Distribution of parvalbumin-immunoreactive neurons in brain correlates with hippocampal and temporal cortical pathology in Creutzfeldt-Jakob disease. *J Neuropathol Exp Neurol* 56: 1119-1124.

19. Hainfellner J, Budka H (1996) Immunomorphology of human prion diseases, in *Transmissible spongiform encephalopathies: prion diseases*, Court L, Dodet B (eds). Elsevier: Paris. pp. 75-80.

20. Hainfellner JA, Budka H (1999) Disease associated prion protein may deposit in the peripheral nervous system in human transmissible spongiform encephalopathies. *Acta Neuropathol (Berl)* 98: 458-460.

21. Hainfellner JA, Wanschitz J, Jellinger K, Liberski PP, Gullotta F, Budka H (1998) Coexistence of Alzheimer-type neuropathology in Creutzfeldt-Jakob disease. *Acta Neuropathol (Berl)* 96: 116-122.

22. Head MW, Farquhar C, Mabbott NA, Fraser J (2001) Transmissible spongiform encepahlopathies: pathogenic mechanisms and strategies for therapeutic intervention. *Expert Opinion on Therapeutic Targets* 5: 569-585.

23. Heidenhain A (1929) Klinische und anatomische Untersuchungen über eine eigenartige Erkrankung des Zentralnervensystems im Praesenium. *Z ges Neurol Psychiat* 118: 49-114.

24. Heppner FL, Musahl C, Arrighi I, Klein MA, Rulicke T, Oesch B, Zinkernagel RM, Kalinke U, Aguzzi A (2001) Prevention of scrapie pathogenesis by transgenic expression of anti-prion protein antibodies. *Science* 294: 178-182.

25. Hill AF, Butterworth RJ, Joiner S, Jackson G, Rossor MN, Thomas DJ, Frosh A, Tolley N, Bell JE, Spencer M, King A, Al-Sarraj S, Ironside JW, Lantos PL, Collinge J (1999) Investigation of variant Creutzfeldt-Jakob disease and other human prion diseases with tonsil biopsy samples. *Lancet* 353: 183-189.

26. Hope J (2000) Prions and neurodegenerative diseases. *Curr Opin Genet Dev* 10: 568-574.

27. Ironside JW, McCardle L, Hayward PA, Bell JE (1993) Ubiquitin immunocytochemistry in human spongiform encephalopathies. *Neuropathol Appl Neurobiol* 19: 134-140.

28. Jacobi C, Zerr I, Arlt S, Otto M, Poser S (2000) Cerebro-spinal fluid pattern in patients with definite Creutzfeldt-Jakob disease. *J Neurol* 247: S14.

29. Jakob A (1921) Über eigenartige Erkrankungen des Zentralnervensystems mit bemerkenswertem anatomischen Befunde (Spastische Pseudosklerose-Encephalomyelopathie mit disseminierten Degenerationsherden). *Z ges Neurol Psychiat* 64: 147-228.

30. Kascsak RJ, Fersko R, Pulgiano D, Rubenstein R, Carp RI (1997) Immunodiagnosis of prion disease. *Immunol Invest* 26: 259-268.

31. Kitamoto T, Muramoto T, Mohri S, Doh-Ura K, Tateishi J (1991) Abnormal isoform of prion protein accumulates in follicular dendritic cells in mice with Creutzfeldt-Jakob disease. *J Virol* 65: 6292-6295.

32. Korth C, May BC, Cohen FE, Prusiner SB (2001) Acridine and phenothiazine derivatives as pharmacotherapeutics for prion disease. *Proc Natl Acad Sci U S A* 98: 9836-9841.

33. Kovács GG, Head M, Hegyi I, Bunn T, Flicker H, Hainfellner JA, McCardle L, László L, Jarius C, Ironside J, Budka H (2002) Immunohistochemistry for the prion protein: comparison of different monoclonal anti-

bodies in human prion disease subtypes. *Brain Pathol* 12: 1-11.

34. Kretzschmar HA, Ironside JW, DeArmond SJ, Tateishi J (1996) Diagnostic criteria for sporadic Creutzfeldt-Jakob disease. *Arch Neurol* 53: 913-920.

35. Liberski P, Budka H (1993) An overview of neuropathology of the slow unconventional virus infections, in *Light and electron microscopic neuropathology of slow virus disorders*, Liberski P (ed). CRC Press: Boca Raton FL. pp. 111-149.

36. Liberski PP, Budka H (1999) Neuroaxonal pathology in Creutzfeldt-Jakob disease. *Acta Neuropathol (Berl)* 97: 329-334.

37. Liberski PP, Budka H, Sluga E, Barcikowska M, Kwiecinski H (1992) Tubulovesicular structures in Creutzfeldt-Jakob disease. *Acta Neuropathol (Berl)* 84: 238-243.

38. Liberski PP, Yanagihara R, Wells GA, Gibbs CJ, Jr., Gajdusek DC (1992) Comparative ultrastructural neuropathology of naturally occurring bovine spongiform encephalopathy and experimentally induced scrapie and Creutzfeldt-Jakob disease. *J Comp Pathol* 106: 361-381.

39. Mabbott NA, Bruce ME, Botto M, Walport MJ, Pepys MB (2001) Temporary depletion of complement component C3 or genetic deficiency of C1q significantly delays onset of scrapie. *Nat Med* 7: 485-487.

40. Mabbott NA, Mackay F, Minns F, Bruce ME (2000) Temporary inactivation of follicular dendritic cells delays neuroinvasion of scrapie. *Nat Med* 6: 719-720.

41. Macchi G, Abbamondi AL, di Trapani G, Sbriccoli A (1984) On the white matter lesions of the Creutzfeldt-Jakob disease. Can a new subentity be recognized in man? *J Neurol Sci* 63: 197-206.

42. Miele G, Manson J, Clinton M (2001) A novel erythroid-specific marker of transmissible spongiform encephalopathies. *Nat Med* 7: 361-364.

43. Mizutani T, Okumura A, Oda M, Shiraki H (1981) Panencephalopathic type of Creutzfeldt-Jakob disease: primary involvement of the cerebral white matter. *J Neurol Neurosurg Psychiatry* 44: 103-115.

44. Otto M, Wiltfang J, Cepek L, Neumann M, Mollenhauer B, Steinacker P, Ciesielczyk B, Schulz-Schaeffer W, Kretzschmar H, Poser S (2002) Tau protein and 14-3-3 protein in the differential diagnosis of Creutzfeldt-Jakob disease. *Neurology* 58: 192-197.

45. Palmer MS, Dryden AJ, Hughes JT, Collinge J (1991) Homozygous prion protein genotype predisposes to sporadic Creutzfeldt-Jakob disease. *Nature* 352: 340-342.

46. Pan T, Colucci M, Wong BS, Li R, Liu T, Petersen RB, Chen S, Gambetti P, Sy MS (2001) Novel differences between two human prion strains revealed by two-dimensional gel electrophoresis. *J Biol Chem* 276: 37284-37288.

47. Parchi P, Capellari S, Chen SG, Petersen RB, Gambetti P, Kopp N, Brown P, Kitamoto T, Tateishi J, Giese A, Kretzschmar H (1997) Typing prion isoforms. *Nature* 386: 232-234.

48. Parchi P, Castellani R, Capellari S, Ghetti B, Young K, Chen SG, Farlow M, Dickson DW, Sima AA, Trojanowski JQ, Petersen RB, Gambetti P (1996) Molecular basis of phenotypic variability in sporadic Creutzfeldt-Jakob disease. *Ann Neurol* 1996: 767-778.

49. Parchi P, Giese A, Capellari S, Brown P, Schulz-Schaeffer W, Windl O, Zerr I, Budka H, Kopp N, Piccardo P, Poser S, Rojiani A, Streichemberger N, Julien J, Vital C, Ghetti B, Gambetti P, Kretzschmar H (1999) Classification of sporadic Creutzfeldt-Jakob disease based on molecular and phenotypic analysis of 300 subjects. *Ann Neurol* 46: 224-233.

50. Parchi P, Zou W, Wang W, Brown P, Capellari S, Ghetti B, Kopp N, Schulz-Schaeffer WJ, Kretzschmar HA, Head MW, Ironside JW, Gambetti P, Chen SG (2000) Genetic influence on the structural variations of the abnormal prion protein. *Proc Natl Acad Sci U S A* 97: 10168-10172.

51. Park TS, Kleinman GM, Richardson EP (1980) Creutzfeldt-Jakob disease with extensive degeneration of white matter. *Acta Neuropathol (Berl)* 52: 239-242.

52. Poser S, Mollenhauer B, Kraubeta A, Zerr I, Steinhoff BJ, Schroeter A, Finkenstaedt M, Schulz-Schaeffer WJ, Kretzschmar HA, Felgenhauer K (1999) How to improve the clinical diagnosis of Creutzfeldt-Jakob disease. *Brain* 122: 2345-2351.

53. Prusiner SB (1998) Prions. *Proc Natl Acad Sci U S A* 95: 13363-13383.

54. Puoti G, Giaccone G, Rossi G, Canciani B, Bugiani O, Tagliavini F (1999) Sporadic Creutzfeldt-Jakob disease: co-occurrence of different types of PrPsc in the same brain. *Neurology* 53: 2173-2176.

55. Ribadeau-Dumas J, Escourolle R (1974) The Creutzfeldt-Jakob syndrome: a neuropathological and electron microscopic study, in *Neurology*, Subirana A, Espalader JM (eds). Elsevier: Amsterdam. pp. 316-329.

56. Richardson EP, Jr., Masters CL (1995) The nosology of Creutzfeldt-Jakob disease and conditions related to the accumulation of PrP^{CJD} in the nervous system. *Brain Pathol* 5: 33-41.

57. Saborio GP, Permanne B, Soto C (2001) Sensitive detection of pathological prion protein by cyclic amplification of protein misfolding. *Nature* 411: 810-813.

58. Salazar AM, Masters CL, Gajdusek DC, Gibbs CJ, Jr. (1983) Syndromes of amyotrophic lateral sclerosis and dementia: relation to transmissible Creutzfeldt-Jakob disease. *Ann Neurol* 14: 17-26.

59. Schmerr MJ, Jenny AL, Bulgin MS, Miller JM, Hamir AN, Cutlip RC, Goodwin KR (1999) Use of capillary electrophoresis and fluorescent labeled peptides to detect the abnormal prion protein in the blood of animals that are infected with a transmissible spongiform encephalopathy. *J Chromatogr A* 853: 207-214.

60. Schroter A, Zerr I, Henkel K, Tschampa HJ, Finkenstaedt M, Poser S (2000) Magnetic resonance imaging in the clinical diagnosis of Creutzfeldt-Jakob disease. *Arch Neurol* 57: 1751-1757.

61. Schulz-Schaeffer WJ, Tschoke S, Kranefuss N, Drose W, Hause-Reitner D, Giese A, Groschup MH, Kretzschmar HA (2000) The paraffin-embedded tissue blot detects PrP(Sc) early in the incubation time in prion diseases. *Am J Pathol* 156: 51-56.

62. Shaked GM, Shaked Y, Kariv-Inbal Z, Halimi M, Avraham I, Gabizon R (2001) A protease-resistant prion protein isoform is present in urine of animals and humans affected with prion diseases. *J Biol Chem* 276: 31479-31482.

63. Suenaga T, Hirano A, Llena JF, Ksiezak-Reding H, Yen SH, Dickson DW (1990) Ubiquitin immunoreactivity in kuru plaques in Creutzfeldt-Jakob disease. *Ann Neurol* 28: 174-177.

63a. Tagliavini F, Forloni G, D'Ursi P, Bugiani O, Salmona M (2001) Studies on peptide fragments of prion proteins, in *Advances in Priotein Chemistry* vol. 57, Caughey B (ed.). Academic Press: San Diego, CA, USA. pp. 171-202.

64. Taraboulos A, Jendroska K, Serban D, Yang SL, DeArmond SJ, Prusiner SB (1992) Regional mapping of prion proteins in brain. *Proc Natl Acad Sci U S A* 89: 7620-7624.

65. Van Everbroeck B, Pals P, Martin JJ, Cras P (1999) Antigen retrieval in prion protein immunohistochemistry. *J Histochem Cytochem* 47: 1465-1470.

66. Wientjens D, Davanipour Z, Hofman A, Kondo K, Matthews W, Will R, van Duijn C (1996) Risk factors for Creutzfeldt-Jakob disease: a reanalysis of case-control studies. *Neurology* 46: 1287-1291.

67. Will R, Ironside J, Zeidler M, Cousens S, Estibeiro K, Alperovitch A, Poser S, Pocchiari M, Hofman A, Smith P (1996) A new variant of Creutzfeldt-Jakob disease in the UK. *Lancet* 347: 921-925.

68. World Health Organization, Human transmissible encephalopathies, in *Weekly Epidemiological Record*. 1998. p. 361-365.

69. Worrall BB, Rowland LP, Chin SS-M, Mastrianni JA (2000) Amyotrophy in prion diseases. *Arch Neurol* 57: 33-38.

70. Zeidler M, Gibbs CJ, Meslin F, *WHO manual for strengthening diagnosis and surveillance of Creutzfeldt-Jakob disease*. 1998, Geneva: WHO.

71. Zerr I, Pocchiari M, Collins S, Brandel JP, de Pedro Cuesta J, Knight RS, Bernheimer H, Cardone F, Delasnerie-Laupretre N, Cuadrado Corrales N, Ladogana A, Bodemer M, Fletcher A, Awan T, Ruiz Bremon A, Budka H, Laplanche JL, Will RG, Poser S (2000) Analysis of EEG and CSF 14-3-3 proteins as aids to the diagnosis of Creutzfeldt-Jakob disease. *Neurology* 55: 811-815.

Familial Creutzfeldt-Jakob Disease

Piero Parchi
Sabina Capellari
Shu G. Chen
Pierluigi Gambetti

bp	base pair
CJD	Creutzfeldt-Jakob disease
EEG	electroencephalography
fCJD	familial Creutzfeldt-Jakob disease
FFI	fatal familial insomnia
GSS	Gerstmann-Sträussler-Scheinker syndrome
PrP	prion protein
PrP^{res}	protease resistant prion protein
PSWC	periodic sharp-wave complex
sCJD	sporadic Creutzfeldt-Jakob disease

Definition

Genetic or familial Creutzfeldt-Jakob disease (fCJD) comprises 5 to 10% of all human prion diseases and is associated with mutations in the prion protein gene (*PRNP*). fCJD is associated with at least 20 distinct genetic mutations with varying degrees of prevalence and penetrance (Figure 1). They are all transmitted in an autosomal dominant manner and include point mutations, deletion and insertion mutations, the last ones being characterised by the presence of 24 base pairs (bp) extrarepeats located between codon 51 and 91. As a group, fCJDs span the clinical and histopathological spectrum of sporadic Creutzfeldt Jakob disease (sCJD) for the age at onset, duration, clinical presentation and electroencephalographic (EEG) changes. The histopathology also overlaps extensively between the 2 forms. While spongiform degeneration is present in all cases, there is considerable variation in the severity of the astrogliosis and neuronal loss. Plaques containing the prion protein (PrP) in a non-amyloid conformation are rare, and to date the amyloid PrP plaques called kuru plaques have only been observed in the fCJD associated with one mutation (86). Mounting evidence indicates that, in addition to the pathogenic mutation, the type of protease resistant prion protein (PrP^{res}) and the codon 129 genotype act as major determinants of the disease phenotype as they do in sCJD. Consequently, distinct fCJD phenotypes can be observed in subjects carrying the same *PRNP* mutation, but having a different genotype at codon 129 and/or PrP^{res} type. In this chapter, fCJD phenotypes are presented in relation to their prevalence. Phenotypes that are relatively common are described individually and in detail while the others are summarised. Other forms of inherited prion diseases are discussed in the chapters on fatal familial insomnia and Gerstmann-Sträussler-Scheinker syndrome.

Historical Annotations

The first case of fCJD was reported in 1924 by Kirschbaum (57). However, the discovery that this case was familial and belonged to a large kindred was only reported later by Meggendorfer (53, 70, 102). In 1995, the D178N *PRNP* mutation with valine at codon 129 (D178N-129V haplotype) was demonstrated in archival tissue from this family (60).

In 1973, Gajdusek, Gibbs and their colleagues demonstrated the transmissibility of fCJD (95) and established, for the first time, that a disease could be both inherited and infectious. They postulated that the affected subjects carried a genetically determined susceptibility to an infection (66). Subsequently, the "protein only" hypothesis (91), largely promoted by Prusiner and collaborators, has provided a novel molecular basis for the transmissibility of the same disease by infection or genetic inheritance.

Phenotypes Associated with Genetci CJD

The E200K-129M haplotype. *Epidemiology.* This is by far the most common fCJD haplotype. The largest cluster occurs among Jews of Libyan and Tunisian origin (54). The E200K-129M haplotype has also been identified in other large clusters of patients with fCJD in Slovakia and Chile (6, 7, 44), as well as in individual families or in cases without a history of fCJD in Poland (6, 38), the United States (3), the United Kingdom (25, 107), France (63), Japan (51), Italy (28), Germany (108), and Spain (27).

Characteristics of the prion protein. In all subjects examined to date PrP^{res} showed the gel mobility pattern of PrP^{res} type 1, with a relative molecular weight of 21 kDa (Figure 2). The proteinase K cleavage sites were also identical to those of PrP^{res} type 1 of

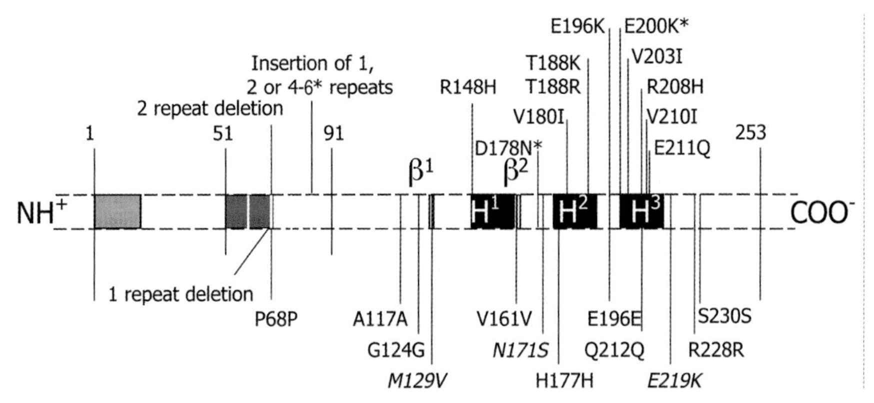

Figure 1. *Diagrammatic representation of the prion protein with pathogenic mutations associated with familial Creutzfeldt-Jakob disease (fCJD) (upper part) and polymorphisms (lower part).* Polymorphisms resulting in amino acid change are shown in italics; silent polymorphisms are unitalicized. * indicates mutations with two or more haplotypes. β^1 and β^2 indicate the regions of the prion protein with β-sheet conformation. H^1-H^3 indicates the regions with α-helical conformation, NH$^+$; N-terminus; COO$^-$: C-terminus.

sCJD, which most commonly occurs at residue 82 (72, 83, 85, 103). However, the ratio of the 3 major PrP^{res} bands, which correspond to the PrP glycoforms, is significantly different. In CJDE200K-129M, the diglycosylated and monoglycosylated forms are the most and least abundant, respectively (72, 81, 85). In contrast, in sCJD the monoglycosylated band is the most abundant (83) (Figure 2). Furthermore, diglycosylated forms form a band on the gel that is more spread out than that formed by PrP^{res} type 1 from sCJD (15, 34). This change is due to the effect of the E200K mutation on the glycosylation of residue 197 (15).

Clinical and pathological features. The clinical features of CJDE200K-129M are comparable to those of the most common sCJD subtype (MM1). In one large series, the mean age at onset was 62 years and the mean duration 5 months (55). In another series of 65 patients, age at onset was 59 years, and the mean duration 7 months (100). No significant difference in both age at onset and disease duration was observed between patients who have methionine and those with valine at codon 129 in the normal *PRNP* allele (32).

As in the most common sCJD, presenting signs may be variable and include cognitive impairment and psychiatric changes (80-83% of patients), cerebellar signs (43-55%), visual signs (19%) and myoclonic jerks (12%) (6, 55). All patients eventually develop dementia as well as other cognitive and psychiatric disturbances; 73% develop myoclonus, 79% cerebellar signs, and 40% seizures (6). The typical EEG activity with periodic sharp-waves complexes (PSWCs) is found in 74 to 76% of CJDE200K-129M, as compared with approximately 80% of the sCJD MM1 (6, 83). The only feature of the CJDE200K-129M phenotype which appears to distinguish this phenotype is the frequent involvement of the peripheral nervous system, which is rare in the course of sCJD. Both motor and sensory peripheral neuropathies may be present, and are often accompanied by protein elevation in the cerebrospinal fluid (2, 21, 74).

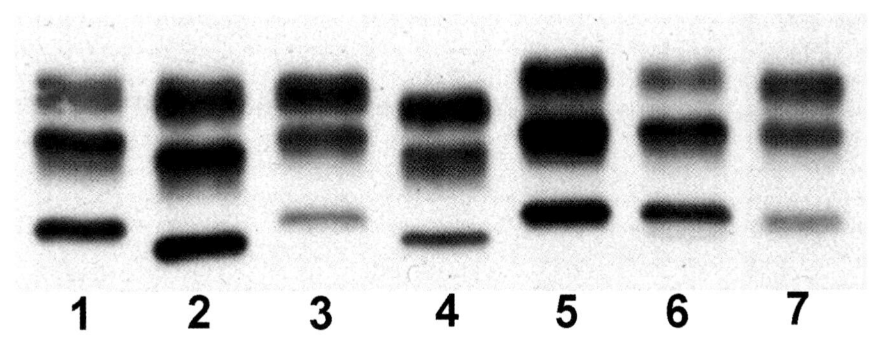

Figure 2. *Immunoblot of profile of PrP^{res} in sporadic CJD and fCJD with PrP^{res} type 1 or 2.* Lane 1: sCJD 129MM, PrP^{res} type 1; lane 2: sCJD 129VV, PrP^{res} type 2; lane 3: fCJD E200K-129M, PrP^{res} type 1; lane 4: fCJD E200K-129V, PrP^{res} type 2; lane 5: fCJD 144bp-Insert-129M, PrP^{res} type 1; lane 6: fCJD V210I-129M, PrP^{res} type 1; lane 7: fCJD D178N-129V, PrP^{res} type 1. Note the under-representation of the unglycosylated, 21kDa, isoform in fCJD E200K-129M, E200k-129V and D178N-129V.

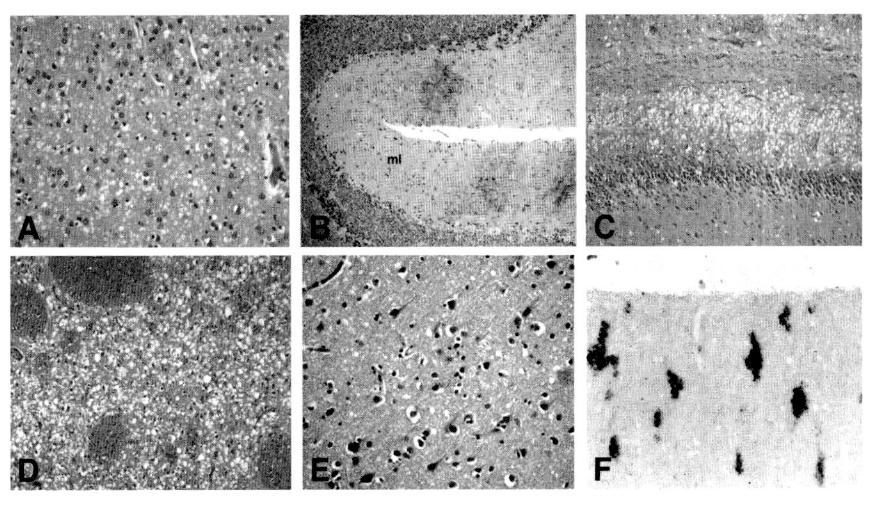

Figure 3. *Histopathology of fCJD.* **A.** Typical spongiform degeneration in the cerebral cortex of fCJD E200k-129M (H&E). **B.** Synaptic pattern of PrP deposition in the molecular layer (ml) of the cerebellum of fCJD E200K-129M (PrP IHC with the monoclonal antibody 3F4). **C.** Severe spongiform degeneration in the fascia dentata of the hippocampus in fCJD D178N-129V (H&E). **D.** Severe spongiform degeneration in the caudate nucleus in fCJD D178N-129V (H&E). **E.** Mild spongiform degeneration despite 7 years of progressive dementia in the cerebral cortex of fCJD with 144bp insertion-129M (H&E). **F.** PrP patches in the molecular layer of the cerebellum in fCJD with 144bp insertion-129M (PrP IHC with the monoclonal antibody 3F4).

The histological changes associated with CJDE200K-129M are also very similar to those of the sporadic CJD MM1 phenotype and are invariably characterised by spongiform degeneration, astrogliosis and neuronal loss in the absence of amyloid plaques (Table 1, Figure 3). These lesions are of variable severity and mainly involve the cerebral cortex, striatum, medial thalamus and cerebellum (83). Immunostaining consistently shows the "synaptic" pattern (Figure 3), occasionally associated with the "coarse" pattern (83). The peripheral neuropathy is both axonal and demyelinating and is characterised by segmental demyelination (2, 21, 74).

The E200K-129V haplotype. *Epidemiology.* This haplotype has been originally described in a family from Austria (45). Since then, 4 additional CJD subjects, from unrelated families, have been identified (84, 93). All but 2 of these subjects carried valine in the normal *PRNP* allele.

Characteristics of the prion protein. Brain extracts from the 5 patients showed PrP^{res} type 2 (45, 84, 93) (Figure 2). The glycoform ratio of PrP^{res}

	Clinical phenotype	Pathological phenotype	PrPSc
E200K-129M	Like sporadic CJD MM1. Atypical signs such as supranuclear palsy, spastic paresis, and peripheral neuropathy in some cases.	Like sporadic CJD MM1.	Type 1B
E200K-129V	Rapidly progressive dementia, early ataxia, late appearance of myoclonus and periodic sharp-waves complexes on the EEG	Similar to sporadic CJD VV2.	Type 2B
D178N-129V	Onset with cognitive impairment, depression, irritability and abnormal behavior. Later, ataxia, dysarthria or aphasia, tremor and myoclonus. EEG without PSWCs.	Frontal, temporal and entorhinal cortices and striatum show most severe pathology; thalamus is relatively spared; cerebellum and brain stem are spared.	Type 1B
V210I-129M	Like sporadic CJD MM1	Like sporadic CJD MM1	Type 1A
T183A-129M	Onset with behavioural disturbances and memory impairment. Later progressive dementia with aggressive behaviour, hyperorality, verbal stereotypes and often parkinsonian signs. EEG without PSWCs.	Spongiform degeneration and atrophy in the cerebral cortex and basal ganglia. PrP positive only in the putamen with a plaque-like pattern and in the molecular layer of the cerebellum where it is diffuse and punctate.	Not Published
V180I-129M	Like sporadic MM1 but with a longer duration.	Similar to sporadic CJD MM1	Not Published
M232R-129M	Rapidly progressive dementia with visual signs or ataxia, and myoclonus. EEG without PSWCs	Similar to sporadic CJD MM1	Type 1
1-4 INS-129M	Like sporadic CJD MM1	Like sporadic CJD MM1	Type 1A
5,6 INS- 129M	Onset with personality changes and abnormal behavior, memory decrease or confusion. Later, ataxia, speech impairments with dysarthria or aphasia, myoclonus, tremor or other involuntary movements, spasticity, and seizures. Typical PSWCs in some cases.	Variable degree of spongiform degeneration in all but two cases, in which only gliosis and neuronal loss were reported. Predominant involvement of the occipital lobe and relative sparing of the hippocampus and brain stem. PrP-patches in the molecular layer of the cerebellum.	Type 1A

Table 1. Clinical and pathological features and scrapie prion phenotype of the major forms of familial Creutzfeldt-Jakob disease.

was similar of that found in the E200K-129M haplotype (45, 84, 93).

Clinical and pathological features. Although an insufficient number of cases is available to draw definitive conclusions, some features of the disease in these patients indicate that the phenotype linked to this haplotype is different from that of the E200K-129M haplotype and is similar of that described in the sporadic CJD VV type 2 subjects (81, 83). These include early ataxia, the late appearance of myoclonus and PSWCs on the EEG, as well as the predominant PrP^{res} accumulation in the cerebellum associated with the presence of PrP^{res} focal deposits.

The D178N-129V haplotype. *Epidemiology.* Eight kindreds have been reported to date: 4 from the United States (8, 39, 40, 84), 2 from France (8, 10, 39, 40, 105), one from Finland (8, 36, 39, 40, 46, 58) and one from Germany (60). Of the 4 kindreds identified in the United States, 3 are of Hungarian-Rumanian, Dutch and French-Canadian origins, respectively, (8, 39, 40), while one is unpublished (Parchi and Gambetti unpublished data). The German kindred, originally reported in 1930, was recently shown to have the CJD178-129V haplotype (60, 70). Finally, 2 unrelated cases of Russian and Yugoslavian origin have been observed in Israel (96).

Characteristics of the prion protein. In the 7 cases examined to date, PrP^{res} has uniformly shown the type 1 pattern of electrophoretic mobility (72, 81, 85) (Figure 2). The glycoform ratio of PrP^{res} is characterised by a marked under-representation of the unglycosylated form that accounts for approximately 20% of the total while the intermediate and highly glycosylated forms are similarly represented (72, 81, 84).

Clinical and pathological features. The mean age at onset and the duration of the disease are influenced by the genotype at codon 129 of the normal allele. The average age at onset is 39 years (range: 26-47) in the 129 valine homozygotes, and 49 years (range: 45-56) in heterozygous patients (40). Similarly, the mean duration of symptoms is 14 months (range: 9-18) in the homozygous and 27 months (range: 7-51) in heterozygous patients (40). Clinical signs are fairly consistent and apparently independent of the zygosity at codon 129. Presentation is characterised by cognitive impairment, especially memory decrease, often associated with depression, irritability and abnormal behavior (8). Ataxia, speech impairments with dysarthria or aphasia, tremor and myoclonus are common signs during the course of the disease. EEG examination invariably reveals generalised slow wave activity without PSWCs (8).

There is apparently no difference in the histopathology between codon 129 homozygous and heterozygous subjects; however, the number of subjects examined at autopsy in which codon 129 is known is limited. The common changes of this fCJD subtype are spongiform degeneration associated with prominent astrogliosis, often in the form of gemistocytic astrocytes, and variable degrees of neuronal loss

(82). The topography of these lesions is consistent and fairly distinctive. The involvement of the cerebral cortex is widespread, but frontal and temporal cortices are generally more severely affected than the occipital cortex. Within the hippocampal region, these changes are especially prominent in the subiculum and entorhinal cortex, while spongiform degeneration is often present in the fascia dentata (Figure 3). Among the subcortical structures, the putamen and the caudate nucleus show severe spongiform degeneration with variable degrees of astrogliosis (Figure 3); the thalamus is minimally or moderately affected with spongiform degeneration and gliosis while the cerebellum is spared and minimal or no pathology is seen in the brain stem. PrP immunostaining shows the synaptic pattern which is usually weak despite the severe spongiform degeneration, as well as small focal deposits (82, unpublished data). In conclusion, the phenotype of this subtype of fCJD shows similarities with the VV1 sCJD with which it shares the type of PrP^{res} and, at least in the VV homozygotes, the codon 129 genotype (83).

The V210I-129M haplotype. *Epidemiology.* The V210I-129M haplotype has only been reported in 21 affected subjects (17, 31, 50, 68, 89, 90, 94, 99, 108). The observation that most of these subjects did not have a positive family history for the disease, combined with the finding of asymptomatic carriers of the mutation in relative advanced age, indicate that the V210I mutation has low penetrance.

Characteristics of the prion protein. Brain extracts from 13 subjects showed PrP^{res} type 1 (17, 68, 81) (Figure 2). The glycoform ratio of PrP^{res} was indistinguishable from that of the sCJD MM1 subjects. Thus, at variance with the E200K and D178N mutations, the V210I substitution does not affect the glycosylation of the protein.

Clinical and pathological features. Among 13 of the reported cases the age at onset varied between 48 and 70 years, and the disease duration between 3 and 8 months. Both parameters do not seem to be affected by the genotype at codon 129 of the normal allele. Adequate clinical data are only available for 9 subjects (31, 50, 68, 89, 90, 94, 99). The presentation included memory loss, behavioral and gait disturbances, sudden sensory and motor hemiparesis, clumsiness, dystonic movements and dysarthria. Common signs during the evolution of the illness were dementia, myoclonus, dysarthria, cerebellar signs, and akinetic mutism. The EEG showed the typical PSWCs in all 6 subjects that have been examined (31, 50, 68, 90). The 7 cases examined at autopsy revealed spongiform degeneration and astrogliosis of cerebral cortex, striatum, thalamus, and molecular layer of the cerebellum (31, 50, 68, 90, 94).

The T183A-129M haplotype. *Epidemiology.* This haplotype has been originally reported in one Brazilian kindred of Spanish and Italian origin (76, 77). Since then, 3 additional subjects belonging to families from the United States, Germany, and Venezuela have been reported (13, 18, 108).

Characteristics of the prion protein. The PrP^{res} characteristics have not been described.

Clinical and pathological features. Among the reported cases the mean age at onset was 44 years, and the mean duration 3.7 years. The disease seems to be shorter (2-year course) in one homozygous than in one heterozygous subject (9 years). Behavioural disturbances are the predominant presenting symptoms associated with memory impairment in half of the cases. They are followed by rapidly progressive dementia with aggressive behaviour, hyperorality, verbal stereotypes and often parkinsonian signs, which are clinical signs similar to those of frontotemporal dementia. The EEG failed to demonstrate PSWCs even in advanced stages.

Main histological features include widespread spongiform degeneration and atrophy in the cerebral cortex and basal ganglia. Immunostaining for PrP is positive only in the putamen where it has a plaque-like pattern and in the molecular layer of the cerebellum where it is diffuse and punctate.

Inherited CJD associated with M232S-129M and the V180I-129M. *Epidemiology.* These 2 haplotypes have only been observed in Japanese subjects (48, 49, 56).

Characteristics of the prion protein. The PrP^{res} gel pattern of the M232S-129M haplotype is unusual since it apparently lacks the high molecular weight glycoform (48). The characteristics of PrP^{res} associated with the V180-129M haplotype have not been reported.

Clinical and pathological features. In CJDV180I-129M, the age at onset varies between 66 and 81 years and the duration between 1 and 2 years. The only subject examined in detail presented with cognitive impairment, especially memory impairment, followed by akinetic mutism, pyramidal and extrapyramidal signs and myoclonus. None of the patients demonstrated PSWCs on the EEG. Typical spongiform degeneration was present in the cerebral cortex, basal ganglia and thalamus. Neuronal loss and astrogliosis were observed in the cerebral cortex. PrP immunostaining of the gray matter was weak and diffuse.

Clinical and pathological findings associated to CJD M232S-129M have been reported in detail in 3 cases (49). Age at onset ranged between 55 and 70 years and duration between 4 and 24 months. Common presenting signs were memory and gait disturbances followed by myoclonus and mutism at more advanced stages. A typical EEG with PSWCs was observed in all cases. The histopathology was characterised by widespread spongiform degeneration, astrogliosis and neuronal loss in variable degrees regardless of the disease duration. The thalamus showed the most severe spongiform degeneration, especially in the dorsomedial nucleus. Neuronal loss was severe in the basal ganglia while the spongiform degeneration was minimal.The cerebral cortex showed moderate spongiform degeneration with moderate to severe astrogliosis and neuronal loss. All three lesions were present in the brain stem; the cerebellum lacked spongiform degeneration but showed neuronal loss and gliosis (49). The PrP immunoreactivity was widespread in cerebrum and spinal cord with more intense immunostaining in the cerebral cortex, especially the hippocampus, and was of the punctate type with no plaque-like PrP deposits (49).

Other rare haplotypes. *Epidemiology.* Altogether the rare *PRNP* haplotypes probably represent less than 5% of all genetic CJD cases. Moreover, they have been often described in single subjects lacking any family history. Linkage analysis is unavailable for these haplotypes and therefore it is currently unknown whether they are pathogenic mutations. To date these rare mutations include the following: I213M, G142S (Laplanche personal communication), Q160S (30), T188R (108), R208H (16,67), T188K (30), T188A (26), E196K, V203I, E211Q (61, 87), P238S (108), R148H (86). Finally, the deletion of 2 octapeptide repeats has also been linked to CJD (4, 14).

Characteristics of the prion protein. In this group the characteristics of the PrP^{res} have only been studied in the subject with the R208H mutation (16, 67), and in one of those carrying the double octapeptide deletion (14). In all cases PrP^{res} showed the physicochemical properties of PrP^{res} type 1.

Clinical and pathological features. Subjects of this group showed a disease with the clinical and pathological features of the typical sporadic CJD MM1 phenotype, with the only exception of the 2 carrying the double deletion mutation who showed a dementia of longer duration (12-18 months) (4, 14).

Inherited prion disease with insertional mutations. The *PRNP* gene contains 4 repeated octapeptides between codons 51 and 91. While deletions of a single repeat is a common polymorphism found in the 1 to 2.5% of the general population (20,62,80), insertions of one to 9 extra repeats have been associated with apparently sporadic as well as familial forms of human prion diseases (Table 1). The disease phenotype associated with the insertion mutations is very variable. Increasing evidence indicates that in addition to the codon 129 genotype and the PrP^{res} type, the size of the extrarepeat insertion significantly influences the disease phenotype. The current available data indicate that 3 groups of subjects can be identified according to the length of the insertion mutation: *i)* patients with 4 or fewer octapetide inserts who show phenotypes virtually indistinguishable from the sCJD subtypes, *ii)* patients with 5 to 7 repeats who also usually show a CJD phenotype but often with an earlier age at onset and a much slower progression than the sCJD subtypes, and *iii)* patients with 8 or 9 extra-repeats who show a Gerstmann-Straussler-Scheinker (GSS) phenotype with widespread amyloid deposition (for this group, refer to the chapter on GSS).

Epidemiology. Since the first report of a six 24-bp extra repeat insert in a British family with atypical dementia (79), CJD affected subjects carrying one to nine 24-bp extra repeat insertions have been reported in the United States (11, 12, 19, 23, 35, 41, 42, 43, 73), Europe (24, 29, 59, 64, 65, 75, 78, 92, 97, 101, 104) and Japan (52,71). Currently, 20 families are known, including 24 subjects who were diagnosed at autopsy. In 16 families the repeat expansion was coupled with the methionine codon at position 129, whereas in 4 the inserts were coupled with the valine codon.

Characteristics of the prion protein. PrP^{res} type 1 was detected in all 4 subjects examined to date who carried insertions of 4, 5, or 6 extrarepeat insertions coupled with methionine at codon 129 (12, 84) (Figure 2). The glycoform ratio of the protein was also comparable to that of the PrPres of sCJD MM1 (81).

Clinical and pathological features. A 1-octapeptide repeat insertion has only been reported in a 73-year-old man who died after a rapidly progressive encephalopathy characterised by dizziness, visual agnosia evolving to cortical blindness, cerebellar ataxia, dementia, diffuse myoclonus and akinetic mutism. Diffuse PSWCs were observed on the EEG. No autopsy was performed (64). Similarly, a 2-octapeptide 48bp insertion has been described in a 58-year-old female who also showed a rapidly progressive myoclonic dementia of 3 months duration indistinguishable from the sCJD129 MM1 phenotype. PSWCs were recorded by EEG also in this case, and the neuropathologic examination revealed the typical regional distribution of lesions of the sCJD MM1 phenotype (64). Two CJD affected subjects carrying a 4-octapeptide (96bp) insert have been described (11, 12). Both patients were in their 50s and had a mean duration of symptoms of 4 months. In both cases, the classical clinical, electroencephalographic and histopathologic features of the typical CJD phenotype were present. At variance with sCJD MM1, however, numerous patches of PrP immunoreactivity, often running perpendicular to the leptomeningeal surface, were seen in the molecular layer of the cerebellum. No family history for CJD was reported in either case.

In subjects carrying 5- to 8-octapeptite (120-168bp) inserts associated with 129MM, the clinical presentation is usually characterised by cognitive impairment, especially memory decrease or confusion, often preceded by personality changes and abnormal behavior (75,106). Gait ataxia or visual signs are also sometime present at onset. Ataxia, speech impairments with dysarthria or aphasia, myoclonus, tremor or other involuntary movements, spasticity, and seizures are all common signs during the course of the disease. Typical PSWCs were recorded in most cases.

Neuropathologic examination revealed a variable degree of spongiform degeneration (Figure 3) in all but 2 cases, in which only astrogliosis and neuronal loss where reported. The relative severity of the lesions in the various brain regions often showed the profile of the sporadic CJD MM1 phenotype with predominant involvement of the occipital lobe and relative sparing of the hippocampus and brain stem. PrP-patches in the molecular layer of the cerebellum (Figure 3) were seen in all cases in which the immunohistochemistry was performed. This futher supports the notion that the latter feature is linked to methionine at codon 129 and remains the most useful diagnostic tool to distinguish this subgroup of human prion disease.

Differential Diagnosis

Familial CJD may be more challenging than sCJD especially because of the disease duration, which can be very long, and, along with the clinical signs can make fCJD more similar to the atypical dementias, such as the frontal lobe dementias, than to sCJD. This is the case with fCJD T183A-129M as well as fCJD associated with long insert mutations. However, once fCJD is suspected, sequencing of the *PRNP* gene will definitely clarify this diagnosis. *PRNP* sequencing should be carried in all patients with probable or definite CJD, as well as in those with a positive family history of dementia and a clinical diagnosis of fronto-temporal dementia, atypical dementia or even Alzheimer's disease, once the known pathogenic mutations in the PS1, PS2, APP, or tau genes have been ruled out.

Pathogenesis

According to the prevalent hypothesis, the central event in the pathogenesis of all forms of prion diseases, ie, inherited, sporadic or acquired by infection, is the conversion of a prion protein isoform that is predominantly soluble into PrP^{res} that is predominantly insoluble and infectious (91). The conversion of normal PrP to PrP^{res} is thought to be a spontaneous event in sporadic prion diseases, possibly due to an error of the cell machinery that makes and modifies proteins, including PrP. In prion diseases acquired by infection, the conversion of the endogenous, normal PrP is thought to result from the interaction with the exogenous PrP^{res}. There is strong evidence that several *PRNP* mutations linked to inherited prion diseases (32, 37, 67, 92) destabilise the mutated PrP facilitating its conversion into PrP^{res} (15, 33, 88). The destabilising effect is likely to vary from one mutation to the other providing a reasonable explanation for the different penetrance of *PRNP* mutations. It has been reported that almost all patients carrying the E200K-129M haplotype become symptomatic during the course of their life (33). In contrast, the majority of patients with the V210I-129M haplotype remain free of symptoms. Another variable in the pathogenesis of inherited prion diseases is the role of PrP^{C}, ie, the non-mutated PrP, in the conversion process that generates PrP^{res}. While in CJD D178N-129V only mutated PrP undergoes conversion to form PrP^{res}, in CJD V210I-129M PrP^{res} is formed by both mutated and non-mutated PrP, presumably because the V210I-129M PrP can converts PrP^{C}, whereas this does not happen in CJD D178N-129V (22). Furthermore, the non mutated PrP becomes insoluble, but not protease resistant, in affected subjects with the E200K-129M haplotype (33). Unexpectedly, the participation of the non-mutated PrP in the conversion process does not correlate with the shorter disease duration which one would expect since the conversion to PrP^{res} of both mutated and non-mutated PrP should result in the presence of a larger quantity of PrP^{res}. The mechanisms by which the various *PRNP* mutations facilitate PrP^{res} formation remain to be clarified.

Treatment

As stated in other chapters (9), while no effective therapies currently exist for prion diseases, a variety of compounds have been shown to inhibit PrP^{res} accumulation in cell free and in vitro model systems and to prolong the incubation period in experimental animal models of prion disease (1, 5, 47). One of the many challenges of treating sporadic neurodegenerative diseases is the early diagnosis so that treatment can be started when damage to the brain tissue is limited. This is especially important in prion diseases that often have a rapid course. Genetic analysis offers the opportunity to establish the diagnosis long before the disease becomes symptomatic when the treatment could prevent the disease phenotype to occur. It is also conceivable that prenatal or even pre-fertilisation diagnosis may eradicate inherited prion diseases and other inherited diseases altogether.

References

1. Aguzzi A, Glatzel M, Montrasio F, Prinz M, Heppner FL (2001) Interventional strategies against prion diseases. *Nat Rev Neurosci* 2: 745-749.

2. Antoine JC, Laplanche JL, Mosnier JF, Beaudry P, Chatelain J, Michel D (1996) Demyelinating peripheral neuropathy with Creutzfeldt-Jakob disease and mutation at codon 200 of the prion protein gene. *Neurology* 46: 1123-1127.

3. Bertoni JM, Brown P, Goldfarb LG, Rubenstein R, Gajdusek DC (1992) Familial Creutzfeldt-Jakob disease (codon 200 mutation) with supranuclear palsy. *JAMA* 268: 2413-2415 .

4. Beck JA, Mead S, Campbell TA, Dickinson A, Wientjens DP, Croes EA, Van Duijn CM, Collinge J (2001) Two-octapeptide repeat deletion of prion protein associated with rapidly progressive dementia. *Neurology* 57: 354-356.

5. Brown P (2001) The pathogenesis of transmissible spongiform encephalopathy: routes to the brain and the erection of therapeutic barricades. *Cell Mol Life Sci* 58: 259-265.

6. Brown P, Goldfarb LG, Gibbs CJ Jr, Gajdusek DC (1991) The phenotypic expression of different mutations in transmissible familial Creutzfeldt-Jakob disease. *Eur J Epidemiol* 7: 469-476.

7. Brown P, Gálvez S, Goldfarb LG, Nieto A, Cartier L, Gibbs CJ Jr, Gajdusek DC (1992) Familial Creutzfeldt-Jakob disease in Chile is associated with the codon 200 mutation of the PRNP amyloid precursor gene on chromosome 20. *J Neurol Sci* 112: 65-67.

8. Brown P, Goldfarb LG, Kovanen J, Haltia M, Cathala F, Sulima M, Gibbs CJ Jr, Gajdusek DC (1992) Phenotypic characteristics of familial Creutzfeldt-Jakob disease associated with the codon 178Asn PRNP mutation. *Ann Neurol* 31: 282-285.

9. Budka H, Head M W, Ironside J W, Gambetti P, Parchi P, Tagliavini F, Zeidler M (2003) Sporadic Creutzfeldt-Jakob disease. Chapter 6, this volume.

10. Buge A, Escourolle R, Brion S, Rancurel G, Hauw JJ, Mehaut M, Gray F, Gajdusek DC (1978) Maladie de Creutzfeldt-Jakob familiale – Étude clinique et

anatomique de trois cas sur huit répartis sur trois générations. Transmission au singe écureuil. *Rev Neurol (Paris)* 134: 165-181.

11. Campbell TA, Palmer MS, Will RG, Gibb WRG, Luthert PJ, Collinge J (1996) A prion disease with a novel 96-base pair insertional mutation in the prion protein gene. *Neurology* 46: 761-766.

12. Capellari S, Parchi P, Landis DD, Petersen R.B, Julien J, Gambetti P (1997) Prion encephalopathy with octapeptide insertions in PRNP: a study of three new families. *Neurology* 48: 5035.

13. Capellari S, Parchi P, Bennett D, Petersen RB, Gambetti P, Cochran E (1999) First North American report of the T183A mutation in the prion protein gene: clinical, pathological, and biochemical analysis of one case. *Neurology* 52 (suppl 2) A324.

14. Capellari S, Parchi P, Wolff BD, Campbell J, Atkinson R, Posey DM, Petersen RB, Gambetti P (2002) Creutzfeldt-Jakob disease associated with a deletion of two repeats in the prion protein gene. *Neurology* 59: 1628-1630.

15. Capellari S, Parchi P, Russo CM, Sanford J, Sy MS, Gambetti P, Petersen RB (2000) Effect of the E200K mutation on prion protein metabolism. Comparative of a cell model and human brain. *Am J Pathol* 157: 613-622.

16. Capellari S, Ladogana A, Volpi G, Roncaroli F, Sità D, Baruzzi A, Pocchiari M, Parchi P (2001). First report of the R208H-129MM haplotype in the prion protein gene in an European subject with CJD. *J Neurol Sci* 22: S109.

17. Cardone F, Liu QG, Petraroli R, Ladogana A, D'Alessandro M, Arpino C, Di Bari M, Macchi G, Pocchiari M (1999) Prion protein glycotype analysis in familial and sporadic Creutzfeldt-Jakob disease patients. *Brain Res Bull* 49: 429-433.

18. Cardozo J, Caruso G, Molina O, Cardozo D, Chen S, Sirko-Osadsa DA, Wang W, Xie Z, Gambetti P (2000) Familial transmissible spongiform encephalopathy with the T183A mutation on the prion protein gene (PRNP). *J Neuropathol Exp Neurol* 56: 433.

19. Cervenakova L, Goldfarb LG, Brown P, Kenney K, Cochran EJ, Bennett DA, Roos R, Gajdusek DC (1995) Three new PRNP genotypes associated with familial Creutzfeldt-Jakob disease. Abstract. *Am J Hum Genet* 57: A209.

20. Cervenakova L, Brown P, Piccardo P, Cummings JL, Nagle J, Vinters HV, Kaur P, Ghetti B, Chapman J, Gajdusek DC, Goldfarb L (1996) 24-nucleotide deletion in the PRNP gene: analysis of associated phenotypes. *Transmissible Subacute Spongiform Encephalopathies: Prion Diseases*, L. Court, B. Dodet (eds), Paris, Elsevier, pp. 433-444 .

21. Chapman J, Brown P, Goldfarb LG, Arlazoroff A, Gajdusek DC, Korczyn AD (1993) Clinical heterogeneity and unusual presentations of Creutzfeldt-Jakob disease in Jewish patients with the PRNP codon 200 mutation. *J Neurol Neurosurg Psychiatry* 56: 1109 -1112.

22. Chen SG, Parchi P, Brown P, Capellari S, Zou W, Cochran EJ, Vnencak-Jones CL, Julien J, Vital C, Mikol J, Lugaresi E, Autilio-Gambetti L, Gambetti P (1997) Allelic origin of the abnormal prion protein isoform in familial prion diseases. *Nature Med* 3: 1009-1015.

23. Cochran EJ, Bennett DA, Cervenakova L, Kenney K, Bernard B, Foster NL, Benson DF, Goldfarb LG, Brown P (1996) Familial Creutzfeldt-Jakob disease with a five-repeat octapeptide insert mutation. *Neurology* 47: 727-733.

24. Collinge J, Brown J, Hardy J, Mullan M, Rossor MN, Baker H, Crow TJ, Lofthouse R, Poulter M, Ridley R, Owen F, Bennett C, Dunn G, Harding AE, Quinn N, Doshi B, Roberts GW, Honavar M, Janota I, Lantos PL (1992) Inherited prion disease with 144 base pair gene insertion. *Brain* 115: 687-710.

25. Collinge J, Palmer MS, Campbell T, Sidle KC, Carroll D, Harding A (193) Inherited prion disease (PrP lysine 200) in Britain: two case reports. *Brit Med J* 306: 301-302.

26. Collins S, Boyd A, Fletcher A, Byron K, Harper C, McLean CA, Masters CL (2000) Novel prion protein gene mutation in an octogenarian with Creutzfeldt-Jakob disease. *Arch Neurol* 57: 1058-1063.

27. Coria F, Cuadrado N, Rubio I, Del Ser T, Canton R, Nos C (1995) Genetics of spongiform encephalopathies in Spain: preliminary data. *Fifth Meeting of the European Neurological Society*, Munich 17-21 June, abstract 227.

28. D'Alessandro M, Petraroli R, Ladogana A, Pocchiari M (1998) High incidence of Creutzfeldt-Jakob disease in rural Calabria. *Lancet* 352: 1989-1990.

29. Duchen LW, Poulter M, Harding AE (1995) Dementia associated with a 216 base pair insertion in the prion protein gene. *Brain* 116: 555-567.

30. Finckh U, Muller-Thomsen T, Mann U, Eggers C, Marksteiner J, Meins W, Binetti G, Alberici A, Hock C, Nitsch RM, Gal A (2000) High prevalence of pathogenic mutations in patients with early-onset dementia detected by sequence analyses of four different genes. *Am J Hum Genet* 66:110-117.

31. Furukawa H, Kitamoto T, Hashiguchi H, Tateishi J (1996) A Japanese case of Creutzfeldt-Jakob disease with a point mutation in the prion protein gene at codon 210. *J Neurol Sci* 141: 120-122.

32. Gabizon R, Rosenmann H, Meiner Z, Kahana I, Kahana E, Shugart Y, Ott J, Prusiner SB (1993) Mutation and polymorphism of the prion protein gene in Libyan Jews with Creutzfeldt-Jakob disease. *Am J Hum Genet* 53: 828-835.

33. Gambetti P, Goldfarb L, Gabizon R, Montagna P, Lugaresi E, Piccardo P, Petersen RB, Parchi P, Chen SG, Capellari S, Ghetti B (1999) Inherited prion diseases. In: *Prion Biology and Diseases*, Cold Springs Harbor Laboratory Press, pp. 509-583.

34. Gabizon R, Telling G, Meiner Z, Halimi M, Kahana I, Prusiner SB (1996) Insoluble wild-type and protease-resistant mutant prion protein in brains of patients with inherited prion disease. *Nature Med* 2: 59-64.

35. Goldfarb LG, Brown P, McCombie WR, Goldgaber D, Swergold GD, Wills PR, Cervenakova L, Baron H, Gibbs CJ, Gajdusek DC (1993). Transmissible familial Creutzfeldt-Jakob disease associated with five, seven and eight extra octapeptide coding repeats in the PRNP gene. *Proc Natl Acad Sci U S A* 88: 10926-10930.

36. Goldfarb LG, Haltia M, Brown P, Nieto A, Kovanen J, McCombie WR, Trapp S, Gajdusek DC (1991) New mutation in scrapie amyloid precursor gene (at codon 178) in Finnish Creutzfeldt-Jakob kindred. *Lancet* 337: 425.

37. Goldfarb L, Korczyn A, Brown P, Chapman J, Gajdusek DC (1990) Mutation in codon 200 of scrapie amyloid precursor gene linked to Creutzfeldt-Jakob disease in Sephardic Jews of Libyan and non-Libyan origin. *Lancet* 336: 637-638.

38. Goldfarb LG, Brown P, Mitrova E, Cervenakova L, Goldin L, Korczyn AD, Chapman J, Galvez S, Cartier L, Rubenstein R, Gajdusek DC (1991) Creutzfeldt-Jacob disease associated with the PRNP codon 200Lys mutation: an analysis of 45 families. *Eur J Epidemiol* 7: 477-486.

39. Goldfarb LG, Brown P, Maltia M, Cathala F, McCombie WR, Kovanen J, Cervenakova L, Goldin L, Nieto A, Godec MS, Asher DM, Gajdusek DC (1992) Creutzfeldt-Jakob disease cosegregates with the codon 178Asn PRNP mutation in families of European origin. *Ann Neurol* 31: 274-281, 1992.

40. Goldfarb LG, Petersen RB, Tabaton M, Brown P, LeBlanc AC, Montagna P, Cortelli P, Julien J, Vital C, Pendlebury WW, Haltia M, Willis PR, Hauw JJ, McKeever PE, Monari L, B Schrank, Swergold GD, Autilio-Gambetti L, Gajdusek C, Lugaresi E, Gambetti P (1992) Fatal familial insomnia and familial Creutzfeldt-Jakob disease: disease phenotype determined by a DNA polymorphism. *Science* 258: 806-808.

41. Goldfarb LG, Brown P, Vrbovska A, Baron H, McCombie WR, Cathala F, Gibbs CJ, Gajdusek DC (1992) An insert mutation in the chromosome 20 amyloid precursor gene in a Gerstmann-Sträussler-Scheinker family. *J Neurol Sci*111: 189-194.

42. Goldfarb LG, Brown P, McCombie WR, Goldgaber D, Swergold GD, Wills PR, Cervenakova L, Baron H, Gibbs CJ, Gajdusek DC (1991) Transmissible familial Creutzfeldt-Jakob disease associated with five, seven and eight extra octapeptide coding repeats in the PRNP gene. *Proc Natl Acad Sci U S A* 88: 10926-10930.

43. Goldfarb LG, Cervenokava L, Brown P, Gajdusek DC (1996) Genotype-phenotype correlations in familial spongiform encephalopathies associated with insert mutations. *Transmissible Subacute Spongiform Encephalopathies: Prion Diseases* (eds. Court L. and Dodet B.), Elsevier, Paris, pp. 425-431.

44. Goldfarb LG, Mitrova E, Brown P, Toh BH, Gajdusek DC (1990) Mutation in codon 200 of scrappie amyloid protein gene in two clusters of Creutzfeldt-Jakob disease in Slovakia. *Lancet* 334: 514-515.

45. Hainfellner JA, Parchi P, Kitamoto T, Jarius C, Gambetti P, Budka H (1999) A novel phenotype in familial Creutzfeldt-Jakob disease: prion protein gene E200K mutation coupled with valine at codon 129 and type 2 protease-resistant prion protein. *Ann Neurol* 45:812-816.

46. Haltia M, Kovanen J, Van Crevel H, Bots GT, Stefanko S (1979) Familial Creutzfeldt-Jakob disease. *J Neurol Sci* 42: 381-389.

47. Head MW, Farquhar C, Mabbott NA, Fraser J (2001) Transmissible spongiform encephalopathies: pathogenic mechanisms and strategies for therapeutic intervention. *Expert Opinion on Therapeutic Targets* 5: 569-585.

48. Hitoshi S, Nagura H, Yamanouchi H, Kitamoto T (1993) Double mutations at codon 180 and codon 232 of the PRNP gene in an apparently sporadic case of Creutzfeldt-Jakob disease. *J Neurol Sci* 120: 208-212.

49. Hoque MZ, Kitamoto T, Furukawa H, Muramoto T, Tateishi J (1996) Mutation in the prion protein gene at codon 232 in Japanese patients with Creutzfeldt-Jakob disease: a clinicopathological, immunohistochemical and transmission study. *Acta Neuropathol* 92: 441-446.

50. Huang N, Marie SKN, Kok F, Nitrini R (2001) Familial Creutzfeldt-Jakob disease associated with a point mutation at codon 210 of the prion protein gene. *Arq Neuropsiquiatr* 59: 932-935.

51. Inoue I, Kitamoto T, Doh-ura K, Shii H, Goto I, Tateishi J (1994) Japanese family with Creutzfeldt-Jakob disease with codon 200 point mutation of the prion protein gene. *Neurology* 44: 299-301.

52. Isozaki E, Miyamoto K, Kagamihara Y, Hirose K, Tanabe H, Uchihara T, Oda M, Nagashima T (1994) CJD presenting as frontal lobe dementia associated with a 96 base pair insertion in the prion protein gene (in Japanese). *Dementia* 8: 363-371.

53. Jakob H, Pyrkosch W, Strube H (1950) Die erbliche Form der Creutzfeldt-Jakobschen Krankheit. (Familie Backer). *Arch Psychiat Nervenkrank* 184: 653-674.

54. Kahana E, Milton A, Braham J, Sofer D (1974) Creutzfeldt-Jakob disease: focus among Libyan Jews in Israel. *Science* 183: 90-91.

55. Kahana E, Zilber N, Abraham M (1991) Do Creutzfeldt-Jakob disease patients of Jewish Libyan origin have unique clinical features? *Neurology* 41: 1390-1392.

56. Kitamoto T, Tateishi J (1994) Human prion disease with variant prion protein. *Phil Trans R Soc Lond B* 343: 391-398.

57. Kirschbaum WR (1924) Zwei eigenartige Erkrankungen des Zentralnervensystems nach Art der spatischen Pseudosklerose (Jakob). *Z Neurol Pyschiat* 92: 175-220.

58. Kovanen J, Haltia M (1988) Descriptive epidemiology of Creutzfeldt-Jakob disease in Finland. *Acta Neurol Scand* 77: 474-480.

59. Krasemann S, Zerr I, Weber T, Poser S, Kretzschmar H, Hunsmann G, Bodemer W (1995) Prion disease associated with a novel nine octapeptide repeat insertion in the PRNP gene. *Mol Brain Res* 34: 173-176b.

60. Kretzschmar HA, Neumann M, Stavrou D (1995) Codon 178 mutation of the human prion protein gene in a German family (Backer family): sequencing data from 72-year old celloidin-embedded brain tissue. *Acta Neuropathol* 89: 96-98.

61. Ladogana A, Almonti S, Petraroli R, Giaccaglini E, Ciarmatori C, Liu QG, Bevivino S, Squitieri F, Pocchiari M (2001) Mutation of the PRNP gene at codon 211 in familial Creutzfeldt-Jakob disease. *Am J Med Genet* 103: 133-137.

62. Laplanche JL, Chatelain J, Launay JM, Gazengel C, Vidaud M (1990) Deletion in prion protein gene in a Moroccan family. *Nucleic Acids Res* 18: 6745.

63. Laplanche JL, Delasnerie-Laupretre N, Brandel JP, Chatelain J, Beaudry P, Alperovitch A, Launay JM (1994) Molecular genetics of prion diseases in France. *Neurology* 44: 2347-2351.

64. Laplanche J, Delasnerie-Laupretre N, Brandel JP, Dussaucy M, Launay JM (1995) Two novel insertions in the prion protein gene in patients with late-onset dementia. *Hum Mol Gen* 4: 1109-1111.

65. Laplanche JL, Hachimi KH, Durieux I, Thuillet P, Defebvre L, Delasnerie-Laupretre N, Peoc'h K, Foncin JF, Destee A (1999) Prominent psychiatric features and early onset in an inherited prion disease with a new insertional mutation in the prion protein gene. *Brain* 122: 2375-2386.

66. Masters CL, Gajdusek DC,Gibbs CJ Jr (1981) The familial occurrence of Creutzfeldt-Jakob disease and Alzheimer's disease. *Brain* 104: 535-558.

67. Mastrianni JA, Iannicola C, Myers RM, DeArmond S, Prusiner SB 81996) Mutation of the prion protein gene at codon 208 in familial Creutzfeldt-Jakob disease. *Neurology* 47: 1305-1312.

68. Mastrianni JA, Capellari S, Telling GC, Han D, Bosque P, Prusiner SB, DeArmond SJ 82001) Inherited prion disease caused by the V210I mutation: Transmission to transgenic mice. *Neurology* 57: 2198-2205.

69. Medori R, Tritschler HJ, LeBlanc A, Villare F, Manetto V, Chen HY, Xue R, Leal S, Montagna P, Cortelli P, Tinuper P, Avoni P, Mochi M, Baruzzi A, Hauw JJ, Ott J, Lugaresi E, Autilio-Gambetti L, Gambetti P (1992) Fatal familial insomnia is a prion disease with a mutation at codon 178 of the prion gene. *New Eng J Med* 326: 444-449.

70. Meggendorfer F (1930) Klinische und genealogische Beobachtungen bei einem Fall von spastischen Pseudokosklerose Jakobs. *Z Neurol Psychiat* 128: 337-341.

71. Mizushima S, Ishii K, Nishimaru T (1994) A case of presenile dementia with a 168 base pair insertion in prion protein gene. (in Japanese). *Dementia* 8: 380-390.

72. Monari L, Chen SG, Brown P, Parchi P, Petersen RB, Mikol J, Gray F, Cortelli P, Montagna P, Ghetti B, Goldfarb LG, Gajdusek DC, Lugaresi E, Gambetti P, Autilio-Gambetti L (1994) Fatal familial insomnia and familial Creutzfeldt-Jakob disease: Different prion proteins determined by a DNA polymorphism. *Proc Natl Acad Sci U S A* 91: 2839-2842.

73. Moore RC, Xiang F, Monaghan J, Han D, Zhang Z, Edstrom L, Anvret M, Prusiner SB (2001) Huntington disease phenocopy is a familial prion disease. *Am J Hum Genet* 1385-1388.

74. Neufeld MY, Josiphov J, Korczyn AD (1992) Demyelinating peripheral neuropathy in Creutzfeldt-Jakob disease. *Muscle & Nerve* 15: 1234-1239.

75. Nicholl D, Windl O, de Silva R, Sawcer S, Dempster M, Ironside JW, Estibeiro JP, Yuill GM, Lathe R, Will RG (1995) Inherited Creutzfeldt-Jakob disease in a British family associated with a novel 144 base pair insertion of the prion protein gene. *J Neurol Neurosurg Psychiatry* 58: 65-69.

76. Nitrini R, Rosemberg S, Passos-Bueno MR, da Silva LS, Iughetti P, Papadopoulos M, Carrilho PM, Caramelli P, Albrecht S, Zatz M, LeBlanc A (1997) Familial spongiform encephalopathy associated with a novel prion protein gene mutation. *Ann Neurol* 42:138-146.

77. Nitrini R, Teixeira da Silva LS, Rosemberg S, Caramelli P, Carrilho PE, Iughetti P, Passos-Bueno MR, Zatz M, Albrecht S, LeBlanc A (2001) Prion disease resembling frontotemporal dementia and parkinsonism linked to chromosome 17. *Arq Neuropsiquiatr* 59: 161-164.

78. Oda T, Kitamoto T, Tateishi J, Mitsuhashi T, Iwabuchi K, Haga C, Oguni E, Kato Y, Tominaga I, Yanai K, Kashima H, Kogure T, Hori K, Ogino K (1995) Prion disease with 144 base pair insertion in a Japanese family line. *Acta Neuropathol* 90: 80-86.

79. Owen F, Poulter M, Lofthouse R, Collinge J, Crow TJ, Risby D, Baker HF, Ridley RM, Hsiao K, Prusiner SB (1989) Insertion in prion protein gene in familial Creutzfeldt-Jakob disease. *Lancet* 1: 51-52.

80. Palmer MS, Mahal SP, Campbell TA, Hill AF, Sidle KCL, Laplanche JL, Collinge J (1993) Deletions in the prion protein gene are not associated with CJD. *Human Molec Genet* 2: 541-544.

81. Parchi P, Castellani R, Capellari S, Ghetti B, Young K, Chen SG, Farlow M, Dickson DW, Sima AAF, Trojanowski JQ, Petersen RB, Gambetti P (1996) Molecular basis of phenotypic variability in sporadic Creutzfeldt-Jakob disease. *Ann Neurol* 39: 669-680.

82. Parchi P, Giese A, Capellari S, Brown P, Schulz-Schaeffer W, Windl O, Zerr I, Budka H, Kopp N, Piccardo P, Poser S, Rojiani A, Streichemberger N, Julien J, Vital C, Ghetti B, Gambetti P, Kretzschmar H (1996) Creutzfeldt-Jakob disease associated with the 178Asn mutation in the prion protein gene: Neuropathological and molecular features. *J Neuropathol Exp Neurol* 55: 121.

83. Parchi P, Giese A, Capellari S, Brown P, Schulz-Schaeffer W, Windl O, Zerr I, Budka H, Kopp N, Piccardo P, Poser S, Rojiani A, Streichemberger N, Julien J, Vital C, Ghetti B, Gambetti P, Kretzschmar H (1999) Classification of sporadic Creutzfeldt-Jakob disease based on molecular and phenotypic analysis of 300 subjects. *Ann Neurol* 46: 224-233.

84. Parchi P, Capellari S, Brown P (1999) Molecular and clinico-pathologic phenotypic variability in genetic Creutzfeldt-Jakob disease. *Neurology* 52 (suppl 2): A323.

85. Parchi P, Zou W, Wang W, Brown P, Capellari S, Ghetti B, Kopp N, Schulz-Schaeffer WJ, Kretzschmar HA, Head MW, Ironside JW, Gambetti P, Chen SG (2000) Genetic influence on the structural variations of the abnormal prion protein. *Proc Natl Acad Sci U S A* 97: 10168-1017.

86. Pastore M, Castellani RJ, Chin S, Hua Z, Bell K, Chin SS, Gambetti P (2002) Creutzfeldt-Jakob desease associated with the novel R148H prion protein gene mutation. *J Neuropathol Exp Neurol* 61: 491.

87. Peoc'h K, Manivet P, Beaudry P, Attane F, Besson G, Hannequin D, Delasnerie-Laupretre N, Laplanche

JL (2000) Identification of three novel mutations (E196K, V203I, E211Q) in the prion protein gene (PRNP) in inherited prion diseases with Creutzfeldt-Jakob disease phenotype. *Hum Mutat* 15: 482.

88. Petersen RB, Parchi P, Richardson SL, Urig CB, Gambetti P (1996) Effect of the D178N mutation and the codon 129 polymorphism on the metabolism of the prion protein. *J Biol Chem* 271: 1266-1268.

89. Piccardo P, Dlouhy SR, Young K (1999) Creutzfeldt Jakob disease (CJD) with prion protein gene (PRNP) V210I mutation. *J Neuropathol Exp Neurol* 58: 166.

90. Pocchiari M, Salvatore M, Cutruzzola F, Genuardi M, Allocatelli CT, Masullo C, Macchi G, Alema G, Galgani S, Xi YG, Petraroli R, Silvestrini MC, Brunori M. (1993) A new point mutation of the prion protein gene in Creutzfeldt-Jakob disease. *Ann Neurol* 34: 802-807.

91. Prusiner SB (1999) Development of the Prion Concept. In: *Prion Biology and Diseases.* Prusiner SB (ed), Cold Springs Harbor Laboratory Press, pp. 67-112.

92. Poulter M, Baker HF, Frith CD, Leach M, Lofthouse R, Ridley RM, Shah T, Owen F, Collinge J, Brown G, Hardy J, Mullan MJ, Harding AE, Bennett C, Doshi R, Crow TH (1992) Inherited prion disease with 144 base pair gene insertion. 1. Genealogical and molecular studies. *Brain* 115: 675-685.

93. Puoti G, Rossi G, Giaccone G, Awan T, Lievens PM, Defanti CA, Tagliavini F, Bugiani O (2000) Polymorphism at codon 129 of PRNP affects the phenotypic expression of Creutzfeldt-Jakob disease linked to the E200K mutation. *Ann Neurol* 48: 269-270.

94. Ripoll L, Laplanche JL, Salzmann M, Jouvet A, Planques B, Dussaucy M, Chatelain J, Beaudry P, Launay JM (1993) A new point mutation in the prion protein gene at codon 210 in Creutzfeldt-Jakob disease. *Neurology* 43: 1934-1938.

95. Roos R, Gajdusek DC, Gibbs CJ (1973) The clinical characteristics of transmissible Creutzfeldt-Jacob disease. *Brain* 96: 1-20.

96. Rosenmann H, Vardi J, Finkelstein Y, Chapman J, Gabizon R (1998) Identification in Israel of 2 Jewish Creutzfeldt-Jakob disease patients with a 178 mutation at their PrP gene. *Acta Neurol Scand* 97: 184-187.

97. Rossi G, Giaccone G, Giampaolo L, Iussich S, Puoti G, Frigo M, Cavaletti G, Frattola L, Bugiani O, Tagliavini F (2000) Creutzfeldt-Jakob disease with a novel four extra-repeat insertional mutation in the PrP gene. *Neurology* 55: 405-410.

98. Sadeh M, Chagnac Y, Goldhammer Y (1990) Creutzfeldt-Jakob disease associated with peripheral neuropathy. *Isr J Med Sci* 26: 220-222.

99. Shyu WC, Hsu YD, Kao MC, Tsao WL (1996) Panencephalitic Creutzfeldt-Jakob disease in a Chinese family. Unusual presentation with PrP codon 210 mutation and identification by PCR-SSCP. *J Neurol Sci* 143: 176-180.

100. Simon ES, Kahana E, Chapman J, Treves TA, Gabizon R, Rosenmann H, Zilber N, Korczyn AD (2000) Creutzfeldt-Jakob disease profile in patients homozygous for the PRNP E200K mutation. *Ann Neurol* 47: 257-260.

101. Skworc KH, Windl O, Schulz-Schaeffer WJ, Giese A, Bergk J, Nagele A, Vieregge P, Zerr I I, Poser S, Kretzschmar HA (1999) Familial Creutzfeldt-Jakob disease with a novel 120-bp insertion in the prion protein gene. *Ann Neurol* 46: 693-700.

102. Stender A (1930) Weitere Beitrage zum Kapitel "Spastische Pseudosklerose Jakobs." *Z Neurol Psychiat* 128: 528-543.

103. Taratuto AL, Piccardo P, Reich EG, Chen SG, Sevlever G, Schultz M, Luzzi AA, Rugiero M, Abecasis G, Endelman M, Garcia AM, Capellari S, Xie Z, Lugaresi E, Gambetti P, Dlouhy SR, Ghetti B (2002) Insomnia associated with thalamic involvement in E200k Creutzfeldt-Jakob disease. *Neurology* 58: 362-367.

104. van Gool WA, Hensels GW, Hoogerwaard EM, Wiezer JHA, Wesseling P, Bolhuis PA (1995) Hypokinesia and presenile dementia in a Dutch family with a novel insertion in the prion protein gene. *Brain* 118: 1565-1571.

105. Vallat JM, Dumas M, Corvisier N, Leboutet MJ, Loubet A, Dumas P, Cathala F (1983) Familial Creutzfeldt-Jakob disease with extensive degeneration of white matter. *J Neurol Sci* 61: 261-275.

106. Vital C, Gray F, Vital A, Parchi P, Capellari S, Petersen RB, Ferrer X, Jarnier D, Julien J, Gambetti P (1998) Prion encephalopathy with insertion of octapeptide repeats: the number of repeats determines the type of cerebellar deposits. *Neuropathol Appl Neurobiol* 24:125-130.

107. Windl O, Dempster M, Estibeiro JP, Lathe R, de Silva R, Esmonde T, Will R, Springbett A, Campbell TA, Sidle KC, Palmer MS, Collinge J (1996) Genetic basis of Creutzfeldt-Jakob disease in the United Kingdom: a systematic analysis of predisposing mutations and allelic variation in the PRNP gene. *Hum Genet* 98: 259-264.

108. Windl O, Giese A, Schulz-Schaeffer W, Zerr I, Skworc K, Arendt S, Oberdieck C, Bodemer M, Poser S, Kretzschmar HA (1999) Molecular genetics of human prion diseases in Germany. *Hum Genet* 105:244-252.

Iatrogenic Prion Disorders

Maura N. Ricketts
Paola Pergami

CJD	Creutzfeldt-Jakob disease
GSS	Gerstmann-Straussler-Scheinker
hGH	human growth hormone
PrP	prion protein
sCJD	sporadic CJD
TSE	transmissible spongiform encephalopathy
vCJD	variant CJD

Definition

Creutzfeldt-Jakob disease (CJD) following exposure to infectious material through the use of human cadaveric-derived pituitary hormones, dural and corneal homografts, and contaminated neurosurgical instruments. CJD can also occur after oral exposure to contaminated human brain (chapter 6. 5) or bovine spongiform encephalopathy tainted products (chapter 6.2.4).

Synonyms and Historical Annotations

A letter written by Hadlow (16) likening kuru with scrapie, a transmissible disease of sheep, prompted Gajdusek and Gibbs to inoculate primates with materials taken from the brains of patients with kuru, leading to the discovery that kuru was transmissible (13). The similarity of the neuropathology of kuru and CJD led to a parallel experiment that demonstrated the infectivity of brain tissue of persons dying from CJD (14) and subsequent discovery of the first cases of iatrogenic CJD.

Epidemiology

Incidence and prevalence. Iatrogenic transmission is a rare event. Approximately 250 episodes of iatrogenic CJD have been identified (9). Almost all have been as a result of exposure to contaminated neurosurgical instruments during neurosurgical exposures, cadaveric dura mater implanted onto the surface of the brain (one commercial product, Lyodura, has been identified more frequently than any other), and inoculated cadaver extracted human growth hormone (hGH) (Table 1). Human exposure potential as opposed to and distinct from transmission is wide; however, transmission has been confirmed in only specific and limited circumstances, as described below. The evidence supporting a causal relationship between CJD and pericardial graft on a perforated eardrum (25), and after liver transplant (12) remains weak or absent. No reports of human TSE transmission from dental exposures have been identified. The hazard of transfusion transmission of human TSEs, and consequent concerns regarding the infectivity of blood deserves consideration; however, transfusion transmission of sporadic CJD (sCJD) is unlikely (7). Standard measures in handling blood or bloody tissues do not require modification to avoid sCJD. However, regarding vCJD, some countries with sufficient resources are revising their infection control guidelines (notably the United Kingdom) and blood donation guidelines to avoid this theoretical risk.

Sex and age distribution. In dural cases, the mean age at onset is 37.7-years-old, with male to female ratio of 1:1.18. The growth hormone cases are generally children, with a mean age at onset of 9.6 years and a male to female ratio of 1:0.26 (19).

Risk factors. Homozygosity of the PrP gene at codon 129 is over-represented in CJD and it has been suggested that infection occurs more easily when molecules with identical amino acid sequences are involved (22), and the incubation period may be shorter. However, investigation is ongoing and the epidemiologic evidence is inconsistent (9).

	Surgical procedures				Hormone therapy	
	Dura mater grafts	Surgical instruments	Stereotactic EEG needles	Corneal transplants	Growth hormone	Gonadotropin
Argentine	1					
Australia	4				1	4
Austria	1					
Brazil					1	
Canada	4					
Croatia	1					
France	8	1			74	
Germany	4			1		
Holland	2				1	
Italy	4					
Japan	67			1		
New Zealand	1				5	
Spain	6					
Switzerland	1		2			
Thailand	1					
United Kingdom	6	4			35	
United States	3			1	22	
Total	114	5	2	3	139	4

Table 1. Number of published cases of iatrogenic CJD. With permission from Brown P, Preece M, Brandel J-P et al. (2000) Iatrogenic Creutzfeldt-Jakob disease at the millennium. *Neurology* 55:1075-1081.

Infectivity category	Tissues, secretions, and excretions
High infectivity	Brain Spinal cord Eye
Low infectivity	CSF Kidney Liver Lung Lymph nodes/spleen Placenta
No detectable infectivity	Adipose tissue Adrenal gland Gingival tissue Heart muscle Intestine Peripheral nerve Prostate Skeletal muscle Testis Thyroid gland Blood Tears Nasal mucous Saliva Sweat Serous exudate Milk Semen Urine Faeces

Table 2. Estimated distribution of infectivity in the human body (5).

Clinical Features

The incubation period for iatrogenic CJD can be long—up to 30 years and never less than 12 months. However, the incubation period after intracerebral exposure is shorter (12-28 months) when compared to peripheral exposures (5-30 years for growth hormone, median 12 years). Additionally, the route of infection seems to influence the clinical presentation, with usually cerebellar onset in peripheral infections (including dura mater implants onto the brain surface) and usually dementing onset in intracerebral infections (9).

Neuropathology

The neuropathological features of most dural cases are similar to those of sporadic CJD (20, 21). One case has also been described with the panencephalitic form of the disease (28). A distinct subtype has now been described with florid plaques similar to those observed in variant CJD (18, 24). Growth-hormone related cases show the typical features of CJD. The changes are often severe, resulting in cerebral and cerebellar atrophy. In addition, there is massive loss of cerebellar granule cells and kuru-type plaques throughout the brain (6, 21). Immunohistochemical staining also shows extensive PrP deposits in the spinal cord (15).

Biochemistry

The prion banding pattern in iatrogenic CJD is similar to that of sporadic cases and both isoforms are represented (23). A suggestion was made that iatrogenic disease due to peripheral inoculation may be associated with a distinct PrP isoform, but this result has not been reproduced (11, 23)

Differential Diagnosis

Some cases of CJD associated with dural transplants have been shown to have florid plaques similar to those seen in variant CJD, as mentioned above. Care should be taken to differentiate those cases from vCJD. Western blots are invaluable to demonstrate the presence of the unique isoform present in vCJD or the usual Type 1 or Type 2 banding patterns seen in sporadic and iatrogenic CJD. For further details, see chapter 6.2.4 on vCJD and chapter 6.2.1 on sCJD.

Pathogenesis

Investigations conducted using brain and other tissues of persons with sporadic, familial, iatrogenic CJD, and GSS into non-human primates demonstrated that infectivity was present in a number of human tissues although clearly concentrated in some (8). Table 2 assigns tissues to high, low and no detectable infectivity levels, however, it is important to note that the grading was based upon the frequency with which infectivity was detected rather than upon quantitative assays of the level of infectivity, for which data are incomplete (27). In addition, some of the categorization was based upon experimentally infected animals. Scrapie (not CJD) has been transmitted via dental pulp and blood only in experimental animals (17). To date, sCJD is the only human TSE linked to iatrogenic transmission. While the rarity of non-sCJD (less than 1 per 10 million population) and consequent extremely rare iatrogenic exposures contributes to this, it is possible there are variations in transmission potentials. There is a growing body of evidence supporting concerns that the risk of iatrogenic vCJD may be higher than for other human TSEs. Specifically, vCJD is known to be accompanied by detectable PrPSc in peripheral tissues (including at least spleen, appendix, peripheral lymph nodes, dorsal root ganglia, and trigeminal ganglia) (10, 26), unlike the other human TSEs. As a result, measures taken to avoid iatrogenic vCJD may be more stringent that those applied to sCJD.

Infection Control Guidelines

A number of countries and organisations have developed guidelines to prevent transmission of the human TSEs. The well-recognised resistance of the agent to conventional decontamination techniques forces infection control methods to be more stringent, and to provide guidance on situations where the risk is theoretical. The reader can find further information in the guidelines prepared by various organisations (1-5).

Future Directions

Recognition of the role of iatrogenic transmission of CJD provided immediate options to prevent further spread through these routes. Most countries of the world no longer use human derived growth hormone, hence it can be expected that hGH associated CJD will disappear over time. Dura mater-associated CJD can be effectively managed through better donor screening and increasing use of synthetic products; some countries use exclusively synthetic dura mater. Donor screening is the only option available for cornea transplants; however, it is possible to improve transplantation safety for both cornea and dura mater transplants. More difficult to resolve are the problems arising concerning ocular surgery and dental surgery. Infection control guidelines provide recommendations on cleaning exposed equipment; however, some pieces of equipment are unable to tolerate exposure to the heat/chemical combinations required to effectively decontaminate them. Some institutions are opting to discard equipment to avoid the theoretical risks of transmission through certain surgical procedures; in others, the use of disposable instruments have led to medical problems. Clearly, further investigation including experimental work is required to provide clear guidance. Regarding vCJD, the horizon is clouded. The risk of potential secondary transmission has led to extensive changes within the United Kingdom regarding surgical procedures and transfusion policies. Whether these measures will be adopted world-wide will certainly depend upon emerging information about the extent of BSE and vCJD globally.

References

1. Creutzfeldt-Jakob disease and other human transmissible spongiform encephalopathies: guidelines on patient management and infection control. *http://www.health.gov.as/pubhlth/strateg/communic/review*

2. Creutzfeldt-Jakob disease:guidance for healthcare workers. *http://www.doh.gov.uk/cjd/cjd_pubs.htm*

3. Questions and answers regarding Creuztfeldt-Jakob disease infection-control practices. http://*www.cdc.gov/ncidod/diseases/cjd/cjd_inf_ctrl_qa.htm*

4. Transmissible spongiform encephalopathy agents: safe working and the prevention of infection. *http://www.official-documents.co.uk/documents/doh/spongifm/report.htm*

5. WHO infection control guidelines for transmissible spongiform encephalopathies. *http://www.who.int/emc-documents/tse/docs/whocdscsr2003.pdf*

6. Billette de Villemeur T, Gelot A, Deslys J, Dormont D, Duyckaert C, Jardin L, Denni J, Robain O (1994) Iatrogenic Creutzfeldt-Jakob disease in three growth hormone recipients: a neuropathological study. *Neuropath Appl Neurobiol* 20:111-117.

7. Brown P, Cervenakova L, McShane LM, Barber P, Rubenstein R, Drohan WN (1999) Further studies of blood infectivity in an experimental model of transmissible spongiform encephalopathy, with an explanation of why blood components do not transmit Creutzfeldt-Jakob disease in humans. *Transfusion* 39:1169-1178.

8. Brown P, Gibbs C, Rodgers-Johnson P, Asher DM, Sulima MP, Bacote A, Goldfarb LG, Gajdusek DC (1994) Human spongiform encephalopathy: the National Institute of Health series of 300 cases of experimentally transmitted disease. *Ann Neurol* 35:513-529.

9. Brown P, Preece M, Brandel JP, Sato T, McShane L, Zerr I, Fletcher A, Will RG, Pocchiari M, Cashman NR, d'Aignaux JH, Cervenakova L, Fradkin J, Schonberger LB, Collins SJ (2000) Iatrogenic Creutzfeldt-Jakob disease at the millennium. *Neurology* 55:1075-1081.

10. Bruce ME, McConnell I, Will RG, Ironside JW (2001) Detection of variant Creutzfeldt-Jakob disease infectivity in extraneural tissues. *Lancet* 358:208-209.

11. Collinge J, Sidle KCL, Meads J, Ironside J, Hill AF (1996) Molecular analysis of prion strain variation and the aetiology of "new variant" CJD. *Nature* 383:685-690.

12. Creange A, Gray F, Cesaro P, Adle-Biassette H, Duvoux C, Cherqui D, Bell J, Parchi P, Gambetti P, Degos JD (1995) Creutzfeldt-Jakob disease after liver transplantation. *Ann Neurol* 38:269-272.

13. Gajdusek DC, Gibbs CJ, Alpers M (1966) Experimental transmission of a Kuru-like syndrome to chimpanzees. *Nature* 209:794-796.

14. Gibbs CJ, Jr., Gajdusek DC, Asher DM, Alpers MP, Beck E, Daniel PM, Matthews WB (1968) Creutzfeldt-Jakob disease (spongiform encephalopathy): transmission to the chimpanzee. *Science* 161:388-389.

15. Goodbrand I, Ironside J, Nicolson D, Bell J (1995) Prion protein accumulation in the spinal cords of patients with sporadic and growth hormone associated Creutzfeldt-Jakob disease. *NeurosciLett* 183:127-130.

16. Hadlow W (1959) Scrapie and Kuru. *Lancet* ii:289-290.

17. Ingrosso L, Pisani F, Pocchiari M (1999) Trasmission of the 263K scrapie strain by the dental route. *J Gen Virol* 80:3043-3047.

18. Kimura K, Nonaka A, Tashiro H, Yaginuma M, Shimokawa R, Okeda R, Yamada M (2001) Atypical form of dural graft associated Creutzfeldt-Jakob disease: report of a postmortem case with review of the literature. *J Neurol Neurosurg Psychiatry* 70:696-699.

19. Lang C, Heckmann J, Neundörfer B (1998) Creuztfeldt-Jakob disease via dural and corneal transplants. *J Neurol Sci* 160:128-139.

20. Martinez-Lage JF, Poza M, Sola J, Tortosa JG, Brown P, Cervenakova L, Esteban JA, Mendoza A (1994) Accidental transmission of Creutzfeldt-Jakob disease by dural cadaveric grafts. *J Neurol Neurosurg Psychiatry* 57:1091-1094.

21. Mikol J (1999) Acquired forms of Creutzfeldt-Jakob disease. *Clin Exp Pathol* 47:145-151.

22. Palmer MS, Dryden AJ, Hughes JT, Collinge J (1991) Homozygous prion protein genotype predisposes to sporadic Creutzfeldt-Jakob disease. *Nature* 352:340-342.

23. Parchi P, Capellari S, Chen SG, Petersen RB, Gambetti P, Kopp N, Brown P, Kitamoto T, Tateishi J, Giese A, Kretzschmar H (1997) Typing prion isoforms. *Nature* 386:232-234.

24. Shimizu S, Hoshi K, Muramoto T, Homma M, Ironside JW, Kuzuhara S, Sato T, Yamamoto T, Kitamoto T (1999) Creutzfeldt-Jakob disease with florid-type plaques after cadaveric dura mater grafting. *Arch Neurol* 56:357-362.

25. Tange RA, Troost D, Limburg M (1990) Progressive fatal dementia (Creutzfeldt-Jakob disease) in a patient who received homograft tissue for tympanic membrane closure. *Eur Arch Otorhinolaryngol* 247:199-201.

26. Wadsworth JD, Joiner S, Hill AF, Campbell TA, Desbruslais M, Luthert PJ, Collinge J (2001) Tissue distribution of protease resistant prion protein in variant Creutzfeldt-Jakob disease using a highly sensitive immunoblotting assay. *Lancet* 358:171-180.

27. WHO, Infection control guidelines for transmissible spongiform encephalopathies. Report of a WHO consultation. 1999, World Health Organization: Geneva

28. Yamada M, Itoh Y, Suematsu N, Matsushita M, Otomo E (1997) Panencephalopathic type of Creutzfeldt-Jakob disease associated with cadaveric dura mater graft. *J Neurol Neurosurg Psychiatry* 63:524-527.

Variant Creutzfeldt-Jakob Disease

James W. Ironside
Mark W. Head
Robert G. Will

BSE	bovine spongiform encephalopathy
PRNP	prion protein gene
PrP	prion protein
sCJD	sporadic Creutzfeldt-Jakob disease
vCJD	variant Creutzfeldt-Jakob disease

Definition

Variant Creutzfeldt-Jakob disease is a novel form of human prion disease first reported in 1996 (41). Most cases have occurred in the United Kingdom, predominantly in young individuals (mean age 27 years at onset) with a relatively long duration of clinical illness (median 14 months), which is characterised by psychiatric symptoms at onset followed by sensory abnormalities, movement disorders (including myoclonus and chorea), and dementia with terminal akinetic mutism. The neuropathology is characterised by the presence of large numbers of florid plaques in the cerebral and cerebellar cortex, spongiform change which is most prominent in the caudate nucleus and putamen, marked posterior thalamic gliosis and extensive deposition of PrP^{res}, particularly in the form of florid plaques, cluster plaques, and amorphous pericellular and perivascular deposits. Biochemically, variant CJD is characterised by a prion protein isotype which resembles that found in bovine spongiform encephalopathy (BSE) in that it has a predominant diglycosylated band on Western blotting, with mobility of the unglycosylated band at around 19kD. All patients in whom genetic investigations have been performed have been methionine homozygotes at codon 129 in the prion protein gene (*PRNP*).

Synonyms and Historical Annotations

The first 2 cases of variant CJD were reported as unusual cases of Creutzfeldt-Jakob disease in teenagers in the United Kingdom (2, 4). Subsequent investigations by the National CJD Surveillance Unit in the United Kingdom over the following 6 months indicated that this was a novel form of human prion disease and the clinical and pathological features in 10 patients were fully described in 1996 as a new variant form of CJD in the United Kingdom (41). Since then, the disorder has become commonly known as variant CJD, and although most cases have occurred in the United Kingdom, there have been small numbers of cases identified in individuals in Europe and North America. Extensive retrospective studies in the United Kingdom and Europe and a detailed study of death certificate data in the United Kingdom has revealed that variant CJD is a novel form of human prion disease; this was accepted at a WHO consultation in 1996 (44).

Epidemiology

Incidence and prevalence. At the time of writing 130 cases of variant CJD have been identified in the United Kingdom, 6 cases in France, one in Italy, one in Ireland, one in Canada, and one in the United States. Since the identification of the first 10 cases from 1995 to 1996, analysis of the incidence of disease onset and death has shown a significant increasing trend in the number of cases since June 2000 (Table 1) (1). This trend does not appear to be maintained throughout 2002, but it is not known whether these rates will change again. Considerable efforts have been made to model the occurrence and likely future numbers of variant CJD cases in the United Kingdom; current estimates range between a few hundred to over 150000 cases (17, 27). There are relatively more cases of variant CJD in northern United Kingdom (Scotland and northern England) in terms of cases per million of the population in comparison with the southern United Kingdom (central and southern England and Wales) (12). Furthermore, a cluster of 5 variant CJD cases has been identified in Leicestershire over a period of 4 years (12). This statistically significant group of cases has been the subject of epidemiological studies, which suggested a common source of exposure to the BSE agent through local butchering practices (9).

The predominant occurrence of variant CJD in the United Kingdom, the country with the highest incidence of bovine spongiform encephalopathy (BSE), suggests a causal link with BSE (41). The most likely hypothesis is dietary exposure through past consumption of BSE-contaminated meat products, but other possibilities include occupational exposure (for example in veterinarians and slaughterhouse workers or butchers who handle BSE-infected carcasses), and exposure to medicinal products in which cattle materials are used.

Sex and age distribution. The age-specific incidence of variant CJD in comparison with sporadic CJD is shown in Figure 1. There seems to be no significant differences in the incidence of this disease in males and

Year	Onsets	Deaths
1994	8	0
1995	10	3
1996	11	10
1997	14	10
1998	17	18
1999	29	15
2000	24	28
2001	16	20
2002	1	17
2003	0	3
Totals	130	124

Table 1. Onsets and deaths of variant CJD cases per annum in UK (to February 2003).

females. Although the mean age at onset and death have remained relatively constant since variant CJD has been identified, the age range of affected patients has widened with the youngest patient developing the illness at age 12 and dying at age 14 years, and the oldest becoming ill and subsequently dying at age 74 years. It is uncertain as to whether this single case in the elderly is truly the first case within this age range or whether other cases will occur in the future (30).

Risk factors. Epidemiological and experimental evidence (reviewed below) have indicated that the transmissible agent from variant CJD is identical to the BSE agent, and resembles the agent identified in other BSE-related illnesses, including feline spongiform encephalopathy and a series of novel spongiform encephalopathies described in exotic ungulates (6, 7). The transmissible agents in all these disorders show similar incubation periods and patterns of brain pathology on transmission to inbred strains of mice or transgenic mice, and also show a similar biochemical profile on Western blot analysis for PrP^{res}. The risk factors for variant CJD are summarised in Table 2. These may be considered as provisional, as a case control study has been set up to identify other risk factors for this disorder. There is no epidemiological evidence to suggest that scrapie (the long-standing prion disease occurring in sheep and goats) is pathogenic for man (5).

Genetics

None of the patients with variant CJD in whom genetic analysis has been undertaken has revealed any pathogenic mutations in the *PRNP* (46). All patients so far have been methionine homozygotes at codon 129 in the *PRNP*, in contrast to the frequency of this genotype in the normal population and in sporadic CJD (Table 3). There is no evidence for familial occurrence of variant CJD. Although experimental studies have suggested that other genes may well influence the

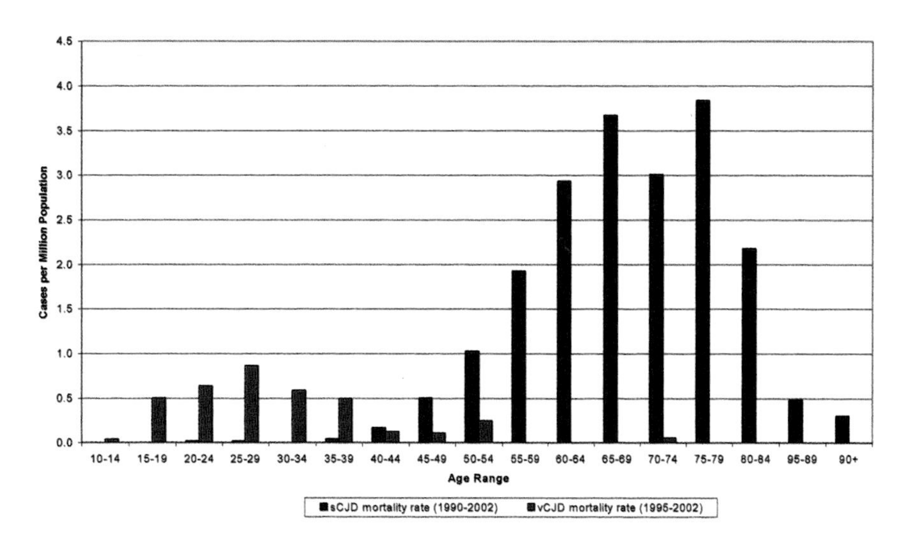

Figure 1. Age distribution of sporadic CJD (blue) and variant CJD (red) patients in the UK, 1990-2002.

occurrence of prion diseases in mammals, the nature of these other genes in humans is unknown. Apolipoprotein E genetic polymorphisms do not seem to be associated significantly with variant CJD.

Clinical Features

Signs and symptoms. Most patients suffer from early and persistent psychiatric symptoms of which the most common are depression, anxiety and withdrawal (42). Patients without frank psychiatric symptoms often exhibit emotional lability for some months before the onset of neurological symptoms and signs (44). Many patients have been thought initially to be suffering from a purely psychiatric disorder and have been treated with psychiatric medication, particularly antidepressants. Clear-cut neurological symptoms usually develop around 6 months after the onset of psychiatric symptoms, but persistent sensory symptoms and forgetfulness have been present from the onset of the illness in a significant minority of cases (42). The most striking of the sensory symptoms is persistent dysaesthesia or paraesthesia which is often painful, including patients suffering from limb pain not associated with other sensory abnormalities. Other early neurological symptoms include dysarthria, dysgeusia and visual abnormalities, including paralysis of upward gaze.

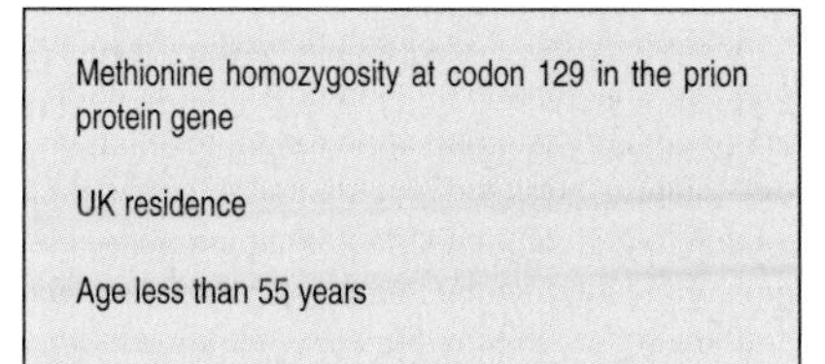
Methionine homozygosity at codon 129 in the prion protein gene

UK residence

Age less than 55 years

Table 2. Risk factors for variant CJD.

Codon 129 genotype (%)	MM	MV	VV
Normal population	37	51	12
Sporadic CJD	74	15	11
Variant CJD	100	0	0

Table 3. Codon 129 *PRNP* genotypes in CJD.

Ataxia is a prominent feature in all cases of variant CJD and involuntary movements have been noted in all cases in which full clinical information is available. Ataxia may develop during the predominantly psychiatric phase and has sometimes been attributed to the complications of medication (42). Severe ataxia with falls occurs in all cases at a later stage in the illness and may be accompanied by a range of involuntary movements including myoclonus, chorea and dystonia. The terminal stages of variant CJD are similar to those of sporadic CJD with progressive cognitive impairment resulting in dementia and often akinetic mutism. Death occurs at a median of 14 months from disease onset (range 6-39 months).

Since the initial clinical features for variant CJD are non-specific, there is a

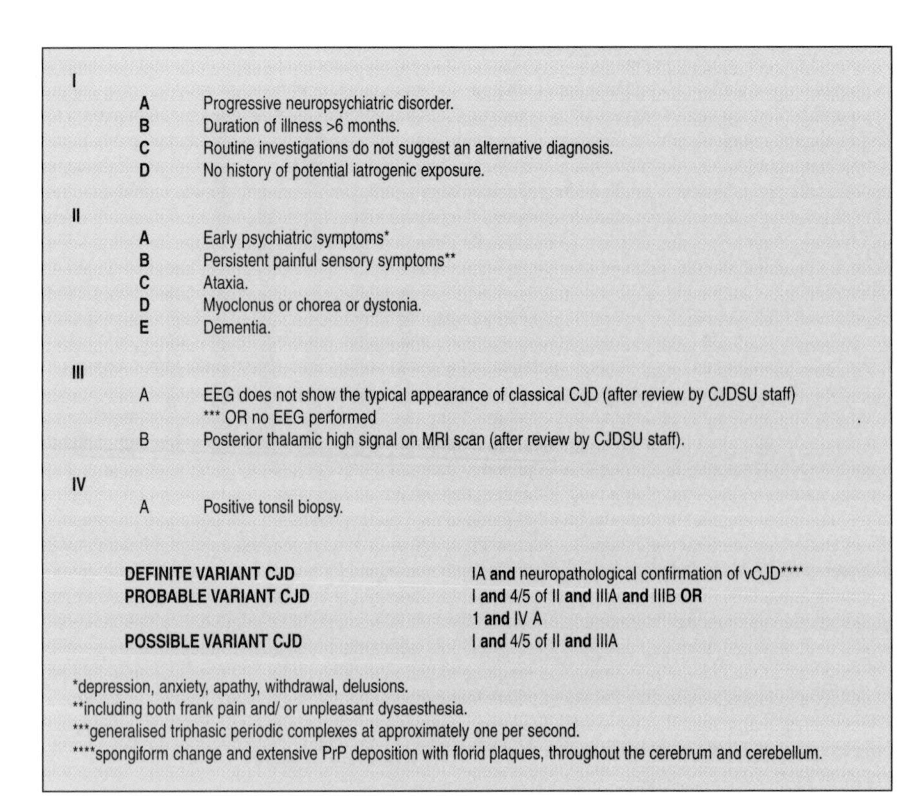

I		
	A	Progressive neuropsychiatric disorder.
	B	Duration of illness >6 months.
	C	Routine investigations do not suggest an alternative diagnosis.
	D	No history of potential iatrogenic exposure.
II		
	A	Early psychiatric symptoms*
	B	Persistent painful sensory symptoms**
	C	Ataxia.
	D	Myoclonus or chorea or dystonia.
	E	Dementia.
III		
	A	EEG does not show the typical appearance of classical CJD (after review by CJDSU staff) *** OR no EEG performed
	B	Posterior thalamic high signal on MRI scan (after review by CJDSU staff).
IV		
	A	Positive tonsil biopsy.

DEFINITE VARIANT CJD	IA and neuropathological confirmation of vCJD****
PROBABLE VARIANT CJD	**I and 4/5 of II and IIIA and IIIB OR 1 and IV A**
POSSIBLE VARIANT CJD	**I and 4/5 of II and IIIA**

*depression, anxiety, apathy, withdrawal, delusions.
**including both frank pain and/ or unpleasant dysaesthesia.
***generalised triphasic periodic complexes at approximately one per second.
****spongiform change and extensive PrP deposition with florid plaques, throughout the cerebrum and cerebellum.

Table 4. Diagnostic clinical criteria for variant CJD.

1. Multiple florid plaques in haematoxylin and eosin-stained sections of the cerebral and cerebellar cortex, with numerous cluster plaques on PrP immunocytochemistry and amorphous pericellular and perivascular PrP accumulation.
2. Severe spongiform change in the caudate nucleus and putamen with perineuronal and periaxonal PrP accumulation.
3. Marked astrocytosis and neuronal loss in the posterior thalamic nuclei.
4. PrP^{res} accumulation in lymphoid tissues throughout the body.
5. Predominance of diglycosylated PrP^{res} in the central nervous system and lymphoid tissues.

Table 5. Pathological diagnostic criteria for variant CJD.

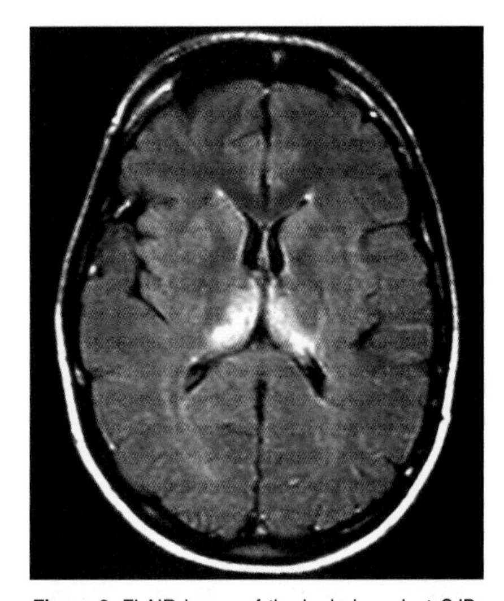

Figure 2. FLAIR image of the brain in variant CJD, showing a bilateral region of high signal in the posterior thalamus (the "pulvinar sign").

wide range of differential clinical diagnosis, which include a range of other neurological disorders with multifocal symptomatology, such as encephalopathy, Alzheimer's disease, vitamin B12 deficiency, cerebrovascular disease, Wilson's disease, corticobasal ganglionic degeneration and cerebral vasculitis. In patients who have died, the most important differential diagnosis is sporadic CJD (42). Other neuropathological diagnoses which have been made in patients with suspected variant CJD include Alzheimer's disease, cerebrovascular disease, cerebral vasculitis, viral encephalitis and limbic encephalitis (42). The current diagnostic criteria for variant CJD incorporate a range of clinical features, investigative findings and laboratory findings including neuropathology, PrP biochemistry and tonsil biopsy (Tables 4, 5) (33). Tonsil biopsy may be particularly helpful in the investigation of patients with suspected CJD in whom the typical MRI changes are not present. However, special precautions are required for performing a tonsil biopsy with the use of disposable surgical instruments and the anaesthetic equipment (the laryngeal air mask). The health and safety procedures for brain biopsy in variant CJD are identical to those for sporadic CJD.

Imaging. Neuroradiological studies have revealed a characteristic abnormality in the posterior thalamus in variant CJD which is best identified on proton density scan images, but is also visible on T-2 weighted magnetic resonance imaging (MRI) scans (Figure 2) (45). This striking abnormality "the pulvinar sign" has a high sensitivity and specificity for variant CJD in the appropriate clinical context, and this finding has been incorporated into the current diagnostic clinical criteria for variant CJD (Table 4) (33). In some cases, the area of high signal extends into the dorsomedial nuclei of the thalamus, and similar changes have also been described around the cerebral aqueduct in the midbrain. Comparative pathological studies have revealed that the abnormal areas identified on MRI scanning have severe neuronal loss with widespread gliosis, mild spongiform change and relatively few amyloid plaques (45). Quantitative studies of the abnormalities in MRI scans in a limited series of variant CJD patients have confirmed these findings (11). Functional imaging has only been employed in a very limited number of patients with variant CJD, with no specific findings (13).

Laboratory findings. Electroencephalography (EEG) studies in variant CJD show non-specific slow wave activity in most cases, but the tracings can be normal even in the presence of unequivocal neurological abnormality(42). None of the EEGs performed in patients with variant CJD show the characteristic periodic triphasic complexes typical of sporadic CJD. Analysis of cerebrospinal fluid (CSF) in variant CJD is normal in terms of the CSF cell count and glucose level, although the protein content may be elevated. Assay of the neuronal protein 14-3-3 is elevated in the CSF in over 80% of cases of sporadic CJD (26). In contrast to sporadic CJD, elevation of CSF 14-3-3 protein is present in only around half the variant CJD cases, making these a less helpful primary investigation (18).

Macroscopy

In most patients with variant CJD there are no macroscopic abnormalities to be identified in the cerebral hemispheres, brainstem or cerebellum (Figure 3) (28). However, in patients with longer duration of clinical illness (over 19 months) there is often cerebellar atrophy (which is most conspicuous in the vermis) with mild cerebral cortical atrophy (often most striking in the primary visual cortex within the occipital lobe). The hippocampi, subcortical white matter, basal ganglia and thalami usually appear normal on macroscopic inspection.

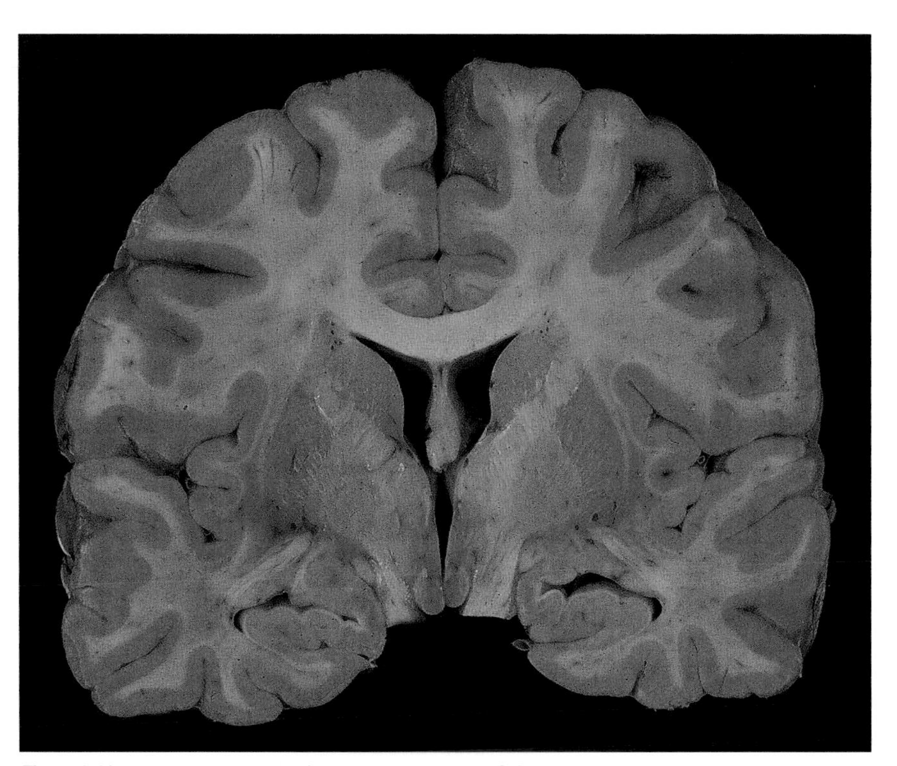

Figure 3. Macroscopic examination of the cerebrum in variant CJD is usually normal

Histopathology

The neuropathological diagnostic criteria for variant CJD are listed in Table 5. Routine histological stains in variant CJD show the characteristic features of a prion disease, with spongiform change, neuronal loss, astrocytosis and amyloid plaque formation (41). The most striking histological feature is the presence of multiple rounded amyloid plaques often with a dense eosinophilic core and a pale radiating fibrillary periphery surrounded by a rim or halo of spongiform change. These lesions have been referred to as florid plaques, and are present in large numbers in the cerebral and cerebellar cortex (Figure 4), particularly in the occipital cortex and occur in large numbers at the depths of gyri (28, 41). Florid plaques are not entirely specific for variant CJD, and have been described in small numbers in a few cases of dura mater associated iatrogenic CJD in Japan (38). Rounded amyloid plaques without surrounding spongiform change can be identified in subcortical grey matter structures including the basal ganglia, thalamus and hypothalamus. These structures however are not present in the brainstem and spinal cord. There is no evidence of an associated amyloid angiopathy. The amyloid plaques stain strongly with PAS and Alcian blue stains, and exhibit argyrophilia. A Gallyas stain will also reveal multiple small amyloid plaques which occur in clusters throughout the cerebral and cerebellar cortex and which are not evident on routine stains. In addition, amorphous fibrillary structures are identified in the cerebral and cerebellar cortex around neurones, occasional astrocytes and in the neuropil adjacent to blood vessels. These pre-amyloid deposits are composed of the disease-associated isoform of PrP. Examination of small numbers of cerebral cortical biopsies performed in patients with variant CJD shows similar but much less extensive features. However, florid plaques were not identified in all biopsies, but small clusters of plaques are consistently present on immunohistochemistry along with the amorphous perineuronal and perivascular PrP deposits.

Spongiform change in variant CJD is consistently most severe in the basal ganglia, particularly in the caudate nucleus and putamen (Figure 4), which contain relatively few amyloid plaques. The thalamus, hypothalamus, brain stem and spinal cord exhibit little spongiform change or amyloid plaque formation. However, severe neuronal loss occurs in the posterior thalamic nuclei (Figure 4), periaqueductal grey matter and colliculi, with a marked accompanying astrocytosis.

Immunohistochemistry and Ultrastructural Findings

The amount of PrP as revealed by immunohistochemistry depends generally on the duration of the clinical illness, with more extensive deposits occurring in patients with a prolonged illness. Immunohistochemistry for PrP stains the large florid plaques and the smaller cluster plaques in the cerebral and cerebellar cortex (Figure 4) (28). In the basal ganglia there is a very different pattern of PrP immunoreactivity with a combined synaptic and pericel-

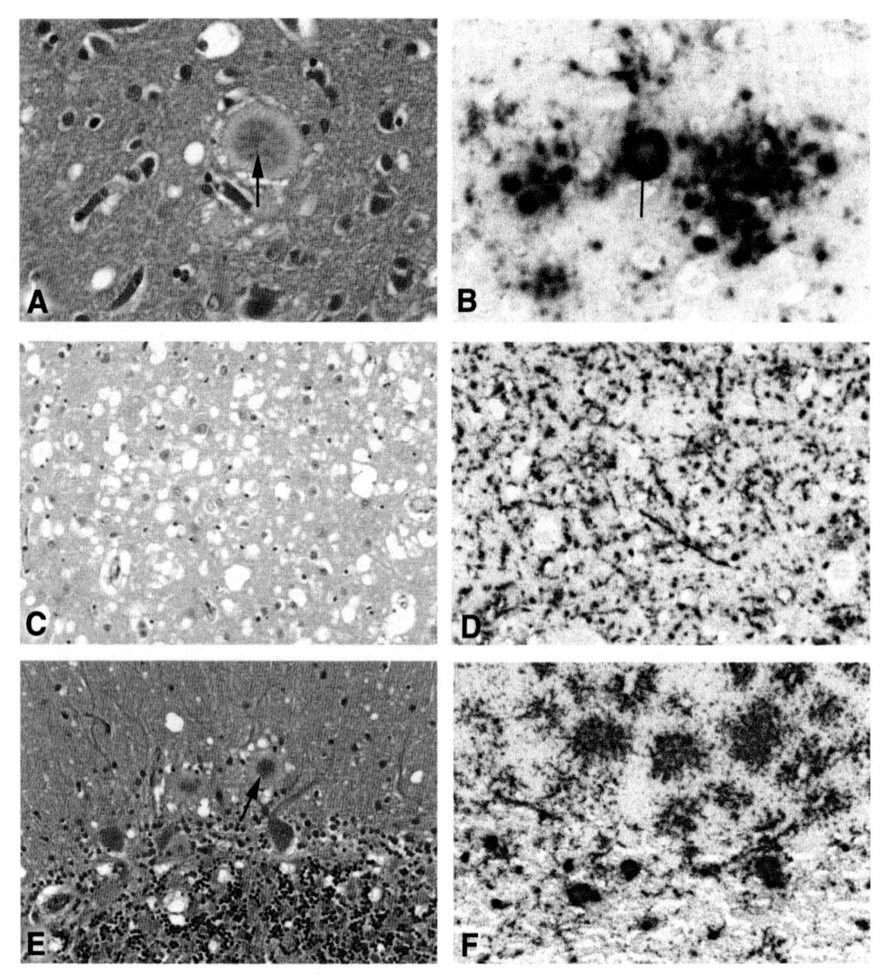

Figure 4. A. Florid plaques in the cerebral cortex, comprising a dense eosinophilic core with a pale fibrillary periphery and surrounding spongiform change. **B.** PrP immunocytochemistry in the cerebral cortex shows strong staining of a florid plaque (centre), with numerous clusters of small plaques in the surrounding grey matter. **C.** Marked spongiform change in the caudate nucleus, with few amyloid plaques. **D.** Immunocytochemistry for PrP shows linear axonal and pericellular positivity in the caudate nucleus. **E.** Florid plaques in the cerebellar molecular layer. **F.** PrP immunocytochemistry in the cerebellum shows staining of the florid plaques and massive pericellular accumulations in the molecular layer. (Figure 4, panels G-L on next page).

lular/periaxonal pattern with linear deposits most evident in the caudate nucleus and putamen (Figure 4). In the thalamus and hypothalamus there is also widespread synaptic positivity with occasional rounded amyloid plaques. Similar PrP deposits are identifiable in the brain stem and in the grey matter of the spinal cord. In the cerebellum, small plaques can identified not only in the granular layer, but occasionally in the adjacent white matter. The dentate nucleus of the cerebellum exhibits strong synaptic and linear periaxonal positivity.

Immunohistochemistry for glial fibrillary acidic protein (GFAP) confirms the presence of marked astrocytosis in the posterior thalamic nuclei (particularly the pulvinar) (Figure 4) and in the midbrain.(28, 45). In the cerebral and cerebellar cortex, GFAP-positive astrocytes are often seen to surround the amyloid plaques. Microglial cells are identified within and around the amyloid plaques on immunohistochemistry for CD68, which also reveals widespread microglial activation in the grey and white matter.

Ultrastructural studies in variant CJD have shown that the florid amyloid plaques measure up to 200 μm and the large clusters may extend up to 1500 μm. The plaques are composed of classical amyloid fibrils with spongiform change at the periphery appearing to represent distended neuritic processes (16). Neuritic dystrophy has also been observed in the cerebellum around amyloid plaques, but paired helical filaments are not present in variant CJD (19). Ultrastructural immunostaining for PrP has shown labelling of amyloid filaments, degenerate neurites and amorphous material around synapses (19).

Immunohistochemistry on tissues outside the central nervous system in variant CJD has revealed positive staining for PrP in lymphoid tissues and some peripheral neural structures (24, 28). The retina, optic nerve, dorsal root ganglia and trigeminal ganglia all exhibit immunocytochemical staining for PrP (Figure 4) and the presence of PrP^{res} has been confirmed by Western blot analysis (22, 24, 28, 40). In addition, there is widespread involvement of the lymphoid tissues with strong staining for PrP within germinal centres in a wide range of lymphoid tissues including the tonsil, lymph nodes, gut-associated lymphoid tissue, spleen and thymus (Figure 4) (28, 40). This has also been confirmed by Western blotting studies in these tissues, which demonstrate the typical PrPres isoform, although tissue-specific differences exist in the relative abundance of the diglycosylated band (21, 40). No other pathological abnormalities are de-tectable within the lymphoid tissues; the presence of infectivity in lymphoid tissues has recently been confirmed in spleen and tonsil by experimental transmission into mice. The widespread involvement of lymphoid tissues in variant CJD is a unique feature in relation to other human prion diseases, and has raised questions concerning the potential infectivity of blood in this disease (39). Attempts at identifying PrP^{res} and demonstrating infectivity in blood by experimental inoculation have so far failed in variant CJD (8) but a recent study of experimental BSE in sheep has resulted in transmission of the disease to a recipient sheep following blood transfusion from a donor animals which were in the preclinical phase of the disease incubation period (24).

Biochemistry

The non-glycosylated protease-resistant core fragment of PrP found in variant CJD is approximately 19 kDa (10, 28, 34). Protein sequencing shows that it has a major N-terminus at serine 97, identical to PrP^{res} from other forms of CJD classified by Western blot as type 2 (35). Most significantly, the PrP^{res} glycoform ratio in variant CJD is characterised by the predominance of the diglycosylated form (Figure 5) (10, 28, 34). Our ongoing analysis (as part of the UK surveillance project for CJD) of over 50 cases of variant CJD has found a consistent PrP^{res} isotype and glycoform ratio, which appears uniform throughout the brain (33). However, none of the above features are absolutely unique to variant CJD (20, 35) and consequently we have argued for caution in the diagnosis of variant CJD on molecular features alone (20, 28). Furthermore, tissue type can have a profound effect on the glycoform ratio of variant CJD PrP^{res}. The glycoform ratio of PrP^{res} found in the tonsil is a further accentuation of the predominantly diglycosylated form found in the corresponding brain (22). Conversely, we have found that the PrP^{res} found in the eye in cases of variant CJD has significantly lower levels of the diglycosylated form than the corresponding brain (21).

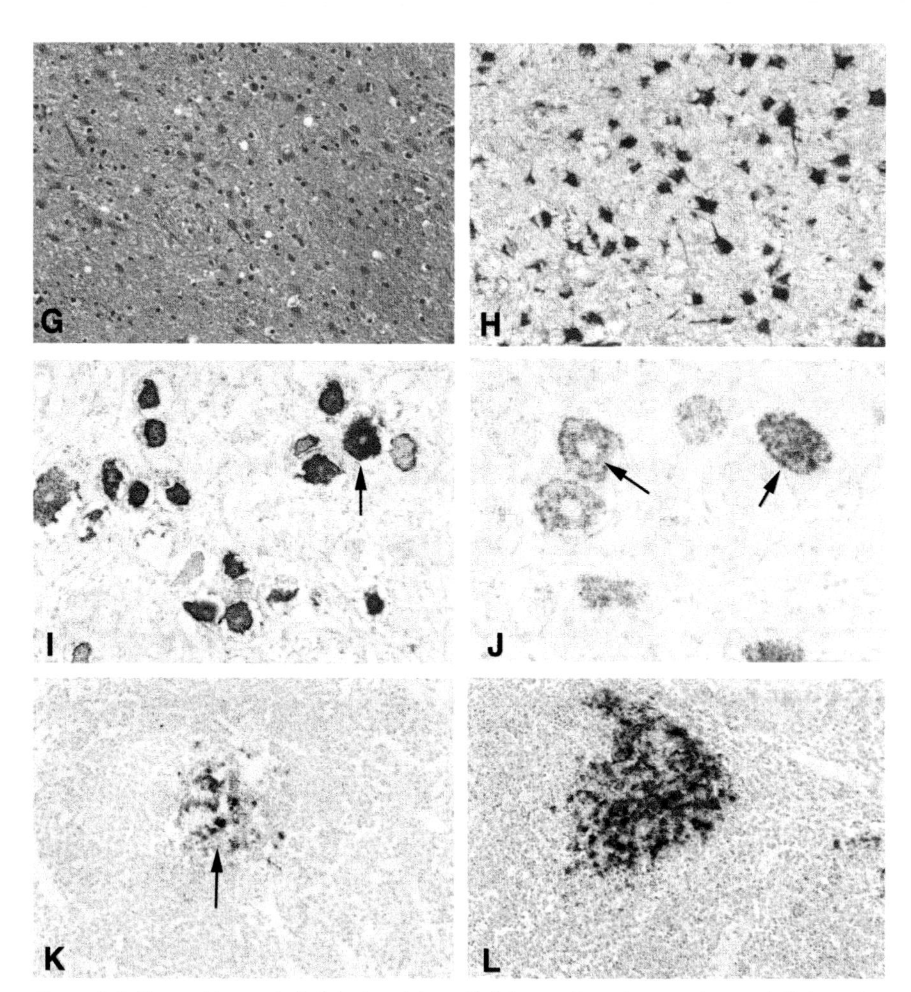

Figure 4. G. Neuronal loss and gliosis in the pulvinar, with little spongiform change and no amyloid plaque formation. **H.** Immunocytochemistry for GFAP shows widespread astrocytosis in the pulvinar. **I.** Positive staining for PrP in ganglion cells and satellite cells in a spinal dorsal root ganglion. **J.** Faint positivity for PrP in ganglion cells within the trigeminal ganglion. **K.** Positive staining for PrP in a germinal centre within a lymphoid follcle in the wall of the appendix (autopsy specimen). **L.** Positive staining for PrP in a germinal centre within the tonsil: follicular dendritic cells and macrophages stain strongly (autopsy specimen).

Differential Diagnosis

The neuropathological diagnostic criteria for vCJD listed in Table 5 should allow a clear distinction from cases of sCJD. As mentioned above, florid plaques are not entirely specific for vCJD and have been described in small numbers in a few cases of dura mater associated iatrogenic CJD in Japan (38).

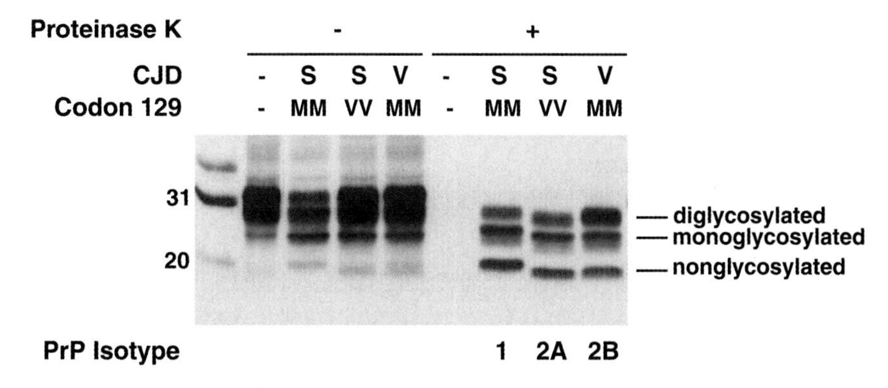

Figure 5. Western blot analysis of prion protein isotype in frontal cortex samples from patients with variant (V) and sporadic (S) CJD and from a patient with an alternative final diagnosis (-). The PRNP codon 129 genotype is shown as MM (methionine homozygote), VV (valine homozygote) or – (undetermined). Samples were analysed prior to (-) or following (+) digestion with proteinase K. The positions of the three protease-resistant glycoforms (di-, mono-, and non-glycosylated PrP^{res}) found in the cases of CJD are indicated, as are the positions of molecular weight markers at 31kDa and 20kDa. The isotype is classified as type 1 (apparent molecular weight ~21kDa) or type 2 (apparent molecular weight ~19kDa). Note that variant CJD sample is characterised by the predominance of the diglycosylated form, and is designated type 2B to distinguish it from the type 2A sCJD sample in which the monoglycosylated form is the most abundant.

Experimental Models

Transmission studies have been a crucial part of establishing a causal link between BSE and variant CJD. Primary transmissions to mice demonstrated that BSE and variant CJD had similar incubation periods and lesion profiles in the brain, which were distinct from those of both scrapie and sporadic CJD (7). In addition, the neuropathological features of BSE transmitted to macaques were found to be very similar to variant CJD, including the presence of florid plaques (29). The PrP^{res} glycoform ratio characteristic of variant CJD was observed in BSE and transmissions of BSE and variant CJD to wild-type and "humanized" mice (10, 23). Since then, transmissions to "bovinized" transgenic mice has confirmed that BSE and variant CJD are indistinguishable on molecular and histopathological grounds (37). Bioassay remains the sole method capable of detecting CJD infectivity and transmissions to mice have been used to demonstrate infectivity in lymphoid tissues in variant CJD (around 1000 fold lower than in brain tissue in this model), while no infectivity was found in plasma and buffy coat preparations (8). In this context, it is interesting to note that the tissue distribution of PrP^{res} in rodents and sheep orally exposed to the BSE agent (15, 31) resembles the tissue distribution of PrP^{res} in variant CJD at end stage disease (22, 40).

Cell culture systems have been developed that can amplify TSE infectivity and maintain strain characteristics (3), but such systems have yet to be applied to the vCJD agent. A fully in vitro, cell-free system has been established that uses PrP^{Sc} from infectious sources to drive the conversion of the normal cellular form of PrP. The system accurately models many aspects of the conversion process seen in vivo, but failed to detect a preference for BSE over scrapie in the conversion of human PrP^{C} (36) Interestingly the same study did show a preference for BSE-driven conversion of codon 129 methionine compared to valine human PrP^{C}, which may in part account for the methionine homozygosity of all cases of variant CJD thus far described.

Pathogenesis

The pathogenetic aspects of variant CJD that potentially differentiate it from other forms of CJD are the agent strain (almost certainly BSE), the route of exposure (presumed to be oral), the involvement of tissues outside the central nervous system and the genotype of susceptible individuals (currently limited to methionine homozygosity at codon 129 of the *PRNP* gene, but possibly including the effects of other, as yet unknown polymorphic loci). Exactly how these factors combine to produce the characteristic neuropathological profile of variant CJD is currently unknown. It is interesting to note that kuru (which probably resulted from oral exposure to a human TSE agent) is distinct from variant CJD even when it occurs in methionine homozygotes (32). One possible explanation for the selective targeting of specific brain areas and neuronal sub-populations is glycan-dependent PrP^{Sc} molecular recognition (14).

Future Directions and Therapy

There are considerable uncertainties of the likely future numbers of variant CJD cases, which reflect the lack of knowledge in several key areas, including the population exposure to the BSE agent, factors affecting individual susceptibility, and the incubation period for variant CJD. Furthermore, if other *PRNP* genotypes are susceptible to BSE, current estimates will have to be revised upwards. Data from kuru and iatrogenic CJD suggest that codon 129 *PRNP* genotype can have a major effect on incubation periods for acquired prion diseases in humans, with heterozygotes having the longest incubation periods. Many of these uncertainties could be at least partly resolved by the development of a preclinical diagnostic test for variant CJD, but this is not currently available. The widespread tissue distribution of infectivity in variant CJD has given rise to concerns that iatrogenic transmission through contaminated surgical instruments, blood transfusion and blood products might occur. Measures have been introduced to reduce the risks of these possibilities on a precautionary basis. The possibility of maternal transmission of variant CJD also exists since many of the patients are within the childbearing age range, and 3 patients have been pregnant during the clinical disease.

The possibly obligate phase of agent replication in the periphery that distinguishes variant CJD from sporadic and familial forms offers an opportunity for the preclinical identification of individuals exposed to the BSE agent. Moreover the peripheral phase of variant CJD offers a therapeutic window, prior to neuroinvasion and the accumulation of irreversible neurological damage.

References

1. Andrews NJ, Farrington CP, Cousens SN, Smith PG, Ward H, Knight RS, Ironside JW, Will RG (2000) Incidence of variant Creutzfeldt-Jakob disease in the UK. *Lancet* 356: 481-482.

2. Bateman D, Hilton D, Love S, Zeidler M, Beck J, Collinge J (1995) Sporadic Creutzfeldt-Jakob disease in a 18-year-old in the UK. *Lancet* 346: 1155-1156.

3. Birkett CR, Hennion RM, Bembridge DA, Clarke MC, Chree A, Bruce ME, Bostock CJ (2001) Scrapie strains maintain biological phenotypes on propagation in a cell line in culture. *EMBO J* 20: 3351-3358.

4. Britton TC, al-Sarraj S, Shaw C, Campbell T, Collinge J (1995) Sporadic Creutzfeldt-Jakob disease in a 16-year-old in the UK. *Lancet* 346: 1155.

5. Brown P, Cathala F, Raubertas RF, Gajdusek DC, Castaigne P (1987) The epidemiology of Creutzfeldt-Jakob disease: conclusion of a 15-year investigation in France and review of the world literature. *Neurology* 37: 895-904.

6. Bruce M, Chree A, McConnell I, Foster J, Pearson G, Fraser H (1994) Transmission of bovine spongiform encephalopathy and scrapie to mice: strain variation and the species barrier. *Philos Trans R Soc Lond B Biol Sci* 343: 405-411.

7. Bruce M, Will R, Ironside J, McConnell I, Drummond D, Suttie A, McCardle L, Chree A, Hope J, Birkett C, Cousens S, Fraser H, Bostock C (1997) Transmissions to mice indicate that "new variant" CJD is caused by the BSE agent. *Nature* 389: 498-501.

8. Bruce ME, McConnell I, Will RG, Ironside JW (2001) Detection of variant Creutzfeldt-Jakob disease infectivity in extraneural tissues. *Lancet* 358: 208-209.

9. Bryant G, Monk P, Final report of the investigation into the Leicestershire cluster of variant Creutzfeldt-jakob disease.*http: //www.leic-ha.org.uk.*

10. Collinge J, Sidle KCL, Meads J, Ironside J, Hill AF (1996) Molecular analysis of prion strain variation and the aetiology of "new variant" CJD. *Nature* 383: 685-690.

11. Coulthard A, Hall K, English PT, Ince PG, Burn DJ, Bates D (1999) Quantitative analysis of MRI signal intensity in new variant Creutzfeldt-Jakob disease. *Br J Radiol* 72: 742-748.

12. Cousens S, Smith PG, Ward H, Everington D, Knight RS, Zeidler M, Stewart G, Smith-Bathgate EA,

Macleod MA, Mackenzie J, Will RG (2001) Geographical distribution of variant Creutzfeldt-Jakob disease in Great Britain, 1994-2000. *Lancet* 357: 1002-1007.

13. de Silva R, Patterson J, Hadley D, Russell A, Turner M, Zeidler M (1998) Single photon emission computed tomography in the identification of new variant Creutzfeldt-Jakob disease: case reports. *Br Med J* 316: 593-594.

14. DeArmond SJ, Qiu Y, Sanchez H, Spilman PR, Ninchak-Casey A, Alonso D, Daggett V (1999) PrPc glycoform heterogeneity as a function of brain region: implications for selective targeting of neurons by prion strains. *J Neuropathol Exp Neurol* 58: 1000-1009.

15. Foster JD, Parnham DW, Hunter N, Bruce M (2001) Distribution of the prion protein in sheep terminally affected with BSE following experimental oral transmission. *J Gen Virol* 82: 2319-2326.

16. Fournier JG, Kopp N, Streichenberger N, Escaig-Haye F, Langeveld J, Brown P (2000) Electron microsocopy of brain amyloid plaques from a patient with new variant Creutzfeldt-Jakob disease. *Acta Neuropathol (Berl)* 99: 637-642.

17. Ghani AC, Ferguson NM, Donnelly CA, Anderson RM (2000) Predicted vCJD mortality in Great Britain. *Nature* 406: 583-584.

18. Green AJ, Thompson EJ, Stewart GE, Zeidler M, McKenzie JM, MacLeod MA, Ironside JW, Will RG, Knight RS (2001) Use of 14-3-3 and other brain-specific proteins in CSF in the diagnosis of variant Creutzfeldt-Jakob disease. *J Neurol Neurosurg Psychiatry* 70: 744-748.

19. Grigoriev V, Escaig-Haye F, Streichenberger N, Kopp N, Langeveld J, Brown P, Fournier JG (1999) Submicroscopic immunodetection of PrP in the brain of a patient with a new-variant of Creutzfeldt-Jakob disease. *Neurosci Lett* 264: 57-60.

20. Head MW, Tissingh G, Uitdehaag BM, Barkhof F, Bunn TJ, Ironside JW, Kamphorst W, Scheltens P (2001) Sporadic Creutzfeldt-Jakob disease in a young Dutch valine homozygote: atypical molecular phenotype. *Ann Neurol* 50: 258-261.

21. Head MW, Northcott V, Rennison K, Ritchie D, McCardle L, Bunn TJ, McLennan NF, Ironside JW, Tullo AB, Bonshek RE (2003) Prion protein accumulation in the eyes of patients with sporadic and variant Creutzfeldt-Jakob disease. *Invest Opthalmol Vis Sci* 44: 342-346.

22. Hill AF, Butterworth RJ, Joiner S, Jackson G, Rossor MN, Thomas DJ, Frosh A, Tolley N, Bell JE, Spencer M, King A, Al-Sarraj S, Ironside JW, Lantos PL, Collinge J (1999) Investigation of variant Creutzfeldt-Jakob disease and other human prion diseases with tonsil biopsy samples. *Lancet* 353: 183-189.

23. Hill AF, Desbruslais M, Joiner S, Sidle KC, Gowland I, Collinge J, Doey LJ, Lantos P (1997) The same prion strain causes vCJD and BSE. *Nature* 389: 448-450, 526.

24. Hill AF, Zeidler M, Ironside J, Collinge J (1997) Diagnosis of new variant Creutzfeldt-jakob disease by tonsil biopsy. *Lancet* 349: 99-100.

25. Hunter N, Foster J, Chang A, McCutcheon S, Parnham D, Eaton S, MacKenzie C, Houston F (2002) Transmission of prion protein diseases by blood transfusion. *J Gen Virol* 83: 2897-2905.

26. Hsich G, Kenney K, Gibbs CJ, Lee KH, Harrington MG (1996) The 14-3-3 brain protein in cerebrospinal fluid as a marker for transmissible spogiform encephalopathies. *N Engl J Med* 335: 924-930.

27. Huillard D'Aignaux J, Cousens S, Smith P (2001) Predictability of the UK variant Creutzfeldt-Jakob disease epidemic. *Science* 294: 1729-1731.

28. Ironside JW, Head MW, Bell JE, McCardle L, Will RG (2000) Laboratory diagnosis of variant Creutzfeldt-Jakob disease. *Histopathology* 37: 1-9.

29. Lasmezas Cl, Deslys JP, Demaimay R, Adjou KT, Lamoury F, Dormont D, Robain O, Ironside J, Hauw JJ (1996) BSE transmission to macaques. *Nature* 381: 743-744.

30. Lorains JW, Henry C, Agbamu DA, Rossi M, Bishop M, Will RG, Ironside JW (2001) Variant Creutzfeldt-Jakob disease in an elderly patient. *Lancet* 357: 1339-1340.

31. Maignien T, Lasmezas Cl, Beringue V, Dormont D, Deslys JP (1999) Pathogenesis of the oral route of infection of mice with scrapie and bovine spongiform encephalopathy agents. *J Gen Virol* 80 (Pt 11): 3035-3042.

32. McLean CA, Ironside JW, Alpers MP, Brown PW, Cervenakova L, Anderson RM, Masters CL (1998) Comparative neuropathology of Kuru with the new variant of Creutzfeldt-Jakob disease: evidence for strain of agent predominating over genotype of host. *Brain Pathol* 8: 429-437.

33. National Creuztfeldt-Jakob Disease Surveillance Unit, University of Edinburg, Department of Infectious and Tropical Diseases London School of Hygiene and Tropical Medicine, Creuztfeldt-Jakob disease Surveillance in the UK. Ninth Annual Report 2000. 2001, National Creuztfeldt-Jakob Disease Surveillance Unit: Edinburgh.

34. Parchi P, Capellari S, Chen SG, Petersen RB, Gambetti P, Kopp N, Brown P, Kitamoto T, Tateishi J, Giese A, Kretzschmar H (1997) Typing prion isoforms. *Nature* 386: 232-234.

35. Parchi P, Zou W, Wang W, Brown P, Capellari S, Ghetti B, Kopp N, Schulz-Schaeffer WJ, Kretzschmar HA, Head MW, Ironside JW, Gambetti P, Chen SG (2000) Genetic influence on the structural variations of the abnormal prion protein. *Proc Natl Acad Sci U S A* 97: 10168-10172.

36. Raymond GJ, Hope J, Kocisko DA, Priola SA, Raymond LD, Bossers A, Ironside J, Will RG, Chen SG, Petersen RB, Gambetti P, Rubenstein R, Smits MA, Lansbury PT, Jr., Caughey B (1997) Molecular assessment of the potential transmissibilities of BSE and scrapie to humans. *Nature* 388: 285-288.

37. Scott MR, Will R, Ironside J, Nguyen HO, Tremblay P, DeArmond SJ, Prusiner SB (1999) Compelling transgenetic evidence for transmission of bovine spongiform encephalopathy prions to humans. *Proc Natl Acad Sci U S A* 96: 15137-15142.

38. Shimizu S, Hoshi K, Muramoto T, Homma M, Ironside JW, Kuzuhara S, Sato T, Yamamoto T, Kitamoto T (1999) Creutzfeldt-Jakob disease with florid-type plaques after cadaveric dura mater grafting. *Arch Neurol* 56: 357-362.

39. Turner ML, Ironside JW (1998) New-variant Creutzfeldt-Jakob disease: the risk of transmission by blood transfusion. *Blood Rev* 12: 255-268.

40. Wadsworth JD, Joiner S, Hill AF, Campbell TA, Desbruslais M, Luthert PJ, Collinge J (2001) Tissue distribution of protease resistant prion protein in variant Creutzfeldt-Jakob disease using a highly sensitive immunoblotting assay. *Lancet* 358: 171-180.

41. Will R, Ironside J, Zeidler M, Cousens S, Estibeiro K, Alperovitch A, Poser S, Pocchiari M, Hofman A, Smith P (1996) A new variant of Creutzfeldt-Jakob disease in the UK. *Lancet* 347: 921-925.

42. Will RG, Zeidler M, Stewart GE, Macleod MA, Ironside JW, Cousens SN, Mackenzie J, Estibeiro K, Green AJ, Knight RS (2000) Diagnosis of new variant Creutzfeldt-Jakob disease. *Ann Neurol* 47: 575-582.

43. World Health Organisation, Report of a WHO consultation on clinical and neuropathological characteristics of the new variant of CJD and other human and animal transmissible spongiform encephalopathies. 1996, World Health Organisation.: Geneva.

44. Zeidler M, Johnstone EC, Bamber RW, Dickens CM, Fisher CJ, Francis AF, Goldbeck R, Higgo R, Johnson-Sabine EC, Lodge GJ, McGarry P, Mitchell S, Tarlo L, Turner M, Ryley P, Will RG (1997) New variant Creutzfeldt-Jakob disease: psychiatric features. *Lancet* 350: 908-910.

45. Zeidler M, Sellar RJ, Collie DA, Knight R, Stewart G, Macleod MA, Ironside JW, Cousens S, Colchester AC, Hadley DM, Will RG, Colchester AF (2000) The pulvinar sign on magnetic resonance imaging in variant Creutzfeldt-Jakob disease. *Lancet* 355: 1412-1418.

46. Zeidler M, Stewart G, Cousens SN, Estibeiro K, Will RG (1997) Codon 129 genotype and new variant CJD. *Lancet* 350: 668.

Gerstmann-Sträussler-Scheinker Disease

Bernardino Ghetti
Orso Bugiani
Fabrizio Tagliavini
Pedro Piccardo

AD	Alzheimer's disease
CJD	Creutzfeldt-Jakob disease
CT	computed tomography
GSS	Gerstmann-Sträussler-Scheinker disease
MRI	magnetic resonance imaging
PK	proteinase K
PRNP	prion protein gene
PrP	prion protein
PrP-CAA	PrP cerebral amyloid angiopathy
SPECT	single photon emission computed tomography

Definition

Gerstmann-Sträussler-Scheinker disease (GSS) is a genetically-determined adult-onset progressive neurodegenerative disease associated with *prion protein* gene (*PRNP*) mutations, which lead to the formation of amyloidogenic degradation products of the prion protein (PrP) (12). The clinical phenotype is characterised by a constellation of signs and symptoms; however, cerebellar ataxia, akinetic parkinsonism, pyramidal signs, and cognitive decline are the most commonly observed, particularly at the onset (12). These clinical characteristics may be present in various combinations and in varying degrees of severity. The central elements of the neuropathologic phenotype are amyloid plaques and diffuse deposits resulting from the accumulation of PrP degradation products. These plaques and deposits are most numerous in the cerebral cortex, basal ganglia, and cerebellar cortex and are associated with nerve cell loss. In addition, the neuronal pathology may vary with the *PRNP* mutation. Biochemically, GSS is characterised by the presence of N- and C-terminal truncated proteinase K (PK) resistant PrP degradation products that range from 7 to 10 kDa (30-32, 35-37).

Prion protein amyloidosis is a term introduced to represent prion diseases that have PrP amyloid accumulation as a central neuropathologic characteristic. Among the familial disorders in this group are GSS, PrP cerebral amyloid angiopathy (PrP-CAA), and some that are associated with insertional mutations involving 24-base pair repeats (15).

Historical Annotation

The clinical and pathologic descriptions of 2 individuals affected with a neurological disorder, which had affected multiple generations of their family (family "H"), were reported in 1912, 1928, and 1936 (4, 10, 11). These individuals presented with cerebellar ataxia, dysdiadochokinesia, and action and intention tremor. Later, they were unable to walk, stand, or even sit upright and had disturbances of speech, swallowing difficulties, lateral and vertical gaze nystagmus, decreased lower extremity reflexes, and bilateral Babinski signs. Changes in personality, specifically irritability, uncontrolled behavior, labile mood, and decreased intellectual performance also appeared. Subsequently, additional members of this family presented similar symptoms. Neuropathologically, Gerstmann et al described atrophy of the cerebral hemispheres and the cerebellar vermis as well as deposits of amorphous material in the cerebellar and cerebral cortices, basal ganglia, and white matter that were reminiscent of the senile plaques seen in Alzheimer's disease (AD) (11). Following Seitelberger's 1981 reexamination of brain tissue from members of the "H" family, he emphasised the similarity of these deposits to kuru plaques and he found a mild to moderate spongiosis (34). Also in 1981, Masters et al reexamined clinicopathologic data from several familial syndromes similar to that in the "H" family (27). He reported that while amyloid deposits were a constant feature, spongiosis was not and that inoculation of brain tissue from some individuals caused a spongiform encephalopathy in the recipient animal. Thus, a relationship between this disorder and the transmissible spongiform encephalopathies, such as Creutzfeldt-Jakob disease (CJD), was found. In 1987, amyloid plaques from an individual with GSS were immunolabeled using antibodies against PrP (22). In 1988, an association between PrP-immunopositive plaques and neurofibrillary tangles was reported in individuals with GSS (13). In 1989, a mutation at codon 102 of the *PRNP* gene was first reported to be associated with GSS and in 1991, the same mutation was found in affected members of the "H" family (9, 23).

Epidemiology

Incidence and prevalence. The most commonly quoted incidence for GSS is 2 to 5 per 100 million people (9). To date, at least 56 families have individuals known to be affected by GSS. These families have been found in Australia, Austria, Canada, Denmark, France, Germany, Hungary, Ireland, Israel, Italy, Japan, Mexico, Poland, the United Kingdom, and the United States. With these countries representing less than 15% of the world's population, an accurate incidence of GSS remains to be determined. This disorder is probably under-diagnosed since it may have a variety of presentations including symptoms such as ataxia, spastic paraparesis, parkinsonism, amyotrophy or dementia. In fact, GSS may mimic olivopontocerebellar atrophy, spinocerebellar ataxia, Parkinson's disease, amyotrophic lateral sclerosis, Huntington's disease, or AD.

Sex and age distribution. The onset of clinical signs and symptoms may occur from late in the second decade to early in the eighth decade of life with a duration of a few months to 12 years.

This disease occurs equally in males and females.

Genetics

GSS is a genetically-determined disease that is inherited in an autosomal dominant pattern with almost 100% penetrance. Linkage analyses helped establish the relationship between GSS and mutations in the *PRNP* gene, which is located on the short arm of chromosome 20 and encodes for PrP (2,5,19,33). Currently, 10 point mutations in the *PRNP* gene are known to be associated with GSS and one with PrP-CAA (Table 1). In addition, a GSS-like phenotype has been seen associated with insertional mutations characterised by 6 to 9 additional 24-base pair repeats. Of the known polymorphisms in the *PRNP* gene, those at codons 129 and 219 have been shown to have an impact on the clinical and pathologic phenotypes (5,8).

Haplotype	Nucleotide Change Normal	Nucleotide Change Disease	Amino Acid Change Normal	Amino Acid Change Disease	Number of Families
P102L-129M	CCG	CTG	Pro	Leu	27
P102L-129M-219K	CCG	CTG	Pro	Leu	1
P102L-129V	CCG	CTG	Pro	Leu	3
P105L-129V	CCA	CTA	Pro	Leu	5
A117V-129V	GCA	GTG	Ala	Val	8
G131V-129M	GGA	GTA	Gly	Val	1
Y145Stop-129M	TAT	TAG	Tyr	stop	1
H187R-129V	CAC	CGC	His	Arg	1
F198S-129V	TTC	TCC	Phe	Ser	3
D202N-129V	GAC	AAC	Asp	Asn	2
Q212P-129M	CAG	CCG	Gln	Pro	1
Q217R-129V	CAG	CGG	Gln	Arg	2
M232T-129?	ATG	ACG	Met	Thr	1

Table 1. Summary of the haplotypes, nucleotide and amino acid changes, and the number of families.

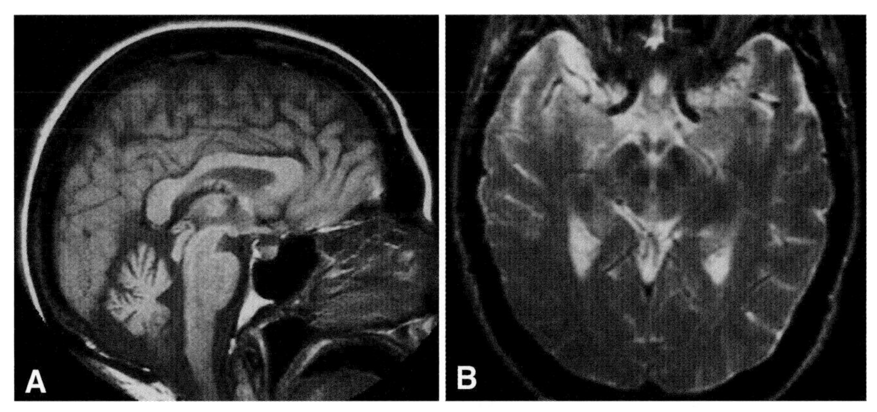

Figure 1. MRI of a patient with GSS. (**A**) T1 weighted image reveals cerebellar atrophy and (**B**) T2 weighted image reveals a reduced signal in the red nucleus and substantia nigra.

Clinical Features

Gerstmann-Sträussler-Scheinker disease. The classic presentation of GSS has progressive cerebellar ataxia and pyramidal signs followed by dementia as the cardinal features; however, there are a number of additional signs and symptoms that may be seen in GSS (6, 9). This phenotypic heterogeneity exists both within and between families with the same mutation. With the discovery of numerous *PRNP* mutations associated with GSS, a haplotype-specific pattern of clinical presentation has been observed. The differences between haplotypes may be the mutation only, the polymorphism only or both.

P102L-129M. This is the most common haplotype of those associated with GSS. The clinical phenotype is characterised by a progressive cerebellar syndrome with ataxia, dysarthria, and incoordination of saccadic movements as well as pyramidal and pseudobulbar signs. In addition, behavioral and cognitive dysfunctions are seen and often evolve into dementia or akinetic mutism. Hyperthermia, tachycardia and hyperhidrosis may occur due to sympathetic hyperactivity. Clinical symptoms start in the fourth to sixth decades of life with a disease duration of a few months to 6 years. In some cases, amyotrophy and an electromyographic pattern of denervation may be seen early in the course of the disease. A computed tomography (CT) may show cerebral and cerebellar atrophy and single photon emission computed tomography (SPECT) may reveal hypoperfusion of the frontal cortex and cerebellum. Myoclonus and pseudoperiodic sharp wave discharges in the electroencephalogram (EEG), characteristics of CJD, are observed in some individuals, which may have a very rapid course ranging from 5 to 9 months with a clinical picture indistinguishable from that of CJD (12, 15).

P102L-129M-219K. The clinical presentation is characterised by either dementia or cerebellar signs. By magnetic resonance imaging (MRI), severe cerebral atrophy was seen in one individual who had cerebellar signs (8).

P102L-129V. The clinical course and duration are different from that associated with the P102L-129M haplotype in that the only individual clinically described had seizures and long tract signs (41). No dementia was present at the time of death, which occurred 12 years after clinical onset.

P105L-129V. Spastic gait, hyperreflexia, and the Babinski sign dominate the picture in the initial stages (21, 40). Extrapyramidal signs such as fine finger tremor and rigidity of limbs may be observed. Paraparesis progresses to tetraparesis and is accompanied by emotional incontinence and dementia. Myoclonus, pseudoperiodic sharp wave discharges in electroencephalography (EEG) or severe cerebellar signs have not been reported. MRI shows

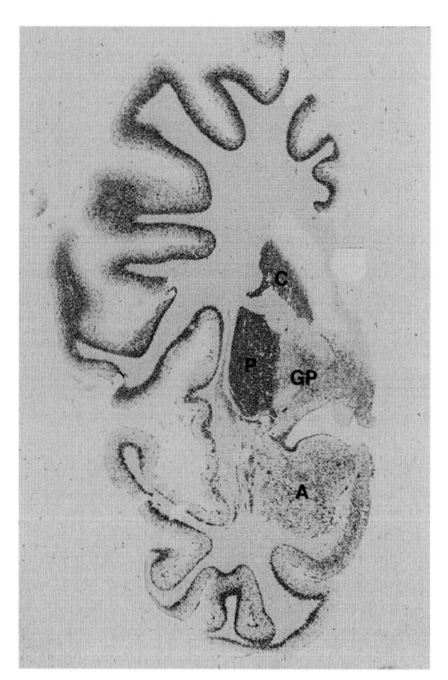

Figure 2. Coronal section of a cerebral hemisphere of a patient with GSS disease reveals PrP-immunoreactivity in the cortex, caudate nucleus (C), putamen (P), globus pallidus (GP) and amygdala (A).

hypointensity of the striatum. Electromyography (EMG) may show denervation, while evoked potentials reveal conduction delays in the posterior funiculus and pyramidal tract. The age at the onset of the clinical signs is in the fourth and fifth decades of life; the duration of the disease ranges from 6 to 12 years (21,40).

A117V-129V. This haplotype is associated with a variety of clinical phenotypes ranging from classic GSS disease to classic AD (26,28,39). In some individuals, marked extrapyramidal signs with parkinsonian features occur early in the course of the disease followed by other neurological symptoms. Additional signs that may be seen include pyramidal signs, amyotrophy, myoclonus, emotional lability and a pseudobulbar syndrome. Behavioral and personality disturbances, such as mood swings, aggressive behavior and paranoia, frequently present long before neurological signs and symptoms. The phenotypic variability observed among affected individuals even occurs within the same family. EEGs are either normal or nonspecifically abnormal, but no pseudoperiodic sharp wave discharges are seen. Results from CT scans vary from normality to moderate cerebral atrophy. The age at onset of clinical signs is in the second to seventh decade of life; the duration ranges from 1 to 11 years.

G131V-129M. Changes in personality, decrease in cognitive performance, apraxia, tremor, and increased deep tendon reflexes are the presenting signs. MRI images show cerebral and cerebellar atrophy. EEGs do not show pseudoperiodic sharp waves. In the late stages, dementia becomes progressively more severe and ataxia develops. The clinical onset is early in the fifth decade of life and the disease has a duration of 9 years (29).

H187R-129V. The clinical phenotype is characterised by early progressive cognitive impairment, cerebellar ataxia and dysarthria followed by myoclonus, seizures and occasionally pyramidal and extrapyramidal signs. Neuroimaging shows a severe, widespread atrophy of the cerebrum and cerebellum. The age at onset is in the fourth to six decade of life with a duration of 7 to 18 years (1).

F198S-129V. A gradual loss of short-term memory, clumsiness in walking evolving into ataxia, bradykinesia, rigidity, mild tremor, dysarthria, and cognitive impairment evolving into dementia are the main clinical characteristics (7). In the early stages of clinical presentation, MRI images show cerebellar atrophy and a reduced signal in the substantia nigra and red nucleus (Figure 1). Signs of cognitive impairment and eye-movement abnormalities may be detected before the onset of clinical symptoms. Psychotic depression has been observed in several patients. The symptoms may progress slowly over 5 years or rapidly over as little as one year. The age at onset of clinical signs ranges from late in the fourth decade to early in the eighth decade of life. Patients homozygous for valine at codon 129 have clinical signs more than 10 years earlier, on average, than heterozygous patients (5). The duration of the disease ranges from 2 to 12 years.

D202N-129V. Cognitive impairment leading to dementia and cerebellar signs are the main clinical features. The age at onset is early in the eighth decade and the duration is 6 years (31).

Q212P-129M. Gradual development of incoordination and slurring of speech are the presenting signs, followed by dysarthria, and ataxia. Dementia is not present. The age at onset is late in the sixth decade and the duration is 8 years (31).

Q217R-129V. The phenotype is characterised by gradual memory loss, progressive gait disturbances, parkinsonism and dementia. The neurological signs may be preceded by episodes of mania or depression that respond to antidepressant medications, lithium and neuroleptics. The age at onset of clinical signs varies from the fifth to seventh decade. The duration of the disease is 2 to 6 years (17,20).

M232T-129M/V. Cerebellar signs and spastic paraparesis are the initial symptoms followed by dementia. The age at onset is in the fifth decade and the duration is 6 years (24-25).

Prion protein cerebral amyloid angiopathy. *Y145STOP-129M.* The clinical phenotype is characterised by memory disturbance, disorientation and a progressive dementia. The EEG does not show pseudoperiodic sharp waves. The age at onset is in the fourth decade and the duration is 21 years (16).

Inherited prion disease with variable phenotypes. *Ins 192bp-129V and Ins 216bp-129M.* The phenotypes associated with the insertional mutations are highly variable; however, individuals with 8 or 9 additional repeats have a GSS-like syndrome characterised by the presence of mental deterioration, cerebellar and extrapyramidal signs. In addition, these individuals often lack the pseudoperiodic sharp wave complexes on EEG examination. It appears that the age at onset and duration of the disease are related to the number of inserted repeats. These specific mutations have an age at onset in the third to sixth decade of life and a disease duration of 5 months to 13 years (9).

Neuropathological Features

The neuropathologic phenotypes associated with GSS vary substantially, not only in morphologic characteristics, but also in the severity; however, the neuropathologic hallmark of GSS is the presence of amyloid plaques in cerebrum and cerebellum deriving from the deposition of PrP degradation products (Figures 2, 3A). In addition, cerebral and cerebellar atrophy is present, however, this may vary from mild to severe (Figure 3B). Frequently, degeneration of the pyramidal tract is also observed in the spinal cord (Figure 4). Phenotypic heterogeneity is witnessed most often between haplotypes, but it is also seen within individuals with the same haplotype (12,15).

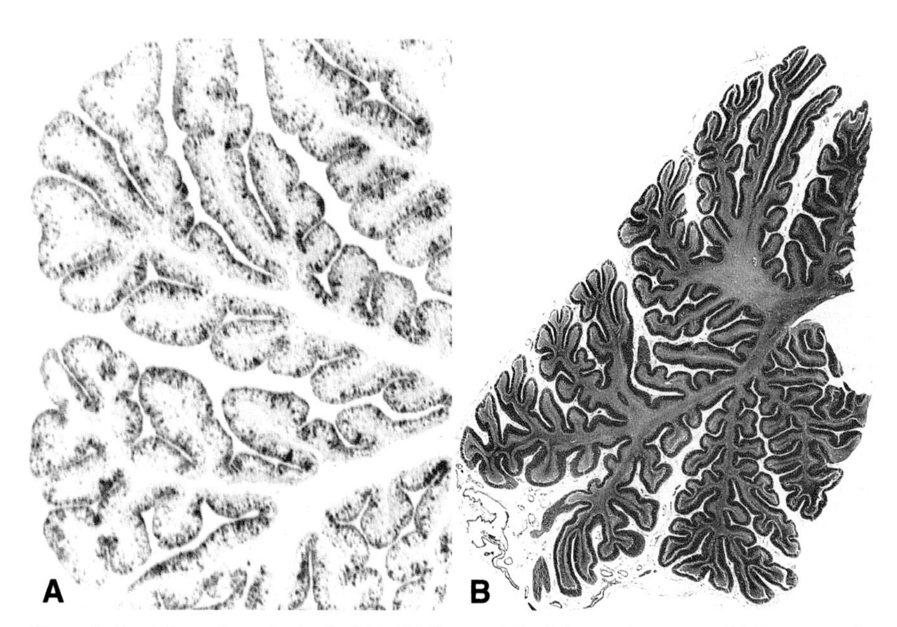

Figure 3. Cerebellum of a patient with GSS. (**A**) The cerebellar folia reveal numerous PrP-immunoreactive plaques. (**B**) The cerebellar vermis is atrophic.

Histopathology, Immunohistochemistry and Ultrastructural Findings

Gerstmann-Sträussler-Scheinker disease. Microscopically, PrP-amyloid plaques and diffuse deposits are associated with moderate to severe neuronal loss and glial proliferation in the cerebral cortex, deep gray nuclei, and cerebellar cortex (Figure 5A-D). Parenchymal PrP-amyloid deposits are birefringent after Congo red stain and strongly fluorescent after thioflavin S treatment (5A). By electron microscopy, the amyloid is composed of bundles of fibrils radiating out from a central core, each fibril measuring 8 to 10 nm in diameter (Figure 6). The core of the amyloid plaque is immunoreactive to antibodies raised against the midregion of PrP, but are unreactive or weakly reactive to antibodies raised against the amino and carboxy terminal regions of PrP. In contrast, there is immunopositivity to antibodies raised against the amino and carboxy terminal regions of PrP in the area adjacent to the amyloid core. Non-fibrillar-PrP deposits appear as diffusely immunolabeled areas in the neuropil (12,15).

P102L-129M. This haplotype is notable for being associated with 2 neuropathologic pictures. The first of these pictures is similar to the typical GSS; the second is a combination of typical GSS features and typical CJD features, namely spongiform degeneration (Figure 7). Unicentric or multicentric PrP plaques are most numerous in the molecular layer of the cerebellum, but they are also found in the cerebral gray matter. Astrocytic proliferation is present in areas with the most severe PrP deposition. Neuronal loss is most severe in the cases with spongiform degeneration (9,11).

P102L-129M-219K. Mild PrP deposition is present in the cerebral and cerebellar cortices as well as the basal ganglia; however, amyloid and spongiform changes are not observed (8).

P102L-129V. There is a moderate to severe loss of fibers in the corticospinal, spinocerebellar, and gracile tracts. In addition, diffuse PrP deposits are present in the substantia gelatinosa. PrP-amyloid plaques are frequently seen in the cerebellar cortex and to a lesser extent in the neocortex. No spongiform degeneration is seen (41).

P105L-129V. PrP-amyloid plaques and diffuse deposits are frequently seen in the neocortex, especially the motor area, striatum, and thalamus, but rarely seen in the cerebellum. Neurofibrillary tangles are seen in some cases and may occur in varying amounts. In addition, axonal loss occurs in the pyramidal tracts. No spongiform changes are seen (21).

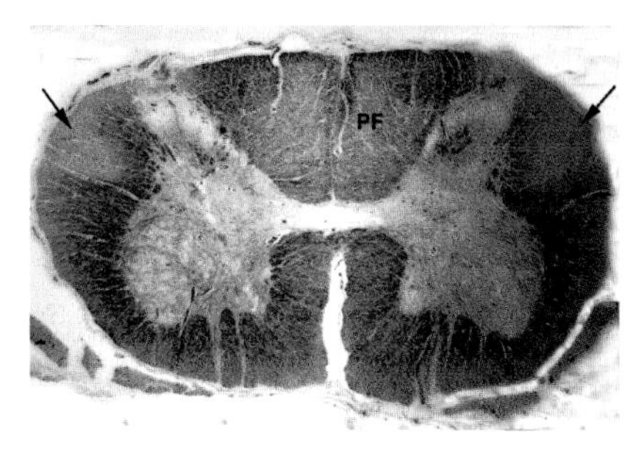

Figure 4. Spinal cord of a patient with GSS shows pallor of myelin stain in the lateral corticospinal tracts (arrows) and in the posterior funicoli (PF).

A117V-129V. Cerebral atrophy is seen in some cases. Variable amounts of PrP-amyloid plaques and diffuse deposits are widespread throughout the cerebral cortex, basal ganglia and thalamus; however, in the cerebellum, they may be absent or present in variable amounts. Pyramidal tract degeneration may be present. Spongiform degeneration may also be seen, but if so, it is focally present in the cerebrum or cerebellum. Neuronal loss, when present, may be severe in the substantia nigra. Neurofibrillary tangles have been seen in individuals that had a long disease duration (26,28).

G131V-129M. PrP-amyloid plaques and diffuse deposits are seen in the cortex and subcortical nuclei as well as in the cerebellum. Neurofibrillary tangles are seen in the Ammon's horn and in

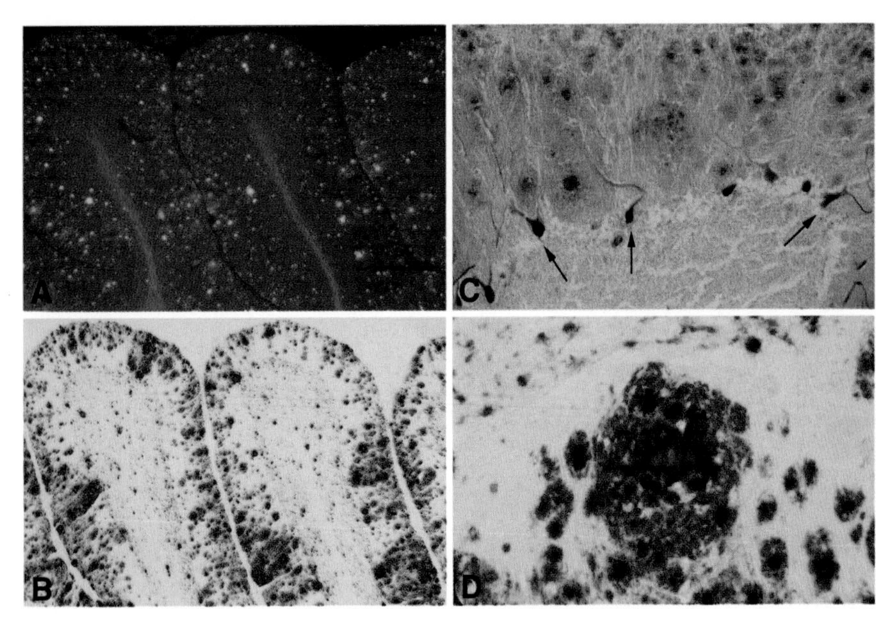

Figure 5. Cerebellar plaques in a patient with GSS associated with the F198S *PRNP* mutation. (**A**) Numerous fluorescent plaques are seen in the molecular and granule cell layers. (**B**) Plaques of various sizes are strongly immunoreactive for PrP. (**C**) PrP-immunoreactive plaques and calcium-binding-protein-immunoreactive Purkinje cells and dendrites are present in the cerebellar cortex. (**D**) Unicentric and multicentric PrP-immunoreactive plaques are seen in the molecular layer. (**A**) Thioflavin S method, (**B and D**) immunohistochemistry using antibodies against PrP (C), double immunohistochemistry using antibodies against PrP and calcium binding protein.

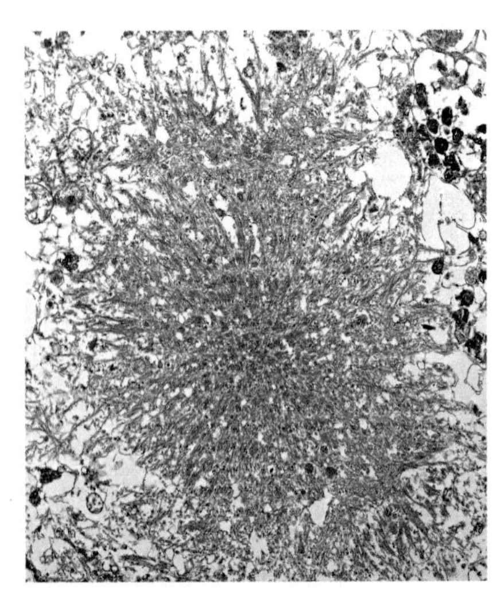

Figure 6. Electron microscopic image of an amyloid plaque from the cerebellar cortex of a patient with GSS.

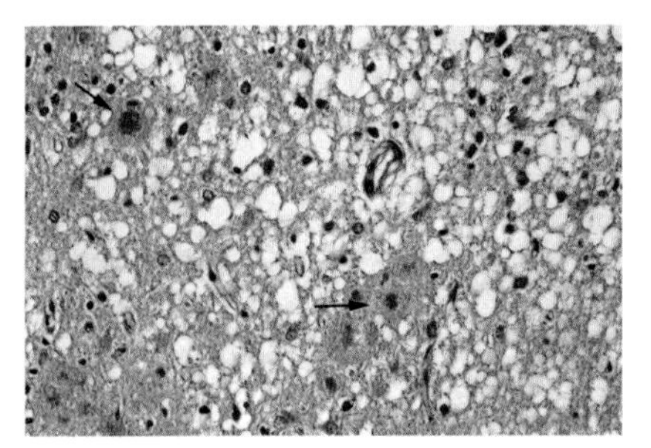

Figure 7. Neocortex of a patient with GSS associated with a P102L *PRNP* mutation shows severe spongiform changes and eosinophilic amyloid plaques (arrows).

the entorhinal cortex. No spongiform degeneration is seen (29).

H187R-129V. PrP deposition is seen in the neocortex, hippocampus and cerebellum with the latter two also having PrP-amyloid plaques. The cortical deposits have a round or elongated, "curly" appearance. Neurofibrillary tangles are also seen in the hippocampus. Atrophy and astrogliosis of the subcortical white matter are present. No spongiform degeneration is seen (3).

F198S-129V. This neuropathologic phenotype is characterised by a severe PrP deposition, in the form of PrP-amyloid plaques and diffuse deposits, and by the presence of numerous neurofibrillary tangles (Figure 8A-C) (18). This PrP deposition is the most severe seen associated with GSS. Unicentric and multicentric PrP-amyloid plaques and diffuse deposits are distributed in varying degrees throughout most gray structures of the cerebrum as well as cerebellum, and midbrain. Amyloid deposition is severe in the frontal, insular, temporal and parietal cortices with the highest concentration of deposits in layers 1, 4, 5, and 6. In the hippocampus, plaques occur predominantly within the stratum lacunosum-moleculare of the CA1 sector and subiculum. Amyloid deposits are surrounded by astrocytes, astrocytic processes and microglial cells. In the neocortex, many amyloid cores are associated with abnormal neurites causing them to appear morphologically similar to neuritic plaques of AD. Neurofibrillary tangles and neuropil threads, which are immunoreactive using antibodies against the tau protein, are found in cortical and subcortical grey nuclei as well as in the midbrain and pons. They are most numerous in areas that have severe PrP-amyloid deposition. Numerous α-synuclein immunopositive Lewy bodies were present in the neocortex of 2 affected members of one family (14). Iron deposition in the globus pallidus, striatum, red nucleus and substantia nigra is seen. Spongiform changes are rarely observed. Some of these neuropathologic characteristics have also been observed in clinically non-symptomatic individuals with this haplotype (12,15).

D202N-129V. Abundant PrP-amyloid deposits are present in the cerebrum and cerebellum and neurofibrillary tangles are seen in the cerebral cortex. No spongiform degeneration is observed (31).

Q212P-129M. PrP-amyloid deposition is mild throughout the central nervous system including the cerebellum, which is significantly less affected than those of individuals with any other GSS associated haplotype. There is degeneration of myelinated fibers in the anterior and lateral corticospinal tracts in the spinal cord. No spongiform degeneration is seen (31).

Q217R-129V. This neuropathologic phenotype, similar to the F198S-129V, is characterised by a severe PrP deposition, in the form of PrP-amyloid plaques and diffuse deposits, and by the presence of numerous neurofibrillary tangles. PrP-amyloid deposits are numerous in the cerebrum and cerebellum. Neurofibrillary tangles are abundant in the cerebral cortex, amygdala, substantia innominata, and thalamus. Lewy bodies may be found in the substantia nigra. No spongiform degeneration is seen (17).

M232T-129M/V. PrP-amyloid plaques and diffuse deposits are seen in the neocortex, subcortical nuclei and cerebellum. It is unclear whether spongiform changes are present (24-25).

Prion protein cerebral amyloid angiopathy. *Y145STOP-129M.* Diffuse atrophy of the cerebrum, dilation of the lateral ventricles, neuronal loss and gliosis are severe. PrP-amyloid deposits are present in the walls of small and medium-sized parenchymal and leptomeningeal blood vessels and in the perivascular neuropil. PrP-amyloid fibrils are seen adjacent to and within the vessel wall (9A-B). Neurofibrillary tangles, neuropil threads and dystrophic neurites are numerous in the cerebral gray matter. These neurofibrillary lesions are immunolabeled using phosphorylation dependent and phosphorylation independent anti-tau antibodies. No spongiform changes are seen (15, 16).

Inherited prion disease with variable phenotypes. *Ins 168bp-129M, Ins 192bp-129V, and Ins 216bp-129M.* The majority of individuals with these haplotypes have a histopathology characterised by PrP-amyloid plaques in the molecular layer of the cerebellum and frequently in the cerebral gray matter. In addition, various degrees of spongiosis, gliosis and neuronal loss may be present in the neocortex (9,14).

Biochemical Features

PrP-amyloid. Studies carried out in F198S, Q217R and A117V have shown that PrP-amyloid filaments are composed of 7 kDa PrP peptides. These peptides extend from residue 85-95 to 148, 152 or 153 in A117V-129V, 81 to 150 in F198S-129V, and 81 to 146 in Q217R-129V. Individuals with the F198S-129V haplotype were also found to have an 11 kDa PrP fibrillogenic peptide spanning residues 58 to 150. Additional studies have shown that these peptides originate only from the mutant allele (35,37).

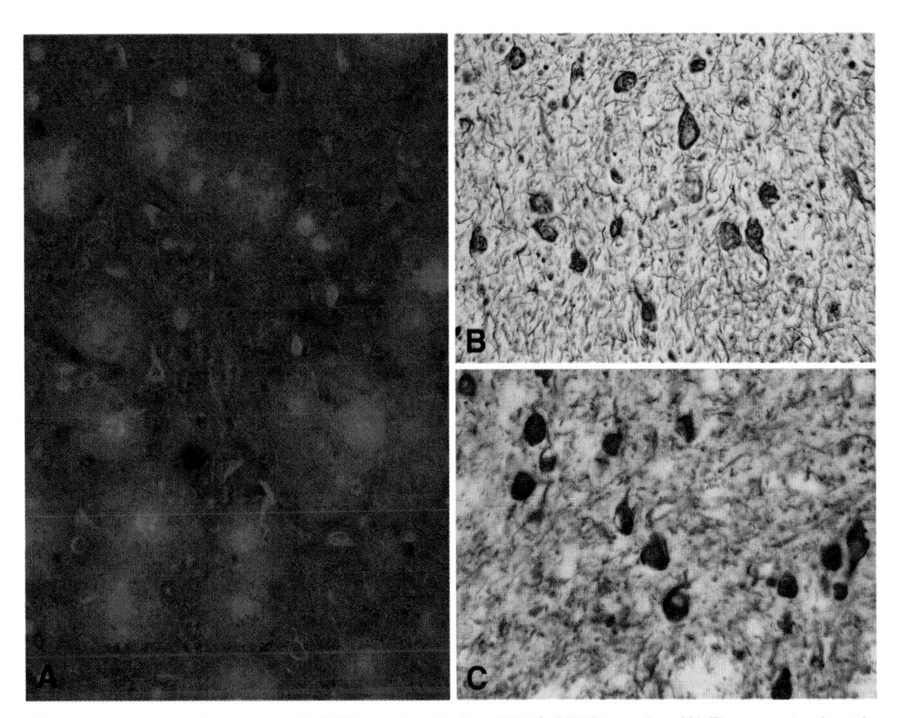

Figure 8. Neocortex of a patient with GSS associated with a F198S *PRNP* mutation. (**A**) Fluorescent unicentric and multicentric plaques as well as numerous neurofibrillary tangles are present in several cortical layers. (**B**) Numerous neurofibrillary tangles and abnormal neurites are shown. (**C**) Tau-immunoreactive neuronal perikarya and neuropil threads are numerous. (**A**) Thioflavin S method, (**B**) Bodian stain, and (**C**) immunohistochemistry using an antibody against the tau protein.

Prion protein. Studies have shown that 7-15 kDa N- and C-cleaved fragments are seen in untreated brain extracts (ie, not digested with proteinase-K (PK) and not deglycosylated). These fragments are non-glycosylated PrP peptides that are partially hydrolyzed by tissue peptidases. Proteinase K digestion and tests of solubility in detergents have been used to analyze the physicochemical properties of PrP (Figure 10A-B). Studies using these methodologies have shown that the lowest molecular weight N- and C-truncated fragments of PrP in PK treated brain extracts are 7 kDa (A117V-129V), 8 kDa (P102L-129M, G131V-129M, F198S-129V, D202N-129V, Q217R-129V), or 10 kDa (Q212P-129M) (31-32). The 8 kDa peptide associated with P102L-129M and F198S-129V have the major N terminus start at residue 78 and 74 respectively (9,30). The 7 kDa fragment associated with A117V-129V, has the major N-terminus cleavage site at residue 90 (30). Since the pattern of digestion depends on the tertiary structure of PrP, these results argue that conformational isomers are present in patients with different disease phenotypes. Another interesting finding is the presence of 21 to 30 kDa fragments in individuals with P102L-129M and spongiform degeneration This pattern was originally described in individuals with CJD (30,32).

Differential Diagnosis

Clinically, GSS may mimic several neurodegenerative diseases. Pathologically, PrP immunohistochemistry is necessary to separate GSS from other non-prion diseases associated with amyloid deposition in the central nervous system. A differential diagnosis between GSS associated with the P102L-129M haplotype and some forms of CJD, including vCJD, may be difficult if carried out only using PrP immunohistochemistry. Western blot and molecular genetic analyses are essential to differentiate between GSS and the various forms of CJD.

Pathogenesis

The pathogenesis of GSS remains largely unknown and no treatment is available. Data suggest that mutations in *PRNP* cause PrP to have an abnor-

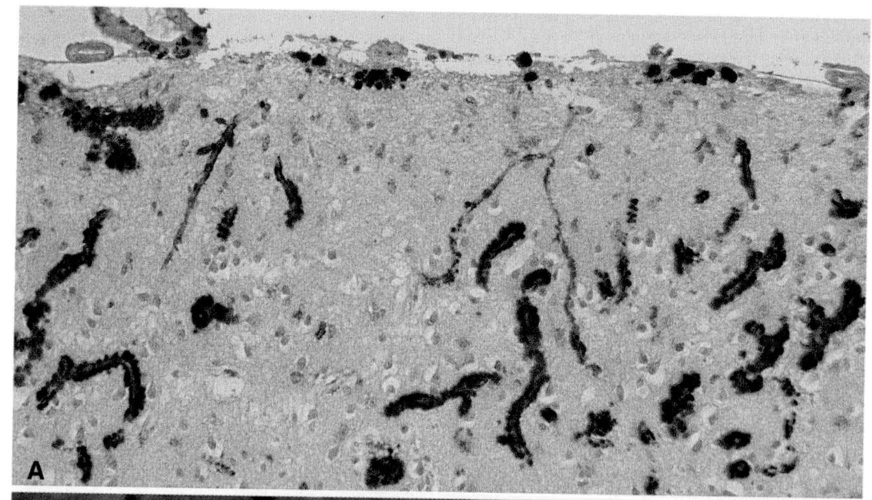

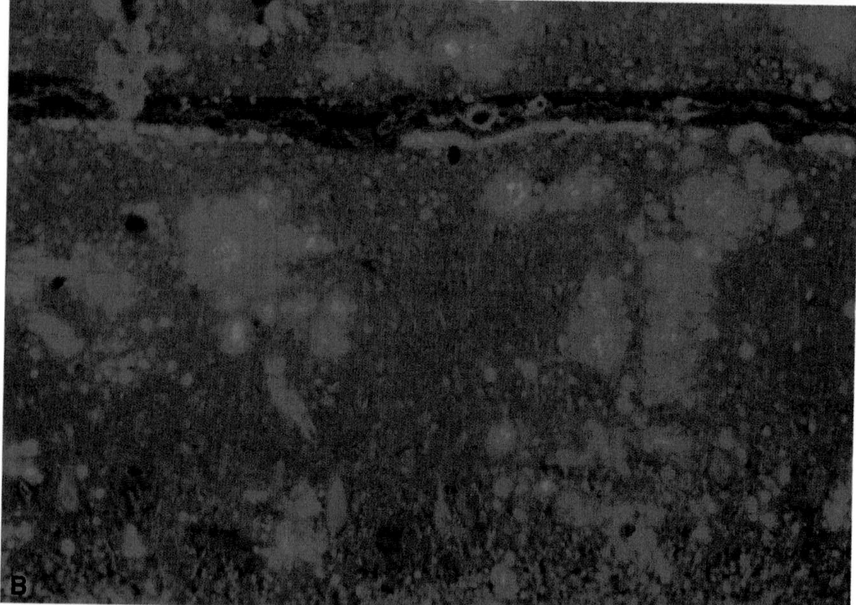

Figure 9. Prion protein cerebral amyloid angiopathy. (**A**) Parenchymal vessels of the cerebral cortex show PrP deposits. (**B**) Vessels of the cerebellar cortex show fluorescent amyloid deposits. (**A**) Immunohistochemistry using an antibody against PrP, (**B**) thioflavin S method.

mal conformation. It is hypothesised that the full-length abnormally conformed PrP is partially degraded by proteases resulting in the formation of amino- and carboxy-terminal-truncated PrP peptides that have high fibrillogenic properties. These peptides accumulate extracellularly leading to the formation of amyloid deposits. In vitro studies have shown that synthetic peptides corresponding to the PrP fragments extracted from brain tissue are readily assembled into amyloid fibrils (38).

Transmission Studies

A spongiform encephalopathy indistinguishable from that seen in CJD, has been transmitted to laboratory animals by intracerebral inoculation of brain extracts of GSS patients with mutation at residue PrP P102L. No transmission has been detected following the inoculation of tissue from patients carrying other GSS mutations. The prevailing hypothesis suggests that transmissibility of prion diseases depends on the interaction between pathologic PrP^{res} (ie, PrP with abnormal tertiary structure) present in the inocula and endogenous PrP (33). The detection of infectivity following the inoculation of tissue obtained from patients with GSS P102L, would indicate that PrP P102L favors the formation of PrP aggregates in the recipient animal and the conversion of endogenous PrP into PrP with abnormal conformation.

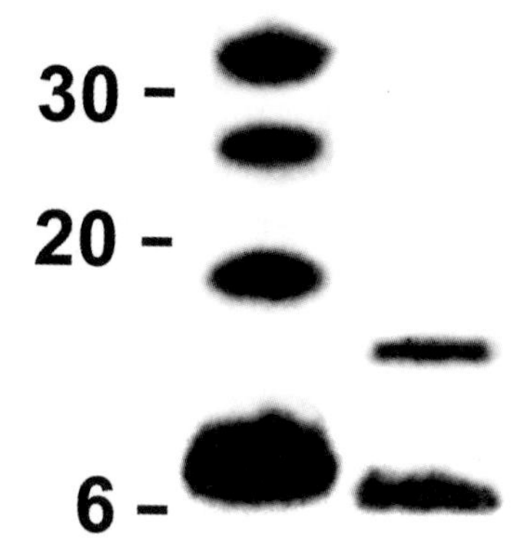

Figure 10. Immunoblot of purified PrP obtained from the frontal cortex of patients with GSS F198S (lane A) and GSS A117V (lane B). Detergent insoluble and PK-resistant PrP isoforms of ca. 32 to 34, 27 to 29, 18 to 19, and 8 kDa are seen in lane A. Detergent insoluble and PK-resistant PrP isoforms of ca. 14 and 7 kDa are seen in lane B. PrP was detected with mAb 3F4 and visualised by enhanced chemoluminescence(ECL).

References

1. Butefisch CM, Gambetti P, Cervenakova L, Park KY, Hallett M, Goldfarb LG (2000) Inherited prion encephalopathy associated with the novel PRNP H187R mutation: a clinical study. *Neurology* 55:517-22

2. Collinge J (2001) Prion diseases of humans and animals: their causes and molecular basis. *Annu Rev Neurosci* 24:519-50

3. Colucci, M, Xie Z, Butefisch CM, Cervenakova L, Wang W, Goldfarb LG, Chen SG, Gambetti P (2000) A novel mutation in the prion protein gene associated with distinct pathology. *Brain Pathol* 10:672

4. Dimitz L (1913) Bericht des Vereines für Psychiatrie und Neurologie in Wien. (Vereinsjahr 1912/13). Sitzung vom 11. Juni 1912. *Jahrb Psychiatr Neurol* 34:384

5. Dlouhy SR, Hsiao K, Farlow MR, Foroud T, Conneally PM, Johnson P, Prusiner SB, Hodes ME, Ghetti B (1992) Linkage of the Indiana kindred of Gerstmann-Sträussler-Scheinker disease to the prion protein gene. *Nat Genet* 1:64-67

6. Farlow MR, Tagliavini F, Bugiani O, Ghetti B (1991) Gerstmann-Sträussler-Scheinker disease. In: *Handbook of Clinical Neurology* PJ Vinken, GW Bruyn, HL Klawans (eds.). JMBV de Jong (Co-Ed.) Elsevier Science Publishers B.V., Amsterdam, The Netherlands, pp. 619-633

7. Farlow MR, Yee RD, Dlouhy SR, Conneally PM, Azzarelli B, Ghetti B (1989) Gerstmann-Sträussler-Scheinker disease: I. Extending the clinical spectrum. *Neurology* 39:1446-1452

8. Furukawa H, Kitamoto T, Tanaka Y, Tateishi J (1995) New variant prion protein in a Japanese family with

Gerstmann-Sträussler syndrome. *Mol Brain Res* 30: 385-388

9. Gambetti P, Petersen RB, Parchi P, Chen SG, Capellari S, Goldfarb L, Gabizon R, Montagna P, Lugaresi E, Piccardo P, Ghetti B (1999) Inherited Prion Diseases. In *Prion Biology and Diseases* SB Prusiner (ed), Cold Spring Harbor Laboratory Press, NY. pp 509-583

10. Gerstmann J (1928) Über ein noch nicht beschriebenes Reflexphanomen bei einer Erkrankung des zerebellaren Systems. *Wiener Med Wochenschr* 78:906-908

11. Gerstmann J, Sträussler E, Scheinker I (1936) Über eine eigenartige hereditär-familiäre Erkrankung des Zentralnervensystems. Zugleich ein Beitrag zur Frage des vorzeitigen lokalen Alterns. *Zeitschrift fur Neurologie und Psychiatrie* 154:736-762

12. Ghetti B, Dlouhy SR, Giaccone G, Bugiani O, Frangione B, Farlow MR, Tagliavini F (1995) Gerstmann-Sträussler-Scheinker disease and the Indiana Kindred. *Brain Pathol* 5:61-75

13. Ghetti B, Farlow M, Conneally M, Azzarelli B, Masters C, Giaccone G, Tagliavini F, Bugiani O (1988) Amyloid plaques and neurofibrillary tangles of Gerstmann-Sträussler-Scheinker Disease. *Neurology* 38 (Suppl. 1):266

14. Ghetti B, Gambetti P (1999) Human Prion Diseases. In *Advances in Cell Aging and Gerontology, Volume 3: Genetic Aberrancies and Neurodegenerative Disorders* MP Mattson (ed.), Jai Press Inc., Greenwich, CT. pp 135-187

15. Ghetti B, Piccardo P, Frangione B, Bugiani O, Giaccone G, Young K, Prelli F, Farlow MR, Dlouhy SR, Tagliavini F (1996) Prion protein amyloidosis. *Brain Pathol* 6:127-145

16. Ghetti B, Piccardo P, Spillantini MG, Ichimiya Y, Porro M, Perini F, Kitamoto T, Tateishi T, Seiler C, Frangione B, Bugiani O et al (1996) Vascular Variant of Prion Protein Cerebral Amyloidosis with Ù-Positive Neurofibrillary Tangles: The Phenotype of the Stop Codon 145 Mutation in PRNP. *Proc Natl Acad Sci U S A* 93:744-748

17. Ghetti B, Tagliavini F, Giaccone G, Bugiani O, Frangione B, Farlow MR, Dlouhy SR (1994) Familial Gerstmann-Sträussler-Scheinker disease with neurofibrillary tangles. *Mol Neurobiol* 8:41-48

18. Ghetti B, Tagliavini F, Masters CL, Beyreuther K, Giaccone G, Verga L, Farlow MR, Conneally PM, Dlouhy SR, Azzarelli B, Bugiani O (1989) Gerstmann-Sträussler-Scheinker disease: II. Neurofibrillary tangles and plaques with PrP-amyloid coexist in an affected family. *Neurology* 39:1453-1461

19. Hsiao K, Baker HF, Crow TJ, Poulter M, Owen F, Terwillinger JD, Westaway D, Ott J, Prusiner SB (1989) Linkage of a prion protein missense variant to Gerstmann-Sträussler syndrome. *Nature* 338:342-345.

20. Hsiao K, Dlouhy SR, Farlow MR, Cass C, Da Costa M, Conneally PM, Hodes ME, Ghetti B, Prusiner SB (1992) Mutant Prion Protein in Gerstmann-Sträussler-Scheinker disease with neurofibrillary tangles. *Nat Genet* 1:68-71

21. Kitamoto T, Amano N, Terao Y, Nakazato Y, Isshiki T, Mizutani T, Tateishi J (1993) A new inherited prion disease (PrP-P105L Mutation) showing spastic paraparesis. *Ann Neurol* 34: 808-813

22. Kitamoto T, Ogomori K, Tateishi J, Prusiner SB (1987) Formic acid pretreatment enhances immunostaining of cerebral and systemic amyloids. *Lab Invest* 57:230-236

23. Kretzschmar HA, Honold G, Seitelberger F, Feucht M, Wessely P, Mehraein P, Budka H (1991) Prion protein mutation in family first reported by Gerstmann, Sträussler, and Scheinker. *Lancet* 337:1160

24. Liberski PP, Barcikowska M, Cervenakova I, Bratosiewicz J, Marczewska M, Brown P, Gajdusek DC (1998) A case of sporadic Creutzfeldt-Jakob disease with a Gerstmann-Sträussler-Scheinker phenotype but no alterations in the PRNP gene. *Acta Neuropathol* 96:425-430

25. Liberski PP, Bratosiewicz J, Barcikowska M, Cervenakova L, Marczewska M, Brown P, Gajdusek DC (2000) A case of sporadic Creutzfeldt-Jakob disease with a Gerstmann-Sträussler-Scheinker phenotype but no alterations in the PRNP gene. *Acta Neuropathol* 100:233-234

26. Mallucci GR, Campbell TA, Dickinson A, Beck J, Holt M, Plant G, de Pauw KW, Hakin RN, Clarke CE, Howell S, Davies-Jones GA, Lawden M, Smith CM, Ince P, Ironside JW, Bridges LR, Dean A, Weeks I, Collinge J (1999). Inherited prion disease with an alanine to valine mutation at codon 117 in the prion protein gene. *Brain* 122:1823-37

27. Masters CL, Gajdusek DC, Gibbs CJ, J. (1981) Creutzfeldt-Jakob disease virus isolations from the Gerstmann-Sträussler syndrome with an analysis of the various forms of amyloid plaque deposition in the virus induced spongiform encephalopathies. *Brain* 104:559-588

28. Nochlin D, Sumi SM, Bird TD, Snow AD, Leventhal CM, Beyreuther K, Masters CL (1989) Familial dementia with PrP-positive amyloid plaques: A variant of Gerstmann-Sträussler syndrome. *Neurology* 39: 910-918

29. Panegyres PK, Toufexis K, Kakulas BA, Brown P, Ghetti B, Piccardo P, Dlouhy SR (2001) A new mutation [G131V] linked to Gerstmann-Sträussler-Scheinker disease. *Arch Neurol* 58:1899-1902

30. Piccardo P, Liepnieks JJ, William A, Dlouhy SR, Farlow MR, Young K, Nochlin D, Bird TD, Nixon RR, Ball MJ, DeCarli C, Bugiani O, Tagliavini F, Benson MD, Ghetti B (2001) Prion proteins with different conformations accumulate in Gerstmann-Sträussler-Scheinker disease caused by A117V and F198S mutations. *Am J Pathol* 158: 2201-2207

31. Piccardo P, Dlouhy SR, Lievens PMJ, Young K, Bird TD, Nochlin D, Dickson DW, Vinters HV, Zimmerman TR, Mackenzie IRA, Kish SJ et al (1998) Phenotypic variability of Gerstmann-Sträussler-Scheinker disease is associated with prion protein heterogeneity. *J Neuropathol Exp Neurol* 57:979-988

32. Piccardo P, Seiler C, Dlouhy SR, Young K, Farlow MR, Prelli F, Frangione B, Bugiani O, Tagliavini F, Ghetti B (1996) Protease K resistant prion protein isoforms in Gerstmann-Sträussler-Scheinker Disease (Indiana kindred). *J Neuropathol Exp Neurol* 55:1157-1163

33. Prusiner SB (1999) An introduction to prion biology and diseases. In *Prion Biology and Diseases* SB Prusiner (ed), Cold Spring Harbor Laboratory Press, NY. Pp 1-67

34. Seitelberger F (1981) Sträussler's disease. *Acta Neuropathol* 7: 341-343

35. Tagliavini F, Lievens PM, Tranchant C, Warter JM, Mohr M, Giaccone G, Perini F, Rossi G, Salmona M, Piccardo P et al (2001) A 7-kDa prion protein (PrP) fragment, an integral component of the PrP region required for infectivity, is the major amyloid protein in Gerstmann-Sträussler-Scheinker disease A117V. *J Biol Chem* 276:6009-6015

36. Tagliavini F, Prelli F, Ghiso J, Bugiani O, Serban D, Prusiner SB, Farlow MR, Ghetti B, Frangione B (1991) The amyloid protein of Gerstmann-Sträussler-Scheinker disease (Indiana kindred) is an 11-Kd degradation product of PrP that starts at position 58 of the cDNA-deduced PrP sequence. *EMBO J* 10:513-519

37. Tagliavini F, Prelli F, Porro M, Rossi G, Giaccone G, Farlow MR, Dlouhy SR, Ghetti B, Bugiani O, Frangione B (1994) Amyloid fibrils in Gerstmann-Sträussler-Scheinker disease (Indiana and Swedish Kindreds) express only PrP peptides encoded by the mutant allele. *Cell* 79:695-703

38. Tagliavini F, Prelli F, Verga L, Giaccone G, Sarma R, Gorevic P, Ghetti B, Passerini F, Ghibaudi E, Forloni G, Salmona M, Bugiani O, Frangione B (1993) Synthetic peptides homologous to prion protein residues 106-147 form amyloid-like fibrils in vitro. *Proc Natl Acad Sci U S A* 90:9678-9682

39. Tranchant C, Dohura K, Warter JM, Steinmetz G, Chevalier Y, Hanauer A, Kitamoto T, Tateishi J (1992) Gerstmann-Sträussler-Scheinker disease in an Alsatian family—Clinical and genetic studies. *J Neurol Neurosurg Psychiatry* 55: 185-187

40. Yamada M, Itoh Y, Inaba A, Wada Y, Takashima M, Satoh S, Kamata T, Okeda R, Kayano T, Suematsu N, Kitamoto T, Otomo E, Matsushita M, Mizusawa . (1999) An inherited prion disease with a PrP P105L mutation: clinicopathologic and PrP heterogeneity. *Neurology* 53:181-8

41. Young K, Clark HB, Piccardo P, Dlouhy SR, Ghetti B (1997) Gerstmann-Sträussler-Scheinker disease with the PRNP P102L mutation and valine at codon 129. *Mol Brain Res* 44:147-150

Fatal Insomnia: Familial and Sporadic

Pierluigi Gambetti
Piero Parchi
Shu G. Chen
Pietro Cortelli
Elio Lugaresi
Pasquale Montagna

CJD	Creutzfeldt-Jakob disease
EEG	electroencephalogram
fCJD	familial Creutzfeldt-Jakob disease
FFI	fatal familial insomnia
FI	fatal insomnia
NMR	nuclear magnetic resonance
NREM	non-rapid eye movement
PET	positron emission tomography
PK	protein kinase
PRNP	human prion protein gene
sFI	sporadic fatal insomnia

Definition

Fatal insomnia (FI) is a transmissible prion disease characterized by alterations of the sleep-wake cycle, dysautonomia and motor signs, associated with thalamic atrophy (20, 33). FI occurs either in familial form that is linked to a point mutation in the prion protein gene (*PRNP*) and is known as fatal familial insomnia (FFI), or, more rarely, in sporadic form, named sporadic fatal insomnia (sFI) (25, 33).

Synonyms and Historical Annotations

The clinical and pathological features of FFI were first reported by Lugaresi, Gambetti and co-workers in 1986 (20). Subsequently, these investigators have defined in detail clinical, electrophysiological, imaging and neuropathological features (3, 4, 6, 36, 39-41, 44) as well as the molecular characteristics including the mutation in *PRNP*, the peculiar genotype determined by the codon 129 polymorphism and the characteristics of the protease-resistant scrapie prion protein (PrP^{res}) (1, 2-4, 13, 22, 27, 31, 36, 38-41, 44).

Sporadic FI was definitely established in 1999 (33). Prior to the discovery of FFI, familial and sporadic cases with histopathological features resembling those of FFI had occasionally been reported under the term of thalamic dementia, thalamic degeneration or thalamic form of Creutzfeldt-Jakob disease (CJD) (22-24, 38). Using modern diagnostic techniques some of these familial and sporadic cases indeed have been shown to have the same genotype and PrP^{res} characteristics as those of FFI and sFI, respectively (33, 38).

Epidemiology

Incidence and prevalence. To date, at least 26 presumably unrelated kindreds, which comprise 55 cases affected by FFI, have been published (9, 15, 47). They include continental European kindreds, American kindreds of European ancestry, and a Japanese kindred. Although overall rare, FFI is the third most common familial prion disease around the world and the most common in Germany (51). Nine well-characterised cases of sFI are on record to date (25, 33, 43).

Sex and age distribution. FFI equally affects both sexes at an age that ranges from 36 to 62 years (28).

Genetics

FFI is remarkable because, at variance with most genetic diseases, its phenotype is linked not only to a mutated codon but also to a second polymorphic codon, which in itself is not pathogenic (Figure 1). The pathogenic mutation linked to FFI is located at codon 178 of *PRNP*, is transmitted in an autosomal dominant manner and results in the substitution of aspartic acid with asparagine in PrP (D178N) (26). The D178N mutation is also linked to another familial prion disease, which is phenotypically similar to CJD and is referred to as familial CJD^{178} ($fCJD^{178}$) (13). The linkage of 2 phenotypically distinct diseases to the same mutation, referred to as phenotypic heterogeneity, was commonly considered to result from the modifying effect of environmental factors, another gene or the paternal or maternal origin of the mutation (46).

Separate sequencing of the 2 alleles in FFI and $fCJD^{178}$ demonstrated that the D178N mutation is aligned on the same allele with either one of 2 differ-

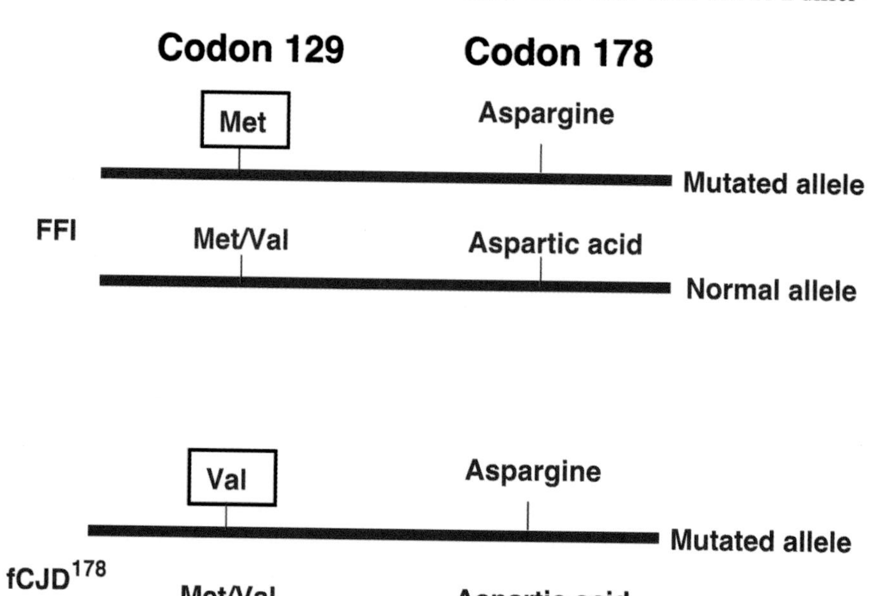

Figure 1. *Diagram of the haplotypes in FFI and* $fCJD^{178}$.

ent codons at position 129, the site of a common methionine/valine polymorphism (2, 12). In fCJD[178] patients, the D178N mutation is aligned with the codon 129, which specifies valine (D178N-129V haplotype), in FFI patients the mutation is aligned with the methionine codon at position 129 (D178N-129M) (12). Furthermore, since by virtue of the polymorphism, the normal allele carries either the methionine or valine codon at position 129, each of the FFI and fCJD178 patient populations comprises patients who are either homozygous or heterozygous at codon 129 (Figure 1) (12). The homozygous (methionine /methionine) FFI patients have on average a shorter disease duration than the heterozygous (methionine/valine) patients (12). Moreover, homozygous and heterozygous subjects differ slightly in the clinical and pathological features (28). Therefore, codon 129 plays a 2-fold role in determining the phenotypic heterogeneity of the D178N mutation: on the mutant allele it determines the phenotype (either FFI or fCJD[178]) of the 2 diseases associated with the D178N mutation; on the normal allele it specifies disease duration (or severity) and some additional features of each of the 2 diseases. A similar mechanism has been demonstrated in other familial prion diseases and might also play a role in other neurodegenerative conditions (14, 49).

Clinical Features

Signs and symptoms. The course is quite variable but, as mentioned above, the variability of the disease duration as well as of the clinical presentation, albeit not the age at onset, is at least in part related to codon 129. FFI patients homozygous at codon 129 had a disease duration of 12 ± 4 months whereas the duration was 21 ± 15 months in heterozygous patients (29). Clinical signs of FFI involve 3 major activities: *i)* wake and sleep, *ii)* autonomic, and *iii)* motor. Insomnia is often an early symptom presenting with drowsiness, frequent arousals, apathy and enacted dreams, and is rapidly progressive especially in homozygous patients. Sleep disturbances are usually associated from the beginning with autonomic alterations, in the form of mild pyrexia, increased salivation and diaphoresis, mild blood pressure elevation and increased heart rate. Impotence may occur early. Motor signs are generally more prominent in the heterozygous patients and include diplopia, dysarthria, dysphagia and gait abnormalities. Myoclonus, spontaneous and evoked, is always found in FFI unassociated with EEG paroxysms. Patients have brisk tendon reflexes and a Babinski sign. Occasional seizures preferentially affect heterozygous patients.

Imaging. Computed tomography and magnetic resonance imaging are unrevealing. Positron emission tomography with [18F]2-fluoro-2-deoxy-D-glucose (PET) shows prominent and nearly selective hypometabolism of the thalamus bilaterally, with variable involvement of the cingulate gyrus in 129 homozygous patients with short disease duration (4, 36). In heterozygous patients with longer disease duration, the cerebral cortex, basal ganglia and cerebellum are also involved even at relatively early stages of the disease. PET studies point to the thalamic hypometabolism as the hallmark of FFI, which is accompanied by the involvement of the cerebral cortex, cerebellum and basal ganglia at later stages of the disease. Whether this more widespread involvement relates to the temporal progression of the disease, or instead is present from the onset in the heterozygous patients, remains to be seen.

Laboratory studies. *Polysomnography.* Electroencephalographic (EEG) background activity becomes progressively flattened and slow, and true periodic activity characteristic of CJD is remarkably absent in homozygous patients but it may appear in advanced stages of the disease in heterozygous patients (28). In typical cases, the 24-hour EEG recording shows a continuous oscillation between the activity of normal wakefulness and desynchronised theta activity (subwakefulness). As the disease progresses, EEG activities typical of Non rapid eye movement (Nrem) sleep (spindles and K complexes) are lost, and slow-wave sleep may disappear completely. Rem sleep may initially remain normal or display a pathologically preserved muscle tone, with simple gesturing or dream enactment. The total sleep time is drastically reduced and the cyclic organization of sleep lacks the orderly transition between sleep stages (44).

Autonomic and endocrine systems. Plasma catecholamines are increased, and cortisol is persistently high in the presence of remarkably normal or even reduced corticotropin levels. Blood pressure and heart rate are also persistently elevated, and their oscillations progressively decline in advanced stages. The nocturnal elevation of somatotropin disappears in parallel with the loss of deep sleep, while prolactin and melatonin circadian oscillations are lost only in the final stages of the disease (40, 41). Overall, there is an unbalanced autonomic control with preserved parasympathetic function but increased background and stimulated orthosympathetic activities (3).

Neuropsychology. Attention and vigilance are progressively impaired along with the working memory, which manifests with difficulty in manipulating and temporally ordering events. The IQ remains remarkably normal (6, 7). Overall, the vigilance abnormalities best define FFI as a confusional-oneiric state, rather than a true dementing disease.

Macroscopy

The gross appearance of the brain is unremarkable except for cases with over 30-month duration, which show widespread atrophy of cerebrum and cerebellum (24).

Histopathology

The invariable and distinctive feature of FFI is the severe atrophy of the anterior ventral, medio-dorsal and pulvinar thalamic nuclei with loss of 80 to 90% of the neurons and 2- to 3-fold

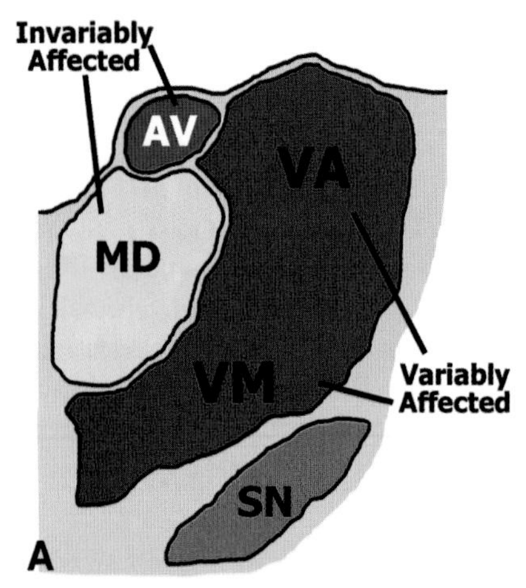

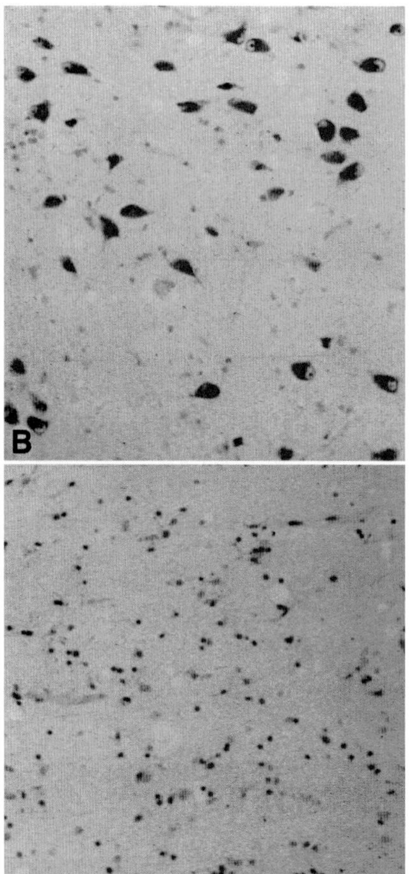

Figure 2. A. Diagrammatic representation of major thalamic nuclei (MD: medial dorsal; AV; anteroventral; VA ventral anterior; VM: ventral medial). **B** and **C**: Histopathology of the MD nucleus of the thalamus showing severe neuronal loss and gliosis in FFI (**C**) compared to age-matched control (**B**).

increase in astroglial cells while spongiosis is absent (Figure 2) (8, 20, 22, 31). Other thalamic nuclei are less and inconsistently affected. Atrophy of the inferior olives is the second common change. Moderate astrogliosis in the periaqueductal gray matter of the mid brain and in the hypothalamus without a visually detectable neuronal loss is also a common finding. While the thalamus, hypothalamus and midbrain are similarly affected in all patients, the presence and degree of histopathological changes in the cerebral cortex are a function of the disease duration, which, in turn, as mentioned above, is largely related to the genotype at *PRNP* codon 129. Cases that come to autopsy between 7 and 10 months from the clinical onset only display focal spongiform degeneration in the entorhinal cortex, and minimal astrogliosis in the deep layers of the cerebral neocortex. In cases of over 10-month disease duration, progressive spongiform degeneration and, to a lesser extent, gliosis and neuronal loss, affect the cerebral neocortex. These lesions are mild and focal in subjects with 11 to 18 month duration, and become widespread beyond 20 months. The cerebellar cortex shows minimal neuronal loss and astrogliosis. Recent findings indicate that serotoninergic neurons are selectively decreased in the raphe nuclei and that neuronal loss in FFI is the result of apoptosis (5, 50).

In conclusion, thalamic atrophy is the histopathological hallmark of FFI, while the severity of the histopathological lesions in the neocortex and in the limbic cortex is directly related to the disease duration. Therefore, lesions generally are limited to the thalamus in homozygous subjects while they also affect the cerebral cortex in the heterozygous subjects (31).

Immunohistochemistry

Immunohistochemistry on paraffin sections fails to detect the scrapie prion protein (PrP^{res}) in any brain region except for the cases of very long duration (31).

Biochemistry

Immunoblot has demonstrated that the amount and distribution of PrP^{res} only partially match the severity and topography of the histological lesions (31). For example, in cases with disease duration of up to 11 months, very little or no PrP^{res} is present in the cerebral neocortex where there is no significant pathology, whereas relatively large amounts are present in the thalamus, which is markedly affected (31). However, significant amounts of PrP^{res} are also present in the limbic regions and brain stem although the pathology is minimal in these regions. Furthermore, the kinetics of PrP^{res} accumulation varies between the cerebral cortex and subcortical structures such as the thalamus and brainstem. While in the cerebral cortex the amount of PrP^{res} increases progressively with the disease duration, in the thalamus and brain stem it remains constant (31). Overall, the amount of PrP^{res} in FFI is 5 to 10 times less than that in typical sporadic CJD and can be difficult to detect in the neocortex in cases of short duration unless larger amount of proteins are immunoblotted (33). Since the amount of PrP^{res} is known to correlate with the severity of spongiform degeneration, this finding provides a reasonable explanation for the lack of significant spongiosis in FFI (31).

Two general features that distinguish PrP^{res} species associated with human prion diseases are the size of the PrP fragment resistant to protease treatment and the ratio of the 3 glycoforms (11). Following treatment with proteinase K (PK), PrP^{res} generates 2 types of protease-resistant fragments with distinct sizes and electrophoretic patterns due to the cleavage of PrP^{res} at different sites (27, 30, 32, 35). PrP^{res} type 1 generates a PK-resistant fragment that has a relative molecular mass of 21 kDa and the primary cleavage site at residue 82; PrP^{res} type 2 fragment has a relative molecular mass of 19 kDa and the primary cleavage site at residue 97 (27, 30, 32, 35). The different sizes are likely to reflect the different conformation of the 2 PrP^{res} types. Furthermore, it has been shown that the PrP types are at least partially specified by the *PRNP* genotype and that they are often associated with different pathologies. FFI is characterised by the presence in the brain tissue of PrP^{res} type 2 of 19 kDa, while $fCJD^{178}$ is associated with PrP^{res} type 1 of 21 kDa. Therefore, the different codon at position 129, methionine in FFI and valine in CJD^{178}, appears to act as a determinant of the PrP^{res} conformation (Figure 3). Furthermore, the glycoform ratio of the PrP^{res} type 2 associated with FFI also is distinctive because it is characterised by a marked under representation of the unglycosylated form (29). In the frontal cortex, the percent distribution of the diglycosylated, monoglycosylated and unglycosylated forms is 58, 37 and 5, respectively, which makes the relative amount of unglycosylated form present in FFI the lowest of all familial prion diseases (27).

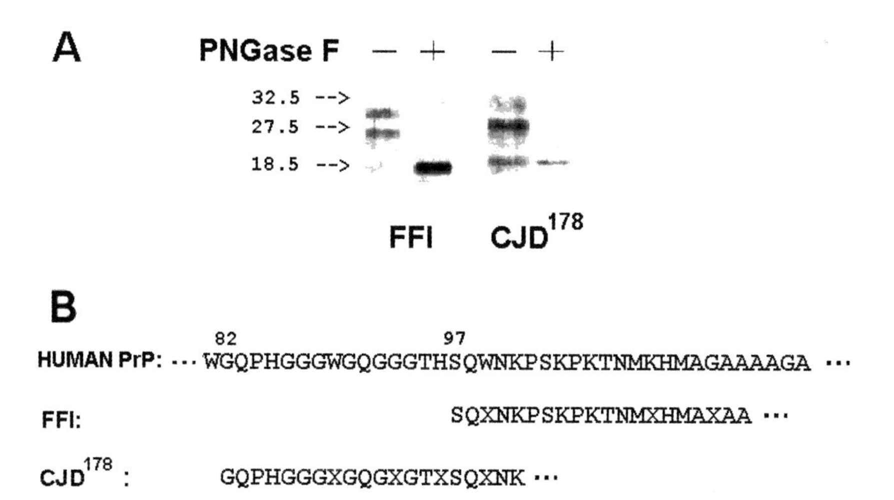

Figure 3. *Characterisation of PK-resistant PrP^{res} in brains of subjects with FFI and CJD^{178}.* **A.** Silver staining of purified PK-resistant PrP^{res} type 2 in FFI and PrP^{res} type 1 in CJD^{178}. Three PrP glycoforms (PNGase F-) are present at different ratio that upon deglycosylation (PNGase F+) reduce to one fragment with the size of approximately 19 kDa (type 2) in FFI and 21 kDa (type 1) in CJD^{178}. **B.** Analysis of PK cleavage site of PrP^{res} in FFI and CJD^{178} by N-terminal sequencing. When aligned with the predicted human PrP sequence (top), the PrP^{res} type 2 in FFI shows an N-terminus consistent with the PK cleavage site at residue 97 (middle), while type 1 PrP^{res} in CJD^{178} (bottom) shows an N-terminus derived from the PK cleavage at residue 82. The N-terminal sequencing was carried out using automated Edman degradation, which sometimes gives ambiguous signals at certain residues (X) in this particular experiment.

Differential Diagnosis

The clinical and polysomnographic features of FFI are quite distinctive, especially in the 129 homozygous patients. In 129 heterozygous patients, the longer disease course, the less prominent sleep-wake disturbance and more evident motor abnormalities require differentiation from the other prion diseases, especially $fCJD^{178}$. Conditions that clinically mimic sFI, in particular the characteristic sleep disturbance, are the Morvan's syndrome, a rare autoimmune disease with antibodies against voltage-gated K channels, limbic encephalitis, and alcohol or tranquillizers withdrawal syndrome (delirium tremens) (18, 19, 45). However, the clinical course and the pathology of these conditions are very different from those of FFI and sFI.

Experimental Models

FFI has been transmitted to receptive transgenic mice expressing a chimera mouse-human PrP carrying methionine in position 129 (48). Following intracerebral inoculation of brain homogenate from FFI-affected subjects, transgenic animals developed a prion disease that mimicked to some extent FFI as for the distribution of the lesions and of PrP^{res}. Furthermore, the PrP^{res} formed by these mice specifically reproduced the type of the PrP^{res} associated with FFI in humans (type 2). This experiment has demonstrated that FFI is a transmissible prion disease and that the PrP^{res} type 2 associated with FFI fulfils the characteristics of a distinct prion species or "strain" since it is associated with a distinct histopathological phenotype that is stable upon transmission (48).

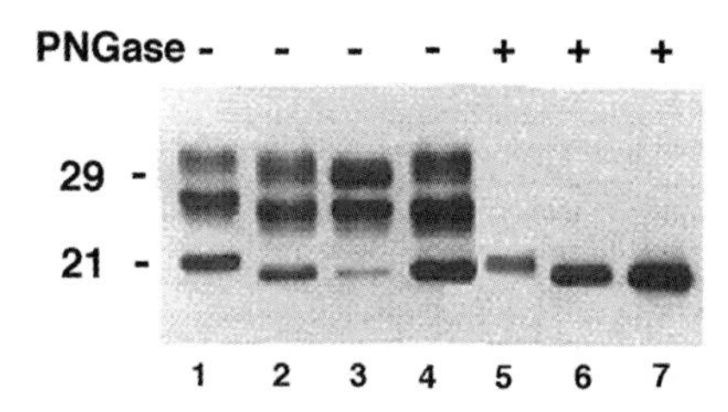

Figure 4. Immunoblot of PK-treated PrP^{res} from sCJD associated with PrP^{res} type 1 and 2 (lanes 1 and 2, respectively), FFI (lane 3) and sFI (lane 4), with the three glycoforms (lanes 1-4) and following removal of the glycans with PNGase (lanes 5-7). Note the under representation of the unglycosylated form in FFI and the different gel mobility between PrP^{res} type 1 (lanes 1 and 5) and type 2 (lanes 2-4 and 6, 7).

Pathogenesis

Data from transfected human neuroblastoma cells carrying the FFI *PRNP* genotype indicate that the D178N mutation results in the destabilization of the mutated PrP that is partially corrected by the glycosylation (37). Therefore, only the glycosylated forms reach the cell surface whereas the mutated PrP lacking the glycans is degraded in intracellular compartments. The preferential degradation of the unglycosylated mutated PrP form suggests that the striking under representation of this form, a distinctive feature of the PrP^{res} associated with FFI, is due to the unavailability of this form for conversion to PrP^{res} rather than preferential conversion of the glycosylated forms. This conclusion is supported by three lines of evidence: *i)* the unglycosylated form of the D178N mutated PrP is also under represented in FFI brains validating the finding obtained from the FFI cell model; *ii)* in FFI, PrP^{res} more likely reflects the glycoform ratio of the mutated PrP because only the mutated PrP (not both mutated and normal as in other familial prion diseases) is converted to PrP^{res}; and *iii)* the PrP^{res} present in sFI, which lacks the D178N mutation, the unglycosylated form is not under represented and is similar to that of other sporadic prion diseases (1, 33, 37).

Nuclear magnetic resonance (NMR) studies have shown that residues 178 and 129 are relatively close in the 3-dimensional structure of recombinant PrP (16, 17, 42). This finding has led to the hypothesis that the perturbation caused by the D178N mutation differs as a function of the residue at position 129 providing the structural basis for the segregation of FFI and fCJD[178] with the 2 distinct haplotypes D178N-129M and D178N-129V, respectively (16, 42).

According to the prevalent hypothesis, mutated PrP that is unstable and has distinctive characteristics would invariably undergo spontaneous conversion to a distinct PrP^{res} isoform or strain that then directs the expression of the FFI phenotype (10). In sFI, PrP^{res} with strain characteristics similar to those of the PrP^{res} associated with FFI would be generated by spontaneous conversion of the normal PrP. As mentioned above, the conclusion that the PrP^{res} associated with FFI and sFI is a distinct prion strain is supported by the experiments of transmission to mice.

A compelling hypothesis holds that sleep impairment in FFI and sFI is due to the severe neuronal loss in medial dorsal and anterior ventral thalamic nuclei that disconnects the limbic cortex from the brain stem and leads to a generalized activation syndrome characterized by inability to sleep associated with autonomic and motor activation (19, 21). However, it must be kept in mind that in FFI and sFI the presence of the mutated PrP and PrP^{res} in the brain of FFI and sFI patients is widespread and goes far beyond the thalamus. Therefore, other mechanisms and brain locales cannot be excluded.

Sporadic Fatal Insomnia

The 9 proven cases of sFI reported to date have clinical, polysomnographic, and pathological features similar to those of FFI (25, 33, 43). The mean age at onset and the duration vary between 36 and 70 years and 15 and 30 months, respectively. The clinical presentation includes ataxia, impaired cognition, dysautonomia and sleep disturbances. Cognitive and motor impairments, such as dysarthria, myoclonus, tremor as well as pyramidal and extrapyramidal signs, appear later in the course. Sleep disturbances and dysautonomia are present in the majority of the cases. EEG recording is non-specific. Polysomnographic recording carried out in one case was indistinguishable from that of FFI (43).

At gross inspection the brain may reveal mild atrophy of frontal lobes. As in FFI, the histological hallmark is loss of neurons and gliosis in thalamic nuclei with no spongiform degeneration. The medial dorsal, anterior ventral, lateral dorsal and pulvinar nuclei are generally more affected than other thalamic nuclei. The cerebral neocortex shows focal spongiform degeneration and astrogliosis in the frontal, parietal and temporal lobes while the occipital cortex is generally less affected. Except for the entorhinal cortex that is affected by moderate spongiform degeneration, astrogliosis and mild neuronal loss, the hippocampal formation is spared. The basal ganglia are also unaffected while the cerebellum generally shows a moderate degree of atrophy of the dentate nucleus and of the cortex with the presence of "torpedoes." In the brain stem, there is consistent atrophy of the inferior olives as well as astrogliosis of the periaqueductal gray and of the tectum.

Immunostaining for PrP^{res} is unrewarding as in FFI. It is only occasionally positive in the lower temporal and entorhinal cortices.

Genetically sFI is very homogeneous. Although the *PRNP* D178N mutation is lacking, all the cases examined to date are homozygous for methionine at codon 129 (25, 33, 43). As in FFI, PrP^{res} associated with sFI is of type 2 and is present in very low amounts. However, at variance with FFI, PrP^{res} of sFI does not show the under representation of the unglycosylated form. The glycoform ratio expressed as percent distribution of the diglycosylated, monoglycosylated and unglycosylated forms is 26:40:34, similar to that of sporadic CJD (33). The different PrP^{res} glycoform ratio is a consistent finding helpful in distinguishing sFI from FFI on immunoblot. One sFI case has been transmitted to transgenic mice expressing a mouse-human PrP with methionine in position 129. Affected mice developed a disease characterized by the presence of PrPSc type 2 as in the donor and a histopathology and PrP^{res} distribution similar to that of FFI (25).

Future Directions

At least 3 important issues related to the pathogenesis of FFI and sFI remain unresolved: *i)* the contribution of the sleep impairment to the rapidity of the disease course; *ii)* the mechanism leading to the selective involvement of the thalamus with neuronal loss and gliosis but not spongiosis, which is the most common change in prion diseases; and *iii)* how amounts of PrP^{res} that are much lower than those of other prion diseases may be associated with a disease that is so severe and has such a wide range of signs. Animal models may help to clarify these issues.

In summary, the importance of FFI goes far beyond its prevalence, for several reasons. First, it has introduced a novel and distinctive phenotype into the group of human prion diseases widening the phenotypic spectrum of these diseases. Second, it has brought about the discovery of a novel genetic mechanism that explains the clinical and pathological variability of familial diseases linked to the same genetic mutation. Third, it has led to the identification of the 2 major forms of scrapie prion protein in human prion diseases. Fourth, because FFI is the first well-characterised hereditary disease associated with alterations of the sleep-wake cycle and other circadian rhythms, it offers a unique model to study clinically and experimentally mechanisms of sleep regulation.

References

1. Chen SG, Parchi P, Brown P, Capellari S, Zou W, Cochran EJ, Vnencak-Jones CL, Julien J, Vital C, Mikol J, Lugaresi E, Autilio-Gambetti L, Gambetti P (1997) Allelic origin of the abnormal prion protein isoform in familial prion diseases. *Nat Med* 3: 1009-1015.

2. Collinge J, Palmer MS, Dryden AJ (1991) Genetic predisposition to iatrogenic Creutzfeldt-Jakob disease. *Lancet* 337: 1441-1442.

3. Cortelli P, Parchi P, Contin M, Pierangeli G, Avoni P, Tinuper P, Montagna P, Baruzzi A, Gambetti PL,

Lugaresi E (1991) Cardiovascular dysautonomia in fatal familial insomnia. *Clin Auton Res* 1: 15-21.

4. Cortelli P, Perani D, Parchi P, Grassi F, Montagna P, De Martin M, Castellani R, Tinuper P, Gambetti P, Lugaresi E, Fazio F (1997) Cerebral metabolism in fatal familial insomnia: relation to duration, neuropathology, and distribution of protease-resistant prion protein. *Neurology* 49: 126-133.

5. Dorandeu A, Wingertsmann L, Chrétien F, Delisle MB, Vital C, Parchi P, et al (1998) Neuronal Apoptosis in Fatal Familial Insomnia. *Brain Pathol* 8: 531-537.

6. Gallassi R, Morreale A, Montagna P, Cortelli P, Avoni P, Castellani R, Gambetti P, Lugaresi E (1996) Fatal familial insomnia: behavioral and cognitive features. *Neurology* 46: 935-939.

7. Gallassi R, Morreale A, Montagna P, Gambetti P, Lugaresi E (1992) "Fatal familial insomnia": neuropsychological study of a disease with thalamic degeneration. *Cortex* 28: 175-187.

8. Gambetti P, Parchi P, Petersen RB, Chen SG, Lugaresi E (1995) Fatal Familial Insomnia and Familial Creutzfeldt-Jakob Disease: Clinical, Pathological and Molecular Features. *Brain Pathol* 5: 43-51.

9. Gambetti P, Lugaresi E (1998) Conclusions of the Symposium. *Brain Pathol* 8: 571-575.

10. Gambetti P, Petersen RB, Parchi P, Chen SG, Capellari S, Goldfarb L, Gabizon R, Montagna P, Lugaresi E, Piccardo P, Ghetti B (1999) Inherited prion diseases. In *Prion Biology and Diseases* (Prusiner SB, ed), pp. 509-583, Cold Springs Harbor Laboratory Press, New York, NY

11. Gambetti P, Parchi P, Capellari S, Russo C, Tabaton M, Teller JK, Chen SG (2001) Mechanisms of phenotypic heterogeneity in prion, Alzheimer and other conformational diseases. *Journal of Alzheimer's Disease* 3: 87-95.

12. Goldfarb LG, Brown P, Goldgaber D (1989) Patients with Creutzfeldt-Jakob disease and kuru lack the mutation in the PRNP gene found in Gerstmann-Sträussler Scheinker syndrome, but they show a different double-allele mutation in the same gene. *Am J Hum Gen* 45: (Supplement): A189.

13. Goldfarb LG, Petersen RB, Tabaton M, Brown P, LeBlanc AC, Montagna P, Cortelli P, Julien J, Vital C, Pendelbury WW, et al (1992) Fatal familial insomnia and familial Creutzfeldt-Jakob disease: disease phenotype determined by a DNA polymorphism. *Science* 258: 806-808.

14. Hainfellner JA, Parchi P, Kitamoto T, Jarius C, Gambetti P, Budka H (1999) A novel phenotype in familial Creutzfeldt-Jakob disease: prion protein gene E200K mutation coupled with valine at codon 129 and type 2 protease-resistant prion protein. *Annals of Neurology* 45(6): 812-816.

15. Harder A, Jendroska K, Kreuz F, Wirth T, Schafranka C, Karnatz N, Theallier-Janko A, Dreier J, Lohan K, Emmerich D, Cervos-Navarro J, Windl O, Kretzschmar HA, Nurnberg P, Witkowski R (1999) Novel twelve-generation kindred of fatal familial insomnia from Germany representing the entire spectrum of disease expression. *Am J Med Genet* 87: 311-316.

16. James TL, Liu H, Ulyanov NB, Farr-Jones S, Zhang H, Donne, DG, Kaneko K, Groth D, Mehlhorn I, Prusiner SB, Cohen FE (1997) Solution Structure of a 142-Residue Recombinant Prion Protein Corresponding to the Infectious Fragment of the Scrapie Isoform. *Proc Natl Acad Sci U S A* 94: 10086-10091.

17. Liemann S., Glockshuber R (1999) Influence of amino acid substitutions related to inherited human prion diseases on the thermodynamic stability of the cellular prion protein. *Biochemistry* 38(11): 3258-3567.

18. Liguori R, Vincent A, Avoni P, Plazzi G, Baruzzi A, Carey T, Gambetti P, Lugaresi E, Montagna P (2001) Morvan's syndrome: peripheral and central nervous system and cardiac involvement with antibodies to voltage-gated potassium channels. *Brain* 124: 2417-2426.

19. Lugaresi E, Provini (2001) Agrypnia Excitata Clinical Features and Pathophysiological Implication. *Sleep Medicine Reviews* 5: 313-322.

20. Lugaresi E, Medori R, Montagna P, Baruzzi A, Cortelli P, Lugaresi A, Tinuper P, Zucconi M, Gambetti P (1986) Fatal familial insomnia and dysautonomia with selective degeneration of thalamic nuclei. *N Engl J Med* 315: 997-1003.

21. Lugaresi E, Tobler I, Gambetti P, Montagna P (1998) The pathophysiology of Fatal Familial Insomnia. *Brain Pathol* 8: 521-526.

22. Manetto V, Medori R, Cortelli P, Montagna P, Tinuper P, Baruzzi A, Rancurel G, Hauw JJ, Vanderhaegen JJ, Mailleux P, et al (1992) Fatal familial insomnia: clinical and pathologic study of five new cases. *Neurology* 42: 312-319.

23. Martin JJ (1975) Thalamic degeneration. In *Handbook of Clinical Neurology*, Vinken PJ, Bruyn GW (eds). North-Holland Publishing Company: Amsterdam. Volume 21 pp. 587-604.

24. Martin JJ, Yap M, Nei IP, Tan TE (1983) Selective thalamic degeneration - Report of a case with memory and mental disturbances. *Clin Neuropathol* 2: 156-162.

25. Mastrianni JA, Nixon R, Layzer R, Telling GC, Han D, DeArmond SJ, Prusiner SB (1999) Prion protein conformation in a patient with sporadic fatal insomnia. *N Engl J Med* 340: 1630-1638.

26. Medori R, Tritschler HJ, LeBlanc A, Villare F, Manetto V, Chen HY, Xue R, Leal S, Montagna P, Cortelli P, et al (1992) Fatal familial insomnia, a prion disease with a mutation at codon 178 of the prion protein gene. *N Engl J Med* 326: 444-449.

27. Monari L, Chen SG, Brown P, Parchi P, Petersen RB, Mikol J, Gray F, Cortelli P, Montagna P, Ghetti B, et al (1994) Fatal familial insomnia and familial Creutzfeldt-Jakob disease: different prion proteins determined by a DNA polymorphism. *Proc Natl Acad Sci U S A* 91: 2839-2842.

28. Montagna P, Cortelli P, Avoni P, Tinuper P, Plazzi G, Gallassi R, Portaluppi F, Julien J, Vital C, Delisle MB, Gambetti P, Lugaresi E (1998) Clinical Features of Fatal Familial Insomnia: Phenotypic Variability in Relation to a Polymorphism at Codon 129 of the Prion Protein Gene. *Brain Pathol* 8: 515-520.

29. Padovani A, D'Alessandro M, Parchi P, Cortelli P, Anzola GP, Montagna P, Vignolo LA, Petraroli R, Pocchiari M, Lugaresi E, Gambetti P (1998) Fatal familial insomnia in a new Italian kindred. *Neurology* 51: 1491-1494.

30. Parchi P, Castellani R, Capellari S, Ghetti B, Young K, Chen SG, Farlow M, Dickson DW, Sima AA, Trojanowski JQ, Petersen RB, Gambetti P (1996) Molecular basis of phenotypic variability in sporadic Creutzfeldt-Jakob disease. *Ann Neurol* 39(6): 767-778.

31. Parchi P, Castellani R, Cortelli P, Montagna P, Chen SG, Petersen RB, Lugaresi E, Autilio-Gambetti L, Gambetti P (1995) Regional distribution of protease-resistant prion protein in Fatal Familial Insomnia. *Ann Neurol* 38: 21-29.

32. Parchi P, Capellari S, Chen SG, Petersen RB, Gambetti P, Kopp N, Brown P, Kitamoto T, Tateishi J, Giese A, Kretzschmar H (1997) Typing prion isoforms. *Nature* 386: 232-234.

33. Parchi P, Capellari S, Chin S, Schwarz HB, Schecter NP, Butts JD, Hudkins P, Burns DK, Powers JM, Gambetti P (1999) A subtype of sporadic prion disease mimicking fatal familial insomnia. *Neurology* 52: 1757-1763.

34. Parchi P, Capellari S, Gambetti P (2000) Intracerebral distribution of the abnormal isoform of the prion protein in sporadic Creutzfeldt-Jakob disease and fatal insomnia. *Microsc Res Tech* 50: 16-25.

35. Parchi P, Zou W, Wang W, Brown P, Capellari S, Ghetti B, Kopp N, Schulz-Schaeffer WJ, Kretzschmar HA, Head MW, Ironside JW, Gambetti P, Chen SG (2000) Genetic influence on the structural variations of the abnormal prion protein. *Proc Natl Acad Sci U S A* 97: 10168-10172.

36. Perani D, Cortelli P, Lucignani G, Montagna P, Tinuper P, Gallassi R, Gambetti P, Lenzi GL, Lugaresi E, Fazio F (1993) [18F]FDG PET in fatal familial insomnia: the functional effects of thalamic lesions. *Neurology* 43: 2565-2569.

37. Petersen RB, Parchi P, Richardson SL, Urig CB, Gambetti P (1996) Effect of the D178N mutation and the codon 129 polymorphism on the metabolism of the prion protein. *J Biol Chem* 271: 12661-12668.

38. Petersen RB, Tabaton M, Berg L, Schrank B, Torack RM, Leal S, Julien J, Vital C, Deleplanque B, Pendlebury WW, Drachman D, Smith TW, Martin JJ, Oda M, Montagna P, Ott J, Autilio-Gambetti L, Lugaresi E, Gambetti P (1992) Analysis of the prion gene in thalamic dementia. *Neurology* 42: 1859-1863.

39. Portaluppi F, Cortelli P, Avoni P, Vergnani L, Contin M, Maltoni P, Pavani A, Sforza E, degli Uberti EC, Gambetti P, et al (1994) Diurnal blood pressure variation and hormonal correlates in fatal familial insomnia. *Hypertension* 23: 569-576.

40. Portaluppi F, Cortelli P, Avoni P, Vergnani L, Maltoni P, Pavani A, Sforza E, Degli Uberti EC, Gambetti P, Lugaresi E (1994) Progressive disruption of the circadian rhythm of melatonin in fatal familial insomnia. *J Clin Endocrinol Metab* 78: 1075-1078.

41. Portaluppi F, Cortelli P, Avoni P, Vergnani L, Maltoni P, Pavani A, Sforza E, Manfredini R, Montagna P, Roiter I, et al (1995) Dissociated 24-hour patterns of

somatotropin and prolactin in fatal familial insomnia. *Neuroendocrinology* 61: 731-737.

42. Riek R, Wider G, Billeter M, Hornemann S, Glockshuber R, Wüthrich K (1998) Prion protein NMR structure and familial human spongiform encephalopathies. *Proc Natl Acad Sci U S A* 95: 11667-11672.

43. Scaravilli F, Cordery RJ, Kretzschmar H, Gambetti P, Brink B, Fritz V, Temlett J, Kaplan C, Fish D, An SF, Schulz-Schaeffer WJ, Rossor MN (2000) Sporadic fatal insomnia: a case study. *Ann Neurol* 48: 665-668.

44. Sforza E, Montagna P, Tinuper P, Cortelli P, Avoni P, Ferrillo F, Petersen R, Gambetti P, Lugaresi E (1995) Sleep-wake cycle abnormalities in fatal familial insomnia. Evidence of the role of the thalamus in sleep regulation. *Electroencephalogr clin Neurophysiol* 94: 398-405.

45. Silber MH, Nippoldt TB, Karnes PS, Goerss JB, Patel T, Kane L (1995) Morvan's fibrillary chorea resembling fatal familial insomnia. *Sleep Res* 24: 431.

46. Steel M (1993) Genetics: Polymorphism, proteins and phenotypes. *Lancet* 341: 212-213.

47. Tabernero C, Polo JM, Sevillano MD, Munoz R, Berciano J, Cabello Baez B, Ricoy JR, Carpizo R, Figols J, Cuadrado N, Claveria LE (2000) Fatal familial insomnia: clinical, neuropathological, and gene description of a Spanish family. *J Neurol Neurosurg Psychiatry* 68: 774-777.

48. Telling GC, Parchi P, DeArmond SJ, Cortelli P, Montagna P, Gabizon R, Mastrianni J, Lugaresi E, Gambetti P, and Prusiner SB (1996) Evidence for the conformation of the pathologic isoform of the prion protein enciphering and propagating prion diversity. *Science* 274: 2079-2082.

49. Walker RH, Friedman J, Weiner J, Hobler R, Gwinn-Hardy K, Adam A, DeWolfe J, Gibbs R, Baker M, Farrer M, Hutton M, and Hardy J. A Family with a Tau P301L Mutation Presenting with Parkinsonism. *Parkinsonism Related D* 9: 121-123.

50. Wanschitz J, Kloppel S, Jarius C, Birner P, Flicker H, Hainfellner JA, Gambetti P, Guentchev M, Budka H (2000) Alteration of the serotonergic nervous system in Fatal Familial Insomnia. *Ann Neurol* 48: 788-791.

51. Windl O, Giese A, Schulz-Schaeffer W, Zerr I, Skworc K, Arendt S, Oberdieck C, Bodemer M, Poser S, Kretzschmar HA (1999) Molecular genetics of human prion diseases in Germany. *Hum Genet* 105: 244-252.

Kuru

Catriona A. McLean

Definition

Prion disease transmitted through the practise of cannibalistic feasting.

Synonyms and Historical Annotations

Kuru is the prototypic iatrogenic human TSE. It occurred in the Fore linguistic group and their neighbours in the Eastern Highlands of New Guinea (1) in an epidemic that started in the 1940s. It is presumed that the disease was transmitted via an original case of sporadic CJD with the abnormal prion protein being recycled within this confined environment due to the practise of cannibalistic feasting by family and community members of the deceased. By 1957 over 200 new cases per year were being registered with a mean incubation period estimated at 12 years. Affected women and children predominated. Brain and internal organ funerary practice was delegated to women and children, hence increasing their transmission risk. The Australian Government put an end to the practice of cannibalistic feasting in 1956 with a subsequent decline and disappearance of the disease over the ensuing 40 years. Analyses of clinical, epidemiological, pathological and limited molecular studies utilising the extraordinary records and reports that commenced in the 1950s and the tissue stored with such insight by the early researchers has provided important information into iatrogenic transmission of PrP^{CJD}. The latter issue has been thrust into contemporary relevance by the initial cases of vCJD.

Genetics

Analyses of codon 129 of kuru has shown M-V, M-M and V-V genotypes (3, 5, 8, 9). More recent studies have shown those patients with an M/M genotype were preferentially affected (9, 10, 12) and those with M/V and V/V genotypes appeared to be predisposed to a lower risk of disease development and longer incubation times.

Clinical Features

The onset of disease ranged from 5 years to over 60 years with a mean duration of illness being 12 months, commencing with subtle loss of coordination and progressing within weeks to postural instability, dysarthria and generalised "shivering tremors." With progressive ataxia, the patients became sedentary with worsening ataxia and tremors associated with emotional lability and choreoathetotic involuntary movements, progressing to death from malnutrition. Unlike sporadic CJD, dementia was not a dominant feature.

Macroscopy

Macroscopic brain examination reveals cerebellar atrophy, the cerebrum and basal ganglia showing no macroscopic pathology.

Histopathology

Microscopy reveals a relatively homogeneous topographical distribution of spongiform change in all kuru cases (Figure 1). Spongiform change is present in laminae 3-5, prominently in the cingulate gyrus, with minimal involvement of occipital cortex and insular gyri. All laminae in the subiculum show prominent spongiform change (2, 4, 6, 7, 10, 11). The hippocampus is unaffected in some studies (5-7, 10) with no evidence of spongiform change or neuronal loss in CA1, 2, or 3, or the dentate gyrus. However, severe changes have been reported in CA1 in 2 kuru cases (8). The putamen and caudate nuclei show prominent and severe spongiform change, with occasional putamenal neurons showing intraneuronal vacuoles. A lesser degree of spongiform change is noted in the thalamus in all cases, with the medial nuclei appearing more affected than the lateral nuclei.

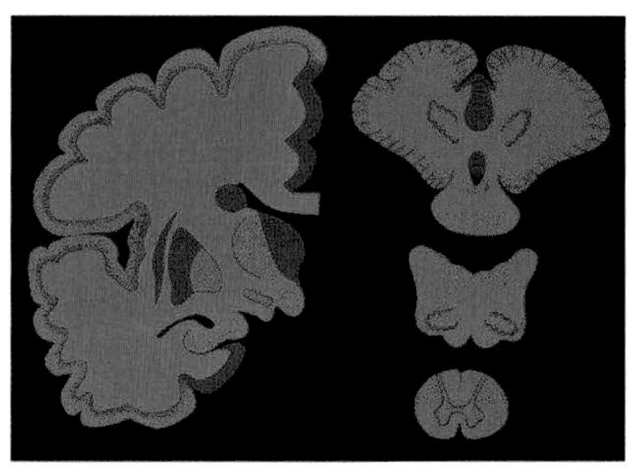

Figure 1. Topographic distribution and intensity of spongiform change in kuru, as indicated by intensity of colour.

The cerebellar molecular layer shows prominent spongiform change with intense molecular and granular

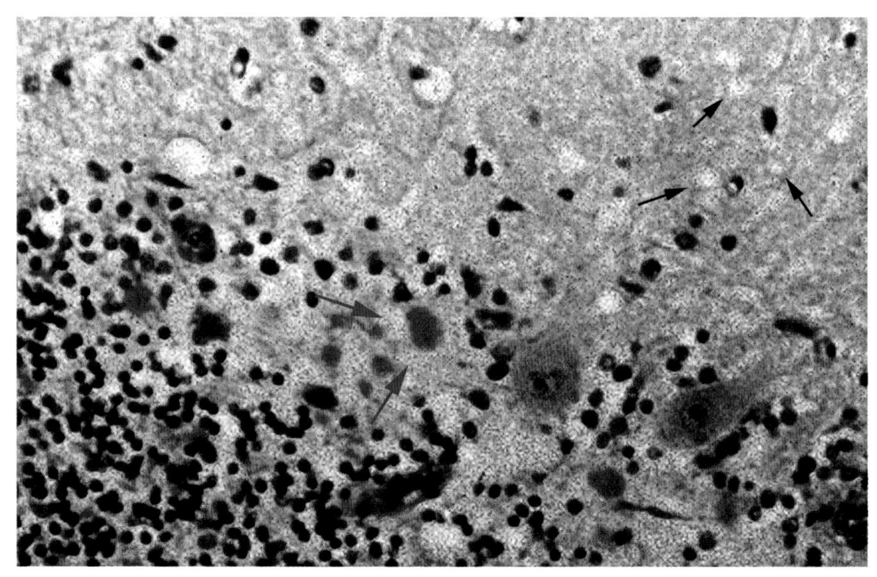

Figure 2. Kuru cerebellum showing spongiform change in the molecular layer (dark arrows) and a multicentric amyloid plaque centred on the granular layer (blue arrows). H & E. ×400.

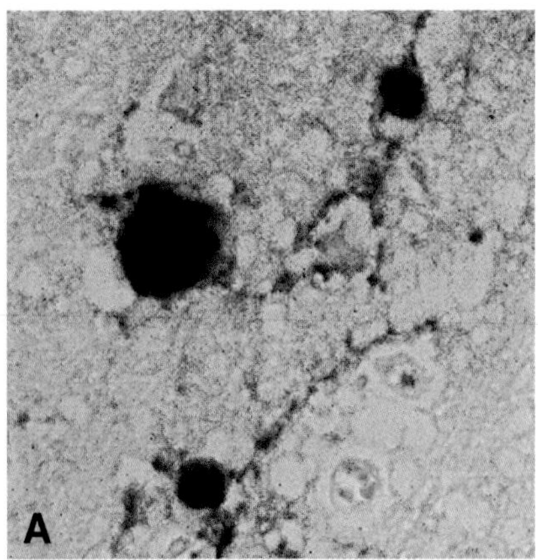

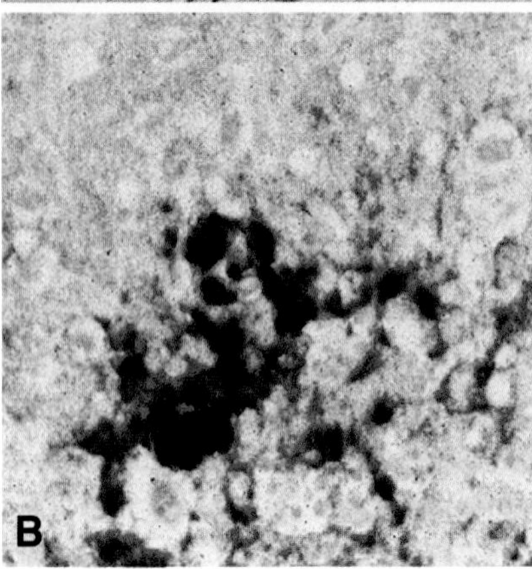

Figure 3. A. Kuru PrP immunoreactive plaques and perineuronal and dendritic PrP in the cortex. **B.** Irregular multi-centric cerebellar granular layer plaques (PrP [3F4 Senetec™]). ×400.

layer gliosis, associated with granular cell and variable Purkinje cell loss. Within the midbrain, minor depigmentation of the neurons of the substantia nigra is seen. Spongiform change is moderate to severe in the periaqueductal grey matter and colliculi, and was associated with moderate gliosis. Minor spongiosis and gliosis are seen in the basis pontis, central tegmental area and inferior olivary nucleus in the pons and medulla. Within the spinal cord available, neuronal preservation is apparent with minimal evidence of gliosis and minor spongiform change in the substantia gelatinosa. Plaques are seen by haematoxylin and eosin stains within the granular layer of the cerebellum with occasional plaques in the molecular layer (Figure 2). Plaques are PAS positive and argyrophilic and uniformly present in cerebellum. Kuru plaques are rarely seen in the cortex and putamen.

Immunohistochemistry and Ultrastructural Findings

By immunocytochemistry, variation in both the form and distribution of PrP within different brain areas in kuru is seen, although the changes seen in each area are relatively constant from case to case. The main forms of PrP deposition are synaptic, plaque and perineuronal. Plaques vary in size up to 30 μm in size and are mostly unicentric, with occasional groups of smaller plaques (Figure 3A, B). Within the cingulate, insular and entorhinal gyri, PrP immunostaining shows a weak lamina 3-5 synaptic pattern with perineuronal PrP outlining large pyramidal cells and their dendrites (5, 10) Scattered, infrequent plaques are seen in all laminae. The subiculum shows an intense synaptic pattern in all laminae with sparse perineuronal staining, but there is no PrP deposition in the pyramidal layer and dentate gyrus of the hippocampus. Within the basal ganglia and thalamus a faint synaptic pattern is seen in most cases, with scattered to moderate numbers of small PrP plaques.

The cerebellum shows a pronounced plaque and synaptic deposition localised to the granular layer with only infrequent molecular layer plaques. Within the brainstem and spinal cord, synaptic PrP of varying degree is seen in the substantia nigra, periaqueductal grey matter, colliculi, basis pontis and central tegmental area, the inferior olivary nucleus, and the spinal grey matter with emphasis on the substantia gelatinosa. Specific cranial nerve nuclei are not affected although very small PrP deposits are present in the adjacent parenchyma. Linear PrP is seen in some transverse white matter tracts with a very occasional plaque. The relatively homogeneous phenotype of kuru resembles the sporadic CJD phenotype seen in cases with a type-2 PrP^{Sc} (13).

Biochemistry

Western blot studies of 2 kuru cases have also revealed a type-2 PrP^{Sc} (12). These findings are evidence for transmission of a similar strain of agent, supporting the hypothesised indexed sporadic CJD case at the commencement of the epidemic.

References

1. Alpers M (1968) Kuru, Implications of its transmissibility for the interpretation of its changing epidemiological pattern. In *The Central Nervous System Models of Neurological Diseases*, Bailey O, Smith D (eds). Williams and Wilkins: Baltimore. pp. 234-251.

2. Beck E, Daniel PM (1979) Kuru and Creutzfeltd-Jakob disease: Neuropathological lesions and their significance. In *Slow Transmissible Diseases of The Nervous System*, Prusiner SB, Hadlow, WJ. (eds). Academic Press: New York. pp. 253-270.

3. Cervenakova L, Goldfarb LG, Garruto R, Lee HS, Gajdusek DC, Brown P (1998) Phenotype-genotype studies in kuru: implications for new variant Creutzfeldt-Jakob disease. *Proc Natl Acad Sci U S A* 95:13239-13241.

4. Fowler M, Robertson E (1958) Observations on Kuru. III Pathological features in five cases. *Australasian Ann Med* 8:16-26.

5. Hainfellner JA, Liberski PP, Guiroy DC, Cervenakova L, Brown P, Gajdusek DC, Budka H (1997) Pathology and immunocytochemistry of a kuru brain. *Brain Pathol* 7:547-553.

6. Kakulas B, Lecours A, Gajdusek DC (1967) Further observations on the pathology of Kuru. *J Neuropathol Exp Neurol* 26:85-97.

7. Klatzo I, Gajdusek DC, Zigas V (1959) Pathology of Kuru. *Lab Invest* 8:799-847.

8. Lantos PL, Bhatia K, Doey LJ, al-Sarraj S, Doshi R, Beck J, Collinge J (1997) Is the neuropathology of new variant Creutzfeldt-Jakob disease and kuru similar? *Lancet* 350:187-188.

9. Lee HS, Brown P, Cervenakova L, Garruto RM, Alpers MP, Gajdusek DC, Goldfarb LG (2001) Increased susceptibility to Kuru of carriers of the PRNP 129 methionine/methionine genotype. *J Infect Dis* 183:192-196.

10. McLean CA, Ironside JW, Alpers MP, Brown PW, Cervenakova L, Anderson RM, Masters CL (1998) Comparative neuropathology of Kuru with the new variant of Creutzfeldt-Jakob disease: evidence for strain of agent predominating over genotype of host. *Brain Pathol* 8:429-437.

11. Neumann M, Gajdusek DC, Zigas V (1964) Neuropathological findings in exotic neurologic disorders among natives of the highlands of New Guinea. *J Neuropathol Exp Neurol* 486-507.

12. Parchi P, Capellari S, Chen SG, Petersen RB, Gambetti P, Kopp N, Brown P, Kitamoto T, Tateishi J, Giese A, Kretzschmar H (1997) Typing prion isoforms. *Nature* 386:232-234.

13. Parchi P, Castellani R, Capellari S, Ghetti B, Young K, Chen SG, Farlow M, Dickson DW, Sima AA, Trojanowski JQ, Petersen RB, Gambetti P (1996) Molecular basis of phenotypic variability in sporadic Creutzfeldt-Jakob disease. *Ann Neurol* 1996:767-778.

In Vivo and In Vitro Models of Prion Disease

Moira Bruce
David Westaway

BSE	bovine spongiform encephalopathy
CJD	Creutzfeldt-Jakob disease
PCR	polymerase chain reaction
PMCA	protein mis-folding cyclic amplification
PrP	prion protein
TSE	transmissible spongiform encephalopathy
vCJD	new variant Creutzfeldt-Jakob disease

Animal Models

Sporadic, variant, and some familial forms of Creutzfeldt Jakob disease (CJD) have been shown to be transmissible to experimental animals. Some of these studies have been in primates, which have the advantage of being genetically, physiologically and anatomically closer to humans than other laboratory animals, but these investigations have been limited in scale. Far more information on the biology of these diseases has come from studies in rodents infected with isolates derived from human and animal transmissible spongiform encephalo-pathies (TSEs) (also known as, prion diseases), in particular mice or hamsters infected with scrapie.

Studies in mice and hamsters. In mice and hamsters infected with TSE agents, as in the human diseases, a range of neuropathological changes is apparent (14). The most characteristic feature, pathological accumulation of PrP, occurs predominantly as diffuse or granular deposits in the neuropil, often in association with specific neuronal groups or individual neurons (6). Focal PrP accumulations, in the form of amyloid plaques, are prominent in some models, ranging from subtle local infiltrates of the neuropil to very large structures similar to those seen in Gerstmann-Sträussler-Scheinker syndrome (GSS). In certain models they may be surrounded by a halo of vacuoles, reminiscent of the "florid" plaques of new variant CJD (vCJD) (34). Both amyloid plaques and diffuse PrP pathology appear to involve accumulation of the protein extracellularly, at the surface of neurons or their processes (23). Another prominent pathological feature in rodents is usually a vacuolation of neurons, neuropil and, sometimes, white matter tracts. In some models a profound loss of neurons is obvious in highly structured areas of the CNS, for example, in the hippocampus (4, 5) or retina (15). These neurodegenerative changes are accompanied by an activation of astrocytes and microglia.

There are many different TSE models in rodents, defined by the strain of TSE agent and the strain of mouse or hamster. The spectrum of neuropathology seen in any particular model is remarkably predictable, with vacuolation and abnormal PrP accumulation being targeted precisely to particular brain areas (6). There are, however, dramatic differences between models in the prominence and regional targeting of the different types of lesions, depending mainly on the strain of infecting agent, but also on genetic factors of the host, including PrP genotype. This neuropathological diversity has been exploited in agent strain typing studies, in which the severity and distribution of vacuolar changes in infected mice, together with incubation periods, are used to identify the TSE strain (7). Applying these strain typing methods to transmissions of CJD to mice has demonstrated that vCJD patients, but not sporadic CJD patients, are infected with the bovine spongiform encephalopathy (BSE) agent (8).

In rodent TSE models, although the time-scales are long (months or even years), the timing of the development of neuropathology and subsequent clinical disease in any particular model is remarkably predictable. This allows detailed serial studies of disease progression and effects of intervention. Time-course studies in mouse scrapie models have demonstrated abnormal distributions of PrP relatively early in the incubation period, with vacuolar changes appearing later (24). Neuronal loss occurs by apoptosis (31) and is preceded by structural abnormalities, for example a loss of synapses and dendritic spines (4, 5, 24). As neuronal structural pathology and markers for the early stages of apoptosis may be detected before abnormal PrP accumulation (22), it seems unlikely that the neurodegenerative changes are simply secondary to pathological PrP accumulation. Recent studies have shown that, even at a late stage, neurons can be rescued. In one study, in a mouse scrapie model that shows retinal degeneration, injecting basic fibroblast growth factor into the eye led to a significant protection of retinal photoreceptors (15). In another study in mice, loss of hippocampal pyramidal neurons was reduced by PrP-deficient foetal brain grafts (4, 5). These observations are encouraging in that they suggest that late-stage therapies may have a place in the human TSEs.

Rodent scrapie models are also proving useful in defining routes of spread of infection from remote sites in the body to the CNS. For example, evidence for transport of infection to the CNS by peripheral nerves has come from time-course studies of hamsters that have been fed scrapie agent (35). The first sites of pathological PrP accumulation within the CNS in this model suggest that infection spreads to the CNS by 2 distinct routes, via the vagus to the brain and via the splanchnic nerve to the spinal cord.

Studies in transgenic mice. Manipulation of the PrP gene in transgenic mice has provided important insights into disease processes in the TSEs (45, 48). Transgenic mice have been produced either by introducing multiple copies of the PrP transgene into the mouse genome, or by replacing the endogenous PrP gene with a mutant allele integrated at its correct position on the chromosome (commonly known as a "knock-in" mutation).

Mice in which the PrP gene has been disrupted by gene targeting (PrP knockout mice) are resistant to TSE challenge, showing no evidence of replication in tissues and no signs of neuropathology or clinical disease (9, 32, 42). On the other hand, mice over-expressing mouse PrP have shorter incubation periods than wild-type mice infected with the same TSE agent, making them useful animals for assaying infectivity (11, 13). A range of transgenes has now been introduced into mice to explore the influence of PrP on susceptibility, pathogenesis and pathology of the TSEs. The effects of transgenes are often greater when expressed in the absence of endogenous mouse PrP.

Transgenic models have been developed for some familial human TSEs by introducing the relevant mutation into the mouse PrP gene. The most extensively studied of these so far is a proline to leucine mutation at codon 101 of the mouse PrP gene, equivalent to the GSS-associated mutation at codon 102 of the human gene. Transgenic mice over-expressing this mutant protein develop spontaneous neurological disease with vacuolation and amyloid plaques (21). The age at which the mice become ill is reduced and the severity of the pathology increased when the transgene is expressed on a PrP knockout background (46). Transgenic mice expressing lower levels of the mutant PrP do not develop clinical disease or neuropathology within their lifespan (20, 33); however, recently it has been shown that introduction of the mutation into mice by gene substitution changes the susceptibility or incubation period seen on challenge with a number of different TSE isolates (1). Another form of GSS, linked with an alanine to valine mutation at codon 117, results in neurodegeneration associated with the accumulation of an aberrant trans-membrane form of PrP ("CtmPrP"), rather than the protease-resistant forms usually seen in TSEs. This disease has been modeled in transgenic mice with mutations that increase the proportion of trans-membrane forms of the protein, resulting in spontaneous neurodegeneration (16). On the other hand, no neurodegeneration is seen in mice over-expressing PrP with a glutamate-to-lysine mutation at codon 199, equivalent to a mutation at codon 200 of the human gene linked to familial CJD (46).

Transgenic mice expressing PrP genes from a range of species are being used to explore the factors governing the transmissibility of TSEs between species and to provide more efficient bioassays. Early studies in mice carrying hamster transgenes, challenged with mouse- or hamster-passaged scrapie, suggested that the efficiency of transmission depends on the degree of similarity between donor and recipient PrPs (36, 44). Some subsequent experiments in transgenic mice have supported the general applicability of this hypothesis, whilst others have not. For example, sporadic CJD is difficult to transmit to wild-type mice, but is more readily transmitted to mice carrying a human PrP gene, or a chimaeric mouse/ human PrP gene (8, 18, 47). These observations provide a practical system for bioassaying infectivity in tissues from patients with sporadic CJD. On the other hand, vCJD is an exception to this general rule in that it is more readily transmitted to wild-type mice than to mice expressing human PrP, even though there is a mismatch between mouse and human PrP (18). Transmissibility can therefore depend on factors other than simple sequence homology between donor and recipient PrPs, but these other factors are not yet understood.

Transgenic approaches have also been useful in investigations of TSE neuropathology. For example, PrP expression has been restricted to particular cell types by introducing transgenes that are under the control of cell or tissue-specific promoters. Thus, TSE-challenged mice in which PrP synthesis is restricted to either neurons or astrocytes can replicate infectivity in their brains and go on to develop neuropathology similar to that seen in wild-type mice (39, 40). Another approach has been to graft foetal neural tissue from mice over-expressing PrP into the brains of PrP knockout mice (3). When the graft is infected with a TSE agent, it develops typical severe TSE pathology. Although the graft produces very high levels of pathological PrP, the adjacent PrP-deficient brain tissue remains normal, suggesting that normal PrP expression is required for neurodegeneration. PrP over-expressing neural grafts have also been used as indicators for the spread of infection within and to the brain, in studies investigating which cells are required for transport and whether they need to express PrP (48).

In Vitro Models

Although small animal models of experimental prion disease are able to capture a remarkable number of features of natural diseases, the very accuracy of these systems in exhibiting extended incubation times and multicellular pathogenesis is a logistic encumbrance. Incisive biochemical insights into prion replication mechanisms and rapid prion bioassays cannot come from these models because of their intrinsic cellular and molecular complexity, and their slow tempo. More likely these needs will be met by cell-free systems. Another possibility is chronically infected tissue culture cells, which might be considered as an intermediate between mice and test-tubes. Such systems have been in use for over a decade, but also have drawbacks including low-infectious titres and lack of compelling cellular pathology that mimics changes seen in the brain (10, 37, 38, 43). Accordingly, it is of interest to consider the current status in vitro systems for addressing prion replication. As will be seen, these systems have a degree of specialization and, depending upon their components, may be geared towards addressing prion infections or familial prion disease.

The first cell-free system was pioneered by Byron Caughey and coworkers (12, 28). In essence this comprises a radiolabeled supply of semipurified PrP^C that is denatured and incubated with cold protease-resistant PrP ("PrP^{res}") that is able to drive synthesis of radiolabeled PrP^{res}. The system exhibits specificity in a number of parameters pertaining to in vivo situations (2, 29). Recent effort has gone into reducing the molar excess of PrP^{res} needed to drive the conversion reaction (now approaching 1:1) (19), although the gold standard of proving the generation of infectivity (which is not necessarily equivalent to protease-resistant PrP (17) remains an active area of research.

Rather than use PrP^{Sc} to drive alterations in the folding of a recombinant PrP substrate, another type of system involves the use of PrP peptide fragments (26, 27). The first iterations of these experiments, while producing biophysical traits such as protease-resistance and elevated β-sheet content reminiscent of authentic PrP^{Sc} again appear to fall short of the mark of producing infectivity. Second generation versions of these experiments have closed the gap towards the end-points seen in prion diseases in vivo. Here, synthetic peptides encompassing a GSS codon 102 mutation were injected in asymptomatic Tg mice expressing a low level of a P101L *Prnp* transgene (Tg[MoPrP,P101L]196/*Prnp*$^{0/0}$ mice: mouse PrP numbering scheme, codon 101 is equivalent to codon human 102). Whereas injected peptide pre-configured into a β-sheet conformation produced clinical disease in the Tg mice at an elapsed time 360±30 days, batches of peptide in a "non β-sheet" conformation failed to produce disease (25, 30). Clinical disease in peptide-inoculated mice was marked by spongiform change and deposition of amyloid deposits. Although a low level of infectivity in the brains of Tg(MoPrP,P101L)196/*Prnp*$^{0/0}$ "recipient" mice precludes the conclusion that these experiments reflect a chemical synthesis of prion infectivity, they indicate progress towards this goal.

The third system is entitled protein mis-folding cyclic amplification (PMCA) (41). The process consists of incubating a brain homogenate containing native PrP^C with a supply PrP^{Sc}. Subsequent to the incubation the reaction is sonicated (to fragment putative heteromeric assemblies of PrP^C and PrP^{Sc}) to increase the number of "seeds" for further rounds of conversion proceeding from incubation with fresh substrate, ie, brain-derived PrP^C. The method can therefore be seen as akin to a protein version of the polymerase chain reaction (PCR) for amplifying nucleic acid sequences. Intuitively, PMCA appears to be an important conceptual breakthrough and suggests the ability of robotic PMCA to amplify trace amounts of prion infectivity in a time-scale of a few days. On the other hand, experimental details are scant, and PCR-like problems of sample carry-over will presumably have to be dealt with, as will the expectation that PMCA amplifies not just protease-resistant PrP, but also prion infectivity, as measured in conventional bioassays.

Conclusion

In contrast to the situation of even a decade ago, there are now both in vitro and in vivo systems to assay and dissect the process of prion replication and the pathogenesis of TSEs. It is not overly optimistic to assume that further refinements of these model systems will lead to better methods to diagnose, control and understand these worrisome diseases.

References

1. Barron RM, Thomson V, Jamieson E, Melton DW, Ironside J, Will R, Manson JC (2001) Changing a single amino acid in the N-terminus of murine PrP alters TSE incubation time across three species barriers. *Embo J* 20: 5070-5078.

2. Bessen RA, Kocisko DA, Raymond GJ, Nandan S, Lansbury PT, Caughey B (1995) Non-genetic propagation of strain-specific properties of scrapie prion protein. *Nature* 375: 698-700.

3. Brandner S, Isenmann S, Raeber A, Fischer M, Sailer A, Kobayashi Y, Marino S, Weissmann C, Aguzzi A (1996) Normal host prion protein necessary for scrapie-induced neurotoxicity. *Nature* 379: 339-343.

4. Brown D, Belichenko P, Sales J, Jeffrey M, Fraser JR (2001) Early loss of dendritic spines in murine scrapie revealed by confocal analysis. *Neuroreport* 12: 179-183.

5. Brown KL, Brown J, Ritchie DL, Sales J, Fraser JR (2001) Fetal cell grafts provide long-term protection against scrapie induced neuronal loss. *Neuroreport* 12: 77-82.

6. Bruce ME, McBride PA, Farquhar CF (1989) Precise targeting of the pathology of the sialoglycoprotein, PrP, and vacuolar degeneration in mouse scrapie. *Neurosci Lett* 102: 1-6.

7. Bruce ME, McConnell I, Fraser H, Dickinson AG (1991) The disease characteristics of different strains of scrapie in Sinc congenic mouse lines: implications for the nature of the agent and host control of pathogenesis. *J Gen Virol* 72: 595-603.

8. Bruce ME, Will RG, Ironside JW, McConnell I, Drummond D, Suttie A, McCardle L, Chree A, Hope J, Birkett C, Cousens S, Fraser H, Bostock CJ (1997) Transmissions to mice indicate that 'new variant' CJD is caused by the BSE agent. *Nature* 389: 498-501.

9. Bueler H, Fischer M, Lang Y, Bluethmann H, Lipp HP, DeArmond SJ, Prusiner SB, Aguet M, Weissmann C (1992) Normal development and behaviour of mice lacking the neuronal cell- surface PrP protein. *Nature* 356: 577-582.

10. Butler DA, Scott MR, Bockman JM, Borchelt DR, Taraboulos A, Hsiao KK, Kingsbury DT, Prusiner SB (1988) Scrapie-infected murine neuroblastoma cells produce protease-resistant prion proteins. *J Virol* 62: 1558-1564.

11. Carlson GA, Ebeling C, Yang SL, Telling G, Torchia M, Groth D, Westaway D, DeArmond SJ, Prusiner SB (1994) Prion isolate specified allotypic interactions between the cellular and scrapie prion proteins in congenic and transgenic mice. *Proc Natl Acad Sci U S A* 91: 5690-5694.

12. Caughey B (2000) Formation of protease-resistant prion protein in cell-free systems. *Curr Issues Mol Biol* 2: 95-101.

13. Fischer M, Rulicke T, Raeber A, Sailer A, Moser M, Oesch B, Brandner S, Aguzzi A, Weissmann C (1996) Prion protein (PrP) with amino-proximal deletions restoring susceptibility of PrP knockout mice to scrapie. *Embo J* 15: 1255-1264.

14. Fraser H (1993) Diversity in the neuropathology of scrapie-like diseases in animals. *Br Med Bull* 49: 792-809.

15. Fraser JR, Brown J, Bruce ME, Jeffrey M (1997) Scrapie-induced neuron loss is reduced by treatment with basic fibroblast growth factor. *Neuroreport* 8: 2405-2409.

16. Hegde RS, Mastrianni JA, Scott MR, DeFea KA, Tremblay P, Torchia M, DeArmond SJ, Prusiner SB, Lingappa VR (1998) A transmembrane form of the prion protein in neurodegenerative disease. *Science* 279: 827-834.

17. Hill AF, Antoniou M, Collinge J (1999) Protease-resistant prion protein produced in vitro lacks detectable infectivity. *J Gen Virol* 80: 11-14.

18. Hill AF, Desbruslais M, Joiner S, Sidle KC, Gowland I, Collinge J, Doey LJ, Lantos P (1997) The same prion strain causes vCJD and BSE. *Nature* 389: 448-450, 526.

19. Horiuchi M, Caughey B (1999) Specific binding of normal prion protein to the scrapie form via a localized domain initiates its conversion to the protease-resistant state. *Embo J* 18: 3193-3203.

20. Hsiao KK, Groth D, Scott M, Yang SL, Serban H, Rapp D, Foster D, Torchia M, Dearmond SJ, Prusiner SB (1994) Serial transmission in rodents of neurodegeneration from transgenic mice expressing mutant prion protein. *Proc Natl Acad Sci U S A* 91: 9126-9130.

21. Hsiao KK, Scott M, Foster D, Groth DF, DeArmond SJ, Prusiner SB (1990) Spontaneous neurodegeneration in transgenic mice with mutant prion protein. *Science* 250: 1587-1590.

22. Jamieson E, Jeffrey M, Ironside JW, Fraser JR (2001) Activation of Fas and caspase 3 precedes PrP accumulation in 87V scrapie. *Neuroreport* 12: 3567-3572.

23. Jeffrey M, Goodsir CM, Bruce M, McBride PA, Scott JR, Halliday WG (1994) Correlative light and electron microscopy studies of PrP localisation in 87V scrapie. *Brain Res* 656: 329-343.

24. Jeffrey M, Halliday WG, Bell J, Johnston AR, MacLeod NK, Ingham C, Sayers AR, Brown DA, Fraser JR (2000) Synapse loss associated with abnormal PrP precedes neuronal degeneration in the scrapie-infected murine hippocampus. *Neuropathol Appl Neurobiol* 26: 41-54.

25. Kaneko K, Ball HL, Wille H, Zhang H, Groth D, Torchia M, Tremblay P, Safar J, Prusiner SB, DeArmond SJ, Baldwin MA, Cohen FE (2000) A synthetic peptide initiates Gerstmann-Straussler-Scheinker (GSS) disease in transgenic mice. *J Mol Biol* 295: 997-1007.

26. Kaneko K, Peretz D, Pan KM, Blochberger TC, Wille H, Gabizon R, Griffith OH, Cohen FE, Baldwin MA, Prusiner SB (1995) Prion protein (PrP) synthetic peptides induce cellular PrP to acquire properties of the scrapie isoform. *Proc Natl Acad Sci U S A* 92: 11160-11164.

27. Kaneko K, Wille H, Mehlhorn I, Zhang H, Ball H, Cohen FE, Baldwin MA, Prusiner SB (1997) Molecular properties of complexes formed between the prion protein and synthetic peptides. *J Mol Biol* 270: 574-586.

28. Kocisko DA, Come JH, Priola SA, Chesebro B, Raymond GJ, Lansbury PT, Caughey B (1994) Cell-free formation of protease-resistant prion protein. *Nature* 370: 471-474.

29. Kocisko DA, Priola SA, Raymond GJ, Chesebro B, Lansbury PT, Jr., Caughey B (1995) Species specificity in the cell-free conversion of prion protein to protease-resistant forms: a model for the scrapie species barrier. *Proc Natl Acad Sci U S A* 92: 3923-3927.

30. Laws DD, Bitter HM, Liu K, Ball HL, Kaneko K, Wille H, Cohen FE, Prusiner SB, Pines A, Wemmer DE (2001) Solid-state NMR studies of the secondary structure of a mutant prion protein fragment of 55 residues that induces neurodegeneration. *Proc Natl Acad Sci U S A* 98: 11686-11690.

31. Lucassen PJ, Williams A, Chung WC, Fraser H (1995) Detection of apoptosis in murine scrapie. *Neurosci Lett* 198: 185-188.

32. Manson JC, Clarke AR, Hooper ML, Aitchison L, McConnell I, Hope J (1994) 129/Ola mice carrying a null mutation in PrP that abolishes mRNA production are developmentally normal. *Mol Neurobiol* 8: 121-127.

33. Manson JC, Jamieson E, Baybutt H, Tuzi NL, Barron R, McConnell I, Somerville R, Ironside J, Will R, Sy MS, Melton DW, Hope J, Bostock C (1999) A single amino acid alteration (101L) introduced into murine PrP dramatically alters incubation time of transmissible spongiform encephalopathy. *Embo J* 18: 6855-6864.

34. McBride PA, Bruce ME, Fraser H (1988) Immunostaining of scrapie cerebral amyloid plaques with antisera raised to scrapie-associated fibrils (SAF). *Neuropathol Appl Neurobiol* 14: 325-336.

35. McBride PA, Schulz-Schaeffer WJ, Donaldson M, Bruce M, Diringer H, Kretzschmar HA, Beekes M (2001) Early spread of scrapie from the gastrointestinal tract to the central nervous system involves autonomic fibers of the splanchnic and vagus nerves. *J Virol* 75: 9320-9327.

36. Prusiner SB, Scott M, Foster D, Pan KM, Groth D, Mirenda C, Torchia M, Yang SL, Serban D, Carlson GA, et al. (1990) Transgenetic studies implicate interactions between homologous PrP isoforms in scrapie prion replication. *Cell* 63: 673-686.

37. Race R (1991) The scrapie agent in vitro. *Curr Top Microbiol Immunol* 172: 181-193

38. Race RE, Fadness LH, Chesebro B (1987) Characterization of scrapie infection in mouse neuroblastoma cells. *J Gen Virol* 68: 1391-1399.

39. Race RE, Priola SA, Bessen RA, Ernst D, Dockter J, Rall GF, Mucke L, Chesebro B, Oldstone MB (1995) Neuron-specific expression of a hamster prion protein minigene in transgenic mice induces susceptibility to hamster scrapie agent. *Neuron* 15: 1183-1191.

40. Raeber AJ, Race RE, Brandner S, Priola SA, Sailer A, Bessen RA, Mucke L, Manson J, Aguzzi A, Oldstone MB, Weissmann C, Chesebro B (1997) Astrocyte-specific expression of hamster prion protein (PrP) renders PrP knockout mice susceptible to hamster scrapie. *Embo J* 16: 6057-6065.

41. Saborio GP, Permanne B, Soto C (2001) Sensitive detection of pathological prion protein by cyclic amplification of protein misfolding. *Nature* 411: 810-813.

42. Sakaguchi S, Katamine S, Shigematsu K, Nakatani A, Moriuchi R, Nishida N, Kurokawa K, Nakaoke R, Sato H, Jishage K et al (1995) Accumulation of proteinase K-resistant prion protein (PrP) is restricted by the expression level of normal PrP in mice inoculated with a mouse-adapted strain of the Creutzfeldt-Jakob disease agent. *J Virol* 69: 7586-7592.

43. Schatzl HM, Laszlo L, Holtzman DM, Tatzelt J, DeArmond SJ, Weiner RI, Mobley WC, Prusiner SB (1997) A hypothalamic neuronal cell line persistently infected with scrapie prions exhibits apoptosis. *J Virol* 71: 8821-8831.

44. Scott M, Groth D, Foster D, Torchia M, Yang SL, DeArmond SJ, Prusiner SB (1993) Propagation of prions with artificial properties in transgenic mice expressing chimeric PrP genes. *Cell* 73: 979-988.

45. Telling GC (2000) Prion protein genes and prion diseases: studies in transgenic mice. *Neuropathol Appl Neurobiol* 26: 209-220.

46. Telling GC, Haga T, Torchia M, Tremblay P, DeArmond SJ, Prusiner SB (1996) Interactions between wild-type and mutant prion proteins modulate neurodegeneration in transgenic mice. *Genes Dev* 10: 1736-1750.

47. Telling GC, Scott M, Mastrianni J, Gabizon R, Torchia M, Cohen FE, DeArmond SJ, Prusiner SB (1995) Prion propagation in mice expressing human and chimeric PrP transgenes implicates the interaction of cellular PrP with another protein. *Cell* 83: 79-90.

48. Weissmann C, Raeber AJ, Shmerling D, Aguzzi A, Manson C (1999) Knockouts, transgenics, and transplants in prion research. In *Prion Biology and Disease*, SB Prusiner (eds). Cold Spring Harbor Laboratory Press: Cold Spring Harbor. pp. 273-305

CHAPTER 7

Frontotemporal Degeneration

Chapter Editor: Catherine Bergeron

7.1 Introduction to Frontotemporal Degeneration 340

7.2 Frontotemporal Lobar Degeneration 342

Frontotemporal Degeneration: Introduction

Catherine Bergeron
James Lowe

FTD	frontotemporal degeneration
FTLD-MND	frontotemporal lobar degeneration with motor neurone disease
FTLD-U	frontotemporal lobar degeneration with ubiquitin-only-immunoreactive neuronal changes

Clinically defined frontotemporal dementias, once all subsumed under the diagnosis of Pick's disease, account for between 10 to 15% of all cases of dementia and are now recognised to be caused by a variety of pathological conditions. The term Pick's disease is now used in relation to a specific pathological form of neurodegenerative disease (chapter 3.4).

The history of frontotemporal dementia and the origins for its eventual pathological separation from that recognised as Pick's disease goes back to the mid-70s when Tissot et al published a monograph based on the detailed clinical and pathological study of 32 cases of degenerative dementias other than Alzheimer's disease (12). A summary of this work was also published in the English language (4). On the basis of their histological findings, Tissot et al classified their 32 cases in 3 distinct groups termed Pick's disease type A (neuronal loss and gliosis, Pick bodies and swollen neurons, 10 cases), type B (neuronal loss and gliosis with swollen neurons only, 10 cases) or type C (neuronal loss and gliosis only, 12 cases). At the conclusion of their study, Tissot et al felt that "given the current state of knowledge about Pick's disease, as well as the absence of specific concepts concerning its pathophysiology, it appeared more cautious to maintain the unity of this entity" (12). The term Pick's disease was subsequently commonly used for all disorders characterised by dominant frontal lobe degeneration, neuronal loss and gliosis, independent of the presence or absence of swollen neurons and Pick bodies. Subsequently, several other dementias exhibiting clinical frontotemporal abnormalities were pathologically characterised as corticobasal ganglionic degeneration (1), dementia with swollen chromatolytic neurons (3), frontal lobe degeneration (2), and dementia lacking distinctive histology (6, 7). There was division as to whether clinical or pathological features should define Pick's disease and the suggestion for delineating a "Pick complex" incorporating several pathological forms of disease was promoted (5).

Following study and application of immunohistochemical reagents developed in the 1980s, the frontotemporal dementias were reclassified in 1994 by the Lund and Manchester Groups (11) on the basis of the pattern of neuronal loss and the immunohistochemical profile of pathological changes. The frontal lobe degeneration type was characterized by milder neuronal loss and microvacuolation of the superficial cortical layers. The Pick type incorporated cases with more severe neuronal loss and gliosis, with or without swollen neurons or Pick bodies. The motor neuron disease type was similar to the first group but also featured involvement of the motor system and ubiquitin-immunoreactive inclusions.

In recent years, abnormality of the microtubule associated protein tau has been identified as a central feature of several neurodegenerative diseases and an immunohistochemistry-based reclassification of non-Alzheimer dementias on the basis of tau and ubiquitin immunohistochemistry was proposed (8). It has become apparent that one subgroup of frontotemporal dementias are associated with abnormal deposits of tau protein and are discussed as a tauopathy in chapter 3.

The present chapter covers the more common group of tau-negative frontotemporal degenerations. Their clinical presentation is heterogenous and includes frontotemporal dementia, semantic dementia, primary aphasia, and a corticobasal-like syndrome (10). For this reason, the Working Group on Frontotemporal Dementia and Pick's disease recently recommended that this neuropathological entity be named frontotemporal lobar degeneration (FTLD) (9). The tau-negative degenerations can be subdivided into 3 types on the basis of the presence or absence of tau-negative, ubiquitin positive pathology and evidence of motor neurone disease: *i)* Frontotemporal lobar degeneration with motor neurone disease (FTLD-MND), *ii)* Frontotemporal lobar degeneration with ubiquitin-only-immunoreactive neuronal changes (FTLD-U), and *iii)* Frontotemporal degeneration (FTD)

It is possible that FTLD-MND and FTLD-U represent the same condition. However until definite proof can be provided, and in case they represent different conditions, they are presently distinguished to facilitate further investigation.

References

1. Bergeron C, Davis A,Lang AE (1998) Corticobasal ganglionic degeneration and progressive supranuclear palsy presenting with cognitive decline. *Brain Pathol* 8: 355-365.

2. Brun A (1987) Frontal lobe degeneration of the non-Alzheimer type. I. Neuropathology. *Arch Gerontol Geriatr* 6: 193-208.

3. Clark AW, Manz HJ, White III CL, Lehmann J, Miller D,Coyle JT (1986) Cortical degeneration with swollen chromatolytic neurons: its relationship to Pick's disease. *J Neuropathol Exp Neurol* 45: 268-284.

4. Constantinidis J, Richard J,Tissot R (1974) Pick's disease: histological and clinical correlations. *Eur J Neurol* 11: 208-217.

5. Kertesz A,Munoz D (1998) Pick's disease, frontotemporal dementia, and Pick complex: emerging concepts. *Arch Neurol* 55: 302-304.

6. Knopman D, Mastri A, Frey II W, JH S,Rustan B (1990) Dementia lacking distinctive histologic fea-

tures: a common non-Alzheimer degenerative dementia. *Neurology* 40: 251-256.

7. Knopman DS (1993) Overview of dementia lacking distinctive histology: pathological designation of a progressive dementia. *Dementia* 4: 132-136.

8. Lowe J (1998) Establishing a pathological diagnosis in degenerative dementias. *Brain Pathol* 8: 403-406.

9. McKhann GM, Albert MS, Grossman M, Miller B, Dickson D,Trojanowski JQ (2001) Clinical and pathological diagnosis of frontotemporal dementia: report of the Work Group on Frontotemporal Dementia and Pick's Disease. *Arch Neurol* 58: 1803-1809.

10. Neary D, Snowden JS, Gustafson L, Passant U, Stuss D, Black S, Freedman M, Kertesz A, Robert PH, Albert M, Boone K, Miller BL, Cummings J,Benson DF (1998) Frontotemporal lobar degeneration: a consensus on clinical diagnostic criteria. *Neurology* 51: 1546-54.

11. The Lund and Manchester groups (1994) Clinical and neuropathological criteria for frontotemporal dementia. *J Neurol Neurosurg Psychiatry* 57: 416-418.

12. Tissot R, Constantinidis J,Richard J, *La maladie de Pick*. 1975, Paris: Masson et Cie.

Frontotemporal Lobar Degeneration

James Lowe
Martin Rossor

ALS	amyotrophic lateral sclerosis
CT	computer tomography
DLDH	dementia lacking distinctive histology
EEG	electroencephalogram
FTD	frontotemporal dementias
FTLD	frontotemporal lobar degeneration
FTLD-MND	frontotemporal lobar degeneration with motor neuron disease
FTLD-U	frontotemporal lobar degeneration with ubiquitin-only-immunoreactive neuronal changes
MRI	magnetic resonance imaging
MND	motor neuron disease
PET	positron emission tomography
SPECT	single photon emission computed tomography

Definitions

Now that conditions caused by abnormalities in tau protein have been recognised, FTLD-MND, FTLD-U, and FTD are presently defined on a clinical and pathological basis as the main underlying causes of frontotemporal dementia (22).

Frontotemporal lobar degeneration with motor neurone disease (FTLD-MND). A neurodegenerative disease in which frontotemporal cognitive abnormalities are associated with clinical OR histopathological features of one form of motor neurone disease. When histologically verified, ubiquitin-immunoreactive inclusion bodies characteristic of motor neuron disease are seen in motor neurons together with the appropriate extramotor pathology which is recognised in some cases of motor neurone disease in frontal and temporal cortex.

Frontotemporal lobar degeneration with ubiquitin-only-immunoreactive neuronal changes (FTLD-U). A neurodegenerative disease in which frontotemporal cognitive abnormalities are associated with EITHER neuronal inclusions identical to the extramotor changes recognised in some cases of motor neuron disease OR in which ubiquitin-only immunoreactive neuritic changes are seen in areas of cortical neuronal loss OR in which both such ubiquitin immunoreactive changes are present. There must be absence of clinical AND pathological evidence of motor neurone disease.

Frontotemporal lobar degeneration (FTLD). A neurodegenerative disease in which frontotemporal dementia (FTD) is associated with frontotemporal lobar atrophy histologically characterised by appropriate regional neuronal loss and astrocytic gliosis and in which pathological investigation, including appropriate immunohistochemistry, has excluded any further present diagnostic refinement.

Synonyms and Historical Annotations

The long-recognised clinical association between motor neurone disease (amyotrophic lateral sclerosis) and cognitive dysfunction (1) has now been associated with the presence of ubiquitin-immunoreactive inclusions in non-motor cortical neurones. Detecting these inclusions is an important part of establishing a diagnosis in this group of diseases.

It is difficult to place some previously published series into the modern classification since the defining criteria, which are based on immunohistochemistry with a panel of antibodies, was not done. It seems likely that some previously published series were composed of a variety of pathological entities. Caution therefore needs to be exercised in the interpretation of cases defined in the absence of appropriate immunohistochemical assessment.

Pathological studies on patients with isolated frontotemporal cognitive abnormalities in which ubiquitin immunohistochemistry reveals the non-motor changes of motor neuron disease (20) immediately suggest a link between these cases of lobar atrophy and the neurodegenerative process underlying motor neuron disease. Unfortunately initial pathological studies did not include examination of the spinal cord, thereby limiting interpretation. More recent anecdotal and published studies that include examination of lower motor neurons now seem to suggest that some patients show subclinical pathological features of motor neurone disease (6, 11).

This is evidence that now supports the hypothesis that such cases might best be regarded as being pathogenetically linked to certain types of motor neurone disease. However, with the small number of published cases it is still essential to attempt to distinguish between cases of lobar atrophy associated with ubiquitin-immunoreactive pathology that are with or without either clinically or pathologically defined motor neuron disease. Testing the hypothesis that FTLD-MND and FTLD-U are part of the same disease spectrum will require further careful clinical and pathological definition. Previous terms and clinicopathological descriptions that overlap with the present suggested classification in this group of diseases are presented in Table 1.

Epidemiology

Incidence and prevalence. There are no reliable data on the prevalence of these non-tau frontotemporal degenerations. In the presenium, FTLD is the most common degenerative cause of dementia after AD. Overall, approximately 10% of early onset dementias have been attributed to frontotemporal dementia but these studies include cases now classified as tauopathies (10). Non-tau forms of FTLD account for about 60% of pathologically confirmed cases (27). Studies on prevalence, age distribution, and clinical features have been based on small series of cases collected by specialists in tertiary referral centres. The general prevalence and characteristics of these diseases in community-based series of dementia remains to be defined.

Age and sex distribution. There appears to be no sex bias in these disorders. Age ranges at onset in published series for FTLD-U are between 53 and 83 with a mean age of around 65 years (11, 14). For FTLD-MND age of onset has been 39 to 77 (4, 24).

Risk factors. There are no known risk factors for these forms of disease. The overlap with pathology of motor neurone disease suggests that there may be an overlap in risk factors for certain types of disease.

Frontotemporal lobar degeneration with motor neurone disease (FTLD-MND)

- Motor neurone disease dementia or dementia with motor neurone disease (MND dementia)
- Amyotrophic lateral sclerosis and dementia (ALS dementia - excluding Guam type)
- Pick's disease combined with motor neurone disease (Cases with no tau pathology)

Frontotemporal lobar degeneration with ubiquitin-only-immunoreactive neuronal changes (FTLD-U) and Frontotemporal degeneration (FTD)

- Motor neurone disease inclusion dementia (MNDID)
- Dementia with ubiquitin-reactive tau-negative inclusions
- Frontal lobe degeneration with ubiquitin neurites
- Primary aphasia with ubiquitinated neurites
- Semantic dementia with ubiquitin-positive tau-negative inclusion bodies
- Dementia with inclusions, tau and synuclein negative, ubiquitinated (ITSNU)
- Frontal lobe degeneration of non-Alzheimer type
- Dementia lacking distinctive histology (DLDH)

Table 1. Previous terms and clinicopathological descriptions that overlap with the present suggested classification in this group of diseases.

Genetics

Approximately 50% of reported series of frontotemporal degeneration are found to have a family history of dementia (25). In many of these series the pedigrees are large, with clear autosomal dominant transmission and with apparent high penetrance. In general, anticipation is not seen (5, 32). Tau gene mutations are not common in patients with frontotemporal dementia (28).

Familial cases of FTLD, FTLD-U, and FTLD-MND are described (9, 14, 15, 18, 31) and 3 genetic loci have been found as follows:

i) Linkage identified in a large Danish family in which the disease gene lies in the pericentromeric region of chromosome 3 (2). The neuropathology in this family reveals neuronal loss and gliosis but without any inclusion bodies, suggesting FTLD.

ii) In a kindred in which patients develop both MND and FTLD or either MND or FTLD alone (FTLD-MND), a genetic locus has been located on chromosome 9q21-q22 (12).

iii) In a family with frontotemporal dementia characterised by ubiquitin-positive, tau-negative inclusions (FTLD-U), linkage to chromosome 17q21-22 has been described but mutations in the tau gene were not found (37). Familial rapidly progressive frontotemporal dementia has been mapped to chromosome 17q12-21 in another family (7).

Clinical Features

Signs and symptoms. The presenting signs and symptoms of frontotemporal degenerations are determined by the topographical distribution of the neuronal loss. Three prototypic clinical syndromes are found in association with the group of frontotemporal degenerations and have been delineated in a consensus meeting by Neary et al (26). These prototypic syndromes are a behavioural syndrome referred to as frontotemporal dementia; progressive non-fluent aphasia; and semantic dementia. The behavioural syndrome is characterised either by a dysexecutive syndrome or a prominent behavioural disturbance with social disinhibition. The non-fluent progressive aphasia is characterised by prominent speech productions deficits and patients ultimately become mute. The patients presenting with semantic dementia are characterised by relative preservation of episodic memory but a profound impairment of semantic memory. This distinction draws upon the difference between episodic or autobiographical memory, which allows us to recall our personal day-to-day events. By contrast semantic memory informs our understanding of meaning both verbal and visual. Many patients with frontotemporal degenerations may have well-preserved autobiographical or episodic memory early in the course of the disease even in the presence of significant semantic memory impairments. The original prototypic cases of semantic memory impairment described by Warrington (35) were subsequently found to have ubiquitin positive tau negative inclusion bodies, but in the absence of involvement of brainstem or spinal cord motor nuclei (FTLD-U) (30). It is not possible to predict reliably the likely underlying neuropathology on the basis of the clinical presentation.

Signs of anterior horn cell dysfunction may emerge and can appear before, coincidentally, or after the development of cognitive changes. Some patients presenting with cognitive abnormalities develop extra pyramidal and pyramidal syndromes later in the course of the illness. Patients with motor-neurone disease inclusions, which involve the brainstem motor nuclei or anterior horn cells may present with or develop additional features of motor-neurone disease. In general, these are largely lower motor-neurone signs and symptoms with less involvement of pyramidal tracts. Characteristically, fasciculations are seen proximally in the upper limb deltoid muscles, in contrast to the widespread fasciculations seen with

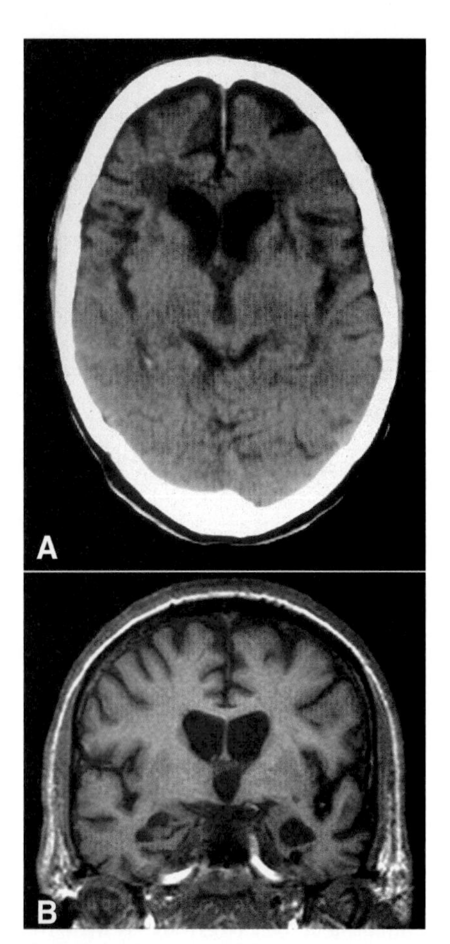

Figure 1. A. CT scan showing frontotemporal atrophy with ventricular dilatation. B. MRI scan showing marked temporal lobe atrophy.

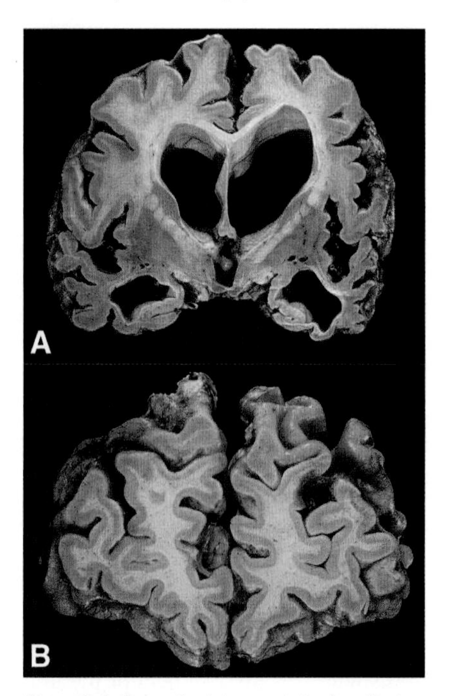

Figure 2. A. Severe frontotemporal atrophy with atrophy of basal ganglia and ventricular dilatation. B. Note superior accentuation of frontal atrophy in this case.

classical motor-neurone disease or ALS. Importantly, patients may be seen with pathologically-confirmed ubiquitin positive tau negative motor-neurone disease inclusion bodies in the absence of clinical involvement of motor nuclei in life (11, 14).

Disease duration in FTLD-U is 4 to 12 years which contrasts with the shorter disease duration described in cases with FTLD-MND which is around 1 to 6 years (mean 2.5) (16). This difference may be explained by the rapid development of fatal complications, such as respiratory failure, secondary to clinical motor system involvement. Patients who present with cognitive problems and subsequently develop MND typically develop motor symptoms between 6 to 26 months of the onset of cognitive decline (23, 34).

It is likely that the future pathological characterisation of other forms of circumscribed cortical atrophy will be characterised by these forms of pathology.

Imaging. Functional imaging with PET and SPECT and structural imaging with CT and MRI will show the characteristic frontal and temporal distribution of pathology (Figure 1). This can be strikingly asymmetric in some instances.

Laboratory findings. In general, laboratory investigations are uninformative. The EEG is characteristically normal when compared with Alzheimer's disease. In particular patients with frontal predominance may have an entirely normal EEG whereas those with predominant temporal lobar atrophy may show an excess of slow waves, which may lateralise.

EMG may confirm anterior horn cell involvement in cases with MND but this may be less prominent than the fasciculation that can sometimes be observed. Nerve conduction is normal.

Macroscopy

Macroscopic changes in FTLD-U, FTLD-MND and FTLD appear similar (Figure 2). The brain weight is generally reduced. Cerebral cortical atrophy is almost always present and typically most severe in frontal and temporal lobes with shrinkage of gyri and widening of sulci. The hippocampus and adjacent mesial temporal lobe structures can be severely atrophic. There is associated dilatation of the ventricular system. Atrophy may be asymmetrical and this has been especially noted in cases associated with aphasia. Cerebral cortical atrophy is of variable severity. In some cases affected cortex shows a pattern of "knife-blade" atrophy with thinning of the cortical ribbon and loss of underlying white matter. In other cases atrophy is more modest. There may be atrophy of the basal ganglia, especially the head of the caudate nucleus. There may be pallor of the substantia nigra, but the pigment in the locus ceruleus is usually preserved. The cerebellum and brain stem are generally unremarkable. In cases associated with motor neurone disease the spinal cord may show macroscopic features of this condition, including atrophy of the anterior roots and discoloration of the lateral funiculus.

Histopathology

Using conventional techniques histological changes in atrophic cerebral cortex in FTLD-U, FTLD-MND and FTLD appear similar. Histopathological examination of areas of atrophic cerebral cortex shows neuronal loss and microvacuolation, associated with astrocytic gliosis. In most instances the neuronal loss and astrocytic gliosis are present in the outer cortical layers, centred on layer 2 (Figure 3). In cases associated with severe atrophy there is transcortical neuronal loss associated with microvacuolation giving an appearance sometimes termed status spongiosus (Figure 3). A small number of swollen cortical neurones may be present and may be detected using antibodies to alpha B crystallin. If swollen neurons are numerous in the convexity cortex, it should suggest the possibility of corticobasal degeneration, and if they are abundant in the limbic lobe, it is important to exclude argyrophilic grain disease. Myelin pallor may be seen in white matter underlying atrophic cortical areas. Cell loss from the substantia nigra may be seen. It is essential that conventional histological examination is accompanied by immunohistochemical assessments. Immunostaining for tau protein and alpha synuclein are not positive: such findings would prompt a diagnosis of either a tauopathy or synucleinopathy (chapters 3 and 4).

The defining features of FTLD-U and FTLD-MND are seen on anti-ubiquitin immunostaining. Ubiquitin immunoreactive neuronal cytoplasmic inclusions as seen in some forms of classical motor neurone disease may be present in neurons in outer cortical layers of frontal and temporal lobes as well as in the granule cells of the hippocampal dentate gyrus (13) (Figure 4). Inclusions may also be seen in other areas including the basal ganglia, motor cortex, and the cingulate gyrus. These neuronal inclusions vary in morphology from dot-like structures through rounded inclusions to crescentic structures that partly surround the nucleus (Figures 5). Ubiquitin-immunoreactive neuronal nuclear inclusions have been described in a small number of cases. These appear as rounded or rod-shaped bodies (Figure 6) (29, 36). Ubiquitin-immunoreactive neuritic changes may be seen in areas of cortical atrophy, generally present in areas of microvacuolation. This may be the only type of ubiquitin-reactive structure present, especially when there has been severe neuronal loss. Neurites appear as thin, wispy tapering structures (17, 33) (Figure 7).

In cases associated with motor neurone disease, histological changes associated with that condition may be seen including appropriate regional neuronal loss, ubiquitin-immunoreactive cytoplasmic neuronal inclusions in motor neurons or tract degenerations. Such changes may be apparent even when there have been no clinical features of motor neurone disease.

If no inclusions are noted following immunostaining for anti-ubiquitin and

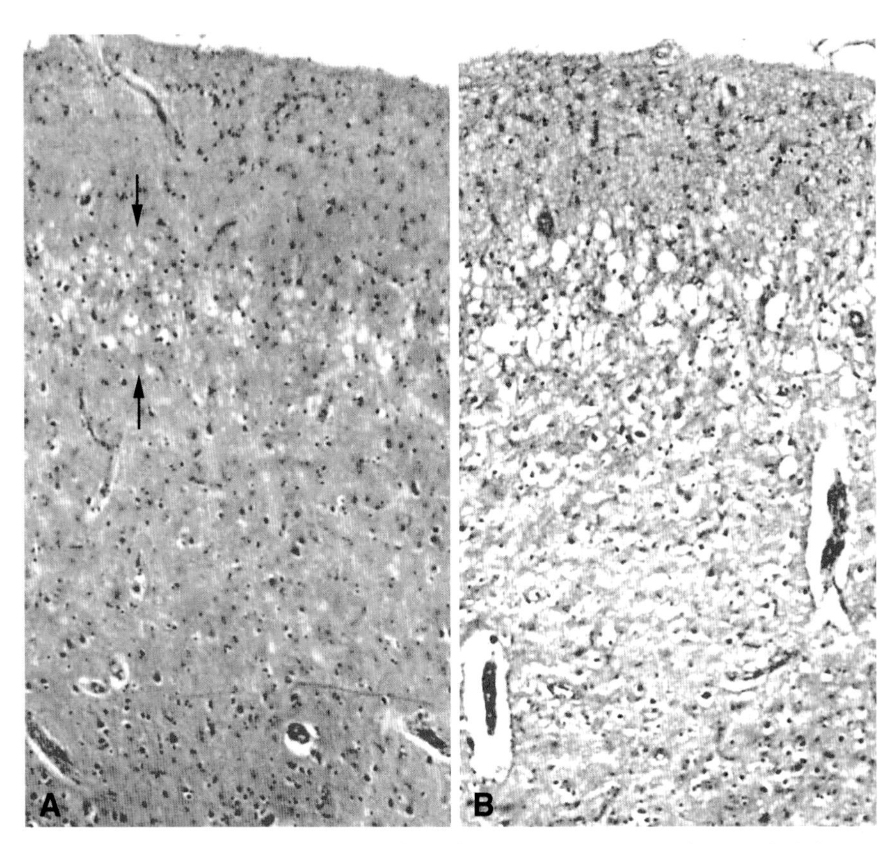

Figure 3. A. Microvacuolation centered on layer 2 (arrows). **B.** In advanced disease there is transcortical microvacuolation with neuronal loss and astrocytic glosis.

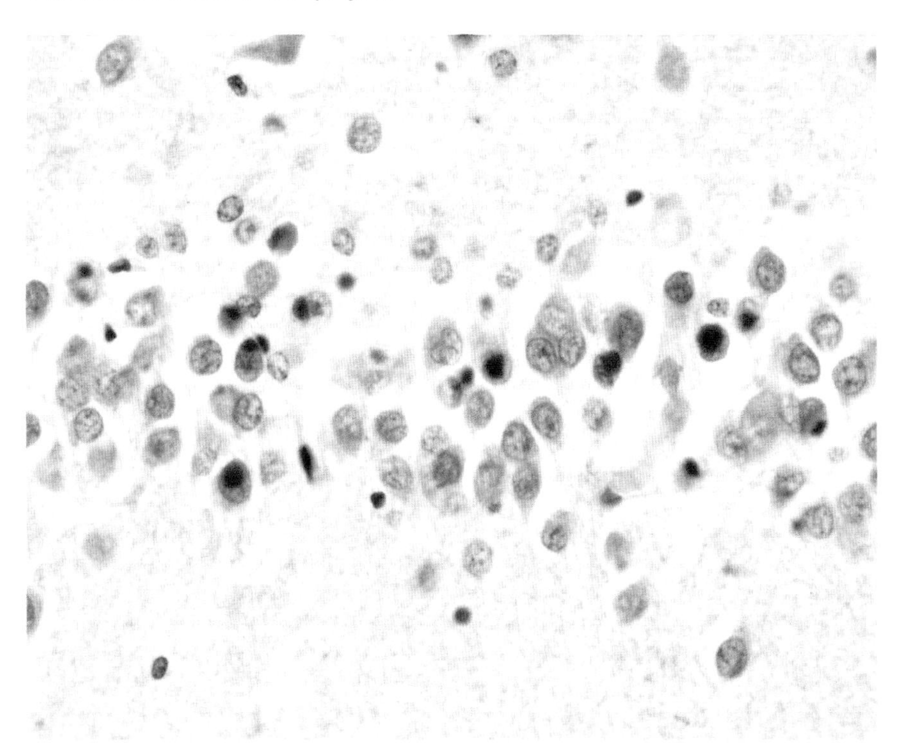

Figure 4. Ubiquitin-immunoreactive inclusions in dentate granule cells.

in the absence of tau or alpha synuclein-positive pathological structures or any other specific neuropathology a diagnosis of fronotemporal lobar degeneration is appropriate. This is a diagnosis based on the presence of appropriate regional cortical atrophy with neuronal loss and astrocytic glio-

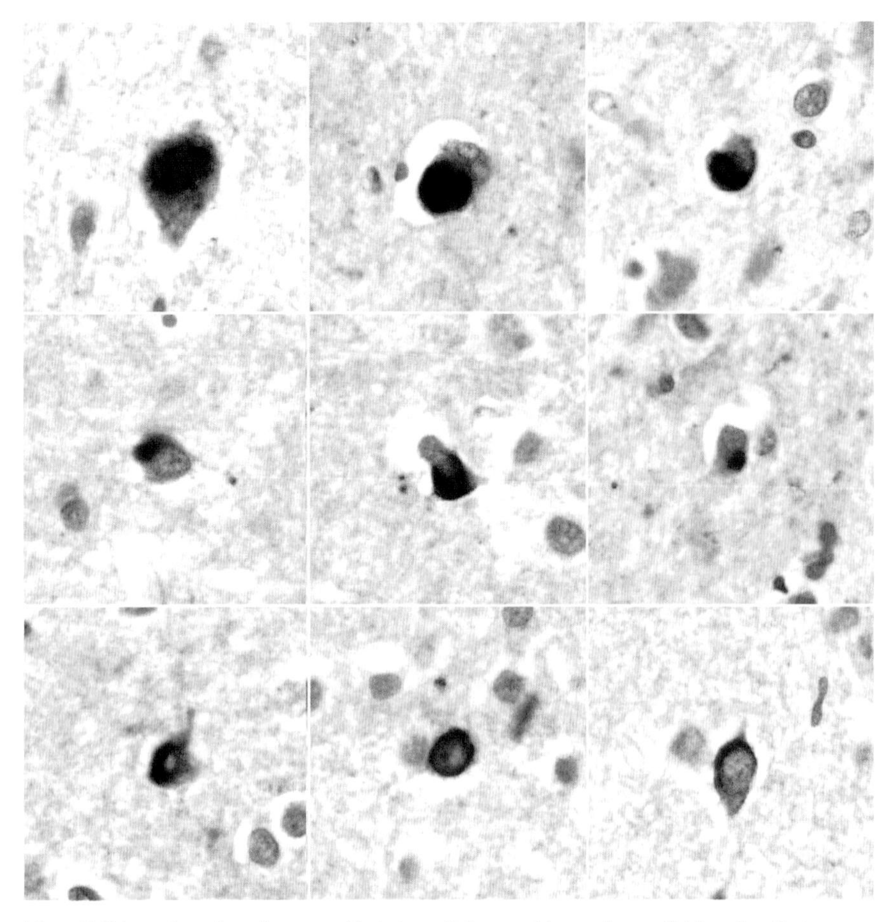

Figure 5. This montage shows the range of inclusions which are mainly seen in superficial small cortical neurons or in the dentate gyrus granule cells.

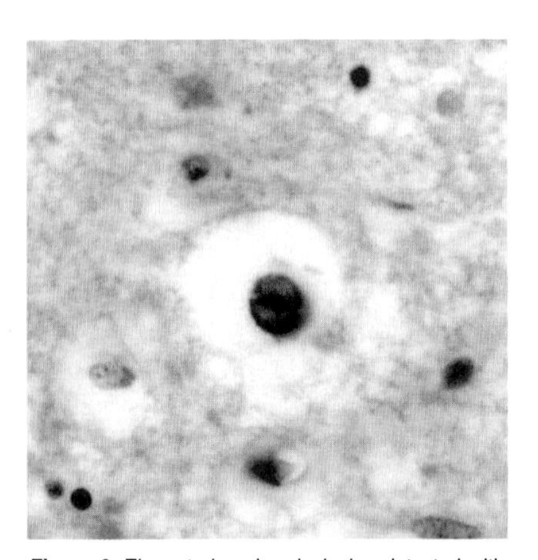

Figure 6. Elongated nuclear inclusion detected with anti-ubiquitin.

sis and in which pathological investigation, including appropriate immunohistochemistry, has excluded any further present diagnostic refinement.

Recently, 5 cases of early-onset dementia have been described characterised by the presence of neurofilament-positive inclusions. The inclusions were immunoreactive to antibodies to NFP, weakly ubiquitin-immunoreactive and non-reactive for α-synuclein and tau. The relationship of these cases to the group of FTLD remains to be determined (3).

Biochemistry

Characterisation of inclusions has not revealed a protein associated with ubiquitin in these forms of disease. Based on analogies with other ubiquitin-filament diseases it will be predicted that one or more proteins will be associated with both inclusions and neuritic change in both sporadic and familial cases and that mutation in the gene coding for these proteins will explain a proportion of familial cases.

An interesting observation has been made in one series described as DLDH that there is reduced expression of tau protein (37), not confirmed in another study (29).

Differential Diagnosis

Diagnosis should only be made in the context of the histological interpretation of a panel of antibodies for phospho-tau, ubiquitin, and alpha synuclein supplemented by assessment using stains sensitive for the pathology of Alzheimer's disease. Cases must be defined, in part, by the exclusion of tau pathology that would otherwise place them into the category of one of the tauopathies. Immunostaining for alpha B crystallin is helpful in defining the presence of swollen neurons, although finding these at present does not appear to have any diagnostic significance.

Given the age for some of these patients, coincidental Alzheimer-type pathology may be encountered. In the presence of significant Alzheimer-type pathology, the diagnosis should be viewed with caution.

The term "Pick's disease associated with motor neurone disease" should now be reserved for cases where there is defined tau pathology in the form of Pick bodies in association with changes of motor neurone disease.

There are currently 7 main clinical syndromes associated with this ubiquitin-only-immunoreactive type of pathology. These are typical motor neurone disease (MND), frontotemporal dementia with MND, pure frontotemporal dementia, semantic dementia, progressive non-fluent aphasia, akinetic rigid syndrome, and corticobasal syndrome (8, 21, 30). Case reports of lobar atrophy outside frontal or temporal regions, in association with relevant clinical syndromes, in which immunohistochemistry shows ubiquitin-only neuronal inclusions or ubiquitin-only immuno-reactive neuritic changes are now starting to be anecdotally noted.

Pathogenesis

The pathogenesis of the disorders discussed in this section is as yet unknown. The ubiquitin system is clearly involved in the biogenesis of inclusion bodies. The inclusions in FTLD-MND and in FTLD-U do not appear to conform to a pattern of aggresomal response, but would fit

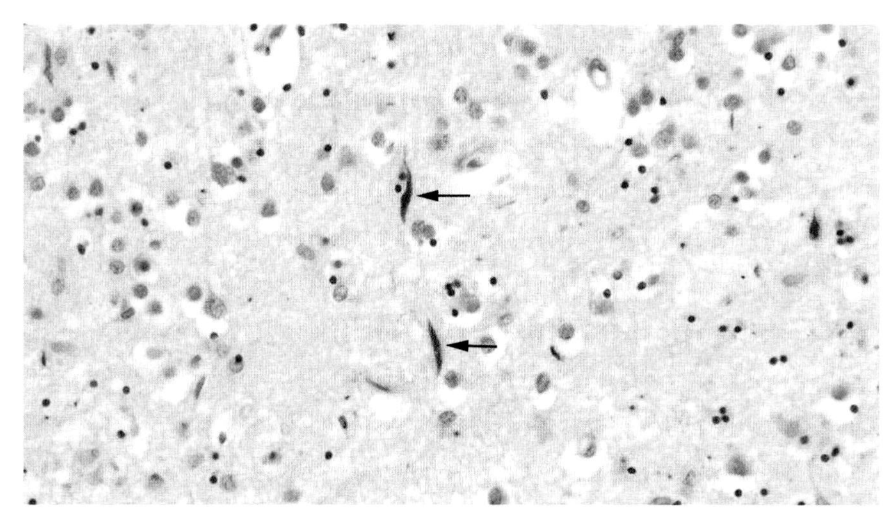

Figure 7. Ubiquitin-immunoreactive neurites with long, tapering profiles (arrows) seen in affected cortical areas.

into the category of a ubiquitin protein catabolic disease (19).

Future Directions and Therapy

The relationship between frontotemporal lobar degeneration with motor neurone disease (FTLD-MND) and frontotemporal lobar degeneration with ubiquitin-only-immunoreactive neuronal changes (FTLD-U), which are both characterised by the presence of similar ubiquitin-immunoreactive, tau-negative neuronal inclusions remains to be determined. The identification of specific protein accumulations in inclusions and the underlying genetic predispositions in familial forms of the disease are important immediate goals for research. It is likely that the future directions emerging from the genetics and pathology of familial motor neurone disease will overlap with a subset of cases described in this category of disease. The diagnostic categories of FTLD-U and FTLD-MND are therefore best regarded as temporary categories, which will be subject to future diagnostic refinement.

It is likely that new forms of neurodegeneration will be defined based on the discovery of new specific protein accumulations or genetic linkages. Given that FTLD is presently defined by several negative findings, the study of such cases is likely to reveal new diagnostic subgroups. The diagnostic category of FTLD is therefore also best regarded as a temporary category that is subject to future diagnostic refinement. For example, a form associated with neuronal small, spherical neurofilament positive, tau and alpha synuclein-negative, ubiquitin weakly positive inclusions has been presented in abstract form at scientific meetings and remains to be characterised.

The recognition of a small number of cases of frontotemporal lobar degeneration with ubiquitin-only-immunoreactive neuronal changes (FTLD-U) or frontotemporal lobar degeneration with motor neurone disease (FTLD-MND) with brainstem Lewy body pathology has been noted. Such cases warrant careful study in case they can be defined as a specific subset associated with distinctive molecular risk factors.

There is a need to define the incidence and prevalence of these forms of dementia outside specialist referral practice. Comparisons between previous studies have been hampered by inconsistent application of immunochemical investigations and use of differing pathological terminologies.

References

1. Bak TH, Hodges JR (2001) Motor neurone disease, dementia and aphasia: coincidence, co-occurrence or continuum? *Journal of Neurology* 248: 260-270.

2. Brown J (1998) Chromosome 3-linked frontotemporal dementia. *Cellular and Molecular Life Sciences* 54: 925-927.

3. Cairns N, Perry R, Jaros E, Lowe J, Skellerud K, Duyckaerts C,Cruz-Sanchez F (2002) A new dementia: Neurofilament inclusion body dementia. *J Neuropathol Exp Neurol* 61: 451.

4. Caselli RJ, Windebank AJ, Petersen RC, Komori T, Parisi JE, Okazaki H, Kokmen E, Iverson R, Dinapoli RP, Graff-Radford NR (1993) Rapidly progressive aphasic dementia and motor neuron disease. *Ann Neurol* 33: 200-207.

5. Chow TW, Miller BL, Hayashi VN, Geschwind DH (1999) Inheritance of frontotemporal dementia. *Archives of Neurology* 56: 817-822.

6. Cooper PN, Jackson M, Lennox G, Lowe L, Mann DM (1996) Brain-stem inclusions in motor neuron disease-type dementia. *Archives of Neurology* 53: 836.

7. Froelich S, Basun H, Forsell C, Lilius L, Axelman K, Andreadis A, Lannfelt L (1997) Mapping of a disease locus for familial rapidly progressive frontotemporal dementia to chromosome 17q12-21. *Am J Med Genet* 74: 380-385.

8. Grimes DA, Bergeron CB, Lang AE (1999) Motor neuron disease-inclusion dementia presenting as cortical-basal ganglionic degeneration. *Mov Disord* 14: 674-680.

9. Gunnarsson L, Dahlbom K, Strandman E (1991) Motor neuron disease and dementia reported among 13 members of a single family. *Acta Neurologica Scandinavica* 84: 429-433.

10. Gustafson L, Brun A, Passant U (1992) Frontal lobe degeneration of non-Alzheimer type. *Baillieres Clinical Neurology* 1: 559-582.

11. Holton JL, Révész T, Crooks R, Scaravilli F (2001) Evidence for pathological involvement of the spinal cord in motor neuron disease-inclusion dementia. *Acta Neuropathologica* 103: 221-227.

12. Hosler BA, Siddique T, Sapp PC, Sailor W, Huang MC, Hossain A, Daube JR, Nance M, Fan C, Kaplan J, Hung WY, McKennaYasek D, Haines JL, Pericak Vance MA, Horvitz HR, Brown RH (2000) Linkage of familial amyotrophic lateral sclerosis with frontotemporal dementia to chromosome 9q21-q22. *Jama* 284: 1664-1669.

13. Ince PG, Lowe J, Shaw PJ (1998) Amyotrophic lateral sclerosis: current issues in classification, pathogenesis and molecular pathology. *Neuropathology and Applied Neurobiology* 24: 104-117.

14. Jackson M, Lennox G, Lowe J (1996) Motor neurone disease-inclusion dementia. *Neurodegeneration* 5: 339-350.

15. Kertesz A, Kawarai T, Rogaeva E, St George Hyslop P, Poorkaj P, Bird TD, Munoz DG (2000) Familial frontotemporal dementia with ubiquitin-positive, tau-negative inclusions. *Neurology* 54: 818-827.

16. Kew J, Leigh N (1992) Dementia with motor neurone disease. *Baillieres Clinical Neurology* 1: 611-626.

17. Kinoshita A, Tomimoto H, Tachibana N, Suenaga T, Kawamata T, Kimura T, Akiguchi I, Kimura J (1996) A case of primary progressive aphasia with abnormally ubiquitinated neurites in the cerebral cortex. *Acta Neuropathol* (Berl) 92: 520-524.

18. Kovari E, Leuba G, Savioz A, Saini K, Anastasiu R, Miklossy J, Bouras C (2000) Familial frontotemporal dementia with ubiquitin inclusion bodies and without motor neuron disease. *Acta Neuropathol* (Berl) 100: 421-426.

19. Layfield R, Alban A, Mayer RJ, Lowe J (2001) The ubiquitin protein catabolic disorders. *Neuropathology and Applied Neurobiology* 27: 171-179.

20. Lowe J (1994) New pathological findings in amyotrophic lateral sclerosis. *J Neurol Sci* 124 Suppl: 38-51.

21. Lowe J (1999) The diseases characterized by ubiquitinated ALS inclusions and neurites. *Neuropathol Appl Neurobiol* 25: 24-25.

22. McKhann G, Albert M, Grossman M, Miller B, Dickson D, Trojanowski J (2001) Clinical and pathological diagnosis of frontotemporal dementia: report of the Work Group on frontotemporal dementia and Pick's disease. *Arch Neurol* 58: 1803-1809.

23. Mitsuyama Y (1984) Presenile dementia with motor neuron disease in Japan: clinico-pathological review of 26 cases. *J Neurol Neurosurg Psychiatry* 47: 953-959.

24. Mitsuyama Y (2000) Dementia with motor neuron disease. *Neuropathology* 20: S79-81.

25. Neary D (1990) Non Alzheimer's disease forms of cerebral atrophy. *J Neurol Neurosurg Psychiatry* 53: 929-931.

26. Neary D, Snowden JS, Gustafson L, Passant U, Stuss D, Black S, Freedman M, Kertesz A, Robert PH, Albert M, Boone K, Miller BL, Cummings J, Benson DF (1998) Frontotemporal lobar degeneration: a consensus on clinical diagnostic criteria. *Neurology* 51: 1546-1554.

27. Neary D, Snowden JS, Mann DM (2000) Classification and description of frontotemporal dementias. *Ann N Y Acad Sci* 920: 46-51.

28. Poorkaj P, Grossman M, Steinbart E, Payami H, Sadovnick A, Nochlin D, Tabira T, Trojanowski JQ, Borson S, Galasko D, Reich S, Quinn B, Schellenberg G, Bird TD (2001) Frequency of tau gene mutations in familial and sporadic cases of non-Alzheimer dementia. *Archives of Neurology* 58: 383-387.

29. Rosso SM, Kamphorst W, de Graaf B, Willemsen R, Ravid R, Niermeijer MF, Spillantini MG, Heutink P, van Swieten JC (2001) Familial frontotemporal dementia with ubiquitin-positive inclusions is linked to chromosome 17q21-22. *Brain* 124: 1948-1957.

30. Rossor MN, Revesz T, Lantos PL, Warrington EK (2000) Semantic dementia with ubiquitin-positive tau-negative inclusion bodies. *Brain* 123 (Pt 2): 267-276.

31. Savioz A, Kovari E, Anastasiu R, Rossier C, Saini K, Bouras C, Leuba G (2000) Search for a mutation in the tau gene in a Swiss family with frontotemporal dementia. *Experimental Neurology* 161: 330-335.

32. Stevens M, van Duijn CM, Kamphorst W, de Knijff P, Heutink P, van Gool WA, Scheltens P, Ravid R, Oostra BA, Niermeijer MF, van Swieten JC (1998) Familial aggregation in frontotemporal dementia. *Neurology* 50: 1541-1545.

33. Tolnay M, Probst A (1995) Frontal lobe degeneration: novel ubiquitin-immunoreactive neurites within frontotemporal cortex. *Neuropathology and Applied Neurobiology* 21: 492-497.

34. Vercelletto M, Ronin M, Huvet M, Magne C, Feve JR (1999) Frontal type dementia preceding amyotrophic lateral sclerosis: a neuropsychological and SPECT study of five clinical cases. *Eur J Neurol* 6: 295-299.

35. Whiteley A, Warrington E (1978) Selective impairment of topographical memory: a single case study. *J Neurol Neurosurg Psychiatry* 41: 575-578.

36. Woulfe J, Kertesz A, Munoz DG (2001) Frontotemporal dementia with ubiquitinated cytoplasmic and intranuclear inclusions. *Acta Neuropathol (Berl)* 102: 94-102.

37. Zhukareva V, Vogelsberg Ragaglia V, Van Deerlin VM, Bruce J, Shuck T, Grossman M, Clark CM, Arnold SE, Masliah E, Galasko D, Trojanowski JQ, Lee VM (2001) Loss of brain tau defines novel sporadic and familial tauopathies with frontotemporal dementia. *Ann Neurol* 49: 165-175.

CHAPTER 8

Motor Neuron Disorders

Chapter Editor: Hidehiro Mizuzawa

8.1 Amyotrophic Lateral Sclerosis 350

8.2 Primary Lateral Sclerosis 369

8.3 Spinal Muscular Atrophy 372

Amyotrophic Lateral Sclerosis

Shinsuke Kato
Pamela Shaw
Clare Wood-Allum
P. Nigel Leigh
Christopher Shaw

AChE	acetylcholin esterase
AGE	advanced glycation endproducts
ALS	amyotrophic lateral sclerosis
ApoE	apolipoprotein E
Ast-HI	astrocytic hyaline inclusion
BI	basophilic inclusion
CCS	copper chaperonce for SOD1
CIDP	chronic inflammatory demyelinating neuropathy
CML	carboxymethyl lysine
CT	computer tomography
DTI	diffusion tensor imaging
EAAT	excitatory amino acid transporter
EMG	electromyography
FALS	familial amyotrophic lateral sclerosis
FTD	fronto-temporal dementia
^{1}H-MRS	proton magnetic resonance spectroscopy
HMSN	hereditary motor and sensory neuropathy
IBM	inclusion body myositis
LBHI	Lewy body-like hyaline inclusion
LMN	lower motor neurone
MMN	multifocal motor neuropathy
MND	motor neurone disease
MRI	magnetic resonance imaging
NFCI	neurofilamentous conglomerate inclusion
NF-H	neurofilament heavy chain
PET	positron emission tomography
PBP	progressive bulbar palsy
PMA	progressive muscular atrophy
PUMNS	probable UMN signs
RHI	round hyaline inclusion
UMN	upper motor neurone
SALS	sporadic amyotrophic lateral sclerosis
SLI	skein-like inclusion
SOD	superoxide dismutase

Definition

Amyotrophic lateral sclerosis (ALS) also known as motor neurone disease (MND) is a progressive disorder characterised by degeneration of motor neurones of the motor cortex, brainstem and spinal cord. In addition to neuronal loss, motor neurones often have characteristic ubiquitin immunoreactive inclusions in the perikarya and dystrophic axons (76, 103, 106, 110, 121, 135). Clinically, this relatively selective degeneration of upper and lower motor neurones is associated with progressive wasting and weakness of skeletal muscles leading to death from respiratory failure in the absence of respiratory support. Concepts on the nosology of ALS have evolved over nearly 200 years, and the terms ALS and MND cover a variety of clinical syndromes. It is now clear from genetics that the molecular basis of ALS is complex, and that many presumably convergent mechanisms lead to the phenotype of ALS. ALS may therefore be considered a syndrome rather than a single disease entity.

Synonyms and Historical Annotations

The first descriptions of ALS certainly precede the classical descriptions of Charcot and colleagues (178). Charles Bell in Edinburgh described a patient with progressive motor weakness associated with degeneration of the anterior half of the spinal cord. Cruveilhier (40) likewise lectured about such cases, and recognised that the syndrome was associated with atrophy of the anterior spinal nerve roots. Aran (13) clearly described what was later designated as ALS, although he described his cases as "progressive muscular atrophy." He included familial cases. At that time, as Rowland (145) points out, semiology was rudimentary and the distinction between upper and lower motor neurone signs was not made clinically.

Charcot defined the syndrome of adult onset progressive muscular wasting as a disease of the spinal motor neurones, rather than a primary disease of muscle (30, 145). In addition, Charcot recognised the importance of corticospinal tract degeneration in the pathological process. He introduced the term "la Sclérose Amyotrophique Latérale." It was soon recognised that the syndrome of progressive bulbar palsy (PBP; described by Duchenne in 1860 [47]) fell within the rubric of ALS. It took longer for the syndrome of progressive muscular atrophy (PMA) to be included within the ALS concept, and to this day there remains a debate about the nosology of adult-onset pure lower motor neurone syndromes (179). No doubt this reflects the heterogeneous nature of PMA although 70 to 80% of patients presenting with PMA will turn out to have ALS as defined pathologically.

On the basis of pathological studies, Déjerine (45) proposed that ALS, PBP and PMA should be considered as an entity. This unitary concept was developed by the British neurologist Russell Brain who used the term motor neurone disease (MND) to include ALS, PBP and PMA. Currently, the terms ALS and MND are used interchangeably.

Epidemiology

Incidence and prevalence. The incidence of amyotrophic lateral sclerosis is about 1 to 3 per 100000 per year and the point prevalence rates have been estimated at 4 to 6 per 100 000 (56, 176). The most reliable estimates derive from population-based studies in which capture-recapture methods are used for ascertainment. There is no conclusive evidence that the incidence of ALS is increasing. The prevalence can be expected to rise somewhat with the increased age of western populations, and also, in part, with the introduction of better treatments.

The incidence of ALS is similar worldwide with the exception of some high risk areas such as the island of Guam, parts of the Kii peninsula of Japan, and parts of Western New Guinea (96, 136, 182). In these regions the disease is atypical and associated with dementia, parkinsonism and neurofibrillary tangles in many brain regions (66, 68, 119). The previously high incidence in these areas may now be falling to levels more typical of the rest of the world (67, 119, 141, 183). The lifetime risk of ALS in most parts of the world where accurate figures are available is about 1 in 1000. This estimate is derived from death certification, so may be an underestimate.

Sex and age distribution. The incidence rises until it peaks around 75 years of age, although the distribution is bi-modal for sex, the incidence being somewhat higher in elderly women compared to men. In familial ALS the mean age of onset is about a decade earlier. The male to female ratio in sporadic ALS is 3:2 but this approaches 1:1 after the menopause because of an over-representation of women with bulbar onset (95, 187). It is interesting that male predominance is particularly marked in some lower motor neurone variants (PMA) such as the "flail arm" or "man in a barrel" syndrome, where it is nearly 10 times more common in men than women (73).

Risk factors. Other than increasing age, the 2 main risk factors for developing ALS are gender and family history (41). Although associations have been detected in various studies between ALS and various environmental factors, taken overall, epidemiological studies have failed to identify consistent and statistically robust associations between ALS and environmental risk factors, although trauma, toxins, viral infections such as poliomyelitis, exercise, and occupation have all been weakly associated with ALS (29, 32, 51, 126, 127, 165, 169).

Genetics

Although most ALS is sporadic, in 5 to 10% of cases a family history is apparent. Most commonly the family history suggests an autosomal dominant disorder, although sibling pairs, and small kindreds are more frequently encountered than large and extensive kindreds, suggesting incomplete penetrance. Juvenile onset autosomal recessive and X-linked forms of familial ALS have been identified but these are rare (Table 1). Twenty percent of familial cases of ALS show mutations in the gene on chromosome 21 that encodes the free radical scavenging enzyme Cu/Zn superoxide dismutase (SOD1) (142). More than 100 mutations in the SOD1 gene have been detected (35, 152). In addition, mutations of SOD1 are found in 2 to 3% of apparently sporadic cases. Most of these are point missense mutations, but some introduce a stop codon and lead to production of truncated protein (7, 35, 133, 140).

Type of ALS	Inheritance	Linkage and OMIM number	Gene/protein	References
Familial ALS	AD	21q22.1-22.2 ALS1	SOD1	(43, 139, 140, 142)
Juvenile familial ALS/HSP (Predominantly spastic quadriparesis; some LMN signs in one family)	AR	2q33-2q35 ALS2	Alsin	(58, 63, 188)
Familial ALS (~80% of families)	AD	Unknown ALS3	Unknown	
Juvenile-onset ALS (Slowly progressive childhood or adolescent onset UMN and LMN syndrome)	AD	9q34 ALS4	Unknown	(138)
Juvenile onset familial ALS/HSP	AR	15q15-15q22 ALS5	Unknown	(64)
Familial ALS	AD	18q21 ALS6	Unknown	(59)
X-linked dominant familial ALS	X-linked	X centromere ALSX	Unknown	(162)
Familial ALS with frontotemporal dementia	AD	9q 21-q22	Unknown	(71)
Familial ALS (Variable penetrance, typical ALS)	AD	16q	Unknown	(146)
Brown-Vialetto-Van Laere disease (Juvenile onset MND with sensorineural deafness)	AR	Unknown	Unknown	
Familial amyotrophy with FTDP-17	AD	17q21-17q22	Tau	(112, 124, 185)

Table 1. Genetically determined forms of ALS.

The ALS phenotype associated with SOD1 gene mutations is diverse, ranging from an aggressive disease, fatal within 2 years of onset such as the A4V mutation (42, 43, 81) to slowly progressive forms such as the Scandinavian form of autosomal recessive ALS associated with homozygous D90A mutations (5, 9-11). With these exceptions, heterogeneity is apparent both within and between families.

The SOD1 protein is widely expressed in cells throughout the body. The major function of the enzyme is to convert intracellular superoxide radicals into hydrogen peroxide, which is in turn removed by the action of other free radical scavenging enzymes. Although the mechanism whereby SOD1 mutations cause ALS is uncertain, there is compelling evidence that mutant SOD1 acquires a toxic gain of function. First, it is apparent that ALS patients carrying SOD1 gene mutations may have normal or near normal levels of SOD1 enzyme activity. Second, mice transgenic for mutant human SOD1 may have normal or high levels of SOD1 enzyme activity and yet develop motor neurone degeneration. Third, all disease-causing mutations known are either point missense mutations or truncation mutations. In other words, in every known case mutant

Syndrome	Main clinical features	Prognosis	References
Classical ('Charcot') ALS	Usually limb (spinal) onset of weakness; bulbar involvement usual; combined UMN and LMN signs; M:F ratio 3:2	Median survival 3-4 years	(31, 178)
Progressive bulbar palsy (PBP)	Onset with dysarthria followed by progressive speech and swallowing difficulties; limb involvement usually follows within months but may be delayed for several years; M:F ratio 1:1 (PBP relatively more common in older women)	Median survival 2-3 years	(47)
Progressive muscular atrophy (PMA)	Almost always limb onset; >50% develop UMN signs; ~85% develop bulbar symptoms eventually; heterogeneous condition but majority are ALS; M:F ratio 3-4:1	Median survival ~5 years; some long survivors (>10 years)	(13)
"Flail arm" syndrome	A syndrome of predominantly LMN weakness of both arms; UMN signs develop in 50-70%; often slow progression; pathology is that of ALS	M:F ratio 9:1; prognosis may be better than in typical ALS; syndrome may be more common in Africans and Asians	(73, 84, 175)
"Flail leg" syndrome; "pseudo-polyneuritic" form of ALS	A syndrome of progressive leg weakness, predominantly LMN	Slow progression	
Monomelic motor neurone disease	Rare ALS variant with slowly progressive focal (upper or lower limb UMN and LMN) syndrome. Rare LMN form most common in Asia (monomelic juvenile onset amyotophy; Hirayama's syndrome, does not generalise and pathology is unknown)	Juvenile onset form is progressive over months or several years and then stabilises	(54, 69)
Primary lateral sclerosis (PLS)	Clinically progressive pure upper motor neuron syndrome; after 5 years rare to convert to ALS, but may do so	20 years +	(24, 101, 137)

Table 2. Clinical syndromes of ALS and related disorders.

protein is produced. There are no known null mutations and SOD1 knockout mice develop normally.

The leading hypotheses for the toxic gain of function include abnormal handling of intracellular free radical species leading to increased generation of hydrogen peroxide and peroxynitrite; the formation of toxic intracellular aggregates; and toxicity resulting from cytosolic release of copper and/or zinc ions.

In addition to the genes and genetic loci mentioned in Table 1, several genes coding for proteins that might play a part in neuronal degeneration have been implicated as causing ALS, modifying its course, or acting as risk factors.

Isolated point mutations have been identified in the genes coding for the glial excitatory amino acid transporter 2 (EAAT2), cytochrome oxidase, and APEX nuclease (62). Possible disease modifying factors include apolipoprotein E (120, 163), and survival motor neurone (SMN) protein (37) and the hypoxia response element of the vascular endothelium growth factor (VEGF) promotor gene (132). However, the statistical associations are weak and (for apolipoprotein E at least) of doubtful validity. More robust is the association of sporadic ALS with mutations of the gene coding for the neurofilament heavy chain, NFH (6, 50). About 1% of patients with apparently sporadic ALS carry mutations (mostly deletions) in the C-terminal region of NFH bearing KSP (lysine-serine-proline) repeat sequences. These are phosphorylation sites, and phosphorylation is thought to be important in NF function (2, 115). Perturbations of NF function lead to motor neurone degeneration in transgenic mouse models (80). Taken together, these findings support the notion that abnormal NF function is important in motor neurone disorders.

Recently, a rare form of juvenile onset ALS has been linked to mutations in a gene on chromosome 2q33 termed alsin (58, 188). The predicted protein structure of alsin has domains homologous to GTPase regulatory proteins. Both the types of mutations and the pattern of inheritance suggest that motor neurone degeneration is likely to be due to a loss of function of alsin.

Clinical Features

Signs and symptoms. As noted above, ALS comprises several clinical syndromes (Table 2) including progressive bulbar palsy (PBP), classical Charcot ALS and progressive muscular atrophy (PMA). Within these categories we can also recognise clinical variants including a progressive, mainly LMN syndrome of leg weakness (the "flail leg" syndrome) and a characteristic syndrome of progressive upper limb weakness and wasting that has variously been termed the "flail arm syndrome," progressive amyotrophic brachial diplegia or the "man in a barrel" syndrome (73, 91, 148, 175). The ALS variant was probably first recognised by Vulpian (52, 181) and by Gowers (55).

Most patients with ALS present with functional changes related to focal muscle weakness. For patients with PBP this almost always takes the form of dysarthria. Dysphagia is usually a later symptom. With limb onset ALS, typical presentations include difficulty with opposition grip (turning an ignition key, for example), opening bottle tops, and managing buttons. If proximal muscles are affected first, patients may notice difficulty carrying bags, reaching for objects on shelves, and dressing. Leg weakness often manifests as an asymmetrical foot drop. If spasticity is marked, patients may complain of stiffness and flexor spasms as well as weakness. Only 2 to 3% of patients present with respiratory failure due to early involvement of the diaphragm. Some of these individuals are only diagnosed after having emergency tracheostomy and assisted ventilation.

Severe or unusually frequent cramps are common and often precede the onset of weakness by months or even several years. Fasciculations are usually noticed by doctors rather than patients, but occasionally can be obtrusive enough to attract the attention of the patient. Sensory symptoms are not uncommon, but sensory signs should trigger further investigation for an alternative diagnosis.

The typical signs of ALS include wasting, usually focal initially, but gradually becoming more widespread; fasciculations, which must be distinguished from other benign muscle twitches; weakness, which begins focally and tends to spread to involve contiguous spinal segments, and which represents the effects of both UMN and LMN damage; changes in the tendon reflexes; and a positive Babinski sign. UMN signs are very variable, and in PMA (by definition) they are absent. The tendon reflexes are abnormally brisk at some time during the evolution of the disease in about 85% of cases, but the definition of what is brisk, normal or depressed is often problematic. The term "Probable UMN Signs" (PUMNS) has been used to indicate that a preserved tendon reflex in a wasted and weak muscle may be presumed to reflect an UMN component. UMN signs tend to be more prominent in patients with PBP, and in a group of patients who present with a progressive spastic paraparesis and who develop LMN signs some months or even years later. They present a difficult diagnostic group.

Primary lateral sclerosis (PLS) is a clinically "pure" upper motor neurone syndrome (137) (chapter 8.3). Electrophysiological studies indicate that there are minor degrees of anterior horn cell involvement (101) and rarely a syndrome of ALS develops after many years (24).

About 25% of patients present with bulbar symptoms and 75% with limb onset. Of the latter, about a quarter present with arm weakness, about a quarter with leg weakness, and the remainder with various combinations of arm and leg weakness (168). A bulbar presentation is associated with worse prognosis, and a higher proportion of older women, so the sex ratio is about equal, in contrast to limb onset ALS where men predominate in a ratio of about 3:2. Bulbar-onset ALS is characterised by the pseudobulbar syndrome, comprising emotional lability, spastic dysarthria, brisk facial, snout and jaw reflexes, and varying degrees of nasality due to palatal weakness. Bulbar onset patients also tend to have more significant cognitive impairment (1) although subtle frontal and memory deficits are not restricted to this group.

About 5% of patients develop (or may present with) dementia of frontotemporal type (FTD), the ALS-dementia syndrome (74, 93, 117, 125, 184). Although 30 to 40% of ALS patients have subtle cognitive abnormalities (usually of frontal lobe type) on neuropsychological testing (1, 92), only a minority of these patients progress to clinical FTD. Some patients develop extrapyramidal features, often in association with the ALS-dementia syndrome (74). The Guam ALS-parkinsonism-dementia syndrome and the similar syndrome encountered in the Kii peninsula of Japan are clearly distinct from the ALS-dementia syndrome both clinically and pathologically (119). A syndrome of progressive supranuclear palsy, dementia, and in a few cases, ALS has been described on Guadeloupe (26). As in the Guam syndrome, this is a tauopathy, although the LMN pathology of the Guam and Guadeloupe syndromes features ubiq-

Genetically determined forms of motor neurone disorder
- Familial ALS/MND
- Brown-Vialetto-Van Laere syndrome (early onset bulbar and spinal ALS with sensorineural deafness)
- Fazio-Londe syndrome (infantile progressive bulbar palsy)
- Hexosaminidase deficiency
- Hereditary spastic paraplegia (many forms, including ALS2, ALS4)
- Spinal muscular atrophy (SMA)
- Proximal childhood and later onset forms of SMA (types 1-4), SMN gene-related
- Distal SMA (various forms)
- Adult-onset proximal SMA (unrelated to SMN gene mutations)
- Juvenile or adult onset laryngeal and distal SMA (Harper Young syndrome)
- X-linked bulbar and spinal muscular atrophy (Kennedy's disease)
- Hereditary Motor and Sensory Neuropathy (predominantly motor forms)
- Multisystem disorders with occasional anterior horn cell involvement (e.g., SCA3)
- Algrove syndrome
- Apparently sporadic (idiopathic) forms of motor neurone disorder with SOD1 mutations?

Sporadic ALS and variants
- Progressive bulbar palsy; limb onset ALS; progressive spinal muscular atrophy
- Segmental spinal muscular atrophy (flail arm and flail leg syndromes)
- Primary lateral sclerosis
- Distal sporadic focal spinal muscular atrophy ("Hirayama syndrome")
- Atypical juvenile onset ALS in South India ("Madras" form of ALS)
- Western Pacific and other similar forms of ALS (Guam, Kii peninsula, New Guinea)
- Guadeloupe PSP-Dementia-ALS syndrome

Multiple system atrophy with anterior horn cell degeneration

Progressive supranuclear palsy with anterior horn cell degeneration

Corticobasal ganglionic degeneration with anterior horn cell degeneration

Acquired forms of motor neurone disorder
- HTLV-1 associated myelopathy (HAM)
- HIV-associated ALS syndrome
- Creutzfeldt-Jacob disease (amyotrophic forms)
- Multifocal motor neuropathy
- Acute poliomyelitis
- Lead, mercury toxicity
- Neurolathyrism (due to *lathyrus sativa*, containing β-oxalyl-L-aminoacid, BOAA)
- Konzo (due to toxic cyanogenic cassava)
- Radiation myelopathy (eg cervical and lumbosacral radiculopathy)
- Post-polio progressive muscular atrophy syndrome
- Autoimmune disorders (eg Sjögren's disease)
- Endocrinopathy (Hyperthyroidism, hyperparathyroidism, hypoglycaemia)

Table 3. Motor neurone disorders.

Diagnostic Criteria for ALS (21)
Definite ALS
UMN signs and LMN signs in 3 regions
Probable ALS
UMN signs and LMN signs in 2 regions with at least some UMN signs rostral to LMN signs
Probable ALS – Laboratory supported
UMN signs in 1 or more region and LMN signs defined by EMG in at least 2 regions
Possible ALS
UMN signs and LMN signs in 1 region (together), or UMN signs in 2 or more regions UMN and LMN signs in 2 regions with no UMN signs rostral to LMN signs
UMN signs: clonus, Babinski sign, absent abdominal skin reflexes, hypertonia, loss of dexterity. LMN signs: atrophy, weakness. If only fasciculation: search with EMG for active denervation. Regions reflect neuronal pools: bulbar, cervical, thoracic and lumbosacral

Table 4. Summary of revised El Escorial diagnostic criteria.

uitin-immunoreactive inclusions, not tau-positive neurofibrillary tangles.

Imaging. Although abnormalities of MRI signal have been detected in the motor cortex and in the corticospinal tracts on MRI, no specific or reliable diagnostic MRI marker for ALS has emerged. Neuroimaging with MRI or occasionally CT myelography serve mainly to exclude other disorders. MRI modalities such as proton magnetic resonance spectroscopy (^{1}H-MRS) and diffusion tensor imaging (DTI) may hold promise as diagnostic tools (105). Positron emission tomography (PET) and single photon emission tomography (SPET) may show altered brain function in patients with ALS-dementia, but overall PET remains a research tool (105).

Laboratory findings. Unfortunately there is no specific diagnostic test for ALS, and the diagnosis depends upon careful clinical evaluation and investigation to exclude other conditions (Tables 2, 3). The creatine kinase serum level may be raised, but is seldom higher than four times the upper limit of normal. Examination of the spinal fluid is usually not helpful, although the total protein may be a little raised. The presence of a significantly raised protein or cell count suggests the need for further investigation to exclude an ALS mimic, such as meningeal infiltration with lymphoma, or (in LMN syndromes) a motor variant of chronic inflammatory demyelinating neuropathy (CIDP).

EMG supports the clinical diagnosis of ALS if there is evidence of active and chronic partial denervation in at least 2 of 4 body regions. In practice, one can be confident of the diagnosis of bulbar onset ALS (PBP) even if the initial EMG fails to show clear evidence of denervation in several regions, providing there are the characteristic UMN and LMN signs in the cranial region, and investigations have excluded other diagnostic possibilities. In LMN syndromes it is important to search carefully for conduction block, a characteristic feature of MMN. Conduction block is demonstrated if there is a significant drop in the amplitude of the compound motor action potential with distal compared to more proximal stimulation of motor nerves and proximal nerve roots (18, 100, 129).

Differential Diagnosis of ALS

In 1998, a conference at Airlie House revisited the 1994 El Escorial criteria for the diagnosis of ALS (21) (Table 4). These research criteria have been validated pathologically (21) and clinically (177), although agreement between observers using the criteria is poor (14).

In order to make a formal diagnosis of ALS under the research criteria there must be: *i)* Evidence of lower motor neurone (LMN) degeneration by clinical, electrophysiological or neuropathological examination; *ii)* Evidence of upper motor neurone (UMN) degeneration by clinical examination, and *iii)* progressive spread of symptoms and signs within a region or to other regions as determined by history or examination. In addition, there must not be: *i)* Electrophysiological and/or pathological evidence of other disease processes that might explain the signs of LMN and or/UMN degeneration, or *ii)* neuroimaging evidence of other disease processes that might explain the observed clinical and electrophysiological signs.

The Airlie House criteria are stringent and designed more for screening candidates for research trials than for clinical practice. Clinical diagnosis rests on careful assessment, supplemented by electrophysiology, imaging, blood tests and sometimes muscle biopsy to exclude other diagnoses. Conditions included in the differential diagnosis may be termed ALS-mimic syndromes if they occur due to other pathologies and ALS with laboratory abnormalities of unknown significance (ALS-LAUS) if they are associated with abnormal laboratory findings that may be related to the motor dysfunction. Patients who meet ALS criteria, but who develop additional features such as extrapyramidal features or dementia, which are not demonstrably due to another pathology, are included as ALS-plus syndromes. In practice, clinical suspicion of a diagnosis of ALS may be present at a stage before the patient meets the formal diagnostic criteria, and other potentially more treatable pathologies should be excluded.

Since the initial symptoms are often non-specific, and because ALS is rare in community practice, family practitioners often refer patients with ALS initially to specialists in otorhinolaryngology, rheumatology, or orthopaedics. The delay from the onset of symptoms to diagnosis averages about 14 months. Analysis of prognostic factors shows that earlier diagnosis is associated with worse prognosis probably reflecting more aggressive disease (177).

Between 5 and 27% of patients in whom ALS is diagnosed initially may

Final diagnosis	Characteristic features	Distinguishing diagnostic features and investigations
Cerebral lesions	Focal motor cortex lesions very rarely mimic ALS, but frontal lesions with co-existent cervical or lumbosacral root damage may cause confusion; questionable entity of parietal wasting	MRI/CT; no EMG evidence of widespread chronic partial denervation (CPD) in limbs
Skull base lesions	Lower cranial nerve signs (bulbar symptoms and signs; wasting of tongue, often asymmetrical); seldom significant long tract signs unless foramen magnum involved in addition	MRI; CT with bone windows; no EMG evidence of CPD in limbs
Cervical spondylotic myelopathy	Progressive limb weakness. Asymmetrical onset; combined UMN and LMN signs in arm(s); spastic paraparesis; occasionally fasciculations in arms	Pain in root distribution, but pain may not be severe and may resolve quickly; often progression followed by clinical stabilisation; no bulbar involvement ; MRI evidence of spinal cord and root compression; no evidence of CPD on EMG (NB: patients may have co-existent lumbosacral motor radiculopathy with lower limb denervation)
Other cervical myelopathies; foramen magnum lesions; intrinsic and extrinsic tumours; syringomyelia	Progressive weakness; foramen magnum lesions and high cervical cord lesions may be associated with focal (C8/T1) wasting; syringomyelia usually associated with LMN signs and dissociated sensory loss	Usually involvement of cerebellar and/or sensory pathways; MRI of head and cervical spine reveal pathology
Conus lesions and lumbosacral radiculopathy	Progressive mixed UMN and LMN syndrome	Usually significant sensory symptoms if not signs; bladder involvement; MRI thoracic and lumbosacral region
Inclusion body myositis	Progressive weakness; bulbar symptoms; sometimes respiratory muscle weakness	Characteristic wasting and weakness of deep fibres of flexor digiti communis, and quadriceps femoris; EMG evidence of myopathy; muscle biopsy as definitive test (rimmed vacuoles)
Multifocal motor neuropathy (MMN)	Focal asymmetrical onset, often upper limb; pure LMN syndrome; may stabilise for months or years; M:F 4:1	Conduction block on nerve conduction studies (NCS); weakness often out of proportion to wasting; improvement with intravenous immunoglobulin (IVIG) in ~70%
Kennedy's disease (X-linked bulbospinal muscular atrophy)	Males symptomatic; slowly progressive bulbar and limb weakness	Family history; fasciculations of facial muscles; gynaecomastia; proximal symmetrical weakness in addition to foot drop; mild sensory neuropathy on NCS; DNA test for CAG repeat mutation in exon 1 of androgen receptor gene

Table 5. Diagnostic errors and most common "ALS mimics."

have other conditions (15, 20, 29, 44, 104) (Tables 3, 5). Some of the conditions that are mistaken for ALS are potentially treatable, and others, while not curable, have a far better prognosis than ALS. The conditions most frequently misdiagnosed as ALS are cervical spondylotic radiculo-myelopathy, thoraco-lumbo sacral disc disease, multi-focal motor neuropathy (MMN), adult onset forms of spinal muscular atrophy, predominantly motor forms of hereditary or acquired motor and sensory neuropathy (HMSN type 2), myasthenia gravis, inclusion body myositis (IBM) and Kennedy's disease. It is particularly important to consider myasthenia gravis in the elderly with predominantly bulbar symptoms and to perform single fibre EMG and to measure anti-acetylcholine and MuSK antibodies (70).

Rarely, Sjögren's disease may mimic ALS. Endocrine disorders such as hyperparathyroidusm may present with weakness and brisk reflexes, and hypoglycaemia with insulinoma may cause wasting of the hand muscles (78). Severe Graves disease (autoimmune hyperthyroidism) may present with muscle weakness, wasting and fasciculation (Basedow's disease). Occasionally the syndrome of post-irradiation lumbosacral radiculopathy (usually following irradiation treatment for testicular cancer or lymphoma) presents with a syndrome of progressive motor weakness of the legs (19). The ALS-dementia syndrome has been regarded by some as a different disease, but this syndrome probably represents a variant of the ALS spectrum (93, 117, 125). ALS has been linked to underlying carcinoma and lymphoma as an autoimmune process (53, 189), but the association is probably fortuitous. Similarly, benign monoclonal gammopathy of unknown significance is not thought to be causally related to ALS.

The syndrome of benign fasciculation is a condition of persistent (although often intermittent and variable) muscle twitching. EMG shows no denervation, and the syndrome does not progress to ALS (17). It may be localised to the leg muscles or generalised. Localised fasciculations of the calf muscles are common and innocent (180). Interestingly, people who carry SOD1 gene mutations do not develop fasciculations or denervation until the onset of clinical symptoms, suggesting that the prodomal phase of ALS is relatively short (3). This is in keeping with clinical observations in sporadic ALS, in which it is rare for cramps and fasciculation to precede the onset of weakness by more than one year.

In summary, although the differential diagnosis of ALS embraces a host of central and peripheral disorders, it is particularly important to identify those (such as spinal cord and root compression and MMN) that are treatable, or even curable (such as myasthenia gravis). Even when no specific treatment is available, accurate diagnosis is essential for counselling and continuing care.

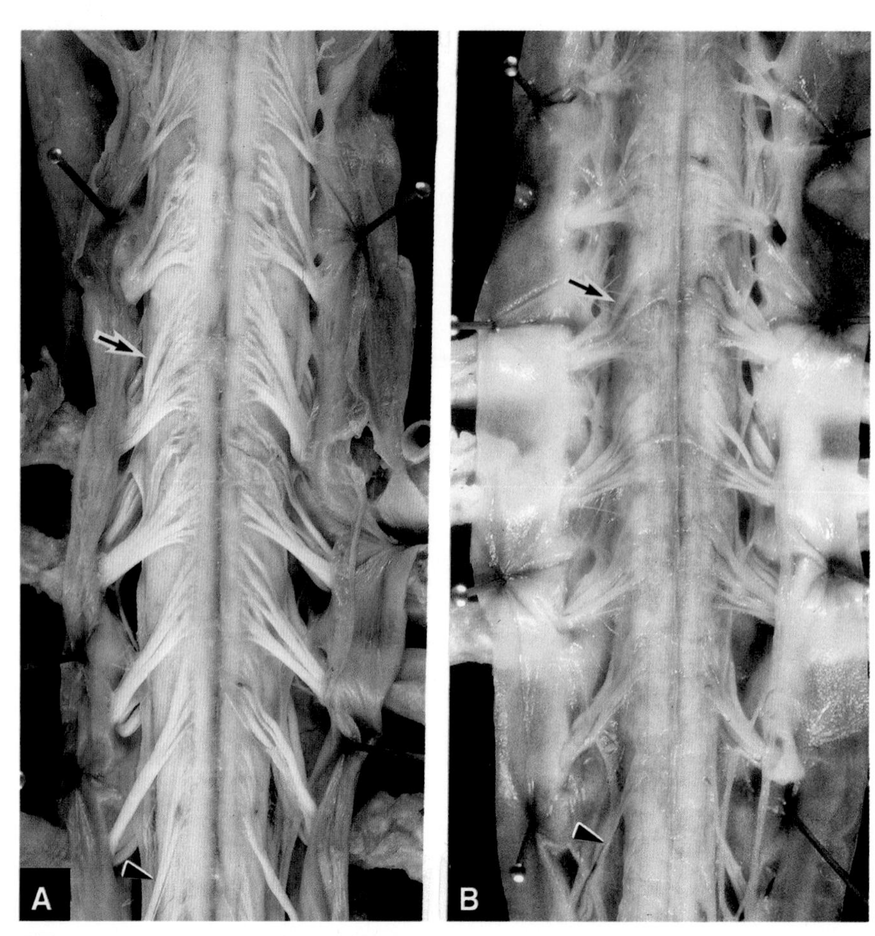

Figure 1. Cervical spinal cords from a normal subject (**A**) and a patient with ALS (**B**). Anterior roots in the ALS patient (**B**) show grayish discoloration and atrophy compared to the normal subject (**A**). The C6 anterior motor root is indicated by an arrow and T2 anterior motor root is marked by an arrowhead. In general, cervical roots are thick, and the T1 root is thinner in caliber while the T2 root is thinner furthermore. This finding is an important procedure to determine the various segments of the spinal cord. The cervical enlargement in the ALS patient (**B**) is also atrophic compared to the normal subject (**A**). ×1.1

Macroscopy

At autopsy, ALS patients show diffuse muscle atrophy and wasting, with reduction in subcutaneous fat. Atrophy affects not only limb muscles, but also intercostal muscles and the diaphragm. The spinal cord is macroscopically atrophic, with the cervical and lumbar enlargements being especially affected (Figure 1). Anterior motor roots show grayish discoloration and atrophy compared with the posterior sensory roots. Certain cranial motor nerves, especially hypoglossal nerves, are also affected. The brain usually reveals no marked changes, although some cases with long duration may have atrophy of the precentral gyrus (Figure 2).

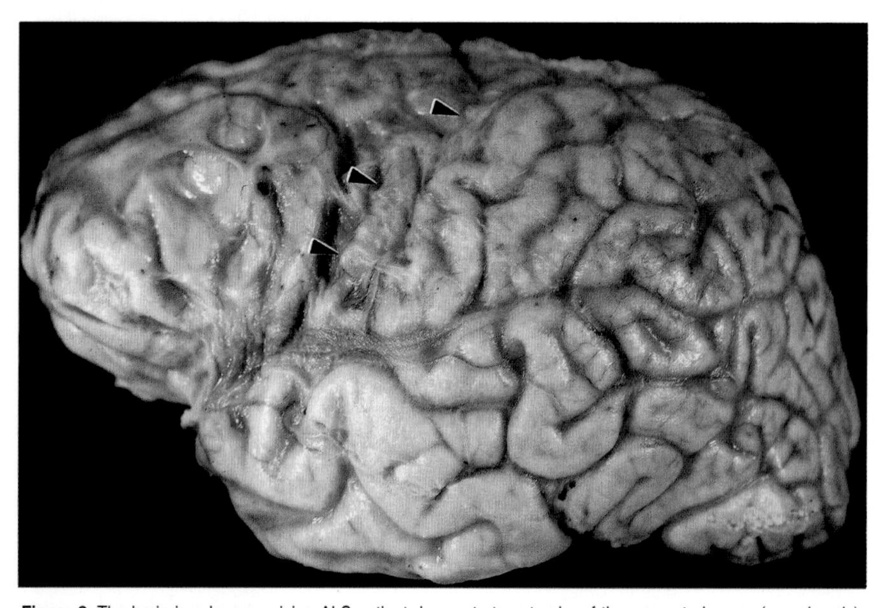

Figure 2. The brain in a long surviving ALS patient demonstrates atrophy of the precentral gyrus (arrowheads). ×0.7

Histopathology

Sporadic ALS. The degenerative changes are mainly restricted to the motor neurone system. There is loss of large anterior horn cells in the spinal cord and motor nuclei in the brain stem, with sparing of oculomotor, trochlear and abducent nuclei, as well as Onufrowicz's nucleus in the spinal cord. Upper motor neurones (Betz cells in the motor cortex) are also affected. Striated muscles demonstrate denervation atrophy.

Degeneration of corticospinal tracts is more apparent within the spinal cord than in the pyramidal tracts in brainstem, diencephalon and cerebrum using conventional myelin stains (Figure 3). On myelin preparations of spinal cords, atrophy of anterior horns, myelin pallor in the anterolateral columns and atrophy of anterior roots are hallmarks of ALS (Figure 3). In contrast, preservation of the posterior columns and spinocerebellar tracts is usual. In the anterolateral columns, there is loss of large myelinated fibres and variable astrocytic gliosis. Tract degeneration is usually associated with lipid-laden macrophages. Loss of these myelinated fibres is more marked in lower than upper spinal cord segments, supporting the hypothesis of a dying back axonal degeneration. In severely affected ALS patients, however, degeneration extends beyond the corticospinal tracts to the spinocerebellar, rubrospinal, and vestibular spinal tracts, so that myelin stains of the spinal cord show diffuse pallor, with still preserved posterior columns (Figure 3).

An essential finding is loss of large anterior horn cells throughout the length of the spinal cord, although neuronal loss is most easily recognised in cervical and lumbar enlargements. In general, anterior horn cell populations are better preserved in lumbar than in cervical segments. The residual motor neurones often show shrinkage, and lipofuscin-filled neurones stand out. Although rare neuronophagia and perivascular lymphocytic cuffing may be seen in cases with very rapid courses, these findings are generally absent.

Characteristic inclusions (Figures 4-6) are frequently detected in sporadic ALS:

i) Bunina bodies (25) are small eosinophilic granular inclusions (2-4 μm in diameter) in the anterior horn cells (Figure 4). They may appear either singly or as a cluster or in a chain-like formation. Bunina bodies stain bright red with H&E, deep blue with phosphotungstic acid hematoxylin, and blue with Luxol fast blue. Bunina bodies are considered a specific histopathological hallmark of ALS. Bunina bodies are observed within the cytoplasm or dendrites of the affected anterior horn cells, but occasionally in normal appearing cells. They have not been detected within axons.

ii) Skein-like inclusions (SLIs) are intracytoplasmic filamentous structures (103). These inclusions are detected with ubiquitin-immunostaining (Figure 5), but not with routine histology or as faintly eosinophilic structures in H&E preparations. SLIs are aggregates of thread-like structures and in a more aggregated form, SLIs show dense collections of filaments, forming a spherical structure.

iii) Round hyaline inclusions (RHIs) are pale eosinophilic inclusions with peripheral halos on H&E (90) (Figure 6). Sometimes, they lack halos and have irregular margins associated with filamentous structures similar to SLIs.

iv) Axonal spheroids are frequently observed in the anterior horn. Carpenter (27) distinguished between larger (over 20 μm in diameter) spheroids and smaller globules. Spheroids are eosinophilic in H&E and markedly argyrophilic in Bielschowsky staining.

v) Basophilic inclusions (BIs) are characteristic of juvenile ALS, which is clinically and histopathologically distinct from classic ALS (131). BIs are large irregular intracytoplasmic basophilic inclusions, that stain light red with methyl green pyronine, reflecting the fact that BIs contain RNA. BIs are not limited to motor neurones, but also found in other systems including the thalamus. There are occasional reports of ALS patients with multisystem degeneration with widespread BIs (97).

Central chromatolysis is characterised by eccentrically placed nuclei and distended, abundant and round cytoplasm. The cytoplasm is slightly eosinophilic or occasionally slightly basophilic. Nissl stains show absence of Nissl bodies.With the use of advanced life support methods, ALS patients may now have longer survival. Although classic descriptions of ALS emphasized pathology confined to the motor neuron system, certain present-day ALS patients with long survival have more widespread pathology. Therefore, there are 2 types in present-day ALS with long survival: typical ALS limited to the motor neurone system and multisystem-degeneration-type ALS (61).

Familial ALS. Familial ALS (FALS) is histopathologically subclassified into 2 types. One type has pathology indistinguishable from sporadic ALS. For example, Bunina bodies are frequently observed. In fact, the original descriptions by the Russian pathologist Bunina (25) was of specif-

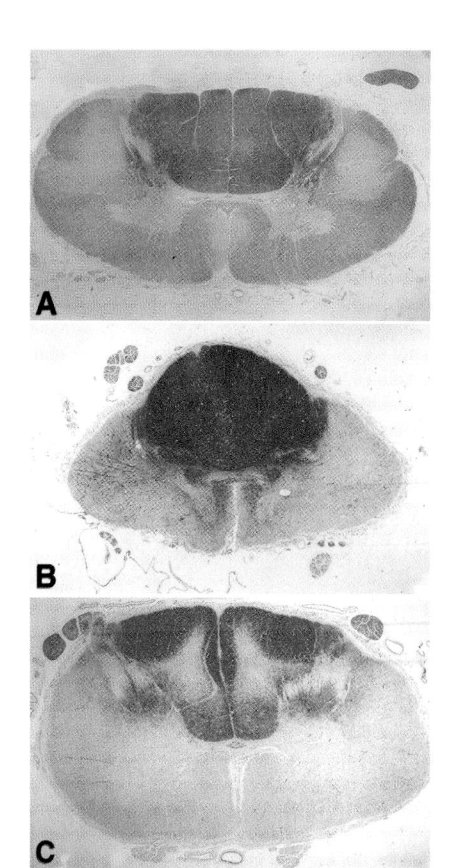

Figure 3. A. A section from the cervical enlargement (C6) shows degeneration of the corticospinal tracts and the anterior roots in ALS. **B.** Section from thoracic segment (T6) of spinal cord of a severely affected ALS patient stained for myelin shows that degeneration extends beyond the corticospinal tracts to the spino-cerebellar, rubrospinal and vestibular spinal tracts, while the posterior column is spared. **C.** The spinal cord from familial ALS (FALS) with a known SOD1 gene mutation shows posterior-column-involvement. Section from lumbar enlargement (L2) shows severe degeneration of the middle root zone of the posterior column, in addition to the other features of sporadic ALS. Klüver-Barrera stain. **A:** ×9.4; **B, C:**

ic inclusion bodies in two FALS patients from two different families.

The other form of FALS is associated with posterior column involvement. Histopathological findings of this form were originally reported by Engel (49). In addition to the pathological features of typical ALS, degeneration of the middle root zone of the posterior column, Clarke's nuclei and posterior spinocerebellar tracts were evident. In 1967, Hirano (67) published further pathological findings, emphasising Lewy body-like hyaline inclusions (LBHIs) in anterior horn cells. Bunina bodies were not observed. Neuronal LBHIs have eosinophilic cores with

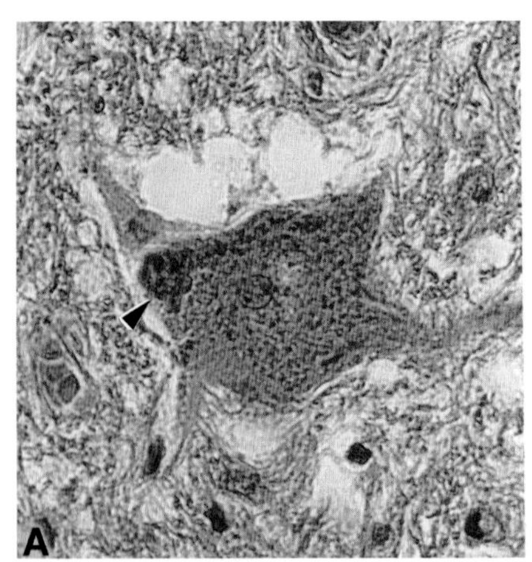
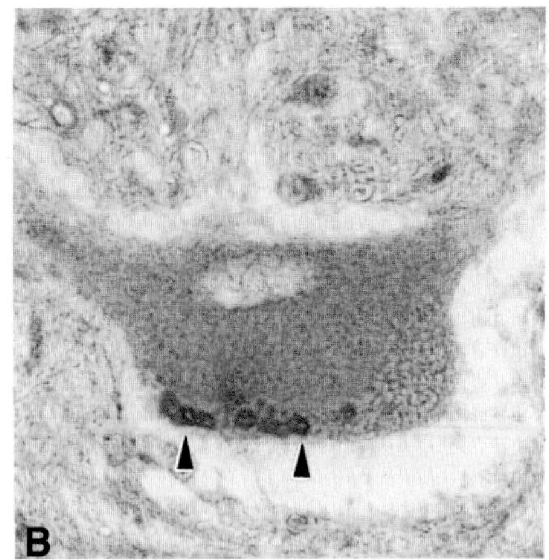
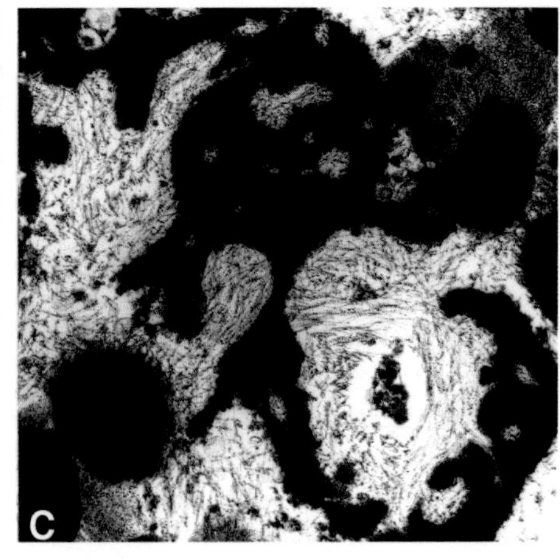

Figure 4. Bunina bodies in an anterior horn cell of ALS (**A**) are small eosinophilic inclusions (2-4 μm in diameter) (arrowhead). **B.** Bunina bodies are positive for cystatin C (arrowheads). **C.** An electron micrograph of a typical Bunina body shows electron-dense amorphous material that contains neurofilaments. **A:** ×610; **B:** ×620; **C:** ×11 200.

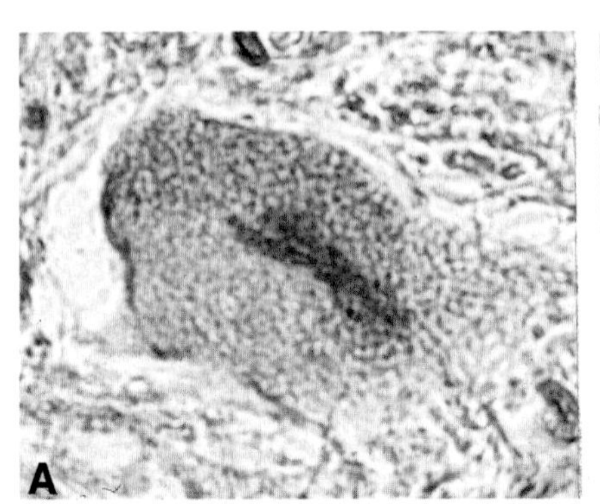
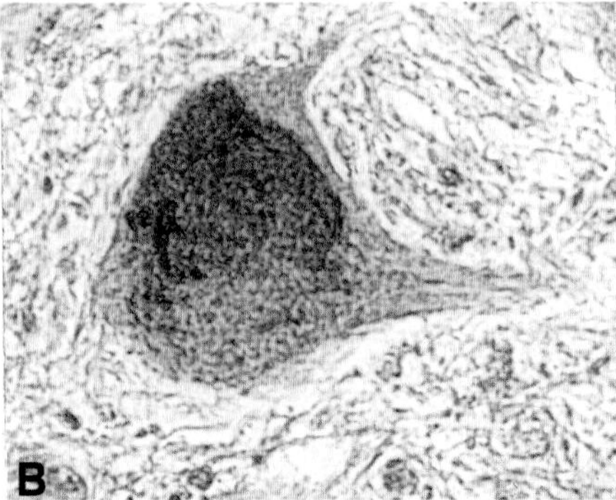
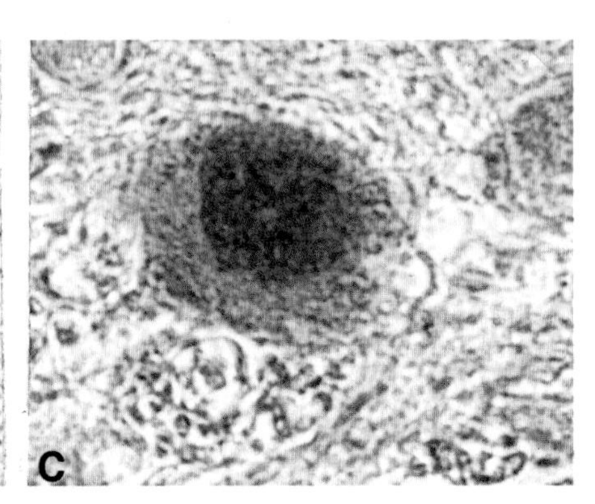

Figure 5. Ubiquitin immunostains show skein-like inclusions (SLIs) in a spinal anterior horn cell (**A**). In (**B**) an aggregated SLI has a dense collection of thread-like filaments. **C.** As the inclusions form dense aggregates, SLIs appear spherical, suggesting an evolution from thread-like structures to spherical structures. **A:** ×850; **B:** ×660 **C:** ×860.

peripheral halos and resemble Lewy bodies.

While there are over 100 different mutations in SOD1 and the SOD1 mutations are found in 20% of FALS patients (81, 90), published neuropathological descriptions of FALS due to SOD1 mutations are limited (Table 6), and there is considerable heterogeneity in those that have been reported. Bunina bodies have not been described in SOD1-related FALS. In addition, many cases have posterior column involvement with neuronal LBHIs. Although neuronal LBHIs are mainly found in motor neurones, some long-surviving FALS cases show widespread degeneration extending beyond the motor neurone system, with LBHIs also in non-motor systems (85, 89).

Another characteristic pathological feature in SOD1-related FALS is slight or minimal corticospinal tract involvement, but severe degeneration of lower motor neurones. In FALS patients with the I113T mutation, neurofilamentous conglomerate inclusions (NFCIs) are almost always observed. NFCIs are less common in sporadic ALS patients (less than 5%) (33). NFCIs are recognized as homogenous, faintly eosinophilic, oval or multi-lobulated inclusions. Although they show strong argyrophilia in Bielschowsky preparations, they are negative for Gallyas-Braak staining unlike neurofibrillary tangles in Alzheimer's disease (33).

Astrocytic hyaline inclusions (Ast-HIs) were first reported by Kato (89). Ast-HIs are observed in long-duration SOD1-related FALS cases (85, 89). Ast-HIs are eosinophilic inclusions and sometimes have cores with pale peripheral halos similar to neuronal LBHIs. Histochemically, most Ast-HIs and neuronal LBHIs are blue-to-violet on Mallory azan or Masson trichrome stains and argyrophilic on Bielschowsky and Gallyas-Braak stains (88, 90).

Immunohistochemistry and Ultrastructural Findings

Bunina bodies can be specifically detected with immunohistochemistry for cystatin C (130), but they do not react with a variety of other antibodies, including ubiquitin. Ultrastructurally, Bunina bodies consist of electron dense, amorphous material that contains tubules or vesicular structures. The amorphous material frequently includes a cytoplasmic island containing neurofilaments and other micro-organelles.

SLIs and RHIs are immunohistochemically positive for ubiquitin, but they are negative for phosphorylated neurofilament protein (pNFP) and SOD1 (118). Ultrastructurally, SLIs are bundles of fibrils with granules, which range in width from approximately 15 nm in segments without granular coating to about 20 nm in segments with granules (97, 118). The bundle sometimes appears to have a central hollow space. In more aggregated forms, SLIs that appear as spherical structures are composed of many bundles of fibrils with granules (118).

RHIs ultrastructurally are composed of 2 major constituents: abnormal fibrils with granules ranging from 15 to 20 nm similar to those in SLIs and 10-nm neurofilaments (90, 118). In RHIs, fibrils with granules are randomly orientated or sometimes form small bundles that are intermixed with neurofilaments, even though RHIs are negative for pNFP. Cellular organelles such as lipofuscin granules and mitochondria are also frequently intermingled within RHIs. They form spherical aggregates without a limiting membrane. An hypothesis for the evolution of inclusions from SLIs to RHIs has been proposed (109).

Axonal spheroids are intensely positive for pNFP. Ultrastructurally, spheroids are composed of bundles of 10-nm neurofilaments. Neurofilament bundles are loosely aggregated and normal cellular organelles such as mitochondria are sometimes observed among the neurofilament bundles. Some spheroids in early stages of ALS are found in proximal axons of normal appearing anterior horn cells, specifically between the distal portion of the initial segment and the first internode of the axon (149).

Electron microscopy of central chromatolytic neurones provide ultrastructural evidence for the displacement of the nucleus and large amounts of lipofuscin granules toward the cell periphery. The cytoplasm contains increased amounts of 10-nm neurofilaments and often mitochondria, as well as scattered fragments of rough endoplasmic reticulum and lysosomes. Like spheroids, central chromatolytic anterior horn cells are immunohistochemically stained with the antibody against pNFP, while the cytoplasm of normal anterior horn cells is usually negative for pNFP. The accumulation of phosphorylated neurofilaments in the cytoplasm of anterior horn cells in ALS patients may be due to impaired axonal transport.

Electron microscopy of BIs reveals a meshwork of 13 to 17 nm thick filaments studded with granules similar to free ribosomes without limiting membrane. Most BIs are negative for ubiquitin, although the inclusions occasionally show ubiquitin-positive granular deposits within them (131).

NFCIs are intensely positive for pNFP. Ubiquitin-immunoreactivity to NFCIs is controversial; most inclusions are negative, but NFCIs may have focal ubiquitin-positive structures within them (33). Ultrastructurally, NFCIs are loosely aggregated, swirled bundles of 10-nm neurofilaments (33). Although the segments of NFCIs often extend into dendrites, they seldom develop into proximal axons. Normal organelles are sometimes seen among bundles of neurofilaments.

Neuronal LBHIs and Ast-HIs in SOD1-mutated FALS patients have strong SOD1 immunoreactivity (85-90). Ultrastructurally, neuronal LBHIs, which consist of filamentous materials, exhibit dense cores with rough peripheral halos and have no limiting membrane. The inclusions are composed of granule-coated fibrils and 10-nm neurofilaments. These granule-coated fibrils are approximately 15 nm wide in the naked parts with no granules and are about 25 nm wide in the widest parts with granules (85, 89). The neurofilaments are mainly located in the periphery and are rarely seen in the central portion. Ast-HIs appear as globular structures that are well demarcated from other cytoplasmic structures, and have no limiting membrane. The major components of Ast-HIs are randomly-oriented fibrils coated with granular materials that have a width ranging from 15 to 25 nm, identical to those of neuronal LBHIs (85,

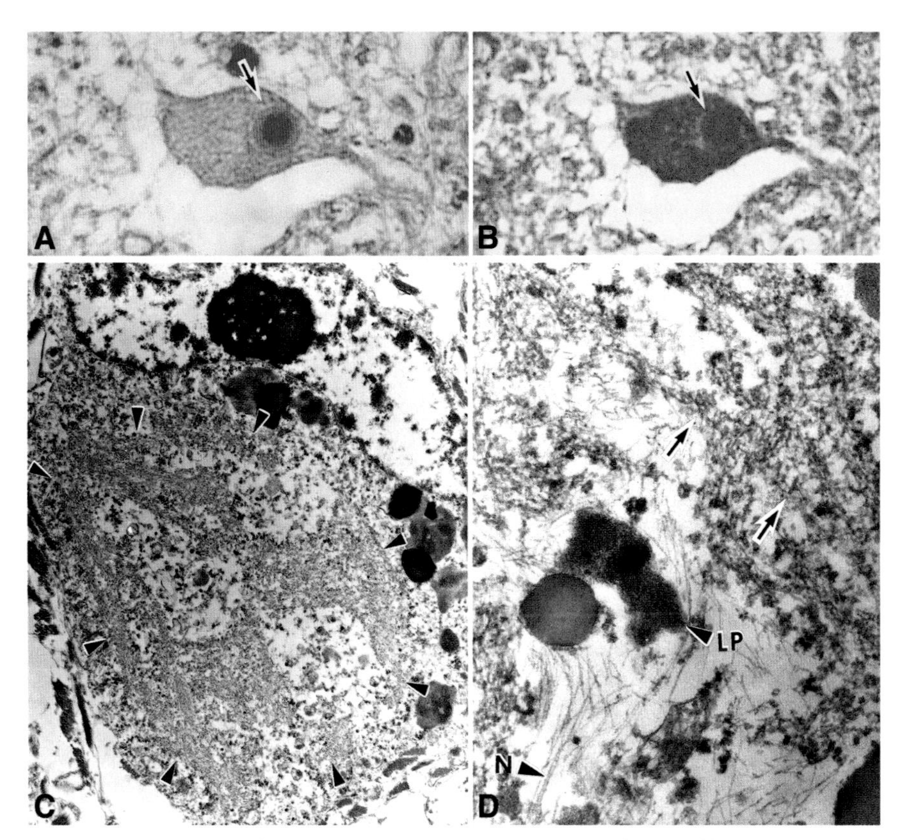

Figure 6. Light micrographs of a round hyaline inclusions (RHI) in sporadic ALS without SOD1 gene mutation. **A.** Typical RHI is a pale eosinophilic spherical structure with a halo (arrow). **B.** The same section as in (A) immunostained by the antibody against SOD1 shows that the RHI is negative for SOD1 (arrow). **C, D.** Electron micrographs of a neuronal RHI. **C.** RHI is formed of fibrils with granules arranged randomly or sometimes as small loosely aggregagated bundles (arrowheads). Cellular organelles are found within the inclusion. **D.** At higher magnification, fibrils with granules of approximately 15-20 nm in diameter comprise the RHI (arrows), with intermingled 10-nm neurofilaments (arrowheads and N) and lipofuscin granules (arrowhead and LP). **A, B:** ×540; **C:** ×4300; **D:** ×17 300. Figures **A, B, C** from Kato et al (90), reproduction with permission from ALS and Other Motor Neuron Disorders. Figure **D** from Kusaka et al (98), reproduction with permission from *Acta Neuropathologica*.

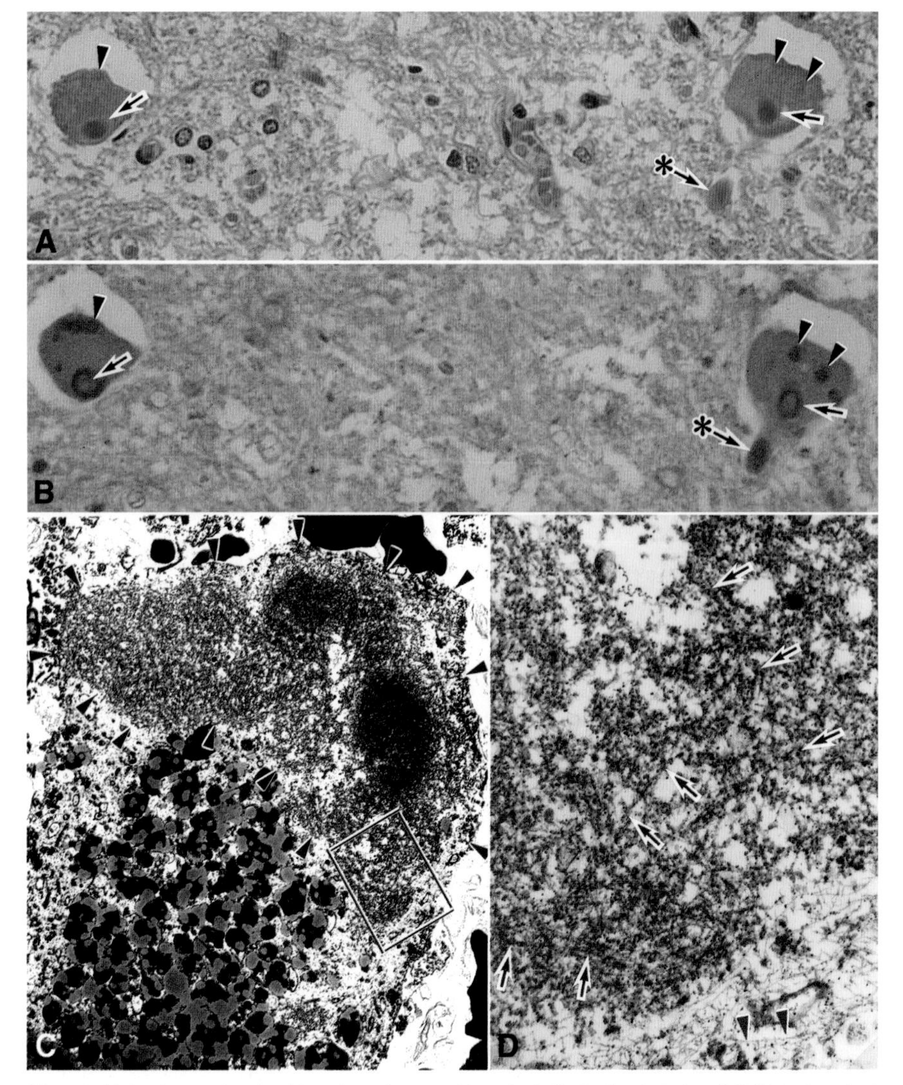

Figure 7. Light micrographs of serial sections of neuronal Lewy body-like hyaline inclusions (LBHIs) in the spinal cord of FALS with SOD1 gene mutation. **A.** Round (arrow) and ill-defined (arrowheads) LBHIs are seen in the cytoplasm of the anterior horn cells. The LBHIs are composed of eosinophilic cores with peripheral halos (arrows). Other LBHIs consist of obscure slightly eosinophilic structures (arrowheads). The proximal neurites have cord-like swelling and a sausage-shaped LBHI (arrow and asterisk). **B.** Immunostaining with the antibody against SOD1 shows labeling of LBHIs, although the immunoreactivity in LBHIs with cores and halos (arrows) is mostly restricted to the halos. The SOD1 immunostaining of ill-defined LBHIs (arrowheads) and an intraneuritic LBHI (arrow and asterisk) is present in the entire inclusions. **C, D.** Electron micrographs of a neuronal LBHI (arrowheads in **C**) in an anterior horn cell show that the major component of the neuronal LBHI are fibrils. The fibrils in the core of the LBHI are more densely aggregated than those in the periphery. **D.** At higher magnification (inset in **C**), the neuronal LBHI is composed of approximately 15 to 25 nm granule-coated fibrils (arrows). In contrast to RHI, organelles such as 10-nm neurofilaments (arrowheads) are mainly located at the periphery of LBHI. **A, B:** ×430; **C:** ×1950; **D:** ×13200.

Figures **A, B** from Kato et al (88), reproduction with permission from Histol Histopathol, Figures **C, D** from Kato et al (89), reproduction with permission from *J Neuropathol Exp Neurol.*

89). Occasionally, small bundles of glial filaments surround the inclusions, or are present within the inclusion-bearing astrocytic cell bodies. The granule-coated fibrils in both inclusions are immunoreactive for SOD1 (85-88). The detailed protein composition of neuronal LBHIs and Ast-HIs has been immunohistochemically studied (85, 86).

Neuronal LBHIs may also express certain neuronal epitopes such as pNFP, non-phosphorylated NFP, synaptophysin and neuron-specific enolase, while Ast-His may express astrocytic markers such as αB-crystallin, metallothionein, glutamine synthetase and S-100 protein. Although the Ast-HIs themselves are not stained by the antibody against glial fibrillary acidic protein (GFAP), the periphery of the Ast-HIs reacts with the anti-GFAP antibody (85-90).

Biochemistry of ALS

No neurochemical changes have been identified in ALS that are equivalent in importance to the dopaminergic deficiency uncovered in Parkinson's disease (155, 160). Some of the neurochemical changes identified may represent a consequence, rather than a cause, of motor neurone loss, but may nevertheless provide important clues to disease pathogenesis. The main biochemical abnormalities identified in ALS are outlined below.

Neurotransmitter systems. Glutamate is the major excitatory neurotransmitter in the human CNS and is responsible for the activation of motor neurones. There is substantial evidence for a dysregulation of the glutamate neurotransmitter system in ALS and for a glutamatergic contribution to motor neurone injury (111, 159). The levels of glutamate in post-mortem CNS tissue in ALS are decreased compared to controls. In contrast, several studies have shown that the level of glutamate in CSF is significantly elevated in ALS (143). Not all groups have confirmed this finding and technical difficulties in measuring glutamate in biological samples may have contributed to differences from different laboratories. Several studies have suggested that the elevation of CSF glutamate may only be present in a subgroup of patients (128, 158). No consensus exists in relation to the levels of plasma glutamate in ALS. Some studies have reported elevation of plasma glutamate, while others have shown a normal profile of plasma amino acids in ALS.

Measurement of the levels of the inhibitory neurotransmitters glycine and GABA have been made in the CSF and serum of ALS patients (155, 160). However, the results have been inconsistent between different studies and

SOD1 mutation	Patient number	Neuronal inclusion	SOD1 aggregation	Bunina body	Corticospinal tract involvement	Posterior column involvement	References
A4V	3	LBHI	+	-	+ (slight)	+	(161)
	5	ICI	ND	ND	-/+ (mild)	+ (asymmetry)	(42)
A4T	1	LBHI	+	-	+ (mild)	+	(170, 171)
G37R	1	LBHI	+	-	+	+	(77)
H46R	1	LBHI	ND	ND	+	+	(147)
H48Q	1	LBHI & SLI	-	-	+ (mild)	minimal	(154)
E100G	1	SLI	-	ND	+	+	(75)
D101N	2	ICHI	ND	ND	-	-	(28)
I113T	1	NFT (brain & brainstem)	ND	ND	+	-	(134)
	1	ICAI	ND	ND	-	ND	(144)
	1	ICAI	+	-	ND	ND	(94)
	1	HC	ND	ND	+	+	(76)
	1	NFCI	-	-	+ (slight)	+	(84)
L126S	1	LBHI	+	-	+	+	(173)
2-bp del	2	LBHI	+	-	+ (slight/marked)	+	(89, 172)
(126)	1	LBHI	+	ND	+	-	(82, 83)
C146R	2	LBHI	+	-	+ (slight)	+	(122, 123)

Table 6. Neuropathology of familial ALS with mutations in SOD1
+, present; -, absent; ND, not described; LBHI, Lewy body-like hyaline inclusion; ICI, intra-cytoplasmic inclusion; SLI, skein-like inclusion; ICHI, intracytoplasmic hyaline inclusion; NFT, neurofibrillary tangle (straight filament); ICAI, intracytoplasmic argyrophilic inclusion (neurofilament accumulation); HC, hyaline conglomerate (with neurofilament epitope); NFCI, neurofilamentous conglomerate inclusion; bp, base pair; del, deletion. Modified from Kato et al (90), reproduction with permission from *ALS and Other Motor Neuron Disorders.*

no clear picture has emerged of significant alterations. Few studies of cholinergic markers have been undertaken in ALS. Increased serum acetylcholinesterase (AChE) has been reported in ALS, but also in other motor neuropathies (60). CSF AChE seems to be similar in ALS patients and controls. Several studies have reported biochemical indices in CSF that may reflect increased activity of the noradrenergic system (190). Serotonin has an excitatory effect on motor neurones, either directly or through interaction with glutamate. No consistent changes in serotonin or its major metabolite 5-hydroxy-indole acetic acid have been reported in CNS tissue or CSF from ALS patients (155, 160).

Markers of oxidative stress. In post-mortem CNS tissue from cases of ALS, markers of oxidative damage to proteins and DNA have been identified and biochemical changes are also present, such as increased expression and activity of free radical scavenging enzymes, which may reflect an attempted compensatory response to the presence of oxidative stress. No significant differences in the levels of a range of anti-oxidants have been found in the CSF or plasma of ALS cases. In CSF an increase in the level of 4-hydroxynonenal, a marker of increased lipid peroxidation and 3-nitrotyrosine, a marker of peroxynitrite-mediated oxidative damage have been reported, though these changes are not disease specific (164, 174). Fibroblasts cultured from the skin of patients with familial or sporadic ALS show increased sensitivity to oxidative insults compared to controls (4).

Cytoskeletal protein alterations. Abnormalities in the expression of neurofilament proteins are a key feature of the molecular pathology of ALS (65). Neuronal spheroids containing neurofilaments are regularly seen in the proximal axons of motor neurones; ubiquitinated inclusions with compact morphology may contain neurofilament epitopes and hyaline conglomerate inclusions seen in some SOD1 related familial ALS cases show strong reactivity for both phosphorylated and non-phosphorylated neurofilament proteins. The expression of neurofilament light mRNA has been reported decreased in motor neurones from cases of ALS (16). One report suggested that the level of neurofilament light in CSF might represent a useful marker for monitoring upper motor neurone degeneration.

Alterations in the ubiquitin-proteasome system. Ubiquitin immunocytochemistry in CNS tissue from patients with ALS has revealed several types of ubiquitinated inclusions as described above. These are considered likely to reflect the presence of ubiquitin-protein conjugates that are resistant to proteolytic degradation.

Inflammatory markers. Evidence is emerging that inflammatory mechanisms may play a role in the progression and propagation of motor neurone degeneration in ALS. The pro-inflammatory cytokines interleukin-6 and interleukin-1β have been reported increased in the CSF and spinal cord respectively of ALS patients compared to controls. The expression of cyclooxygenase type 2 (COX-2), a key enzyme in the synthesis of the prostanoid group of inflammatory mediators such as PGE2, is increased in the spinal cord in ALS and also in transgenic mouse models expressing mutant SOD1 (8).

Miscellaneous neurochemical abnormalities. Multiple other neurochemical studies have been undertaken in ALS including measurements of neuropeptides and metals and trace elements (155, 160). Several studies have reported that the CSF of ALS patients is toxic to neurones in culture (39). The biochemical basis of this toxicity has not been identified though it may be mediated in part by activation of glutamate receptors.

Pathogenesis

Current evidence suggests that multiple interacting factors contribute to motor neurone injury in ALS. The 3 key pathogenetic hypotheses include genetic factors, oxidative stress and glutamatergic toxicity, which may result in damage to critical target proteins such as neurofilaments and organelles such as mitochondria (23, 155, 157). There is ongoing interest in the role played by protein aggregation in motor neurone injury (34). There is also a body of evidence emerging that cell death of motor neurones may occur by a programmed cell death mechanism similar to apoptosis (113, 150). There are cell-specific molecular and biochemical properties that may render motor neurones susceptible to injury (157).

Excitotoxicity. Motor neurones are activated by stimulation of cell surface glutamate receptors. The AMPA (α-amino-3-hydroxy-5-methyl-4-isoxazole propionic acid) subtype of glutamate receptor is responsible for much of the routine fast excitatory neurotransmission, and motor neurones may be particularly susceptible to toxicity via activation of cell surface AMPA receptors. A body of circumstantial evidence has implicated glutamate-mediated toxicity as a contributory factor to motor neurone injury, though it is uncertain whether this is a primary pathophysiological process or secondary to other insults leading to motor neurone failure (111, 159). The key findings are that the expression and function of the major glial glutamate re-uptake transporter protein EAAT2, may be impaired in ALS and that CNS extracellular glutamate and CSF glutamate may be abnormally elevated in at least a proportion of ALS patients. Anti-glutamate therapy with riluzole has some effect in prolonging the survival of patients with ALS (99). In addition clinical studies using positron emission tomography and transcranial magnetic stimulation of the motor cortex have indicated that there is hyperexcitability of the motor system in ALS. Abnormal RNA transcripts for EAAT2 were reported to be present in pathologically affected areas of the CNS from ALS cases as a disease specific change (108). However, subsequent studies have demonstrated that these abnormal splice variants are also present in control tissue.

Oxidative stress. There is particular interest in the role of oxidative stress in ALS (36) given the presence of mutations in a free radical scavenging enzyme SOD1 and studies of post-mortem CNS tissue and CSF from ALS cases that have demonstrated biochemical changes to proteins and DNA which reflect free radical damage. There is also evidence that mitochondrial dysfunction may contribute to motor neurone injury in ALS (114). There are several possible mechanisms of pathogenic mutations in SOD1. They may cause aberrant catalysis by permitting novel substrates access to the active site resulting in the production of damaging hydroxyl radicals or peroxynitrite, capable of injuring many different cellular components. This Copper (Cu^{2+})-mediated catalytic hypothesis is supported by the demonstration of increased protein oxidation as evidenced by carbonyl groups and 3-nitrotyrosine in SOD1 transgenic mice and ALS cases (151, 156). Not all evidence supports this notion. Copper is delivered to SOD1 solely by the copper chaperone for SOD1 (CCS) and without CCS SOD1 is inactive. Cross breeding three different mice expressing SOD1 mutations with CCS knockout mice did not affect their survival, implying that toxicity is independent of Cu^{2+}-mediated catalysis (35, 167).

Protein aggregation. The characteristic ubiquitinated inclusions of motor neurones, in some patients with SOD1 mutations, may be composed of protein aggregates of SOD1 and neurofilaments. SOD1 aggregation is unlikely to be essential in the pathogenesis of all ALS since most sporadic and familial cases do not have SOD1 immunoreactive inclusions (76, 153, 159). Likewise, perikaryal aggregation of neurofilaments is not a common feature of sporadic ALS (76) although accumulation of neurofilaments within proximal axonal swellings (spheroids) is a common, albeit non-specific, feature of ALS.

It has been postulated that cellular aggregates could lead to cellular toxicity in one of 3 ways: *i)* by sequestration of other proteins required for normal motor neurone function; *ii)* by reducing the availability of chaperone proteins required for the folding and function of other essential intracellular proteins; and *iii)* by reducing the proteasome activity needed for degradation of damaged proteins (34). However, as in the case of protein aggregates in other neurodegenerative diseases, it remains uncertain at present whether the aggregates play an important role in disease pathogenesis; whether they represent harmless bystanders or whether they could actually exert a beneficial effect by sequestering abnormal intracellular proteins.

Apoptosis. The evidence that motor neurones may die in ALS by programmed cell death has been reviewed (150). Examination of spinal cord tissue from patients with ALS has shown evidence of internucleosomal DNA fragmentation; apoptotic morphology of degenerating motor neurones; increased expression of certain apoptosis related molecules including Le^y antigen and prostate apoptosis response 4 protein as well as increases in the activities of the apoptosis effectors caspases 1 and 3. Several studies have also provided evidence for an alteration in the balance and subcellular compartmental localisation of pro- and anti-apoptotic members of the Bcl-2 family of proteins in the spinal cord of ALS cases in a direction favouring apoptosis (113). The evidence from human tissue is supplemented by studies in cellular and animal models of SOD1-related familial ALS. For example, there is evidence of DNA laddering, increased expression and activation of caspase 1 and 3 in the spinal cords of G93A SOD1 mice, along with alterations in the balance of key members of the Bcl-2 family of proteins in a direction favouring apoptosis. Intraventricular administration of a broad spectrum caspase inhibitor in these mice delays disease onset and prolongs survival (107).

Other pathogenetic hypotheses. Other pathogenetic hypotheses for ALS include the potential contributions of exogenous toxins, viral infection and immune-mediated mechanisms that have been reviewed elsewhere (12, 166).

Experimental Models of ALS

Several natural models of motor neurone degeneration occur in mice and other animals (46). Examples include the Wobbler mouse, the Mnd mouse and hereditary canine spinal muscular atrophy. However, none of these animal diseases closely resembles human ALS.

The discovery that SOD1 mutations are the cause of ~20% of familial ALS has allowed generation of several strains of transgenic mice expressing mutant human SOD1 (57). These mice develop a disease that closely resembles human ALS both clinically and pathologically. They have been used to test multiple therapeutic compounds and some positive findings have emerged from these studies (Table 7). Potentially important pathophysiological changes have been observed in these mice including impaired axonal transport, increased calcium concentrations in motor nerve terminals and early pathological changes affecting the mitochondria of motor neurones which precede clinical manifestations of the disease (186). Cross breeding strategies have identified genetic factors which may modulate mutant SOD1 related motor neurone injury, including the beneficial effect resulting from over-expression of the anti-apoptotic molecule Bcl-2 and from concomitant manipulation of neurofilament protein expression.

Mice with motor neurone pathology have also been generated by overexpressing human neurofilament proteins and by mutation in neurofilament light (38, 79, 102). A new mouse model of ALS was also serendipitously developed by mutating the promotor region of the vasoactive endothelial growth factor (VEGF), a molecule which has been shown to be important in cellular response to hypoxia and which also appears to be a trophic factor for motor neurones (132).

Other experimental models which have yielded important insights into the pathogenesis of ALS in recent years include embryonic primary motor neurone cultures from rats and mice; motor neuronal cell lines which can be propagated in culture to yield sufficient material for biochemical analyses; and neonatal murine spinal cord slice explants which have the advantages that motor neurones retain some of their normal connectivity with other cell groups and can also be kept alive for several months in vitro (48).

Therapy and Future Directions

The identification of a disease marker of ALS would represent a major advance, reducing diagnostic uncertainty and allowing the early administration of neuroprotective therapy. In attempting to identify a robust serum or CSF metabolic marker of ALS, it will be necessary to take into account that the disease comprises multiple subgroups of patients. At present therapy can be divided into symptomatic treatment and neuroprotective treatment aimed at retarding disease progression.

Many of the symptomatic therapies currently recommended by clinicians have not been assessed in rigorous controlled trials. The evidence base for many of these therapies has recently been reviewed by an American Academy of Neurology taskforce (116). Recent advances in supportive care for patients with ALS include the development of specialist clinics, with input from multidisciplinary teams, the availability of hospice care for patients in the late stages of the disease, as well as improvements in the management of nutritional and respiratory problems. Multiple recent therapeutic trials of potential neuroprotective drugs have been undertaken in patients with ALS, including anti-glutamate, antioxidant and neurotrophic agents. To date only the anti-glutamate agent riluzole has been shown to have a reproducible, though modest, effect in prolonging the survival of patients with ALS (99).

Vitamin E
Riluzole
Gabapentin
Penicillamine
Creatine
Janus kinase 3 inhibitor
Polyamine or putrescine modified catalase
Ginseng root
Lyophilised red wine
GDNF
Adenovirus delivered Bcl-2
N-acetyl-L-cysteine
Lysine acetylsalicylate
Trientine + ascorbate
Genistein
Caspase inhibitor

Table 7. Neuroprotective therapies in SOD1 transgenic mouse models of ALS.

In the next few years, progress is likely to be made in further elucidating the molecular mechanisms of motor neurone injury and death in ALS. It can be anticipated that further genetic mutations associated with familial ALS will be identified as well as genetic susceptibility factors for the sporadic form of the disease. The use of cellular and animal experimental models will lead to increased understanding of the sequential molecular events leading to motor neurone degeneration and to the identification of new neuroprotective strategies. Future therapy for patients with ALS may well involve a cocktail of drugs aimed at different mechanisms contributing to the biochemical cascade of motor neurone injury. Anti-glutamate drugs, anti-oxidants, drugs stabilising mitochondrial function, anti-apoptotic agents, drugs modifying the inflammatory response, inhibitors of protein aggregation and possibly the use of gene therapy and stem cells may all have a role to play in therapy.

References

1. Abrahams S, Goldstein LH, Al-Chalabi A, Pickering A, Morris RG, Passingham RE, Brooks DJ, Leigh PN (1997) Relation between cognitive dysfunction and pseudobulbar palsy in amyotrophic lateral sclerosis. J Neurol Neurosurg Psychiatry 62: 464-472.

2. Ackerley S, Grierson AJ, Brownlees J, Thornhill P, Anderton BH, Leigh PN, Shaw CE, Miller CC (2000) Glutamate slows axonal transport of neurofilaments in transfected neurons. *J Cell Biol* 150: 165-176.

3. Aggarwal A, Nicholson G (2002) Detection of preclinical motor neurone loss in SOD1 mutation carriers using motor unit number estimation. *J Neurol Neurosurg Psychiatry* 73: 199-201.

4. Aguirre T, Van Den Bosch L, Goetschalckx K, Tilkin P, Mathijs G, Cassiman JJ, Robberecht W (1998) Increased sensitivity of fibroblasts from amyotrophic lateral sclerosis patients to oxidative stress. *Ann Neurol* 43: 452-457.

5. Al-Chalabi A, Andersen PM, Chioza B, Shaw C, Sham PC, Robberecht W, Matthijs G, Camu W, Marklund SL, Forsgren L, Rouleau G, Laing NG, Hurse PV, Siddique T, Leigh PN, Powell JF (1998) Recessive amyotrophic lateral sclerosis families with the D90A SOD1 mutation share a common founder: evidence for a linked protective factor. *Hum Mol Genet* 7: 2045-2050.

6. Al-Chalabi A, Andersen PM, Nilsson P, Chioza B, Andersson JL, Russ C, Shaw CE, Powell JF, Leigh PN (1999) Deletions of the heavy neurofilament subunit tail in amyotrophic lateral sclerosis. *Hum Mol Genet* 8: 157-164.

7. Al-Chalabi A, Leigh PN (2000) Recent advances in amyotrophic lateral sclerosis. *Curr Opin Neurol* 13: 397-405.

8. Almer G, Guegan C, Teismann P, Naini A, Rosoklija G, Hays AP, Chen C, Przedborski S (2001) Increased expression of the pro-inflammatory enzyme cyclooxygenase-2 in amyotrophic lateral sclerosis. *Ann Neurol* 49: 176-185.

9. Andersen PM, Forsgren L, Binzer M, Nilsson P, Ala-Hurula V, Keranen ML, Bergmark L, Saarinen A, Haltia T, Tarvainen I, Kinnunen E, Udd B, Marklund SL (1996) Autosomal recessive adult-onset amyotrophic lateral sclerosis associated with homozygosity for Asp90Ala CuZn-superoxide dismutase mutation. A clinical and genealogical study of 36 patients. *Brain* 119: 1153-1172.

10. Andersen PM, Nilsson P, Ala-Hurula V, Keranen ML, Tarvainen I, Haltia T, Nilsson L, Binzer M, Forsgren L, Marklund SL (1995) Amyotrophic lateral sclerosis associated with homozygosity for an Asp90Ala mutation in CuZn-superoxide dismutase. *Nat Genet* 10: 61-66.

11. Andersen PM, Nilsson P, Keranen ML, Forsgren L, Hagglund J, Karlsborg M, Ronnevi LO, Gredal O, Marklund SL (1997) Phenotypic heterogeneity in motor neuron disease patients with CuZn- superoxide dismutase mutations in Scandinavia. *Brain* 120: 1723-1737.

12. Appel SH, Alexianu M, Engelhardt JI et al(2000) Involvement of immune factors in motor neuron injury in amyotrophic lateral sclerosis. In *Amyotrophic lateral sclerosis*, RH Brown, V Meininger, M Swash (Eds). Martin Dunitz Ltd: London. pp. 309-326.

13. Aran FA (1850) Recherches sur une maladie non encore décrite du systemé musculaire (atrophie musculair progressive). *Arch Gen Med* 14: 5-35, 172-214.

14. Beghi E, Balzarini C, Bogliun G, Logroscino G, Manfredi L, Mazzini L, Micheli A, Millul A, Poloni M, Riva R, Salmoiraghi F, Tonini C, Vitelli E (2002) Reliability of the El Escorial diagnostic criteria for amyotrophic lateral sclerosis. *Neuroepidemiology* 21: 265-270.

15. Belsh JM, Schiffman PL (1990) Misdiagnosis in patients with amyotrophic lateral sclerosis. *Arch Intern Med* 150: 2301-2305.

16. Bergeron C, Beric-Maskarel K, Muntasser S, Weyer L, Somerville MJ, Percy ME (1994) Neurofilament light and polyadenylated mRNA levels are decreased in amyotrophic lateral sclerosis motor neurons. *J Neuropathol Exp Neurol* 53: 221-230.

17. Blexrud MD, Windebank AJ, Daube JR (1993) Long-term follow-up of 121 patients with benign fasciculations. *Ann Neurol* 34: 622-625.

18. Bouche P, Moulonguet A, Younes-Chennoufi AB, Adams D, Baumann N, Meininger V, Leger JM, Said G (1995) Multifocal motor neuropathy with conduction block: a study of 24 patients. *J Neurol Neurosurg Psychiatry* 59: 38-44.

19. Bowen J, Gregory R, Squier M, Donaghy M (1996) The post-irradiation lower motor neuron syndrome neuronopathy or radiculopathy? *Brain* 119: 1429-1439.

20. Bromberg M (1999) Accelerating the diagnosis of amyotrophic lateral sclerosis. *Neurologist* 5: 63-74.

21. Brooks BR, Miller RG, Swash M, Munsat TL (1999) El Escorial revisited: revised criteria for the diagnosis of amyotrophic lateral sclerosis. *Amyotroph Lateral Scler Other Motor Neuron Disord* 1: 293-299.

22. Brooks BR, Miller RG, Swash M, Munsat TL (2000) El Escorial revisited: revised criteria for the diagnosis of amyotrophic lateral sclerosis. *Amyotroph Lateral Scler Other Motor Neuron Disord* 1: 293-299.

23. Brown RH, Jr., Robberecht W (2001) Amyotrophic lateral sclerosis: pathogenesis. *Semin Neurol* 21: 131-139.

24. Bruyn RP, Koelman JH, Troost D, de Jong JM (1995) Motor neuron disease (amyotrophic lateral sclerosis) arising from longstanding primary lateral sclerosis. *J Neurol Neurosurg Psychiatry* 58: 742-744.

25. Bunina TL (1962) On intracellular inclusions in familial amyotrophic lateral sclerosis. *Korsakov J Neuropathol Psychiat 62:* 1293-1299.

26. Caparros-Lefebvre D, Sergeant N, Lees A, Camuzat A, Daniel S, Lannuzel A, Brice A, Tolosa E, Delacourte A, Duyckaerts C (2002) Guadeloupean parkinsonism: a cluster of progressive supranuclear palsy-like tauopathy. *Brain* 125: 801-811.

27. Carpenter S (1968) Proximal axonal enlargement in motor neuron disease. *Neurology* 18: 841-851.

28. Cervenakova L, Protas, II, Hirano A, Votiakov VI, Nedzved MK, Kolomiets ND, Taller I, Park KY, Sambuughin N, Gajdusek DC, Brown P, Goldfarb LG (2000) Progressive muscular atrophy variant of familial amyotrophic lateral sclerosis (PMA/ALS). *J Neurol Sci* 177: 124-130.

29. Chancellor AM, Slattery JM, Fraser H, Warlow CP (1993) Risk factors for motor neuron disease: a case-control study based on patients from the Scottish Motor Neuron Disease Register. *J Neurol Neurosurg Psychiatry* 56: 1200-1206.

30. Charcot J-M (1874) De la sclérose latérale amyotrophique. *Prog Med* 2: 325-327, 341-342, 453-455.

31. Charcot J-M, Joffroy A (1869) Deuxcas d'atrophie musculaire progressive avec lésions de la substance grise et de faisceaux antérolatéraux de la moelle épinière. *Arch Physiol Norm Pathol* 1; 2; 3: 1; 354-357; 352; 628-649: 353; 744-757.

32. Chio A (2000) Risk factors in the early diagnosis of ALS: European epidemiological studies. *Amyotroph Lateral Scler Other Motor Neuron Disord* 1 Suppl 1: S13-S18.

33. Chou SM, Wang HS, Taniguchi A (1996) Role of SOD-1 and nitric oxide/cyclic GMP cascade on neurofilament aggregation in ALS/MND. *J Neurol Sci* 139 Suppl: 16-26.

34. Cleveland DW, Liu J (2000) Oxidation versus aggregation—how do SOD1 mutants cause ALS? *Nat Med* 6: 1320-1321.

35. Cleveland DW, Rothstein JD (2001) From Charcot to Lou Gehrig: deciphering selective motor neuron death in ALS. *Nat Rev Neurosci* 2: 806-819.

36. Cookson MR, Shaw PJ (1999) Oxidative stress and motor neurone disease. *Brain Pathol* 9: 165-186.

37. Corcia P, Mayeux-Portas V, Khoris J, de Toffol B, Autret A, Muh JP, Camu W, Andres C (2002) Abnormal SMN1 gene copy number is a susceptibility factor for amyotrophic lateral sclerosis. *Ann Neurol* 51: 243-246.

38. Cote F, Collard JF, Julien JP (1993) Progressive neuronopathy in transgenic mice expressing the human neurofilament heavy gene: a mouse model of amyotrophic lateral sclerosis. *Cell* 73: 35-46.

39. Couratier P, Hugon J, Sindou P, Vallat JM, Dumas M (1993) Cell culture evidence for neuronal degeneration in amyotrophic lateral sclerosis being linked to glutamate AMPA/kainate receptors. *Lancet* 341: 265-268.

40. Cruveilhier J (1953) Sur le paralysie musculaire, progressive, atrophique. *Bull Acad Med* 18: 490-501; 546-583.

41. Cruz DC, Nelson LM, McGuire V, Longstreth WT, Jr. (1999) Physical trauma and family history of neurodegenerative diseases in amyotrophic lateral sclerosis: a population-based case-control study. *Neuroepidemiology* 18: 101-110.

42. Cudkowicz ME, McKenna-Yasek D, Chen C, Hedley-Whyte ET, Brown RH, Jr. (1998) Limited corticospinal tract involvement in amyotrophic lateral sclerosis subjects with the A4V mutation in the copper/zinc superoxide dismutase gene. *Ann Neurol* 43: 703-710.

43. Cudkowicz ME, McKenna-Yasek D, Sapp PE, Chin W, Geller B, Hayden DL, Schoenfeld DA, Hosler BA, Horvitz HR, Brown RH (1997) Epidemiology of muta-

tions in superoxide dismutase in amyotrophic lateral sclerosis. *Ann Neurol* 41: 210-221.

44. Davenport RJ, Swingler RJ, Chancellor AM, Warlow CP (1996) Avoiding false positive diagnoses of motor neuron disease: lessons from the Scottish Motor Neuron Disease Register. *J Neurol Neurosurg Psychiatry* 60: 147-151.

45. Déjerine J (1883) Etude anatomique et clinique sur la paralysie labio-glosso-laryngée. *Arch Physiol Norm Pathol* 2: 180-227.

46. Doble A, Kennel P (2000) Animal models of amyotrophic lateral sclerosis. *Amyotroph Lateral Scler Other Motor Neuron Disord* 1: 301-312.

47. Duchenne G (1860) Paralysie musculaire progressive de la langue, du voile du palais et des lèvres. *Arch Gén Méd* 16: 283-296; 431-445.

48. Elliott JL (1999) Experimental models of amyotrophic lateral sclerosis. *Neurobiol Dis* 6: 310-320.

49. Engel WK, Kurland LT, Klatzo I (1959) An inherited disease similar to amyotrophic lateral sclerosis with a pattern of posterior column involvement. An intermediate form ? *Brain* 82: 203-220.

50. Figlewicz DA, Krizus A, Martinoli MG, Meininger V, Dib M, Rouleau GA, Julien JP (1994) Variants of the heavy neurofilament subunit are associated with the development of amyotrophic lateral sclerosis. *Hum Mol Genet* 3: 1757-1761.

51. Forsgren L, Almay BG, Holmgren G, Wall S (1983) Epidemiology of motor neuron disease in northern Sweden. *Acta Neurol Scand* 68: 20-29.

52. Gamez J, Cervera C, Codina A (1999) Flail arm syndrome of Vulpian-Bernhart's form of amyotrophic lateral sclerosis. *J Neurol Neurosurg Psychiatry* 67: 258.

53. Gordon PH, Rowland LP, Younger DS, Sherman WH, Hays AP, Louis ED, Lange DJ, Trojaborg W, Lovelace RE, Murphy PL, Latov N (1997) Lymphoproliferative disorders and motor neuron disease: an update. *Neurology* 48: 1671-1678.

54. Gourie-Devi M, Suresh TG, Shankar SK (1984) Monomelic amyotrophy. *Arch Neurol* 41: 388-394.

55. Gowers W (1886-1888) A manual of diseases of the nervous system. Churchill: England.

56. Group SMNDR (1992) The Scottosh motor neuron disease register: a prospective study of adult onset motor neuron disease in Scotland. Methodology, demography and clinical features of incidence cases in 1989. *J Neurol Neurosurg Psychiatry* 55: 536-541.

57. Gurney ME, Pu H, Chiu AY, Dal Canto MC, Polchow CY, Alexander DD, Caliendo J, Hentati A, Kwon YW, Deng HX et al (1994) Motor neuron degeneration in mice that express a human Cu,Zn superoxide dismutase mutation. *Science* 264: 1772-1775.

58. Hadano S, Hand CK, Osuga H, Yanagisawa Y, Otomo A, Devon RS, Miyamoto N, Showguchi-Miyata J, Okada Y, Singaraja R, Figlewicz DA, Kwiatkowski T, Hosler BA, Sagie T, Skaug J, Nasir J, Brown RH, Jr., Scherer SW, Rouleau GA, Hayden MR, Ikeda JE (2001) A gene encoding a putative GTPase regulator is mutated in familial amyotrophic lateral sclerosis 2. *Nat Genet* 29: 166-173.

59. Hand CK, Khoris J, Salachas F, Gros-Louis F, Lopes AA, Mayeux-Portas V, Brewer CG, Brown RH, Jr., Meininger V, Camu W, Rouleau GA (2002) A novel locus for familial amyotrophic lateral sclerosis, on chromosome 18q. *Am J Hum Genet* 70: 251-256.

60. Hartikainen P, Reinikainen KJ, Soininen H, Sirvio J, Soikkeli R, Riekkinen PJ (1992) Neurochemical markers in the cerebrospinal fluid of patients with Alzheimer's disease, Parkinson's disease and amyotrophic lateral sclerosis and normal controls. *J Neural Transm Park Dis Dement Sect* 4: 53-68.

61. Hashizume Y, Yoshida M, Murakami N (1993) Clinicopathological study of two respirator-assisted long survival cases of amyotrophic lateral sclerosis. *Neuropathology* 13: 237-241.

62. Hayward C, Colville S, Swingler RJ, Brock DJ (1999) Molecular genetic analysis of the APEX nuclease gene in amyotrophic lateral sclerosis. *Neurology* 52: 1899-1901.

63. Hentati A, Bejaoui K, Pericak-Vance MA, Hentati F, Speer MC, Hung WY, Figlewicz DA, Haines J, Rimmler J, Ben Hamida C et al (1994) Linkage of recessive familial amyotrophic lateral sclerosis to chromosome 2q33-q35. *Nat Genet* 7: 425-428.

64. Hentati A, Ouahchi K, Pericak-Vance MA, Nijhawan D, Ahmad A, Yang Y, Rimmler J, Hung W, Schlotter B, Ahmed A, Ben Hamida M, Hentati F, Siddique T (1998) Linkage of a commoner form of recessive amyotrophic lateral sclerosis to chromosome 15q15-q22 markers. *Neurogenetics* 2: 55-60.

65. Hirano A (1991) Cytopathology of amyotrophic lateral sclerosis. *Adv Neurol* 56: 91-101.

66. Hirano A, Kurland LT, Krooth RS, Lessel S (1961) Parkinsonism-dementia complex, an endemic disease on the island of Guam. 1. Clinical features. *Brain* 84: 642-661.

67. Hirano A, Kurland LT, Sayre GP (1967) Familial amyotrophic lateral sclerosis. A sub-group characterized by posterior and spinocerebellar tract involvement and hyaline inclusions in the anterior horn cells. *Arch Neurol* 16: 232-243.

68. Hirano A, Malamud N, Kurland LT (1961) Amyotrophic lateral sclerosis and parkinsonism-dementia on Guam. 11 Pathological features. *Brain* 84: 662-679.

69. Hirayama K, Tomonaga M, Kitano K, Yamada T, Kojima S, Arai K (1987) Focal cervical poliopathy causing juvenile muscular atrophy of distal upper extremity: a pathological study. *J Neurol Neurosurg Psychiatry* 50: 285-290.

70. Hoch W, McConville J, Helms S, Newsom-Davis J, Melms A, Vincent A (2001) Auto-antibodies to the receptor tyrosine kinase MuSK in patients with myasthenia gravis without acetylcholine receptor antibodies. *Nat Med* 7: 365-368.

71. Hosler BA, Siddique T, Sapp PC, Sailor W, Huang MC, Hossain A, Daube JR, Nance M, Fan C, Kaplan J, Hung WY, McKenna-Yasek D, Haines JL, Pericak-Vance MA, Horvitz HR, Brown RH, Jr. (2000) Linkage of familial amyotrophic lateral sclerosis with frontotemporal dementia to chromosome 9q21-q22. *JAMA* 284: 1664-1669.

72. Howland DS, Liu J, She Y, Goad B, Maragakis NJ, Kim B, Erickson J, Kulik J, DeVito L, Psaltis G, DeGennaro LJ, Cleveland DW, Rothstein JD (2002) Focal loss of the glutamate transporter EAAT2 in a transgenic rat model of SOD1 mutant-mediated amyotrophic lateral sclerosis (ALS). *Proc Natl Acad Sci U S A* 99: 1604-1609.

73. Hu MT, Ellis CM, Al-Chalabi A, Leigh PN, Shaw CE (1998) Flail arm syndrome: a distinctive variant of amyotrophic lateral sclerosis. *J Neurol Neurosurg Psychiatry* 65: 950-951.

74. Hudson AJ (1981) Amyotrophic lateral sclerosis and its association with dementia, parkinsonism and other neurological disorders: a review. *Brain* 104: 217-247.

75. Ince PG, Shaw PJ, Slade JY, Jones C, Hudgson P (1996) Familial amyotrophic lateral sclerosis with a mutation in exon 4 of the Cu/Zn superoxide dismutase gene: pathological and immunocytochemical changes. *Acta Neuropathol (Berl)* 92: 395-403.

76. Ince PG, Tomkins J, Slade JY, Thatcher NM, Shaw PJ (1998) Amyotrophic lateral sclerosis associated with genetic abnormalities in the gene encoding Cu/Zn superoxide dismutase: molecular pathology of five new cases, and comparison with previous reports and 73 sporadic cases of ALS. *J Neuropathol Exp Neurol* 57: 895-904.

77. Inoue K, Sato Y, Shimada K, Fujimura H, Sakoda S (2001) *An autopsy case of familial amyotrophic lateral sclerosis with Gly37Arg substitution in superoxide dismutase 1.* Presented at 42nd annual meeting of Japanese Society of Neurology, Tokyo.

78. Jaspan JB, Wollman RL, Bernstein L, Rubenstein AH (1982) Hypoglycemic peripheral neuropathy in association with insulinoma: implication of glucopenia rather than hyperinsulinism. Case report and literature review. *Medicine (Baltimore)* 61: 33-44.

79. Julien JP (1999) Neurofilament functions in health and disease. *Curr Opin Neurobiol* 9: 554-560.

80. Julien JP (2001) Amyotrophic lateral sclerosis. unfolding the toxicity of the misfolded. *Cell* 104: 581-591.

81. Juneja T, Pericak-Vance MA, Laing NG, Dave S, Siddique T (1997) Prognosis in familial amyotrophic lateral sclerosis: progression and survival in patients with glu100gly and ala4val mutations in Cu,Zn superoxide dismutase. *Neurology* 48: 55-57.

82. Kadekawa J, Fujimura H, Ogawa Y, Hattori N, Kaido M, Nishimura T, Yoshikawa H, Shirahata N, Sakoda S, Yanagihara T (1997) A clinicopathological study of a patient with familial amyotrophic lateral sclerosis associated with a two base pair deletion in the copper/zinc superoxide dismutase (SOD1) gene. *Acta Neuropathol (Berl)* 94: 617-622.

83. Kadekawa J, Fujimura H, Yanagihara T, Sakoda S (2001) A clinicopathological study of patient with familial amyotrophic lateral sclerosis associated with a two-base pair deletion in the copper/zinc superoxide dismutase (SOD1) gene. *Acta Neuropathol (Berl)* 101: 415.

84. Katayama S, Watanabe C, Noda K, Ohishi H, Yamamura Y, Nishisaka T, Inai K, Asayama K, Murayama S, Nakamura S (1999) Numerous conglomerate inclusions in slowly progressive familial amyotrophic

lateral sclerosis with posterior column involvement. *J Neurol Sci* 171: 72-77.

85. Kato S, Hayashi H, Nakashima K, Nanba E, Kato M, Hirano A, Nakano I, Asayama K, Ohama E (1997) Pathological characterization of astrocytic hyaline inclusions in familial amyotrophic lateral sclerosis. *Am J Pathol* 151: 611-620.

86. Kato S, Horiuchi S, Liu J, Cleveland DW, Shibata N, Nakashima K, Nagai R, Hirano A, Takikawa M, Kato M, Nakano I, Ohama E (2000) Advanced glycation endproduct-modified superoxide dismutase-1 (SOD1)- positive inclusions are common to familial amyotrophic lateral sclerosis patients with SOD1 gene mutations and transgenic mice expressing human SOD1 with a G85R mutation. *Acta Neuropathol (Berl)* 100: 490-505.

87. Kato S, Nakashima K, Horiuchi S, Nagai R, Cleveland DW, Liu J, Hirano A, Takikawa M, Kato M, Nakano I, Sakoda S, Asayama K, Ohama E (2001) Formation of advanced glycation end-product-modified superoxide dismutase-1 (SOD1) is one of the mechanisms responsible for inclusions common to familial amyotrophic lateral sclerosis patients with SOD1 gene mutation, and transgenic mice expressing human SOD1 gene mutation. *Neuropathology* 21: 67-81.

88. Kato S, Saito M, Hirano A, Ohama E (1999) Recent advances in research on neuropathological aspects of familial amyotrophic lateral sclerosis with superoxide dismutase 1 gene mutations: neuronal Lewy body-like hyaline inclusions and astrocytic hyaline inclusions. *Histol Histopathol* 14: 973-989.

89. Kato S, Shimoda M, Watanabe Y, Nakashima K, Takahashi K, Ohama E (1996) Familial amyotrophic lateral sclerosis with a two base pair deletion in superoxide dismutase 1 gene: multisystem degeneration with intracytoplasmic hyaline inclusions in astrocytes. *J Neuropathol Exp Neurol* 55: 1089-1101.

90. Kato S, Takikawa M, Nakashima K, Hirano A, Cleveland DW, Kusaka H, Shibata N, Kato M, Nakano I, Ohama E (2000) New consensus research on neuropathological aspects of familial amyotrophic lateral sclerosis with superoxide dismutase 1 (SOD1) gene mutations: inclusions containing SOD1 in neurons and astrocytes. *Amyotroph Lateral Scler Other Motor Neuron Disord* 1: 163-184.

91. Katz JS, Wolfe GI, Andersson PB, Saperstein DS, Elliott JL, Nations SP, Bryan WW, Barohn RJ (1999) Brachial amyotrophic diplegia: a slowly progressive motor neuron disorder. *Neurology* 53: 1071-1076.

92. Kew JJ, Goldstein LH, Leigh PN, Abrahams S, Cosgrave N, Passingham RE, Frackowiak RS, Brooks DJ (1993) The relationship between abnormalities of cognitive function and cerebral activation in amyotrophic lateral sclerosis. A neuropsychological and positron emission tomography study. *Brain* 116: 1399-1423.

93. Kew JJM, Leigh PN (1992) Dementia with motor neuron disease. In *Baillière's Clinical Neurology: Unusual Dementias*, M Rossor (eds). Baillière Tindall: London. pp. 611-626.

94. Kokubo Y, Kuzuhara S, Narita Y, Kikugawa K, Nakano R, Inuzuka T, Tsuji S, Watanabe M, Miyazaki T, Murayama S, Ihara Y (1999) Accumulation of neurofilaments and SOD1-immunoreactive products in a patient with familial amyotrophic lateral sclerosis with I113T SOD1 mutation. *Arch Neurol* 56: 1506-1508.

95. Kondo K (1995) Epidemiology of motor neuron disease. In *Motor Neuron Disease: Biology and Management*, PN Leigh, M Swash (eds). Springer-Verlag: London, UK. pp.19.

96. Kurland LT, Mulder DW (1954) Epidemiologic investigations of amyotrophic lateral sclerosis: 1. Preliminary report on geographic distribution, with special reference to the Mariana Islands, including clinical and pathological observations. *Neurology* 4: 355-378.

97. Kusaka H, Hirano A (1999) Cytopathology of the motor neuron. In *Motor Disorders*, Younger DS (ed). Lippincott Williams & Wilkins: Philadelphia. pp. 93-101.

98. Kusaka H, Imai T, Hashimoto S, Yamamoto T, Maya K, Yamasaki M (1988) Ultrastructural study of chromatolytic neurons in an adult-onset sporadic case of amyotrophic lateral sclerosis. *Acta Neuropathol* 75: 523-528.

99. Lacomblez L, Bensimon G, Leigh PN, Guillet P, Meininger V (1996) Dose-ranging study of riluzole in amyotrophic lateral sclerosis. Amyotrophic Lateral Sclerosis/Riluzole Study Group II. *Lancet* 347: 1425-1431.

100. Le Forestier N, Chassande B, Moulonguet A, Maisonobe T, Schaeffer S, Birouk N, Baumann N, Adams D, Leger JM, Meininger V, Said G, Bouche P (1997) Multifocal motor neuropathies with conduction blocks. 39 cases. *Rev Neurol (Paris)* 153: 579-586.

101. Le Forestier N, Maisonobe T, Piquard A, Rivaud S, Crevier-Buchman L, Salachas F, Pradat PF, Lacomblez L, Meininger V (2001) Does primary lateral sclerosis exist? A study of 20 patients and a review of the literature. *Brain* 124: 1989-1999.

102. Lee MK, Marszalek JR, Cleveland DW (1994) A mutant neurofilament subunit causes massive, selective motor neuron death: implications for the pathogenesis of human motor neuron disease. *Neuron* 13: 975-988.

103. Leigh PN, Anderton BH, Dodson A, Gallo JM, Swash M, Power DM (1988) Ubiquitin deposits in anterior horn cells in motor neurone disease. *Neurosci Lett* 93: 197-203.

104. Leigh PN, Ray-Chaudhuri K (1994) Motor neuron disease. *J Neurol Neurosurg Psychiatry* 57: 886-896.

105. Leigh PN, Simmons A, Williams S, Williams V, Turner M, Brooks D (2002) Imaging: MRS/MRI/PET/SPECT: summary. *Amyotroph Lateral Scler Other Motor Neuron Disord* 3: S75-S80.

106. Leigh PN, Whitwell H, Garofalo O, Buller J, Swash M, Martin JE, Gallo JM, Weller RO, Anderton BH (1991) Ubiquitin-immunoreactive intraneuronal inclusions in amyotrophic lateral sclerosis. Morphology, distribution, and specificity. *Brain* 114: 775-788.

107. Li M, Ona VO, Guegan C, Chen M, Jackson-Lewis V, Andrews LJ, Olszewski AJ, Stieg PE, Lee JP, Przedborski S, Friedlander RM (2000) Functional role of caspase-1 and caspase-3 in an ALS transgenic mouse model. *Science* 288: 335-339.

108. Lin CL, Bristol LA, Jin L, Dykes-Hoberg M, Crawford T, Clawson L, Rothstein JD (1998) Aberrant RNA processing in a neurodegenerative disease: the cause for absent EAAT2, a glutamate transporter, in amyotrophic lateral sclerosis. *Neuron* 20: 589-602.

109. Lowe J (1994) New pathological findings in amyotrophic lateral sclerosis. *J Neurol Sci* 124 Suppl: 38-51.

110. Lowe J, Lennox G, Jefferson D, Morrell K, McQuire D, Gray T, Landon M, Doherty FJ, Mayer RJ (1988) A filamentous inclusion body within anterior horn neurones in motor neurone disease defined by immunocytochemical localisation of ubiquitin. *Neurosci Lett* 94: 203-210.

111. Ludolph AC, Meyer T, Riepe MW (2000) The role of excitotoxicity in ALS—what is the evidence? *J Neurol* 247 Suppl 1: I7-16.

112. Lynch T, Sano M, Marder KS, Bell KL, Foster NL, Defendini RF, Sima AA, Keohane C, Nygaard TG, Fahn S et al (1994) Clinical characteristics of a family with chromosome 17-linked disinhibition-dementia-parkinsonism-amyotrophy complex. *Neurology* 44: 1878-1884.

113. Martin LJ (1999) Neuronal death in amyotrophic lateral sclerosis is apoptosis: possible contribution of a programmed cell death mechanism. *J Neuropathol Exp Neurol* 58: 459-471.

114. Menzies FM, Ince PG, Shaw PJ (2001) Mitochondrial involvement in amyotrophic lateral sclerosis. *Neurochemistry International* in press.

115. Miller CC, Ackerley S, Brownlees J, Grierson AJ, Jacobsen NJ, Thornhill P (2002) Axonal transport of neurofilaments in normal and disease states. *Cell Mol Life Sci* 59: 323-330.

116. Miller RG, Rosenberg JA, Gelinas DF, Mitsumoto H, Newman D, Sufit R, Borasio GD, Bradley WG, Bromberg MB, Brooks BR, Kasarskis EJ, Munsat TL, Oppenheimer EA (1999) Practice parameter: the care of the patient with amyotrophic lateral sclerosis (an evidence-based review): report of the Quality Standards Subcommittee of the American Academy of Neurology: ALS Practice Parameters Task Force. *Neurology* 52: 1311-1323.

117. Mitsuyama Y (1984) Presenile dementia with motor neuron disease in Japan: clinico- pathological review of 26 cases. *J Neurol Neurosurg Psychiatry* 47: 953-959.

118. Mizusawa H, Nakano I, Ohama E, Kuroda S, Wakayama I, Kihira T, Hirano A (1996) Ubiquitinated intracytoplasmic inclusions in motor neurons of amyotrophic lateral sclerosis. In *Amyotrophic Lateral Sclerosis: Progress and Perspectives in Basic Research and Clinical Application*, Nakano I, Hirano A (eds). Elsevier Science: Amsterdam. pp. 1-5.

119. Morris HR, Al-Sarraj S, Schwab C, Gwinn-Hardy K, Perez-Tur J, Wood NW, Hardy J, Lees AJ, McGeer PL, Daniel SE, Steele JC (2001) A clinical and pathological study of motor neurone disease on Guam. *Brain* 124: 2215-2222.

120. Moulard B, Sefiani A, Laamri A, Malafosse A, Camu W (1996) Apolipoprotein E genotyping in sporadic amyotrophic lateral sclerosis: evidence for a major influence on the clinical presentation and prognosis. *J Neurol Sci* 139 Suppl: 34-37.

121. Murayama S, Mori H, Ihara Y, Bouldin TW, Suzuki K, Tomonaga M (1990) Immuno-cytochemical and ultrastructural studies of lower motor neurons in amyotrophic lateral sclerosis. *Ann Neurol* 27: 137-148.

122. Murayama S, Namba E, Nishiyama K, Kitamura Y, Morita T, Nakashima K, Ishida T, Mizutani T, Kanazawa I (1997) Molecular pathological studies of familial amyotrophic lateral sclerosis. *Neuropathology* 17 (Suppl): 219.

123. Murayama S, Ookawa Y, Mori H, Nakano I, Ihara Y, Kuzuhara S, Tomonaga M (1989) Immunocytochemical and ultrastructural study of Lewy body-like hyaline inclusions in familial amyotrophic lateral sclerosis. *Acta Neuropathol* 78: 143-152.

124. Nasreddine ZS, Loginov M, Clark LN, Lamarche J, Miller BL, Lamontagne A, Zhukareva V, Lee VM, Wilhelmsen KC, Geschwind DH (1999) From genotype to phenotype: a clinical pathological, and biochemical investigation of frontotemporal dementia and parkinsonism (FTDP-17) caused by the P301L tau mutation. *Ann Neurol* 45: 704-715.

125. Neary D, Snowden J (1996) Frontotemporal dementia: nosology, neuropsychology, and neuropathology. *Brain Cogn* 31: 176-187.

126. Nelson LM, Matkin C, Longstreth WT, Jr., McGuire V (2000) Population-based case-control study of amyotrophic lateral sclerosis in western Washington State. II. Diet. *Am J Epidemiol* 151: 164-173.

127. Nelson LM, McGuire V, Longstreth WT, Jr., Matkin C (2000) Population-based case-control study of amyotrophic lateral sclerosis in western Washington State. I. Cigarette smoking and alcohol consumption. *Am J Epidemiol* 151: 156-163.

128. Niebroj-Dobosz I, Janik P (1999) Amino acids acting as transmitters in amyotrophic lateral sclerosis (ALS). *Acta Neurol Scand* 100: 6-11.

129. Nobile-Orazio E (1996) Multifocal motor neuropathy. *J Neurol Neurosurg Psychiatry* 60: 599-603.

130. Okamoto K (1993) Bunina bodies in amyotrophic lateral sclerosis. *Neuropathology* 13: 193-199.

131. Okamoto K, Fujita Y, Aizawa H, Kusaka H, Mihdra B (2001) Basophilic cytoplasmic inclusions in amyotrophic lateral sclerosis. In *Molecular Mechanism and Therapeutics of Amyotrophic Lateral Sclerosis*, Abe K (ed). Elsevier Science: Amsterdam. pp. 21-26.

132. Oosthuyse B, Moons L, Storkebaum E, Beck H, Nuyens D, Brusselmans K, Van Dorpe J, Hellings P, Gorselink M, Heymans S, Theilmeier G, Dewerchin M, Laudenbach V, Vermylen P, Raat H, Acker T, Vleminckx V, Van Den Bosch L, Cashman N, Fujisawa H, Drost MR, Sciot R, Bruyninckx F, Hicklin DJ, Ince C, Gressens P, Lupu F, Plate KH, Robberecht W, Herbert JM, Collen D, Carmeliet P (2001) Deletion of the hypoxia-response element in the vascular endothelial growth factor promoter causes motor neuron degeneration. *Nat Genet* 28: 131-138.

133. Orrell RW, Figlewicz DA (2001) Clinical implications of the genetics of ALS and other motor neuron diseases. *Neurology* 57: 9-17.

134. Orrell RW, King AW, Hilton DA, Campbell MJ, Lane RJM, de Belleroche JS (1995) Familial amyotrophic lateral sclerosis with a point mutation of SOD-1: intrafamilial heterogeneity of disease duration associated with neurofibrillary tangles. *J Neurol Neurosurg Psychiatry* 59: 266-270.

135. Piao Y-S, Wakabayashi K, Kakita A, Yamada M, Hayashi S, Morita T, Ikuta F, Oyanagi K, Takahashi H (2003) Neuropathology with clinical correlations of sporadic amyotrophic lateral sclerosis: 102 autopsy cases examined between 1962 and 2000. *Brain Pathol* 12: 10-22.

136. Plato CC, Garruto RM, Fox KM, Gajdusek DC (1986) Amyotrophic lateral sclerosis and parkinsonism-dementia on Guam: a 25-year prospective case-control study. *Am J Epidemiol* 124: 643-656.

137. Pringle CE, Hudson AJ, Munoz DG, Kiernan JA, Brown WF, Ebers GC (1992) Primary lateral sclerosis. Clinical features, neuropathology and diagnostic criteria. *Brain* 115: 495-520.

138. Rabin BA, Griffin JW, Crain BJ, Scavina M, Chance PF, Cornblath DR (1999) Autosomal dominant juvenile amyotrophic lateral sclerosis. *Brain* 122: 1539-1550.

139. Radunovic A, Leigh PN (1996) Cu/Zn superoxide dismutase gene mutations in amyotrophic lateral sclerosis: correlation between genotype and clinical features. *J Neurol Neurosurg Psychiatry* 61: 565-572.

140. Robberecht W (2000) Genetics of amyotrophic lateral sclerosis. *J Neurol* 247: 2-6.

141. Rodgers-Johnson P, Garruto RM, Yanagihara R, Chen KM, Gajdusek DC, Gibbs CJ, Jr. (1986) Amyotrophic lateral sclerosis and parkinsonism-dementia on Guam: a 30-year evaluation of clinical and neuropathologic trends. *Neurology* 36: 7-13.

142. Rosen DR, Siddique T, Patterson D, Figlewicz DA, Sapp P, Hentati A, Donaldson D, Goto J, O'Regan JP, Deng HX et al (1993) Mutations in Cu/Zn superoxide dismutase gene are associated with familial amyotrophic lateral sclerosis. *Nature* 362: 59-62.

143. Rothstein JD, Tsai G, Kuncl RW, Clawson L, Cornblath DR, Drachman DB, Pestronk A, Stauch BL, Coyle JT (1990) Abnormal excitatory amino acid metabolism in amyotrophic lateral sclerosis. *Ann Neurol* 28: 18-25.

144. Rouleau GA, Clark AW, Rooke K, Pramatarova A, Krizus A, Suchowersky O, Julien JP, Figlewicz D (1996) SOD1 mutation is associated with accumulation of neurofilaments in amyotrophic lateral sclerosis. *Ann Neurol* 39: 128-131.

145. Rowland LP (2001) How amyotrophic lateral sclerosis got its name: the clinical-pathologic genius of Jean-Martin Charcot. *Arch Neurol* 58: 512-515.

146. Ruddy DM, Parton MJ, Al-Chalabi A, Lewis C, Leigh PN, Powell JF, Siddique T, Meyjes EP, Baas F, de Jong V, Shaw CE (2003) Two families with familial amyotrophic lateral sclerosis are linked to a novel locus on chromosome 16q. Unpublished observations.

147. Saida K, Ohi N, Nabeshima K, Asada Y, Kumamoto K, Matsukura S (1999) An autopsy case of familial amyotrophic lateral sclerosis with a His(46)Arg substitution in exon 2 of Cu/Zn-superoxide dismutase gene. *Clin Neurol* (Japanese abstract) 39: 287.

148. Sasaki S, Iwata M (2000) Immunocytochemical and ultrastructural study of the motor cortex in patients with lower motor neuron disease. *Neurosci Lett* 281: 45-48.

149. Sasaki S, Maruyama S (1992) Increase in diameter of the axonal initial segment is an early change in amyotrophic lateral sclerosis. *J Neurol Sci* 110: 114-120.

150. Sathasivam S, Ince PG, Shaw PJ (2001) Apoptosis in amyotrophic lateral sclerosis: a review of the evidence. *Neuropathol Appl Neurobiol* 27: 257-274.

151. Shaw CE, al-Chalabi A, Leigh N (2001) Progress in the pathogenesis of amyotrophic lateral sclerosis. *Curr Neurol Neurosci Rep* 1: 69-76.

152. Shaw CE, Enayat ZE, Chioza BA, Al-Chalabi A, Radunovic A, Powell JF, Leigh PN (1998) Mutations in all five exons of SOD-1 may cause ALS. *Ann Neurol* 43: 390-394.

153. Shaw CE, Enayat ZE, Powell JF, Anderson VER, Radunovic A, Al-Sarraj S, Leigh PN (1997) Familial amyotrophic lateral sclerosis. Molecular pathology of a patient with a SOD1 mutation. *Neurology* 49: 1612-1616.

154. Shaw CE, Enayat ZE, Powell JF, Anderson VER, Radunovic A, Al-Sarraj S, Leigh PN (1997) Familial amyotrophic lateral sclerosis: molecular pathology of a patient with a SOD1 mutation. *Neurology* 49: 1612-1616.

155. Shaw PJ (2000) Biochemical Pathology. In *Amyotrophic lateral sclerosis*, RH Brown, V Meininger, M Swash (eds). Martin Dunitz Ltd: London. pp. 113-144.

156. Shaw PJ (2001) Mechanisms of cell death and treatment prospects in motor neuron disease. *Hong Kong Med J* 7: 267-280.

157. Shaw PJ, Eggett CJ (2000) Molecular factors underlying the selective vulnerability of motor neurones to neurodegeneration in amyotrophic lateral sclerosis. *J Neurol* 247: 17-27.

158. Shaw PJ, Forrest V, Ince PG, Richardson JP, Wastell HJ (1995) CSF and plasma amino acid levels in motor neuron disease: elevation of CSF glutamate in a subset of patients. *Neurodegeneration* 4: 209-216.

159. Shaw PJ, Ince PG (1997) Glutamate, excitotoxicity and amyotrophic lateral sclerosis. *J Neurol* 244 Suppl 2: S3-14.

160. Shaw PJ, Williams R (2000) Serum and cerebrospinal fluid biochemical markers of ALS. *Amyotroph Lateral Scler Other Motor Neuron Disord* 1 Suppl 2: S61-67.

161. Shibata N, Hirano A, Kobayashi M, Siddique T, Deng HX, Hung WY, Kato T, Asayama K (1996) Intense superoxide dismutase-1 immunoreactivity in intracytoplasmic hyaline inclusions of familial amyotrophic lateral sclerosis with posterior column involvement. *J Neuropathol Exp Neurol* 55: 481-490.

162. Siddique T. Unpublished observations.

163. Siddique T, Pericak-Vance MA, Caliendo J, Hong ST, Hung WY, Kaplan J, McKenna-Yasek D, Rimmler JB, Sapp P, Saunders AM, Scott WK, Siddique N, Haines JL, Brown RH (1998) Lack of association between apolipoprotein E genotype and sporadic

amyotrophic lateral sclerosis. *Neurogenetics* 1: 213-216.

164. Smith RG, Henry YK, Mattson MP, Appel SH (1998) Presence of 4-hydroxynonenal in cerebrospinal fluid of patients with sporadic amyotrophic lateral sclerosis. *Ann Neurol* 44: 696-699.

165. Strickland D, Smith SA, Dolliff G, Goldman L, Roelofs RI (1996) Physical activity, trauma, and ALS: a case-control study. *Acta Neurol Scand* 94: 45-50.

166. Strong MJ (2000) Exogenous neurotoxins. In *Amyotrophic lateral sclerosis*, RH Brown, V Meininger, M Swash (eds). Martin Dunitz Ltd: London. pp. 289-308.

167. Subramaniam JR, Lyons WE, Liu J, Bartnikas TB, Rothstein J, Price DL, Cleveland DW, Gitlin JD, Wong PC (2002) Mutant SOD1 causes motor neuron disease independent of copper chaperone-mediated copper loading. *Nat Neurosci* 5: 301-307.

168. Swash M (2000) Clinical features and diagnosis of amyotrophic lateral sclerosis. In *Amyotrophic lateral sclerosis*, RH Brown, V Meininger, M Swash (eds). Martin Dunitz: London, UK. pp. 3-30.

169. Swingler RJ, Fraser H, Warlow CP (1992) Motor neuron disease and polio in Scotland. *J Neurol Neurosurg Psychiatry* 55: 1116-1120.

170. Takahashi H (1995) Familial amyotrophic lateral sclerosis with or without mutation of the Cu/Zn superoxide dismutase gene. *No To Shinkei* 47: 535-541.

171. Takahashi H, Makifuchi T, Nakano R, Sato S, Inuzuka T, Sakimura K, Mishina M, Honma Y, Tsuji S, Ikuta F (1994) Familial amyotrophic lateral sclerosis with a mutation in the Cu/Zn superoxide dismutase gene. *Acta Neuropathol* 88: 185-188.

172. Takahashi K, Nakamura H, Okada E (1972) Hereditary amyotrophic lateral sclerosis. Histochemical and electron microscopic study of hyaline inclusions in motor neurons. *Arch Neurol* 27: 292-299.

173. Takehisa Y, Ujike H, Ishizu H, Terada S, Haraguchi T, Tanaka Y, Nishinaka T, Nobukuni K, Ihara Y, Namba R, Yasuda T, Nishibori M, Hayabara T, Kuroda S (2001) Familial amyotrophic lateral sclerosis with a novel Leu126Ser mutation in the copper/zinc superoxide dismutase gene showing mild clinical features and Lewy body-like hyaline inclusions. *Arch Neurol* 58: 736-740.

174. Tohgi H, Abe T, Yamazaki K, Murata T, Ishizaki E, Isobe C (1999) Remarkable increase in cerebrospinal fluid 3-nitrotyrosine in patients with sporadic amyotrophic lateral sclerosis. *Ann Neurol* 46: 129-131.

175. Tomik B, Nicotra A, Ellis CM, Murphy C, Rabe-Hesketh S, Parton M, Shaw CE, Leigh PN (2000) Phenotypic differences between African and white patients with motor neuron disease: a case-control study. *J Neurol Neurosurg Psychiatry* 69: 251-253.

176. Traynor BJ, Codd MB, Corr B, Forde C, Frost E, Hardiman O (1999) Incidence and prevalence of ALS in Ireland, 1995-1997: a population- based study. *Neurology* 52: 504-509.

177. Turner MR, Bakker M, Sham P, Shaw CE, Leigh PN, Al-Chalabi A (2002) Prognostic modelling of therapeutic interventions in amyotrophic lateral sclerosis. *Amyotroph Lateral Scler Other Motor Neuron Disord* 3: 15-21.

178. Tyler HR, Shefner J (1991) Amyotrophic lateral sclerosis. *Handb Clin Neuro* 15: 169-215.

179. Van den Berg-Vos RM, Visser J, Franssen H, de Visser M, de Jong JMBV, Kalmijn S, Wokke JHJ, Van den Berg LH Sporadic lower motor neuron disease with adult onset: classification of subtypes. *Brain* in press.

180. van der Heijden A, Spaans F, Reulen J (1994) Fasciculation potentials in foot and leg muscles of healthy young adults. *Electroencephalogr Clin Neurophysiol* 93: 163-168.

181. Vulpian A (1886) Maladies du systéme nervaux (moelle épinière)., (Eds). Octave Doin: Paris. pp. p 436.

182. Waring S (1994) *Amyotrophic lateral sclerosis and parkinsonism demential complex of Guam: descriptive epidemiology, secular trends and birth cohort effects in incidence 1950-1989.* Houston School of Public Health: Houston; University of Texas.

183. Wiederholt WC (1999) Neuroepidemiologic research initiatives on Guam: past and present. *Neuroepidemiology* 18: 279-291.

184. Wightman G, Anderson VE, Martin J, Swash M, Anderton BH, Neary D, Mann D, Luthert P, Leigh PN (1992) Hippocampal and neocortical ubiquitin-immunoreactive inclusions in amyotrophic lateral sclerosis with dementia. *Neurosci Lett* 139: 269-274.

185. Wilhelmsen KC, Lynch T, Pavlou E, Higgins M, Nygaard TG (1994) Localization of disinhibition-dementia-parkinsonism-amyotrophy complex to 17q21-22. *Am J Hum Genet* 55: 1159-1165.

186. Wong PC, Pardo CA, Borchelt DR, Lee MK, Copeland NG, Jenkins NA, Sisodia SS, Cleveland DW, Price DL (1995) An adverse property of a familial ALS-linked SOD1 mutation causes motor neuron disease characterized by vacuolar degeneration of mitochondria. *Neuron* 14: 1105-1116.

187. Worms PM (2001) The epidemiology of motor neuron diseases: a review of recent studies. *J Neurol Sci* 191: 3-9.

188. Yang Y, Hentati A, Deng HX, Dabbagh O, Sasaki T, Hirano M, Hung WY, Ouahchi K, Yan J, Azim AC, Cole N, Gascon G, Yagmour A, Ben-Hamida M, Pericak-Vance M, Hentati F, Siddique T (2001) The gene encoding alsin, a protein with three guanine-nucleotide exchange factor domains, is mutated in a form of recessive amyotrophic lateral sclerosis. *Nat Genet* 29: 160-165.

189. Younger DS, Rowland LP, Latov N, Hays AP, Lange DJ, Sherman W, Inghirami G, Pesce MA, Knowles DM, Powers J et al (1991) Lymphoma, motor neuron diseases, and amyotrophic lateral sclerosis. *Ann Neurol* 29: 78-86.

190. Ziegler MG, Brooks BR, Lake CR, Wood JH, Enna SJ (1980) Norepinephrine and gamma-aminobutyric acid in amyotrophic lateral sclerosis. *Neurology* 30: 98-101.

Primary Lateral Sclerosis

Michael Swash

ALS	amyotrophic lateral sclerosis
EMG	electro myography
LMN	lower motor neurone
PLS	primary lateral sclerosis
PMA	progressive muscular atrophy
SNAP	sensory nerve action potential amplitude
UMN	upper motor neurone

Definition

Primary lateral sclerosis (PLS) is a nonfamilial, clinical syndrome characterised by features consistent with pathology limited to the upper motor neurone (19).

Synonyms and Historical Annotations

PLS was initially described by Erb (5), but its nosology has been frequently disputed subsequently (5, 19, 22). PLS is usually regarded as a syndrome within the clinical spectrum of other motor neurone diseases, a spectrum that includes Charcot's amyotrophic lateral sclerosis (ALS), progressive bulbar palsy, and progressive muscular atrophy (PMA) (19). In PLS, ALS and progressive bulbar palsy signs of corticospinal tract involvement are prominent, leading to a clinical debate as to whether PLS is a discrete entity or represents a form of ALS with especially prominent corticospinal signs. In the rare essential form of PLS, corticospinal signs are not only predominant, but may be the only feature of the syndrome.

Epidemiology

Incidence and prevalence. While a number of epidemiologic studies have addressed the indicence and prevalence of ALS, similar studies are not available for PLS.

Sex and age disribution. It has been suggested that PLS is more common in men than women, but this has not been addressed in a rigorous large-scale study. In one small series the median age of onset was 50 and median disease duration was 19 years (18). Life expectancy is not easily predicted, but cases of up to 35 years duration have been recorded (12).

Genetics and Risk Factors

PLS has almost invariably been reported as a sporadic disorder; however, in reports of families with familial ALS it has often been noted that the phenotype is variable, and patients have been described within individual families expressing phenotypes consistent with ALS, PMA and even PLS (4, 16). Environmental risk factors for PLS are unknown.

Infantile onset forms of spastic paraparesis with clinical features of PLS have been linked to the same locus as the locus for juvenile ALS on chromosome 2 (2q33-35) and deletion and splice site mutations were identified in the *alsin* gene in some, but not all cases (6, 21).

Clinical Features

There is a progressive motor deficit, with marked spasticity, that is relatively symmetrical, and involves all 4 limbs, the axial muscles, and the bulbar musculature. Dysarthria is often prominent, and there may be dysphagia, but muscular atrophy is not a feature, and fasciculations are not present. The spasticity is accompanied by marked rigidity at rest, suggesting involvement of non-corticospinal motor pathways. Released laughter and crying may be prominent, reflecting pseudobulbar signs. The syndrome is not uniform, since a number of other features have been described. For example, urinary incontinence has been reported in about a third of cases, particularly in cases older than 45 years at onset, in whom there were pseudobulbar signs (12), and mild atrophy of hand muscles, and of quadriceps, has often been noted (13, 14, 19). Abnormal somatosensory evoked potentials were noted in 11 of the 20 patients studied by Le Forestier et al (13, 14), and in 2 of these patients there were abnormalities of ocular movements.

Imaging. Pringle et al (19) described a distinctive MRI appearance in the brain in PLS, with atrophy of the precentral gyrus. The lateral sulcus was unusually prominent in PLS; however, this finding has not been confirmed by others (13, 14, 19), who have pointed out that frontal and motor cortex atrophy is frequent in ALS.

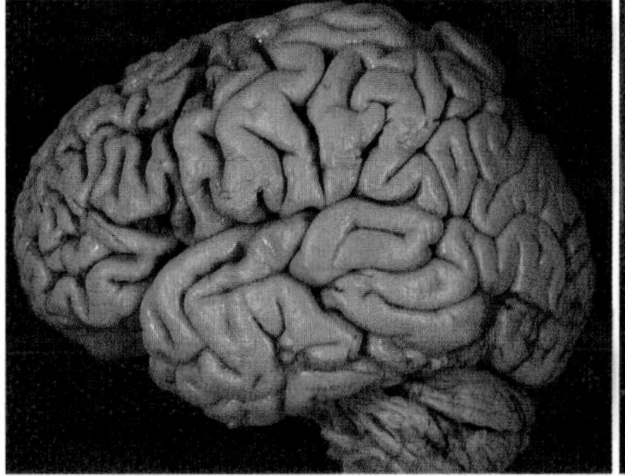
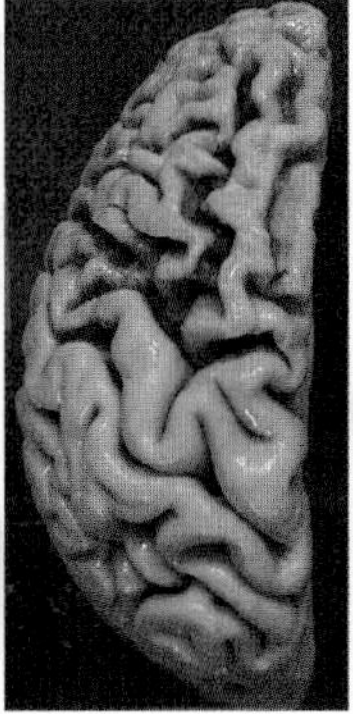
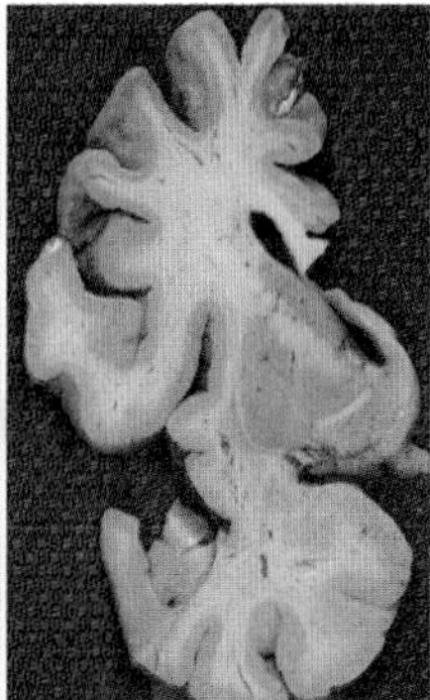

Figure 1. Gross appearance of brain in PLS. Note atrophy of precentral and premotor gyri with preservation of temporal, parietal and occipital lobes. View of brain from dorsal aspect clearly shows motor and premotor atrophy. On coronal sections there is thinning of the cortical ribbon in the superior frontal gyrus, attenuation of frontal white matter and thinning of the corpus callosum. Illustration kindly provided by Dr Dennis W. Dickson.

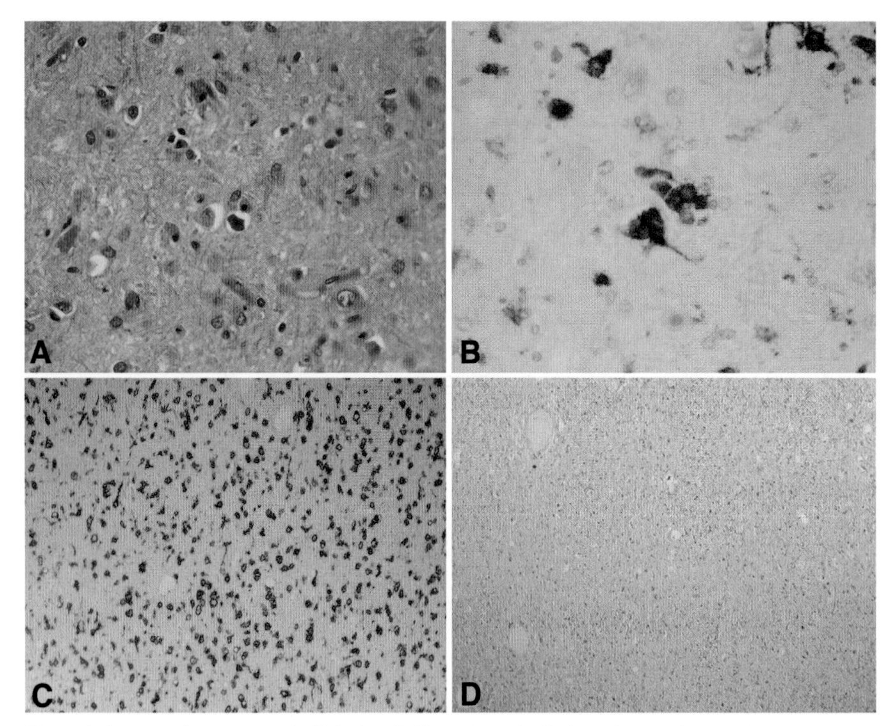

Figure 2. Sections of motor cortex in PLS show fibrillary astrocytic gliosis as clusters of macrophages in layer V. Betz cells are decreased. **A.** Section stained for microglia (HLA-DR) reveals clusters of macrophages in motor cortex. **B.** White matter beneath motor cortex has many macrophages (**C**) and myelin staining pallor on Luxol fast blue (**D**). Photo: Dr Dennis W. Dickson.

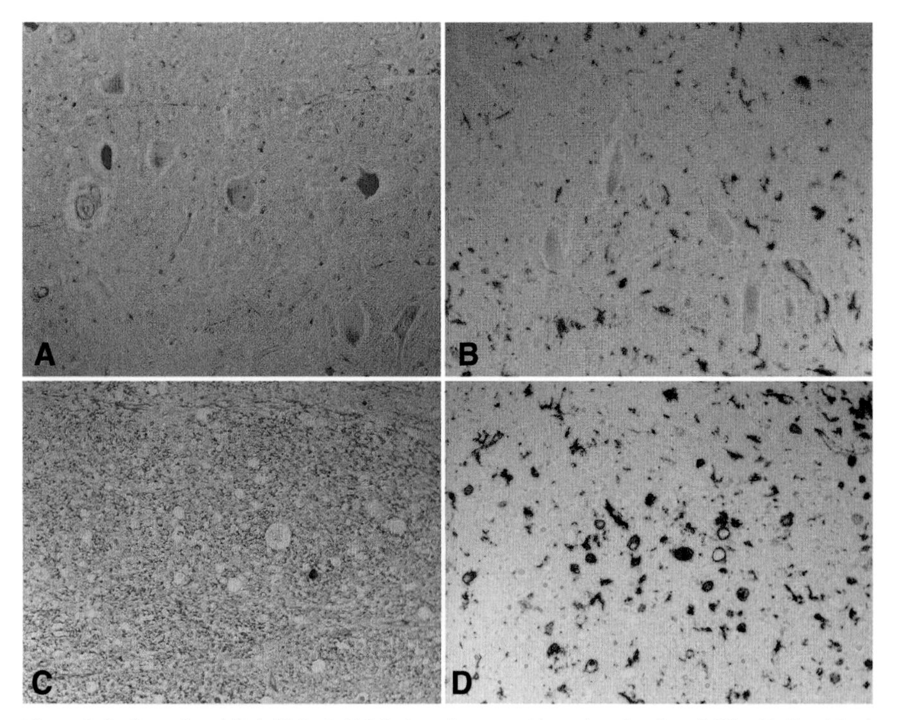

Figure 3. Sections of medulla in PLS. **A.** Relatively well-preserved hypoglossal nucleus (LFB) with **B.** minimal microglial activation. In contrast the medullary pyramid has myelin vacuolation **C.** with many lipid-laden macrophages **D.** Photo: Dr Dennis W. Dickson.

Positron emission tomography (PET) studies of cortical blood flow and of diazepam receptor density, as a measure of cell loss, have revealed abnormalities in the frontal opercular, precentral gyri, and in the anterior cingulate region in both ALS (1, 9, 10) and in PLS (13). Cognitive abnormalities, consistent with frontal lobe dysfunction, have been recognised in ALS (1), and in PLS (13).

The corticospinal and corticobulbar pathways in the brain show hyperintensity in T2 and proton density MR images in PLS and ALS. This hyperintensity probably correlates with Wallerian degeneration in these pathways. The abnormality is more prominent when corticospinal signs are prominent. In the later stages there are imaging abnormalities in the white matter of the centrum semiovale, and in the middle third of the corpus callosum, representing degenerating transcallosal motor fibres (17).

Laboratory findings. The presence of EMG evidence of lower motor neurone (LMN) involvement in most reported cases (12-14, 18, 19) suggests that PLS is not a discrete neurological disorder, but an extreme form of ALS in which clinical involvement is strikingly upper motor neurone (UMN) in type (13, 14, 19). Fasciculations were observed in 6 of 9 patients followed serially over several years (14). In addition, subtle sensory abnormalities, particularly reduction in sensory nerve action potential amplitude (SNAP) in sural nerve studies, have been reported in 2 to 75% of patients (14).

Macroscopy

Atrophy of the precentral gyrus and premotor frontal cortex has been described in some, but not all cases.

Histopathology

Descriptions of the histopathology of PLS are available from early reports, and from the more recent revival of interest in the syndrome. Loss of Betz cells in layer 5, and of pyramidal cells in layers 3 and 5 of the motor cortex, without loss of anterior horn cells or of motor cells in the somatic motor nuclei of the brain stem is the classical feature, but in fact most studies of the CNS pathology have noted some loss of anterior horn cells (3, 4, 16, 18). There was gliosis in layers 3 and 5 of the motor cortex (18). There was no loss of motor neurones in the Onuf nucleus in the sacral cord

(18). In these older studies no Lewy bodies, cytoplasmic swelling, Pick bodies or neurofibrillary tangles were noted in surviving cortical neurones (18). Bunina bodies have also been reported in PLS, consisting of eosinophilic inclusions within neuronal nuclei of anterior horn cells, or in the hypoglossal nucleus (8).

Loss of myelinated fibres in the corticospinal tracts in the brain and in the brainstem and spinal cord was noted in these reports. In several autopsy reports of PLS demyelination in the posterior columns in the spinal cord has been reported, perhaps accounting for the abnormal somatosensory evoked potentials (7, 18, 22). Similar findings have often been noted in ALS (3, 4, 8).

Immunohistochemistry

Immunohistochemistry with ubiquitin antibodies reveals, ubiquitinated cytoplasmic neuronal inclusions in some lower motor neurones, as in ALS (15), and in cortical neurones in a distribution typical of ALS dementia (8, 11, 20). These observations indicate the likely close pathogenetic relationship of ALS, PLS and frontotemporal degeneration.

Pathogenesis and Future Directions

The overlap clinically and pathologically between ALS, PLS and frontotemporal degeneration suggest that these clinical syndromes probably represent clinical heterogeneity within a multisystem degenerative disorder, most often dominated by a combination of UMN and LMN features as in ALS, but sometimes presenting with more or less restricted involvement of the corticospinal tracts, as in PLS, or with frontotemporal dementia (8). The data are consistent, therefore, with the concept that PLS is not a distinct disease, but an extreme form of the syndrome of ALS. Future studies are warranted to explore this relationship.

References

1. Abrahams S, Goldstein LH, Kew JJ, Brooks DJ, Lloyd CM, Frith CD et al (1996) Frontal lobe dysfunction in amyotrophic lateral sclerosis; a PET study. *Brain* 119: 2105-2120.

2. Beal MF, Richardson EP (1981) Primary lateral sclerosis; a case report. *Arch Neurol* 38: 630-637.

3. Brownell B, Oppenheimer DR, Hughes JT (1970) The central nervous system in motor neurone disease. *J Neurol Neurosurg Psych* 33: 338-357.

4. Castaigne P, Lhermitte F, Cambier J, Escourolle R, Le Bigot P (1972) Etude neuropathologique de 62 observations de sclerose laterale amyotrophique; discussions nosologique. *Revue Neurologie (Paris)* 127: 401-414.

5. Erb WH (1875) Über einen wenig bekannten Spinalen Symptomencomplex. *Berliner Klinischen Wockenschrift* 12: 357-359.

6. Eymard-Pierre E, Lesca G, Dollet S, Santorelli FM, di Capua M, Bertini E, Boespflug-Tanguy O (2002) Infantile-onset ascending hereditary spastic paralysis is associated with mutations in the alsin gene. *Am J Hum Genet* 71: 518-527.

7. Fisher CM (1977) Pure spastic paralysis of corticospinal origin. *Canad J Neurol Sci* 4: 251-258.

8. Ince PG (2000) Neuropathology, in *Amyotrophic Lateral Sclerosis*, Brown RH, Meininger V, Swash M, Editors, Martin Dunitz Publishers, London, Chapter 5: 83-112.

9. Kew JJ, Goldstein LH, Leigh PN, Abrahams S, Cosgrave N, Passingham RE et al (1993) The relationship between abnormalities of cognitive function and cerebral activation in amyotrophic lateral sclerosis. *Brain* 116: 1399-1423.

10. Kew JJ, Leigh PN, Playford ED, Passingham RE, Goldstein LH, Frackowiak RS et al (1993) Cortical function in amyotrophic lateral sclerosis. *Brain* 116: 655-680.

11. Konagaya M, Sakai M, Matsuoka Y et al (1998) Upper motor neuron predominant degeneration with frontal and temporal lobe atrophy. *Acta Neuropathologica* 96: 532-536.

12. Kuipers-Upmeijer J, de Jager AEJ, Hew JM, Snoek JW, van Weerden TW (2001) Primary lateral sclerosis: clinical, neurophysiological and magnetic resonance findings. *J Neurol Neurosurg Psychiatr* 71: 615-620.

13. Le Forestier N, Maisonobe T, Piquard A, Rivaud S, Crevier-Buchman L, Salachas F, Pradat PF, Lacomblez L, Meininger V (2001) Does primary lateral sclerosis exist? A study of 20 patients and a review of the literature. *Brain* 124: 1989-1999.

14. Le Forestier N, Maisonobe T, Spelle L, Lesort A, Salache F, Lacomblez L, Samson Y, Bouche P, Meininger V (2001) Primary lateral sclerosis: further clarification. *J Neurol Sci* 185: 95-100.

15. Leigh PN, Anderton BH, Dodson A, Gallo J-M, Swash M, Power DM (1988) Ubiquitin deposits in anterior horn cells in motor neurone disease. *Neurosci Lett* 93: 197-203.

16. Mackay RP (1963) Course and prognosis in amyotrophic lateral sclerosis. *Arch Neurol* 8: 117-127.

17. Pioro EP (2000) Imaging in amyotrophic lateral sclerosis in *Amyotrophic Lateral Sclerosis*, Brown RH, Meininger V, Swash M, Editors, Martin Dunitz Publishers, London, Chapter 10: 187-210.

18. Pringle CE, Hudson AJ, Munoz DG, Kiernan JA, Brown WF, Ebers GC (1992) Primary lateral sclerosis: the clinical features, neuropathology and diagnostic criteria. *Brain* 115: 495-520.

19. Swash M, Desai J, Misra VP(1999) What is primary lateral sclerosis? *J Neurol Sci* 170: 5-10.

20. Watanabe R, Iino M, Honda M et al (1997) *Neuropathology* 17: 220-224.

21. Yang Y, Hentati A, Deng HX, Dabbagh O, Sasaki T, Hirano M, Hung WY, Ouahchi K, Yan J, Azim AC et al (2001) The gene encoding alsin, a protein with three guanine-nucleotide exchange factor domains, is mutated in a form of recessive amyotrophic lateral sclerosis. *Nat Genet* 29: 160-165.

22. Younger DS, Chou S, Hays AP. Lange DJ, Emerson R, Brin M, Rowland LP (1988) Primary lateral sclerosis; a clinical diagnosis re-emerges. *Arch Neurol* 45: 1304-1307.

Spinal Muscular Atrophy

Brian N. Harding

Bu	bulbar
Bg	basal ganglia
Cba	cerebellar atrophy
Cbh	cerebellar hypoplasia
CK	creatine kinase
Coch	cochlea
DRG	dorsal root ganglion
EMG	electro myography
NAIP	neuronal apoptosis inhibitory protein gene
NCV	nerve conduction velocity
Sc	spinal cord
SMA	spinal muscular atrophy
SMNI	survival motor neuron gene

Definition and Classification

Progressive degeneration of lower motor neurons (in spinal cord and often also brainstem) characterises this heterogeneous group of degenerative disorders that together constitute the second most frequently lethal genetic disorder of childhood.

Classification and nomenclature remain problematic, the most useful being based on a combination of type of inheritance, age of onset, distribution of weakness and clinical progression. This chapter is principally concerned with the most common childhood forms of proximal, recessively inherited spinal muscular atrophy (SMA), the acute early onset type 1 SMA or Werdnig-Hoffman disease, the chronic infantile type II SMA or arrested Werdnig-Hoffman disease, and the chronic childhood type III SMA or Kugelberg-Welander disease. These 3 disorders all result from homozygous deletions in the *SMN1* gene at chromosome 5q13.

Epidemiology

The incidence of SMA1 is 1 in 20 000 live births, and the gene carrier frequency is 1 in 60 to 80. The gene carrier frequency of the chronic forms of SMA is 1 in 76 to 111 (14).

Genetics

Genetic linkage studies have mapped all 3 types of SMA to chromosome 5q11.2-13.3, thus facilitating prenatal diagnosis. In this region of the chromosome, which is especially prone to large scale deletions, 4 genes have been identified: the survival motor neuron (*SMN1*) gene, the neuronal apoptosis inhibitory protein (*NAIP*) gene, the *p44* gene and the *H4F5* gene. These genes are duplicated as telomeric and centromeric copies that have very subtle differences, but it has been found that only deletions of the telomeric *SMN* designated *SMN1* or *SMNt* causes SMA.

Homozygous *SMN1* deletions are found in all 3 types of SMA; a small proportion has subtle point mutations, micro-deletions or insertions. In normal control subjects *SMN1* is always present, but the centromeric form *SMN2* though occasionally absent is not pathogenic.

The presence of *SMN1* deletions in all 3 types of SMA and the rare occurrence of asymptomatic members of SMA families having the same haplotype as affected family members suggest the operation of modifier genes. Two have been implicated. *NAIP* can reduce neuronal apoptosis under experimental conditions, and two-thirds of SMA type I patients have large deletions which include the telomeric form of *NAIP*, compared with <5% of types II and III. A second potential modifier gene is *SMN2*, the centromeric form of *SMN*. The observation that there are more copies of *SMN2* in chromosomes from the chronic forms of SMA than in chromosomes of type 1 SMA provides a correlation between genotype and phenotype and has given rise to the suggestion that gene conversion rather than deletion is the underlying defect in SMA II and III (16).

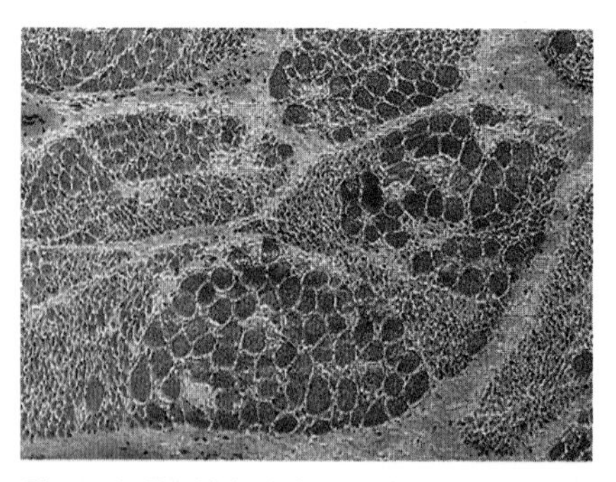

Figure 1. Established changes in the quadriceps muscle of a 1-year-old child with SMA type II. There are large groups of small rounded fibres, mostly type 1, and larger type 2 fibres individually or in groups. H&E.

Clinical Features

Type I. There is prenatal onset in about one third of cases, heralded by reduced fetal movements, with proximal limb weakness and areflexia at birth, progressing rapidly within a few weeks to symmetric paralysis. This includes axial muscles especially in the neck, intercostal muscles resulting in a characteristic lateral flattening of the thorax and quadriparesis with some preservation of distal muscles. Respiration is performed by the diaphragm, which is spared until late in the disease. Retrognathia, preservation of eye movements and an alert look give a characteristic facial appearance.

Deep tendon reflexes are absent, tongue fasciculation is common, but there is no sensory loss, sphincter disturbance or pyramidal tract signs. In the vast majority, death occurs within 18 months of birth from respiratory insufficiency precipitated by intercurrent infection and swallowing difficulties. Those with neonatal onset often succumb within 3 months.

The EMG shows neurogenic changes with spontaneous rhythmical activity or fibrillations in many, as well as polyphasic potentials. Nerve conduction velocity (NCV) may be normal or reduced. Serum CK levels are usually normal. With the advent of genetic diagnosis, muscle biopsy is becoming an infrequent investigation.

Type II. Onset is insidious after 3 months of age and a normal early motor development, with failure to stand and to acquire a normal sitting position, as there is excessive spinal curvature. Although slowly progressive weakness and wasting become widespread though may plateau around 2 years. Deep tendon reflexes are abolished, fasciculations obvious, intercostal involvement present in half the patients but swallowing remains intact. Contractures and deformities are common in childhood, particularly hip dislocation and kyphoscoliosis, with risk of respiratory complication. Survival may only be 18 months or extended into adulthood. The EMG is similar to type I but fasciculation is common and pseudomyotonic discharges may be observed.

Type III. In addition to recessive inheritance, sporadic occurrence is not uncommon. Onset between infancy and early childhood is almost imperceptible, as parents may not notice the thinness and weakness of the proximal muscles of the legs. On examination there is a positive Gowers manoeuvre, wasting of proximal muscles and absent knee jerks which other tendon reflexes are preserved. Waddling gait and calf hypertrophy may give a resemblance to muscular dystrophy. There is very slow progression involving distal lower limbs and proximal upper limb musculature, with pes cavus, and coarse hand tremor. Many patients lead relatively normal lives. Serum CK may be moderately elevated and secondary myopathic features in muscle biopsies may make differentiation from dystrophy difficult, but the EMG is usually diagnostic.(1)

Muscle Pathology

The effects of deafferentation on involved muscles vary with the patient's age. In neonates the classical changes of group atrophy or angulated fibres may not be present. One observes scattered small fibres throughout the fascicles—they may be type 1 fibres reminiscent of congenital fibre type disproportion, or alternatively small type 2 fibres. From 6 weeks of age, one finds the typical changes of neurogenic atrophy, including large groups of atrophic fibres, mostly type 2 fibres with scattered type 1 fibres interspersed with larger often hypertrophic type 1 fibres singly or in groups. With immunocytochemistry the larger fibres express slow myosin exclusively, while the small fibres co-express fetal, slow and fast myosins suggesting that they may have become denervated before they are fully mature.

Similar changes are present in both type I and type II SMA. In patients with chronic disease endomysial connective tissue may be markedly increased and with fatty infiltration give appearances reminiscent of congenital muscular dystrophy, but unlike congenital muscular dystrophy the small fibres are mostly type 2. In type 3 SMA the pathology is more variable with less atrophy and fibre type grouping. With longstanding disease myopathic changes increase the resemblance to dystrophy.

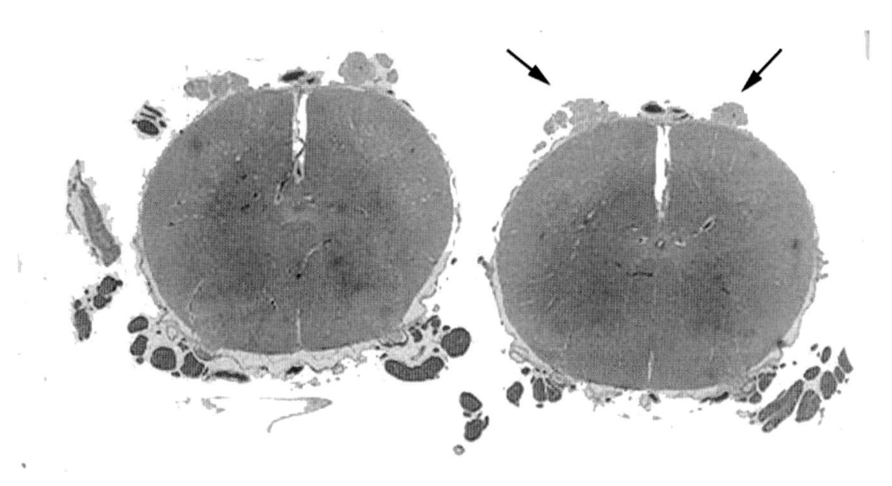

Figure 2. Low power view of segments of the lumbar cord. Anterior roots are atrophic (arrows) and the horns are poorly cellular. H&E.

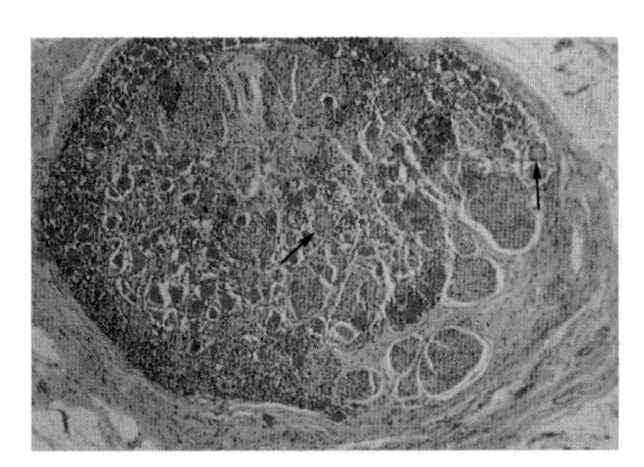

Figure 3. Chromatolytic sensory neurons in a dorsal root ganglion. Examples indicate by an arrow. H&E.

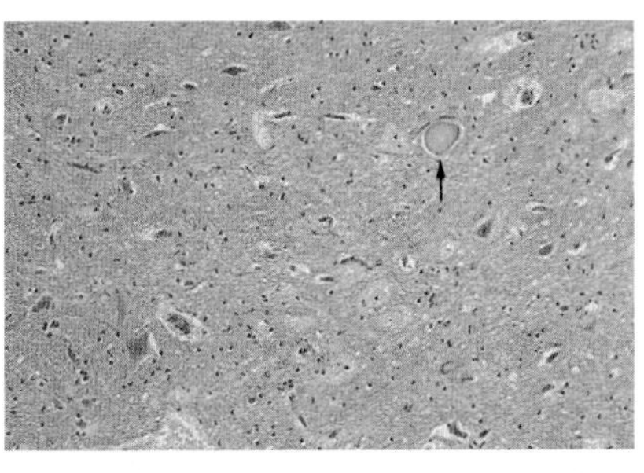

Figure 4. The anterior horn at a high cervical level shows a very reduced number of motoneurons, gliosis and one ballooned chromatolytic cell (arrow). H&E.

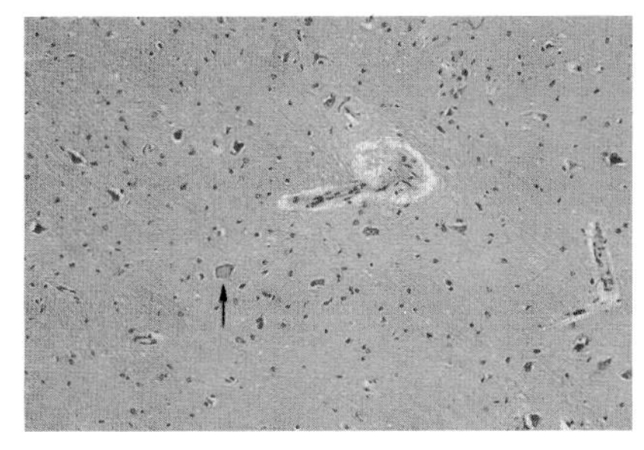

Figure 5. Chromatolysis, neuronal loss and gliosis are present also in the thalamus. H&E.

Macroscopic Neuropathology

Autopsy reports are virtually confined to SMA type 1. The brain appears normal externally, but dissection of the spinal cord reveals thin gray anterior roots.

Microscopic Neuropathology

Anterior horn cell loss and gliosis is usually profound and extensive throughout most levels of the spinal

Type	Inheritance	Presentation	Duration (years)	Pathology Usual	Pathology Occasional
SMA	AR (AD)	early hypotonia	2	Sc Bu Th	DRG
Distal infantile SMA with diaphragmatic paralysis	AR	early diaphragmatic weakness	1	Sc Bu Th	
SMA with cerebellar hypoplasia	AR	hypotonia at birth, mental retardation	2	Sc Bu Cbh	Th
SMA with cerebellar atrophy	AR	hypotonia at birth	1	Sc Bu Cba	Bg
Fazio-Londe	AR & AD	bulbar weakness	1-5	Bu Sc	Cba Th Bg
Brown-Vialetto-van Laere	AR	nerve deafness, lower cranial nerve palsies	1-30	Coch Bu Sc	Cba

Table 1. Differential diagnosis of lower motor neuron disorders in childhood.

cord, but in the early stages of the more acute examples, one may observe ballooning and chromatolysis, microglial activation and occasionally neuronophagia. Bulbar motoneurones, dorsal root ganglion sensory cells and Clarke's column can be affected, while chromatolytic neurons are regularly seen in the thalamus (a useful diagnostic pointer when the spinal cord is unavailable for examination).

Differential Diagnosis

In neonatal muscle biopsies, type 1 fibre atrophy is also a feature of myotonic dystrophy or nemaline myopathy, and also congenital fibre type disproportion. At the other end of the spectrum older patients with longstanding disease may have markedly myopathic changes resembling congenital muscular dystrophy requiring immunocytochemical study with a panel of sarcolemmal markers.

Neuropathological differential diagnosis is aimed at discriminating the rarer forms and variants of lower motor neuron disorder (Table 1).

Animal Models

Clinical evidence suggests that SMA type I may begin in utero when the neuromuscular axis is immature, a situation that can to some extent be reproduced in the neonatal rat where the neuromuscular system matures later than man. Cutting the unmyelinated rat sciatic nerve at birth causes motor neurons to die, though not 4 weeks later when motor neurons are mature and at the time when Schwann cells start to produce ciliary neurotrophic factor, which has been shown to delay cell death occurring after axotomy and in a hereditary mouse model of motoneuron disease. Axotomy in the immature rat is not followed by reinnervation, and after a few weeks the muscle has a similar appearance to that of human SMA type I (16).

Of the small number of hereditary motoneuron disorders in animals thus far examined, the distal-proximal gradient of involvement points towards axonopathy rather than primary neuronal disease unlike in human SMA. Spontaneous mutations in the single *Smn* gene in mice have yet to be detected with motoneuron disorders. Homozygous *Smn* knockout mice are not viable following massive apoptosis in the early blastocyst while heterozygotes display a mild spinal muscular atrophy (17). More recent models involving *SMN2* transgenes or conditional deletion of mouse *Smn* exon 7 are still at an early stage of phenotypic characterisation.

Pathogenesis

Much controversy has attended the morphogenetic basis of SMA, the underlying degenerative process in motoneurons and the pathogenetic relationship between neuron and muscle degeneration. Is the ballooning merely a manifestation of chromatolysis similar to that resulting from loss of synaptic target or a dying-back axonopathy, or is it evidence for an intrinsic disturbance? Reduced synaptophysin expression in anterior horns (7, 21) may indicate loss of pre-synaptic terminals, but this does not distinguish between primary motoneuron degeneration and loss of its peripheral target. On the other hand, immunohistochemical studies of ballooned motoneurons have demonstrated accumulations of ubiquitinated degradation products in the centre of the perikaryon (12) displacing phosphorylated neurofilaments to the periphery where glycosylation may be abnormally reduced, promoting abnormal neurofilament assembly, neuron-glia adhesion and failure of synapse formation (3).

Is the process of cell death apoptosis or necrosis? The 2 principal candidate genes for SMA located in the deleted region of chromosome 5q13, *SMN* and *NAIP*, both have anti-apoptotic properties (8). Recently Simic et al (18) have presented convincing morphological and TUNEL evidence for apoptosis as well as loss of bcl-2 and up-regulation of p53 immunostaining in spinal motoneurons from children with genetically confirmed SMA type I in addition to describing morphological changes of necrotic cell death.

The integrity of the neuron-muscle unit may also be compromised by the loss of *SMN* within muscle cells. Coculture systems of cloned human muscle satellite cells and fibroblasts with embryonic rat spinal cord form innervated myotubes. Myofibres derived from SMA I and II patients degenerate 1 to 3 weeks after innervation, but this degeneration can be prevented by adding 50% cloned satellite cells from normal donors indicating an important role for muscle cells in the establishment and degeneration of the neuromuscular junction and a potential target for therapy (6).

Atypical Forms of SMA

This is a group of rare disorders with early onset and rapidly fatal course not linked to deletions of chromosome 5q (15).

Distal infantile SMA with diaphragmatic paralysis. Unlike SMA I, there is congenital or early onset of diaphragmatic paralysis or weakness and muscle wasting initially restricted to the distal parts of the limbs. (2,11). The pathology is indistinguishable from SMA.

SMA with cerebellar hypoplasia, SMA with cerebellar atrophy. SMA with cerebellar hypoplasia (5, 9) and SMA with cerebellar atrophy (*syn.* infantile neuronal degeneration) (13, 19) have a congenital onset, often arthrogryposis, severe mental retardation and evidence of slowed motor conduction velocity, with rapid course. Major cerebellar pathology mark out these two possibly related familial disorders.

Bulbospinal Muscular Atrophy of Childhood

Brown-Vialetto-van Laere syndrome; Bulbar hereditary neuropathy type 1 (BHN 1). This rare recessively inherited disorder presents late in childhood or adolescence with bilateral neural deafness and vestibular areflexia, then later involvement of cranial nerves resulting in facial palsy dysarthria and dysphagia; although the course is slow, death may result from swallowing problems and respiratory insufficiency. There are degenerative changes in auditory and vestibular pathways as well as bulbar cranial nerve nuclei and anterior horns (4, 20).

Fazio-Londe disease; Bulbar hereditary neuropathy type 2 (BHN 2). Dominant inheritance is exceptional. Most cases are recessive, either with early onset before 2 years of respiratory symptoms and stridor, and rapid fatal progression, or a later onset of dysarthria dysphagia and facial weakness with protracted clinical course of many years. The few neuropathological reports consistently describe widespread degeneration of motor cranial nerve nuclei through the brainstem, worst caudally but extending to the III nuclei, and usually anterior horn cell degeneration, with variable involvement of cerebellum thalamus and basal ganglia (10).

References

1. Aicardi J (1998).Diseases of the motor neuron 20: 699-711. In *Diseases of the Nervous System in Childhood*, Edit by Aicardi J, 2nd ed. MacKeith Press: London.

2. Bertini E, Gadisseux JL, Palmieri G, Ricci E, Di-Capua M, Ferriere G, Lyon G (1989) Distal infantile spinal muscular atrophy associated with paralysis of the diaphragm: a variant of infantile spinal muscular atrophy. *Am J Med Genet* 33: 328-335.

3. Chou SM, Wang HS (1997) Aberrant glycosylation/phosphorylation in chromatolytic motoneurons of Werdnig-Hoffmann disease. *J Neurol Sci* 152:198-209.

4. Gallai V, Hockaday JM, Hughes JT, Lane DJ, Oppenheimer DR, Rushworth G (1981) Ponto-bulbar palsy with deafness (Brown-Vialetto-Van Laere syndrome). *J Neurol Sci* 50: 259-275.

5. Goutières F, Aicardi J, Farkas E (1977) Anterior horn cell disease associated with pontocerebellar hypoplasia in infants. *J Neurol Neurosurg Psych* 40: 370-378.

6. Guettier-Sigrist S, Coupin G, Braun S, Warter JM, Poindron P (1988) Muscle could be the therapeutic target in SMA treatment. *J Neurosci Res* 53: 663-669.

7. Ikemoto A, Hirano A, Matsumoto S, Akiguchi I, Kimura J (1996) Synaptophysin expression in the anterior horn of Werdnig-Hoffmann disease. *J Neurol Sci* 136: 94-100.

8. Iwahashi H, Eguchi Y, Yasuhara N, Hanafusa T, Matsuzawa Y, Tsujimoto Y (1997) Synergistic anti-apoptotic activity between Bcl-2 and SMN implicated in spinal muscular atrophy. *Nature* 390: 413-417.

9. Kamoshita S, Takei Y, Miyao M, Yanagisawa M, Kobayashi S, Saito K (1990) Pontocerebellar hypoplasia associated with infantile motor neuron disease (Norman's disease). *Pediatric Pathology* 10: 133-142.

10. McShane MA, Boyd S, Harding B, Brett EM, Wilson J (1992) Progressive bulbar paralysis of childhood: a reappraisal of Fazio-Londe disease. *Brain* 115: 1889-1900.

11. Mellins RB, Hays AP, Gold AP, Berdon WE, Bowdler JD (1974) Respiratory distress as the initial manifestation of Werdnig-Hoffmann disease. Pediatrics 53: 33-40.

12. Murayama S, Bouldin TW, Suzuki K (1991) Immunocytochemical and ultrastructural studies of Werdnig-Hoffmann disease. *Acta Neuropathol (Berl)* 81: 408-417.

13. Norman RM, Kay JM (1965) Cerebello-thalamo-spinal degeneration in infancy: an unusual variant of Werdnig-Hoffmann Disease. *Arch Dis Childhood* 40: 302-308.

14. Pearn J (1980) Classification of spinal muscular atrophies. *Lancet* 1: 919-922.

15. Rudnik Schoneborn S, Forkert R, Hahnen E, Wirth B, Zerres K (1996) Clinical spectrum and diagnostic criteria of infantile spinal muscular atrophy: further delineation on the basis of SMN gene deletion findings. *Neuropediatrics* 27: 8-15.

16. Schmalbruch H, Haase G (2001) Spinal muscular atrophy: present state. *Brain Pathol* 11: 231-247.

17. Schrank B, Gotz R, Gunnersen JM, Ure JM, Toyka KV, Smith AG, Sendtner M (1997) Inactivation of the survival motor neuron gene, a candidate gene for human spinal muscular atrophy, leads to massive cell death in early mouse embryos. *Proc Natl Acad Sci U S A* 94: 9920-9925.

18. Simic G, Seso-Simic D, Lucassen PJ, Islam A, Krsnik Z, Cviko A, Jelasic D, Barisic N, Winblad B, Kostovic I, et al (2000) Ultrastructural analysis and TUNEL demonstrate motor neuron apoptosis in Werdnig-Hoffmann disease. *J Neuropathol Exp Neurol* 59: 398-407.

19. Steimann GS, Rorke LB, Brown MJ (1980) Infantile neuronal degeneration masquerading as Werdnig-Hoffmann disease. *Annals Neurology* 8: 317-324.

20. Summers BA, Swash M, Schwartz MS, Ingram DA (1987) Juvenile-onset bulbospinal muscular atrophy with deafness: Vialetta-van Laere syndrome or Madras-type motor neuron disease? *J Neurol* 234: 440-442.

21. Yamanouchi Y, Yamanouchi H, Becker LE (1996) Synaptic alterations of anterior horn cells in Werdnig-Hoffmann disease. *Pediatr Neurol* 15: 32-35.

CHAPTER 9

Other Neurodegenerative Disorders

Chapter Editor: Peter L. Lantos

9.1 Introduction: Other Neurodegenerative Diseases 378

9.2 Inherited Amyloidoses and Neurodegeneration: Familial British Dementia and Familial Danish Dementia 380

9.3.1 Neuroaxonal Dystrophies 386

9.3.2 Infantile Neuroaxonal Dystrophy (Seitelberger Disease) 390

9.3.3 Neurodegeneration with Brain Iron Acculation, Type 1 (Hallervorden-Spatz Disease) 394

9.4 Familial Encephalopathy with Neuroserpin Inclusion Bodies 400

9.5 Neuronal Intranuclear Inclusion Disease 404

Other Neurodegenerative Disorders: Introduction

Peter L. Lantos

FENIB	familial encephalopathy with neuroserpin bodies
FBD	familial British dementia
FDD	familial Danish dementia
NAD	neuroaxonal dystrophy
NIID	neuronal intranuclear disease

The last section of this book covers 4 different neurodegenerative diseases, and unlike the previous sections, these disorders are unrelated: they are not linked by shared clinical symptomatology, similar neuropathological manifestations, common biochemical lesions, or even the same genetic abnormality. In fact, these conditions have nothing in common except that none can be classified with those previously described that conveniently fall into well-defined groups based on shared morphological, biochemical, or molecular genetic lesions. Moreover, they are rare, not only by the epidemiological yardstick of Alzheimer's disease, but also by the more modest incidence of Pick's disease or multiple system atrophy.

Nonetheless, they are important both from theoretical and practical points of view. Although rare, they may give insight into the pathogenesis of more common conditions. Practising neuropathologists should be aware enough of their existence to consider them, when appropriate, in the complex and often treacherous field of differential diagnosis of neurodegenerative disorders. There are 4 diseases, or more precisely, 4 groups in this section: inherited amyloidoses, familial enceph-alopathy with neuroserpin inclusions, neuroaxonal dystrophies, and the neuronal nuclear inclusion disease.

Familial British dementia (FBD) and familial Danish dementia (FDD) are inherited amyloidoses associated with neurodegeneration. Both show an autosomal dominant mode of inheritance with distinct mutations in the recently identified *BRI2* or *ITM2B* gene. The amyloidogenic peptides, ABri in FBD and ADan in FDD, have been biochemically characterised to be composed of 34 amino acids, sharing 22 amino acid long *N*-terminal sequences. The deposition of these abnormal peptides in the brain and cerebral vasculature is associated with degenerative changes of the grey matter and vascular damage to the white matter. Although the 2 disorders share many common morphological features, there are also differences, and it is tempting to compare the overall clinicopathological features with those of Alzheimer's disease. Although the differences are striking, there is a fundamental similarity: the deposition of an abnormal protein. This raises interesting and controversial issues of pathogenesis, since it could apparently lend further support to the so-called amyloid cascade hypothesis of Alzheimer's disease. Whether FBD and FDD will give additional insight into the cellular mechanism of Alzheimer's disease—particularly molecular—remains to be established.

While inherited amyloidoses are genetically well-defined, neuroaxonal dystrophies (NAD) cover an heterogeneous group of diseases based on a morphological common denominator: the presence of abnormal axonal swellings or "spheroids." The underlying pathogenetic mechanisms vary, and 3 groups can be conveniently distinguished: physiological, primary, and secondary NAD. The physiological form, an ageing phenomenon, may appear as early as the end of the first decade of life to increase with age, and may be responsible for some of the neurological impairment associated with ageing. Secondary NAD usually develops as a non-specific change in a variety of neurological disorders as diverse as Parkinson's disease, chronic alcoholism, and cystic fibrosis. It is primary NADs in which the formation of axonal abnormalities is the core pathology. The 2 commonest are infantile neuroaxonal dystrophy (Seitelberger's disease) and neurodegeneration with brain iron accumulation, type I (previously known as Hallervorden-Spatz disease).

The histological hallmark of all NADs is the widespread presence of dystrophic axons in the central, peripheral, and autonomic nervous systems. They are spherical, eosinophilic, and argyrophilic structures with a rather indiscriminate immunoreactivity for neurofilament proteins, ubiquitin, superoxide dismutase, and synucleins. Electron microscopy shows these abnormal axons to contain a wide range of cytoplasmic organelles, probably with altered structures. Recent important developments in our understanding of NADs include the discovery of mutations in neurodegeneration with brain iron accumulation, type I, the clarification of the immunohistochemical phenotypes of abnormal axons and the construction of mutant mice to provide suitable experimental models.

Familial encephalopathy with neuroserpin inclusion bodies (FENIB) is a recently described, extremely rare neurodegenerative disease. It has an autosomal dominant inheritance pattern linked to mutations in the *SERPINI1* gene that, in turn, encodes the *ser*in *p*roteinase *in*hibitor, neuroserpin, expressed in neurons. The pathognomonic histological lesions, the so-called Collins bodies, are round, eosinophilic cytoplasmic inclusions up to 50 μm to be found in neurons in the grey matter of the CNS and in the dorsal root ganglia of the spinal cord. They are argyrophilic, PAS positive, diastase resistant, and positively immunostain with antibodies to neuroserpin. In the electron microscope they appear to be composed of osmiophilic globlules with an amorphous or finely granular structure. Thus, Collins bodies, being different from inclusions of other neurodegenerative diseases, provide a reliable diagnostic hallmark of FENIB. The clinical symptomatology ranges from presenile dementia, through epilepsy with dementia, to progressive myoclonus.

The last disorder in this section is neuronal intranuclear disease (NIID). It is rare, and since its first description in 1980, only some 30 cases have been reported throughout the world. The neuropathological diagnosis is secured by the ubiquitous presence of well demarcated, round, eosinophilic inclusions in neuronal nuclei. Their size is usually 2 to 6 μm, although larger ones may also occur. Moreover, occasional, smaller inclusions of 1 to 2 μm in diameter are also present in astrocytic nuclei. The antigenic profile of these inclusions is of interest: while ubiquitin positive, they do not react with antibodies to most cytoskeletal proteins, including tau and other components of neurofilaments. Nonetheless, ultrastructurally they are composed of randomly distributed filaments of about 8 to 10 μm in diameter.

Although most of the above disorders are rare and relatively recently described, we have already accumulated a considerable amount of information about their phenotypic manifestations, both clinical and neuropathological, their molecular genetics, histological hallmark lesions, and the biochemistry of the abnormal proteins that may characterise these conditions. Investigation of more cases will produce much needed further knowledge of their pathogenesis.

Inherited Amyloidoses and Neurodegeneration: Familial British Dementia and Familial Danish Dementia

Tamas Revesz
Jorge Ghiso
Gordon T. Plant
Janice L. Holton
Blas Frangione

FBD	familial British dementia
FDD	familial Danish dementia
GSS	Gerstmann-Sträussler-Scheinker syndrome

Definition

Familial British dementia (FBD) and familial Danish dementia (FDD) are inherited forms of cerebral amyloidosis, characterised by widespread cerebral amyloid angiopathy and deposition of extracellular protein aggregates in combination with severe neurofibrillary degeneration (5, 6, 11, 12). FBD is one of the "dementia and spasticity" syndromes (7), in which cerebellar ataxia is also a common feature. Dementia and ataxia, preceded by the development of cataracts and hearing loss early in the disease process, characterise FDD. Both diseases show an autosomal dominant mode of inheritance, and are associated with distinct mutations of the recently identified *BRI2* gene also known as *ITM2B* gene (9, 15, 16). Proteolytic processing of the mutated precursor proteins, which are elongated in both diseases due to the specific genetic alterations, leads to the release of the newly created amyloidogenic peptides, ABri in FBD and ADan in FDD (15, 16).

Synonyms and Historical Annotation

FBD is the most recent term (15) given for the description of a rare familial disease, clinically characterised by gradually progressive dementia, spastic tetraparesis and ataxia (8, 11). The condition was originally described by Worster-Drought et al as familial presenile dementia with spastic paralysis in 1933 (18). The pathological description of the disease that followed a few years later is the earliest English language description of cerebral amyloid angiopathy (17), although it was not until some years later that re-examination of the cases by the same authors confirmed the vascular changes as amyloid angiopathy. This condition has been quoted with other terms in the literature, such as atypical Alzheimer's disease, Gerstmann-Sträussler-Scheinker syndrome (GSS), a form of familial amyloid angiopathy, and hereditary spastic paraparesis (10, 11).

FDD, an autosomal dominantly inherited disease with a clinical presentation suggestive of ocular, auditory and central nervous system involvement, was first described by Strömgren et al under the term of heredopathia ophthalmo-oto-encephalica in members of a single pedigree living northeast of Århus, Denmark (13, 14).

Epidemiology

Incidence and prevalence. Both conditions are rare; FBD has been identified in 3 pedigrees, 2 of which may be related (unpublished data). The data about the original family have repeatedly been updated and information about 9 generations dating back to the late-18th century is now available (8, 11). This pedigree includes 35 historical cases, 52 living descendants at risk of developing the disease, and also 6 living affected patients. FDD has so far been described in a single pedigree with 13 affected members with a further 2 probably affected individuals (6).

Sex and age distribution. In FBD the median age of onset of the disease is 48 years (range from 40-60), the median age at death is 56 years (range from 48-70). The mean duration of illness is 9 years. Males and females are approximately equally affected (8).

In 10 cases of FDD in which information is available, the median age of onset of the visual symptoms is 27 years (range from 10-46), while the median age at death is 58 years (range from 34-62). Males and females are equally affected (6, 13, Hans Brandgaard, personal communication).

Risk factors. Apart from the genetic risk described below, there are no other known risk factors in either disease.

Genetics

It has been demonstrated that a T→A mutation of the stop codon of the recently discovered *BRI2* gene, located on the long arm chromosome 13, is associated with FBD (15). The wild type *BRI2* gene encodes a type II, single-spanning transmembrane protein (BriPP), which is composed of 266 amino acids, while the extended mutated precursor protein has 277 amino acids (ABriPP). Cleavage of the C-terminal 34 amino acids of the mutated precursor protein generates a fragment, amyloid-Bri or ABri, which is deposited as amyloid in leptomeningeal and parenchymal blood vessels as well as in parenchymal plaques. It also forms preamyloid lesions in many areas of the central nervous system (Figure 1) (5, 15).

FDD is associated with a 10-nt duplication (TTT AAT TTG T), occurring between codons 265 and 266, which is one codon before the normal stop codon of the *BRI2* gene. This results in a frame-shift in the gene sequence and, by abolishing the normal stop codon, the production of a 277 amino acid long, extended precursor protein (ADanPP) (16). The amyloidogenic peptide, amyloid-Dan or ADan, similar to ABri, consists of 34 amino acids, although these have a different sequence at the C-termimus, and is deposited as amyloid in leptomeningeal and cerebral blood vessels as well as parenchymal lesions, which are most frequently preamyloid (6, 16) (Figure 1).

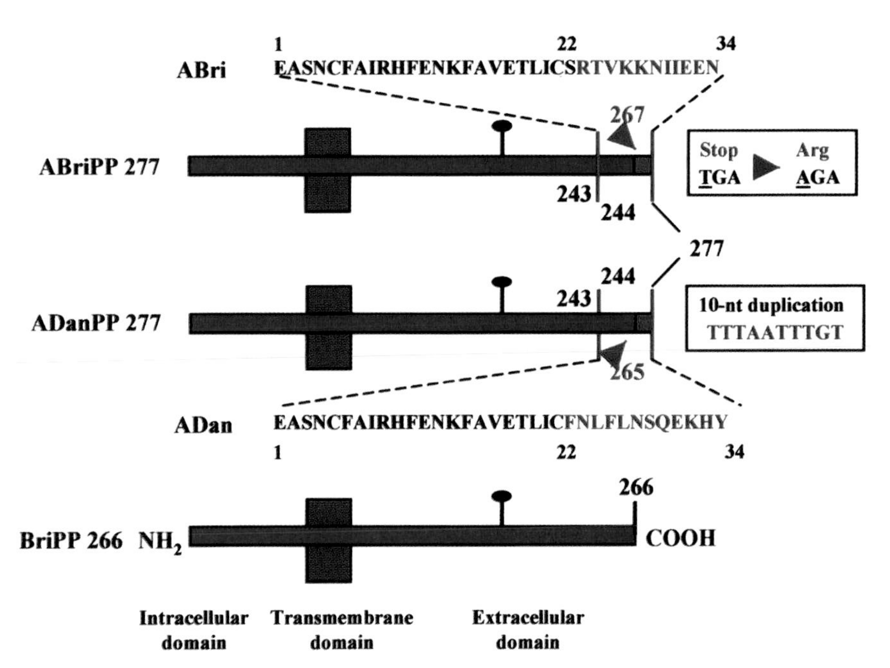

Figure 1. Genetic defects, amyloid precursor proteins and amyloid peptides in familial British dementia and familial Danish dementia.

Clinical Features

Symptoms and signs. In FBD the most consistent neuropsychological finding at an early stage is isolated memory loss. Affected individuals often complain of headaches, and there is usually evidence of personality change, psychological problems, and sleep disturbances. With the progression of the disease, cerebellar ataxia and spastic paraplegia are characteristic. Brainstem signs, pseudo-bulbar palsy, and dysarthria are common, and stroke-like episodes may be present. Patients progress to a chronic vegetative state, become mute, unresponsive, tetraplegic, and doubly incontinent. In contrast to other familial cerebrovascular amyloidoses, cerebral haemorrhage is relatively rare (8, 11).

In FDD visual disturbance is the earliest symptom as patients develop cataracts usually before the age of 30. This may be followed by other ocular disorders such as haemorrhages. The visual abnormality is severe, resulting in greatly impaired vision or blindness. Ten to twenty years after the beginning of the ocular symptoms the patients develop severe to total perceptive loss of hearing. Cerebellar ataxia usually starts after age 40, followed by psychiatric disturbance and progressive dementia (1, 6, 13, 16).

Neuroimaging. MRI scans of patients with FBD show hyperintensities in the cerebral white matter from an early stage of the disease. These are most pronounced around the frontal and occipital horns of the lateral ventricles. Infarcts and atrophy of the corpus callosum are also common (Figure 2A).

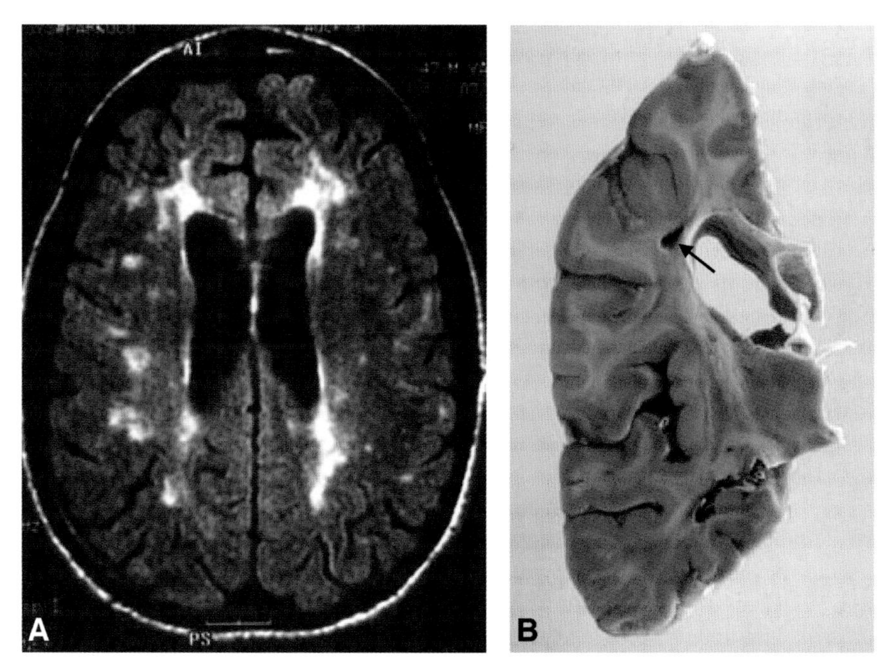

Figure 2. Neuroimaging and macroscopic findings in familial British dementia. **A.** FLAIR MRI showing extensive white matter high signal intensities. **B.** Atrophied deep white matter with a lacunar infarct.

Neuroimaging studies in FDD show the presence of white matter changes, which are similar to those seen in FBD (10).

Laboratory findings. *Blood tests.* Blood samples of at risk individuals may be used for genetic testing. In affected individuals of the British pedigree, the mutation introduces an *XbaI* restriction site, which is absent in normal controls and individuals carrying the Danish mutation. In those with the Danish disease gel electrophoresis of PCR-amplified genomic DNA fragments reveals an extra band due to the 10-nt duplication. DNA sequence analysis of amplified DNA fragments confirms the characteristic T→A mutation of the stop codon and 10-nt duplication between codons 265 and 266 in FBD and FDD, respectively (15, 16).

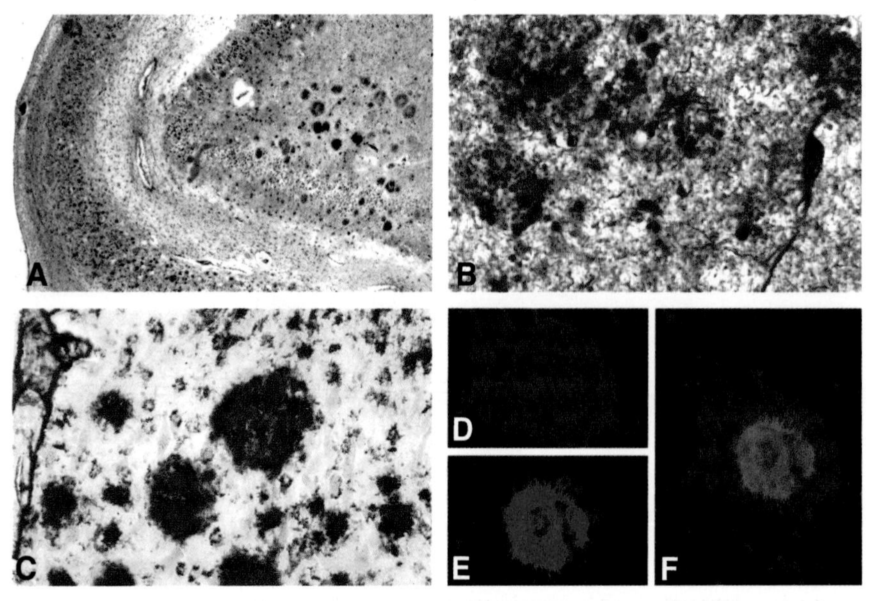

Figure 3. Histological features of familial British dementia. **A.** Argyrophilic "large plaques," "small plaques" and neurofibrillary tangles in the hippocampus. **B.** Tau-positive neurofibrillary tangles, neuropil threads and abnormal neurites in the amygdala. **C.** Hippocampal amyloid plaques showing strong immunoreactivity for ABri. **D-F.** Spinal cord blood vessel with amyloid is immunoreactive for ABri (**D**) and positive with thioflavin S (**E**) (confocal microscopy, **F**: combined image).

In cases with FBD a soluble form of ABri has been shown to be present in the circulation with an estimated concentration around 20 ng/ml (3). No similar data are available as yet in patients with FDD.

CSF, EEG and other investigations. Data of patients with FBD suggest that both examination of the cerebrospinal fluid and EEG, which most frequently shows a diffuse, non-specific abnormality, are unhelpful in the diagnosis.

In cases with FDD, detailed ophthalmological testing reveals posterior subcapsular cataract and retinal neovascularisations leading to vitreous haemorrhages and neovascular glaucoma. Electroretinography shows decreased amplitude of the rod and cone responses and extinguished oscillatory potential (1).

Macroscopy

Information about the macroscopic pathology is available in 7 cases of FBD. The brain weight, which is known in 5 cases, varies between 1120 g and 1400 g, and a thickening of the leptomeninges over the frontal lobes is often described. The lateral and third ventricles are moderately enlarged and diffuse cerebral atrophy may also occur. The cerebral cortex is usually well-preserved, while the deep white matter, including the corpus callosum, is reduced in bulk and shows patchy greyish discolouration with scattered lacunar infarcts (Figure 2B). The hippocampi are atrophied in some cases. While the lentiform and caudate nuclei are usually well-preserved, the thalamus, which may contain lacunar infarcts, may be reduced in size. In the majority of the cases the brainstem is normal, while the cerebellum may show vascular lesions. The spinal cord usually appears normal, although in one case the cord was reported to be reduced in size with areas of the lateral columns showing greyish discolouration.

Macroscopic changes have been documented only in a small number of cases of FDD with the brain weights, available in 2 cases, varying between 1220 g and 1438 g. The leptomeninges are thickened; a degree of cortical atrophy together with some dilatation of the lateral ventricles is seen and the hippocampi may be small. The hemispheric white matter is reduced in bulk and may contain focal perivascular grey, translucent areas. The cerebellum and spinal cord show evidence of atrophy, and the cranial and spinal roots have been noted to be thin and firm.

Histopathology

FBD is characterised by deposition of amyloid in the blood vessels as well as in the parenchyma in combination with neurofibrillary degeneration. The structures most affected by amyloid deposition are the hippocampus and cerebellum. The widespread amyloid angiopathy affects leptomeningeal and parenchymal grey and white matter vessels of nearly all central nervous system areas, including the cerebrum, cerebellum, brainstem and the spinal cord (Figure 3D, E, F). There are only a few sites spared, and such structures include the striatum and the substantia nigra. The majority of the affected blood vessels has a diameter of less than 300 μm and capillary involvement is also present in some of the affected anatomical regions (5). Amyloid deposition around a significant proportion of blood vessels, which has been described as perivascular plaques, is also a feature. Cerebellar degeneration due to severe cerebral amyloid angiopathy and parenchymal, often perivascular, amyloid deposition is characteristic. In the cerebrum parenchymal amyloid plaques as well as neurofibrillary degeneration are most severe in limbic structures (Figure 3A, B). The hippocampal amyloid plaques are of 2 types; large plaques, up to 150 μm in diameter are often seen in the CA4 subregion of the hippocampus, while smaller amyloid plaques with a diameter of up to 30 μm are characteristic in the CA1 subregion and the subiculum (Figure 3A, C). Amyloid plaques are relatively rare in neocortical areas. Neurofibrillary tangles and neuropil threads are numerous in the limbic structures and a proportion of the amyloid plaques is associated with argyrophilic abnormal neurites. White matter degeneration similar to that found in Binswanger's subcortical arteriosclerotic encephalopathy, presumably due to severe cerebral amyloid angiopathy, is a feature. The retinal blood vessels also show extensive amyloid deposition (5). A striking astrocytic response together with an activated microglial reaction is associ-

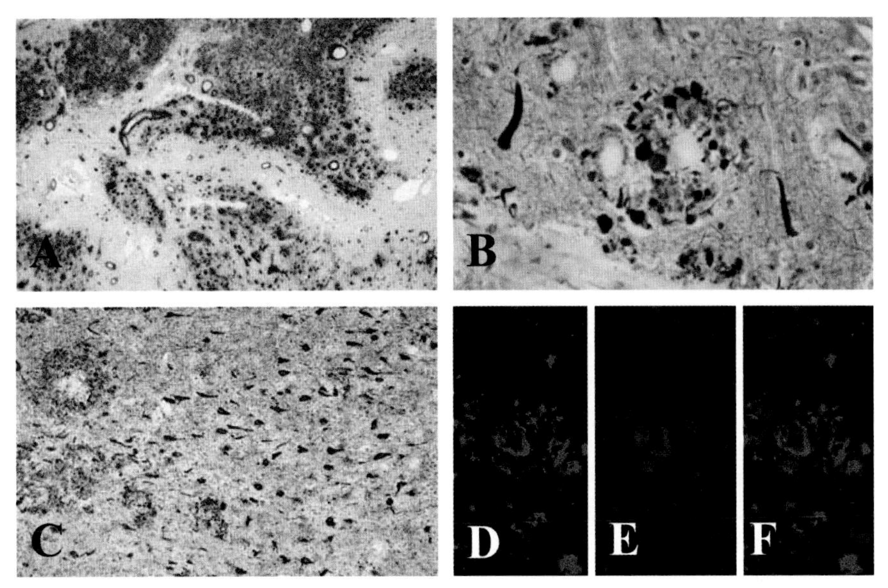

Figure 4. Histological features of familial Danish dementia. **A.** Extensive deposition of ADan in the hippocampus. **B, C.** Argyrophilic and tau positive neurofibrillary tangles and neuropil threads in the hippocampus; abnormal neurites only around amyloid laden blood vessels. **D-F.** Codeposition of Aβ (**D**) and ADan (**E**) (confocal microscopy, **F**: combined image).

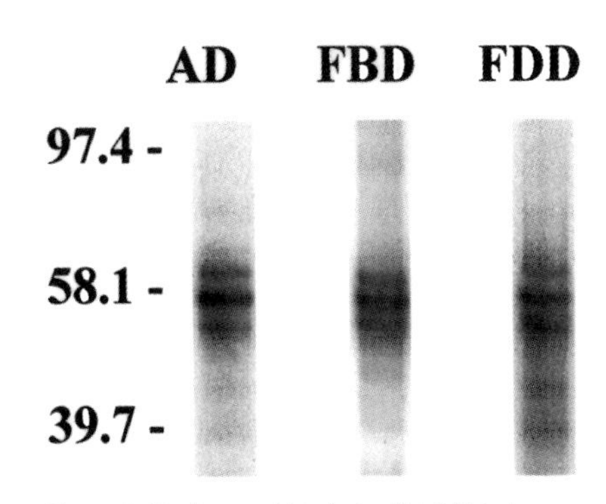

Figure 5. Tau immunoblots in familial British dementia (FBD) and familial Danish dementia (FDD). In both diseases there is a triplet electrophoretic migration pattern, identical to that seen in Alzheimer's disease (AD).

ated with the vascular and parenchymal amyloid deposits in FBD.

Although the microscopic findings in FDD are, in general, similar to those of FBD, there are also noteworthy differences between the 2 diseases (Figure 4A-F). *i)* In FDD, although abundant preamyloid lesions are present (see below), hippocampal argyrophilic, amyloid plaques are absent and the numerous abnormal neurites that are present, are formed only around blood vessels with amyloid angiopathy (Figure 4B). *ii)* The cerebral cortices are more extensively affected by protein deposits and neurofibrillary pathology in FDD than in FBD. *iii)* Perivascular plaque formation in the cerebellum, which is a prominent feature of FBD, is less severe in FDD. *iv)* The retinal pathology, including amyloid angiopathy and parenchymal damage, is more severe in FDD than in FBD (1, 6).

Clinicopathological correlations. In FBD, the hippocampal, limbic pathology explains the prominent and early amnesic syndrome and, together with the extensive white matter changes, accounts for the dementia. The severe cerebellar degeneration correlates with the ataxia and the white matter pathology explains the spastic paraparesis.

The ocular presentation in FDD is associated with subcapsular cataract, retinal neovascularisation resulting in vitreous haemorrhages and neovascular glaucoma (1). Investigation of the eye shows amyloid in retinal blood vessels and parenchyma and evidence of previous haemorrhages with severe parenchymal damage. At present the mechanism of hearing loss in FDD is largely unknown. The severe degeneration of limbic structures and involvement of the cerebral cortices by neurofibrillary degeneration in combination with Binswanger-type white matter changes explain the dementia syndrome, while the cerebellar degeneration accounts for the ataxia.

Immunohistochemistry and Ultrastructural Findings

The blood vessels affected by amyloid deposition (Congo red and Thioflavin S positive deposits) are positively stained with antibodies specifically recognising the mutated extensions of ABri and ADan in FBD and FDD, respectively (Figures 3C, D, 4A, D). In FBD the anti-ABri antibody also stains the different hippocampal, limbic plaque types and the parenchymal amyloid plaques in the cerebellum and other structures. In FDD the parenchymal deposition of ADan, is also extensive, although the protein aggregates are primarily of preamyloid nature (Congo red and Thioflavin S negative deposits). Immunoelectron microscopic examination of the vascular and parenchymal lesions also confirms that ABri and ADan can be deposited in both fibrillar (amyloid) and non-fibrillar (preamyloid) configurations.

In both conditions, neurofibrillary tangles are composed ultrastructurally of typical paired helical filaments (PHFs) and are immunohistochemically indistinguishable from neurofibrillary tangles in Alzheimer's disease (12) (Figure 3B, 4C).

ABri immunohistochemistry shows that ABri is also deposited in blood vessels and parenchyma of systemic organs (3). Data are not available in FDD cases yet.

A feature of all cases with FDD so far examined is the presence of various degrees of Aβ peptide deposition, either in combination with ADan or alone, in blood vessels and in brain parenchyma (Figure 4D-F). The Aβ parenchymal deposition, similar to that of ADan, most severely affect the limbic structures, but is also seen in neocortical areas where it is more severe than deposition of ADan. The cause and significance of the codeposition of ADan and Aβ are not clear at present.

Biochemistry

The origin of the amyloidogenic subunits, ABri and ADan deposited in the central nervous system as amyloid and preamyloid, remains to be investigated.

In both FBD and FDD, furin-like proteolytic processing of the mutated precursor proteins generates characteristic 4 kDa amyloidogenic fragments, ABri and ADan, respectively, which form amyloid fibrils and preamyloid lesions. ADan and ABri are both 34 amino acids in length and share common 22 amino acid long N-terminal sequences (Figure 1). However, the 2 amyloidogenic peptides have unique C-termini composed of 12 amino acids, which allow their recognition by "disease specific" antibodies (15, 16). Amyloid isolated from leptomeningeal deposits shows that both ABri and ADan are highly polymerised and have post-translationally modified N-termini (pyroglutamate) (15). Synthetic peptides homologous to the ABri sequence are able to mimic in vitro the in vivo properties of ABri in that they show a high tendency for polymerisation and formation of amyloid-like fibrils under physiological conditions (2, 4).

In both FBD and FDD, Western blotting shows that insoluble, hyperphosphorylated tau has a triplet electrophoretic migration pattern, which is indistinguishable from that of PHF-tau in Alzheimer's disease (5, 6) (Figure 5).

Differential Diagnosis

The major clinical differential diagnosis of FBD and FDD includes atypical Alzheimer's disease with spastic paraparesis, GSS, primary progressive multiple sclerosis, spinocerebellar ataxia with cognitive impairment, olivo-ponto-cerebellar atrophy, Binswanger's disease, and CADASIL (8). In the pathological differential diagnosis, other hereditary cerebral amyloid angiopathies can be considered, including: hereditary cerebral haemorrhage Dutch type (APP gene), hereditary cerebral haemorrhage Icelandic type (cystatin C gene), oculoleptomeningeal amyloidosis (transthyretin gene), a form of GSS associated with a premature stop codon mutation with amyloid angiopathy and neurofibrillary degeneration (prion protein gene), and also familial Alzheimer's disease (APP, PS1 and PS2 genes), especially atypical Alzheimer's disease with spastic paraparesis and cotton wool plaques (PS1 gene). The amyloid angiopathy in both FBD and FDD is more widespread than in the other hereditary cerebral amyloid angiopathies and affects most parts of the central nervous system (5, 6, 11). This feature together with the characteristic plaque morphology in cases of the British pedigree (12) are important indicators of the pathological diagnosis. Furthermore, with the use of specific antibodies, recognising ABri and ADan, a specific pathological diagnosis can be made even before genetic information is available for the pathologist.

Pathogenesis

The mechanism of neurofibrillary degeneration in the *BRI2* gene-related conditions is not known. The close topographic association of both ABri and ADan lesions with tau pathology is, however, in keeping with the hypothesis that ABri and ADan-mediated neurotoxicity, similar to that of Aβ in Alzheimer's disease, is likely to be of primary importance in the neurodegenerative process (5, 6).

Future Directions and Therapy

As FBD and FDD both share important morphological features with Alzheimer's disease, future studies of transgenic animal models are awaited. As both ABri and ADan are newly created peptides due to disease-specific mutations and are not present in normal individuals, such models may provide direct evidence for the link between cerebral amyloid deposition and neurodegeneration.

Genetic counselling is available for individuals at risk for developing the disease, but no therapy is currently available. Future success of new therapeutic approaches, aiming at lowering cerebral Aβ load in Alzheimer's disease by immunisation or pharmacological means, may facilitate the design of similar therapies for patients suffering from other cerebral amyloidoses including FBD and FDD.

References

1. Bek T (2000) Ocular changes in heredo-oto-ophthalmo-encephalopathy. *Br J Ophthalmol* 84:1298-1302.

2. El Agnaf OM, Sheridan JM, Sidera C, Siligardi G, Hussain R, Haris PI, Austen BM (2001) Effect of the disulfide bridge and the C-terminal extension on the oligomerization of the amyloid peptide ABri implicated in Familial British Dementia. *Biochemistry* 40:3449-3457.

3. Ghiso J, Holton J, Miravelle L, Calero M, Lashley T, Vidal R, Houlden H, Wood N, Neubert T, Rostagno A, Plant G, Revesz T, Frangione B (2001) Systemic amyloid deposits in familial British dementia. *J Biol Chem* 276: 43909-43914.

4. Ghiso J, Vidal R, Rostagno A, Miravalle L, Holton JL, Mead S, Revesz T, Plant G, Frangione B (2000) Amyloidogenesis in familial British dementia is associated with a genetic defect on chromosome 13. *Ann N Y Acad Sci* 920:84-92.

5. Holton JL, Ghiso J, Lashley T, Rostagno A, Guerin CJ, Gibb G, Houlden H, Ayling H, Martinian L, Anderton BH, Wood NW, Vidal R, Plant G, Frangione B, Revesz T (2001) Regional Distribution of Amyloid-Bri Deposition and Its Association with Neurofibrillary Degeneration in Familial British Dementia. *Am J Pathol* 158:515-526.

6. Holton JL, Lashley T, Ghiso J, Braendgaard H, Vidal R, Guerin CJ, Gibb G, Hanger DP, Rostagno A, Anderton BH, Strand C, Ayling H, Plant G, Frangione B, Bojsen-Moller M, Revesz T (2002) Familial Danish dementia: a novel form of cerebral amyloidosis associated with deposition of both amyloid-Dan and amyloid-beta. *J Neuropathol Exp Neurol* 61: 254-267.

7. Masters CL, Beyreuther K (2001) The Worster-Drought syndrome and other syndromes of dementia with spastic paraparesis: the paradox of molecular pathology. *J Neuropathol Exp Neurol* 60:317-319.

8. Mead S, James-Galton M, Revesz T, Doshi RB, Harwood G, Pan EL, Ghiso J, Frangione B, Plant G (2000) Familial British dementia with amyloid angiopathy: early clinical, neuropsychological and imaging findings. *Brain* 123:975-991.

9. Pittois K, Deleersnijder W, Merregaert J (1998) cDNA sequence analysis, chromosomal assignment and expression pattern of the gene coding for integral membrane protein 2B. *Gene* 217:141-149.

10. Plant GT, Esiri MM (1997) Familial cerebral amyloid angiopathies. In *The Neuropathology of Dementia*. Esiri MM, Morris JH (eds). University Press: Cambridge. pp. 260-276.

11. Plant GT, Revesz T, Barnard RO, Harding AE, Gautier-Smith PC (1990) Familial cerebral amyloid angiopathy with nonneuritic amyloid plaque formation. *Brain* 113:721-747.

12. Revesz T, Holton JL, Doshi B, Anderton BH, Scaravilli F, Plant GT (1999) Cytoskeletal pathology in familial cerebral amyloid angiopathy (British type) with

non-neuritic amyloid plaque formation. *Acta Neuropathol (Berl)* 97:170-176.

13. Strömgren E (1981) Heredopathia ophthalmo-oto-encephalica. In *Handbook of Clinical Neurology*. Vinken PJ, Bruyn GW (eds). North-Holland Publishing Company: Amsterdam. pp. 150-152.

14. Strömgren, E, Dalby A, Dalby MA, Ranheim B (1970) Cataract, deafness, cerebellar ataxia, psychosis and dementia: A new syndrome. *Acta Neurol Scand* (Suppl 43) 46:261-262.

15. Vidal R, Frangione B, Rostagno A, Mead S, Revesz T, Plant G, Ghiso J (1999) A stop-codon mutation in the BRI gene associated with familial British dementia. *Nature* 399:776-781.

16. Vidal R, Revesz T, Rostagno A, Kim E, Holton JL, Bek T, Bojsen-Moller M, Braendgaard H, Plant G, Ghiso J, Frangione B (2000) A decamer duplication in the 3' region of the BRI gene originates an amyloid peptide that is associated with dementia in a Danish kindred. *Proc Natl Acad Sci U S A* 97:4920-4925.

17. Worster-Drought C, Greenfield JG, McMenemey WH (1940) A form of familial presenile dementia with spastic paralysis (including the pathological examination of a case). *Brain* 63:237-254.

18. Worster-Drought C, Hill TR, McMenemey WH (1933) Familial presenile dementia with spastic paralysis. *J Neurol Psychopathol* 14:27-34.

Neuroaxonal Dystrophies

Kurt A. Jellinger
John Duda

BTB	broad complex, tramtrack and brick-a-brack
CT	computer tomography
GFAP	glial fibrillary acidic protein
GAN	giant axonal dystrophy or neuropathy
HDSL	hereditary diffuse leukoencephalopathy with spheroids
IF	intermediate filaments
INAD	infantile neuroaxonal dystrophy
NAD	neuroaxonal dystrophy
NS	nervous system
TYRO	tyrosine kinase binding protein

Definition

Neuroaxonal dystrophies (NADs) (21) includes a group of rare sporadic or familial neurodegenerative disorders of undetermined aetiology (Table 1), clinically presenting with progressive neuropsychiatric dysfunctions in different age groups and morphologically characterised by the occurrence of axon swellings ("spheroids") in the central, peripheral and autonomous nervous systems, composed of structured material and associated with other neuropathological findings (Table 2).

Infantile neuroaxonal dystrophy (Seitelberger's disease) and late infantile, juvenile and rare adult NAD are presented in chapter 9.3.2. Hallervorden-Spatz disease (Neurodegeneration with brain iron accumulation, type I) is described in chapter 9.3.3. The remaining types (Table 1) are introduced in the following paragraphs.

Physiological and Secondary NAD

The development of NAD is a common morphological finding in certain parts of the CNS and may account for some of the neurological decline seen with ageing. Physiological NAD is seen in the gracile and cuneate nuclei, zona reticulata of substantia nigra, and medial globus pallidus from the age of about 10 years (21). The age related incidence of NAD in the first 4 decades in the gracile nucleus ranges from 9 to 13% and increases with age to almost 100% over the age of 80 years (10). Similar changes are seen in sympathetic ganglia with ageing (13, 20). NAD predominantly in the gracile nucleus related to dying-back axonal changes is also seen in aged dogs, rats, and monkeys (7).

NAD may also occur as a symptomatic phenomenon in other disorders, either as accentuation of the severity or a more widespread distribution of physiological NAD. Increased intensity of physiological NAD in the pallido-nigral system, often associated with accumulation of iron-lipofuscin containing pigment in dystrophic axons and glia, is seen in Parkinson disease, Parkinson-dementia-ALS complex on Guam, multiple system atrophy, and chronic alcoholism. Development of widespread NAD with or without pallidonigral pigmentation may be seen in cystic fibrosis, mucoviscidosis, congenital biliary artresia, neuronal storage diseases, eg, Niemann-Pick type C, Zellweger syndrome, neurolipidoses, Wilson's disease, vitamin E deficiency (also in experimental animals), anticancer chemotherapy, HTLV-1 infection, and after long-term demyelination in experimental allergic encephalomyelitis (13, 18, 23).

Giant Axonal Neuropathy

Giant axonal dystrophy or neuropathy (GAN) is an autosomal recessive neurodegenerative disorder affecting both the peripheral and central nervous systems due to mutations of the gene encoding gigaxonin, a new member of the cytoskeletal BTB/kelch repeat family, encoded to chromosome 16q24.1 (1, 3-6, 12). It is clinically characterised by the development of chronic distal polyneuropathy during childhood, areflexia, ataxia, nystagmus, mental retardation, dysarthria, and rare optic nerve atrophy, kinky or curly hair, and skeletal abnormalities. Cranial CT and MRI show diffuse demyelination or atrophy of the brain (15).

Morphologically, axonal spheroids are found in dorsal columns and their nuclei, in the corticospinal tracts, middle cerebellar peduncle, basal ganglia, deep cortex, and cerebral and cerebellar white matter associated with astrogliosis. In subependymal, subpial, and periventricular areas, numerous Rosenthal fibres are seen, and pseudotumourous proliferation of astrocytes can obstruct the aqueduct and fourth ventricle. Ultrastructurally, the axonal swellings of 50 to 100 μm diameters, in contrast to the spheroids in INAD, are composed of densely packed neurofilaments with increased diameter and reduced numbers of lateral processes. In between, electron dense granular material is found (Figure 1). GAN corresponds to a generalised disorganisation of the cytoskeletal inter-

1. Physiological NAD, as part of normal or pathological brain ageing
2. Secondary (symptomatic) NAD occurring as a "reactive" process in other conditions
3. Primary NAD: Diseases in which the main pathology is NAD:
    a. Infantile neuroaxonal dystrophy (Seitelberger's disease), Chapter 9.3.2
    b. Late infantile, juvenile and rare adult NAD
    c. Neuroaxonal leukodystrophy
    d. Hallervorden-Spatz disease (Neurodegeneration with brain iron accumulation, type I), Chapter 9.3.3
    e. Nasu-Hakola disease
    f. Giant axonal dystrophy

Table 1. Different types of neuroaxonal dystrophy.

Type thal	Onset (years)	Death (years)	Heredity	Principal neurological symptoms: Muscular hypotonia	Pyramidal tract signs	Cerebellar symptoms	Extra-pyramidal symptoms	Psychomotor retardation (dementia)	Optic nerve atrophy	Principal neuropathological findings: Localized spheroids	Status dysmyelin-isation	Iron pigment in basal ganglia	Lipid depos-ition globus pallidus	Cerebral atrophy	Rosen- fibres
Generalized form															
Infantile	< 1	6-11	} autosomal recessive	++	++	+	(+)	++	+	CNS, periph. & auton. NS	++	–	+	++	–
Late infantile	1-2	8-12	} sporadic	–	++	–	+	++		localized and/or disseminated	+	(+)	(+)	(+)	–
Juvenile	9-21	21-38	}	(+)	++	+	+	+	–	CNS, periph. NS	+	+	(+)	++	–
Giant axonal dystrophy	1-3 (-6)	5-30	autosomal recessive	++	+	+	–	+	(+)	CNS – disseminated	–	(+)	–	+	+
Neuroaxonal leuko-dystrophy	Adults (24-50)		autosomal dominant	–	+	(+)	++	++	–	cer. white matter, cortex	–	–	–	–	–
Localized form															
Hallervorden-Spatz-disease	7-12	12-40	autosomal, recessive, sporadic	(+)	+	(+)	++	+	(+)	globus pall., subst. nigra	–	++	(+)	(+)	–

Table 2. Principal neurological symptoms and neuropathological findings of primary neuroaxonal dystrophies.

mediate filaments (IFs) to which neurofilaments belong, as abnormal aggregation of multiple tissue specific IFs has been reported; vimentin in endothelial cells, pericytes, Schwann cells, perineural cells, melanocytes, Langerhans cells, cultured skin fibroblasts, and glial fibrillary acidic protein (GFAP) in astrocytes. Keratin IFs also seem to be altered in hairs.

The gene encoding gigaxonin, a ubiquitously expressed protein composed of an amino terminal BTB domain followed by 6-kelch repeats, which are predicted to adopt a β-propelled shape, has been found in a series of mutations in GAN patients (4, 12). Distantly related proteins sharing a similar domain organisation have various functions associated with the cytoskeleton (1), predicting that gigaxonin is a novel and distinct cytoskeletal protein that may represent a general pathological target for other neurodegenerative disorders with alterations in the neurofilament network. GAN and INAD are considered overlap diseases in a spectrum of intermediate pathology with various organelles participating in the temporal evolution of the disease process (14).

Neuroaxonal Leukodystrophy and Nasu-Hakola Disease

Hereditary diffuse leukoencephalopathy with spheroids (HDLS) is an autosomal dominant progressive disease with variable age at onset, which was described in multiple members of a large Swedish pedigree in 1984 (2). Only a few other patients have been reported (8, 24, 25). Recent case reports concern a father and his daughter, and an unrelated patient (22). Clinical history with disease consisted of an adult-age onset (24-50 years) neurological deterioration with signs of frontal lobe dysfunction, epilepsy, spasticity, ataxia, and mild extrapyramidal symptoms. MRI showed cerebral atrophy and patchy white matter changes, most pronounced in frontal and frontoparietal areas with extension through the posterior limb of the internal capsule into the pyramidal tracts of

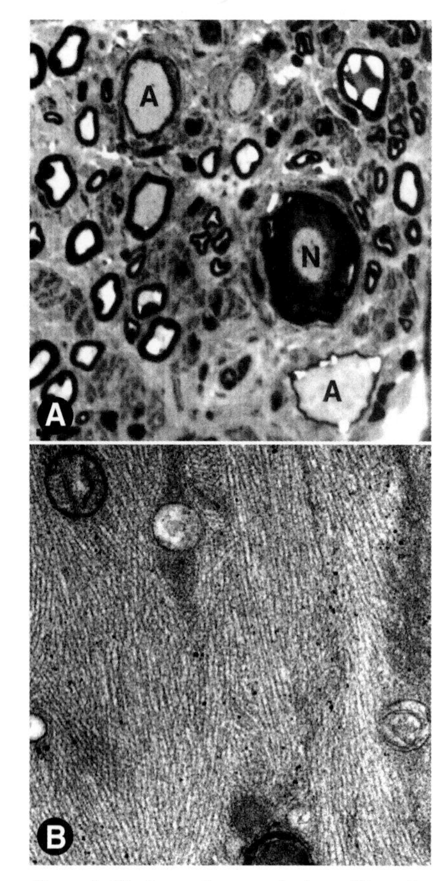

Figure 1. *Giant axonal neuropathy in an 11 months old girl (sural nerve).* **A.** The axons (A) are extremely distended and some of the myelin sheeths are extremely thin, a few others are thickened (N). Toluidin blue ×670. **B.** The giant axon contains densely packed neurofilaments. ×38 000. These illustrations kindly provided by J. M.Schröder, Aachen, Germany.

the brainstem. Autopsy in 3 patients revealed a leukoencephalopathy with frontoparietal and frontal preponderance, destruction of axons, and numerous axonal spheroids in the abnormal white matter. Ultrastructurally, the spheroids contained neurofilaments and mitochondria. Cerebral cortex, basal ganglia, and cerebellum were normal apart from marked loss of Purkinje cells.

The combination of leukoencephalopathy and axonal spheroids in the abnormal white matter, apart from HDLS is seen in membranous lipodystrophy or Nasu-Hakola disease, an autosomal recessive disorder characterised by a combination of cystic bone disease, cerebral white matter lesions, and calcium deposition in the basal ganglia leading to progressive dementia of frontal lobe type and extrapyramidal rigidity in the third

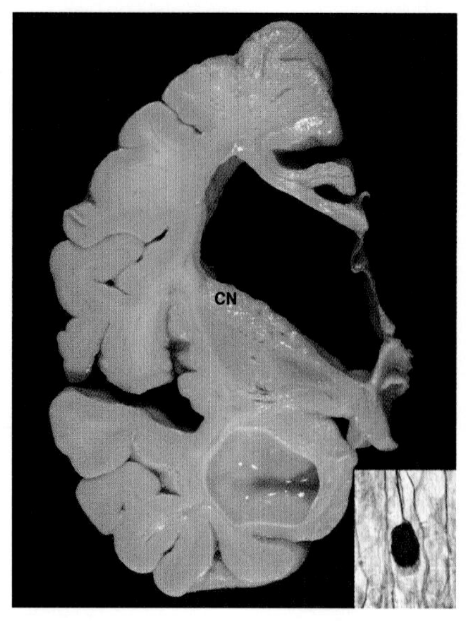

Figure 2. Coronal section of the left hemisphere of a PLOSL patient (Nasu-Hakola disease) shows reduction of the deep frontal and temporal white matter. The cingulate gyrus and corpus callosum are severely affected. The caudate nucleus (CN) is shrunken and the lateral ventricle much enlarged. **Insert:** Axonal spheroid in deep frontal white matter. Holmes silver (width of spheroid: 7.1 μm). This figure kindly provided by M. Haltia, Helsinki, Finland.

decade (9, 11, 17). It is caused by loss-of-function mutations in the gene encoding TYRO protein tyrosine kinase binding protein (TYROBP, formerly DAP12), a transmembrane protein that has been recognised as a key activating signal transduction element in natural killer cells (18). Another type is dermatoleukodystrophy with neuroaxonal spheroids that has an early infantile onset and results in early death (16). With unsuccessful searches for a primary abnormality in lipid metabolism, the pathogenesis of these rare disorders is unknown.

References

1. Adams J, Kelso R, Cooley L (2000) The kelch repeat superfamily of proteins: propellers of cell function. *Trends Cell Biol* 10: 17-24.

2. Axelsson R, Roytta M, Sourander P, Akesson HO, Andersen O (1984) Hereditary diffuse leucoencephalopathy with spheroids. *Acta Psychiatr Scand* Suppl 314: 1-65.

3. Ben Hamida C, Cavalier L, Belal S, Sanhaji H, Nadal N, Barhoumi C, M'Rissa N, Marzouki N, Mandel JL, Ben Hamida M, Koenig M, Hentati F (1997) Homozygosity mapping of giant axonal neuropathy gene to chromosome 16q24.1. *Neurogenetics* 1: 129-133.

4. Bomont P, Cavalier L, Blondeau F, Ben Hamida C, Belal S, Tazir M, Demir E, Topaloglu H, Korinthenberg R, Tuysuz B, Landrieu P, Hentati F, Koenig M (2000) The gene encoding gigaxonin, a new member of the cytoskeletal BTB/kelch repeat family, is mutated in giant axonal neuropathy. *Nat Genet* 26: 370-374.

5. Cavalier L, BenHamida C, Amouri R, Belal S, Bomont P, Lagarde N, Gressin L, Callen D, Demir E, Topaloglu H, Landrieu P, Ioos C, Hamida MB, Koenig M, Hentati F (2000) Giant axonal neuropathy locus refinement to a <590 kb critical interval. *Eur J Hum Genet* 8: 527-534.

6. Flanigan KM, Crawford TO, Griffin JW, Goebel HH, Kohlschutter A, Ranells J, Camfield PR, Ptacek LJ (1998) Localization of the giant axonal neuropathy gene to chromosome 16q24. *Ann Neurol* 43: 143-148.

7. Fujisawa K (1994) Gracile axonal dystrophy in an old (28 years) Japanese monkey: Species-specifity of ultrastructural features and particular pattern of proliferation of smooth endoplasmic reticulum. *Neuropathology* 14: 37-55.

8. Goodman L, DW D (1995) Nonhereditary diffuse leukoencephalopathy with spheroids presenting as early-onset rapidly progressive dementia. *J Neuropathol Exp Neurol* 54: 471.

9. Hakola HP, Puranen M (1993) Neuropsychiatric and brain CT findings in polycystic lipomembranous osteodysplasia with sclerosing leukoencephalopathy. *Acta Neurol Scand* 88: 370-375.

10. Jellinger K (1973) Neuroaxonal Dystrophy: Its natural history and related disorders. In *Progress in Neuropathology*, HM Zimmerman (eds). Grune & Stratton: New York- London. pp. 129-180.

11. Kondo T, Takahashi K, Kohara N, Takahashi Y, Hayashi S, Takahashi H, Matsuo H, Yamazaki M, Inoue K, Miyamoto K, Yamamura T (2002) Heterogeneity of presenile dementia with bone cysts (Nasu-Hakola disease): three genetic forms. *Neurology* 59: 1105-1107.

12. Kuhlenbäumer G, Young P, Oberwittler C, Hünermund G, Schirmacher A, Domschke K, Ringelstein B, Stögbauer F (2002) Giant axonal neuropathy (GAN): case report and two novel mutations in the gigaxonin gene. *Neurology* 58: 1273-1276.

13. Lowe J, Leigh PN (2002) Disorders of movement and system degenerations. In *Greenfield's Neuropathology*, 7th Ed., D Graham, PL Lantos (eds). E. Arnold: London. pp. 389-391..

14. Mahadevan A, Santosh V, Gayatri N, Ratnavalli E, NandaGopal R, Vasanth A, Roy AK, Shankar SK (2000) Infantile neuroaxonal dystrophy and giant axonal neuropathy--overlap diseases of neuronal cytoskeletal elements in childhood? *Clin Neuropathol* 19: 221-229.

15. Malandrini A, Dotti MT, Battisti C, Villanova M, Capocchi G, Federico A (1998) Giant axonal neuropathy with subclinical involvement of the central nervous system: case report. *J Neurol Sci* 158: 232-235.

16. Matsuyama H, Watanabe I, Mihm MC, Richardson EP, Jr. (1978) Dermatoleukodystrophy with neuroaxonal spheroids. *Arch Neurol* 35: 329-336.

17. Paloneva J, Autti T, Raininko R, Partanen J, Salonen O, Puranen M, Hakola P, Haltia M (2001) CNS

manifestations of Nasu-Hakola disease: a frontal dementia with bone cysts. *Neurology* 56: 1552-1558.

18. Paloneva J, Kestila M, Wu J, Salminen A, Bohling T, Ruotsalainen V, Hakola P, Bakker AB, Phillips JH, Pekkarinen P, Lanier LL, Timonen T, Peltonen L (2000) Loss-of-function mutations in TYROBP (DAP12) result in a presenile dementia with bone cysts. *Nat Genet* 25: 357-361.

19. Raine CS, Cross AH (1989) Axonal dystrophy as a consequence of long-term demyelination. *Lab Invest* 60: 714-725.

20. Schmidt RE, Chae HY, Parvin CA, Roth KA (1990) Neuroaxonal dystrophy in aging human sympathetic ganglia. *Am J Pathol* 136: 1327-1338.

21. Seitelberger F (1986) Neuronal Dystrophy: It's relations to aging and neurological diseases. In *Handbook of Clinical Neurology*, PJ Vinken, G Bruyn, W., HL Klawans (eds). Elsevier: Amsterdam. pp. 391-412.

22. van der Knaap MS, Naidu S, Kleinschmidt-Demasters BK, Kamphorst W, Weinstein HC (2000) Autosomal dominant diffuse leukoencephalopathy with neuroaxonal spheroids. *Neurology* 54: 463-468.

23. Walkley SU, Baker HJ, Rattazzi MC, Haskins ME, Wu JY (1991) Neuroaxonal dystrophy in neuronal storage disorders: evidence for major GABAergic neuron involvement. *J Neurol Sci* 104: 1-8.

24. Yazawa I, Nakano I, Yamada H, Oda M (1997) Long tract degeneration in familial sudanophilic leukodystrophy with prominent spheroids. *J Neurol Sci* 147: 185-191.

25.Yamashita, Yamamoto T (2002) Neuroaxonal leukoencephalopathy with axonal spheroids. *Eur Neurol* 48: 20-25.

Infantile Neuroaxonal Dystrophy (Seitelberger Disease)

Kurt A. Jellinger
John Duda

BAEP	brainstem auditory evoked potentials
cMAP	compound muscle action potential
CSF	cerebrospinal fluid
CT	computer tomography
EMG	electro myography
GOT	glutamate oxalacetate transaminase
HSS	Hallervorden-Spatz syndrome
INAD	infantile neuroaxonal dystrophy
LDH	lactate dehydrogenase
MCV	motor conduction velocity
MRI	magnetic ressonance imaging
NAD	neuroaxonal dystrophy
α-NAGA	α-N-acetyl galactosaminidase
SAP	sensory action potential
SCV	sensory conduction velocity
VEP	visual evoked potential

Definition

Infantile neuroaxonal dystrophy (INAD), described by Seitelberger in 1952 (18, 20), is an inherited autosomal recessive condition of infantile onset, characterized by progressive clinical course with weakness, hypotonia and areflexia, leading to tetraplegia, rigidity, spasticity, cerebellar signs, deafness, blindness, and mental deterioration due to multi-systemic involvement and widespread presence of dystrophic axons in the central, peripheral, and autonomic nervous systems. The genetics and basic metabolic defects are unknown.

Epidemiology

INAD is a rather rare disorder for which no incidence and prevalence data are available. The largest available review concerns 13 cases (16). Both sexes are involved with a considerable male predominance. The age at onset ranges from 6 to 24 (mean 15) months; with rare neonatal cases probably having intrauterine onset. Death occurs between the age of 6 and 12 years. Genetic risk factors are consanguinity and positive family history.

Genetics

The disorder is both sporadic and hereditary with sex-independent autosomal recessive trait. Familial cases often involve siblings. No specific chromosomal linkage or mutations are known at present. Molecular markers are missing. An X-chromosomal neonatal variant showed rapid lethal course.

Autosomal recessive NAD due to α-N-acetylgalactosaminidase deficiency due to point mutation at the α-NAGA-Gen (E325K) at chromosome 22q13.1-13.2 has been described in a few children with similar clinical signs and symptoms as INAD (11, 27). However, patients with classical INAD show normal α-NAGA activities, and up to the present, no association of α-NAGA deficiency and INAD has been confirmed (1).

Clinical Features

Signs and symptoms. All published patients had been born after a normal pregnancy and delivery, and had normal early development. Initial/presenting symptoms are slowed psychomotor development or psychomotor regression, occasionally sucking difficulties or vomiting. There is rapid motor and mental deterioration, truncal and neck hypotonia, areflexia and amyotrophy progressing to tetraparesis, accompanied by gait disorders, truncal and gait ataxia, pendular nystagmus, strabism, and deterioration of vision progressing to blindness due to optic nerve atrophy (5). For more detailed information about the signs and symptoms, see Hermann et al (9) and Nardocci et al (16).

Later development shows tetraplegia with signs of peripheral nerve involvement, tetraspasticity, or rigidity with pyramidal signs, often involving the legs earlier and more severely than the arms. Occasionally, mixed central and peripheral motor symptoms are present, with hypotonia and areflexia of the lower, and spasticity and hyperreflexy of the upper extremities. Rare early symptoms are reduced reaction to pain and segmental sensory disturbances on the trunk and extremities, dysphagia, deafness and loss of vestibular reactions. Pigmentary retinopathy and red macular spot are missing. Rare seizures of partial or generalized type or myoclonus are rare, as are extrapyramidal symptoms including choreiform, athetoid, perioral or buccofacio-lingual hyperkinesias, and dyskinetic movements (12). The progressive course leads to loss of voluntary movements, tetraplegia, rigidity, dysphagia, bladder and bowel incontinence and terminal decerebrate posture with limb contractures, areactivity towards the environment, and bulbar syndrom. Death results from intercurrent complication between 6 and 15 years of age.

Imaging. Farina et al (4) have described the neuroradiological findings in 11 patients. Cranial CT in early stages of disease is often normal; in later stages it reveals signs of progressive cerebral or cerebellar atrophy. MRI studies are initially normal, but later show cerebral atrophy and cerebellar atrophy mainly involving the inferior part of the vermis; T2-weighted images show signal hyperintensity in the cerebellar cortex, rarely in the dentate nuclei. Additional findings are hyperintensity in posterior periventricular white matter, thinning of the optic chiasm, and large cisterna magna. Occasionally, pallidonigral hypointensity is observed (21). MR spectroscopy showed increased lactate and choline/creatine ratio in the basal ganglia, with reduced N-acetylaspartate/creatine ratio which may be of diagnostic value (15).

Laboratory findings. The clinical spectrum and diagnostic criteria including laboratory findings have been described by Nardocci et al (16). Blood and urine chemistry, electrolytes, liver enzymes, and CSF are usually unremarkable except for rare

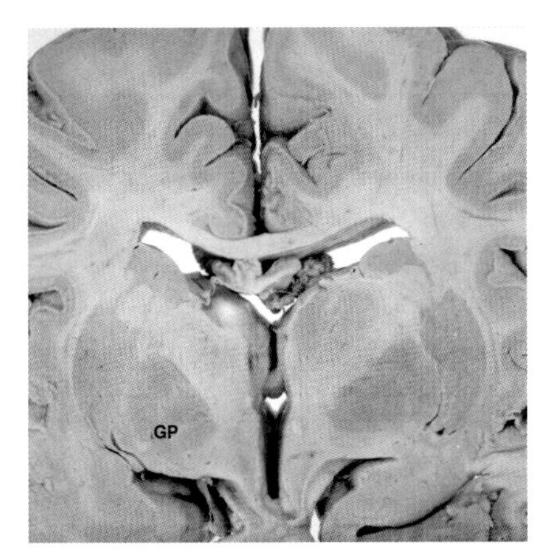

Figure 1. Infantile neuroaxonal dystrophy with enlarged pale globus pallidus (GP).

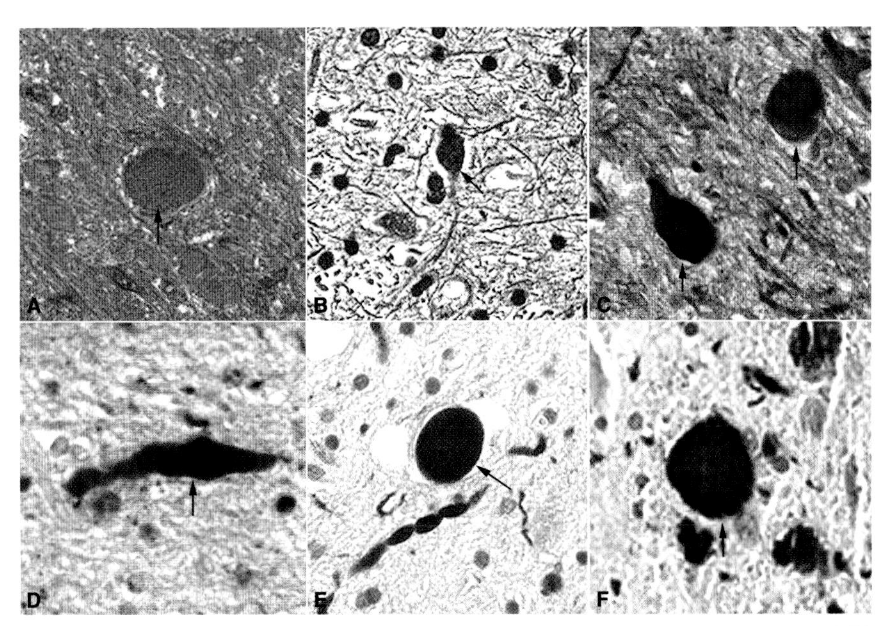

Figure 2. Neuroaxonal spheroids (arrows) are demonstrated with a variety of methods including staining with (**A**) eosin, (**B**) silver stains (Bodian silver stain, as well as immunohistochemistry with antibodies against neurofilaments (**C**, neurofilament light chain, (**D**) ubiquitin, (**E**) α-synuclein, and (**F**) hyperphosphorylated tau.

increases of LDH and transaminases in serum and CSF. Electroencephalography in infants under 2 years of age may be normal; later it shows a slow background activity with fast (14-22 Hz) rhythm (FRs) in both the sleeping and waking states, evident mainly on the anterior leads, with absent reaction to eye opening and photostimulation. Under hyperventilation, slowing of the curves occurs, indicating isolation of the cortex from subcortical centres Some children never show the typical fast EEG pattern during follow-up. Epileptiform activity consisting of paroxysmal focal and multifocal, spike-wave discharges, or BNS variants may be present.

Electromyography in later stages is either normal or shows signs of partial denervation of anterior horn type. Nerve conduction studies are normal or show reduced lower limb cMAPs; others show reduced MCVs and SCVs combined with severely reduced cMAPs and SAPs.

Electroretinograms are usually normal. VEPs are often abnormal, with altered early and/or late components, or cannot be elicited. BAEPs are normal or show increased latencies, while in some children no responses could be evoked.

Late-infantile and Juvenile Forms

A rare late-infantile sporadic or familial form with autosomal recessive inheritance, after unremarkable early development, at 2 to 6 years of age presents with disturbance of psychomotor development, autism, progressive gait disorders, spasticity of rigidity, ataxia, nystagmus, visual disorders, seizures, and myelonic epilepsy, but lacks hyperkinesias and other symptoms typical for HSS. Late stages show dementia and contractures, occasionally with predominant psychiatric symptoms (23). Death occurs between 6 and 23 years of age.

Other rare patients between 9 and 21 years of age present with disorders of gait, speech and vision, cerebellar ataxia, spasticity or athetoid hyperkinesias, psychotic symptoms, dyskinesia, blindness, cranial nerve disordes, and progressive dementia (17). Neuropathology in both types reveals generalized NAD with typical ultrastructure of the spheroids, cerebellar atrophy, and only mild pallido-nigral hyperpigmentation. Lewy bodies in melanized brainstem nuclei and neocortex, and neurofibrillary tangles have been reported (8).

Some adults develop changes of personality, disorders of memory and gain, apraxia, rigidity, dysarthria, and dementia. The brain, in addition to mild brownish colour of the internal pallidum, reveals multiple axonal spheroids and gliosis in cerebral and cerebellar white matter, cortex, basal ganglia, and cerebellum. The axonal swellings are immunoreactive to antibodies against neurofilament proteins, and ultrastructurally show accumulation of 10 nm filaments (14). All these disorders of postinfantile onset are considered transitional forms between generalized NAD and localized NAD with hyperpigmentation (19).

Macroscopy

The brain shows atrophy of the cerebral hemispheres with ventricular dilatation and cerebellar atrophy. The globus pallidus is pale and enlarged (Figure 1), while in children dying after the 4 years of age, it shows a rusty-brownish discoloration which is consistent in late-infantile cases.

Histopathology

The histological hallmark is disseminated presence of dystrophic axonal swellings (spheroids) in central, peripheral, and autonomous nervous systems. These are eosinophilic structures of 20 to 120 μm diameter usually well-stained by silver techniques (Figure 2); the smaller spheroids are immunorective for neurofilament proteins, ubiquitin, superoxide dismutase, amyloid precursor protein (APP), and in some disorders, for synucleins (6).

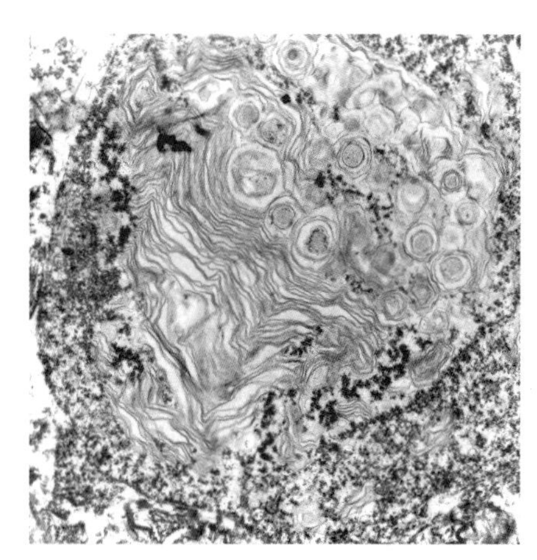

Figure 3. Infantile neuroaxonal dystrophy, boy aged 5 years. Electron microscopy of axonal spheroid showing multilamellated bodies, tubulovasicular profiles and mitochondria. Original magnification ×35 000.

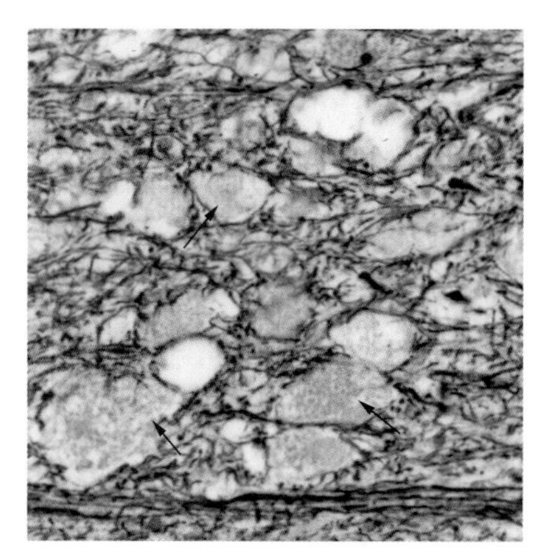

Figure 4. Infantile neuroaxonal dystrophy. Multiple axonal spheroids and spongy changes in globus pallidus. Bodian ×150.

Ultrastructurally, the distended axon contains an accumulation of mitochondria, lysosomal dense, multilamellated bodies, membrane-bound vesicles, tubulovesicular profiles of soft endoplasmic reticulum, amorphous matrix amterial, and few neurofilaments (Figure 3). Areas affected by NAD show associated astrocytosis and accumulation of lipids or iron-containing pigment depending on the age of the affected subject.

In INAD, predilective involvement occurs in the brainstem, cerebellar cortex, thalamus, globus pallidus, substantia nigra, and spinal cord; less often in the cerebral cortex, hypothalamus, cerebral white matter, red nucleus, hypophysis, infundibulu, neurophypophysis, and myenteric plexus of the colon. There is localized or diffuse atrophy of the cerebellar cortex and optic nerves, and spongy neuropil changes in severely involved areas (Figure 4). The globus pallidus and reticular part of substantia nigra that are enlarged due to accumulation of spheroids show deposition of neutral lipids (pallidal fat; lipophanerosis) or defective myelination (status dysmyelinisatus). Rare diffuse demyelination and gliosis of cerebral and cerebellar white matter are associated with degeneration of the corticospinal and spinobulbar, optic and olfactory systems. Axonal spheroids are also seen in peripheral and autonomous nerves, motor endplates, conjunctiva, tooth pulp, and additionally, in muscle biopsies (6, 25). Schwann cells of peripheral nerves contain membranotubular profiles and other abnormal organelles. Autopsy in rare cases showed glycolipid storage in the liver and kidney, in histiocytes of spleen and lymph nodes, and in thyroid and thymus; however, in general, there are no indications for neurovisceral storage disorder.

NAD type II is a rare intermediate form mainly involving girls with protracted clinical course, morphologically showing generalized occurrence of axonal spheroids like in INAD and pallido-nigral hyperpigmentation similar to the Hallervorden-Spatz syndrome (HSS) (10). A recently reported familial disorder revealed INAD with perineuronal argyrophilic bodies (13).

Biochemistry

Reduction of cerebrosides, fatty acids, phospholipids, and cholesterol in brain tissue is due to non-specific myelin damage. Gray matter shows decreased gangliosides, glycoproteins, and neuronal polypeptides due to loss of neurofilaments in dystrophic axons. Choline acetyltransferase, acetyl cholinesterase, and glutamate dehydrogenase are reduced (26).

Differential Diagnosis

Psychomotor retardation in early infancy associated with gait and visual disturbances, missing reaction to pain and a combination of hypotonia, areflexia and pyramidal signs, particularly when occurring in families at risk, are suspect of INAD. This can be supported by increased LDH and GOT levels in serum and CSF, EMG signs of anterior horn involvement, neuroimaging data, proton MR spectroscopy showing lactate spectra in basal ganglia, and further invasive diagnostic procedures (ie, biopsies of skin, conjunctiva, tooth pulp, or rectum) with demonstration of dystrophic axons in both infantile and juvenile forms.

Differential diagnosis of INAD includes leukodystrophies, in partiuclar metachromatic, sudanophilic, and globoid cell types, neurolipidoses, spongy dystrophies, Leigh's disease, spinal muscular atrophies, perinatal brain damage, and other encephalopathies. For juvenile and adult forms, the differential diagnostic parameters of HSS are to be considered.

Experimental Models

Endogenous NAD in animals has been reported in horses, sheep, rats, rabbits, cats, and dogs (24, 28) and several inherited diseases of domestic animals (2). Among dogs, NAD most frequently affects young Rottweilers (3) showing dystrophic axons in dorsal horns of spinal cord, gracile, cuneate, vestibular, and other brainstem nuclei, with abnormal expression of synaptic vesicle-associated presynaptic plasma membrane, cytosolic proteins, and α-synuclein. Since these proteins participate in the trafficking, docking and fusion of the synaptic vesicle to the plasma membrane, disruption of axonal transport in dystrophic axons is suggested (22).

A model of INAD could be an autosomal recessive disorder in C6-deficient rats clinically presenting with subacute motor neuropathy, morphologically showing multiple axon spheroids in CNS grey matter and peripheral nerves. Ultrastructural findings with tubulovesicular material, dense bodies, and aggregates of parallel membranes are similar to those in human NAD (7). Other models are various mouse mutants of neurodegenerations with dystrophic axons in mice (lnd, gnd, and vmd), located on chromosome 7 that show lumbosacral, vestibular, or generalized NAD (2). In view of animal models of NAD caused by vitamin E deficiency, it has been proposed that malabsorption of tocopherol may have a pathogenic role in some cases of symptomatic NADs (14).

References

1. Bakker HD, de Sonnaville ML, Vreken P, Abeling NG, Groener JE, Keulemans JL, van Diggelen OP (2001) Human alpha-N-acetylgalactosaminidase (alpha-NAGA) deficiency: no association with neuroaxonal dystrophy? *Eur J Hum Genet* 9:91-96.

2. Bronson RT, Sweet HO, Spencer CA, Davisson MT (1992) Genetic and age related models of neurodegeneration in mice: dystrophic axons. *J Neurogenet* 8:71-83

3. Christman CL (1992) Neurological diseases of rottweilers: Neuroaxonal dystrophy and leukoencephalomalacia. *J Small Anim Pract* 33:500-504

4. Farina L, Nardocci N, Bruzzone MG, D'Incerti L, Zorzi G, Verga L, Morbin M, Savoiardo M (1999) Infantile neuroaxonal dystrophy: neuroradiological studies in 11 patients. *Neuroradiology* 41:376-380.

5. Ferreira RC, Mierau GW, Bateman JB (1997) Conjunctival biopsy in infantile neuroaxonal dystrophy. *Am J Ophthalmol* 123:264-266.

6. Galvin JE, Giasson B, Hurtig HI, Lee VM, Trojanowski JQ (2000) Neurodegeneration with brain iron accumulation, type 1 is characterized by alpha-, beta-, and gamma-synuclein neuropathology. *Am J Pathol* 157:361-368.

7. Giannini C, Monaco S, Kirschfink M, Rother KO, Lorbacher de Ruiz H, Nardelli E, Bonetti B, Salviati A, Zanette GP, Rizzuto N (1992) Inherited neuroaxonal dystrophy in C6 deficient rabbits. *J Neuropathol Exp Neurol* 51:514-522.

8. Hayashi S, Akasaki Y, Morimura Y, Takauchi S, Sato M, Miyoshi K (1992) An autopsy case of late infantile and juvenile neuroaxonal dystrophy with diffuse Lewy bodies and neurofibrillary tangles. *Clin Neuropathol* 11:1-5.

9. Hermann W, Barthel H, Reuter M, Georgi P, Dietrich J, Wagner A (2000) Hallervorden-Spatz disease: findings in the nigrostriatal system. *Nervenarzt* 71:660-665.

10. Jellinger K (1999) Neuroaxonale Dystrophien. In *Neurologie in Praxis und Klinik*, DG Hopf HC, Diener HC, Reichmann H (eds). G. Thieme: Stuttgart. pp. 962-970

11. Keulemans JL, Reuser AJ, Kroos MA, Willemsen R, Hermans MM, van den Ouweland AM, de Jong JG, Wevers RA, Renier WO, Schindler D, Coll MJ, Chabas A, Sakuraba H, Suzuki Y, van Diggelen OP (1996) Human alpha-N-acetylgalactosaminidase (alpha-NAGA) deficiency: new mutations and the paradox between genotype and phenotype. *J Med Genet* 33:458-464.

12. Koeppen AH, Dickson AC (2001) Iron in the Hallervorden-Spatz syndrome. *Pediatr Neurol* 25:148-158

13. LaVaute T, Smith S, Cooperman S, Iwai K, Land W, Meyron-Holtz E, Drake SK, Miller G, Abu-Asab M, Tsokos M, Switzer R, 3rd, Grinberg A, Love P, Tresser N, Rouault TA (2001) Targeted deletion of the gene encoding iron regulatory protein-2 causes misregulation of iron metabolism and neurodegenerative disease in mice. *Nat Genet* 27:209-214.

14. Lowe J, Leigh PN (2002) Disorders of movement and system degenerations. In *Greenfield's Neuropathology*, 7th Ed. D Graham, PL Lantos (eds). E. Arnold: London. pp. 389-391.

15. Mader I, Krageloh-Mann I, Seeger U, Bornemann A, Nagele T, Kuker W, Grodd W (2001) Proton MR spectroscopy reveals lactate in infantile neuroaxonal dystrophy (INAD). *Neuropediatrics* 32:97-100.

16. Nardocci N, Zorzi G, Farina L, Binelli S, Scaioli W, Ciano C, Verga L, Angelini L, Savoiardo M, Bugiani O (1999) Infantile neuroaxonal dystrophy: clinical spectrum and diagnostic criteria. *Neurology* 52:1472-1478.

17. Ramaekers VT, Lake BD, Harding B, Boyd S, Harden A, Brett EM, Wilson J (1987) Diagnostic difficulties in infantile neuroaxonal dystrophy. A clinicopathological study of eight cases. *Neuropediatrics* 18:170-175.

18. Seitelberger F (1952) *Eine unbekannte Form von infantiler Lipoid-Speicher-Krankheit des Gehirns*. Presented at Proceedings, First International Congress of Neuropathology, Rome

19. Seitelberger F (1986) Neuronal Dystrophy: It's relations to aging and neurological diseases. In *Handbook of Clinical Neurology*, PJ Vinken, G Bruyn, W., HL Klawans (eds). Elsevier: Amsterdam. pp. 391-412

20. Seitelberger F, Gross H (1957) Über eine spätinfantile Form der Hallervorden-Spatzschen Krankheit. II. Mitteilung Histochemische Befunde. Erörterung der Nosologie. *Dtsch Z Nervenheilk* 176:104-125

21. Simonati A, Trevisan C, Salviati A, Rizzuto N (1999) Neuroaxonal dystrophy with dystonia and pallidal involvement. *Neuropediatrics* 30:151-154

22. Sisó S, I F, M P (2001) Juvenile neuroaxonal dystrophy in a rottweiler: Accumulation of synaptic proteins in dystrophic axons. *Acta Neuropathol*, (in press) 102

23. Sugiyama H, Hainfellner JA, Schmid-Siegel B, Budka H (1993) Neuroaxonal dystrophy combined with diffuse Lewy body disease in a young adult. *Clin Neuropathol* 12:147-152.

24. Summers B, JF C, A dL (1995) *Veterinary Neuropathology*: Mosby, St. Louis, Baltimore, Berlin, Boston, Carlsbad, Chicago, London, Madrid, Naples, New York, Philadelphia, Sydney, Tokyo, Toronto.

25. Wakai S, Asanuma H, Tachi N, Ishikawa Y, Minami R (1993) Infantile neuroaxonal dystrophy: axonal changes in biopsied muscle tissue. *Pediatr Neurol* 9:309-311.

26. Wisniewski K, Czosnek H, Wisniewski HM, Soifer D, Ramos PL, Kim KS, Iqbal K (1982) Reduction of neuronal specific protein and some neurotransmitters in the infantile neuroaxonal dystrophy (INAD). *Neuropediatrics* 13:123-129.

27. Wolfe DE, Schindler D, Desnick RJ (1995) Neuroaxonal dystrophy in infantile alpha-N-acetylgalactosaminidase deficiency. *J Neurol Sci* 132:44-56.

28. Zhang JH, Sampogna S, Morales FR, Chase MH (1998) Age-related intra-axonal accumulation of neurofilaments in the dorsal column nuclei of the cat brainstem: a light and electron microscopic immunohistochemical study. *Brain Res* 797:333-338.

Neurodegeneration with Brain Iron Acculation, Type 1 (Hallervorden-Spatz Disease)

Kurt A. Jellinger
John Duda

CSF	cerebrospinal fluid
CT	computer tomography
EMG	electro myography
HSD	Hallervorden-Spatz disease
HSS	Hallervorden-Spatz syndrome
INAD	Infantile neuroaxonal dystrophy
MCV	motor conduction velocity
NAD	neuroaxonal dystrophy
NBIA-1	neurodegeneration with brain iron accumulation, type I
OMIM	Online Mendelian Inheritance in Man. *http://www.ncbi.nlm.nih.gov/omim*
PKAN	pantothenate kinase associated neurodegeneration
SEP	sensory evoked potential

Definition

Hallervorden-Spatz disease (HSD) is a rare familial and sporadic progressive autosomal recessive neurodegenerative condition in which extrapyramidal movement disorders are associated with a combination of neuroaxonal dystrophy and iron accumulation in the basal ganglia. It is caused by a novel pantothenate kinase gene (*PKAN2*) (606157) linked to chromosome 20p12.3-p13 (33, 40, 41).

Synonyms and Historical Annotations

The syndrome was described in 1922 by Hallervorden and Spatz (11) in a sibship of 12, in which 5 sisters showed increasing dysarthria, progressive dementia, and at autopsy, a brown discoloration of the globus pallidus and substantia nigra. Due to recent historical discussions, the syndrome was recently renamed "Neurodegeneration with brain iron accumulation type I" (NBIA 1) (2), and due to recent molecular genetic findings, it has been added to pantothenate kinase-associated neurodegenerations (PKAN) (9a, 41).

Epidemiology

HSD is a rare disorder with around 100 published cases for which no incidence or predominance data are available. It concerns all ethnic groups with almost equal involvement of both sexes. In addition to familial forms with involvement of brothers and sisters, sporadic and atypical cases are known. Risk factors are consanguinity in families and missense mutations in *PANK2* gene.

Genetics

Using homozygosity mapping in a large Amish family, Taylor (33) mapped HSD to 20p13-p12.3. Analysis of other families from New Zealand, Australia, Spain, and Italy supported linkage to this region with a total maximum 2-point load score of 13.75 at theta=0.0 for one polymorphic micro-satellite marker. Homozygosity in the Amish family and recombinant haplotypes in 3 of the other families suggested that the gene involved is located in a 4-cM interval between D20S906 and D20S116. There is locus heterogeneity for the disorder, although one Japanese family did not show linkage to this region, suggesting the existence of another locus.

Using linkage analysis of an extended Amish pedigree, Zhou et al (41) narrowed the critical interval on chromosome 20p13 to a 1.4-Mb interval that contained 21 known or predicted genes. In the index family, they identified a 7-bp deletion (606157.0001) in the coding sequence of a gene called *PANK2*, that is homologue to murine pantothenate kinase-1 (28b). Additional missense and null mutations were identified in 32 of 38 individuals with classic HSS. Mutations on both alleles could be accounted for in 22 of these 32 subjects. DNA from individuals with atypical PKAN also demonstrated missense mutations in *PANK2*. These individuals have later onset, evidence of increased basal ganglia iron and diverse phenotypes including early onset Parkinson disease, severe intermittent dystonia, stuttering with palilalia or facial ticks with repetitive hair caressing.

One consanguineous family with pigmentary retinopathy and late-onset dystonia but without radiological evidence of brain iron accumulation even into their 30s carried a homozygous missense mutation (606157.0007). In the group studied, most mutations were unique with a notable exception of the gly411-to-art mutation (606157.0002) which was present in both classical and atypical individuals (OMIM #234200, updated 09/18/2002). A new member of the glia-derived neurotrophic factor (GDNF) receptor family was discovered at chromosome 20p12.3-13 which is glycosyl-phosphatidylinositol linked and maintains conserved cystein residues but lacks the sequence corresponding to exons 2 and 3 in other family members. Mutation analysis in patients with HSD revealed 2 potentially significant amino changes but failed to identify mutation in other 10 (41).

A workshop on pantothenate kinase associated neurodegenerations (HSD) at Munich, April 19, 2002, revealed 21 *PKAN2* mutations among 65 European patients (T. Kloppstock, personal communication). Pantothenate kinase is a rate-determining enzyme in coenzyme A biosynthesis (28a).

A previously unknown, dominantly inherited, late-onset basal ganglia disease, variably presenting with extrapyramidal features similar to those of Huntington's disease or parkinsonism was mapped, by linkage analysis, to chromosome 19q13.3. This chromosome contains the gene for ferritin light polypeptide (PTS) with an adenine insertion at position 460-461 that is predicted to alter carboxy-terminal residues of the gene product. Brain histochemistry disclosed abnormal mutation of ferritin and iron, while the patients showed low serum ferritin levels. The same mutation was found in 5 apparently unrelated subjects with similar extrapyramidal symptoms. Since an abnormality in ferritin strongly indicates a primary function for iron in the pathogenesis of this new disease, the name "neuroferritinopathy" was proposed (6). Similar changes may be associated with a pathological phenotype of Rb2(-/-) mice due to targeted deletion of the gene encoding iron regulator protein-2 misregulation in iron metabolism and neurodegenerative disease (18).

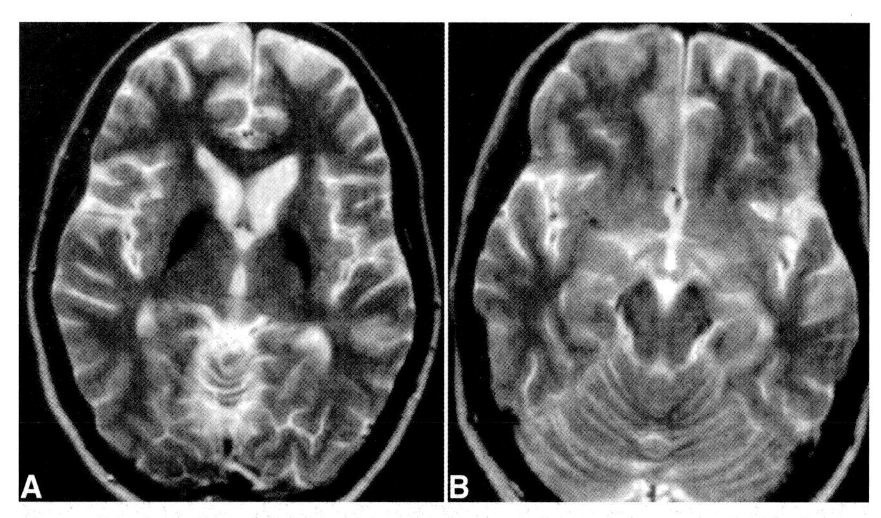

Figure 1. Hallervorden-Spatz disease. T2 weighted MRI shows a marked decrease in signal intensity in the globus pallidus (**A**) and substantia nigra (**B**), and mild frontal atrophy.

Clinical Features

Signs and symptoms. Familial cases often show similar clinical phenotype with similar onset and symptoms, while sporadic cases reveal considerable variation in clinical symptoms and progress. According to the onset of the disorder, one distinguishes (12, 15, 30): *i)* infantile forms with onset in the first year of life, *ii)* late-infantile cases with onset between the age of 2 and 5 years; duration in both types is up to 10 years with death occurring between the age of 8 and 16 years; *iii)* juvenile "classic" HSD with onset between 7 and 15 years of age and duration of 6 to 30 years, death supervening between 12 and 36 years; the duration increases with the age at onset, and *iv)* adult or late cases with onset between the age of 22 and 64 years, duration between 3 months and 13 years with death up to the age of 70 years.

Recent studies suggest that HSD can develop at any age, and that the phenotype should be extended to include late onset parkinsonism (28a).

The disease presents with slowly progressive gait disorders, stiffness, and cramps in the legs; muscular hypotonia rarely progresses into rigidity. Occasional presenting signs are clubfoot, stuttering, speech and visual disorders. Often, delay of psychomotor development antedates neurological symptoms, which may be related to inborn mental retardation or perinatal injury.

Hyperkinesias occur in about half of the classical cases, rarely in infantile and late-infantile patients. They include choreic, athetotic, and dystonic disorders, variable tremor in extremities and face with grimacing, rolling eye and tongue movements, occasional rest tremor. Steady or intervallary dystonias are frequent, myoclonus is rare or may occur in terminal states. Ballism or parkinsonism with rest tremor was observed in late cases. Rigidity and hyperkinesias often progress to face, tongue, and eye muscles and cause dysarthria, dysphagia and bizarre eye movements.

In addition to hyperreflexia with and without plantar reflexes, often there are spastic pareses and amyotrophies in the legs. Seizures as initial or late symptoms are rare. Other symptoms include ataxia, nystagmus, visual disorders, or optic nerve atrophy (3). Additional acanthocytosis, retinitis pigmentosa, and tapetoretinal degeneration may be present. Progressive mental deterioration with or without memory disorders may finally lead to dementia. In late stages the dyskinesias decrease and are replaced by rigid stiffness and contractures, dysphagia, loss of reactivity, and death. Some cases with typical neuropathology show atypical clinical course: early-infantile onset presenting with psychomotor retardation or seizures, followed by progressive rigidity or spasticity often without dyskinesias, ataxia, and visual disturbances terminating in stiffness and dementia. In rare adult cases, speech disorders, ataxia and seizures are followed by rigidity, athetosis, torsion dystonia, tremor, and myoclonus, or an akinetic-rigid parkinsonian syndrome with or without dementia, rarely as early onset dementia or late onset chorea (10) or rarely as early onset dementia with later motor manifestations or movement disorders (5, 19).

Laboratory data. Blood chemistry including copper and iron contents, excretion of amino acids and iron in urine and CSF are unremarkable. CSF may show increased non-protein-bound iron. Acanthocytosis, sea-blue histiocytes in the bone marrow and curvilinear inclusions in lymphocytes have been observed in single cases (32). Electroencephalography is often abnormal with non-specific changes. EMG may show rigidospasticity or fasciculations. Abnormal somatosensory evoked potentials (SEPs) may indicate sensory loss due to dorsal column dysfunction (23).

Imaging. Neuroimaging is of great importance in arriving at a diagnosis in life. Cranial CT and MRI reveal atrophy of the cerebral hemispheres, cerebellum and brainstem with dilated ventricles. CT shows high signal lesions in

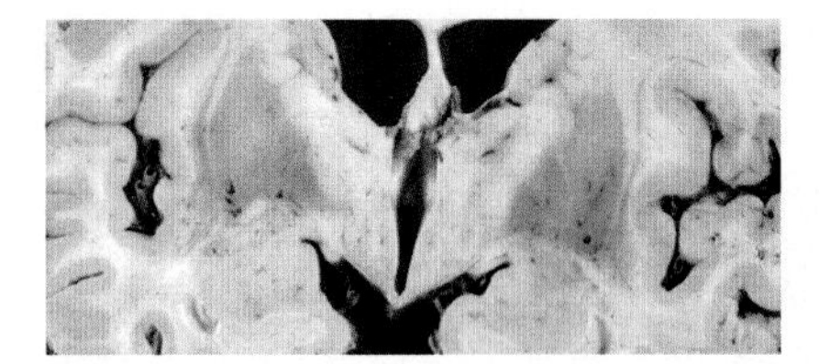

Figure 2. Hallervorden-Spatz disease. Mild discoloration of the globus pallidus.

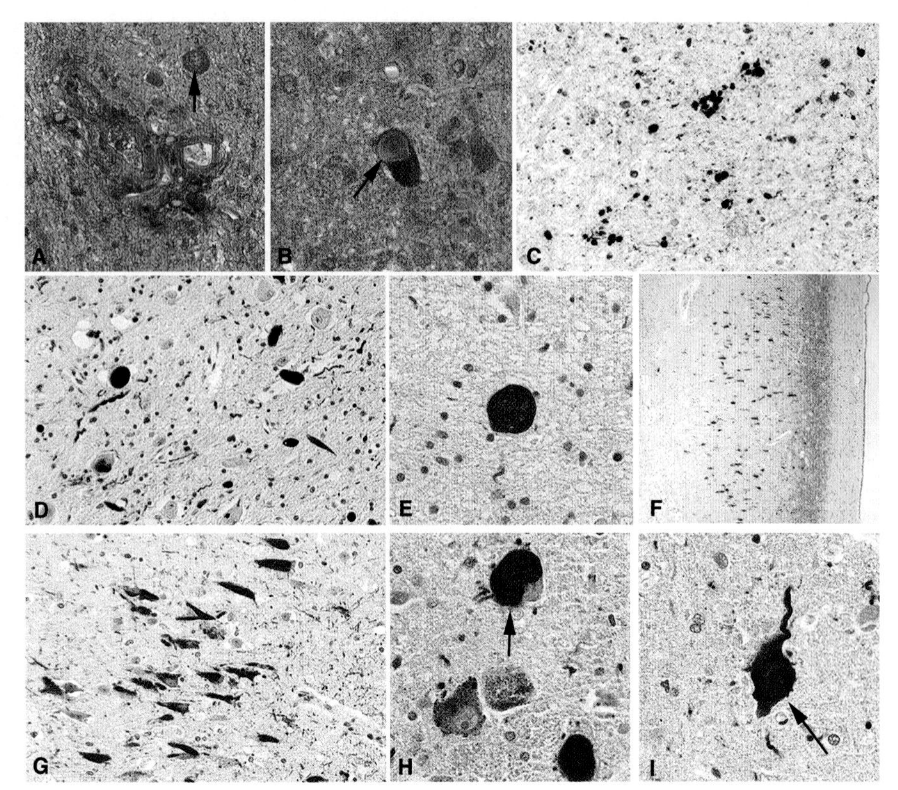

Figure 3. Hallervorden-Spatz disease. Haematoxylin and eosin staining readily reveals brownish deposits of iron (**A**), neuroaxonal spheroids (A, arrow) and Lewy bodies (**B**). Iron staining of globus pallidus also reveals the iron deposits (**C**, Gomori stain). Immunohistochemistry for α-synuclein readily reveals neuroaxonal spheroids, dystrophic neurites, glial cytoplasmic inclusions and Lewy bodies (**D**) as well as neuroaxonal spheroids that resemble the grumous degeneration of Tretiakoff (**E**). Immunostaining for hyperphosphorylated tau reveals numerous neurofibrillary tangles (**F, G**) as well as globose tangle-like inclusions (**H, I**).

the globus pallidus on both sides, while MRI in T-2 weighted images shows a marked decreased intensity in the globus pallidus and substantia nigra (Figure 1) consistent with increased iron and ferritin content, and a small hyperintensive area in the internal segment corresponding to gliosis and vacuolation of tissue. This "eye-of-the-tiger" signal is of great diagnostic value particularly in the late-infantile form (1, 27), but is also seen in atypical familial cases with acanthocytosis and retinitis pigmentosa (22). Decreased iron uptake into the basal ganglia is seen after intravenous application of ^{59}Fe (32) while CIT and IBZM-SPECT, in contrast to Parkinson disease and multisystem atrophy, are both normal in HSD (13). PET studies revealed no pallidal abnormalities, but showed significant hypoperfusion of the head of the caudate nucleus, pons, and cerebellar vermis with normal dopaminergic function of the basal ganglia, suggesting that lesions are not confined to the globus pallidus (4).

Macroscopy

The brain may show mild atrophy of cerebral hemispheres and cerebellum, with shrinkage and rust-brown discoloration of the globus pallidus and pars reticularis of substantia nigra (Figure 2).

Histopathology

The key pathology involves the pallido-nigral system with accumulation of iron-containing pigment, demyelination (status dysmyelinisatus), and in later stages, neuron loss and astrogliosis associated with axonal spheroids predominantly but not exclusively involving the medial globus pallidus and substantia nigra pars reticulata. The external globus pallidus is typically spared. The granular pigment, consisting of iron, lipofuscin and neuromelanin is present within neurones, some spheroids, astrocytes, microglial cells, whilse some appear free in the neuropil, often around small vessels (Figure 3). Spheroids may also be seen in the corpus subthalamicum, striatum, thalamus, brainstem tegmentum, cerebral cortex, and the spinal cord.

Infantile and late-infantile cases also show deposition of neutral fat and glycolipids in the enlarged globus pallidus. In rare cases the lesions are restricted to the globus pallidus without involvement of substantia nigra. Widespread cortical and brainstem-type Lewy body pathology has been encountered in several adult patients with HSD (Figure 3) reinforcing the link with cases described as late onset neuroaxonal dystrophy (NAD) (2, 8, 24, 29, 37). In other cases there have been associated neurofibrillary tangles (7, 36).

In contrast to infantile neuroaxonal dystrophy (INAD), the peripheral nerves are rarely involved, the motor end plates are free. Muscle pathology rarely includes fibre splitting, myeloid structures, and dense bodies (21). The eye may show degeneration of photoreceptors and accumulation of melanin in the pigmented cells of the retina (34). Similar fine granular pigment was also found in hepatocytes. Bone marrow biopsy has demonstrated sea-blue histiocytes and osmiophilic inclusions have been described in lymphocytes, suggesting that HSD is a systemic disorder (32, 42).

Immunohistochemistry and Ultrastructural Findings

Axonal spheroids have been shown to contain immunoreactive neurofilament proteins (37), ubiquitin, superoxide dismutase (26), amyloid precursor protein (APP), and α-synuclein (8, 24, 25, 37) (Figure 3) as well as β- and γ-synuclein (8). Axonal spheroids are immunoreactive for tau and very strongly for ferritin and for stainable iron-II (DAB-enhanced Perls' reaction) (14). Double labelling of ferritin, as an indirect marker of intracellular iron and phosphorylated neurofilament protein revealed close proximity of ferritin-reactive microglial and oligodendroglial processes to tightly packed axons, suggesting that a primary axonal disorder allows the seepage of iron into the axoplasm, although iron may also contribute to axonal damage (17).

In addition to spheroids, other characteristic lesions include glial cytoplasmic inclusions (35), Lewy body-like intraneuronal inclusions (2, 8, 24, 37), and dystrophic neurites (35, 37). Whereas in late onset HSD, tau pathology has been demonstrated, consisting of both paired helical filaments and straight filaments without amyloid β protein deposition (36). However, recent studies of pallido-nigral spheroids in old rhesus monkeys and baboons (*Papio anumbis*) showed that they were located in swollen astrocytic processes, and thus, were classified as astroglial accumulations of heat shock proteins (38).

Ultrastructural studies of axonal spheroids occurring in presynaptic axon terminals reveal accumulation of amorphous, granular, multilamellated, and dense bodies, mitochondria, and tubulovesicular structures in axoplasm. They are identical with those in generalized and experimental axon dystrophies (30), but are different from those in INAD (21). In the pallido-nigral system, they are associated with melanin-like deposits.

Biochemistry

Late-infantile and adult cases show a 3- to 4-fold increase of iron in the putamen and globus pallidus due to increased uptake of radioactive iron (32) without signs of a generalized disorder of iron metabolism. The globus pallidus shows also significant increase of zinc, copper and calcium. In 2 autopsy cases, marked elevation of cystine and glutathione-cysteine mixed disulphide was associated with reduced activity of cysteine dioxygenase, the enzyme which converts cysteine to cysteine sulphinic acid. It has been suggested that accumulated cysteine may act as a chelating agent and may be responsible for the accumulation of iron (28).

Western blot analysis of HSD brain demonstrated high-molecular weight α-synuclein aggregates in the high-salt-soluble and Triton X-100-insoluble/sodium dodecyl sulphate-soluble fractions. Significantly, the levels of α-synuclein were markedly reduced in the Triton X-100-soluble fractions compared to control brain, and unlike other synucleinopathies, insoluble α-synuclein did not accumulate in the formic acid-soluble fraction (8). The involvement of synucleins in the neuronal, glial, and axonal pathology of HSD may expand the concept of neurodegenerative synucleinopathies, but the mechanisms leading to the conversion of soluble proteins into insoluble aggregates in both neurones and axonal spheroids remain to be elucidated.

Differential Diagnosis

The diagnosis HSD should be reserved for neurodegenerative disorders in adolescence and young adulthood; it is clinically easy in pedigrees with autopsy or biopsy-proven cases, and encompasses a number of distinctive disorders, each having the pallidal triad of iron deposition, axonal spheroids and gliosis. The demonstration of hyperintensity of the globus pallidus and substantia nigra in T-2 weighted MRI images and of the "tiger's eye" signal in the internal pallidum is important for the in vivo diagnosis of HSD. Clinically or pathologically distinct groups include: *i)* female patients with dementia, quadriparesis and neurofibrillary tangles; *ii)* cases with Lewy bodies; and *iii)* those with acanthocytosis and pigmentary retinal degeneration. Sporadic and adult-onset cases show considerable case-to-case variability (12, 15). HSD is to be distinguished from Wilson's disease, idiopathic torsion dystonia, akinetic-rigid forms of juventile Huntington's and Parkinson's diseases, dyskinesias in perinatal and postnatal disorders, subacute sclerosing panencephalitis.

In the patient originally reported as HARP syndrome (12a), Ching et al (4a) demonstrated homozygosity for a C-to-T transition at nucleotide 1111 in exon 5 of the PKAN gene. The mutation changed an arginine codon to a stop codon at amino acid 371 and shortened *PKAN2* by 89 amino acids. It was supected that the patient was the offspring of consanguineous parents becasue they came from the same village of 500 inhabitants. The patient demonstrated severe spasticity and dystonia from early childhood. At age 10, she was shown to have pigmentary retinopathy on funduscopic examination and the "eye of the tiger" sign on brain MRI. Peripheral blood smear and electron microscopy demonstrated marked acanthocytosis that was not due to an intrinsic erthrocyte protein defect. On high-resolution lipoprotein electrophoresis, she demonstrated absence of the pre-beta fraction and normal blood levels of cholesterol, triglycerides, high and low density lipoprotein cholesterol, and apolipoproteins A, B, and E.

HSD is an extrapyramidal syndrome due to a combination of pallido-nigral hyperpigmentation and NAD. It should be distinguished from disorders associated with mineralization of the basal ganglia with or without clinical symptoms similar to HSD, some being primary and other epiphenomena, eg, pallido-nigral atrophy, heredoataxias, Nasu-Hakola disease, atypical parkinsonism (12, 20).

Experimental Models

Mutant mice with a targeted disruption of the gene encoding iron regulatory protein 2(IRP2) have been shown to misregulate iron metabolism in the intestinal mucosa and the central nervous system. In adulthood, Ireb2(-/-) mice develop a movement disorder characterised by ataxia, bradykinesia, and tremor. Significant accumulation of iron in the white matter tracts and nuclei throughout the brain precede the onset of neurodegeneration and movement disorder by many months. Ferric iron accumulated in the cytosol of neurons and oligodendrocytes is in distinctive regions of the brain. Abnormal accumulations of ferritin colocalize with iron accumulation in populations of neurons that degenerate, and iron-laden oligodendrocytes accumulate ubiquitin-positive inclusions (18). Neurodegenerative disease in Ireg2(-/-) mice due to misregulation of iron metabolism may be an animal model for HSD and may contribute to further elucidation of the pathogenesis of this and comparable human neurodegenerative disorders.

Another murine model, the gracile axonal dystrophy mouse, is an autosomal recessive mutant that is characterised by accumulation of axonal spheroids in the gracile nucleus and fascicle, and to a lesser extent, in many other areas of the brain (39). The phenotype, including sensory and motor ataxia, has been found to be due to deletion in the gene for the ubiquitin carboxy-terminal hydrolase 1-1 isoenzyme. While not characterised by iron deposition, further understanding of the pathogenesis of this model may lead to a better understanding of the role of the ubiquitin-proteosomal system in NAD and neurodegeneration.

Pathogenesis

The pathogenesis and molecular basis of all types of NAD are unclear. For INAD and other generalized NADs, disruption of axonal transport due to hitherto unknown causes may be considered, but no molecular markers are available at present. For HSD and related disorders with increased iron deposition in the pallidonigral system, misregulation of iron metabolism due to genetic disruption of iron regulating proteins, as observed in the Ire2(-/-) mouse mutant may be considered, probably associated with oxidative stress and free radical formation causing disturbances of axonal transport (17, 31), while disorders of cysteine metabolism with iron accumulation due to chelate formation have not been confirmed. Recent studies revealed widespread occurrence of α-synuclein immunoreactive inclusions in juvenile and adult onset HSD (2, 8, 24, 37), as well as extensive tau pathology with NFTs, often coexisting with Lewy bodies in the same neurones, the development of which could be related to disturbances of axonal transport caused by axonal swelling/spheroid formation (29) or oxidative damage linked to α-synuclein nitration (9).

Future Directions and Therapy

Future research concerns elucidation of the pathogenic and molecular genetic backgrounds of NAD and iron accumulation in the brain.

A causal treatment of all kinds of NAD is unknown. Symptomatic strategies include administration of levodopa and dopamine agonists which show limited effects on rigid-akinetic movement disorders (15), and stereotactic pallidotomy and botulinum toxin to reduce painful dystonia (16). Trials with iron chelator desferrioxamine and high-dose α-tocopherol (vitamin E) gave negative results. Current treatment and rehabilitation are largely restricted to supportive care and multidisciplinary approaches to improve functional skills, communication, and cognitive strategies.

References

1. Angelini L, Nardocci N, Rumi V, Zorzi C, Strada L, Savoiardo M (1992) Hallervorden-Spatz disease: clinical and MRI study of 11 cases diagnosed in life. *J Neurol* 239: 417-425.

2. Arawaka S, Saito Y, Murayama S, Mori H (1998) Lewy body in neurodegeneration with brain iron accumulation type 1 is immunoreactive for alpha-synuclein. *Neurology* 51: 887-889.

3. Battistella PA, Midena E, Suppiej A, Carollo C (1998) Optic atrophy as the first symptom in Hallervorden-Spatz syndrome. *Childs Nerv Syst* 14: 135-138.

4. Castelnau P, Zilbovicius M, Ribeiro M-J, Hertz-Pannier L, Ogier H, Evrard P (2001) Striatal and pnotocerebellar hypoperfusion in Hallervorden-Spatz syndrome. *Pediatr Neurol* 25: 170-176.

4a. Ching KH, Westaway SK, Gitschier J, Higgins JJ, Hayflick SJ (2002) HARP syndrome is allelic with pantothenate kinase-associated neurodegeneration. *Neurology* 58: 1673-1674.

5. Cooper GE, Rizzo M, Jones RD (2000) Adult-onset Hallervorden-Spatz syndrome presenting as cortical dementia. *Alzheimer Dis Assoc Disord* 14: 120-126.

6. Curtis AR, Fey C, Morris CM, Bindoff LA, Ince PG, Chinnery PF, Coulthard A, Jackson MJ, Jackson AP, McHale DP, Hay D, Barker WA, Markham AF, Bates D, Curtis A, Burn J (2001) Mutation in the gene encoding ferritin light polypeptide causes dominant adult-onset basal ganglia disease. *Nat Genet* 28: 350-354.

7. Eidelberg D, Sotrel A, Joachim C, Selkoe D, Forman A, Pendlebury WW, Perl DP (1987) Adult onset Hallervorden-Spatz disease with neurofibrillary pathology. A discrete clinicopathological entity. *Brain* 110: 993-1013.

8. Galvin JE, Giasson B, Hurtig HI, Lee VM, Trojanowski JQ (2000) Neurodegeneration with brain iron accumulation, type 1 is characterized by alpha-, beta-, and gamma-synuclein neuropathology. *Am J Pathol* 157: 361-368.

9. Giasson BI, Duda JE, Murray IV, Chen Q, Souza JM, Hurtig HI, Ischiropoulos H, Trojanowski JQ, Lee VM (2000) Oxidative damage linked to neurodegeneration by selective alpha- synuclein nitration in synucleinopathy lesions. *Science* 290: 985-989.

9a. Gordon N (2002) Pantothenate kinase-associated neurodegeneration (Hallervorden-Spatz syndrome). *Eur J Paediatr Neurol* 6: 243-247.

10. Grimes DA, Lang AE, Bergeron C (2000) Late adult onset chorea with typical pathology of Hallervorden-Spatz syndrome. *J Neurol Neurosurg Psychiatry* 69: 392-395.

11. Hallervorden J, Spatz H (1922) Eigenartige Erkrankung im extrapyramidalen System mit besonderer Beteiligung des Globus pallidus und der Substantia nigra. Ein Beitrag zu den Beziehungen zwischen diesen beiden Zentren. *Zentralbl Gesamte Neurol* 79: 254-302

12. Halliday W (1995) The nosology of Hallervorden-spatz disease. *J Neurol Sci* 134 Suppl: 84-91.

12a. Higgins JJ, Patterson MC, Papadopoulos NM, Brady RO, Pentchev PG, Barton NW (1992) Hypoprebetalipoproteinemia, acanthocytosis, retinitis pigmentosa, and pallidal degeneration (HARP syndrome). *Neurology* 42: 194-198.

13. Hermann W, Barthel H, Reuter M, Georgi P, Dietrich J, Wagner A (2000) [Hallervorden-Spatz disease: findings in the nigrostriatal system]. *Nervenarzt* 71: 660-665.

14. Ince P (2001) Personal communication.

15. Jellinger K (1999) Neuroaxonale Dystrophien. In *Neurologie in Praxis und Klinik*, DG Hopf HC, Diener HC, Reichmann H (eds). G. Thieme: Stuttgart. pp. 962-970.

16. Justesen CR, Penn RD, Kroin JS, Egel RT (1999) Stereotactic pallidotomy in a child with Hallervorden-Spatz disease. Case report. *J Neurosurg* 90: 551-554.

17. Koeppen AH, Dickson AC (2001) Iron in the Hallervorden-Spatz syndrome. *Pediatr Neurol* 25: 148-158.

18. LaVaute T, Smith S, Cooperman S, Iwai K, Land W, Meyron-Holtz E, Drake SK, Miller G, Abu-Asab M, Tsokos M, Switzer R, 3rd, Grinberg A, Love P, Tresser N, Rouault TA (2001) Targeted deletion of the gene encoding iron regulatory protein-2 causes misregula-

tion of iron metabolism and neurodegenerative disease in mice. *Nat Genet* 27: 209-214.

19. Lechner C, Meisenzahl EM, Uhlemann H, Helber-Bohlen H, Fahndrich E (1999) [Hallervorden-Spatz syndrome. Differential diagnosis of early onset dementia]. *Nervenarzt* 70: 471-475.

20. Lowe J, Lennox G, Leigh PN (1997) Disorders of movement and system degenerations. In *Greenfield's Neuropathology*, D Graham, PL Lantos (eds). E. Arnold: London. pp. 280-366

21. Malandrini A, Bonuccelli U, Parrotta E, Ceravolo R, Berti G, Guazzi GC (1995) Myopathic involvement in two cases of Hallervorden-Spatz disease. *Brain Dev* 17: 286-290.

22. Malandrini A, Fabrizi GM, Bartalucci P, Salvadori C, Berti G, Sabo C, Guazzi GC (1996) Clinicopathological study of familial late-infantile Hallervorden-Spatz disease: a particular form of neuroacanthocytosis. *Childs Nerv Syst* 12: 155-160.

23. Mutoh K, Okuno T, Ito M, Mikawa H (1990) Somatosensory evoked potentials in Hallervorden-Spatz-neuroaxonal- dystrophy complex with dorsal column involvement. *Clin Electroencephalogr* 21: 58-66.

24. Neumann M, Adler S, Schluter O, Kremmer E, Benecke R, Kretzschmar HA (2000) Alpha-synuclein accumulation in a case of neurodegeneration with brain iron accumulation type 1 (NBIA-1, formerly Hallervorden-Spatz syndrome) with widespread cortical and brainstem-type Lewy bodies. *Acta Neuropathol* 100: 568-574.

25. Newell KL, Boyer P, Gomez-Tortosa E, Hobbs W, Hedley-Whyte ET, Vonsattel JP, Hyman BT (1999) Alpha-synuclein immunoreactivity is present in axonal swellings in neuroaxonal dystrophy and acute traumatic brain injury. *J Neuropathol Exp Neurol* 58: 1263-1268.

26. Nishiyama K, Murayama S, Nishimura Y, Asayama K, Kanazawa I (1997) Superoxide dismutase-like immunoreactivity in spheroids in Hallervorden- Spatz disease. *Acta Neuropathol* 93: 19-23.

27. Ostergaard JR, Christensen T, Hansen KN (1995) In vivo diagnosis of Hallervorden-Spatz disease. *Dev Med Child Neurol* 37: 827-833.

28. Perry TL, Norman MG, Yong VW, Whiting S, Crichton JU, Hansen S, Kish SJ (1985) Hallervorden-Spatz disease: cysteine accumulation and cysteine dioxygenase deficiency in the globus pallidus. *Ann Neurol* 18: 482-489.

28a. Racette BA, Perry A, D'Avossa G, Perlmutter JS (2001) Late-onset neurodegeneration with brain iron accumulation type 1: expanding the clinical spectrum. *Mov Disord* 16: 1148-1152.

28b. Rock CO, Karim MA, Zhang YM, Jackowski S (2002) The murine pantothenate kinase (Pank1) gene encodes two differentially regulated pantothenate kinase isozymes. *Gene* 29: 35-43.

29. Saito Y, Kawai M, Inoue K, Sasaki R, Arai H, Nanba E, Kuzuhara S, Ihara Y, Kanazawa I, Murayama S (2000) Widespread expression of alpha-synuclein and tau immunoreactivity in Hallervorden-Spatz syndrome with protracted clinical course. *J Neurol Sci* 177: 48-59.

30. Seitelberger F (1986) Neuronal Dystrophy: It's relations to aging and neurological diseases. In *Handbook of Clinical Neurology*, PJ Vinken, G Bruyn, W., HL Klawans (eds). Elsevier: Amsterdam. pp. 391-412

31. Shoham S, Youdim MB (2000) Iron involvement in neural damage and microgliosis in models of neurodegenerative diseases. *Cell Mol Biol* 46: 743-760.

32. Swaiman KF (1991) Hallervorden-Spatz syndrome and brain iron metabolism. *Arch Neurol* 48: 1285-1293.

33. Taylor T, Litt M, Kramer P, Pandolfo M, Angelini L, Nardocci N, Pineda M, Davies S, Hattori H, Flett PJ, Cilio MR, Bertini E, Hayflick SJ (1996) Homozygosity mapping of Hallervorden-Spatz syndrome to chromosome 20p12.3-p13. *Nat Genet* 14: 479-481.

34. Tripathi RC, Tripathi BJ, Bauserman SC, Park JK (1992) Clinicopathologic correlation and pathogenesis of ocular and central nervous system manifestations in Hallervorden-Spatz syndrome. *Acta Neuropathol* 83: 113-119.

35. Tu PH, Galvin JE, Baba M, Giasson B, Tomita T, Leight S, Nakajo S, Iwatsubo T, Trojanowski JQ, Lee VM (1998) Glial cytoplasmic inclusions in white matter oligodendrocytes of multiple system atrophy brains contain insoluble alpha-synuclein. *Ann Neurol* 44: 415-422.

36. Wakabayashi K, Fukushima T, Koide R, Horikawa Y, Hasegawa M, Watanabe Y, Noda T, Eguchi I, Morita T, Yoshimoto M, Iwatsubo T, Takahashi H (2000) Juvenile-onset generalized neuroaxonal dystrophy (Hallervorden-Spatz disease) with diffuse neurofibrillary and lewy body pathology. *Acta Neuropathol* 99: 331-336.

37. Wakabayashi K, Yoshimoto M, Fukushima T, Koide R, Horikawa Y, Morita T, Takahashi H (1999) Widespread occurrence of alpha-synuclein/NACP-immunoreactive neuronal inclusions in juvenile and adult-onset Hallervorden-Spatz disease with Lewy bodies. *Neuropathol Appl Neurobiol* 25: 363-368.

38. Willwohl D, Kettner M, Braak H, Hubbard GB, Dick EJ, Cox AB, Schultz C (2002) Pallido-nigral spheroids in nonhuman primates: accumulation of heat shock proteins in astroglial processes. *Acta Neuropathol* 103: 276-280.

39. Yamazaki K, Wakasugi N, Tomita T, Kikuchi T, Mukoyama M, Ando K (1988) Gracile axonal dystrophy (GAD), a new neurological mutant in the mouse. *Proc Soc Exp Biol Med* 187: 209-215.

40. Yazawa I, Nakano I, Yamada H, Oda M (1997) Long tract degeneration in familial sudanophilic leukodystrophy with prominent spheroids. *J Neurol Sci* 147: 185-191.

41. Zhou B, Westaway SK, Levinson B, Johnson MA, Gitschier J, Hayflick SJ (2001) A novel pantothenate kinase gene (PANK2) is defective in Hallervorden-Spatz syndrome. *Nat Genet* 28: 345-349.

42. Zupanc ML, Chun RW, Gilbert-Barness EF (1990) Osmiophilic deposits in cytosomes in Hallervorden-Spatz syndrome. *Pediatr Neurol* 6: 349-352.

Familial Encephalopathy with Neuroserpin Inclusion Bodies

Richard L. Davis
George H. Collins

FENIB	familial encephalopathy with neuroserpin inclusion bodies
PME	progressive myoclonic epilepsy
rCBF	regional cerebral blood flow
Serpin	serine proteinase inhibitor
SPECT	single photon emission computed tomography
UPR	unfolded protein response

Definition

FENIB is an autosomal dominant genetic disorder caused by mutations in the *SERPINI1* gene which encodes the neuronally expressed serine proteinase inhibitor neuroserpin (8, 13, 16, 18). Its defining neuropathological feature is the Collins body, a neuronal inclusion described below (7).

Synonyms and Historical Annotations

Cases of this disorder have previously been reported as atypical inclusion body progressive myoclonus epilepsy, myoclonus body disease type II (Dastur), and progressive dementia and epilepsy with "Lafora-like" intraneuronal inclusions (1, 2, 6, 10, 23).

Epidemiology

FENIB appears to be extremely rare. Neither the incidence nor the prevalence has been established. It affects males and females equally, and the age of onset, from the second to the fifth decade of life, is dependent upon the severity of the mutation and the resultant instability of the mutant neuroserpin protein (9).

Genetics

FENIB, a Mendelian disorder with autosomal dominant inheritance, was first established in the study of a large North American kindred involving both sexes in each of 4 generations, and in a small North American kindred with an occurrence in 2 successive generations (7, 8). In both families, mutations in the *SERPINI1* gene were found to segregate with the disease phenotype, and a study of the larger family demonstrated linkage to that gene (8). FENIB is caused by missense mutations which encode amino acid substitutions in the neuroserpin protein in regions which are critical for molecular stability and regulation (8, 9). The known mutations and associated clinical features are summarised in Table 1.

Mutation*,†	Decade of onset	Clinical manifestations	References
T226C **S49P**	Fifth	Dementia, motor unrest, tremor, dystonia, seizures (rarely)	(7, 8)
A235C **S52R**	Second to Third	Focal motor seizures, myoclonus, dementia, dystonia, tremor	(7, 8, 23)
A235C **S52R**	Third	PME, status epilepticus, dementia, dysarthria, nystagmus, hypoalgesia	(20, 22)
A1013G **H338R**	Second	PME, dementia, tremor, dysarthria	(9)
G1175A	Second	PME, status epilepticus, dementia, spasticity, tremor, dysdiadochokinesia, dysarthria, ataxic gait, chorea	(1,9)

Table 1. Summary of FENIB cases.
* Mutation is presented as the base change in the SERPINI1 gene (italics) and the resulting amino acid substitution (bold).
† Two apparently unrelated families carry the S52R mutation and manifest somewhat different clinical syndromes.

Clinical Features

FENIB may present as a presenile dementia or as epilepsy, including progressive myoclonic epilepsy (PME) (3, 6, 7, 20, 23). Dementia always develops in the course of the disease. In the dementia predominant cases, the disease is a slowly progressive disorder characterised by deficits in frontal lobe processes, including attention, concentration, and response regulation, oral fluency, and visuospatial organization but with relative preservation of recall memory. There is motor restlessness and a tendency to perseverate (3). Mild tremor, dystonia, and rarely, seizures may also occur. Alternatively, the disease may begin with seizures, dystonia, and tremor, all of which are responsive to pharmacotherapy, but a progressive dementing process ensues (23). Finally, FENIB may present as PME with intractable seizures and myoclonus progressing to dementia, severe disability, and early death (1, 9, 20). MRI findings are initially normal but progress to diffuse cerebral atrophy in the later stages (1, 3, 20). Early in the course of the dementia-predominant cases, the EEG is normal but SPECT rCBF studies show frontal lobe abnormalities. Later, EEG studies show global slowing and SPECT rCBF reveals patchy flow reduction globally (2). In those cases presenting with epilepsy or PME, EEG studies reveal various epileptiform discharges (1, 20, 23). CSF findings have been found to be within the normal range (23).

Macroscopy

In the dementia predominant cases that have presented thus far to autopsy, the gross examination has revealed little atrophy aside from mild ventricular dilatation, with brain weights within the normal range (7). Cases presenting with PME have demonstrated diffuse atrophy, preferentially affecting the frontal lobe, and brain weights less than 1000 g (1, 20).

Histopathology

The principal finding consists of round, 5 to 50 mm, eosinophilic inclusions (Collins bodies) affecting neurons throughout most of the central nervous grey matter as well as the dorsal root ganglia (Figure 1A) (1, 7, 20). They are rarely seen in the white matter and have not been observed in other organs. They are found throughout layers III to VI of the cerebral cortex, affecting especially the pyramidal neurons of layers III and V. The subcortical grey nuclei as well as the grey matter of the spinal cord are affected to a varying degree but the substantia nigra is markedly involved. In all cases examined to date, the dentate gyrus, cerebellar cortex, and inferior olive have been unaffected. The inclusions appear both free in the neuropil and within neuronal perikarya and processes, often displacing and compressing the nucleus and cytoplasm. In some instances there is no apparent cytoplasm, but only a large inclusion surrounded by a thin, basophilic rim and a nuclear remnant. Smaller and multiple inclusions, however, are seen within otherwise normal appearing cell bodies and dendrites. Collins bodies are strongly PAS positive and diastase resistant (Figure 1B). Bodian silver stains the central portion darkly. The dementia predominant cases show 5 to 10 Collins bodies per 25× objective field, with only slight neuronal loss and mild astrocytosis, predominantly in layers II to III, and a low grade subcortical gliosis (7). In cases presenting with PME, the bodies are far more numerous with more neuronal loss and gliosis (1, 9, 20).

Immunohistochemistry and Ultrastructural Findings

Collins bodies stain specifically with antibodies to the neuroserpin protein (Figure 1C). Some inclusions, especially the smaller ones, are homogeneously positive, while others show a darker periphery. Many neurons in FENIB brains and in age-matched controls show diffuse positivity for neuroserpin easily distinguishable from Collins bodies involving the cell body and its processes (7, 20). Collins bodies appear to be composed entirely of mutant neuroserpin and are not labeled with antibodies directed against other proteins (7, 20, 22). Ultrastructurally, they appear as osmiophilic globules with an amorphous or finely granular composition (Figure 1D). They show little internal structure aside from some speckling with darker material and sometimes a darker core surrounded by a less intensely osmiophilic periphery. The periphery is usually well-delimited, and displaced organelles often appear in the adjacent cytoplasm. A limiting membrane of rough endoplasmic reticulum (ER) is frequently seen (7, 20).

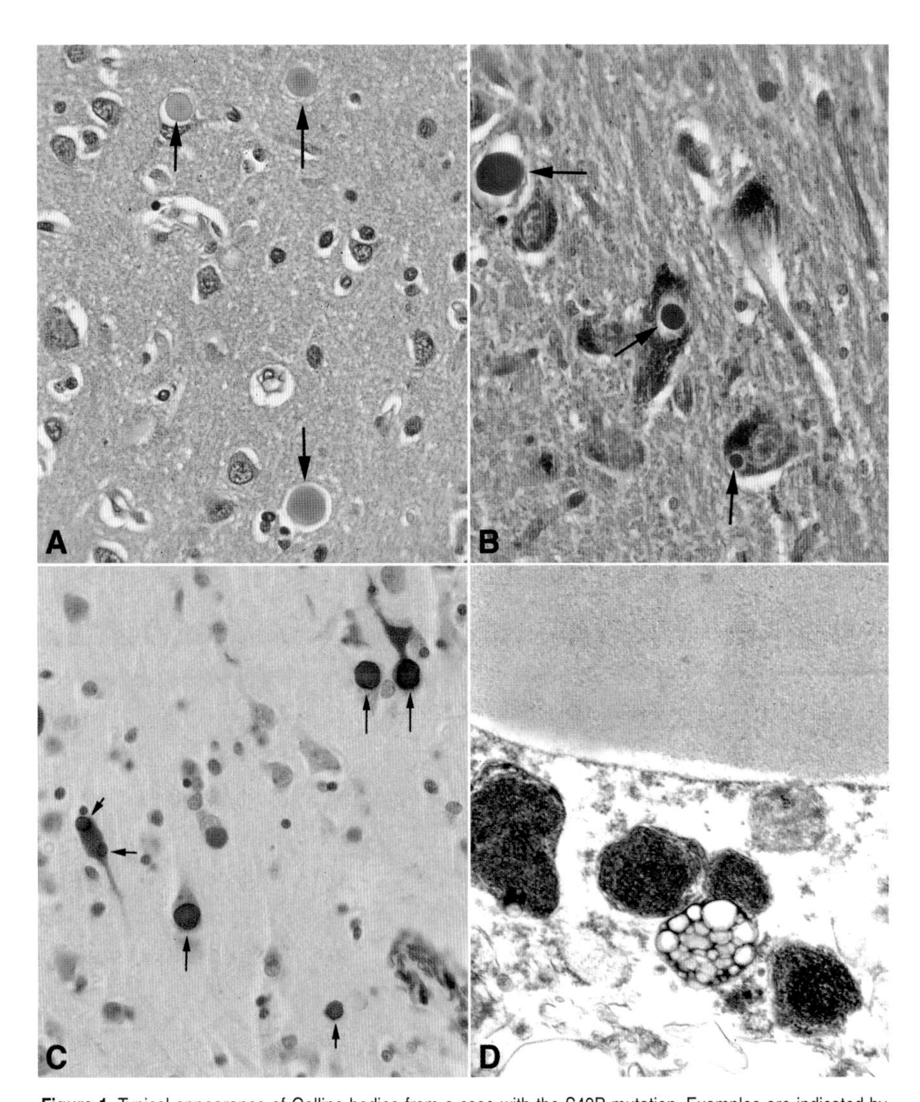

Figure 1. Typical appearance of Collins bodies from a case with the S49P mutation. Examples are indicated by arrows. **A.** Cingulate cortex, H&E, ×400. **B.** Substantia nigra, PAS, ×400. **C.** Occipital cortex, neuroserpin immunohistochemistry, ×400. **D.** Frontal cortex, electron microscopy, original magnification ×20 000.

Biochemistry

Neuroserpin, a glycoprotein that is secreted by axons, inhibits extracellular serine proteinases, especially tissue plasminogen activator. Regulated proteolysis is crucial to the development, maintenance, and plasticity of the nervous system (13, 16). All inhibitory serpins share a common molecular architecture consisting of a compact body dominated by a large, central β sheet and a carboxyl terminal extended reactive center loop (RCL) which encodes the proteinase specificity. The RCL is flexible and can be inserted into the β sheet as an additional strand, either after cleavage by a target proteinase or as an intact loop to form a latent conformation. Loop insertion is precisely controlled by a core of amino acid residues underlying the β sheet, collectively referred to as the shutter region (18, 21). The mutations causing FENIB result in amino acid substitutions which disrupt the shutter region and permit the unregulated and inappropriate insertion of the RCL of one molecule into the β sheet of another in a sequential fashion to give linear polymers which entangle and accumulate within the ER, thus forming Collins bodies (4, 7, 8, 9, 14, 18).

Differential Diagnosis

Neuropathologically, FENIB is readily distinguished from diffuse Lewy body disease by the strong PAS positivity of Collins bodies, by their amorphous, non-filamentous ultrastructure, and by their immunoreactivity with antibodies to neuroserpin. Lafora bodies also show a filamentous ultrastructure and faint eosinophilia. They occur extraneuronally in other body organs and are easily distinguished (7, 20).

Experimental Models

No experimental models currently exist.

Pathogenesis

The intracellular polymerization of mutant neuroserpin protein is well established as the molecular pathogenesis of FENIB (8). The challenge is to understand the cellular pathophysiology and how it relates to the clinical manifestations of the disease. A possible but unlikely explanation is that there is a deficiency of neuroserpin. The fact that affected individuals are developmentally normal and asymptomatic early in life argues against this hypothesis, as does the finding that Collins bodies are composed of only mutant neuroserpin and so do not appear to sequester the wild type protein (22). It is much more probable, as with other autosomal dominant disorders such as Huntington disease, that the mutant protein is itself injurious to neurons (5). The initial accumulation within the ER of polymerized neuroserpin that can neither be exported nor efficiently degraded is likely to induce an ER stress response, ie, the unfolded protein response (UPR) (11). This is a transcriptional response which upregulates a large battery of genes essential to ER function, producing chaperones that promote the folding and export of misfolded proteins, and proteosomal components that eliminate proteins which are terminally misfolded. The UPR also initiates a global attenuation of protein translation (12). Since polymers of neuroserpin are unsatisfactory substrates for either refolding or degradation, their continuing accumulation will likely result in a chronic state of ER stress. This may adversely affect intracellular calcium stores and the processing of other secretory proteins, thereby perturbing cellular homeostasis (17).

Future Directions and Therapy

There is currently no available therapy other than seizure control with anticonvulsants. Prevention or reversal of the course of the disease might be achievable with agents that promote protein folding (chemical chaperones such as dimethyl sulfoxide [DMSO] or glycerol) (15). Less toxic and more specific therapy might be possible by designing small peptides based on the sequence of the RCL which can block or reverse polymer formation. This approach has worked in vitro with other serpins and efforts to develop shorter peptides or mimetics of those peptides which could be effective in vivo are ongoing (19). To provide a more comprehensive understanding of the disease process, cell culture and transgenic models are currently being developed.

References

1. Bergener M, Gerhard L (1970) Myoklonuskorperkrankheit und progressive Myoklonusepilepsie. *Nervenarzt* 41: 166-173.

2. Berkovic SF, So NK, Andermann F (1991) Progressive myoclonus epilepsies: clinical and neurophysiological diagnosis. *J Clin Neurophysiol* 8: 261-274.

3. Bradshaw C, Davis RL, Shrimpton AE, Holohan PD, Rea C, Feiglin D, Kent P, G aC (2001) Cognitive deficits associated with a recently reported familial neurodegenerative disease, FENIB. *Arch Neurol* in press.

4. Briand C, Kozlov SV, Sonderegger P, Grutter MG (2001) Crystal structure of neuroserpin: a neuronal serpin involved in a conformational disease. *FEBS Lett* 505: 18-22.

5. Carrell RW, Lomas DA (1997) Conformational disease. Lancet 350: 134-138.

6. Davis R, Yerby M, Shaw C, Holohan P, Shämpton A, Taturn A, Daucher J, Lawrence D, Gerhard L (2000) Collins bodies and atypieal myoclonus bodies: the neurosperpin connection. *Brain Pathol* 10: 682-683.

7. Davis RL, Holohan PD, Shrimpton AE, Tatum AH, Daucher J, Collins GH, Todd R, Bradshaw C, Kent P, Feiglin D, Rosenbaum A et al (1999) Familial encephalopathy with neuroserpin inclusion bodies. *Am J Pathol* 155: 1901-1913.

8. Davis RL, Shrimpton AE, Holohan PD, Bradshaw C, Feiglin D, Collins GH, Sonderegger P, Kinter J, Becker LM, Lacbawan F, Krasnewich D et al (1999) Familial dementia caused by polymerization of mutant neuroserpin. *Nature* 401: 376-379.

9. Davis RL, Shrimpton AE, Carrell RW, Lomas DA, Gerhard L, Baumann B, Lawrence DA, Yepes M, Kim TS, Ghetti B et al (2002) Association between conformational mutations in neuroserpin and onset and severity of dementia. *Lancet* 359: 2242-2247.

10. Gerhard L, Kryne-Kubat B, Reinhardt V, Horstmann W, Przuntek H (1990) Zur klinischen und morphologischen differential-diagnose der progressiven myoklonusepilepsie bei myoklonuskorperkrankheit (Typ Laföra, Typ Dastur). In *Aktuelle Neuropadiatrie 1989.* Hanefeld F, Rating D, Christen H-J (eds.) Springer-Verlag: Berlin. pp. 56-60.

11. Hampton RY (2000) ER stress response: getting the UPR hand on misfolded proteins. *Curr Biol* 10: R518-521.

12. Harding HP, Zhang Y, Ron D (1999) Protein translation and folding are coupled by an endoplasmic-reticulum- resident kinase. *Nature* 397: 271-274.

13. Hastings GA, Coleman TA, Haudenschild CC, Stefansson S, Smith EP, Barthlow R, Cherry S, Sandkvist M, Lawrence DA (1997) Neuroserpin, a brain-associated inhibitor of tissue plasminogen activator is localized primarily in neurons. Implications for the regulation of motor learning and neuronal survival. *J Biol Chem* 272: 33062-33067.

14. Huntington JA, Pannu NS, Hazes B, Read RJ, Lomas DA, Carrell RW (1999) A 2.6 A structure of a serpin polymer and implications for conformational disease. *J Mol Biol* 293: 449-455.

15. Morello JP, Petaja-Repo UE, Bichet DG, Bouvier M (2000) Pharmacological chaperones: a new twist on receptor folding. *Trends Pharmacol Sci* 21: 466-469.

16. Osterwalder T, Contartese J, Stoeckli ET, Kuhn TB, Sonderegger P (1996) Neuroserpin, an axonally secreted serine protease inhibitor. *Embo J* 15: 2944-2953.

17. Paschen W, Doutheil J (1999) Disturbances of the functioning of endoplasmic reticulum: a key mechanism underlying neuronal cell injury? *J Cereb Blood Flow Metab* 19: 1-18.

18. Silverman GA, Bird PI, Carrell RW, Church FC, Coughlin PB, Gettins PG, Irving JA, Lomas DA, Luke CJ, Moyer RW et al (2001) The serpins are an expanding superfamily of structurally similar but functionally diverse proteins. Evolution, mechanism of inhibition, novel functions, and a revised nomenclature. *J Biol Chem* 276: 33293-33296.

19. Skinner R, Chang WS, Jin L, Pei X, Huntington JA, Abrahams JP, Carrell RW, Lomas DA (1998) Implications for function and therapy of a 2.9 A structure of binary- complexed antithrombin. *J Mol Biol* 283: 9-14

20. Takao M, Benson MD, Murrell JR, Yazaki M, Piccardo P, Unverzagt FW, Davis RL, Holohan PD, Lawrence DA, Richardson R, Farlow MR, Ghetti B (2000) Neuroserpin mutation S52R causes neuroserpin accumulation in neurons and is associated with progressive myoclonus epilepsy. *J Neuropathol Exp Neurol* 59: 1070-1086.

21. Whisstock JC, Skinner R, Carrell RW, Lesk AM (2000) Conformational changes in serpins: I. The native and cleaved conformations of alpha(1)-antitrypsin. *J Mol Biol* 296: 685-699.

22. Yazaki M, Liepnieks JJ, Murrell JR, Takao M, Guenther B, Piccardo P, Farlow MR, Ghetti B, Benson MD (2001) Biochemical characterization of a neuroserpin variant associated with hereditary dementia. *Am J Pathol* 158: 227-233.

23. Yerby MS, Shaw CM, Watson JM (1986) Progressive dementia and epilepsy in a young adult: unusual intraneuronal inclusions. *Neurology* 36: 68-71.

Neuronal intranuclear inclusion disease

Matti Haltia

APP	amyloid precursor protein
GFAP	glial fibrillary acidic protein
MAP	microtubule associated protein
NFP	neurofilament protein
NIID	neuronal intranuclear inclusion disease

Definition of Entity

Neuronal intranuclear inclusion disease is a slowly progressive neurodegenerative disorder characterized by the widespread occurrence of round eosinophilic intranuclear inclusion bodies in the nerve cells of the central and peripheral nervous systems accompanied by neuronal loss. Cases published under this designation probably represent more than one entity (see Differential diagnosis).

Synonyms and Historical Annotations

The disease was first recognized by Sung et al (10), who published a case under the title of "Neuronal intranuclear hyaline inclusion disease." Haltia et al (2) concluded that their 2 cases, the case of Sung et al, and the patients reported by Janota (3) and Michaud and Gilbert (8) under various designations, constituted a new entity for which they proposed the abreviated term neuronal intranuclear inclusion disease (NIID), adopted by many later authors. A familial disease with neuronal intranuclear inclusions, presenting as intestinal pseudo-obstruction, had been described earlier by Schuffler et al (9).

Epidemiology

Incidence and prevalence. NIID is a very rare disorder, and to date only about 30 cases have been published from Europe, North America, Australia and Japan (4).

Sex and age distribution. Both sexes are equally affected. The onset usually is in childhood, most often in the second decade, although a number of adult-onset cases have been reported. In one case the onset was as late as the seventh decade (12).

Risk factors. No environmental risk factors are known.

Genetics

Most cases reported so far are apparently sporadic. However, the disease has occurred in siblings, including 2 affected concordant pairs of female monozygotic twins (2, 4). Two adult sons of one of the twin sisters developed an identical illness, suggesting autosomal dominant inheritance (4). No evidence of an expanded SCA1, SCA2, SCA3, SCA6, SCA7, or atrophin allele has been found (7, 11).

Clinical Features

Signs and symptoms. NIID patients with onset in childhood most often show the features of a multisystem degenerative process of the nervous system. The patients develop ataxia, extrapyramidal signs such as oculogyral crises, tremor and progressive rigidity, lower motor neurone abnormalities, behavioural or cognitive dysfunction. In adult-onset cases dementia may be a prominent feature (12). The disease has a slowly progressive course with duration often exceeding 10 or even 20 years.

Imaging. Neuroimaging may show generalized cerebral and cerebellar atrophy.

Laboratory findings. Consistent abnormalities have not been recorded in routine analyses of the blood or CSF. Electrophysiological studies may show reduced nerve conduction velocities and evidence of muscle denervation (4).

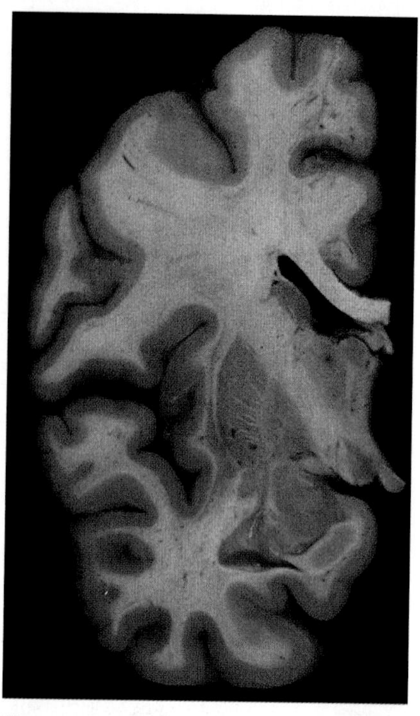

Figure 1. Coronal section of the left cerebral hemisphere of a 22-year-old female NIID patient (brain weight 1020 g). The macroscopic features are unremarkable, apart from slight reduction in the thickness of the cortex.

Macroscopy

The external appearance of the brain may be normal (Figure 1) or there may be slight to moderate generalized cerebral and cerebellar atrophy with widening of the sulci. The brain stem may appear smaller than normal. The cerebral cortical ribbon may be slightly reduced in thickness, while the white matter usually has a normal appearance. The basal ganglia and thalami are unremarkable. The substantia nigra is often severely depigmented (Figure 2). The ventricular system may be enlarged.

Histopathology

The most characteristic light microscopic feature is the almost ubiquitous presence of sharply demarcated round,

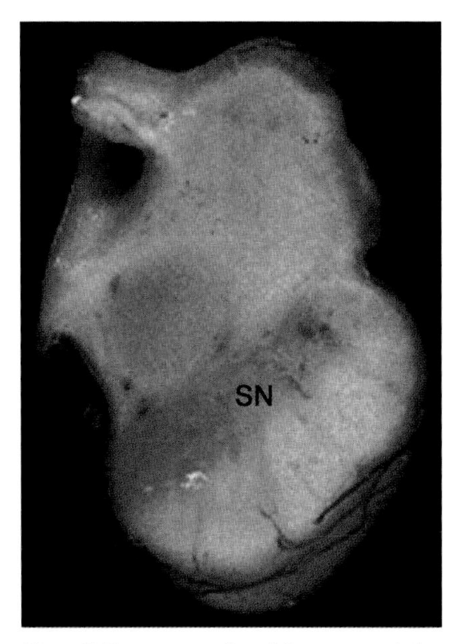

Figure 2. Transverse section of the mesencephalon of the above patient. Note the severe depigmentation of the substantia nigra (SN).

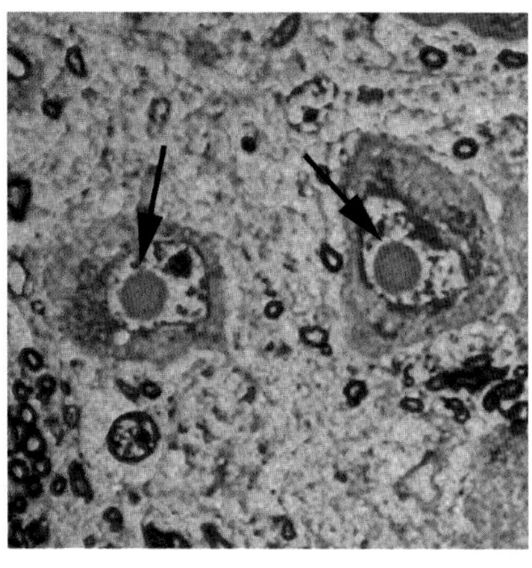

Figure 3. Intranuclear inclusion bodies in 2 neurones (arrows) of the inferior olivary nucleus. Epon section, Richardson stain.

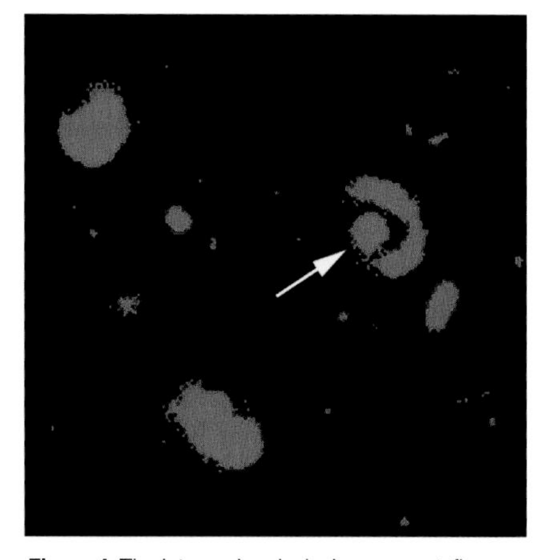

Figure 4. The intranuclear inclusions are autofluorescent in ultraviolet light (unstained paraffin section, one example indicated by an arrow).

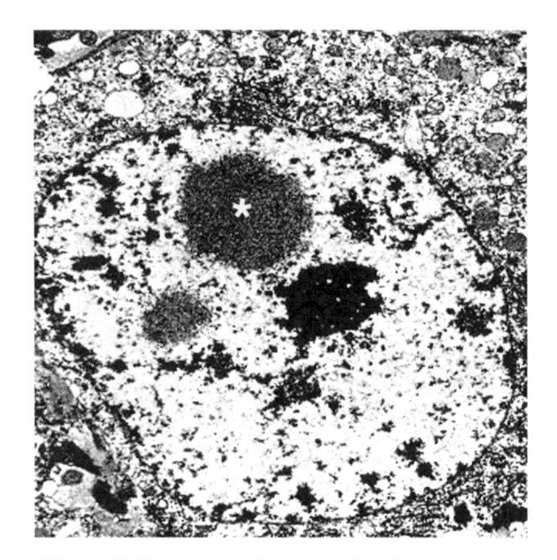

Figure 5. The neuronal intranuclear inclusions are non-membrane bound (star). Electron micrograph.

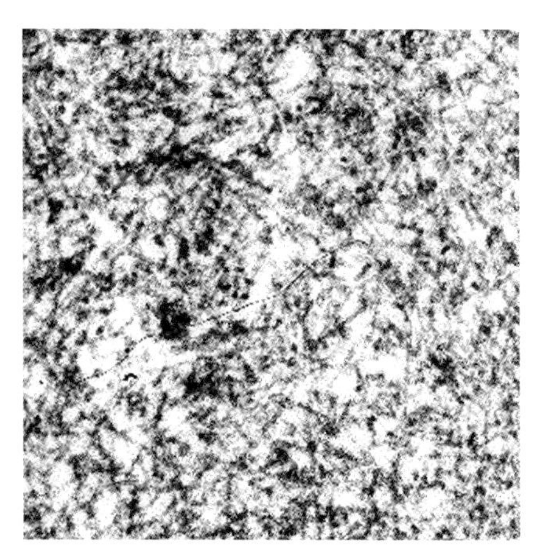

Figure 6. The inclusions show a filamentous ultrastructure. Electron micrograph.

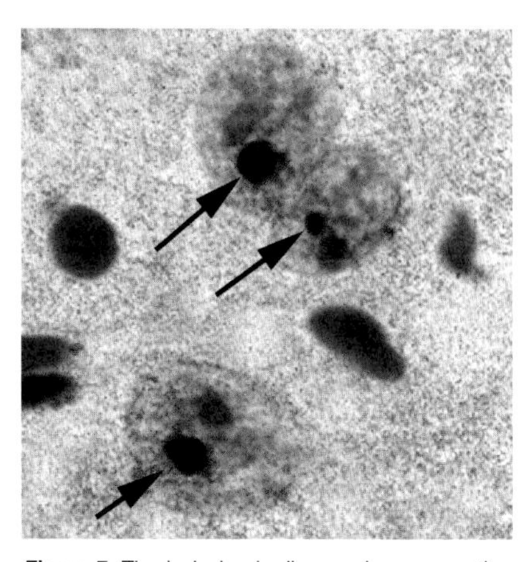

Figure 7. The inclusion bodies are immunoreactive for ubiquitin (frozen section, immunoperoxidase staining, examples indicated by an arrow).

eosinophilic inclusion bodies in the neuronal nuclei at various levels of the central nervous system (Figures 3, 4). These inclusion bodies also occur in the spinal ganglion cells, retina, and less frequently, in the autonomic ganglion cells.

The inclusion bodies usually have a diameter of 2 to 6 μm. However, in certain locations, notably in the basal ganglia and brain stem, the inclusions may be larger, and occupying most of the nucleus. Occasionally, 2 or more inclusions are seen within the same nucleus. Similar tiny intranuclear inclusions, 1 to 2 μm in diameter, may occasionally be seen in astrocytes at high magnification. In addition to the inclusion bodies, there is neuronal loss usually most accentuated in the cerebellar Purkinje cell layer, substantia nigra, inferior olivary nuclei, spinal anterior horns, and the dorsal nuclei of Clarke. In some cases the nigral neurones have been almost completely lost. There is usually only a modest astrocytic or microglial reaction.

Immunohistochemistry and Ultrastructural Findings

By electron microscopy (Figures 5, 6), the intranuclear inclusions are seen as non-membrane bound aggregates of tightly packed randomly oriented filaments, most often about 8 to 10 nm in diameter. The inclusion bodies are autofluorescent in ultraviolet light (Figure 4). In frozen sections they show strong immunostaining with antibodies to ubiquitin (Figure 7), but the immunoreactivity may be equivocal in paraffin sections. The intranuclear inclusions are not immunoreactive with antibodies to tau, MAP5, MAP2, NFP200, NFP160, NFP68, alpha- and beta-tubulin, GFAP, and APP. Occasional inclusion bodies in a NIID patient were reported to contain a polyglutamine epitope (6). Further immunohistochemical observations indicated that certain proteins with long polyglutamine tracts (including ataxin 1 and 3) are recruited into the NIID inclusions (7, 11).

Biochemistry

A severe nigrostriatal dopamine deficiency has been found in a patient with parkinsonian features (5). A marked loss of brain norepinephrine and serotonin was found in the basal ganglia and hypothalamus, while the amino acid and cholinergic neurotransmitter systems were normal or less severely affected.

Differential Diagnosis

The varied interpretations of the early cases (eg, atypical Friedreich's ataxia, multiple system atrophy, juvenile parkinsonism) reflect some of the considerable problems associated with the wide clinical differential diagnosis of NIID. So far, a definite diagnosis can only be established by morphological studies of neural tissue. Apart from a few cases diagnosed by rectal biopsy (1), the diagnosis has been reached at autopsy. Rare cases with additional intranuclear inclusion bodies in a number of extraneural tissues may represent separate conditions. The inclusion bodies in some of these cases have shown a granular rather than filamentous ultrastructure. The relationship between NIID and cases presenting with intestinal pseudo-obstruction (9) remains unsettled.

Experimental Models

No animal models currently exist.

Pathogenesis, Future Directions, and Therapy

The presence in nerve cells of ubiquitinated intranuclear inclusions links NIID with the trinucleotide repeat diseases. The apparent in vivo recruitment of normal proteins with long polyglutamine tracts into the neuronal intranuclear inclusions provides further support to an association of NIID with polyglutamine disorders. However, no evidence of CAG repeat expansions has been found in the respective genes analyzed so far in a few NIID patients. The possibility remains that NIID may be caused by a CAG expansion in an unknown gene, or alternatively, by mutations in a modifying gene predisposing to protein aggregation.

References

1. Goutières F, Mikol J, Aicardi J (1990) Neuronal intranuclear inclusion disease in a child: diagnosis by rectal biopsy. Ann Neurol 27:103-106.

2. Haltia M, Somer H, Palo J, Johnson WG (1984) Neuronal intranuclear inclusion disease in identical twins. Ann Neurol 15:316-321.

3. Janota I (1979) Widespread intranuclear neuronal corpuscles (Marinesco bodies) associated with a familial spinal degeneration with cranial and peripheral nerve involvement. Neuropathol Appl Neurobiol 5:311-317.

4. Kimber TE, Blumbergs PC, Rice JP, Hallpike JF, Edis R, Thompson PD, Suthers G (1998) Familial neuronal intranuclear inclusion disease with ubiquitin positive inclusions. J Neurol Sci 160:33-40.

5. Kish SJ, Gilbert JJ, Chang LJ, Mirchandani L, Shannak K, Hornykiewicz O (1985) Brain neurotransmitter abnormalities in neuronal intranuclear inclusion body disorder. Ann Neurol 17:405-407.

6. Lieberman AP, Robitaille Y, Trojanowski JQ, Dickson DW, Fischbeck KH (1998) Polyglutamine-containing aggregates in neuronal intranuclear inclusion disease. Lancet 351:884.

7. Lieberman AP, Trojanowski JQ, Leonard DG, Chen KL, Barnett JL, Leverenz JB, Bird TD, Robitaille Y, Malandrini A, Fischbeck KH (1999) Ataxin 1 and ataxin 3 in neuronal intranuclear inclusion disease. Ann Neurol 46:271-273.

8. Michaud J, Gilbert JJ (1981) Multiple system atrophy with neuronal intranuclear hyaline inclusions. Report of a new case with light and electron microscopic studies. Acta Neuropathol 54:113-119

9. Schuffler MD, Bird TD, Sumi SM, Cook A (1978) A familial neuronal disease presenting as intestinal pseudoobstruction. Gastroenterology 75:889-898.

10. Sung JH, Ramirez-Lassepas M, Mastri AR, Larkin SM (1980) An unusual degenerative disorder of neurons associated with a novel intranuclear hyaline inclusion (neuronal intranuclear hyaline inclusion disease). A clinicopathological study of a case. J Neuropathol Exp Neurol 39:107-130.

11. Takahashi J, Tanaka J, Arai K, Funata N, Hattori T, Fukuda T, Fujigasaki H, Uchihara T (2001) Recruitment of nonexpanded polyglutamine proteins to intranuclear aggregates in neuronal intranuclear hyaline inclusion disease. J Neuropathol Exp Neurol 60:369-376.

12. Weidenheim KM, Dickson DW (1995) Intranuclear inclusion bodies in an elderly demented woman: a form of intranuclear inclusion body disease. Clin Neuropathol 14:93-99.

Contributors

Dr Hiroaki Adachi
Department of Neurology
Nagoya University
Graduate School of Medicine
Tsurumai-cho 65, Showa-ku
Nagoya JP-466-0065
JAPAN
Phone: +81 52 7442391
Fax: +81 52 7442394

Dr Yves Agid
Fédération de Neurologie
Paris VI University, INSERM U 289
La Salpêtrière l'Hôpital
FR-75651 Cedex 13 Paris
FRANCE
Phone: +33 42 16 17 71
Fax: +33 42 16 19 65

Dr Adriano Aguzzi
Institut für Neuropathologie
Universitätsspital
Schmelzbergstrasse 12
CH-8091 Zürich
SWITZERLAND
Phone: +41 125 52869
Fax: +41 125 54402

Dr Catherine Bergeron
Department of Pathology
Toronto Western Hospital
399 Bathurst Street, EW-512
Toronto ON M5T 2S8
CANADA
Phone: +1 416 978 1877
Fax: +1 416 978 1878

Dr Lars Bertram
Center for Aging, Genetics and Neurodegeneration
Massachusetts General Hospital
Neuroscience Center, Building 149
13th Street
Charlestown MA 02129
UNITED STATES
Phone: +1 617 724 5567
Fax: +1 617 724 1823

Dr Konrad Beyreuther
ZMBH, University of Heidelberg
Im Neuenheimer Feld 282
DE-69120 Heidelberg
GERMANY
Phone: +49 6221 546845
Fax: +49 6221 545891

Dr Heiko Braak
Anatomisches Institut I
Klinikum der J. W. Goethe Universität
Theodor-Stern-Kai 7
DE-60590 Frankfurt/Main
GERMANY
Phone: +49 69 6301 6900
Fax: +49 69 6301 6425

Dr Moira Bruce
Neuropathogenesis Unit
Institute for Animal Health
West Mains Road
Edinburgh EH9 3JF
UNITED KINGDOM
Phone: +44 131 166 75204
Fax: +44 131 166 75204

Dr Herbert Budka
Neurologisches Institut
AKH 4J, PO Box 48
AU-1097 Vienna
AUSTRIA
Phone: +43 1 40400 5500
Fax: +43 1 40400 5511

Dr Orso Bugiani
Instituto Neurologico Carlo Besta
Via Celoria 11
I 20133 Nilan
ITALY
Fax: +39 270 638217
obugiani@istituto-besta.it

Dr Sabina Capellari
Department of Neurological Sciences
University of Bologna
Via Foscolo 7
I-40123 Bologna
ITALY
Phone: +39 51 644228
Fax: +39 51 583054

Dr Shu G. Chen
Institute of Pathology
Case Western Reserve University
2085 Adelbert Road
Cleveland OH 44106
UNITED STATES
Phone: +1 216 368 8925
Fax: +1 216 368 2546
sxc59@po.cwru.edu

Dr H. Brent Clark
Department of Laboratory Medicine & Pathology
University of Minnesota Medical Center
MMC 174
420 Delaware St SE
Minneapolis MN 55455
Phone: +1 612 625 7636
Fax: +1 612 625 0440

Dr George H. Collins
Department of Pathology
SUNY Healt Science Center
766 Irving Avenue
Syracuse NY 13210
UNITED STATES
Phone: +1 315 464 5170
Fax: 315 464 7130

Dr Pietro Cortelli
Instituto di clinica neurologica
dell'Università di Bologna
Via Ugo Foscolo, 7
I-40123 Bologna
ITALY
Phone: +39 51 6442228
Fax: +39 51 583054
cortelli@unibo.it

Dr Richard L. Davis
Department of Pathology
State University of New York Health Science Center
Syracuse NY 13210
UNITED STATES
Phone: +1 315 464 4750
Fax: +1 315 464 7130

Dr Simon Dawson
School of Biomedical Science
Nottingham Medical School
Queen's Medical Centre
Nottingham NG7 2UH
UNITED KINGDOM
Phone: +44 115 970 9369
Fax: +44 115 970 9969

Dr Dennis W. Dickson
Department of Pathology
Neuropathology Laboratory
Mayo Clinic
4500 San Pablo Road
Jacksonville FL- 32224
UNITED STATES
Phone: +1 904 953 7137
Fax: +1 904 953 7117

Dr John Duda
Center for Neurodegenerative Disease Research
University of Pennsylvania School of Medicine
University and Woodland Avenue
Philadelphia PA 19119
UNITED STATES

Dr Charles Duyckaerts
Laboratoire Neuropathologique
R. Escourolle
47 Boulevard de l'Hôpital
FR 75651 Paris
FRANCE
Phone: +33 14 216 1891
Fax: +33 14 423 9828

Dr Blas Frangione
New York University School of Medicine
Tisch Rm 432
550 First Avenue
New York NY 10016
UNITED STATES
Phone: +1 212 263 6751

Dr Perliuigi Gambetti
Institute of Pathology
Case Western Reserve University
2085 Adelbert Road
Cleveland OH 44106
UNITED STATES
Phone: +1 216 368 0587
Fax: +1 216 368 2546

Dr Estifanos Ghebremedhin
Department of Clinical Neuroanatomy
J. W. Goethe-University
Theodor-Stern-Kai 7, Haus 27a
DE 60590 Frankfurt
GERMANY
Phone: +49 69 63016912
Fax +49 69 63016425

Dr Bernardino Ghetti
Department of Pathology & Laboratory Medicine
Medical Sciences Building, A 142
Indiana University Medical Center
635 Barnhill Dr.
Indianapolis IN 46202-5120
UNITED STATES
Phone: +1 317 274 7818
Fax: +1 317 274 4882

Dr Jorge Ghiso
New York University School of Medicine
Department of Pathology
Tisch Hospital, Rm. 432
560 First Avenue
NY 10016 New York
UNITED STATES
Phone: + 1 212 263 7997
Fax: + 1 212 263 6751

Dr Michel Goedert
Medical Research Council
Laboratory of Molecular Biology
Hills Road
Cambridge CB2 2QH
UNITED KINGDOM
Phone: +44 1223 402036
Fax: +44 1223 402197

Dr Matti Haltia
Department of Pathology
Haartsmangaten 3
FIN-00290 Helsingfors
FINLAND
Phone: +358 919 12670
Fax:

Dr Brian N. Harding
Department of Histopathology
Hospital for Sick Children
Great Ormond Street
London WC1N 3JH
UNITED KINGDOM
Phone: +44 207 405 9200
Fax: +44 207 819 1170

Dr John A. Hardy
Laboratory of Neurogenetics
National Institute on Aging
NIH, Building 10, Room 6C103
MSC1589
Bethesda MD20892
UNITED STATES
Phone: +1 01 451 6076

Dr Jean-Jacques Hauw
Laboratoire de Neuropathologie R Escourolle,
Paris VI University, INSERM U 360, Association Claude Bernard
Hôpital de la Salpêtrière
47- bd de l'Hôpital
FR-75651 13 Paris
FRANCE
Phone: 33 142 16 18-80
Fax: +33 144 239828

Dr Mark Head
CJD Surveillance Unit
Western General Hospital
Edinburgh EH4 2XU
UNITED KINGDOM
Phone: +44 131 537 1980
Fax: +44 131 343 1404

Dr John Hedreen
Harvard Brain Tissue Resource Center
McLean Hospital
Belmont MA 02478
UNITED STATES
Phone: +1 617 636 8935
Fax: +1 617 636 8934

Dr James M. Henry
Division of Diagnostic Neuropathology
Armed Force Institute of Pathology
Washington DC 20306-6000
UNITED STATES
Phone: +1 202 782 1620
Fax: +1 202 782 4099

Dr Janice Holton
Department of Molecular Pathogenesis
Queen Square
London WC1N 3BG
UNITED KINGDOM
Phone: +44 207 837 3611
Fax: +44 207 916 9546

Dr Mike Hutton
Mayo Clinic Jacksonville
4500 San Pablo Road
Jacksonville FL 32224
UNITED STATES
Phone: +1 904 953 0159
Fax: +1 904 953 7370

Dr Paul G. Ince
Neuropathology 'E' Floor
Royal Hallamshire Hospital
Glossop Road
Sheffield S10 2JFle/Tyne
UNITED KINGDOM
Phone:
Fax: +44 114 27800591

Dr James Ironside
CJD Surveillance Unit
Western General Hospital
EH4 2XU Edinburgh
UNITED KINGDOM
Phone: +44 131 537 1980
Fax: +44 131 343 1404

Dr Kurt A. Jellinger
L.B. Institut für Klinische Neurobiologie
Kenyongasse 18 / 7
AU-1070 Vienna
AUSTRIA
Phone: +43 1 5266534
Fax: +43 152 38634

Dr Shinsuke Kato
Department of Neuropathology
Institute of Neurology
Tottori University
Nishi-machi 36-1
Yonago JP-683-8504
JAPAN
Phone: +81 859 34 8034
Fax: +81 859 34 8289

Dr Masahisa Katsuno
Department of Neurology
Nagoya University
Graduate School of Medicine
Tsurumai-cho 65, Showa-ku
Nagoya JP-466-0065
JAPAN
Phone: +81 52 744 2391
Fax: +81 52 744 2394

Dr Thomas Klockgether
Department of Neurology
Rheinische Friedrich-Wilhelms-Univerisät
Sigmund Freud Strasse 25
DE-53105 Bonn
GERMANY
Phone: +49 228 287 5726
Fax: +49 228 287 5024

Dr David Knopman
Department of Neurology
Mayo Clinic
200 First Street Southwest
Rochester MN 55905
UNITED STATES
Phone: +1 507 284 2511
Fax: +1 507 284 407

Dr Arnulf H. Koeppen
Department of Neurology
Albany Medical College
VA Medical Center
113 Holland Avenue
New York NY 12208
UNITED STATES
Phone: +1 518 626 6373
Fax: +1 518 626 6369

Dr Jacques Lamarche
Department of Pathology
Center Hospital University Sherbrooke
3001, 12 Ave Nord
Sherbrooke QC J1H 5N4
CANADA
Phone: +1 819 346 1110

Dr Peter Lantos
Institute of Psychiatry
De Crespigny Park
London SE5 8AF
UNITED KINGDOM
Phone: +44 20 8480273
Fax: +441717083895

Dr Robert Layfield
School of Biomedical Science
Nottingham Medical School
Queen's Medical Centre
Nottingham NG7 2UH
UNITED KINGDOM
Phone: +44 115 970 9369
Fax: +44 115 970 9969

Dr Peter Nigel Leigh
Department of Neurology
PO41, AND Building
Institute of Psychiatry
De Crespigny Park
London SE5 8AF
UNITED KINGDOM
Phone: +44 20 78485187
Fax: +44 20 7848 5181

Dr Jada Lewis
Mayo Clinic
4500 San Pablo Road
Jacksonville FL- 32224
UNITED STATES
Phone: +1 904 953 1085
Fax: +1 904 953 7370

Dr Carol F. Lippa
Department of Neurology
MCP Hahnemann University
3300 Henry Avenue, 9th floor
Philadelphia PA 19129
UNITED STATES
Phone: +1 215 849 1645
Fax: +1 215 849 1645

Dr Irene Litvan
Neuroepidemiology Branch
NINDS, NIH
Federal Building, Room 714
Bethesda MD 20814
UNITED STATES
Phone: +1 301 496 1189
Fax: +1 301 496 23 58

Dr James Lowe
Department of Pathology
University of Nottingham Medical School
Clifton Boulevard
Nottingham NG7 2UH
UNITED KINGDOM
Phone: +44 115 970 9269
Fax: +44 115 970 0759

Dr Elio Lugaresi
Instituto di clinica neurologica
dell'Università di Bologna
Via Ugo Foscolo, 7
I-40123 Bologna
ITALY
Phone: +39 51 644 2184
Fax: +39 51 644 2165

Mr Duncan MacRae
Brain Pathology Editorial Office
Section of Neuropathology
UCLA Medical Center, CHS 18-126
Los Angeles, CA 90095
UNITED STATES
Phone: +1 310 267 0543
Fax +1 310 267 0545

Dr Colin L. Masters
Department of Pathology
University of Melbourne
Grattan Street
Victoria 3052 Parkville
AUSTRALIA
Phone: +61 3 9344 5868

Dr R. John Mayer
School of Biomedical Science
Nottingham Medical School
Queen's Medical Centre
Nottingham NG7 2UH
UNITED KINGDOM
Phone: +44 115 970 9369
Fax: +44 115 970 9969

Dr Eileen McGowan
Department of Pathology
Neuropathology Laboratory
Mayo Clinic
4500 San Pablo Road
Jacksonville FL- 32224
UNITED STATES
Phone: +1 904 953 7370
Fax: +1 904 953 632

Dr Ian G. McKeith
Newcastle Upon Tyne
Inst Health Elderly
Newcastle Upon Tyne
Tyne & Wear NE4 6BE
UNITED KINGDOM
Phone: +44 191 256 3011

Dr Catriona A McLean
The Alfred Hospital
Prahran 3181
3050 Melbourne, Vic
AUSTRALIA
Phone: +61 33 927 63150
Fax: +61 3 9276 2899

Dr Yoshikuni Mizuno
Department of Neurology
Juntendo University School of Medicine
2-1-1 Hongo, Bunkyo
Tokyo JP-113-8421
JAPAN
Phone: +81 3 3813 3111
Fax: +81 3 5800 0547

Dr Hidehiro Mizusawa
Department of Neurology
Tokyo Medical and Dental University
Graduate School of Medicine
1-5-45 Yushima, Bunkyo-ku
Tokyo JP-113-8519
JAPAN
Phone: +81 3 5803 5233
Fax: +81 3 5803 0134

Dr Pasquale Montagna
Instituto di clinica neurologica
dell'Università di Bologna
Via Ugo Foscolo, 7
I-40123 Bologna ITALY
Phone: +39 51 6442179
Fax: +39 51 644 2165

Dr Huw R. Morris
Department of Neurology
St.Thomas' Hospital
Lambeth Palace Road
London SE1 7EH
UNITED KINGDOM
Phone: +44 20 8345 6789 #881
Fax: +44 87 0831 8923

Dr Akihiko Nunomura
Department of Psychiatry and Neurology
Asahikawa Medical College
Higashi 2-1-1-1, Midorigaoka 078-8510
Asahikawa
JAPAN
Phone: +81 166 682473
Fax: +81 166 68 2479

Dr Yngve Olsson
Rudbeck Laboratory C5 1 trp
SE-75185 Uppsala
SWEDEN
Phone: +46 18 6113838

Dr Kiyomitsu Oyanagi
Department of Neuropathology
Tokyo Metropolitan Institute for Neuroscience
2-6 Musashidai, Fuchu
Tokyo JP183-8526
JAPAN
Phone: +81 42 325 3881
Fax: +81 42 321 8678

Dr Piero Parchi
Department of Neurological Sciences
University of Bologna
Via Foscolo 7
I-40123 Bologna
ITALY
Phone: +39 51 644 228
Fax: +39 51 583054

Dr Paola Pergami
World Health Organization
Ave Appia 27
CH-1211 Geneva
SWITZERLAND
Phone: 011 41 22 7912381
Fax: 0041 22 791 4893

Dr George Perry
Institute of Pathology
Case Western Reserve University
2085 Adelbert Road
Cleveland OH 44106
UNITED STATES
Phone: +1 216 368 2488
Fax: +1 216 368 8964

Dr Pedro Piccardo
Department of Pathology and Laboratory Medicine
Medical Sciences Building, A 142
Indiana University Medical
Indianapolis IN 46202-5120
UNITED STATES
Phone: +1 317 274 0107
Fax: +1 317 278 2018

Dr Fiona Pickford
Department of Pathology
Neuropathology Laboratory
Mayo Clinic
4500 San Pablo Road
Jacksonville FL- 32224
UNITED STATES
Phone: +1 904 953 7370
Fax: +1 904 953 632

Dr Alphonse Probst
Institut für Pathologie
Abteilung Neuropathologie
Schönbeinstrasse 40
CH-4003 Basel
SWITZERLAND
Phone: +41 61 265 2895
Fax: +41 61 265 3194

Dr Niall Quinn
Institute of Neurology
National Hospital
Queen Square
London WC1N 3BG
UNITED KINGDOM
Phone: +44 171 2785616

Dr Tamas Révész
Department of Molecular Pathogenesis
Institute of Neurology
Queen Square
London WC1N 3BG
UNITED KINGDOM
Phone: +44 207 837 3611 ext: 4232
Fax: +44 207 916 9546

Dr Khosrow Rezvani
School of Biomedical Science
Nottingham Medical School
Queen's Medical Centre
Nottingham NG7 2UH
UNITED KINGDOM
Phone: +44 115 970 9369
Fax: +44 115 970 9969

Dr Maura N. Ricketts
World Health Organization
Ave Appia 27
CH-1211 Geneva
SWITZERLAND
Phone: 41 22 791 3935
Fax: +41 22 791 4893

Dr Yves Robitaille
Department of Pathology
Hopital Sainte Justine
3175 Cote Ste-Catherine
Montreal QC H3T 1C5
CANADA
Phone: +1 514 345 4649
Fax: +1 514 345 4819

Dr Raymond A. C. Roos
Department of Neurology
Leiden University, Medical Centre
Albinusdreef 2, PO Box 9600
NL - 2300 RC Leiden
NETHERLANDS
Phone: +31 71 526 2197
Fax: +31 71 524 8253

Dr Christopher A. Ross
Division of Neurobiology
Department of Psychiatry
Johns Hopkins University
School of Medicine
Ross Research Building, Room 618
Baltimore, MD 21205-2196
UNITED STATES
Phone: +1 410 614 0011
Fax: +1 410 614 0013

Dr Martin Rossor
Dementia Research Group
Institute of Neurology
Queen Square
London WC1N 3BG
UNITED KINGDOM
Phone: +44 20 7829 8773

Dr Kevin A. Roth
Department of Pathology (Neuropathology)
University of Alabama at Birmingham (UAB),
SC 961E
1530 Third Avenue South
Birmingham, AL 35294-0017
UNITED STATES
Phone: +1 4 205 934 5802
Fax: +1 205 934 6700
kroth@path.uab.edu

Dr Christopher Shaw
Department of Neurology
PO41, AND Building
Institute of Psychiatry
De Crespigny Park
SE5 8AF London
UNITED KINGDOM
Phone: +44 20 78485182
Fax: +44 20 7848 5181

Dr Pamela Shaw
Academic Neurology Unit
E Floor, Medical School
University of Sheffield
Beech Hill Road
S10 2RX Sheffield
UNITED KINGDOM
Phone: +44 114 271 3579
Fax: +44 114 276 0095

Dr Mark A. Smith
Institute of Pathology
Case Western Reserve University
2085 Adelbert Road
Cleveland OH 44106
UNITED STATES
Phone: +1 216 368 3670
Fax: +1 216 368 8964

Dr Gen Sobue
Dept of Neurology
Nagoya University
Graduate School of Medicine
Tsurumai-cho 65, Showa-ku
Nagoya JP-466-0065
JAPAN
Phone: +81 52 744 2385
Fax: +81 52 744 2384

Dr Maria Spillantini
Centre for Brain Repair
Forvie Site
University of Cambridge
Robinson Way
Cambridge CB2 2PY
UNITED KINGDOM
Phone: +44 1223 331145
Fax: +44 1223 331174

Dr Ravi Srinivas
Institute of Pathology
Case Western Reserve University
2085 Adelbert Road
Cleveland OH 44106
UNITED STATES
Phone: +1 216 368 3671
Fax: +1 216 368 8964

Dr Michael Swash
Department of Neurology
The Royal London Hospital
London Whitechapel E1 1BB
UNITED KINGDOM
Phone: +44 20 7377 7472
Fax: +4420 7377 7318

Dr Fabrizio Tagliavini
Servizio di Neuropathologica
Instituto Neurologico Carlo Besta
Via Celoria, n 11
IT 20133 Milano
ITALY
Phone: +39 02 239 4384
Fax: +39 02 7063 8217

Dr Hitoshi Takahashi
Department of Pathology
Brain Research Institute
Niigata University
1-757 Asahimachi
Niigata JP- 951-8585
JAPAN
Phone: +81 25 227 0633
Fax: +81 25 227 0817

Dr Rudolph E. Tanzi
Genetics and Aging Research Unit
Center for Aging, Genetics and Neurodegeneration
Massachusetts General Hospital
Neuroscience Center, Building 149
13th Street
Charlestown MA 02129
UNITED STATES
Phone: +1 617 726 6845
Fax: +1 617 724 a949

Dr Marcus Tolnay
Institut für Pathologie
Abteilung Neuropathologie
Schönbeinstrasse 40
CH-4003 Basel
SWITZERLAND
Phone: +41 61 265 2525
Fax: +41 61 265 3194

Dr John Q. Trojanowski
Department of Pathology
University of Pennsylvania School of Medicine
3600 Spruce St., 3rd Floor Maloney
Philadelphia PA 19104-4283
UNITED STATES
Phone: +1 215 662 6399
Fax: +1 215 349 5909

Dr Shoji Tsuji
Department of Pathology
Brain Research Institute
Niigata University
1-757 Asahimachi
JP-951-8585 Niigata 951-8585
JAPAN
Phone: +81 25227 0663
Fax: +81 25 227 0820

Dr David Westaway
Department of Pathology
Toronto Western Hospital
399 Bathurst Street, EW-512
Toronto ON M5T 2S8
CANADA
Phone: +1 416 978 1878
Fax:

Dr Robert Will
CJD Surveillance Unit
Western General Hospital
EH4 2XU Edinburgh
UNITED KINGDOM
Phone: +44 131 332 2117
Fax: +44 131 3431404

Dr Claire Wood-Allum
Academic Neurology Unit
E Floor, Medical School
University of Sheffield
Beech Hill Road
S10 2RX Sheffield
UNITED KINGDOM

Dr Zbigniew K. Wszolek
Department of Neurology
Mayo Clinic Jacksonville
FL 32224 Jacksonville
UNITED STATES
Phone: +1 904 953 0323
wszolek.zbigniew@mayo.edu

Dr Mitsunori Yamada
Department of Pathology
Brain Research Institute
Niigata University
1-757 Asahimachi
Niigata JP- 951-8585
JAPAN
Phone: +81 25 227 0634
Fax: +81 25 227 0817

Dr Martin Zeidler
Department of Clinical Neurosciences
Western General Hospital
Crewe Road
Edinburgh EH4 2XU
UNITED KINGDOM
martinz@globalnet.co.uk

Acknowledgments

Chapter 1.4. The author thanks Dr V. M-Y. Lee, past and current members of the Center for Neurodegenerative Disease Research (CNDR) and collaborators within and outside the University of Pennsylvania for their important contributions to the studies reviewed here. Appreciation also is expressed to the families of the many patients studied over the past decade who have made it possible to pursue the research discussed here. The studies summarized here from the laboratory of the author were supported by grants from the National Institute on Aging of the National Institutes of Health, the Dana Foundation and the Alzheimer's Association. Additional information on the neurodegenerative diseases reviewed here can be obtained by visiting the CNDR website, *http://www.uphs.upenn.edu/cndr/.*

Chapter 2.2. This work was sponsored by grants from the NIMH, NIA (ADRC) and the Alzheimer Association. CIDR is fully funded through a federal contract from the National Institutes of Health to The Johns Hopkins University, Contract Number N01-HG-65403. L. B. is a fellow of the Deutsche Forschungsgemeinschaft (DFG) and the Harvard Center for Neurodegeneration and Repair (HCNR), and A. J. S. is an NIA-NRSA recipient.

Chapter 3.2. Figure 4 is courtesy of Drs Caviness (images L and M), Cheshire (image K), Pooley (image J), Tsuboi (images C-G) and Witte (images H and I) from the Mayo Clinic Jacksonville, Fla and Dr Stoessl (images A and B) from the University of British Columbia, Vancouver, Canada. Figures 14 to 17 are courtesy of the *Journal of Neuropathology and Experimental Neurology.* Supported by Indiana Alzheimer Disease Center (PHS P30 AG 10133), M.H. Udall PD Center for Excellence (NINDS/PHS), and the Tau Program Project (NIA/PHS).

Chapter 3.8. The authors gratefully acknowledge the help of our colleagues in Molecular Biology at the AFIP, Drs J. Taubenberger, A. Reid, and S. McCall. We are also grateful to Ms R. Upshur-Tyree and to Dr E. Mitter-Ferstl for their capable transcription support. The work was partially supported by the Austrian Parkinson Society and the Progressive Supranuclear Palsy Society, Inc., Baltimore, Md.

Chapter 5.3. Dr Koeppen's work is supported by the Department of Veterans Affairs, Washington, D.C.; the National Ataxia Foundation, Minneapolis, Minn; Neurochemical Research, Inc., Glenmont, NY; and a generous donation by the Edith C. Brennan family. Dr Henry L. Paulson provided anti-ataxin-3. The author also acknowledges the technical expertise of Mr Andrew C. Dickson.

Chapter 5.4. The authors wish to extend their appreciation to Stephane Dedelis for skillfull help with computerised photography and panels of microphotographs.

Chapter 6.4. Supported by NIH grants AG14359, AG08012, CDC grant CCU 515004, the Britton Fund. The authors wish to extend their appreciation to Stephane Dedelis for skillfull help with computerised photography and panels of microphotographs.

Chapter 9.2. The authors wish to thank Gordon Plant for providing the MRI scan and Hans Braaendgard for permission to use unpublished material.

Index

6-OHDA model: 215

A
Abeta: 48, 69
Alpha-synuclein: 156
Alpha-synucleinopathy: 190
Alpha2-macroglobulin gene: 40
ALS: 350
Alzheimer's disease: 17, 24, 40, 47, 66, 69, 74
    amyloid angiopathy: 48
    astrocytosis: 55
    CERAD criteria: 58
    clinical features: 27
    clinical stages: 29
    cognitive deficits: 29
    definition: 24
    experimental model: 74
    genetics: 17, 26, 40
    granulo-vacuolar degeneration: 55
    gyral atrophy: 47
    Hirano body: 55
    Khachaturian criteria: 58
    molecular pathogenesis: 69
    neurofibrillary degeneration: 51
    neurofibrillary tangle: 52
    neuronal loss: 55
    neuropathological diagnostic criteria: 58
    NIA-Reagan Institute criteria: 58
    prevalence: 25
    protective factors: 26
    risk factors: 26, 40
    secretase: 69
    senile placque: 48
    spongiform change: 55
    synaptic loss: 55
    therapy: 32
    variants: 66
Amyloid: 48
Amyloid precursor protein: 40, 47, 69, 74
    experimental model: 74
Amyotrophic lateral sclerosis: 350, 369
Bunina body: 357
    experimental models: 363
    genetics: 351
    pathology: 356
    Skein-like inclusion: 357
Apolipoprotein E gene: 40
Apoptosis: 4
Argyrophilic grain dementia: 132
Argyrophilic grain disease: 132
Arrested Werdnig-Hoffman disease: 372
Astrocytic plaques: 118
    corticobasal degeneration: 115
Ataxia associated with vitamin E deficiency: 243
Atypical Alzheimer's disease: 380
    familial British dementia: 380
Autosomal dominant ataxia: 242
Axonal swelling: 391

B
Balooned neuron: 115
    corticobasal degeneration: 115
Basic neurodegenerative processes: 2
Bcl-2: 4
Beta-secretase cleave enzyme gene: 40
BRI2 gene: 380
Brown-Vialetto-van Laere syndrome: 375
Brownell-Oppenheimer variant of CJD: 287
Bulbar hereditary neuropathy: 375
Bulbar muscular atrophy: 275
Bunina body: 357

C
Caspases: 4
CERAD criteria: 58
Chamorro: 137
Coiled body: 133
Cortical cerebellar atrophy: 242
Cortical Lewy body disease: 188
Corticobasal degeneration: 56, 115
Corticobasal ganglionic: 115
Corticonigral degeneration: 115
Creutzfeldt Jakob disease: 335
    experimental models: 335
Creutzfeldt-Jakob disease: 287, 310
    varient Creutzfeldt-Jakob disease: 310

D
Dementia with argyrophilic grains: 132
Dementia with grains: 132
Dementia with Lewy bodies: 188
Dentatorubral-pallidoluysian atrophy: 269
Dentatorubropallidoluysial atrophy: 242
Diffuse Lewy body disease: 188
DSM-IV: 24

E
Early onset ataxia with oculomotor apraxia and hypoalbuminemia: 245
Encephalitis lethargica: 143

F
FALS: 357
Familial British dementia: 380
Familial Creutzfeldt-Jakob disease: 298
Familial Danish dementia: 380
Fatal familial insomnia: 326
Fatal insomnia: 326
Fazio-Londe disease: 375
Filamentous inclusions: 12
Friedreich's ataxia: 242, 257
Frontotemporal dementia: 342
Frontotemporal dementia and parkinsonism: 86
Frontotemporal lobar degeneration: 342
FTDP: 86

G
Genetics: 17
Gerstmann-Sträussler-Scheinker disease: 318
Gerstmann-Sträussler-Scheinker syndrome: 380
    familial British dementia: 380
Glial cell pathology: 2
Glial cytoplasmic inclusion: 156, 203
Globus pallidus: 163
    Parkinson's disease: 163
Granulo-vacuolar degeneration: 55
Guam PDC: 137

H
Heidenhain syndrome: 287
Hereditary spastic paraparesis: 380
    familial British dementia: 380
Heredopathia ophthalmo-oto-encephalica: 380
Hirano body: 55
Huntingtin: 229
Huntington's disease: 17, 229
    genetics: 17, 229

I
Iatrogenic prion disorder: 307
Idiopathic late-onset cerebellar ataxia: 203
Infantile neuronal degeneration: 375
Insulin-degrading enzyme gene: 40
Interleukin-1 alpha gene: 40
ITM2B gene: 380

K
Khachaturian criteria: 58
Kugelberg-Welander disease: 372

L
Lewy body: 156, 159, 188
Lewy body dementia: 188
Lewy body variant of Alzheimer's disease: 188
Locus coeruleus: 160
Low density lipoprotein receptor-related protein-1 gene: 40

M
Machado-Joseph disease: 244
Methamphetamine: 216
Molecular genetics: 17
Motor neurone disease: 350
    Bunina body: 357
    experimental models: 363
    genetics: 351
    pathology: 356
    Skein-like inclusions: 357
MPTP model: 216
Multiple system atrophy: 156, 203
Multisystem degeneration: 203

N
NAD type II: 392
NAIP gene: 372

Neuroaxonal dystrophy: 386, 390
juvenile form: 392
late-infantile form: 392
neuropathological findings: 386, 391
signs and symptoms: 386, 390
Neurofibrillary tangle: 52, 137, 143
Alzheimer's disease: 47
Parkinsonism-dementia complex of Guam: 137
postencephalitic Parkinsonism: 143
Neuroleptic-induced akinesia: 215
NIA-Reagan Institute criteria: 58
Nicastrin gene: 40
NINCDS-ADRDA: 24
Nitric oxide: 8

O

Olivopontocerebellar atrophy: 203, 242
Oxidative mechanisms: 8

P

Pael receptor: 161
Paired helical filament: 82
introduction to the tauopathies: 82
Papp-Lantos inclusion: 156, 203
Paralysis agitans: 159
Parkin: 159
Parkinson's disease: 17, 143, 156, 159, 215
experimental models: 215
genetics: 17
globus pallidus: 163
locus ceruleus: 163
postencephalitic parkinsonism: 143
substantia nigra: 159
Parkinson's disease dementia: 188
Parkinsonism-dementia complex of Guam: 137
Pick's disease: 124
Plaque-only Alzheimer's disease: 66
Postencephalitic Parkinsonism: 143
Presenilin gene: 40
Primary lateral sclerosis: 369
Prion disorders: 282, 287, 298, 307, 310, 318, 326, 335
bovine spongiform encephalopathy: 282
chronic wasting disease: 282
Creutzfeldt-Jakob disease: 282, 287
experimental models: 335
familial Creutzfeld-Jakob disease: 282, 298
fatal familial insomnia: 282, 326
feline spongiform encephalopathy: 282
follicular dendritic cells: 282
Gerstmann-Sträussler-Scheinker disease: 318
Gerstmann-Sträussler-Scheinker syndrome: 282
iatrogenic: 307
iatrogenic Creutzfeldt-Jakob disease: 282
new variant Creutzfeldt-Jakob disease: 282
spontaneous Creutzfeldt-Jakob disease: 282
transmissible mink encephalopathy: 282
transmissible spongiform encephalopathy: 282
variant Creutzfeldt-Jakob disease: 310
Prion protein cerebral amyloid angiopathy: 318
Programmed cell death: 4
Progressive supranuclear palsy: 103
Protein aggregate: 11

R

REM sleep behaviour disorder: 204
Rotenone: 217

S

Seitelberger Disease: 390
Senile dementia of Lewy body type: 188
Senile plaque: 48
amyloid: 48
composition: 53
non-amyloid components: 51
Shy-Drager syndrome: 203
SMN1 gene: 372
SNCA gene: 157
Spheroids: 391
Spinal muscular atrophy: 275, 372
Spinocerebellar ataxia: 242
Spinocerebellar degeneration: 242
Steele, Richardson and Olszewski syndrome: 103
Striatonigral degeneration: 210, 242
Substantia nigra: 159
Parkinson's disease: 159
Superoxide dismutase: 8
Synphylin: 161
Synucleinopathy: 11

T

TaClo: 218
Tau: 132
argyrophilic grain disease: 132
Tau aggregate: 48
Tauopathies: 150
experimental models: 150
Tauopathy: 11, 82, 103, 115, 124, 137, 143
corticobasal degeneration: 115
introduction to the tauopathies: 82
Parkinsonism-dementia complex of Guam: 137
Pick's disease: 124
postencephalitic Parkinsonism: 143
progressive supranuclear palsy: 103
Transcriptional factor LBP-1c/CP2/ LSF gene: 40
Transmissible spongiform encephalopathy: 307
Transmissible spongiform encephalopathy: 310
Trinucleotide repeat disorder: 226
introduction: 226

U

Ubiquitin: 14

V

Variant Creutzfeldt-Jakob disease: 310
Very low density lipoprotein receptor gene: 40
von Economo's encephalitis: 143

W

Werdnig-Hoffman disease: 372